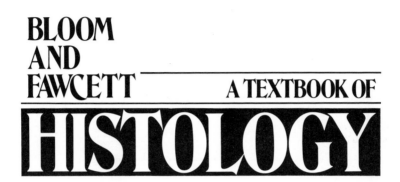

DON W. FAWCETT, M.D.

Hersey Professor of Anatomy, Emeritus
Harvard Medical School
Boston, Massachusetts
Senior Scientist
International Laboratory for Research
on Animal Diseases
Nairobi, Kenya, Africa

ELEVENTH EDITION

1986
W. B. SAUNDERS COMPANY
PHILADELPHIA □ LONDON □ TORONTO □ MEXICO CITY □ RIO DE JANEIRO □ SYDNEY □ TOKYO □ HONG KONG

W. B. Saunders Company: West Washington Square
Philadelphia, PA 19105

Library of Congress Cataloging in Publication Data

Fawcett, Don Wayne, 1917–

A textbook of histology.

At head of title: Bloom and Fawcett.

Rev. ed. of: Textbook of histology/William Bloom,
Don W. Fawcett. 10th ed. 1975.

Includes bibliographies and index.

1. Histology.   I. Bloom, William, 1899–1972. Textbook of
   histology. 10th ed.   II. Title.   III. Title: Histology.

QM551.F34 1986   611'.018   85–8218

ISBN 0–7216–1729–8

Listed here is the latest translated edition of this book together
with the language of the translation and the publisher.

Portuguese (*10th Edition*)—DISCOS CBS Industria e Comercio Ltda., Rio de Janeiro, Brazil

Japanese (*10th Edition*)—Hirokawa Publishing Co., Tokyo, Japan

Spanish (*10th Edition*)—Editorial Labor, S. A., Barcelona, Spain

Italian (*10th Edition*)—Piccin Editore, Padova, Italy

Editor: Dana Dreibelbis
Designer: Terri Siegel
Production Manager: Bob Butler
Manuscript Editor: David Harvey
Illustration Coordinator: Walt Verbitski
Indexer: Susan Thomas

A Textbook of Histology   ISBN   0-7216-1729-8

Last digit is the print number: 9   8   7   6   5   4   3   2   1

Preface

Advances in histology and cytology in the past decade have continued to be impressive, requiring extensive revision of the *Textbook of Histology.* In this period a number of smaller books have appeared that may seem to be more commensurate with the diminishing time allotted to this subject in the curricula of medicine, dentistry, and veterinary science. Nonetheless, we believe that there is still a place for a book that treats this important body of knowledge more thoroughly. The benefits of such a book may extend beyond the immediate needs of students and teachers to the future needs of those engaged in biomedical research.

Research in many areas of biological science is now dominated by "reductionism"—the laudable attempt to understand complex living organisms by studying the properties of their smallest components. The advancing frontier of knowledge has rapidly progressed down to the cell and its subcellular organelles and macromolecules. Much of current research is carried out on a small number of cell types that can be grown in vitro. The contributions of such studies to our understanding of fundamental biological processes have been impressive. But in the longer term, the objective must be to understand not only what cells can do in the controlled environment of the culture vessel, but how cells function in the complex interactive systems that make up the tissues and organs of the body. In the foreseeable future the pendulum will surely swing back from reductionism. When it does, it is hoped that this book will serve as a repository of useful information that would otherwise have to be rediscovered by cellular and molecular biologists when they undertake to apply their knowledge of isolated components to the functioning of the heterogeneous associations of interacting cells characteristic of higher levels of organization in whole animals.

In the productive period embraced by this revision, there have been remarkable advances in our understanding of the structural basis of cell and tissue function. New interpretations of the molecular organization of the cell membrane have been put forward. New filamentous components of the cytoskeleton have been identified and their relationships to each other and to the plasmalemma described. Receptor-mediated endocytosis has been found to be a widespread cellular activity of great physiological importance. Gaps in our understanding of the biosynthesis of proteins have been filled by further elaboration of the signal hypothesis and elucidation of a number of molecular events in the assembly and translocation of the nascent polypeptides. The mechanism of action of hormones and neurotransmitters has been clarified by identification and isolation of many of their receptors. The discovery of a host of new biologically active peptides and their immunocytochemical localization in cells widely dispersed in the gastrointestinal tract and brain has led to recognition of a diffuse endocrine system hitherto overlooked. Atrial cardiac muscle cells have been shown to have an endocrine as well as a contractile mechanical function. The endothelium of arteries has been found to synthesize and release a clotting factor into the blood and the endothelium of the pulmonary vessels has been shown to have surface enzymes that transform or catabolize certain hormones. Functions have been assigned to a number of other cell types previously considered to be relatively inert. Several genetically distinct types of collagen have been identified in the extracellular matrix of connective tissue. Fibronectin and laminin and other new structural proteins have been characterized and their distribution and functions described. Much has been learned about the properties of proteoglycans and their interactions with the fibrous components of the extracellular matrix. Major changes have taken place in interpretation of stem cell kinetics and cell lineages in hemopoesis and the influence of humoral and microenvironmental factors in control of blood cell differentiation.

We have endeavored to incorporate these and many other advances into the book without substantial increase in its length. Outmoded interpretations have been deleted and the sections on histogenesis have been omitted except where essential to an understanding of the structure of the organ. In past editions the opening chapter was devoted to *Methods*, for it was thought desirable to give the student some insight into how new information in this field is acquired. It seems unlikely that curricular time still permits presentation of such material, and the techniques for analysis of structure and function have become so diverse that their exposition, however brief, would occupy a disproportionate fraction of the book. Therefore, the chapter on *Methods* has been omitted from this edition, and those pages have been used to expand and update the material on *The Cell*. This chapter does not presume to cover the burgeoning field of cell biology, but describes briefly the structure and function of the cell organelles, and introduces terminology and concepts needed for an understanding of later chapters.

A special effort has been made to update and improve the sections on the histophysiology of the organs. Histology is a highly visual subject in which illustrations often contribute as much to understanding as the text. As in previous revisions, old photomicrographs and electron micrographs have been replaced by new ones of better quality or more informational content wherever these were available. Approximately 100 figures have been eliminated and 160 added, bringing the total to over 900. For the first time the references for each chapter have been grouped under headings corresponding to those in the text, to facilitate the task for those readers who may wish to consult the literature for more detailed information on specific topics.

All books can be improved, and this book is no exception. I will welcome constructive criticism from knowledgeable colleagues and students, and will depend upon you, my readers, to point out items that need to be changed, added, or deleted. With your help I look forward to a greatly improved next edition.

I am indebted to Helen Deacon in the United States and Doris Churi in Kenya for typing and retyping manuscript, and to Drs. Giuseppina and Elio Raviola for sending countless xeroxes of literature not otherwise available to me in East Africa. The patience of Mr. Dana Dreibelbis, Medical Editor, and others at the W. B. Saunders Company was greatly appreciated.

Don W. Fawcett, M.D.

Contents

THE CELL

The living substance of plants and animals has traditionally been described by the general term *protoplasm*. The smallest unit of protoplasm capable of independent existence is the *cell*. The simplest animals consist of a single cell. The higher animals can be thought of as a colony or complex society of interdependent cells of many kinds, specialized in various ways to carry out the functions essential to survival and reproduction of the animal as a whole. Cells serving the same general function are grouped together and united by varying amounts of intercellular substance to form the basic *tissues* of the body, such as blood, bone, muscle, nervous tissue, connective tissue and so forth. Two or more tissues are usually combined to form the larger functional units called *organs*: e.g, skin, kidney, blood vessels, glands, and so on. Several organs whose functions are interrelated constitute an *organ system*; examples are the respiratory system (comprising the nose, larynx, trachea, and lungs) and the urinary system (composed of the kidneys, ureters, urinary bladder, and urethra).

The etymological derivation of the term *histology* may suggest that this is a subdivision of morphological science that deals only with the tissues, but it is in fact equally concerned with the cellular and extracellular components and the patterns of their association to form organs. In this broader sense histology is synonymous with *microscopic anatomy*. The boundaries of the field were formerly limited by the resolving power of the light microscope. In the past 30 years the increasing use of the electron microscope by histologists has greatly extended the scope of the subject so that it now includes tissue ultrastructure and much of cell biology, and thus embraces biological structure at all levels of organization from the lower limit of direct visual inspection down to the structure of large molecules. For the localization of specific macromolecules and enzymatic activities, the interests of contemporary histologists also extend to histo- and cytochemistry.

THE CELL

Hundreds of microscopically distinguishable kinds of cells are found in the body, but they all have certain structural features in common. This chapter does not refer to a particular cell type but undertakes to describe the structural components of cells in general.

The cell is partitioned into two major compartments: the *nucleus,* composed of *nucleoplasm (karyoplasm),* and the *cytoplasm,* which surrounds the nucleus and makes up the rest of the cell body. Both of these compartments contain structural components of characteristic form and staining properties that can be recognized with the light microscope (Fig. 1–1). On the basis of the generality of their occurrence and certain assumptions as to their functional significance, these have been classified in two categories: *organelles* and *inclusions.*

Organelles are structures common to nearly all cell types and are regarded as metabolically active internal organs carrying out essential specific functions. Inclusions, on the other hand, are considered to be metabolically inert accumulations of metabolites or cell products such as stored carbohydrate, protein or lipid and various crystals, pigment deposits, secretory granules, and the like. In contrast to organelles, inclusions are regarded as dispensable and often temporary constituents of cells. Although the distinction between organelles and inclusions is still useful, the assignment of cell components to these two categories was originally made by histologists at a time when too little was known about their ultrastructure and chemical nature to make a valid judgment as to whether they were metabolically active or

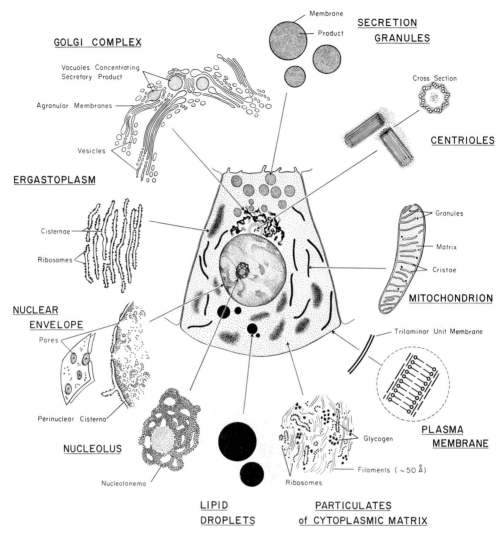

GOLGI COMPLEX

Vacuoles Concentrating Secretory Product

Agranular Membranes

Vesicles

Membrane

Product

SECRETION GRANULES

Cross Section

CENTRIOLES

ERGASTOPLASM

Cisternae

Ribosomes

Granules

Matrix

Cristae

MITOCHONDRION

NUCLEAR ENVELOPE

Pores

Trilaminar Unit Membrane

Perinuclear Cisterna

NUCLEOLUS

Nucleolonema

Glycogen

PLASMA MEMBRANE

Filaments (~50 Å)

Ribosomes

LIPID DROPLETS

PARTICULATES of CYTOPLASMIC MATRIX

Figure 1–1. In the center of this figure is a drawing of the cell and its organelles and inclusions as they appear by light microscopy. Around the periphery are representations of these same components as seen in electron micrographs. What was called ergastoplasm by light microscopists is now called the rough endoplasmic reticulum. The illustration of the plasma membrane encircled by an interrupted line is not directly visualized but represents the bimolecular layer of phospholipids inferred from indirect methods of analysis.

inert, essential or dispensable. As knowledge of cell biology has advanced, the list of cell organelles has lengthened, and the traditional classification of some components as inclusions has become debatable. For example, some pigment granules formerly considered to be inert inclusions are now identified as melanosomes, organelles with a highly organized internal structure and specific enzymatic activity. Similarly, secretory granules formerly regarded as accumulations of stored cell product are now found to be limited by an enzymatically active membrane and hence can qualify as organelles. A number of the fibrillar elements of the cytoplasmic matrix

that escaped detection with the light microscope are not defined as organelles or inclusions but are grouped in a third category: *cytoskeletal components.*

Control of the differentiation and synthetic functions of the cell resides in the nucleus while most of the responding synthetic and metabolic activities are functions of the cytoplasm. The cell organelles and inclusions are suspended in a *cytoplasmic matrix* that appears structureless with the light microscope, but which consists of a fluid phase occupying the interstices of a complex three-dimensional meshwork of fibrillar components constituting the *cytoskeleton.*

Although the organelles visible with the light microscope (mitochondria, Golgi apparatus, ergastoplasm) were originally interpreted as granular or lamellar solid structures, the electron microscope has revealed that these and other newly described organelles are hollow structures bounded by thin membranes of lipid and protein and often having a complex internal structure. One of the most important contributions of electron microscopy has been to make us aware of the importance of compartmentation of the cell by membranes.

Most of the important physiological processes take place at surfaces and interfaces. Hundreds of enzymes that catalyze the chemical transformations occurring in cells are strategically located in the membranes at the interface between the cell and its environment or between the organelles and the cytoplasmic matrix. The internal partitioning of the cytoplasm achieved by membrane-bounded organelles promotes the efficiency of countless complex chemical reactions by amplifying the area of the physiologically active interfaces within the cell. The partitioning of the cytoplasm is also essential to the control mechanisms that govern cell metabolism. The membranes enable the cell to maintain a separation of enzymes and substrates at some times, and at other times to permit their controlled interaction by varying permeability of a particular membrane or the rate of active transport across it. If there were unlimited diffusion and interaction within the cell it would be impossible to maintain the high degree of chemical heterogeneity characteristic of the cytoplasm. Enzymes would attack their substrates, and all the potential interactions of the countless chemical constituents of the cell would race out of control. This does not occur. The cell is able to regulate its activities and to hold in reserve a large repertoire of unexpressed biochemical reactions. It can call each of these into play at the proper time and at the rate appropriate to the needs of the organism as a whole. The fact that this is possible is due in large measure to the prevalence of membrane-bounded organelles in the cytoplasm.

CELL MEMBRANE

The outer boundary of all cells is the *plasmalemma* or *cell membrane*. It is invisible with the light microscope, and in electron micrographs usually appears as a thin dense line 8.5 to 10 nm thick. Although microscopically unimpressive, it is remarkably complex in its molecular organization and carries out many essential functions. It regulates the traffic in ions and macromolecules in and out of the cell. It possesses devices for cell attachment and cell-to-cell communication; antigenic molecules that are the basis of cell recognition and tissue specificity; ion pumps for regulating the internal environment of the cell; receptors for hormones; and mechanisms for generating messenger molecules that activate the cell's physiological responses to stimulation.

In electron micrographs of high magnification, three parallel lines can be discerned in thin sections of the cell membrane—two electron-dense layers (2.5–3.0 nm) separated by an electron-lucent intermediate layer (3.5–4 nm) (Fig. 1–2). With minor dimensional variations, all membranous components of cells have the same appearance. This does not reflect a trilaminar structure at the molecular level, but is a characteristic pattern of binding of the osmium used as a stain for electron microscopy. Membranes are composed of lipids and proteins, some of which possess terminal polysaccharides and hence are glycolipids and glycoproteins. The lipid is responsible for the form and many of the permeability properties of membranes, while their enzymatic activities reside in their protein constituents.

All biological membranes consist of a bimolecular layer of mixed phospholipids oriented with their hydrophilic ends at the outer surfaces and their hydrophobic chains projecting toward the middle of the bilayer. Deposition of osmium in the hydrophilic ends of the phospholipid molecules is believed to result in the two dense lines seen in electron micrographs, while the intervening pale line represents the unstained hydrocarbon chains of the lipid molecules. The *integral proteins* of the membrane occur as globular particles of varying size distributed in the lipid bilayer (Fig. 1–3). They occupy different positions within the bilayer depending on the distribution of the hydrophilic and hydrophobic regions in the protein molecules. Some having their polar amino acids at one end will be exposed on an outer surface and have their nonpolar region in the hydrophobic interior of the membrane. Others with polar regions at either end and a nonpolar segment in the middle extend through the

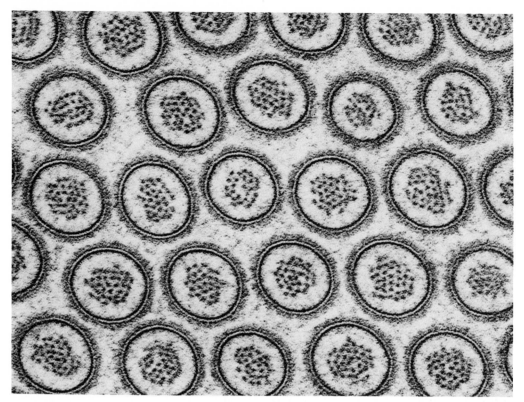

Figure 1–2. Electron micrograph of microvillous processes of an intestinal epithelial cell in cross section. Each microvillus is enclosed by an extension of the cell membrane. The membrane appears trilaminar—two dense layers separated by a light intermediate layer. The dense lines are due to deposition of the osmium stain in the hydrophilic ends of the phospholipid molecules of a bimolecular layer of lipid. The hydrocarbon chains remain unstained and form the light middle line. On the outer aspect of the membrane is a moderately dense surface coat or glycocalyx consisting of terminal polysaccharides of the integral glycoproteins embedded in the lipid bilayer of the membrane. (Micrograph courtesy of Atsushi Ichikawa.)

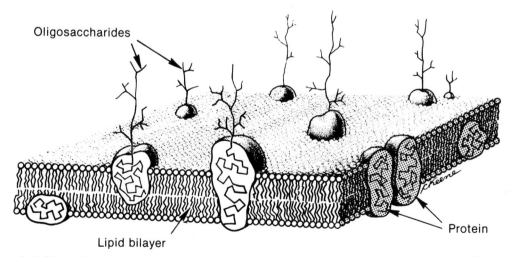

Figure 1–3. Schematic representation of the fluid mosaic model of the cell membrane. Globular protein molecules are positioned in the lipid bilayer at different depths depending on the distribution of their hydrophilic and hydrophobic groups. Some extend entirely through the bilayer (transmembrane proteins). The lipid bilayer is fluid and the integral proteins are free to diffuse laterally within the plane of the membrane if not restrained by binding to peripheral proteins in the underlying cytoplasm. Terminal oligosaccharides of the glycoproteins extend outward contributing to the surface coat or glycocalyx.

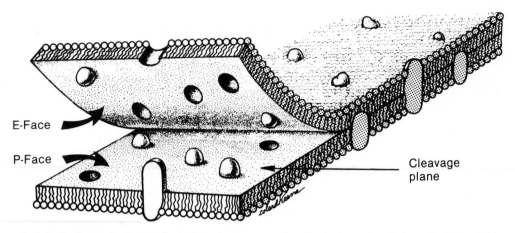

E-Face

P-Face

Cleavage plane

Figure 1–4. In the freeze-fracture method of specimen preparation, the fracture plane follows the hydrophobic region of the membrane exposing two fracture faces—the *E-face,* the inwardly facing outer half, and the *P-face,* the outwardly facing inner half, which usually contains the majority of integral protein particles.

entire thickness of the lipid bilayer and are described as *transmembrane proteins.*

The proteins are not identifiable in thin sections of membranes, but they can be visualized in tissues prepared by the freeze-fracture method. In this procedure, tissues are rapidly frozen in liquid Freon or liquid nitrogen and then cracked under vacuum by impact of a blade cooled to $-196°$ C. The plane of fracture through the frozen tissue preferentially follows the path of least resistance through the hydrophobic region of the lipid bilayer and thus cleaves cell membranes in half, exposing extensive areas of their interior (Fig. 1–4). A replica of the exposed surface is then made by evaporation of a heavy metal, such as platinum, from a source at an acute angle to the fracture surface. Carbon is then deposited uniformly over the surface by evaporation from a separate electrode directly over the specimen, forming a coherent and stable replica of all irregularities on the fracture face. The tissue is then digested away and the replica recovered for examination with the electron microscope.

In such preparations, the cleaved cell membranes present two distinct appearances. The outwardly facing inner half-membrane, called the *P-face,* shows numerous randomly distributed 6- to 9-nm particles that represent the integral membrane proteins (Fig. 1–5). The inwardly facing outer half-membrane, called the *E-face,* is relatively smooth but may contain occasional particles and numerous shallow pits corresponding in distribution to the particles on the opposing P-face. Why the majority of protein particles remain with the inner half-membrane is not clear.

The concentration of particles seen in freeze-fracture replicas of various cellular membranes correlates well with their biochemically determined protein content. Since their distinctive enzymatic properties reside in their proteins, the membranes of very active cell organelles have a higher concentration of membrane particles than those that are metabolically relatively inert.

At body temperature, the lipid bilayer is fluid and many of the integral protein particles are free to move laterally within the plane of the membrane. In freeze-fracture preparations, the seemingly random pattern of particles in unspecialized regions of the plasma membrane gives a misleading impression of uniformity of membrane structure and function over the entire cell. It is known, however, that the luminal, lateral, and basal membranes of many epithelial cells differ in their enzymatic and other properties. Therefore, despite the lateral mobility of some membrane proteins, the cell is able to maintain regional differences in the population of certain specific protein particles. How this is accomplished is not entirely clear, but it is speculated that mobility of some transmembrane proteins is restricted by their binding to *peripheral membrane proteins*—polypeptide polymers in the underlying cytoplasm associated with the inner aspect of the plasma membrane.

In addition to these regional differences in biochemical properties of the cell membrane, which are not reflected in obvious differences in distribution of intramembrane particles, there are local specializations of the membrane for cell-to-cell communication and for

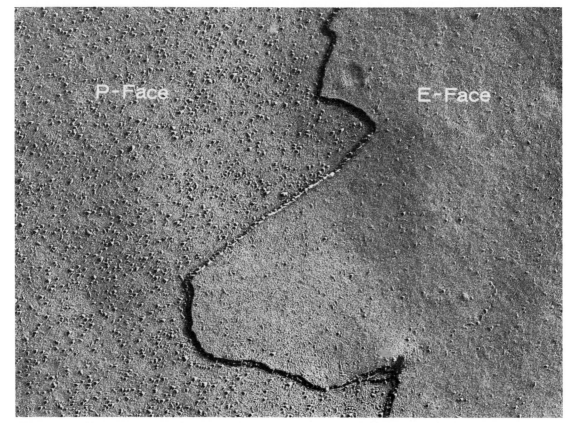

Figure 1–5. Freeze-fracture preparation of the plasma membranes of two adjacent cells. The fracture plane has broken across from one to the other, exposing the E-face of one and the P-face of the other.

cell-to-cell attachment. At these sites, integral protein particles are aggregated into closely packed plaques or into linear arrays that form circumferential bands around the cell apex. These junctional specializations of the membrane will be discussed in more detail in Chapter 2.

The polysaccharide components of the integral glycoproteins and glycolipids project from the outer aspect of the lipid bilayer and contribute to the formation of a carbohydrate-rich *surface coat* or *glycocalyx*. This is present on the free surface of nearly all cells, but is most highly developed on the luminal surface of certain epithelia. It is especially conspicuous on the brush border of the absorptive cells of the intestinal epithelium where it appears as a mat of delicate, branching, 2- to 5-nm polysaccharide filaments. Ionized carboxyl and sulfate groups of the acid polysaccharides give the glycocalyx a strong negative charge, and it avidly binds cationic dyes such as Alcian blue, ruthenium red, and cationic ferritin. This layer acts as a protective mechanical barrier, and its polyanionic prop-

erties probably confer some degree of selectivity with respect to naturally occurring substances that can bind to the cell surface.

ENDOPLASMIC RETICULUM

The cytoplasm of many cell types is permeated by an extensive system of membrane-bounded canaliculi making up the *endoplasmic reticulum*. This organelle consists of a loose network of branching and anastomosing tubules throughout the cytoplasm, but the tubules may be expanded locally into broad flat saccules called cisternae. Where cisternae are abundant they tend to become arranged in parallel array. The endoplasmic reticulum is a closed intracellular canalicular system that does not normally open onto the cell surface. Its limiting membrane is, however, continuous with the outer membrane of the nuclear envelope. Thus, the space between the two nuclear membranes may be considered a perinuclear cistern of the endoplasmic reticulum.

This organelle occurs in two forms: the *rough endoplasmic reticulum* and the *smooth endoplasmic reticulum* (Figs. 1–6, 1–7). In the former the outer surface of the limiting membrane is studded with dense granules of ribonucleoprotein, the *ribosomes,* which are involved in the synthesis of proteins. The newly synthesized protein accumulates in the lumen of the reticulum and is transported through it to the supranuclear region for further processing in the Golgi complex, an organelle concerned with concentrating and packaging cell products for secretion.

The smooth reticulum predominates in cells involved in synthesis of triglycerides, cholestrol, or steroid hormones. The membranes contain a versatile complement of enzymes involved in conjugation, oxidation, and methylation. The smooth reticulum in liver cells plays an important role in synthesis of plasma lipoproteins, and in the metabolism and detoxification of exogenous lipid-soluble drugs. A special form of smooth reticulum, the sarcoplasmic reticulum, surrounds the myofibrils in striated muscle. Here its principal function is the sequestration and release of the calcium ions that control muscular contraction and relaxation (see Chapter 10).

The ribonucleoprotein of the ribosomes is largely responsible for the affinity of the cytoplasm for basic dyes. Aggregations of rough endoplasmic reticulum appear under the light microscope as coarse basophilic bodies of irregular shape and varying size. When cells are homogenized for biochemical analysis, the endoplasmic reticulum is broken up and the membranes of the fragments close to form small ribosome studded vesicles that make up the *microsome fraction* recovered by differential centrifugation (Fig. 1–8). Thus, microsomes, as such, do not occur in the living cell but are fragments of the endoplasmic reticulum resulting from homogenization of cells. If the microsome fraction is treated with lipid solvents to remove the membranes, recentrifugation yields a *ribosome fraction.* Much of our present understanding of the biosynthesis of proteins is based on the study of such fractions. Upon addition of *messenger RNA* (mRNA) and cofactors, microsomes will synthesize specific proteins in vitro.

The ribosomes measure 15 by 25 nm and are composed of a smaller and larger subunit. The small subunit contains a single large molecule of ribonucleic acid (RNA) and some 30 associated small proteins. The larger subunit adjacent to the membrane consists of two molecules of RNA and about 40 associated proteins. Ribosomes may occur singly free in the cytoplasmic matrix but in this form they are nonfunctional. To participate in protein synthesis, they must become associated with a molecule of mRNA, which carries the codons determining the sequence of assembly of amino acids into polypeptides. In synthetically active cells, the great majority of ribosomes occur in clusters of 10 to 20 linked together by their common attachment to a long molecule of mRNA. These assemblies are called *polyribosomes or polysomes.*

Polyribosomes that occur free in the cytoplasm are engaged in synthesis of the integral proteins of the cell. Those that are bound to the membrane of the rough endoplasmic reticulum are involved in synthesis of protein destined for export from the cell as a secretory product. When seen in surface view on the membranes, they appear as beaded chains or rosettes. The connecting strand of mRNA usually cannot be resolved in micrographs of thin sections. The ribosomes bind to receptors in the membrane by their large subunit. The nascent polypeptide chains come off vectorially, extending through the membrane into the lumen of the reticulum. The newly synthesized protein is channeled through the reticulum to the Golgi region where it is transferred in small transport vesicles to the Golgi for further processing and packaging for export. The participation of the rough endoplasmic reticulum in protein synthesis will be considered in greater detail in a subsequent chapter on glands and secretion.

The smooth endoplasmic reticulum has no associated ribosomes and usually takes the form of a closer-meshed three-dimensional network of tubules (Fig. 1–7). Smooth-surfaced cisternae are rarely seen. Where rough and smooth reticulum occur in the same cell they are continuous with one another but represent regional differentiation of the organelle for different functions. The relative proportions of the two vary with the cell type. The rough endoplasmic reticulum is most highly developed in glandular cells synthesizing a large volume of a protein-rich secretory product.

GOLGI COMPLEX

The *Golgi apparatus* or *Golgi complex* is an organelle found in nearly all eukaryotic cells. It is best developed and has been most thor-

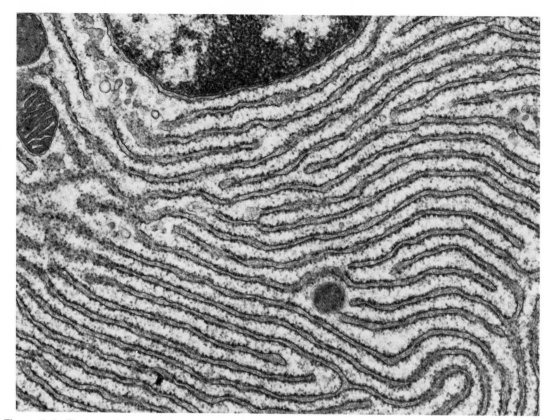

Figure 1–6. Electron micrograph of a portion of a human plasma cell containing an extensive rough endoplasmic reticulum consisting of cisternae studded with ribosomes. The moderately dense material in the lumen of the cisternae represents newly synthesized protein.

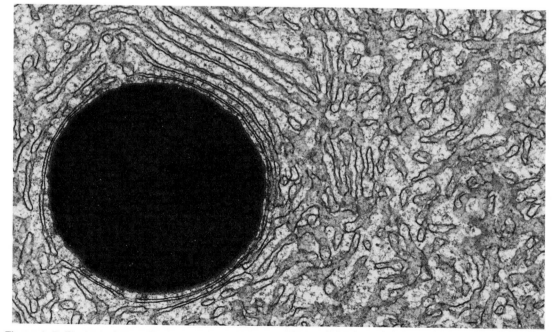

Figure 1–7. Electron micrograph of an area of cytoplasm rich in smooth endoplasmic reticulum. The elements of the reticulum are branching and anastomosing tubules. This form of the organelle is common in cells engaged in steroid synthesis and lipid metabolism. The round dense body is a droplet of lipid.

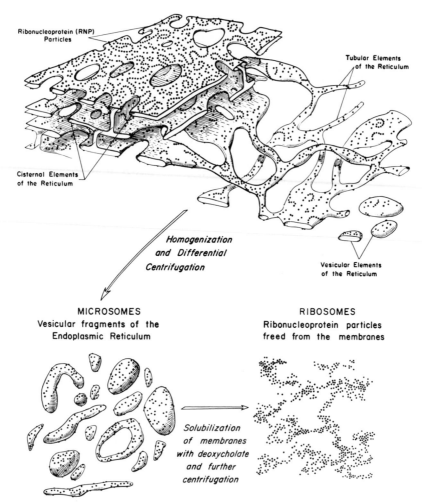

Ribonucleoprotein (RNP)
Particles

Tubular Elements
of the Reticulum

Cisternal Elements
of the Reticulum

Vesicular Elements
of the Reticulum

Homogenization
and Differential
Centrifugation

MICROSOMES
Vesicular fragments of the
Endoplasmic Reticulum

RIBOSOMES
Ribonucleoprotein particles
freed from the membranes

Solubilization
of membranes
with deoxycholate
and further
centrifugation

Figure 1–8. Diagrammatic representation of the three-dimensional configuration of the granular or rough endoplasmic reticulum. When cells are homogenated for biochemical analysis, the reticulum is fragmented into small closed vesicles called *microsomes*. The membranes of the microsome fraction can be solubilized and the *ribosomes* of the reticulum can be recovered by further centrifugation.

oughly studied in glandular cells, where it is the site of concentration, chemical modification, and packaging of the secretory products synthesized on the rough endoplasmic reticulum. It has limited synthetic activity of its own for complex carbohydrates, and plays an important role in renewal of the plasma membrane of the cell and its carbohydrate-rich surface coat.

The organelle is not seen in routine histological preparations, but can be impregnated with silver or osmium by several classical staining procedures developed 75 to 100 years ago. It is also stained by histochemical reactions for localizing certain enzymes.

In electron micrographs, it consists of several membrane-limited flattened saccules or cisternae, stacked in parallel array (Figs. 1–9, 1–10). In section, the lumen of the cisternae is narrow in its central portion but somewhat expanded toward the ends where the profile of the cistern may be interrupted by fenestrations. There is no membrane continuity between the successive cisternae. The cisternae are often curved so that the organelle as a whole has a convex and a concave surface. These curved assemblages of parallel cisternae correspond to the arciform structures seen in stained preparations and called *dictyosomes* by classical cytologists.

A structural and functional polarity is evident in the organization of the Golgi complex. The lumen of the cisternae is narrow at the convex face of the stack and becomes wider in the successive saccules toward the concave face, and in actively secreting glan-

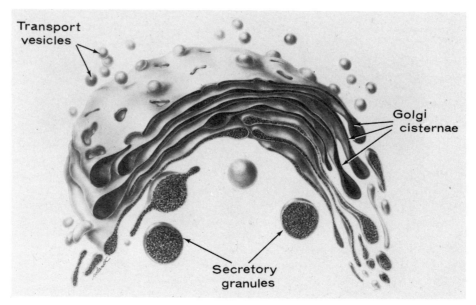

Figure 1–9. Three-dimensional drawing of the Golgi complex sectioned vertically. Small transport vesicles originating from the endoplasmic reticulum are abundant at its convex or forming face. In glandular cells, secretory granules are associated with its concave or maturing face.

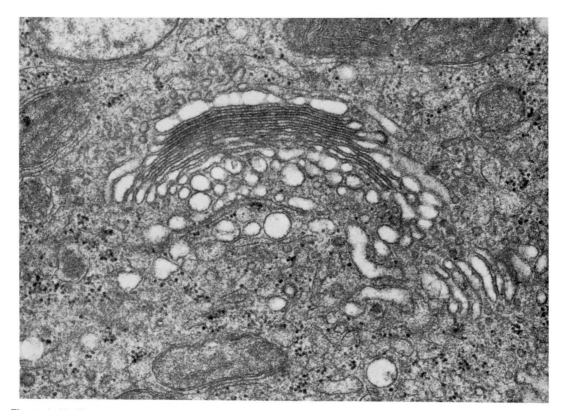

Figure 1–10. Electron micrograph of the Golgi complex of a cell in the epithelium of the vas deferens. (Micrograph courtesy of Daniel Friend.)

dular cells the density of the cisternal contents increases progressively from the outer convex to the inner concave surface. There is also histochemical evidence of regional functional diversity. When subject to prolonged osmication, the metal is deposited preferentially in one or two cisternae at the convex face of the stack. The intermediate cisternae are selectively stained for nicotinamide adenine dinucleotide phosphatase (NADPase), and the reaction product of the histochemical method for thiamine pyrophosphatase is confined to one or two cisternae on the concave inner side of the organelle.

Proteins synthesized on the rough endoplasmic reticulum are transported in small transitional vesicles that bud off from ribosome-free areas of the reticulum near the convex surface of the Golgi complex. The exact destination of these transport vesicles in this organelle is not settled. According to the most widely accepted view, the vesicles fuse with one another to form the outermost cistern of the Golgi (Fig. 1–11A). This saccule with its content of secretory product is thought to progress through the organelle to the opposite face as successive cisternae are formed behind it. The convex side of the stack is therefore called the *forming face* and the concave side the *maturing* or *secretory face*. In this interpretation, all the cisternae in the stack are involved in processing the secretory product. In its transit through the organelle, the protein is concentrated and glycosylated by glycosyl transferases present in the Golgi membranes. Upon reaching the secretory face, the cistern rounds up into a number of small vacuoles containing the concentrated protein. These subsequently coalesce to form a single large *condensing vacuole*. After further concentration of its contents, this vacuole becomes a dense, spherical secretory granule.

This interpretation accounts for the gradient in density of the content of the cisternae from one side of the stack to the other, but it involves a number of assumptions that are yet to be validated. If the transport vesicles budded off from the reticulum are continuously incorporated in the Golgi membranes, then with time the lipid and enzymatic composition of the two organelles should become the same. Biochemical studies provide no evidence of mixing of either the lipid or protein components of the two compartments. To explain the maintenance of their specific properties, it is necessary to assume that membrane proteins characteristic of the reticulum are excluded and those destined for incorporation in the Golgi are clustered in the transitional region from which the transport vesicles arise by budding. Moreover, if the cisternae move through the stack in the continual renewal of the organelle, the consistent regional differences in enzymatic properties demonstrated histochemically would be difficult to explain in an organelle lacking the capacity for protein synthesis.

An alternative interpretation favored by some cell biologists assumes that the transport vesicles go directly from the transitional region of the reticulum to the condensing vacuoles and in certain conditions to the expanded rims of cisternae near the secretory face of the Golgi (Fig. 1–11B). Thus, the bulk of the Golgi complex would be bypassed and would not participate in condensation or modification of the product. Such a scheme would avoid the problem of mixing and dilution of Golgi-specific membrane components by contributions of membrane from the reticulum and would make the maintenance of regional distribution of specific enzymes more understandable. On the other hand, it leaves unexplained the gradient in product density in cisternae from the convex to the concave side of the organelle, and offers no mechanism for replacement of the continual loss of Golgi membrane from the secretory face through formation of the condensing vacuoles. The contradictions in both interpretations remain unresolved, and clearly much remains to be learned about the function of this important organelle in the secretory process and its role in renewal and recycling of components of the plasmalemma.

A group of structures in close proximity to the Golgi complex, but considered by some to be a distinct organelle, is the *Golgi-associated Endoplasmic Reticulum from which Lysosomes form*—commonly referred to by the acronym *GERL*. When glandular cells are staining with the cytochemical method for the enzyme acid phosphatase, the condensing vacuoles, a cistern near the secretory face of the Golgi complex, and contiguous tubules of the endoplasmic reticulum all give a positive reaction. It has been proposed that these structures constitute a specialized complex for the transfer of hydrolases directly from their site of synthesis in the endoplasmic reticulum to lysosomes forming near the inner face of the Golgi. Because condensing vacuoles and im-

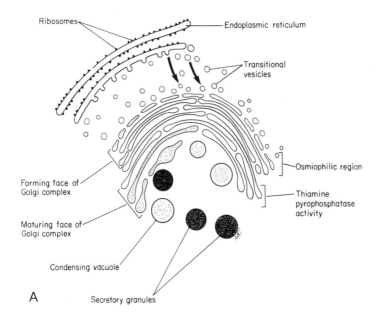

A

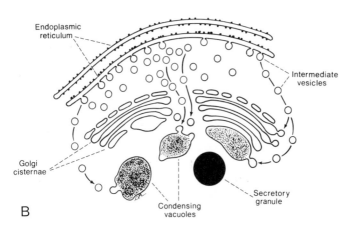

B

Figure 1–11. Alternative interpretations of the path of secretory products through the Golgi complex. *A,* Transport vesicles fuse at convex surface into a cistern, which progresses through the stack as new ones form behind it. *B,* transport vesicles fuse with the periphery of relatively static cisternae or directly with the condensing vacuoles at the secretory face of the organelle. *C,* Transport vesicles fuse directly with condensing vacuoles arising not from the Golgi but from Golgi-associated endoplasmic reticulum (GERL) from which lysosomes also arise.

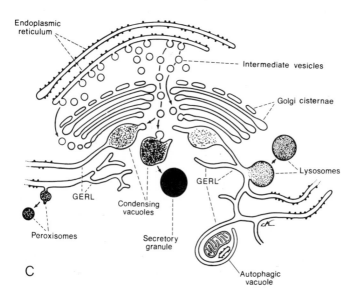

C

mature secretory granules also exhibit phosphatase activity, it is argued that these arise from GERL and not from the Golgi complex (Fig. 1–11C). If this is true, the secretory pathway would bypass the Golgi, and the condensing vacuoles would receive secretory proteins from the reticulum via intermediate vesicles, and hydrolases directly from acid phosphatase–positive elements of the adjacent reticulum. Although this interpretation has recently gained some measure of acceptance, it remains controversial. The Golgi complex has long been assigned a major role in the packaging of secretory product in a membrane capable of fusing with the plasmalemma during exocytosis. The suggestion that condensing vacuoles do not arise from the Golgi but are derived from the GERL, a specialized region of the endoplasmic reticulum, is difficult to bring into accord with the widely accepted view of Golgi function.

MITOCHONDRIA

Mitochondria are the organelles that provide the energy for the biosynthetic and motor activities of cells. They are present in all eukaryotic cells in numbers ranging from a few to several thousand, depending on the energy requirements for the specific functions of the cell.

In living cells, the mitochondria appear as slender rods 0.2 to 0.3 μm in diameter and 2 to 6 μm long. They may be randomly distributed in the cytoplasm or concentrated at sites of high energy utilization. In electron micrographs of thin sections, mitochondria are seen to be limited by a smooth contoured *outer membrane* about 7 nm thick and a slightly thinner *inner membrane* that is generally parallel to the limiting membrane but exhibits a number of slender folds called *cristae,* which project some distance into the interior of the organelle (Fig. 1–12). The cristae are a device for amplifying the surface area of this enzyme-rich membrane to increase the efficiency of the organelle in generating energy. In cells with high energy requirements, the number of cristae in the mitochondria is greater than in cells with less metabolic activity.

The mitochondrial membranes delimit two compartments: a large *intercristal space* com-

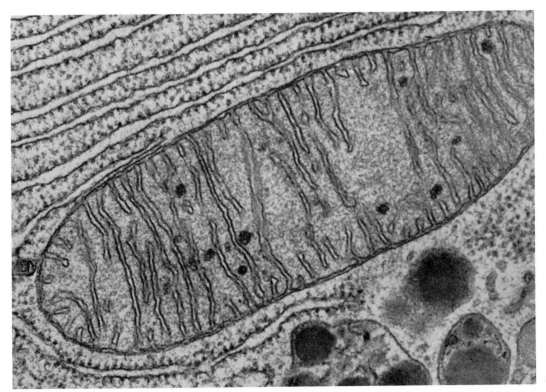

Figure 1–12. Electron micrograph of a typical mitochondrion from the pancreas of a bat, showing the cristae, matrix, and matrix granules. Endoplasmic reticulum is seen at upper left and lysosomes at lower right. (Micrograph courtesy of K. R. Porter.)

prising all of the area within the inner membrane, and a smaller *membrane space* consisting of the narrow cleft between outer and inner membranes and its inward extensions between the leaves of the cristae. These latter clefts are sometimes referred to as *intracristal spaces,* but it is clear that they are not functionally distinct from the rest of the membrane space. This space usually is only 10 to 20 nm across, and because it contains little protein precipitable by chemical fixatives, it generally appears empty in electron micrographs. The large intercristal space, on the other hand, is occupied by a moderately electron dense *mitochondrial matrix.* Although the outer and inner membranes are similar in appearance in electron micrographs of thin sections, they differ in their physiological properties, the outer being freely permeable to small molecules and the inner having the osmotic properties of a semipermeable membrane. The inner membrane also has a distinguishing morphological feature that can be demonstrated only by negative staining of disrupted isolated mitochondria. In such preparations, its inner surface is studded with numerous minute particles. These *inner membrane subunits* consist of a globular head 9 to 10 nm in diameter connected to the underlying membrane by a slender stem 3 to 4 nm thick and about 5 nm long.

The energy-generating function of the mitochondria depends on oxygen and products of the digestion of the protein, carbohydrate, and lipid in the food ingested by the organism. These are delivered to the cell in the form of amino acids (from proteins), glucose (from carbohydrates), and fatty acids (from lipids). A multienzyme system in the mitochondria oxidizes these substrates in a series of chemical reactions called the *tricarboxylic acid cycle* or *Krebs cycle.* The hydrogen atoms removed in the successive steps of oxidation are passed along a chain of respiratory enzyme complexes in the inner mitochondrial membrane and utilized in the conversion of adenosine diphosphate (ADP) to adenosine triphosphate (ATP), the ubiquitous energy-carrying molecule required for transport across membranes, for all synthetic processes throughout the cells, and for the mechanical work involved in the motor activities of cells. The succinoxidase, cytochrome oxidase, and other enzymes concerned with electron transport are in the inner mitochondrial membrane, while the enzymes of oxidative phosphorylation of ADP and hydrolysis of ATP

reside in the inner membrane subunits projecting into the mitochondrial matrix.

Mitochondria are self-duplicating organelles that increase their number by undergoing division that resembles the binary fission of bacteria. Indeed, mitochondria are believed to have evolved from symbiotic bacteria very early in the development of living forms when the earth's atmosphere was still relatively poor in oxygen and most of the primitive unicellular organisms depended on anaerobic fermentation of organic molecules. It is speculated that a small bacterium that had evolved the ability to utilize oxygen invaded a larger anaerobic cell type, and a symbiotic relationship developed with the aerobic symbiont generating energy in return for protection and nutrients from the larger host cell. With the passage of time, the interdependence of the two increased and the parasite became an indispensable cell organelle passed on by the host cell to its progeny. The mitochondria retain a mode division similar to that of their ancestral symbiotic respiring bacteria.

Mitochondria not only have their own DNA, but also have ribosomal RNA, transfer RNA, and messenger RNAs, the informational macromolecules involved in translation of the information encoded in DNA. Their DNA is not enclosed in a nuclear membrane but is visible as loose aggregations of slender filaments in electron-lucent areas of the mitochondrial matrix (Fig. 1–13). When isolated from centrifugal fractions of mitochondria and examined in negatively stained preparations, it closely resembles the DNA of bacteria—a double helix of naked DNA in the form of a circle with a circumference of about 5.5 μm (Fig. 1–14). It differs from the DNA of the cell nucleus in its circular form and in its much lower molecular weight. Although mitochondria have their own genome, they are not genetically self-sufficient. Their DNA consists of only about 15,000 nucleotides and has a very limited coding capacity. It determines the RNA of mitochondrial ribosomes, which are visible as 12-nm granules distributed throughout the matrix, and transfer RNAs, but it makes messenger RNAs that code for only a few elements of the respiratory enzyme complexes in the inner membrane. The nuclear DNA encodes the rest of the inner membrane proteins, those of the outer membrane, and those of the matrix. These proteins are all synthesized on ribosomes in the cytoplasm and imported into

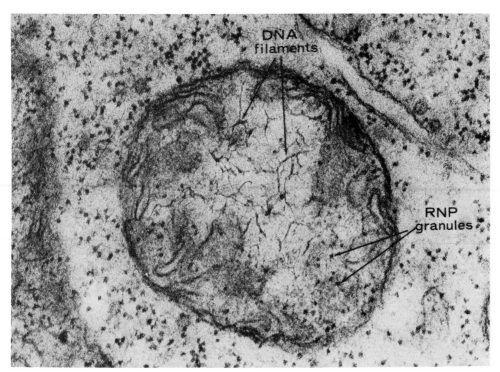

Figure 1–13. Electron micrograph of a mitochondrion from a plant cell showing filaments of DNA and ribosome-like granules of ribonucleoprotein in the matrix. Similar components are demonstrable in mitochondria of animal cells. (Micrograph courtesy of H. Swift.)

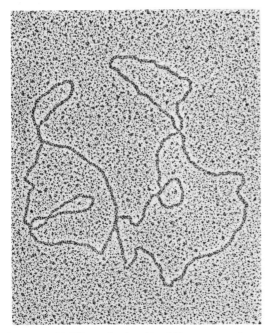

Figure 1–14. When mitochondria of *Xenopus* oocytes are spread upon the surface film of fluid, the organelles are disrupted and the DNA strands can be collected on a specimen grid and examined with the electron microscope. Mitochondrial DNA is in the form of circles 5.6 to 6 μm in contour length. (Micrograph courtesy of I. B. Dawid and D. R. Wolstenholme.)

the mitochondria. All the enzymes needed to replicate DNA and transcribe it into RNA also depend on nuclear genes. Thus, in evolving from free-living bacteria over a billion years, mitochondria have given over to the nucleus and cytoplasm of the host cell the coding and synthesis of most of their structural and functional proteins. Interestingly enough, however, mitochondrial protein synthesis is blocked by antibacterial antibiotics that do not affect synthesis elsewhere in the cell. Although an evolutionary origin of mitochondria from symbiotic bacteria is an attractive speculation, the fact that mitochondrial DNA encodes information in a manner differing somewhat from that of the universal genetic code casts some doubt upon this hypothesis.

The most conspicuous of the matrix components are the *matrix-granules*—dense spherical or irregular bodies 30 to 50 nm in diameter occurring anywhere in the intercristal space but often closely associated with the membranes of the cristae. Their density tends to obscure their internal structure, but in very thin sections they appear to be subdivided by septa into minute loculi or compartments. The composition and function of the matrix granules continues to be a subject of controversy. When calcium or other divalent cations are present in high concentration in the fluid bathing isolated mitochondria, the size and density of the matrix granules is increased. It was initially suggested that these granules function in the internal ionic regulation of the mitochondrion. This interpretation has been weakened by x-ray microanalyses of glutaraldehyde-fixed mitochondria from noncalcifying tissues that failed to reveal calcium in matrix granules. However, when fixed in osmium in the presence of calcium, they bound calcium in detectable amounts. Their affinity for osmium and their membrane-like ultrastructure suggest that their major component is lipid. Biochemical analysis of fractions enriched in matrix granules indicates that they are composed of phospholipoprotein. There is no convincing evidence that the matrix granules in tissues other than bone and cartilage are involved in calcium sequestration in vivo. Their close association with cristae and their membrane-like composition suggest instead that they may play some role in assembly of the mitochondrial inner membrane, but the evidence for this is largely circumstantial.

LYSOSOMES

The lysosome was added to the roster of common cell organelles in 1955 when De-Duve and associates isolated from cell homogenates a fraction of particles, distinct from mitochondria, that were rich in hydrolytic enzymes active at acid pH. Since substrates were accessible to the enzymes only after disruption of the particles or their treatment with surface active agents, it was inferred that they were enclosed by a membrane, and this was subsequently confirmed by electron microscopy. Historically, cell organelles have first been described by microscopists, and their isolation and biochemical characterization followed many years later. But lysosomes went unrecognized by morphologists because, unlike other membrane-bounded organelles, they do not have a consistent and characteristic form. They are a highly heterogeneous group of bodies so diverse in size, shape, and internal organization that no single description encompasses all of their variations.

In general, they are dense bodies 0.25 to 0.5 μm in diameter limited by a membrane.

They may be ovoid or irregular in outline (Fig. 1–15). Their content may be homogeneous or may include aggregations of dense granules in a less dense matrix. They may contain crystalline inclusions or concentric systems of lamellae interpreted as myelin forms of phospholipid. The lysosome cannot be confidently identified from morphological criteria alone. Histochemical demonstration of acid phosphatase or some other hydrolase is required for verification.

Some 50 enzymes have now been identified in lysosomes. These include a number of proteases, glycosidases, nucleases, phosphatases, phospholipases, and sulfatases. The pH optima of nearly all of these are in the acid range. In the normal cell, these hydrolytic enzymes are safely contained within the limiting membrane of the lysosome. In various pathological conditions, however, the permeability of the membrane may be increased, allowing the enzymes to escape and digest or lyse the cell. The term *lysosome* is descriptive of this property.

Cell digestion by lysosomes is not confined to pathological states. Programmed cell death is a normal part of the embryonic development of some organs. Also, in postnatal life, certain organs may undergo massive reduction in volume, as in the regression of the mammary gland after weaning of the offspring. Under these physiological circumstances, lysosomal membranes are somehow altered, permitting escape of acid hydrolases and destruction of the cells.

Lysosomes probably play their most important role in defense of the organism against microbial invasion. Lysosomes are abundant in the cytoplasm of white blood cells and tissue macrophages that are specialized for *phagocytosis*—ingestion of bacteria and other extracellular particles. The lysosomes constitute an intracellular digestive system that enables these cells to break down the ingested material and dispose of the degradation products. When bacteria are engulfed, they are taken into the cell in membrane-bounded *phagocytosis vacuoles* or *phagosomes*. Lysosomes then gather around the phagosome, and their membrane fuses with its membrane, releasing hydrolytic enzymes into the phagosome to kill and digest the ingested bacteria (Fig. 1–16).

Intracellular digestion of extracellular material taken into the cell by phagocytosis is referred to as *heterophagy,* and the phagosomes to which lysosomes have contributed

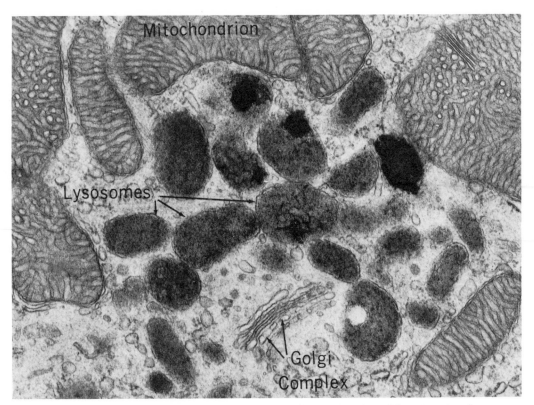

Figure 1–15. Micrograph of a cluster of lysosomes in the Golgi region of a cell from the adrenal cortex.

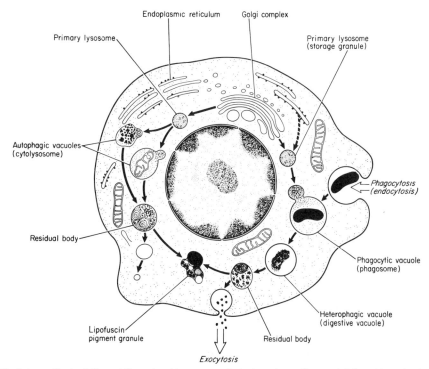

Figure 1–16. Schematic depiction of the role of lysosomes in heterophagy *(lower right)* and in autophagy *(upper left)*. Bacteria may be taken up by phagocytosis; primary lysosomes fuse with these heterophagic vacuoles and their enzymes digest the contents. On the other hand, membranes may be formed around excess organelles or inclusions, and lysosomes then fuse with these autophagic vacuoles. The end products of either process may be recognized in cells as residual bodies or lipofuscin pigment.

their enzymes are described as *heterophagic vacuoles.* Some kinds of ingested material are completely broken down. Others may leave indigestible residues that persist in the form of membrane-bounded structures called *residual bodies.* These vary greatly in the appearance of their content. It has been suggested that cells are capable of divesting themselves of this indigestible matter by *exocytosis*—fusion of the limiting membrane of residual body, with the plasmalemma and discharge of its contents into the extracellular space. This is well documented for amebae, but examples of such behavior in mammalian cells have only rarely been recorded and some cell biologists remain unconvinced of its occurrence.

The lysosomal digestive system of the cell is also involved in the elimination of cell organelles and inclusions in the course of the normal turnover of cell components and in the reorganization of the cytoplasm that is associated with rapid changes in physiological activity. Mitochondria, elements of the endoplasmic reticulum, or secretory granules that are damaged or present in excess of the functional requirements are enveloped in a membrane to form an *autophagic vacuole.* Lysosomes then fuse with this vacuole, releasing into it enzymes that digest its content (Fig. 1–17). This process of controlled degradation of organelles in an otherwise healthy cell is called *autophagy,* in contradistinction to *heterophagy,* which is the digestion of exogenous material imported into the cell by phagocytosis. The residual bodies resulting from the two processes are readily distinguishable. The indigestible residues of autophagic activity that accumulate in cells of aging animals have traditionally been called *wear-and-tear pigment* or *lipofuscin.*

The development of the concept of an intracellular digestive system has led to a proliferation of terms to describe its components. The term *primary lysosomes* is often used for those that have not yet become engaged in digestive activity, and the term *secondary lysosomes* is applied to vacuolar structures that are the sites of current or past digestive activity. The latter term thus encompasses autophagic and heterophagic vacuoles, residual bodies, and lipofuscin pigment deposits.

Some uncertainty prevails as to the mode of formation of primary lysosomes. They are believed to arise in much the same manner as secretory granules, their enzymes being synthesized on the endoplasmic reticulum

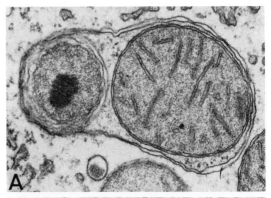

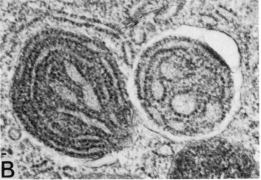

Figure 1–17. Examples of autophagic vacuoles. *A,* A peroxisome and a mitochondrion enclosed in the same vacuole. *B,* Elements of rough endoplasmic reticulum in two adjacent autophagic vacuoles.

and segregated and packaged in the Golgi region. A considerable body of evidence now indicates that they may be formed in a special differentiated region of the endoplasmic reticulum that is closely associated with the secretory face of the Golgi complex—an organelle designated GERL (Fig. 1–11C).

Clinical interest in lysosomes has been stimulated by the discovery that 20 or more rare "storage diseases" of children are due to an inherited defect in the synthesis of lysosomal enzymes (Table 1–1). When a lysosomal enzyme is lacking, its normal substrate accumulates in large membrane-bounded inclusions in the cytoplasm that are, in effect, autophagic vacuoles that are unable to digest their contents. Massive accumulation of such material in the cells of liver and other organs seriously impairs their other functions and leads to early death.

Although lysosomes normally carry out their functions intracellularly, there are situations in which lysosomal enzymes are released from cells. At sites of acute inflammation where leukocytes are actively phagocytizing bacteria, their lysosomal gran-

Table 1–1. INBORN LYSOSOMAL DISEASES

Disease	Substance Accumulating in Cells	Enzyme Defect
Glycogen storage disease II (POMPE)	Glycogen	α-Glucosidase
Gaucher's disease	Glucocerebroside	β-Glucosidase
Niemann-Pick disease	Sphingomyelin	Sphingomyelinase
Krabbe's disease	Galactocerebroside	β-Galactosidase
Metachromatic leukodystrophy	Sulfatide	Sulfatidase
Fabry's disease	Ceramide trihexoside	α-Galactosidase
Tay-Sachs disease	Ganglioside GM$_2$	N-Acetyl-β-glucosaminidase A
Generalized gangliosidoses	Ganglioside GM$_1$	β-Galactosidase
Fucosidosis	H-isoantigen	α-Fucosidase

ules may fuse with a phagosome before its closure and enzymes may escape into the surrounding connective tissue, destroying collagen, elastin, or cartilage matrix. It is now realized that much of the lasting damage to joints, kidney, and lungs following protracted inflammation is a consequence of this leakage of acid hydrolases from phagocytic cells mobilized in the defenses against invading bacteria.

Multivesicular Body

Membrane-bounded vacuoles containing numerous small vesicles are observed in many cell types. These *multivesicular bodies* are stained with histochemical reactions for acid phosphatase and are usually interpreted as a form of lysosome. Their origin and relationship to the more common dense lysosomes remain to be established.

Peroxisome

With centrifugation procedures of improved resolution, it is possible to separate from a crude lysosome fraction a class of particles that lack acid hydrolases but are rich in urate oxidase, D-amino acid oxidase, and catalase. These are called *peroxisomes* because of the ability of two of their enzymes to generate hydrogen peroxide. It has become apparent that these particles correspond to spherical, membrane-limited bodies 0.2 to 0.4 μm in diameter observed by microscopists a decade earlier and called *microbodies*. This old term has now been abandoned in favor of peroxisome. This organelle is found in the cytoplasm of a number of cell types, especially those of the liver and the kidney. In some species, those in the liver contain a dense inclusion, the *nucleoid*, suspended in a homogeneous matrix of lower density (Fig.

1–18). The nucleoids have been isolated and identified as crystals of urate oxidase. The peroxisomes of human liver are devoid of urate oxidase and therefore lack a nucleoid. The matrix of peroxisomes is believed to consist mainly of catalase. Peroxisomes stain selectively and intensely with the diamino benzidine reaction for peroxidase, and this serves to distinguish them from primary lysosomes.

The origin of peroxisomes remains unsettled. Some investigators report that their limiting membrane is continuous at some point on its circumference with that of the smooth endoplasmic reticulum and insist that they

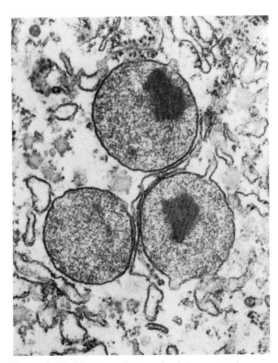

Figure 1–18. Electron micrograph of three peroxisomes from rat liver. Two contain a conspicuous dense nucleoid. (Micrograph courtesy of Daniel Friend.)

arise as evaginations from that organelle. Others believe that their enzymes are synthesized on ribosomes and are released into the cytoplasmic matrix, where they form aggregates that subsequently acquire a membrane.

The function of peroxisomes in the metabolism of the cell is not well understood. Administration of drugs that induce hypocholesterolemia causes a striking increase in the number of hepatic peroxisomes, but this observation has not led to any valid inference as to their function.

ANNULATE LAMELLAE

Some cell types have in their cytoplasm membrane structures that resemble segments of nuclear envelope. These *annulate lamellae* consist of a pair of parallel membranes enclosing a cisternal cavity 30 to 50 nm wide. At regular intervals of 100 to 200 nm, the membranes are continuous with one another around circular fenestrations or pores in the cistern about 50 nm in diameter. These are lined by dense material forming a cylindrical *annulus* within the pore that projects a few nanometers on either side of the pair of membranes. Thus, annulate lamellae are membrane-bounded cisternae traversed by uniformly spaced pore complexes identical in appearance to those of the nuclear envelope (Fig. 1–19). They are frequently stacked in parallel array with the pores of neighboring lamellae in register. At their ends lamellae are often continuous with cisternae of rough endoplasmic reticulum. Annulate lamellae were previously believed to form by delamination from the nuclear envelope but are now known to arise independently in the cytoplasm, often at some distance from the nucleus.

The functional significance of this organelle remains unclear. It has been suggested that the pore complexes of the nuclear envelope may be involved in formation of polyribosomes or in processing subunits of ribosomes and mRNA as these leave the nucleus. It is possible that annulate lamellae may have a comparable function in assembly or activation of informational macromolecules stored in the cytoplasm. The hypothesis derives some indirect support from the fact that annulate lamellae are most consistently found in the early male and female germ cells where there is a long delay between transcription and translation. Also consistent

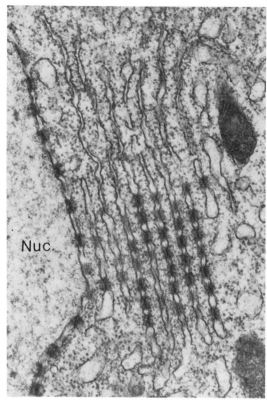

Figure 1–19. Micrograph of annulate lamellae. Notice their close resemblance to the nuclear envelope at left of figure (Nuc.). The lamellae are continuous above with cisternae of rough endoplasmic reticulum. (Micrograph courtesy of S. Ito.)

with this interpretation is the finding that in such cells they are often associated with accumulations of ribonucleoprotein-containing material that may represent deposits of ribosomal subunits or long-lived messenger RNA. Until more evidence becomes available, the function of annulate lamellae will remain conjectural.

CENTRIOLES

In cells that have been suitably stained, a pair of short rods, the *centrioles*, is visible with the light microscope. These are centrally placed in a specially differentiated region of the juxtanuclear cytoplasm called the *centrosome* or *cell center*. In secretory epithelial cells, the centrosome with its pair of centrioles (diplosome) is usually located in the supranuclear cytoplasm and partially surrounded by the Golgi complex. In other epithelial cells, the centrioles may be immediately beneath the plasma membrane at the free surface of the cell.

The centrioles are self-duplicating organelles, ensuring their continuity from one cell generation to the next. Immediately before cell division, they replicate and the two resulting pairs migrate to opposite poles of the nucleus. When the nuclear envelope breaks down and the mitotic spindle forms, a pair of centrioles is found at each pole of the spindle. This association of the centriole with spindle poles suggested that they served as organizing centers or sites of nucleation of the spindle microtubules. It is now known that small dense components of the centrosome called *centriolar satellites* are the microtubule-initiating centers.

In electron micrographs, the centrioles are short cylindrical structures about 0.2 μm in diameter and 0.5 μm long with a dense wall surrounding an electron-lucent central cavity (Fig. 1–20). Embedded in the wall are nine evenly spaced triplet microtubules. Each triplet is set at a constant angle of about 40° to its respective tangent. This oblique orientation of the triplets results in a cross-sectional pattern reminiscent of the vanes of a turbine or the charges of a pyrotechnic "pinwheel" (Fig. 1–20, inset).

When centrioles replicate, they do not divide. The new centriole develops in an end-to-side relationship to a specific region on the preexisting centriole but separated from it by a narrow electron-lucent space. The anlage, called the *procentriole,* is an annular condensation of dense material about the same diameter as a centriole but initially devoid of microtubules. The procentriole elongates by accretion of material to its free end and polymerization of tubulin to form the triplets incorporated in its wall. The newly formed centriole separates from the parent centriole but maintains its perpendicular orientation to it (Fig. 1–21). After duplication the two members of the original diplosome separate and each, with its newly formed daughter centriole, moves to one pole of the division figure. Centrioles are not

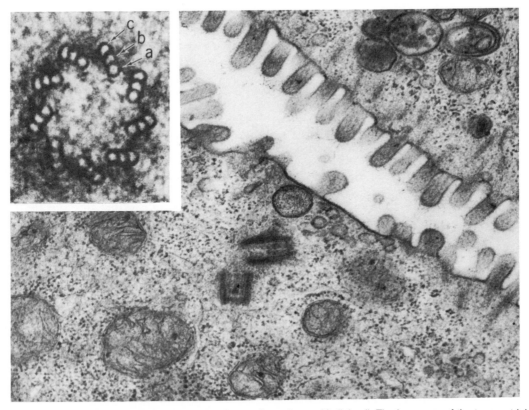

Figure 1–20. Micrograph of a diplosome near the free surface of an epithelial cell. The long axes of the two centrioles are usually perpendicular. (Micrograph courtesy of S. Sorokin.) Inset shows a centriole in cross section at higher magnification. The wall is composed of nine triplet microtubules (with subunits a, b, c). (Micrograph courtesy of J. André.)

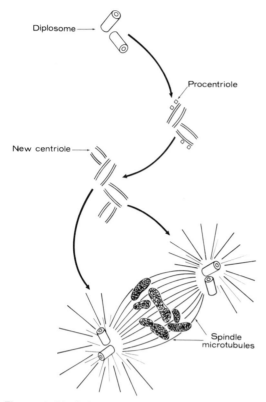

Figure 1–21. Before the onset of cell division, each member of the diplosome becomes a site of nucleation of a new centriole. Its anlage, the procentriole, is a ringlike structure devoid of microtubule elements. It elongates by accretion to its distal end, and microtubules assemble within its wall. Each member of the original diplosome, together with its newly formed daughter centriole, migrates to one pole of the division figure.

essential for mitosis. In plants, acentriolar divisions are common. The association of centrioles with the poles of the spindle appears to have evolved as a device for ensuring that both daughter cells receive a pair of centrioles.

Centrioles are essential for the formation of cilia and flagella. In the cells of ciliated epithelia, the large numbers of centrioles that serve as basal bodies for the cilia do not arise simply by successive replications from the original pair. Another mechanism has evolved for their more rapid generation. Dense spherical bodies of unknown provenance appear in the cytoplasm, and multiple procentrioles arise radially around each of these *procentriole organizers* of *deuterosomes*. When the assembly of multiple centrioles around each deuterosome is completed, they dissociate from it and move to a position

immediately beneath and perpendicular to the apical cell membrane. Two members of each triplet microtubule in the wall of the centriole then become sites of nucleation for rapid polymerization of tubulin to form the doublet microtubules that make up the axoneme of the developing cilium. Elongation of the cilium to its definitive length requires less than 50 minutes. The centrioles thus serve a template function in ciliogenesis, imposing upon the axonemes the ninefold radial symmetry expressed in the arrangement of triplets in their wall. Rootlet-like appendages may develop at the inner ends of each centriole to serve as anchoring devices to stabilize the base of the cilium.

CYTOPLASMIC INCLUSIONS

Glycogen

Carbohydrate is stored in animal cells in the form of the polysaccharide *glycogen*. It is broken down as needed to yield glucose. The enzymatic degradation of glucose in turn provides energy and short-chain carbon skeletons that are reused in the synthesis of various components of protoplasm. The major sites of carbohydrate storage are the liver and skeletal muscle, but glycogen is found in smaller amounts in a great many other cell types.

Glycogen occurs in the form of dense isodiametric 20- to 30-nm particles, often slightly irregular in outline. These so-called *beta particles* of glycogen occur singly in some cell types, while in others they form larger aggregates of varying size called *alpha particles* (Fig. 1–22). Glycogen is usually confined to the cytoplasm but in diabetes and the heritable glycogen storage diseases, it may also accumulate in the nucleus.

Lipid

Cells frequently contain lipid stored as spherical droplets of triglycerides that are liquid at body temperature. In routine histological preparations, the lipid is extracted by the solvents used in dehydration, leaving behind round clear vacuoles. In tissues fixed with glutaraldehyde and osmium tetroxide for electron microscopy, the lipid is preserved as spherical globules varying in density from gray to black, depending in part on

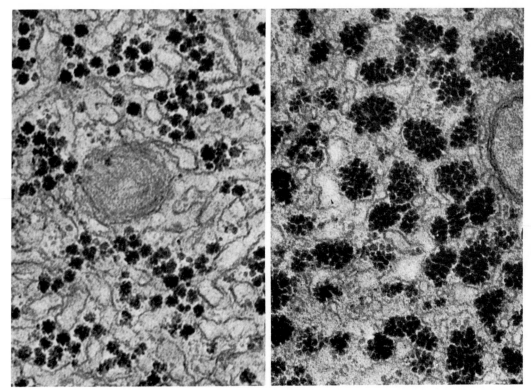

Figure 1–22. Micrographs of liver glycogen of two different species at the same magnification. In the salamander liver (A), the rosettes or alpha particles are considerably smaller than in the hamster (B). In both the glycogen particles are aggregates of smaller subunits.

the degree of unsaturation of the constituent fatty acids (Fig. 1–23).

The lipid droplets serve as an energy store and source of short carbon chains that can be utilized in the synthesis of membranes and other lipid-rich structural components. In fat cells specialized for its storage, lipid in a single very large droplet makes up the bulk of the cell volume. It is also abundant in cells that synthesize and secrete steroid hormones.

Pigment

The principal pigment of mammalian cells is *melanin,* the brown pigment of skin and hair; the choroid, ciliary body, and iris of the eye; and the leptomeninges and substantia nigra of the brain. Melanin is synthesized in specialized cells called *melanocytes,* which arise in the neural crest of the embryo and subsequently migrate to the skin and other sites mentioned above. Melanin is not confined to the melanocytes but may be transferred to the cytoplasm of other cell types that lack the capacity to synthesize melanin. The pigment

occurs complexed with the structural protein of dense ellipsoidal granules about 0.3 μ by 0.7 μ, called *melanosomes* (Fig. 1–24). These form in the Golgi and become distributed in the cytoplasm of melanocytes. When transferred to other cells, especially those of the basal layer of the epidermis, clusters of melanosomes tend to occur enclosed in a limiting membrane derived from the plasmalemma of the donor melanocyte.

More widely distributed in cells throughout the body are deposits of a yellowish-brown substance called *lipofuscin* or *lipochrome pigment* (Fig. 1–25). It occurs in coarse, irregularly shaped granules that exhibit a golden-brown fluorescence in ultraviolet light. They stain lightly with lipid-soluble dyes, but are insoluble in acid and alkali and in most lipid solvents. Lipofuscin deposits are rare in cells from young animals but increase in number with advancing age—an observation that led to their designation as "wear-and-tear pigment." Since the discovery of lysosomes and their digestive properties, lipofuscin deposits have come to be regarded as the end stages

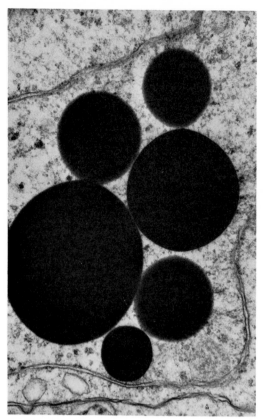

Figure 1–23. Lipid droplets in an electron micrograph of an osmium-fixed cell. After glutaraldehyde fixation, they are less osmiophilic and often appear pale gray.

of autophagic activity—accumulations of undigestible residues not completely degraded by lysosomal hydrolases.

Cells in the liver, spleen, and bone marrow may contain membrane-bounded deposits of a golden-brown, iron-containing pigment, *hemosiderin.* It usually occurs in the cytoplasm of phagocytic cells that participate in the degradation of the hemoglobin of senescent erythrocytes. The amount of this pigment is greatly augmented in diseases that involve an increase in the rate of destruction of the red blood cells. Hemosiderin can be distinguished from lipofuscin and melanin by staining reactions for iron. In electron micrographs, hemosiderin appears as dense masses of 9-nm particles of ferritin, an iron storing protein.

Deposits of lipofuscin and hemosiderin are metabolically inert inclusions. Melanosomes, on the other hand, are rich in the enzyme tyrosinase, which catalyzes the oxidation of tyrosine to dihydroxyphenylalanine, which is an intermediate in the synthesis of melanin. Because of this metabolic activity, melano-

somes are probably more appropriately included among the cell organelles.

Crystalline Inclusions

In a few cell types, conspicuous crystals normally occur free in the cytoplasmic matrix or within the lumen of the endoplasmic reticulum. Most of these have not been isolated and chemically characterized, but their staining and solubility properties suggest that they may be a storage form of protein. Crystals of guanine occur in cells of the epidermis of amphibia, and precisely oriented, rodlike intracellular crystals form a mirror-like layer, the tapetum lucidum, behind the retina of cats. In general, crystalline inclusions as normal cell components are rare, but viruses often form crystalline nuclear or cytoplasmic inclusions in infected cells.

CYTOSKELETON

The term cytoskeleton is now commonly used to describe a structural framework of

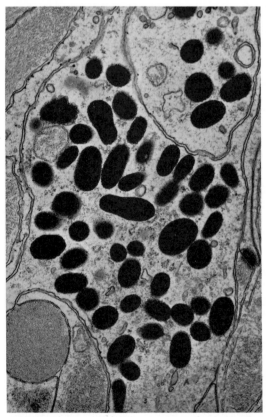

Figure 1–24. Micrograph of portion of an invertebrate melanocyte containing very dense melanosomes. In vertebrates, they are less dense and more fusiform.

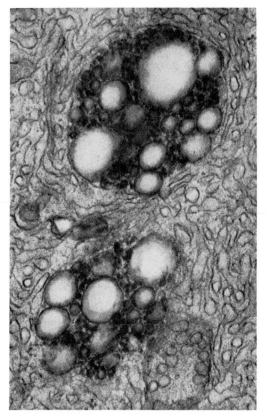

Figure 1–25. Micrograph of two lipofuscin pigment granules in a cell of the human adrenal cortex.

the cell composed of several filamentous components—*microtubules* (25 nm), *microfilaments* (6 nm), *intermediate filaments* (8–10 nm), and a *microtrabecular lattice*. These components of the cytoplasm are visible with the light microscope only when aggregated into coarse bundles. In transmission electron micrographs segments of filaments and microtubules of varying length are seen, but their three-dimensional organization cannot be satisfactorily studied in thin sections. The architecture of the cytoskeleton is best demonstrated in thinly spread cells in culture that have been extracted with non-ionic detergents to remove membranes and soluble matrix components. The general distribution of the several filamentous components of the cytoskeleton can be studied at lower resolution with the light microscope if tissue culture cells are stained with fluorescent antibodies against specific polypeptide subunits of the filaments (Fig. 1–26).

The realization that many of the dynamic processes of cells depend on interactions between the plasma membrane and the cytoskeleton has stimulated intense interest in the filamentous components of the cytoplasm. Maintenance of cell shape; stabilization of cell attachments; endocytosis; movements of local specializations of the cell surface; and

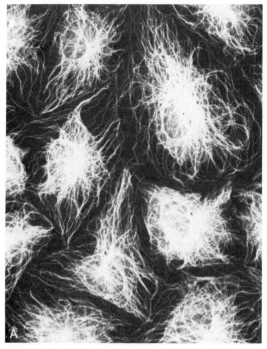

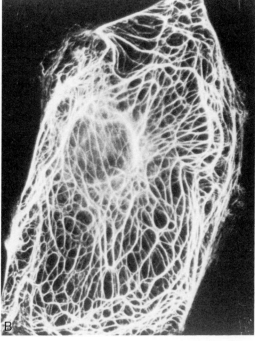

Figure 1–26. Immunofluorescence photomicrographs of cells treated with fluorescein-labeled antibody to cytoskeletal components. *A*, Hamster cells (NIL8) stained for 58K polypeptide of 10 nm filaments. (Micrograph from Hynes, R. O. Cell *13*:151, 1978.) *B*, Epithelial cell (PtK₂) reacted with antibody against prekeratin. (Micrograph from Franke, W. W. Proc. Natl. Acad. Sci. 75:5034, 1978.)

cell motility in general all involve integrated interaction of the cytoskeleton and the cell membrane.

Microtubules

The cytoplasm of most eukaryotic cells contains slender straight microtubules that can be traced in electron micrographs for several micrometers before they pass out of the plane of section (Fig. 1–27). They are circular in transverse section with a diameter of about 25 nm and a wall 5 to 7 nm thick. The cylindrical wall is composed of 13 parallel *protofilaments* having a center-to-center spacing of 5.5 nm. The protofilaments are linear polymers of *tubulin,* a 55,000 M.W. protein that occurs in two forms, α-*tubulin* and β-*tubulin.* These form 110,000 M.W. heterodimers that are subunits of the protofilaments in the wall of the microtubule (Fig. 1–28).

Microtubules may be found anywhere in the cytoplasm and in any orientation, but the majority tend to converge upon the centrosome and often terminate in small dense bodies associated with the centrioles. These *centriolar satellites* serve as nucleation sites for polymerization of tubulin to form microtubules. Developing microtubules exhibit a polarity, tubulin being added preferentially at one end—usually the end away from the initial site of nucleation. The polarity manifested in their directional polymerization is thought to be related to the ability of microtubules to function in promoting directed movements of cytoplasmic organelles.

When tubulin is extracted from brain, the purified preparation contains about 15 per cent of two other proteins of 270,000 and 340,000 M.W. These *microtubule associated proteins* (MAPs) form slender lateral projections that are observed in electron micrographs at regular 32-nm intervals along the length of microtubules. The function of these filamentous projections is not entirely clear, but it is speculated that they may form stabilizing cross links where microtubules are laterally associated in organized arrays as they are in the mitotic spindle.

The number of microtubules present in the cytoplasm varies. They appear to be tran-

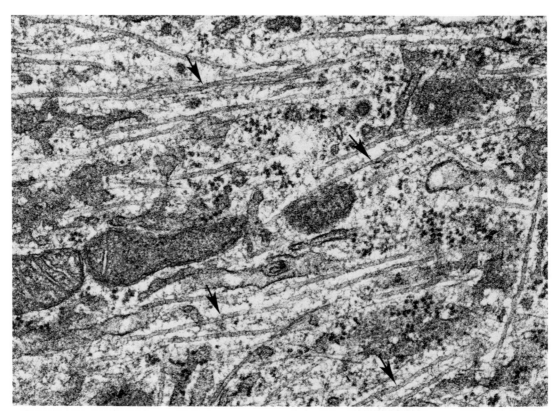

Figure 1–27. Micrograph of the cytoplasm of a Sertoli cell showing numerous microtubules *(at arrows)*. (Micrograph courtesy of W. Vogl.)

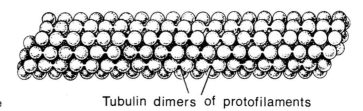

Tubulin dimers of protofilaments

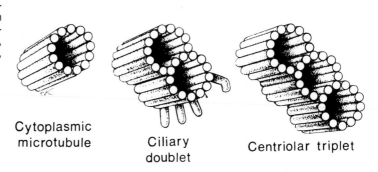

Figure 1–28. Schematic depiction of the linear polymers of tubulin that form the protofilaments in the wall of the microtubule. Below are three configurations in which the protofilaments may be assembled: cytoplasmic singlet microtubule, doublet in ciliary and flagellar axonemes, and triplet in the wall of centrioles.

Cytoplasmic microtubule

Ciliary doublet

Centriolar triplet

sient structures being disassembled, assembled, and redeployed in new patterns as the cytoskeletal requirements of the cell change. Thus, they are believed to be in dynamic equilibrium with a large reserve of their unpolymerized subunits in the cytoplasmic matrix. They are most conspicuous in dividing cells where very large numbers of microtubules are assembled to form the mitotic spindle. Colchicine, a drug that arrests cell division, binds to tubulin, preventing its polymerization to form the microtubules of the spindle.

The relatively ephemeral microtubules of the cell cytoplasm are single tubules with a

circular cross section. However, in the axonemes of cilia and flagella, tubulin polymerizes to form nine *doublets*—pairs of conjoined microtubules that share a segment of the wall of one and therefore have a figure 8 cross section. And in centrioles, the wall is formed of nine *triplets* (Fig. 1–28). Although similar in subunit composition, these doublets and triplets are much more stable than the singlet microtubules of the cytoplasm. In addition to this difference, the doublets possess paired lateral appendages, the *dynein arms* regularly spaced at 24-nm intervals along one member of the doublet. Dynein is a protein with ATPase activity essential for ciliary and flagellar motility.

As major components of the cytoskeleton, microtubules function in maintenance of cell shape, and their directional polymerization and orientation plays a significant role in shape changes. They also participate in movement of particles within the cell by determining the direction along which cytoplasmic streaming occurs. Whether they contribute to the generation of force for translocation of particles remains unsettled. However, in the case of the specialized doublet microtubules of axonemes, it is generally accepted that the dynein arms generate sliding movements responsible for the oscillatory motion of cilia and the propagated waves of bending in flagella.

Microfilaments

The contractile proteins, *actin* and *myosin*, were formerly thought to occur principally

Table 1–2. COMPONENTS AND DISTRIBUTION OF MICROTUBULES

Protein	Peptide Subunit Mol. Wt.	Distribution
Tubulin	55,000 53,000	Mitotic spindle; axonemes of cilia and flagella; cytoplasm of nearly all cell types
Microtubule associated proteins (MAPs)		
MAP$_1$	340,000	Associated with cytoplasmic microtubules of neurons and most other cell types
MAP$_2$	270,000	Associated with cytoplasmic microtubules of neurons and most other cell types

in the myofibrils of striated muscle where they form highly ordered interdigitating sets of filaments that interact to cause muscle shortening. It is now known that both of these proteins are present in nearly all cell types and are responsible for the viscoelastic properties and contractility of the cytoplasm. Indeed, actin is one of the most abundant cellular proteins accounting for 10 to 15 per cent of the total protein.

Demonstration of the distribution of actin within cells depends on its staining with fluo-rescein-labeled antibody or upon use of heavy meromyosin fragments of the myosin molecule that bind specifically to actin filaments, decorating them with regularly spaced barbs that result in a characteristic arrowhead configuration. Both these methods identify as actin, the 6-nm microfilaments seen in electron micrographs of cytoplasm. These filaments are usually widely dispersed and have a sinuous course through the cytoplasm, but in cells grown in vitro they often occur in bundles that are visible with the light microscope and have been called "stress fibers."

Actin extracted from tissues is in the form of globular molecules (G-actin), but under appropriate conditions it will polymerize in vitro to form 6-nm filaments (F-actin). These consist of the globular molecules arranged in a double helix with a pitch length of 37 nm.

Electron micrographs give a misleading impression that microfilaments are present in rather low concentration. This can be attrributed to the fact that actin filaments are dissolved by prolonged exposure to conventional fixatives, or are transformed to networks of very thin microfilaments that usually go undetected in thin sections. When cells are rapidly frozen with liquid helium, deeply etched, and rotary shadowed, their cytoplasm is seen to be crowded with actin filaments. They are present in highest concentration at the periphery of the cell where they form a dense meshwork immediately beneath the plasma membrane. Cytoplasmic organelles are usually excluded from this zone, which was called the *ectoplasm* or *cell cortex* by classical cytologists.

Actin has a dual function in the cell. A cross-linked lattice of actin filaments is the component of the cytoskeleton largely responsibile for the gelatinous consistency of the cytoplasmic matrix, and its local interaction with myosin generates the forces necessary for cell motility.

Myosin filaments are a conspicuous feature of striated and smooth muscle. In nonmuscle cells the forces required for cellular motility are low and in contrast to actin, myosin is a minor protein of the cytoplasm. Moreover, myosin cannot be identified in filamentous form in these cells by conventional light or electron microscopy. It can be detected by fluorescein-labeled antibodies and can be extracted for biochemical analysis.

Whereas actins from different cell types and different species are very similar, myosins vary in molecular size and configuration. They all have in common ATPase activity and the ability to bind reversibly to actin filaments, and they can be induced to form bipolar filaments in vitro. The molecules consist of a rod-shaped "tail" and two globular "heads" that contain the actin-binding sites and ATPase activity. The thick myosin filaments of muscle are 15 μm long and 15 nm wide and are composed of 300 to 400 molecules. The filaments formed in vitro from the myosins of nonmuscle cells are all very much smaller.

The interaction of actin and myosin filaments to generate tension in striated muscle has been thoroughly studied and the mechanism is quite clear (see Chapter 10). However, in nonmuscle cells the arrangement of actin, myosin, α actinin, and tropomyosin in the cytoplasm has not been worked out and the mechanism of their interaction in cell motility is not understood.

Intermediate Filaments

The early studies of the filamentous components of the cytoplasm concentrated upon the microtubules (25 nm) and actin filaments (6 nm) as the principal components of the cytoskeleton. But it soon became apparent that there was another major category of filaments (8–11 nm) present in the cytoplasm of most eukaryotic cells. Because their cross-sectional dimensions fell between those of microtubules and actin, they came to be called *intermediate filaments*. When these were isolated from various cell types and their polypeptides characterized, the intermediate filaments proved to be not a single protein but a family of ultrastructurally similar but chemically distinct filaments composed of subunits of differing molecular weight. Employing fluorescent antibodies raised against their purifed subunits, five major classes of intermediate filaments can now be identified

Table 1–3. COMPONENTS AND DISTRIBUTION OF INTERMEDIATE FILAMENTS

Protein	Peptide Subunit Mol. Wt.	Distribution
Prekeratin	40,000–80,000	Keratinizing and nonkeratinizing epithelia
Vimentin	~52,000	Mesenchymal cells and their derivatives
Desmin	~55,000	Skeletal, cardiac, and smooth muscle
Neurofilament protein	68,000 160,000 210,000	Neurons
Glial fibrillary acidic protein	51,000	Astrocytes

immunocytochemically; *keratins, desmin, vimentin, neurofilaments,* and *glial filaments* (Table 1–3). Most of the cell types in adult animals contain only a single intermediate filament type, but a few contain two types.

Keratin Filaments. Intermediate filaments of this class are characteristic of epithelial cells (Fig. 1–29). They are most abundant in stratified squamous epithelia such as the epidermis where they occupy the bulk of the cytoplasm of the fully differentiated superficial cells. Present in other epithelial cells in smaller numbers, they form bundles of tonofilaments that terminate in desmosomes at sites of cell-to-cell adhesion. Keratin filaments are not found in cells of mesenchymal origin.

Keratins are composed of six or more major polypeptides with molecular weights ranging from 47,000 to 58,000. The solubilized subunits can be repolymerized in vitro to form filaments (8 nm) of the same appearance as the native filaments. Although all keratin filaments are morphologically similar, the keratins in different epidermal tissues and those formed at successive stages of differentiation of the same cell type may differ slightly in the proportions of their several polypeptide subunits.

Desmin Filaments. The cytoskeleton of smooth, skeletal, and cardiac muscle is com-

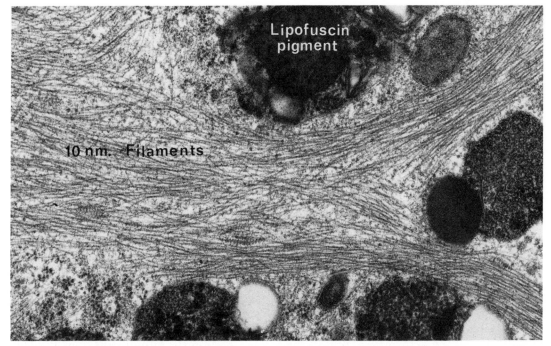

Figure 1–29. Micrograph of an area of cytoplasm from cultured Sertoli cell showing numerous intermediate filaments. The individual filaments are not resolved by the light microscope, but bundles of filaments such as those shown here are visible when treated with fluorescent antibody to filament peptides. (Micrograph courtesy of W. Vogl.)

prised of intermediate filaments of *desmin,* a protein of 50,000 to 55,000 M.W. In striated muscle, a delicate framework of these filaments links the myofibrils together laterally and serves to keep the sarcomeres in register. At each Z band, desmin filaments form a planar network that surrounds the myofibrils and extends laterally to the plasma membrane. In smooth muscle, desmin filaments form a three-dimensional network linking together cytoplasmic dense bodies that are sites of atachment of the actin filaments of the cell's contractile apparatus. The lattice of desmin intermediate filaments is also anchored to dense plaques distributed over the inner aspect of the cell membrane. Thus, in all three types of muscle cells, desmin filaments provide a cytoskeletal framework for attachment and mechanical integration of the contractile proteins.

Vimentin Filaments. Connective tissue fibroblasts and many other cell types derived from the embryonic mesenchyme contain intermediate filaments whose major subunit is a 52,000 M.W. polypeptide called *vimentin.* Although filaments of this type may occur throughout the cytoplasm, they are most consistently in intimate association with the nuclear envelope and may provide the nucleus with mechanical support or stabilize its position in the cell. In cell types that contain more than one kind of intermediate filament, vimentin is always one of them. Thus, it may be associated with desmin in vascular smooth muscle cells; with glial filament acidic protein in astrocytes of the brain; and so forth.

Neurofilaments. Neurofilaments (10 nm) are a conspicuous feature of the perikaryon, dendrites, and axon of nerve cells. They tend to be uniformly spaced and oriented parallel to the long axis of the cell processes. They have thin lateral appendages not found on other intermediate filaments. Neurofilaments consist of three major polypeptides with molecular weights of 210,000, 160,000, and 68,000. They appear to provide internal support for the long nerve cell processes and are probably essential for maintaining the gelated state of the cytoplasm. Freshly extruded axoplasm is a firm gel but rapidly becomes a sol in the presence of Ca^{2+}, which permits proteolytic degradation of the neurofilaments.

Glial Filaments. The intermediate filaments (8 nm) of the nonneuronal cells of the central nervous system—astrocytes, oligodendrocytes, and microglia—consist of *glial fibrillary acidic protein* (GFA), a polypeptide of 51,000 M.W.

The intermediate filaments are morphologically indistinguishable, and to divide them into five types on the basis of immunological differences in their polypeptide subunits may seem to the student an academic exercise of little value, but it has had unexpected applications. Most cell types in the body contain only one of the several kinds of intermediate filaments. Specific antibodies against the major subunits of each are now available. Immunofluorescence microscopy has therefore proved a valuable tool for distinguishing cell types in pathological conditions where morphological criteria alone are inadequate for identification. For example, in malignant tumors the cytological characteristics of the cells may be so altered that it is difficult to determine the tissue of origin. In such cases, immunocytochemical identification of the type of intermediate filaments often makes it possible to determine whether the tumor is of epithelial, mesenchymal, neural, or glial origin.

Microtrabecular Lattice

When thinly spread cells in tissue culture are fixed, dried by the critical point method, and examined with the high-voltage electron microscope, a three-dimensional lattice of slender strands (10–12 nm) is seen throughout the ground substance of the cytoplasm. This provocative observation has led to the suggestion that the cytoplasmic matrix is not a homogeneous protein solution, but a gel with a highly structured *microtrabecular lattice* forming its solid phase, and linking together the other filamentous components and organelles into a single structural and functional unit called the *cytoplast.* The molecular structure and composition of the trabecular lattice have not been worked out in any detail and its existence in the living cell has not yet been accorded general acceptance. Some cell biologists contend that the preparative procedures necessary for its demonstration precipitate soluble proteins of the cytoplasm on a three-dimensional network of actin filaments. On the other hand, those who accept its reality attribute the control of cell shape and cell movement to the integrated functioning of the cytoskeletal elements and the microtrabecular lattice, and speculate that enzymes incorporated in it may be spatially coordinated in such a way as to favor their

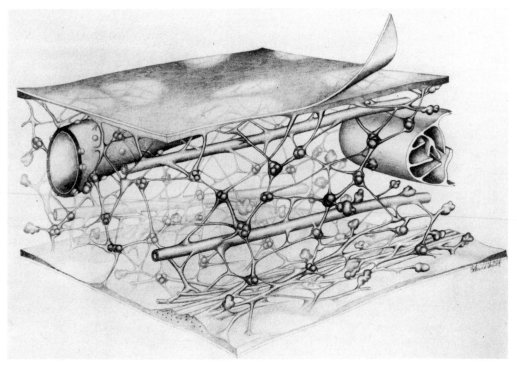

Figure 1–30. Schematic presentation of the microtrabecular lattice in the cytoplasm of a thinly spread cell in culture as interpreted from high-voltage electron micrographs. The trabeculae are joined at thicker nodal points. The lattice is traversed by microtubules, and the trabeculae appear to attach to these and to the cell membrane. (Drawing courtesy of K. R. Porter.)

sequential interaction with their substrates rather than relying on diffusion and random collision. The viscoelastic properties of the ground substance and the directional movements of visible particles within the cytoplasm are consistent with a highly structured matrix, but the concept of a microtrabecular lattice distinct from other filamentous components of the cytoplasm remains controversial.

NUCLEUS

The nucleus stained with hematoxylin or other basic dyes is the most conspicuous organ in the cell. It is centrally situated and usually round or elliptical but, in some cell types, may be deeply infolded or lobulated. *Chromatin,* the nucleoprotein that binds the basic dyes, occurs in aggregations of varying size called *karyosomes.* These are scattered throughout the nucleoplasm but are usually more concentrated at its periphery. The *nucleolus,* a prominent intensely staining nuclear organelle, is centrally or eccentrically placed in the nucleoplasm. In preparations stained by the Feulgen reaction specific for deoxyri-

bonucleic acid (DNA), the chromatin is colored but the nucleolus, which is rich in ribonucleic acid (RNA), is not stained.

The nucleus is the archive of the cell, the repository of its genetic material. Encoded in its DNA is the information necessary for synthesis of all the integral proteins of the cell and all its potential secretory products. It is the source of the informational macromolecules *ribosomal ribonucleic acid (rRNA), messenger ribonucleic acid (mRNA),* and *transfer ribonucleic acid (tRNA),* which direct the protein synthetic activities of the cell cytoplasm.

Nuclear Envelope

The nucleus is enclosed by two parallel membranes that bound a narrow space, the *perinuclear cistern.* The inner and outer membranes are continuous with one another around the *nuclear pore* channels (Fig. 1–31) that traverse the nuclear envelope and provide avenues of communication between the nucleoplasm and cytoplasm. The outer nuclear membrane has associated ribosomes and is occasionally continuous with tubules or cisternae of the endoplasmic reticulum (Fig. 1–31). Thus, the lumen of the perinu-

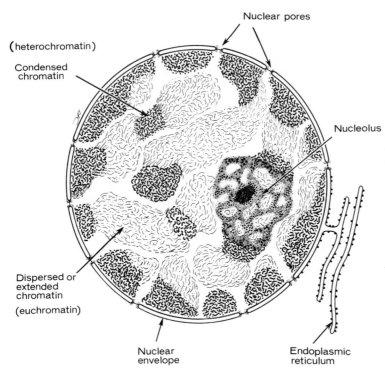

Nuclear pores

(heterochromatin)

Condensed
chromatin

Nucleolus

Dispersed or
extended
chromatin

(euchromatin)

Nuclear
envelope

Endoplasmic
reticulum

Figure 1–31. Schematic interpretation of the state of the chromatin in the interphase nucleus. The condensed portions of the chromosomes (heterochromatin) are thought to be relatively inactive. The extended or uncoiled segments (euchromatin) are sites of active transcription. Also shown is the nuclear envelope delimiting a perinuclear cistern, which is continuous with the endoplasmic reticulum.

clear cistern is continuous with that of an extensive system of membrane-bounded canaliculi in the cytoplasm. The nuclear envelope is therefore regarded as a specialized portion of the cell's endoplasmic reticulum.

The term nuclear pore originally referred only to the membrane-bounded channel from nucleus to cytoplasm; it was subsequently found that there are several discrete, nonmembranous structures associated with the pore. The term *nuclear pore complex* is now used to embrace all constituents of this complex organelle. A hollow cylinder of dense material extending through the pore has long been called the *annulus,* and a thin transverse diaphragm with a central thickening was described as extending across the annulus at its midpoint (Fig. 1–32). By image processing of micrographs of negatively stained pore complexes, the annulus has now been resolved into two distinct coaxial rings attached to the nuclear membranes at the inner and outer rims of the pore, so that one faces the nucleoplasm and the other the cytoplasm. Extending inward from these rings, in the middle of the pore, are eight radially arranged structures called *spokes.* These approach a central spherical granule or *plug.* Together these components correspond to the pore diaphragm and its central thickening described from thin sections of the pore com-

plex. Associated with the perimeter of the ring facing the cytoplasm are eight particles identified as ribosomes (Fig. 1–33).

The structural framework of the complex, consisting of the rings, the spokes, and their connecting links, thus possesses octagonal symmetry around an axis perpendicular to the planes of the membranes. In freeze-fracture replicas, and in negatively stained preparations of the intact nuclear envelope, the pores occasionally have an octagonal outline, presumably imposed by the octagonal symmetry of the associated nonmembranous components. How this highly organized complex functions to permit and regulate the passage of molecules between the nucleus and cytoplasm is not known.

The number and distribution of nuclear pores varies with cell type and in different states of differentiation of the same cell type (Fig. 1–34). Most detailed studies have been carried out on oocytes in which nuclear pores are exceptionally abundant.

On the inner aspect of the nuclear envelope, a thin meshwork of interwoven fine filaments is interposed between the membrane and the peripheral chromatin (Fig. 1–32). This *fibrous lamina* has a supporting function stabilizing the inner nuclear membrane and providing sites of attachment for other structural components of the nucleoplasm. It

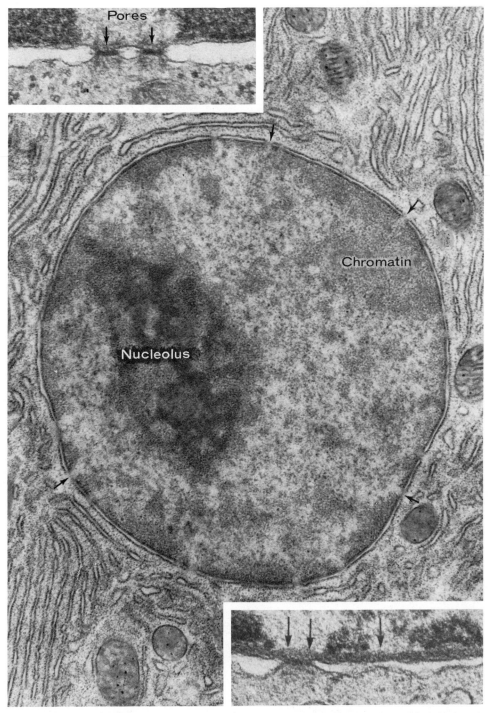

Figure 1–32. Micrograph of a typical nucleus showing a prominent nucleolus and large aggregations of heterochromatin against the nuclear envelope, which is traversed by numerous pores *(at arrows)*. Inset *(upper left)* shows two nuclear pores traversed by pore diaphragms. Inset *(lower right)* shows the fibrous lamina present on the inner aspect of the nuclear envelope.

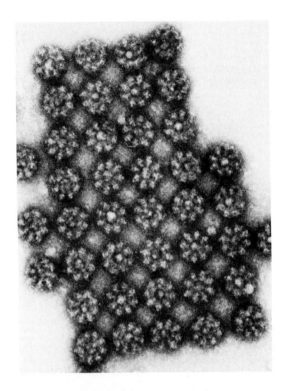

Figure 1–33. Negatively stained preparation of pore complexes isolated from an amphibian oocyte. The central "plug" and eight surrounding "spokes" are clearly visible. Together these comprise subunits of what was formerly called the pore diaphragm in micrographs of thin sections. (Micrograph courtesy of Unwin, P. N. T. Reproduced from The Journal of Cell Biology 93:63, 1982 by copyright permission of The Rockefeller University Press.)

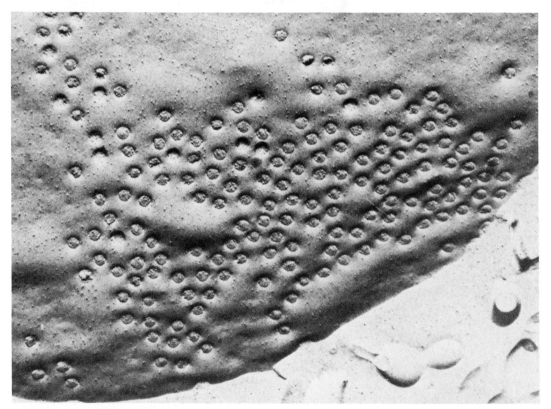

Figure 1–34. Freeze-fracture preparation of a portion of the nuclear envelope of a spermatocyte showing the nuclear pores. In most cell types they are distributed more uniformly over the surface, but in this cell dense aggregations of pores are separated by wide pore-free areas, and the pattern of distribution changes as the cells differentiate into spermatids. (From Fawcett, D. W., and Chemes, H. E. Tissue and Cell 11:147, 1979.)

varies greatly in its thickness in different cell types and in the same cell type in different species, but it is now believed to be a ubiquitous component of the eukaryotic nuclear envelope. It can be isolated as a thin coherent lamina also containing portions of the nuclear pore complexes. It is composed of three major polypeptides with molecular weights between 60,000 and 70,000. When fluorescent antibody against these is applied to cells in culture, the staining is confined to the periphery of the nuclei, suggesting that the fibrous lamina is biochemically distinct from a general structural framework of the nuclear matrix that has been postulated by some cell biologists. When the nuclear envelope is dispersed during cell division, the antigenic polypeptides of the fibrous lamina become diffusely distributed throughout the cytoplasm, and in telophase they become localized at the site of reconstruction of the nuclear envelope around the aggregated chromosomes of the daughter cells. The specific association of these polypeptides with the inner aspect of the nuclear envelope suggests a significant biochemical difference between the inner and outer membranes.

Chromatin

The genetic material of the nucleus is confined to the *chromosomes,* which are seen as discrete rodlike organelles only during one stage of nuclear division. When the nucleus is reformed after division, major segments of the chromosomes become uncoiled and dispersed in the nucleoplasm. In this extended state the genetic material has little or no affinity for histological stains, and in electron micrographs its subunits are indistinguishable from other finely granular and flocculent constituents of the nucleoplasm. Other segments of the chromosomes remain condensed and do bind basic dyes. These stainable portions of the interphase chromosomes constitute the visible *chromatin* of the nucleus. This condensed chromatin is termed *heterochromatin* and the invisible dispersed form is referred to as *euchromatin* (Fig 1–31). Differing degrees of synthetic activity are associated with these two states of aggregation of the genetic material. The euchromatin is the portion being transcribed to direct protein synthesis in the cytoplasm, and the heterochromatin contains that portion of the genome not being expressed. The numerous cell types in the body vary greatly in their range of synthetic activities and in the proportion of chromatin that is in the active dispersed state. The depth and pattern of chromatin staining differs, therefore, from cell type to cell type and may provide useful criteria for their identification.

Analysis of the ultrastructural components of the nucleoplasm progressed less rapidly than that of the cytoplasm. Electron micrographs of the nucleus in thin sections gave no hint of the high degree of order that genetic considerations had led us to expect. Heterochromatin appeared as poorly defined dense aggregations of 20- to 30-nm subunits. Whether these represented small granules of nucleoprotein or cross sections of highly convoluted fibrils could not be determined by study of thin sections. However, if isolated nuclei are disrupted and their content spread on the surface of water, the dissociated chromatin can be picked up on specimen grids, dried, and examined directly. In micrographs of such preparations, the chromatin appears as a tangle of 20- to 30-nm fibrils (Fig. 1–35A). When nuclei are ruptured and spread on the surface of low-salt buffers, the chromatin is dissociated into 10-nm filaments, and if the shearing forces generated in outflow of the chromatin are strong enough, these are further extended and appear as delicate beaded strands composed of regularly repeating discoid subunits about 11 nm in diameter connected by an extremely thin (4-nm) filament interpreted as double-stranded DNA (Fig. 1–35B). The discoid subunits, now called *nucleosomes,* have a core composed of two molecules each of the histones H_4, H_3, H_2A, and H_2B. A segment of DNA, 140 base pairs in length, is coiled around this histone core, and spacer segments of variable length (10–70 base pairs) extend between successive nucleosomes. Histone H_1 is somehow associated with the connecting segments of DNA (Fig. 1–36). When not artificially extended, the nucleosomes and their associated DNA are believed to form the 10-nm filaments seen in micrographs of dissociated chromatin. In their native state, these are helically coiled around a central channel to form the 20- to 30-nm nucleoprotein fibers making up the heterochromatin of the nucleus. The dense subunits seen in thin sections of chromatin, formerly called "granules," are now interpreted as transverse and oblique sections of 20- to 30-nm nucleoprotein fibers.

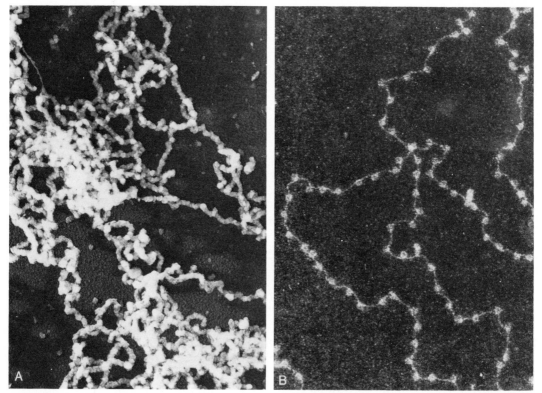

Figure 1–35. *A,* Chromatin from salamander erythrocyte spread upon water, fixed in formalin, critical point dried, and shadowed with carbon-platinum appears as a tangled mass of 20- to 30-nm fibrils. (Micrograph courtesy of H. Ris.)

B, If chromatin fibrils are extended sufficiently by the shear forces generated in the outflow of chromatin, the fibrils uncoil and appear as delicate beaded strands, consisting of nucleosomes connected by segments of double-stranded DNA. (Micrograph courtesy of A. Olins.)

Chromosomes

Chromosomes are the rodlike or threadlike organelles that become visible in the nucleus of cells when all of the chromatin reverts to its condensed form during cell division. The number of chromosomes is constant in all somatic cells and is characteristic for each species. For the human somatic cells, the number is 46—the *diploid* number. The germ cells have half as many, 23—the *haploid* number. At fertilization, the fusion of the haploid sets of chromosomes of the sperm and egg restores the diploid number in the cells of the zygote. Abnormal cells that contain more than two sets of chromosomes are said to be *polyploid.* Cells exhibiting departures from the diploid number that do not involve whole sets of chromosomes are described as *aneuploid.*

Each of the chromosomes in a haploid set has its own characteristic size and shape, and a diploid cell has two chromosomes of each kind forming *homologous pairs,* one member contributed by the sperm and the other by the ovum. One pair, the *sex chromosomes,* differs from the other 22 in males. One member, the *Y chromosome,* is shorter than its partner, the *X chromosome.* Since the homologous pairs separate during formation of the haploid germ cells, the male produces, in equal numbers, spermatozoa containing a Y chromosome and spermatozoa bearing an X chromosome. In humans, the male is the *heterogametic sex* and its chromosome complement is designated 44XY. The female is the *homogametic sex* (44XX) having two X chromosomes and producing ova all containing an X chromosome. Their fertilization by a 22X spermatozoon results in a female offspring (44XX); fertilization by a 22Y spermatozoon results in a male (44XY).

The study of chromosome morphology seemed to be purely of academic interest until it was discovered 25 years ago that the cells of children with mongolism (Down's syndrome) had an extra chromosome. The discovery of a specific chromosomal abnor-

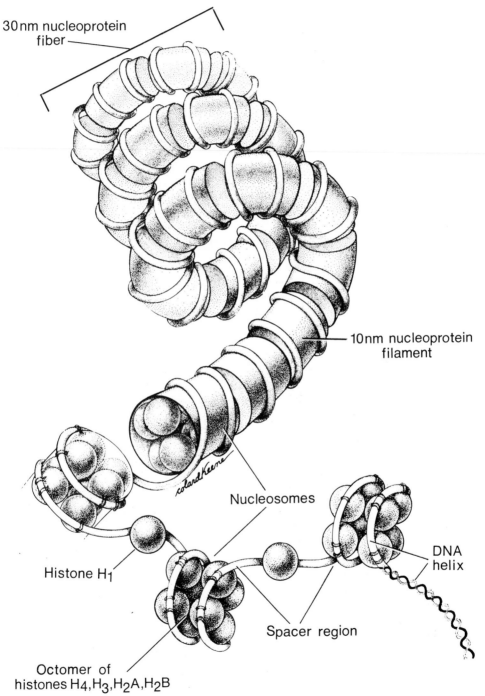

30 nm nucleoprotein fiber

10 nm nucleoprotein filament

Nucleosomes

Histone H$_1$

DNA helix

Spacer region

Octomer of histones H$_4$,H$_3$,H$_2$A,H$_2$B

Figure 1–36. Diagrammatic representation of a 30-nm chromatin fiber showing its postulated helical structure around a central channel. In lower part of figure, the fiber is drawn out to maximal extension to illustrate the nucleosome core of histones with the DNA double helix wrapped around it. Successive nucleosomes are joined by spacer segments of DNA and their associated histone H$_1$. (Figure redrawn after Bradbury, LaRecherche *9*:644, 1978; Worcel, A., and Benyajati, C., The Cell *12*:88, 1977; Olins, A. L., and Olins, D. E. Am. Scientist *66*:704, 1978.)

mality in a common congenital disorder aroused great interest in the examination of human chromosomes. This has led to identification of a growing list of examples of disease states that are associated with visible chromosomal abnormalities. Cytogenetic analysis has now become a routine laboratory procedure on pediatric and obstetrical services of hospitals. It is possible in some instances to diagnose congenital disorders before birth from chromosomal analysis of cells obtained by aspiration of amniotic fluid (amniocentesis). It is necessary, therefore, for students of medicine to acquire some knowledge of the basic terminology of cytogenetics.

Since chromosomes are accessible for analysis only at metaphase of mitotic cell division, a source of dividing cells is needed (Fig. 1–37). Leukocytes separated by centrifugation of a blood sample are cultured for a few days after exposure to phytohemagglutinin, a substance of plant origin that has the property of stimulating proliferation of lymphoblasts. Cultures are then treated with colchicine, a plant alkaloid that blocks the formation of the mitotic spindle and arrests cell division.

This permits accumulation of cells in metaphase of mitotic division. The cultures are then fixed and stained for chromosomal analysis.

The metaphase chromosomes in such preparations each consist of two identical parallel strands, the *chromatids*, joined together at a narrow region, the *primary constriction*. This contains a pale-staining *centromere* or *kinetochore*, which is the site of attachment of the spindle fiber (*fusal microtubules*) to that chromosome. Some chromosomes have another narrow segment, a *secondary constriction*, on one of the arms. The small terminal portion separated from the rest of the chromosome by the secondary constriction is called a *satellite*.

Successful cytogenetic analysis requires that the 23 chromosomes be individually identifiable. Since chromosomes differ in length and in the position of their centromere or primary constriction, these features are useful in their recognition. If the centromere is in the middle and the arms of the chromatids are of about equal length, the chromosome is described as *metacentric*. If the

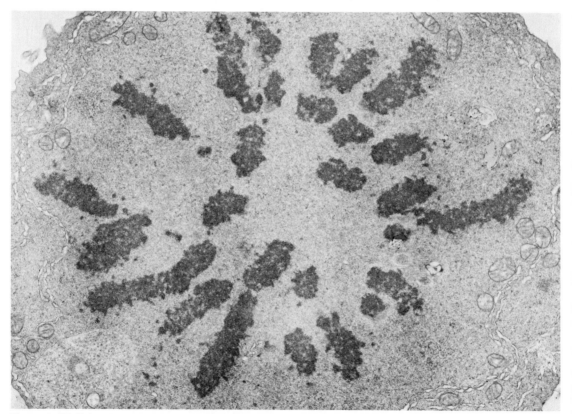

Figure 1–37. Polar view of chromosomes on the equatorial plate of a dividing lymphoblast as seen in an electron micrograph. Micrographs of thin sections are not useful for cytogenetic analysis because whole chromosomes are not included in the section and their relative lengths cannot be determined.

centromere is between the midpoint and one end, the chromosome is said to be *submetacentric*. If it is quite near one end, the chromosome is termed *acrocentric,* and if at the very end, it is *telocentric* (Fig. 1–38).

To facilitate systematic analysis, the chromosomes are cut out of a photomicrograph; the homologous pairs are identified, juxtaposed, and arranged in groups on the basis of differences in length, and position of the centromere (Fig. 1–39). Such an ordered arrangement of the chromosomes of any animal species is referred to as its *karyotype.*

The human karyotype is composed of seven groups within each of which the members are arranged in order of decreasing size. Group A consists of large metacentric chromosomes, numbers 1 to 3; Group B includes large submetacentrics 6 to 12 and the X chromosome; group D includes medium-sized acrocentric chromosomes 13 to 15; Group E consists of short metacentrics 19 and 20; and Group G are very short acrocentrics 21 and 22, and the Y chromosome. Some cytogeneticists include the X and Y chromosomes in groups with autosomes according to their size; others prefer to set them apart as a separate group as in Figure 1–39.

Within the seven groups, it is difficult to identify individual chromosomes by number, but this has been facilitated by staining with a modified Giemsa technique or with a fluorescent quinacrine compound. These methods bring out characteristic patterns of crossbanding that provide additional criteria for identification of individual chromosomes. The hypothetical units of inheritance, the *genes,* are known to be arranged in linear sequence along the length of the chromosomes. Although these cannot be seen with the light microscope, the approximate position of a particular gene (gene locus) can sometimes be described in relation to one of the bands characteristic of that chromosome.

The cytogenetic anomalies of clinical significance involve aneuploidy of one or more chromosomes, loss of a portion of a chromosome (*deletion*), or transfer of a segment to a nonhomologous chromosome (*translocation*). In Down's syndrome, for example, there is an extra chromosome 21 (*trisomy 21*), owing to failure of one of the members of that homologous pair to go to the appropriate spindle pole in meiotic division during formation of one of the gametes. Aneuploidy involving the sex chromosomes may result in *Turner's syndrome,* in which loss of an X chro-

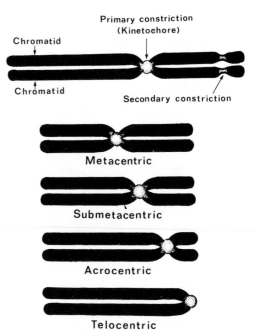

Figure 1–38. Diagram presenting the descriptive terms for chromosomes based on the location of the primary constriction or kinetochore.

mosome (44XO) leads to a phenotypic female whose ovaries are vestigial and usually devoid of germ cells. An extra X chromosome in a phenotypic male (44XXY) results in *Klinefelter's syndrome,* characterized by underdeveloped testicles, sterility, and breast development (gynecomastia).

In the cells of females, one of the X chromosomes remains condensed (heterochromatic) during interphase and appears as a small clump of intensely staining chromatin usually located adjacent to the inner surface of the nuclear envelope. This *sex chromatin* (*Barr body*) is not found in the nuclei of normal males. This sexual dimorphism of the interphase nuclei makes it possible to determine the genetic sex of an individual by light microscopic examination of squamous cells scraped from the inside of the cheek. This simple test is clinically useful in the differential diagnosis of abnormalities of sex development.

Ultrastructure of Chromosomes. Analysis of the ultrastructural organization of chromosomes continues to be one of the more challenging problems in cell biology. Any acceptable model must be compatible with what is known about the replication of the genome, gene transcription, chromatid exchanges, chiasma formation in meiosis, and other well-documented aspects of chromo-

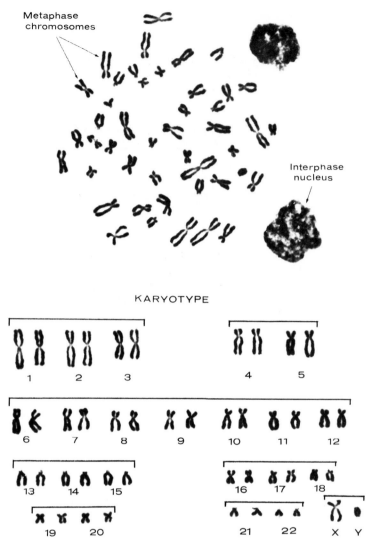

Metaphase
chromosomes

Interphase
nucleus

KARYOTYPE

Figure 1–39. Photomicrograph of human metaphase chromosomes of a dividing lymphoblast *(above)*. In lower half of figure is the human karyotype constructed by cutting out the chromosomes from a photograph like that above and arranging them in groups according to their size and the location of the primary constriction. The 22 pairs of autosomes are identified by number and the six chromosomes by X and Y. (Photomicrograph courtesy of L. Lisco and H. Lisco.)

some behavior. No model proposed for the mammalian chromosome has yet been accorded general acceptance, and current interpretations depend on analogy with the chromosomes of amphibian oocytes, which lend themselves to analysis because of their large size and relative simplicity. They consist of two chromatids each made up of two very long DNA molecules that are folded to form hundreds of symmetrical lateral loops that radiate from the long axis of the chromosome. These lateral loops are responsible for the name "lamp-brush" or "bottle-brush" chromosomes. The loops have been shown to be sites of active RNA synthesis and represent functional units of the DNA molecule called *replicons*. The central axis of the chromosome seems to consist of contracted inactive segments of the DNA molecule.

High-voltage electron microscopic (Fig. 1–40) and biochemical studies on isolated mammalian chromosomes suggest that they too are made up of closely packed 0.5 to 2 μm long loops of nucleoprotein fibers arranged radially around a central axis. The mitotic chromosomes are transcriptionally inactive and the loops consist of the same 20- to 30-nm fibers described above in the heterochromatin of interphase nuclei. When the histones of isolated chromosomes are chemically extracted and the residue spread and examined with the electron microscope, a remarkable transformation is found to have taken place. The DNA of the nucleoprotein loops, now depleted of histones, has uncoiled and extended, forming a broad halo around an axial protein framework that retains the original linear dimension of the chromosome

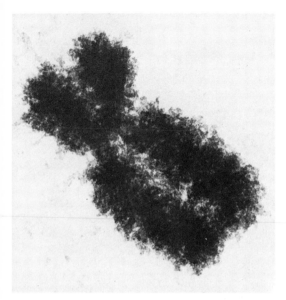

Figure 1–40. Electron micrograph of unsectioned metaphase chromosome from a cultured cell, showing the chromatids, primary constriction, and what appear to be closely packed loops of filaments radially arranged around the long axis of the chromatids. (Micrograph courtesy of H. Ris.)

(Fig. 1–41). The DNA still seems to be in the form of loops but now many times longer (20–24 μm) than when associated with histone and coiled into 20- to 30-nm nucleoprotein fibers.

A typical mammalian cell nucleus 4 to 5 μm in diameter contains a quantity of DNA that if fully extended would be nearly 1 meter in length. Its coiling and condensation into the small volume occupied by the mitotic chromosomes depends on a highly specific association with histones and involves an 8000-fold shortening and compaction. How this orderly process is controlled at each cell division so as to maintain the same chromosomal form and arrangement of genes along their length continues to defy explanation.

Nucleolus

The most conspicuous organelle of the nucleus is the *nucleolus*. It is visible in the living cell as a rounded refractile body eccentrically placed in the nucleus. In histological sections it is intensely stained with basic dyes. Its affinity for basic dyes is due to its content of ribonucleoprotein. It is usually unstained by the Feulgen reaction for deoxyribonucleoprotein but is often surrounded by a rim of reactive *nucleolus-associated chromatin*.

In electron micrographs the nucleolus is quite variable in its appearance from one cell type to another, and within the same cell type its size and organizational pattern may change in different functional states. Common to all, however, is a three-dimensional network of anastomosing dense strands 60 to 80 nm thick, called the *nucleolonema* (Fig. 1–42). It is composed of 12-nm dense granules in a matrix of fine filaments. The nucleolonema exhibits local variations in the state of aggregation of its filamentous component. Regions rich in granules tend to be less dense with the filaments more loosely organized, whereas in segments free of granules the filaments are closely compacted, resulting in greater electron density. The filamentous and granular components of the nucleolonema are ribonucleoprotein. The pale interstices between the meshes of the nucleolonema are occupied by material indistinguishable from the surrounding nucleoplasm. The presence of DNA in some of the interstices can be demonstrated autoradiographically.

The nucleolus disperses during cell division and is reformed in the daughter cells during reconstitution of their nuclei. The nucleolus is reformed at particular sites on one or more of the chromosomes. The *nucleolus organizer region* of the chromosomes is often recognizable with the light microscope as a narrower and less intensely stained segment. These are also called secondary constrictions to distinguish them from the *primary constriction (kinetochore* or *centromere)*, which is the site of attachment of spindle microtubules to the chromosome. The genes coding for ribosomal RNA are located in the nucleolus organizer region, and the nucleolus remains in close topographical relation to this segment of the chromosome.

The number of nucleolus organizer regions in the chromosome set determines the number of nucleoli formed. This number should theoretically be constant for a given species. However, the number actually found may depart somewhat from the expected number. The number in most somatic cells ranges from one to four, but polyploidy may result in multiples of the basic number, and coalescence of nucleoli may result in fewer than the expected number.

The nucleolus is an essential nuclear organelle that functions as a site of processing

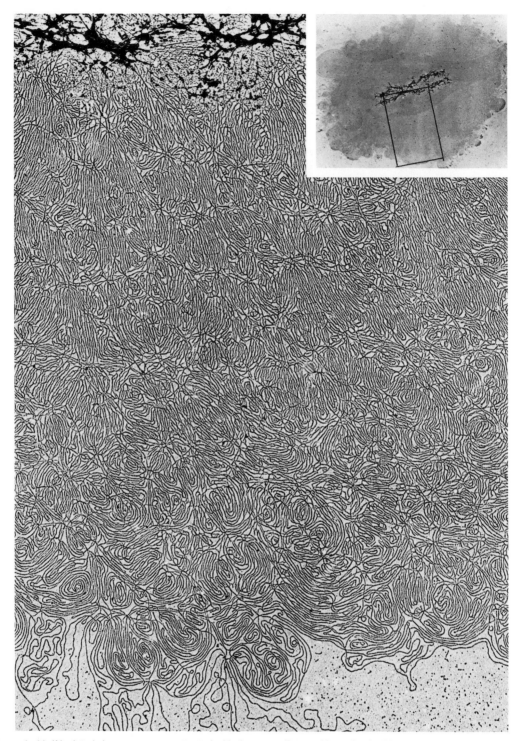

Figure 1–41. If isolated chromosomes are treated with dextran sulfate and heparin, the histones are extracted, permitting the DNA to uncoil forming a broad halo around the core structural proteins. These can be spread upon water and picked up on electron microscope grids *(see inset)*. If an area such as that in the rectangle is examined at higher magnification, the halo is revealed as a labyrinthine pattern of 4-nm filaments of DNA. (Micrograph from Paulsen, J. R., and U. K. Laemmli. Cell *12*:817, 1977.)

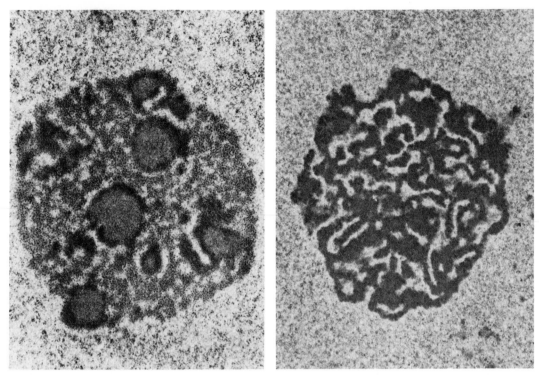

Figure 1–42. Electron micrographs of nucleoli from two different cell types illustrating variations in the reticular pattern of the nucleolonema.

and partial assembly of subunits of the ribosomes. Biochemical analyses of isolated nucleoli have identified three major classes of RNA with sedimentation constants of 45S, 35S, and 28S. Labeled precursors are incorporated most rapidly into the 45S fraction and appear later in the others. It is believed that ribosomal RNAs are first synthesized as long 45S molecules that subsequently undergo cleavage to yield smaller fragments. Among these an 18S RNA combines with specific proteins and passes rapidly into the cytoplasm where it is incorporated into the smaller subunits of the ribosomes. A 35S fragment conjugated with protein forms small particles that may correspond to the granular component seen in electron micrographs of the nucleolonema. The 35S RNA is ultimately cleaved to yield a 28S RNA, which is incorporated with its associated proteins into the large subunit of the ribosomes.

Destruction of the nucleolus of living cells by bombardment with a laser beam results in cessation of incorporation of RNA precursors into ribosomes. In a mutant of the African frog *Xenopus,* development of embryos that lack nucleoli is arrested at an early stage because of their inability to synthesize ribosomal RNA. Thus, it is apparent that the protein-synthetic activities of the cytoplasm are dependent on the functional integrity of the nucleolus.

CELL ACTIVITIES

Having defined the principal structural components of the cell, it may facilitate discussion of tissue and organ functions in later chapters if certain activities common to most cell types are briefly described here.

Cell Division

Growth, renewal, and repair in all multicellular organisms depend on formation of new cells by repeated division of preexisting cells. Two processes of *cell division* are distinguished, *mitosis,* which occurs in somatic cell types, and *meiosis,* which takes place only in the development of germ cells in the ovary and testis. The two have many features in common but differ in the behavior of the chromosomes during the early stages of division. Two events occur in succession in the course of cell division—division of the nucleus (*karyokinesis*), and division of the cytoplasm (*cytokinesis*).

Mitosis. Mitotic division results in distribution of identical copies of the original cell's genome to the two daughter cells. Before the onset of division the DNA is replicated so that the cell enters mitosis with double the normal diploid complement. Cell division extends over a period of 30 to 60 minutes in mammals but may take considerably longer in cold-blooded vertebrates. The period between successive episodes of cell division is called *interphase.* The continuous train of events in mitosis is arbitrarily divided, for descriptive purposes, into four stages—*prophase, metaphase, anaphase,* and *telophase.*

During interphase the only structure visible in the living nucleus is the nucleolus, but in stained preparations a few clumps of chromatin can be seen in the nucleoplasm, usually concentrated around the periphery adjacent to the nuclear envelope. Except for these condensed segments, the chromosomes are in the extended euchromatic state and are not visually identifiable. After replication of the DNA the euchromatic regions condense, so that the chromosomes become visible in both living and fixed material as slender threadlike structures pursuing a meandering course throughout the nucleoplasm (Figs. 1–43, 1–44).

The first appearance of the chromosomes marks the beginning of prophase (Fig. 1–43D, E, F). Throughout this stage they continue to condense, becoming shorter and thicker. Each consists of two parallel strands called *chromatids* joined to one another at the *centromere* or *kinetochore,* a constricted segment common to both. Other events occurring during prophase include disappearance of the nucleoli; migration of the centrioles (which replicate just before onset of division) to opposite poles; and the breakdown of the nuclear envelope. Disappearance of the nuclear envelope marks the end of prophase.

Metaphase begins with the alignment of the chromosomes in the same plane in the middle of the cell to form the *equatorial plate* (Fig. 1–43H). This ordered assembly of the chromosomes is associated with the development of the *mitotic spindle*—a fusiform array of microtubules extending between the centrioles located at the poles of the division figure. Some of these microtubules go from pole-to-pole as the *continuous fibers* of the spindle while others, called the *chromosomal fibers,* extend only from the poles to the kinetochore of each chromosome.

Anaphase is initiated by division or reduplication of the kinetochore of the chromosomes so that each chromatid has its own. The sister chromatids, no longer attached, are then free to migrate to opposite poles of the spindle as separate chromosomes (Fig. 1–43I, J). During these anaphase movements of the chromosomes, the kinetochore regions to which the microtubules attach usually lead and the arms trail behind. The mechanism of anaphase movements is still a subject of debate. The chromosomal fibers appear to shorten, possibly by depolymerization of the microtubules at their polar ends, while the continuous fibers appear to lengthen, moving the spindle poles apart. It is not yet clear whether movement of the chromosomes depends solely upon changes in length of the two sets of microtubules by polar addition of tubulin to one and depolymerization of the other, or whether there is a sliding mechanism involving interaction of chromosomal and continuous microtubules and their displacement relative to one another. In either case, at the end of anaphase, the two groups of chromosomes are clustered at the spindle poles.

At telophase, segments of nuclear envelope begin to reform around the chromosomes, and these uncoil and extend, losing their stainability except in those regions destined to remain condensed as the heterochromatin of the interphase nucleus. Nucleoli are reformed and the initially discontinuous segments of nuclear envelope coalesce to form a complete perinuclear cistern (Fig. 1–43L–O). With these events, karyokinesis is concluded and the two identical daughter nuclei have attained their interphase appearance.

While the reconstitution of the nuclei is in progress, a constriction of the cytoplasm occurs midway between them. This *cleavage furrow* deepens until it encounters a bundle of the continuous fibers of the spindle. The cell bodies of the two daughter cells remain connected for a short time in telophase by a slender cytoplasmic bridge filled with spindle microtubules that are held together at their midpoint by dense amorphous material, which is visible with the light microscope as a dark dot called the *midbody.* After a brief delay the microtubules depolymerize, the spindle bridge gives way at one side of the midbody, and the two halves retract into their respective daughter cells to complete cytokinesis.

The precise replication of the DNA prior to cell division, and the longitudinal splitting

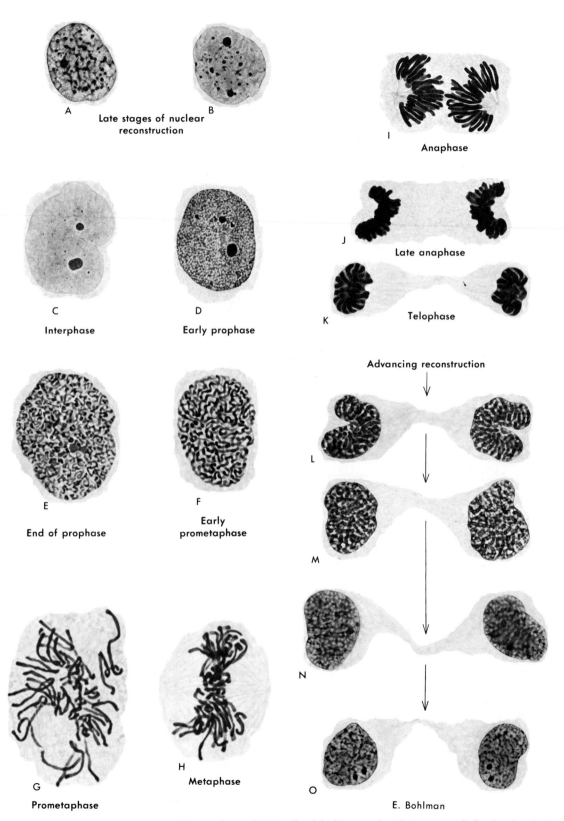

Figure 1–43. Drawings of changes in mitosis of mesothelial cells of *Amblystoma* in culture as seen in fixed and stained material. Compare with phase-contrast photomicrographs of living cells in Figure 1–44.

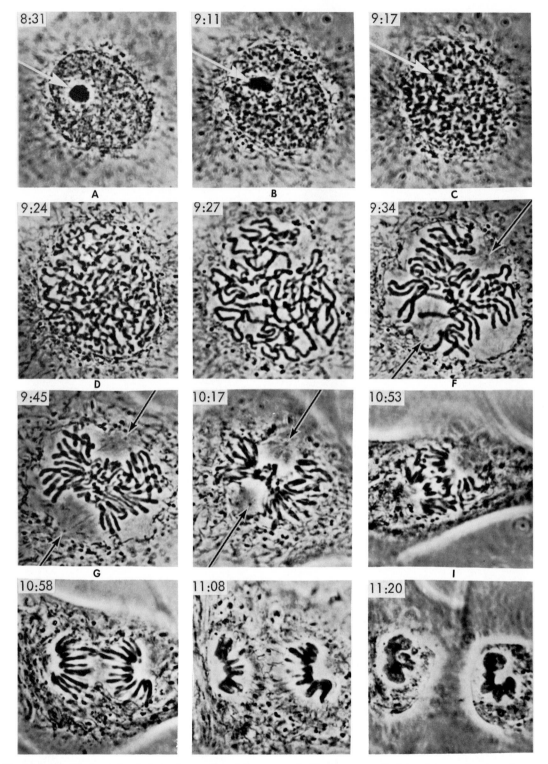

Figure 1–44. Phase-contrast photomicrographs of the same *Amblystoma* mesothelial cell in successive stages of mitosis. Large white arrow points to the nucleolus: black arrows indicate centrioles. *A* to *E,* Prophase; *F, G, H,* metaphase; *I, J, K,* anaphase; *L,* telophase. The duration of three hours is much longer than required for mitosis in warm-blooded vertebrates.

of each chromosome into two identical chromatids, which separate and are distributed to opposite poles, ensures that the daughter cells are of the same genetic make-up as the cell from which they were derived.

Meiosis. Meiosis occurs early in the development of ova and spermatozoa, and consists of two successive divisions with only one replication of the chromosomes. It results in separation of the two members of each pair of homologous chromosomes in the first division, thus reducing the chromosomes in each daughter cell to half the normal number. The second meiotic division involves separation of the two chromatids of each chromosome and results in four nuclei with half the normal number of chromosomes. The gametes that differentiate following meiosis are thus described as *haploid,* and when a male and female gamete unite at fertilization, the normal diploid number of chromosomes is restored in the fertilized egg, now called the *zygote.*

Meiosis is characterized by a very long prophase, which is divided into five stages. In the earliest of these, called *leptotene,* the chromosomes become visible as long, thin, single strands. In *zygotene,* the homologous chromosomes begin to come together in close lateral apposition with corresponding sites along their length in register. This pairing is also referred to as *synapsis.* The chromosomes then begin to coil, becoming shorter and thicker in *pachytene.* In this stage, because of the close apposition of homologues, the chromosomes may appear to be present in only the haploid number. The pairs are referred to as *bivalents.*

In *diplotene,* the paired chromosomes separate along their length. Their coiled nature is evident, and it becomes apparent that each is split longitudinally. Each bivalent therefore consists of four *chromatids.* At certain points along their length, the homologous half-chromosomes cross one another and exchange segments. The sites of crossing are called *chiasmata* and are the morphological expression of the genetic phenomenon of *crossing over.* The shortening and thickening of the chromosomes continues and they tend to clump in the center. The nucleolus, which remained during earlier stages of prophase, begins to fragment in diplotene and later disappears altogether.

In *metaphase,* the nuclear envelope is dispersed and the spindle forms as it does in mitosis. The bivalents gather on the meta-phase plate. The kinetochore of the bivalents does not divide as it does in mitosis. Consequently, in *anaphase* of the first meiotic division, whole chromosomes, not sister chromatids, separate and move to the opposite poles.

The nuclei in mammals are reconstituted in *telophase* for a brief interval, but in some other taxa the chromosomes may proceed directly into the events of the second division without full reconstitution of the nucleus. In the second meiotic division, the haploid nuclei divide by a mechanism essentially identical to that seen in mitosis. The chromosomes split longitudinally, the kinetochores divide, and sister chromatids move to opposite poles, resulting in formation of four cells with haploid nuclei. The reduction in chromosome number occurs in the first meiotic division. Therefore, this is also called the *reductional division,* while the second is called the *equational division.*

The biological significance of meiosis is twofold. It ensures constancy of chromosome number from generation to generation by producing haploid gametes whose fusion restores the original diploid number. It also provides for genetic variability upon which evolution depends. The members of each pair of homologous chromosomes in the diploid spermatogonia and oogonia come from the two parents of the individual. As a result of the exchange of segments between homologous chromosomes in prophase of the first meiotic division, the chromatids emerging are different genetically from the chromosomes that entered meiosis. The randomness of distribution of the homologues to the daughter nuclei during reduction division contributes further to the genetic diversity of the gametes.

Cell Cycle

The frequency of cell division varies greatly among the many cell types in the body. In some tissues (nervous tissue, cardiac muscle), the cells are very long-lived and there is no cell division in postnatal life to replace those lost through age or injury. In other organs such as the liver, there is normally a very slow renewal with cell divisions seen only rarely. However, after removal of part of the organ, the remaining cells are stimulated to proliferate rapidly until the original volume of liver has been restored. In a number of epithelia such as those of the gastrointestinal tract and the skin where there is a continual loss of fully differentiated superficial cells, a population of relatively undifferentiated cells retains the capacity for rapid proliferation and provides for continual replacement commensurate with the rate of cell loss.

For cell types that proliferate rapidly in vivo or in vitro with a constant doubling time, it is possible to define a repeating sequence of biochemical and morphological events known as the *cell cycle.* The key biochemical event of the cycle is replication of the strands of DNA that form the chromosomes. This occurs during interphase while the chromosomes are in the extended condition, and it is not attended by any microscopically visible change in the cell nucleus. DNA replication can be detected, however, by autoradiography following administration of radiolabeled thymidine, a precursor that is incorporated into the newly synthesized DNA molecules. The period of DNA synthesis extends over

30 to 40 per cent of the cycle length and is referred to as the *S-phase.* It is followed by a short *G_2-phase,* occupying 10 to 15 per cent of the cycle during which other preparations for division take place. The succeeding *M-phase* includes the visible morphological events of mitosis. This is followed by the *G_1-phase,* a period of active RNA and protein synthesis during which the daughter cells increase in size. It extends for 30 to 40 per cent of the cycle length (Fig. 1–45). The duration of the cell cycle varies with the cell type and animal species. In rapidly proliferating cells of laboratory rodents, it may be only one third of the cycle length of the same cell type in humans.

The study of these phases in synchronized cultures has made important contributions to our understanding of the molecular biology of cell proliferation and growth, but it is important to note that these definitions require that the cells of the population are rapidly growing, with a constant doubling

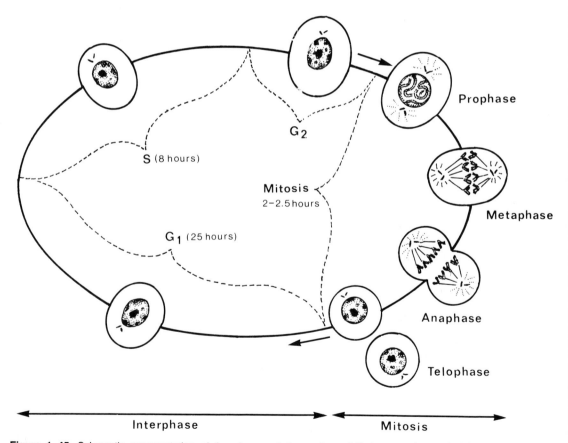

Figure 1–45. Schematic representation of the phases of the cycle and their approximate duration in the case of proliferating bone cells with a cycle length of 25 hours. Cycle length varies greatly among different cell types, G_1 being the most variable phase. (Redrawn after Junqueira, L. C., and Carneiro, J. Basic Histology. Lange Medical Publishers, 1983.)

time. This type of growth is seldom found in normal adult tissues. Cells may remain for weeks or months in interphase and then undergo one or more division cycles. Some authors refer to these long phases of rest as a G_0-*phase*, but this is not properly a part of the cell division cycle.

Cell Motility

All cells are capable of some degree of motility. Free cells that are not organized into compact tissues wander through interstices in the connective tissues of the body with an active ameboid locomotion. Where cells are in close contact as in epithelia, their motility may be limited to changes of surface configuration by extension and retraction of microvilli, and to streaming movements within the cytoplasm that continually alter the distribution of their organelles. Even such relatively sessile cell types undergo changes of shape, rounding up at the onset of division and forming a cleavage furrow during cytokinesis, and then returning to their original form. During repair after injury, they migrate and flatten to cover denuded areas of the basal lamina.

Exploration of the mechanisms of locomotion and of the streaming movements that occur within cells has proved to be one of the most challenging problems in cell biology, and some understanding of its molecular basis is only beginning to emerge. Ameboid movements of migratory cells have been most thoroughly studied. In such cells there is an actin-rich cortical zone of cytoplasm that has a gel-like consistency. The initial event in movement appears to involve local conversion of the gel to a sol, making this a weak point. Contraction of the cortex at the other end of the cell forces the solated cytoplasm forward, extending a blunt process or pseudopod that adheres to the substrate in a more advanced position while the contracting tail region detaches. The process is repeated with extension of a new pseudopod, and the cell, thus slowing, crawls over the substrate.

The movement may be random, or its direction may be determined by extracellular signals such as the topography of the substrate, or by diffusible chemical signals in the medium called *chemotactic* agents. In *chemotaxis*, pseudopods are induced at the site of contact with the attractant and the cell continues to move up the concentration gradient of the chemotactic agent. In the most thoroughly studied example, the ameboid stage of the fungus *Dictyostelium*, the chemotactic substance is cyclic AMP. A number of the white blood cells of mammals respond to chemotactic agents liberated at sites of tissue injury or bacterial invasion. The chemical characterization of the attractant for these cells is still incomplete.

Connective tissue cells and epithelial cells in culture have a different behavior. They spread and flatten against the substrate. Their thin, advancing end forms thin folds or ruffles that exhibit an active undulating motion while the rest of the cell remains quiescent. This ruffling edge advances over the surface and the cell body follows. In neurons in culture, the cell body remains at the site of initial adherence and the active ruffling portion moves away, drawing out very long slender processes simulating the axons and dendrites of such cells in the brain. Thus, the shape and pattern of movement of cells is not determined entirely by environmental stimuli but also depends on endogenous determinants for particular cell lineages. Where the endogenous determinants are located in the cell; how they are transmitted to daughter cells; or how they exercise their control over cell form are unknown.

Information is now rapidly accumulating on the structural components determining cell form, and on the changes induced by extrinsic stimuli. The architecture of the cytoskeleton can be revealed in three dimensions by detergent extraction of the membranes and soluble components of the cytoplasm followed by examination of the unextracted filamentous framework in stereo micrographs. The several categories of cytoplasmic filaments can be identified *in situ* by their decoration with specific monoclonal antibodies. The organization of the cytoskeleton can be altered experimentally by drugs that prevent or promote the polymerization of tubulin to form microtubules. Drugs are available that similarly affect the polymerization and depolymerization of actin that takes place in gel-sol transformation and in assembly of contractile associations of actin and myosin. Polypeptides that cross-link actin and stabilize the cytoskeletal lattice have been identified and others that mediate the attachment of actin to integral proteins of the cell membrane—a linkage essential to any mode of cell locomotion.

Although at present we are still in the stage of analyzing motile behavior and compiling a catalogue of the visible components and of the macromolecules involved, these descriptive and analytic approaches may soon provide the basis for valid explanations of cell motility.

Endocytosis

Endocytosis is a general term applied to the bulk uptake of materials by cells. Fluid is taken in from the extracellular environment by local invagination of the plasma membrane followed by fusion of the neck of the invagination to form a closed, fluid-filled vacuole. This is then separated from the cell membrane and moved into the cytoplasm. This process is called *pinocytosis* (drinking by cells). All eukaryotic cells probably engage in this activity, but in varying degrees.

Solid particles may be taken into cells by formation of pseudopods, blunt processes of the cell surface that progressively elongate and ultimately encircle the object. Fusion of the tips of the engulfing pseudopods beyond the particle then detaches a membrane-bounded vacuole from the plasmalemma, carrying the ingested matter into the cytoplasm. This mechanism for ingestion of solid objects, 1 μm or more in diameter, is called *phagocytosis* (eating by cells). Although some epithelial cells are capable of phagocytosis, it is most highly developed in white blood cells and tissue macrophages, which are specialized for defense of the organism against microbial invasion. Cells exhibiting this activity are referred to as *phagocytes*. They not only ingest and destroy invading microorganisms, but also play an important role in tissue maintenance by disposing of dead cells and cellular debris. For example, some 3×10^{11} senescent red blood cells are removed from the blood each day and destroyed by the phagocytic cells in the spleen.

Living cells and normal extracellular elements are generally immune to phagocytosis, but degenerating cells with altered membranes and tissue components whose proteins are partially denatured are readily ingested. Most nonpathogenic bacteria are rapidly phagocytized. On the other hand, a number of pathogenic bacteria have capsules that resist binding to the surface of phagocytes. Their ingestion requires the presence of *immune globulin* (antibody) produced by cells of the body's immune system, and/or the presence of a protein constituent of blood plasma called *complement*. These substances bind to the capsule of pathogenic bacteria, making them vulnerable to ingestion by ensuring their attachment to specific receptors in the membranes of phagocytes.

Phagocytosis is considered to occur in two steps: (1) *attachment,* which involves binding of ligands on the particle to receptors in the membrane of the phagocyte; and (2) *interiorization* of the particle. In the case of pathogenic bacteria referred to above, the immune globulin (IgG) and a component of complement (C_3) bind selectively to the surface of the bacterium and serve as *ligands,* which interact with specific *receptors* (Fc) on the membrane of the phagocytic cell (Fig. 1–46). This attachment phase of the process can occur at 1° to 3° C in vitro and thus is not energy dependent. Interiorization, however, requires expenditure of energy. At the point of initial contact, a zipper-like process of ligand-to-receptor binding is initiated and spreads laterally, tightly apposing the cell membrane to the surface of the particle. This interaction is believed to generate a signal that results in assembly of actin filaments and myosin in the cell cortex, leading to formation of pseudopods. Their extension increases the area of contact with the bacterium, entailing further ligand-receptor binding, which in turn induces more extensive aggregation of contractile proteins. This self-propagating process continues until the tightly adhering pseudopods meet and fuse beyond the bacterium to complete its enclosure in a *phagocytic vacuole* or *phagosome.* Discharge of lysosomal hydrolytic enzymes into the vacuole and activation of other bactericidal mechanisms of the cell then results in destruction of the invader.

In addition to receptors for IgG and C_3, some phagocytes evidently have nonspecific receptors that enable them to ingest a variety of nonbacterial foreign particles without the cooperation of the immune system.

In pinocytosis, imbibition of fluid occurs in vacuoles of two size categories whose formation involves somewhat different activities of the cell surface. In *macropinocytosis*, sizeable droplets of fluid (0.5–1.5 μm) that are visible by phase-contrast microscopy are enveloped by thin, undulating folds (*lamellipodia*) on the cell surface and are drawn into the cytoplasm. In *micropinocytosis*, fluid is taken up in minute invaginations of the cell membrane that bud off to form vesicles visible only in electron micrographs.

Two functionally distinct forms of micro-

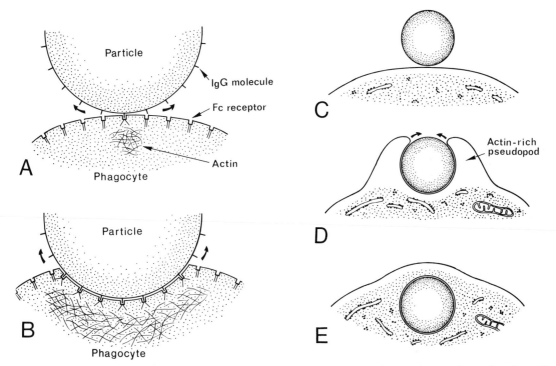

Figure 1–46. Schematic representation of the mechanism of phagocytosis. In the attachment phase, ligands on the surface of the particle bind to receptors on the phagocyte membrane. Progressive circumferential binding spreads from the site of initial contact, "zippering" the membranes together. This triggers polymerization of actin in the underlying cytoplasm and extension of engulfing pseudopods that bring the phagocyte membrane into contact for binding around the entire circumference of the particle. When the pseudopods meet and fuse, interiorization is complete.

pinocytosis are recognized: *fluid-phase pinocytosis* and *adsorptive* or *receptor-mediated pinocytosis*. In the former, fluid, solutes, and submicroscopic particulates in suspension are taken up in small vesicles whose limiting membrane is unspecialized (Fig. 1–47). This process is *nonselective*. The latter is *selective* in that certain substances are bound to specific receptors clustered in areas of the membrane that then invaginate to form pits and later detach as free vesicles in the cytoplasm. The luminal aspect of these vesicles has a visible surface coat and the cytoplasmic surface is

enclosed in a basket-like lattice composed mainly of an 180,000 M.W. protein called *clathrin* (Fig. 1–48). The presence of the clathrin basket gives the *coated vesicles* of receptor-mediated pinocytosis a characteristic spiny appearance that serves to distinguish them from the *smooth vesicles* of fluid-phase pinocytosis.

Nonselective, fluid-phase pinocytosis is apparently a device for imbibition of fluid and solutes or for their transport across epithelia. Receptor-mediated endocytosis is now a subject of intense interest because of its potential

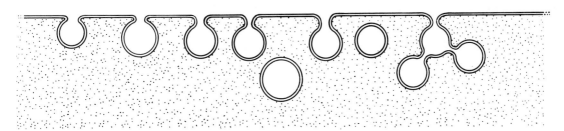

Figure 1–47. In fluid-phase micropinocytosis, minute invaginations of the cell membrane detach and move into the cytoplasm as smooth vesicles. In some epithelia they may transport materials across the cell. In endothelium, chains of communicating vesicles may form transient channels from lumen to cell base. This form of pinocytosis is nonselective.

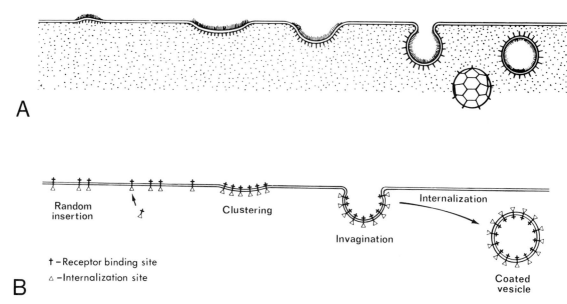

A

B

t – Receptor binding site

△ – Internalization site

Figure 1–48. *A,* In receptor-mediated pinocytosis the vesicles are lined by a thin carbohydrate-rich cell coat and their cytoplasmic surface is enclosed in a basket-like lattice of clathrin.

B, Receptors are randomly distributed in the cell membrane. Binding of specific macromolecules causes clustering of the receptors, and this portion of the membrane forms a coated pit that subsequently separates from the membrane as a coated vesicle. (Redrawn and modified from Goldstein et al. Nature *279*:679, 1979.)

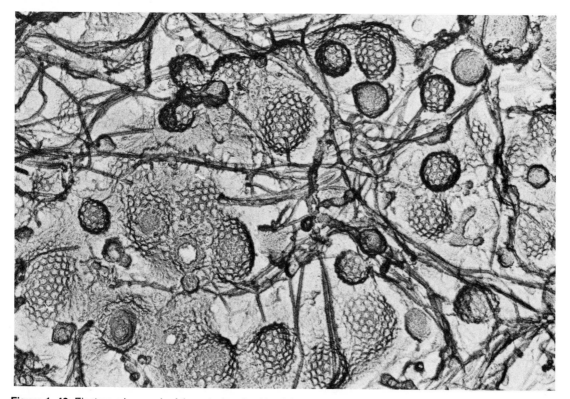

Figure 1–49. Electron micrograph of the cytoplasmic side of the plasmalemma of a liver cell prepared by rapid-freezing, fracturing, and deep-etching. Filaments in the cortical cytoplasm are visible and the clathrin lattice of many forming coated pits and vesicles. (Micrograph courtesy of N. Hirokawa and J. Heuser.)

physiological importance in selective uptake of nutritional and regulatory proteins (e.g., hormones such as insulin and transport proteins such as transferrin). There is also strong evidence for the involvement of clathrin-coated vesicles in retrieval and recycling of membrane added to the plasmalemma during release of glandular secretions and neurotransmitters.

Exocytosis

The term *exocytosis* describes the release of secretory products of the cell into the extracellular compartment. The product of glandular cells is accumulated and concentrated in spherical granules or vesicles in the Golgi region of the cell. They are enclosed in a membrane that is capable of fusing with the apical plasma membrane. The secretory product of such cells may be stored for some time in secretory granules. When the cell receives an appropriate stimulus, the granules move to the surface and their membrane fuses with the plasmalemma, permitting their contents to flow out. The product thus leaves the cell without creating any breach in the cell membrane. The membrane of the secretory granules that is added to the plasma membrane during exocytosis is subsequently recovered in small vesicles that invaginate, bud off, and are recycled through the Golgi complex. This stimulus-dependent exocytosis is best exemplified in glandular cells that produce and release large volumes of secretion. Many other cell types form products that are not significantly concentrated in the Golgi or stored in conspicuous secretory granules, but are released continuously in minute vesicles that fuse with the plasmalemma. The vesicles involved in this stimulus-independent exocytosis are morphologically indistinguishable from pinocytosis vesicles. The secretory activity of such cells went unrecognized until synthesis and release of their products was detected in studies employing radiolabeled precursors.

REFERENCES

General

Brachet, J., and A. E. Mirsky: The Cell: Biochemistry Physiology, Morphology. Vols. I to VI. New York, Academic Press, 1959–1964.

Busch, H. B., ed.: The Cell Nucleus. 3 vols. New York, Academic Press, 1974.

Fawcett, D. W.: The Cell. 2nd ed. Philadelphia, W. B. Saunders Co., 1981.

Flickinger, C. J., J. C. Brown, H. C. Kutchai, and J. W. Ogilvie: Medical Cell Biology. Philadelphia, W. B. Saunders Co., 1979.

Karp, G.: Cell Biology. New York, McGraw-Hill Book Co., 1979.

Watson, J. D., ed.: Organization of the Cytoplasm. Cold Spring Harbor Symp. Quant. Biol. Vol. 46, 1982.

Cell Membrane

Branton, D.: Freeze-etching studies of membrane structure. Trans. R. Soc. Lond. (Biol.) 261:133, 1971.

Finian, J. B.: The development of ideas on membrane structure. Subcell. Biochem. 1:363, 1977.

Hendler, R. W.: Biological membrane ultrastructure. Physiol. Rev. 51:66, 1971.

Ito, G.: The surface coat of enteric microvilli. J. Cell Biol. 27:475, 1965.

Marchesi, V. T., H. Furtlmayr, and M. Tomita: The red cell membrane. Annu. Rev. Biochem. 45:667, 1976.

Rambourg, A., M. Neutra, and C. P. Leblond: Presence of a cell coat rich in carbohydrates at the surface of cells in the rat. Anat. Rec. 154:41, 1966.

Singer, S. J.: Molecular organization of membranes. Annu. Rev. Biochem. 43:805, 1974.

Singer, S. J., and G. L. Nicholson: The fluid-mosaic model of the structure of the cell membranes. Science 175:720, 1972.

Steck, T. L.: The organization of proteins in human red blood cell membrane. J. Cell Biol. 62:1, 1974.

Endoplasmic Reticulum

Blöbel, G., and B. Dobberstein: Transfer of proteins across membranes. I. Presence of proteolytically processed and unprocessed nascent immunoglobulin light chains on membrane-bound ribosomes of murine myeloma. J. Cell Biol. 67:835, 1975.

Blöbel, G., and B. Dobberstein: Transfer of proteins across membranes. II. Reconstitution of functional rough microsomes from heterologous components. J Cell Biol. 67:852, 1975.

Palade, G. E.: A small particulate component of the cytoplasm. J. Biophys. Biochem. Cytol. 1:59, 1955.

Palade, G. E., and K. R. Porter: Studies on the endoplasmic reticulum. I. Its identification in cells in situ. J Exp. Med. 100:641, 1954.

Porter, K. R.: Observations on a submicroscopic basophilic component of the cytoplasm. J. Exp. Med. 97:727, 1953.

Redman, C. M., and D. D. Sabatini: Vectorial discharge of peptides released by puromycin from attached ribosomes. Proc. Natl. Acad. Sci. USA 56:608, 1966.

Sabatini, D. D., and G. Blöbel: Controlled proteolysis of nascent polypeptides in liver cell fractions. II. Location of the polypeptides in rough microsomes. J. Cell Biol. 45:146, 1970.

Sabatini, G. G., Y. Tashiro, and G. E. Palade: On the attachment of ribosomes to microsomal membranes. J. Mol. Biol. 19:503, 1966.

Smooth Endoplasmic Reticulum

Cardell, R., R. S. Bodenhausen, and K. R. Porter: Intestinal triglyceride absorption in the rat. J. Cell Biol. 34:123, 1967.

Christensen, A. K., and G. W. Gillim: Correlation of fine structure and function in steroid secreting cells with emphasis on those of gonads. In Kerns, K. W., ed.: The Gonads. New York, Appleton-Century-Crofts, 1969.

Dallner, G., and L. Ernster: Subfractionation and composition of microsomal membranes. A review. J. Histochem. Cytochem. *16*:611, 1968.

Jones, A. L., and D. W. Fawcett: Hypertrophy of the agranular reticulum in hamster liver induced by phenobarbital. (With a review of the functions of this organelle in liver.) J. Histochem. Cytochem. *14*:215, 1966.

Jones, A. L., N. B. Ruderman, and H. G. Herrera: Electron microscopic and biochemical study of lipoprotein synthesis in isolated perfused rat liver. J. Lipid. Res. *8*:429, 1967.

Porter, K. R., and G. E. Palade: Studies on the endoplasmic reticulum. III. Its form and distribution in striated muscle cells. J. Biophys. Biochem. Cytol. *3*:269, 1958.

Porter, K. R., and E. Yamada: Studies on the endoplasmic reticulum. V. Its form and differentiation in pigment epithelial cells of frog retina. J. Biophys. Biochem. Cytol. *8*:161, 1960.

Remmer, H., and H. J. Merker: Effect of drugs on the formation of smooth endoplasmic reticulum and drug metabolizing enzymes. Ann. N.Y. Acad. Sci. *123*:79, 1963.

Golgi Complex

Bearns, H. W., and R. G. Kessel: The Golgi apparatus: structure and function. Int. Rev. Cytol. *23*:209, 1968.

Bennett, G., C. P. Leblond, and A. J. Haddad: Migration of glycoproteins from Golgi apparatus to the surface of various cell types as shown by radioautography after labelled fucose injection. J. Cell Biol. *60*:258, 1974.

Farquhar, M. G., and G. E. Palade: The Golgi apparatus (complex)—1954–1981—from artefact to center stage. J. Cell Biol. *91*:(Suppl.) 77, 1981.

Fleischer, B., G. Fleischer, and H. Ogawa: Isolation and characterization of Golgi membranes from bovine liver. J. Cell Biol. *43*:59, 1967.

Jamieson, J. D.: Role of the Golgi complex in the intracellular transport of secretory proteins. In Clementi, F., and B. Ceccarelle, eds.: Advances in Cytopharmacology. Vol. 1. New York, Raven Books, Abelard–Schuman, 1971.

Neutra, M., and C. P. Leblond: The Golgi apparatus. Sci. Am. *220*:100, 1969.

Novikoff, P. M., A. B. Novikoff, N. Quintana, and J. J. Hauw: Golgi apparatus, GERL, and lysosomes of neurons in rat dorsal root ganglia. J. Cell Biol. *50*:859, 1971.

Whaley, W. G.: The Golgi Apparatus. New York, Springer-Verlag, 1975.

Mitochondria

Dawid, I. B., and D. R. Wolstenholme: The structure of the frog oocyte mitochondrial DNA. In Slater, E. C., J. M. Tager, S. Papa, and E. Quagliarello, eds.: Biochemical Aspects of Biogenesis of Mitochondria. Bari, Italy, Adriatica Editrice, 1968.

Grivell, L. A.: Mitochondrial DNA. Sci. Am. *248*:60, 1983.

Kalf, G. F.: Deoxyribonucleic acid in mitochondria and its role in protein synthesis. Biochemistry *3*:1702, 1964.

Larson, W. J.: Genesis of mitochondria in insect fat body. J. Cell Biol. *47*:373, 1970.

Lehninger, A. L.: The Mitochondrion. New York, W. B. Benjamin, 1964.

Nass, M. M. K., and S. Nass: Intramitochondrial fibers with DNA characteristics. Fixation and electron staining reactions. J. Cell Biol. *19*:593, 1963.

Palade, G.: An electron microscope study of mitochondrial structure. J. Histochem. Cytochem. *1*:188, 1953.

Peachey, L. D.: Electron microscopic observations on the accumulation of divalent cations in intramichondrial granules. J. Cell Biol. *20*:95, 1964.

Rabinowitz, M., J. Sinclair, L. DeSalle, R. Haselhorn, and H. H. Swift: Isolation of deoxyribonucleic acid from mitochondria of chick embryo heart and liver. Proc. Natl. Acad. Sci. USA *53*:1126, 1964.

Reich, E., and D. J. Luck: Replication and inheritance of mitochondrial DNA. Proc. Natl. Acad. Sci. USA *55*:1600, 1966.

Sinclair, J. H., and B. V. Stevens: Circular DNA filaments from mouse mitochondria. Proc. Natl. Acad. Sci. USA *56*:508, 1966.

Tandler, B., and C. L. Hoppel: Division of giant mitochondria during recovery from cuprizone intoxication. J. Cell Biol. *56*:266, 1973.

Tedeschi, H.: Mitochondria: Structure, Biogenesis and Transducing Function. Cell Biology Monographs, Vol. 4. Vienna, Springer-Verlag, 1976.

Lysosomes

Allison, A.: Lysosomes and disease. Sci. Am. *217*:62, 1967.

Davies, P., and A. C. Allison: Secretion of macrophage enzymes in relation to the pathogenesis of chronic inflammation. In Nelson, D. S., ed.: Immunobiology of the Macrophage. New York, Academic Press, 1976.

DeDuve, C. Lysosomes. Sci. Am. *208*:5, 1963.

DeDuve, C., and R. Wattiaux: Function of lysosomes. Annu. Rev. Physiol. *28*:435, 1966.

Dingle, J. T., and H. B. Fell, eds.: Lysosomes in Biology and Pathology. Vols. I and II. Amsterdam, North Holland Publishing Co., 1969.

Hirsch, J. G.: Cinematographic observations on granule lysis in polymorphonuclear leukocytes during phagocytosis. J. Exp. Med. *116*:827, 1962.

Koloday, E. H.: Lysosomal storage diseases. N. Engl. J. Med. *294*:1217, 1976.

Weissmann, G.: Leukocytes as secretory organs of inflammation. Hosp. Pract. *13*:53, 1978.

Weissmann, G., R. B. Zurier, P. J. Spieler, and I. M. Goldstein: Mechanisms of lysosomal enzyme release from leucocytes exposed to immune complexes and other particles. J. Exp. Med. *134*:149s, 1971.

Peroxisomes

DeDuve, C., and P. Baudhuin: Peroxisomes. Physiol. Rev. *46*:323, 1966.

Fahimi, H. D.: Cytochemical localization of peroxidase activity in rat hepatic microbodies. J. Histochem. Cytochem. *16*:547, 1968.

Goldman, B. M., and G. Blobel: Biogenesis of peroxisomes. Intracellular site of synthesis of catalase and uricase. Proc. Natl. Acad. Sci. USA *75*:5066, 1978.

Novikoff, P. M., and A. B. Novikoff: Peroxisomes in absorptive cells of mammalian small intestine. J. Cell Biol. *53*:532, 1972.

Reddy, J. K., and T. P. Krishnahantha: Hepatic peroxisome proliferation: induction by two novel compounds structurally unrelated to chlofibrate. Science 190:787, 1975.

Tiukada, T., Y. Mochuzuki, and S. Fujiwara: The nucleoids of rat liver cell microbodies. J. Cell Biol. *28*:449, 1966.

Annulate Lamellae

Kessel, R. G.: Annulate lamellae. J. Ultrastr. Res. Suppl. *10*:1, 1968.

Kessel, R. G.: Origin, differentiation, distribution and possible functional role of annulate lamellae during spermatogenesis in *Drosophila melanogaster*. *J. Ultrastr. Res.* 75:72, 1981.

Kessel, R. G.: Fibrogranular bodies, annulate lamellae, and polyribosomes in the dragonfly oocyte. J. Morphol. *176*:171, 1983.

Centrioles

Anderson, R. G. W., and R. M. Brenner: The formation of basal bodies in the *Rhesus* monkey oviduct. J. Cell Biol. *50*:10, 1971.

Fulton, C.: Centrioles. *In* Reinert, J., and H. Ursprung, eds.: Origin and Continuity of Cell Organelles. New York, Springer-Verlag, 1971.

Sorokin, S.: Reconstruction of centriole formation and ciliogenesis in mammalian lungs. J. Cell Sci. *3*:207, 1968.

Steinman, R. M.: An electron microscopic study of ciliogenesis in developing epidermis and trachea in embryos of *Xenopus*. Am. J. Anat. *122*:19, 1968.

INCLUSIONS

Glycogen

Fawcett, D. W.: Identification of particulate glycogen and ribonucleoprotein in electron micrographs. J. Histochem Cytochem. *6*:95, 1958.

Revel, J. P., L. Napolitano, and D. W. Fawcett: Identification of glycogen in electron micrographs of thin tissue sections. J. Biophys. Biochem. Cytol. *8*:575, 1960.

Lipid

Cushman, S. W.: Structure-function relationships in the adipose cell. I. Ultrastructure of the isolated adipose cell. J. Cell Biol. *46*:326, 1970.

Napolitano, L.: The differentiation of white adipose tissue. J. Cell Biol. *18*:663, 1963.

Pigment

Björkerud, S.: The isolation of lipofuscin granules from bovine cardiac muscle. J. Ultrastr. Res. Suppl. *5*:5, 1963.

Fitzpatrick, T. B., and G. Szabo: The melanocyte: cytology and cytochemistry. J. Invest. Dermatol. *32*:197, 1959.

Mann, D. M. A., and P. O. Yates: Lipochrome pigments—their relationship to aging in the human nervous system. I. Lipofuscein content of nerve cells. Brain *97*:481, 1974.

Stekler, B. L., D. Mark, A. S. Mildvan, and M. V. Gee: Rate and magnitude of age pigment accumulation in human myocardium. J. Gerontol. *14*:430, 1959.

Szabo, G.: The biology of the pigment cell. *In* Bittar, E. B., and N. F. Bittar, eds.: Biological Basis of Medicine. Vol. 6. New York, Academic Press, 1969.

Crystals

Hamilton, D. W., D. W. Fawcett, and A. K. Christensen: The liver of the slender salamander, *Batrachoseps attenuatus*. I. The structure of its crystalline inclusions. Z. Zellforsch. Mikroskop. Anat. *70*:347, 1966.

Nagano, T.: Some observations on the fine structure of

the Sertoli cell of human testis. Z. Zellforsch. Mikroskop. Anat. *73*:89, 1966.

Nagano, T., and I. Otsuki: Reinvestigation of the fine structure of Reinke's crystal in the human testicular interstitial cell. J. Cell Biol. *51*:148, 1971.

CYTOSKELETON

Microtubules

Binder, L. I., and J. L. Rosenbaum: The in vitro assembly of flagellar outer doublet tubulin. J. Cell Biol. *79*:500, 1978.

Burnside, B.: The form and arrangement of microtubules: an historical, primarily morphological review. Ann. N.Y. Acad. Sci. *253*:14, 1975.

Haimo, L. T., and J. L. Rosenbaum: Cilia, flagella, and microtubules. J. Cell Biol. *91*:125s, 1981.

Murphy, D. B., and G. B. Borisy: Association of high molecular weight proteins with microtubules and their role in microtubule assembly in vitro. Proc. Natl. Acad. Sci. USA 72:2696, 1975.

Olmsted, J. B., and G. B. Borisy: Microtubules. Annu. Rev. Biochem. *42*:507, 1973.

Taylor, E.: The mechanism of colchicine inhibition of mitosis. I. Kinetics of inhibition and the binding of H^3-colchicine. J. Cell Biol. *25*:145, 1965.

Tilney, L. G.: Origin and continuity of microtubules. *In* Reinert, J., and H. Ursprung, eds.: Origin and Continuity of Cell Organelles. New York, Springer-Verlag, 1971.

Filaments

Fujiwara, K., and T. D. Pollard: Fluorescent antibody localization of myosin in the cytoplasm cleavage furrow and mitotic spindle of human cells. J. Cell Biol. *23*:243, 1976.

Gard, D., and E. Lazarides: The synthesis and distribution of desmin and vimentin during myogenesis *in vitro*. Cell *19*:263, 1980.

Hynes, R. U., and A. T. Destree: 10 nm filaments in normal and transformed cells. Cell *13*:151, 1978.

Lazarides, E.: Intermediate filaments as mechanical integrators of cellular space. Nature *283*:249, 1980.

Osborn, M., N. Geisler, G. Shaw, G. Sharp, and K. Weber: Intermediate filaments. Cold Spring Harbor Symp. Quant. Biol. *LXVI:* 413, 1981.

Shelanski, M. L., and R. K. Liem: Neurofilaments. J. Neurochem. *33*:5, 1979.

Small, J. V., and A. Sobiesek: Studies on the function and composition of the 10 nm filaments of vertebrate smooth muscle. J. Cell Biol. *23*:243, 1977.

Sun, T. T., C. Shih, and H. Green: Keratin cytoskeletons in epithelial cells of internal organs. Proc. Natl. Acad. Sci. USA 76:2813, 1979.

Microtrabecular Lattice

Penman, S., D. G. Capco, E. G. Fey, P. Chatterjee, T. Rieter, S. Ermish, and K. Wan: The three dimensional structural networks of cytoplasm and nucleus: function in cells and tissue. Modern Cell Biol. *2*:385, 1983.

Porter, K. R., and J. B. Tucker: The ground substance of the living cell. Sci. Am. *244*:40, 1981.

Wolosowick, J. J., and K. R. Porter: Microtrabecular lattice of the cytoplasmic ground substance: artifact or reality? J. Cell Biol. *82*:114, 1979.

Nuclear Envelope and Fibrous Lamina

Aaronson, R. P., and G. Blöbel: On the attachment of the nuclear pore complex. J. Cell Biol. *62*:746, 1974.

Fawcett, D. W.: On the occurrence of a fibrous lamina on the inner aspect of the nuclear envelope in certain cells of vertebrates. Am. J. Anat. *119*:129, 1966.

Francke, W. W.: Structure, biochemistry, and functions of the nuclear envelope. Int. Rev. Cytol. (Suppl. 4)72, 1974.

Gerace, L., A. Blum, and G. Blöbel: Immunocytochemical localization of the major polypeptides of the nuclear pore complex–lamina fraction. Interphase and mitotic distribution. J. Cell Biol. *79*:546, 1978.

Krohne, G., W. W. Franke, and U. Schur: The major polypeptides of the nuclear pore complex. Exp. Cell Res. *116*:85, 1978.

Maul, G. C.: The nuclear and cytoplasmic pore complex structure, dynamics, distribution and evolution. Int. Rev. Cytol. (Suppl. 6)76, 1977.

Unwin, P. N. T., and R. A. Milligan: A large particle associated with the perimeter of the nuclear pore complex. J. Cell Biol. *93*:63, 1982.

Chromatin

Bradbury, E. M.: La chromatine. Recherche *9*:644, 1978.

Hozier, J., M. Renz, and R. Niels: The chromosome fiber: evidence for an ordered superstructure of nucleosomes. Chromosoma *62*:301, 1977.

Kornberg, R.: Structure of chromatin. Annu. Rev. Biochem. *46*:931, 1977.

Olins, D. E., and A. L. Olins: Nucleosomes: the structural quantum of chromosomes. Am. Scientist *66*:704, 1978.

Worcel, A., and C. Benyajati: Higher order coiling of DNA in chromatin. Cell *12*:83, 1977.

Chromosomes

Gall, J. G.: On the submicroscopic structure of chromosomes. Brookhaven Symp. in Biol. *8*:17, 1956.

Laemmle, U. K., S. M. Cheng, K. W. Adolf, J. R. Paulson, J. A. Brown, and W. R. Baumbach: Metaphase chromosome structure: the role of non-histone proteins. Cold Spring Harbor Symp. Quant. Biol. *42*:35, 1977.

Marsden, M. P. F., and U. K. Laemmli: Metaphase chromosome structure: evidence for a radial loop model. Cell *17*:849, 1979.

Paulsen, J. P., and U. K. Laemmli: The structure of histone depleted metaphase chromosomes. Cell *12*:817, 1977.

Ris, H., and D. Kubai: Chromosome structure. Annu. Rev. Genet. *4*:263, 1970.

Stubblefield, E.: The structure of mammalian chromosomes. Int. Rev. Cytol. *35*:1, 1973.

Nucleolus

Brown, D. D., and J. B. Gurdon: Absence of ribosomal RNA synthesis in the anucleolate mutant of *Xenopus laevis*. Proc. Natl. Acad. Sci. USA *51*:39, 1964.

Hay, E. D.: The structure and function of the nucleolus in developing cells. *In* Dalton, A. J., and F. Haguenau, eds.: The Nucleus. Vol. 3. New York, Academic Press, 1968.

Hay, E. D., and J. B. Gurdon: The fine structure of the nucleolus in normal and mutant *Xenopus* embryos. J. Cell Sci. *2*:151, 1967.

Miller, O. L.: Structure and composition of peripheral nucleoli of salamander oocytes. Natl. Cancer Inst. Monogr. *23*:53, 1966.

Perry, R. P.: Role of the nucleolus in ribonucleic acid metabolism and other cellular processes. Natl. Cancer Inst. Monogr. *18*:325, 1964.

CELL DIVISION AND CELL CYCLE

Bajer, A., and J. Mole-Bajer: Architecture and function of the mitotic spindle. Adv. Mol. Biol. *1*:213, 1971.

Baserga, R., and F. Weibel: The cell cycle of mammalian cells. Int. Rev. Exp. Pathol. 7:1, 1969.

Inoue, S.: Cell division and the mitotic spindle. J. Cell Biol. (Suppl.) *93*:131s, 1981.

Inoue, S., and H. Ritter: Dynamics of mitotic spindle organization and function. *In* Inoue, S., and R. E. Stephens, eds.: Molecules and Cell Movement. New York, Raven Press, 1975.

Leblond, C. P., and B. E. Walker: Renewal of cell populations. Physiol. Rev. *36*:255, 1956.

Mazia, D.: The cell cycle. Sci. Am. *230*:54, 1964.

McIntosh, J. P., P. K. Hepler, and D. G. Van Wie: Model for mitosis. Nature *224*:659, 1969.

Rappaport, R.: Cytokinesis in animal cells. Int. Rev. Cytol. *31*:301, 1972.

Cell Motility

Allen, R. A.: Cell Motility. J. Cell Biol. (Suppl.) *93*:148s, 1981.

Pollard, T. D.: Cytoplasmic contractile proteins. J. Cell Biol. (Suppl.) *93*:156s, 1981.

Endocytosis

Allison, A. C., and P. Davies: Mechanisms of endocytosis and exocytosis. Symp. Soc. Exp. Biol. *28*:419, 1974.

Goldstein, J. L., R. G. W. Anderson, and M. S. Brown: Coated pits, coated vesicles, and receptor mediated endocytosis. A review. Nature *279*:679, 1979.

Gordon, S., and Z. A. Cohn: The macrophage. Int. Rev. Cytol. *36*:171, 1973.

Griffin, F. M., J. A. Griffin, J. F. Leider, and S. C. Silverstein: Studies on the mechanism of phagocytosis. J. Exp. Med. *142*:1263, 1975.

Hirsch, J. G.: Phagocytosis. Annu. Rev. Microbiol. *19*:339, 1965.

Kanaseki, T., and K. Kadota: The vesicle in a basket. A morphological study of coated vesicles isolated from the nerve endings of guinea pig brain. J. Cell Biol. *42*:202, 1969.

Pearse, B. M. F.: Clathrin: a unique protein associated with the intracellular transfer of membrane by coated vesicles. Proc. Natl. Acad. Sci. USA *73*:1255, 1976.

Roth, T. F., J. A. Cutting, and S. B. Atlas: Protein transport: a selective membrane mechanism. J. Supramol. Struct. *4*:527, 1976.

Silverstein, S. C., R. M. Steinman, and Z. A. Cohn: Endocytosis. Annu. Rev. Biochem. *46*:669, 1977.

Exocytosis

Jamieson, J. D.: Transport and discharge of exportable proteins in pancreatic exocrine cells: *in vitro* studies. *In* Bronner, F., and Kleinzeller, A., eds.: Current Topics in Membranes and Transport. New York: Academic Press, 1972.

Jamieson, J. D.: Membranes and secretion. Hosp. Pract. *8*:71, 1973.

2

EPITHELIUM

In the past decade, increasing emphasis has been placed on the biology of the cell, often to the neglect of higher levels of organization. Much of the research in this field is now done upon a small number of cell types that can be grown in isolation in vitro. Valuable as those studies are, the student should be aware that isolated cells are seldom encountered in the body. The great majority are assembled in coherent groupings bound together by cell junctions and extracellular matrix to form *tissues*. Each of the tissues is specialized for a particular function and has a distinctive pattern of organization.

The first chapter was devoted to the cell—the fundamental unit of living matter. This chapter, and four following, will present the identifying characteristics of the basic tissues—*epithelium, connective tissue, blood, muscular tissue,* and *nervous tissue*. Later chapters will describe the patterns in which these tissues are combined to form the larger functional units called *organs*.

Epithelium is a tissue composed of cells in close apposition over a large portion of their surface and with little or no intercellular substance. In its simplest form an epithelium consists of a single coherent layer of identical cells covering an external, or lining an internal, surface. But the cells may differentiate into two or more functionally distinct types to meet specific local requirements, and may take on various shapes and become arranged in multiple layers. Several categories of epithelia are defined and assigned different terms to lend precision and consistency to the descriptive literature of histology and pathology (Fig. 2–1). It is of some importance therefore for students to learn the classification and terminology of the several kinds of epithelia.

Origin and Distribution of Epithelium

Two of the primary germ layers of the early embryo, the *ectoderm* and *endoderm*, are epithelial, and most of the epithelial organs of the body are derived from these germ layers. For example, the epidermis of the skin and the epithelium of the cornea, which together cover the entire external surface of the body, develop from the ectoderm. By invagination and proliferation, this outer covering epithelium gives rise to tubes or solid cords that form the glandular appendages of the skin–the sudoriparous, sebaceous, and mammary glands. Similarly, the alimentary tract is lined by epithelium of endodermal origin, and liver, pancreas, gastric glands, and intestinal glands all arise in the embryo by invagination, proliferation, and specialization of epithelial outgrowths from the lining of the primitive gut. Each *exocrine gland* of the adult communicates with an internal cavity or an external surface by way of ducts that open onto the epithelium of the inner or outer surface layer from which it developed during embryonic life. The *endocrine glands,* on the other hand, usually lose their connection with the surface epithelium from which they originally develop.

In addition to the epithelial structures that develop from the ectoderm and endoderm, there are a few organs composed of epithelia that arise from mesoderm. Examples are the kidney and the lining of the male and female reproductive tracts.

The linings of the peritoneal cavity and of other serous cavities, and the linings of blood and lymph vessels, are all derivatives of mesenchyme. These are in all respects typical epithelia but it is convenient and customary to refer to the lining of blood and lymph vessels as *endothelium* and to the lining of serous cavities as *mesothelium*.

Epithelia are specialized for many different functions—*absorption, secretion, transport, excretion, protection,* and *sensory reception.* Those that form the outer surface of the body are adapted for protection of the organism against mechanical damage and loss of moisture. They also play a role in sensory recep-

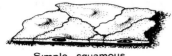

Simple squamous

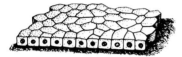

Simple cuboidal

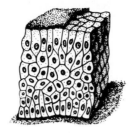

Stratified columnar

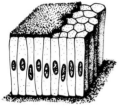

Simple columnar

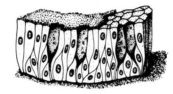

Pseudostratified columnar

Figure 2–1. Drawings illustrating the shape and arrangement of cells in the principal types of epithelium.

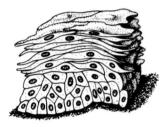

Stratified squamous

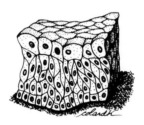

Transitional

tion, containing nerve endings that provide the warning of pain that make the organism avoid injury. Others contain neural elements, such as taste buds and olfactory cells, specialized to function as chemical receptors. All substances received or given off by the body must traverse an epithelium; thus, many of the epithelia lining internal surfaces are modified for absorption or secretion. Those concerned with secretion may contain only scattered individual secretory cells, or the epithelium may give rise to a gland in which most of the cells are specialized for elaboration of a particular product. Other epithelia, concerned with excretion, become modified to increase their efficiency in transport of solutes and water or in elimination of substances from the body.

CLASSIFICATION OF EPITHELIA

Epithelia are named and classified according to the number of cell layers and the shape of the cells. If there is one layer of cells the epithelium is described as *simple;* if there are two or more layers it is said to be *stratified.* The superficial cells can usually be described as *squamous, cuboidal,* or *columnar.* Thus, a single layer of flat cells is a *simple squamous epithelium.* A single layer of tall prismatic cells is a *simple columnar epithelium.* The corresponding multilayered epithelia are called *stratified squamous epithelium* and *stratified columnar epithelium.*

Within the same general category of epithelium the cells may or may not have motile cell processes called *cilia* on their free surfaces. In the interest of more precise description, it is customary to make note of this surface specialization in naming the epithelium. When such a border is present, the tissue is described as a *ciliated simple columnar epithelium* or a *ciliated stratified columnar epithelium.* Similarly in stratified squamous epithelium, the superficial cells in some cases accumulate in their cytoplasm the fibrous protein *keratin* and are reduced to scalelike lifeless residues of cells. To distinguish such epithelia from others in which the superficial cells do not undergo this change, it is customary to describe them as *keratinized stratified squamous epithelium.*

Among the simple columnar epithelia one category is described as *pseudostratified* because the cells are so arranged that the nuclei occur at two or more levels and the epithelium thus appears to be stratified. However, it can be shown by maceration that there is actually only one layer, all the cells being fixed to the basal lamina (basement membrane) but only some of them reaching the free surface. In truly stratified epithelia, only the cells of the lowermost layer are in contact with the substrate.

Among the stratified epithelia there are two types that cannot adequately be described by reference to the shape of their surface cells. These are the *transitional epithelium* of the urinary tract and the *germinal epithelium* of the male gonad. Their distinguishing characteristics will be described later.

Simple Squamous Epithelium

Thin platelike cells are arranged in a single layer and adhere closely to one another by their edges (Fig. 2–1). When examined in surface view, especially after the cell limits are stained with silver nitrate, a characteristic mosaic pattern is seen (Fig. 2–2). The individual cells have polygonal or irregular wavy outlines. In sections perpendicular to the epithelium the cells, in profile, appear as plump spindles or thin rectangles (Fig. 2–3). Because of the large area covered by each flattened cell, a given plane of section will pass through the nucleus of only a fraction of the cells transected.

Epithelia of this variety are found on the inner surface of the wall of the membranous labyrinth and on the inner surface of the tympanic membrane of the inner ear; in the parietal layer of Bowman's capsule and in the thin segment of the loop of Henle in the kidney; in the rete testis; and in the smallest

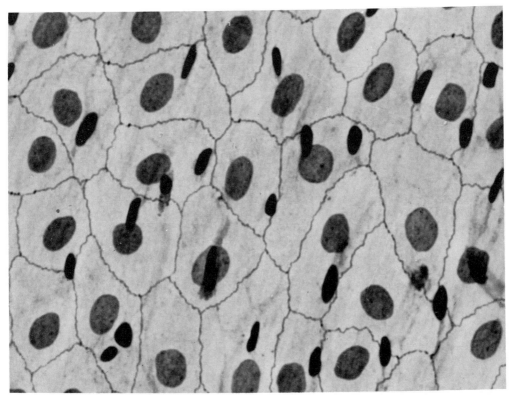

Figure 2–2. A thin spread of guinea-pig mesentery treated with silver nitrate and subsequently stained with May-Grünwald and Giemsa stains. The limits of the simple squamous mesothelial cells have been blackened by the silver, revealing their polygonal outlines. The large oval nuclei are those of the mesothelial cells. The darker ellipsoidal nuclei are those of fibroblasts beneath the mesothelium.

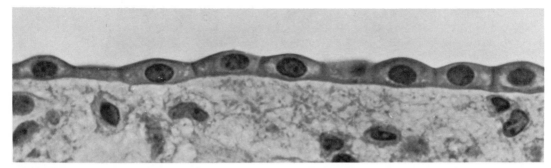

Figure 2–3. Epithelium of a collecting duct of the dog kidney is flattened to form a thick squamous epithelium here, but the cells in other species may be cuboidal.

excretory ducts of many glands. Also included in this category are the *mesothelium* lining the pleural, peritoneal, and other serous cavities and the *endothelium* lining the walls of the blood and lymph vessels.

Simple Cuboidal Epithelium

On surface view this epithelium also appears as a mosaic of small, usually hexagonal polygons, and in vertical section the sheet of cells appears as a row of square or rectangular profiles (Fig. 2–1).

Epithelium of this kind is found in many glands, as in the thyroid; on the free surface of the ovary; on the choroid plexus; on the capsule of the lens; in the ducts of glands, and as the pigmented epithelium of the retina. Secreting epithelia in the terminal portions of many glands can often be placed in this class, although the cells of glandular acini or tubules are usually pyramidal rather than cuboidal.

Simple Columnar Epithelium

Sections parallel to the surface of this type of epithelium present a mosaic pattern much like that in other simple epithelia, but one in which the polygonal outlines of the cells are considerably smaller (Fig. 2–1). In sections perpendicular to the surface the rectangular outlines of the cells may be only a little taller than those of cuboidal epithelium (Fig. 2–4A), or they may be very tall and slender, standing upright like columns or fence palings (Fig. 2–4C). In many examples of columnar epithelium, all the nuclei are at approximately the same level (Fig. 2–4E). Simple columnar epithelium lines the surface of the digestive tract from the cardia of the stomach to the anus and is also common in the excretory ducts of many glands. Ciliated

simple columnar epithelium (Figs. 2–4E and 2–5) is found in the uterus and oviducts, in the bronchi of the lung, in some of the paranasal sinuses, and in the central canal of the spinal cord.

Stratified Squamous Epithelium

The epithelial sheet is thick, and a vertical section shows the cells to vary in shape from base to free surface (Figs. 2–4E, 2–6). The layer next to the basal lamina consists of plump cuboidal or even columnar cells with rounded or beveled upper ends. Above this basal layer are additional layers of irregularly polyhedral cells. The nearer to the free surface they occur, the more the cells are flattened (Fig. 2–6.). The superficial layers are composed of thin squamous cells.

Epithelium of this kind is found in the epidermis, the mouth, the esophagus, part of the epiglottis, the conjunctiva, the cornea, and the vagina and in a portion of the female urethra. When stratified squamous epithelium occurs on the exposed outer surface of the body, the superficial cells have lost their nuclei and the cytoplasm has been largely replaced by the scleroprotein *keratin*. The cells are dry, devitalized, scalelike structures. Such epithelium is described as *keratinized stratified squamous epithelium*. On the inner moist surfaces of the body, the superficial cells of this type of epithelium are viable nucleated elements, not unlike the deeper lying cells except for their shape. In these sites the tissue is described as a *nonkeratinized stratified squamous epithelium* (Fig. 2–4F).

Stratified Columnar Epithelium

The deeper layer or layers consist of small, irregularly polyhedral cells that do not reach the free surface. The superficial cells are

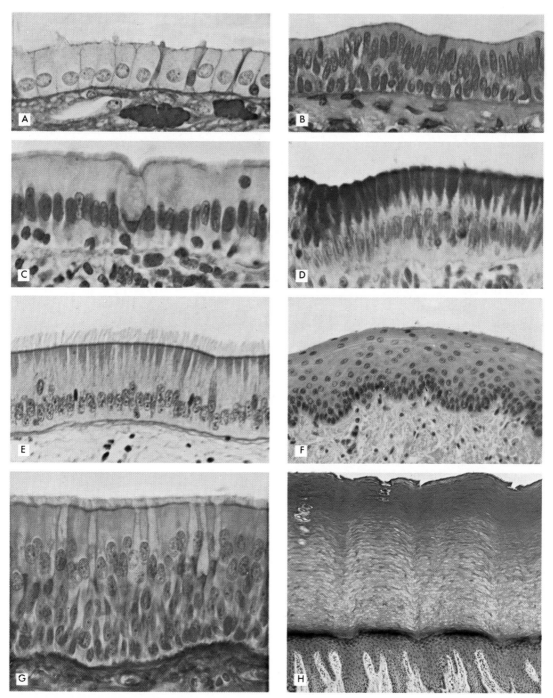

Figure 2–4. Photomicrographs of various types of epithelium. *A,* Simple low columnar epithelium of the papillary duct of the dog kidney. Mallory trichrome stain.

B, Stratified columnar epithelium from a large salivary gland duct. Mallory-azan stain.

C, Simple columnar epithelium from the intestinal mucosa of a cat. The epithelium has a striated border. Notice the presence of a single goblet cell among the columnar cells. Heidenhain's azan stain.

D, Simple columnar epithelium of mucous cells from the stomach. The mucus is stained a deep magenta. PAS-hematoxylin stain.

E, Simple ciliate columnar epithelium from the typhlosole of a mollusc. Notice the long cone of rootlets extending from the basal bodies of the cilia downward into the apical cytoplasm. Chrome alum-hematoxylin-phloxine stain.

F, Stratified squamous epithelium from the esophagus of a macaque. Hematoxylin and eosin stain.

G, Ciliated pseudostratified columnar epithelium from the human trachea. Mallory-azan stain.

H, Keratinized stratified squamous epithelium of the epidermis of the sole of the foot. Notice the very thick superficial stratum of fully keratinized devitalized cells.

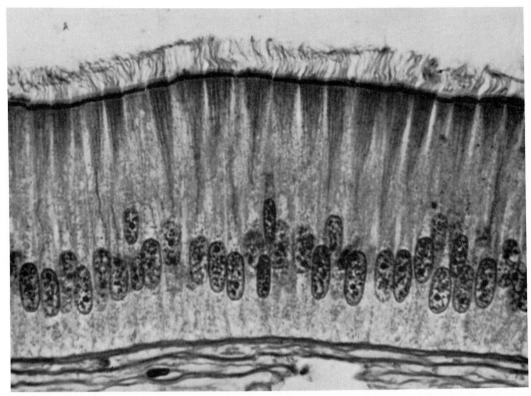

Figure 2–5. Simple columnar ciliated epithelium from the alimentary tract of a fresh water muscle. Notice the dark row of ciliary basal bodies just beneath the free surface of the cells and the cones of fibrous rootlets that extend downward from the basal bodies into the apical cytoplasm. Observe also the distinct "basement membrane" upon which the epithelium rests.

columnar in form. Stratified columnar epithelium is relatively uncommon. It is found in the fornix of the conjunctiva, in the cavernous urethra, in some small areas of the anal mucous membrane, in the pharynx, on the epiglottis, and in the large excretory ducts of some glands (Figs. 2–1, 2–4B, 2–7). *Ciliated stratified columnar epithelium* is found on the nasal surface of the soft palate, in the larynx, and transiently in the fetal esophagus.

Pseudostratified Columnar Epithelium

In pseudostratified columnar epithelium, all the cells are in contact with the basal lamina but not all of them reach the surface (Fig. 2–1). The cells are quite variable in shape: some have fairly broad attachment at the base, narrow rapidly, and extend upward through only a fraction of the thickness of the epithelium. Others extend throughout the thickness of the epithelium, but are widest near the free surface and have long slender processes that extend downward between the basally situated cells to attach to the basal lamina. Since the nucleus in both categories is in the widest portion of the cell, nuclei are found aligned at two or more levels in this class of epithelium, giving a specious appearance of stratification—hence the term pseudostratified.

Pseudostratified epithelium occurs in the large excretory ducts of the parotid and several other glands and in the male urethra. *Ciliated pseudostratified columnar epithelium* lines the greater part of the trachea and bronchi (Fig. 2–4G), the eustachian tube, a part of the tympanic cavity, and the lacrimal sac.

Transitional Epithelium

This was originally interpreted as an intermediate or transitional form between stratified squamous and columnar epithelium. The term *transitional epithelium* persists, even though its implication of change from one type to another is no longer considered appropriate. This kind of epithelium varies greatly in appearance depending on the con-

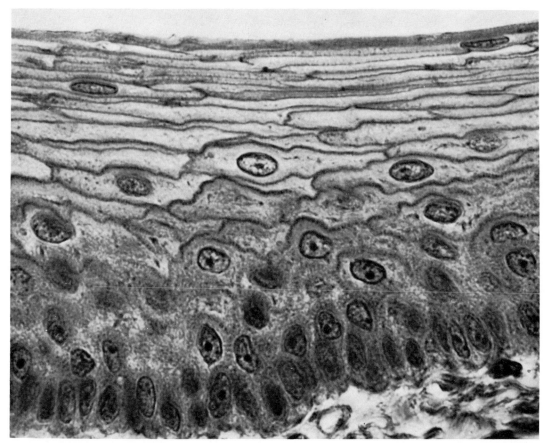

Figure 2–6. Photomicrograph of stratified squamous epithelium from the gingiva of a kitten. Observe the darker-staining cuboidal cells of the basal layer and the progressive flattening of cells in the more superficial layers.

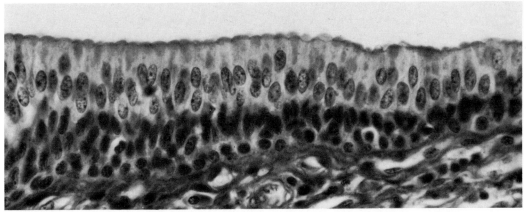

Figure 2–7. Photomicrograph of stratified columnar epithelium from the human male urethra. Notice the columnar form of the superficial layer of cells and the multiple layers of nuclei not attributable to obliquity of section.

ditions under which it is fixed. It is found lining the urinary bladder, which is subject to great changes owing to emptying and distention. In the contracted condition it consists of many cell layers (Fig. 2–1 and 2–8). The deepest cells have a cuboidal or even a columnar shape; above these are several layers of irregularly polyhedral cells, and the superficial layer consists of large cells with a characteristic rounded free surface. In the stretched condition the interrelations of the cells change to accommodate to the distention of the organ, and usually only two layers can then be distinguished—a superficial layer of large squamous elements over a layer of more or less cuboidal cells. This type of epithelium is characteristic of the mucosa of the excretory passages of the urinary system from the renal calyces to the urethra and is sometimes called *uroepithelium*.

The classification of epithelia that has been presented here applies primarily to the higher vertebrates. Other categories would be necessary to describe adequately the patterns of cell association found in invertebrates and lower vertebrates. In the adult mammal a given type of epithelium is char-

acteristic of the particular organ, and under normal conditions it does not change. However, in chronic inflammation or in the development of tumors one type of epithelium may change into another, a process called *metaplasia*. For example, under certain pathological conditions the ciliated pseudostratified epithelium of the bronchi may change to stratified squamous epithelium—a change described as *squamous metaplasia*. A similar transformation can be induced experimentally. If one nostril of a dog is closed surgically, the greater evaporative loss of moisture that accompanies the increased ventilation through the remaining nasal passage causes its pseudostratified ciliated columnar epithelium to transform into stratified squamous epithelium.

SPECIALIZATIONS OF EPITHELIA

A fundamental property of epithelial cells is their inherent tendency to maintain extensive contacts with one another and thus to

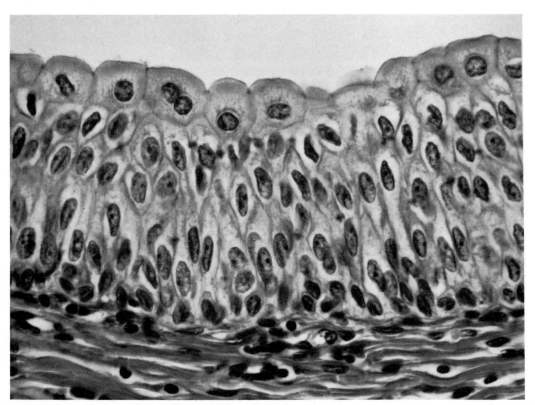

Figure 2–8. Photomicrograph of stratified transitional epithelium from the renal pelvis of a monkey, showing the characteristic superficial layer of large rounded cells, often binucleate.

form coherent sheets covering surfaces and lining cavities. As structural correlates of this property, there are specializations of the plasmalemma on the lateral surfaces of the cells that serve to maintain close cell-to-cell contact. The free surfaces of the superficial cells may also be modified in various ways to increase the efficiency of the epithelium in carrying out the functions of absorption or transport. Because all substances entering or leaving the body must traverse an epithelium in a direction perpendicular to its surface, the cells are structurally and functionally *polarized*—i.e., the distal end, toward the free surface, differs from the proximal end, toward the underlying connective tissue. This polarity is evident not only in the specialization of the respective surfaces but also in the arrangement of organelles in the interior of the cell. The centrosome and Golgi apparatus are usually in an adluminal or supranuclear position. An imaginary line passing through the centrosome and the center of the nucleus defines the *cell axis,* and this is usually vertical or perpendicular to the basement lamina. The long filamentous mitochondria of columnar epithelia tend to be oriented parallel to the cell axis and are often mobilized in greater numbers in the apical cytoplasm.

The evidence of cell polarity is less obvious in stratified squamous epithelia, which are more concerned with protection than with absorption or secretion. In these, the surface specializations for cell attachment are especially well developed, and the cytoplasm contains a conspicuous internal reinforcement or *cytoskeleton* composed of filaments, aggregated in bundles, to form *tonofibrils* visible with the light microscope. Such an internal supporting framework is not a prominent feature of columnar epithelia, but in many of these there is a *terminal web*, consisting of a feltwork of fine filaments immediately beneath the free surface, where it apparently provides for stiffening and mechanical support for the striated or ciliated border of the epithelium.

Specializations for Cell Attachment and Communication

Adjacent epithelial cells cohere so tightly that a relatively strong mechanical force must be applied to separate them. According to the traditional interpretation, a thin layer of an interstitial substance between cells acted as an adhesive. This hypothetical substance was referred to as the *intercellular cement.* It was stainable by the periodic acid–Schiff reaction and hence appeared to have a carbohydrate component. It also was a site of selective deposition of metallic silver when tissues immersed in silver nitrate solution were subsequently exposed to sunlight. This method was often used to demonstrate the cell boundaries of epithelia (Fig. 2–2).

Certain epithelial cells, particularly those of epidermal stratified squamous epithelium, appeared with the light microscope to adhere to one another by many small processes distributed over the entire cell surface. These seemed to extend from cell to cell and were called "intercellular bridges." Between the bridges a labyrinthine system of expanded intercellular spaces called *interfacial canals* was described. At the midpoint of each bridge was a densely staining dot called a *desmosome.* Some histologists insisted that there was protoplasmic continuity from cell to cell through the bridges, but others interpreted the desmosomes as special sites of attachment at end-to-end junctions of short processes on the neighboring cells. With special preparative procedures, desmosomes could also be demonstrated on the lateral surfaces of columnar epithelial cells that had no obvious intercellular bridges.

The nature of the contacts between epithelial cells was greatly clarified with the advent of electron microscopy. In micrographs of simple squamous, cuboidal, and columnar epithelia, the lateral membranes of adjacent cells are usually separated by a clear intercellular cleft only 15 to 20 nm wide. If this space is occupied in vivo by an intercellular substance, it is extracted during specimen preparation. The existence of an adhesive "intercellular cement" has not been substantiated, but some authors would assign such a role to the recently described glycoprotein cell product, fibronectin. In columnar absorptive epithelia the lateral cell membranes often diverge toward the base, creating wider intercellular spaces. The existence of an extensive system of interfacial canals in stratified squamous epithelia is confirmed in electron micrographs.

On the boundary between adjacent columnar epithelial cells, immediately subjacent to their free surface, dark dots can be seen with the light microscope in vertical sections, or dense bars in horizontal subtangential sections. In the latter they appear to form a continuous band around the polygonal perimeter of each cell. These were formerly called *terminal bars* and were interpreted as local accumulations of intercellular cement. They were assumed to seal or close the intercellular spaces at the free surface of the epithelium.

Electron microscopy now permits a more precise definition of the contact surface specializations of epithelia.

Zonula Occludens or Tight Junction. Where terminal bars were seen with the light

microscope in columnar epithelia, the electron microscope reveals a *junctional complex* consisting of three distinct components—the *zonula occludens,* the *zonula adherens,* and the *macula adherens* or *desmosome.* Immediately below the free surface of the epithelium is the zonula occludens, a region of surface specialization where the membranes of adjoining cells converge and appear to fuse (Fig. 2–9). Within this region, which may occupy 0.1 to 0.3 μm of the lateral cell

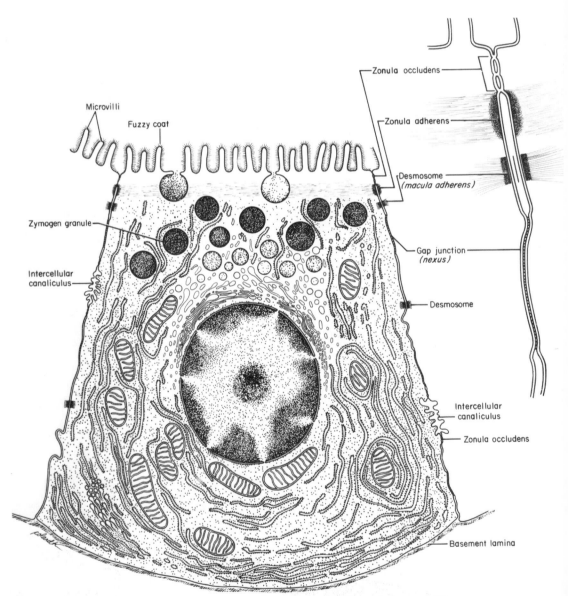

Figure 2–9. Drawing of a typical epithelial cell illustrating the basement lamina, microvilli on the free surface, desmosomes on the lateral surfaces, and a juxtaluminal junctional complex. The latter consists of a zonula occludens, zonula adherens, and macula adherens. In addition a gap junction is depicted near the junctional complex. These communicating junctions may occur anywhere on the opposing lateral surfaces of epithelial cells. (Drawing from Hay, E., *In* Greep, R. O., ed.: Histology. 2nd ed. New York, McGraw-Hill Book Co., 1965.)

boundary, there may be multiple sites of fusion separated by short regions in which the opposing membranes are separated by 10 to 15 nm. This juxtaluminal region of membrane fusion extends in a belt around the perimeter of the cell and serves to close the intercellular space.

When this region is examined in freeze-cleaved preparations, it presents a very distinctive reticular pattern (Fig. 2–10). Each membrane appears to contain straight, rod-like structures that branch and join to form a rectilinear network of ridges on the P-face and a complementary pattern of shallow grooves on the E-face of the cleaved membrane. These intramembranous rods are believed to coincide with the lines of membrane fusion seen in this region of the cell membrane in thin sections.

As a consequence of the obliteration of the intercellular space along these circumferential bands at the apex of the cells, large molecules cannot traverse the epithelium from the lumen via an intercellular route. Occluding junctions of this kind are especially important in a transporting epithelium such as that of the gallbladder (see Chapter 27). They make it possible for the cells to pump solute actively through their lateral membranes into the intercellular cleft below the zonula occludens, creating there a stand-ing osmotic gradient that serves to move water across the epithelium, thereby concentrating the luminal contents.

The zonula occludens also has a mechanical role in maintaining the structural integrity of the epithelium. The cells are more firmly attached in this region of membrane fusion than anywhere else on their surface.

The Zonula Adherens. On the epithelial cell boundaries just below the zonula occludens, the membranes diverge to a distance of 15 to 20 nm. The opposing unit membranes are reinforced on their cytoplasmic surface by a dense mat of fine filamentous material that forms a continuous band around the cell parallel to the zonula occludens (Fig. 2–9). This junctional element is not identifiable in freeze-cleaved preparations because there seems to be no specialization within the plane of the membrane that distinguishes this from other parts of the plasmalemma. The associated condensation of cytoplasmic filaments has ill-defined limits, and in some epithelia it blends with a transverse zone of filament-rich cytoplasm called the *terminal web*. No structural elements are seen traversing the intercellular space at the zonula adherens and the nature of the forces that hold the membranes more tightly together at this site is not known. Nevertheless, as the name implies, the structure is generally

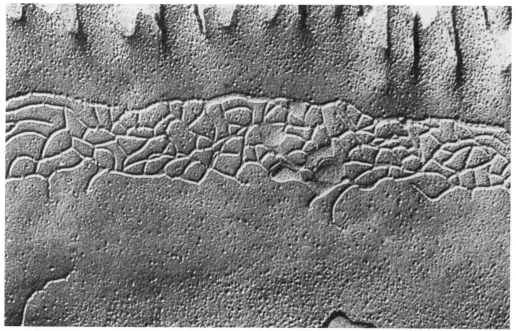

Figure 2–10. Electron micrograph of a freeze-fracture replica of the zonula occludens of intestinal epithelium. A reticular pattern of anastomosing intramembrane strands is seen on the P-face of the cleaved lateral cell membrane just below the brush border. (Micrograph courtesy of J. P. Revel.)

believed to be a band of firm adhesion between neighboring cells.

Owing to the affinity of its filamentous component for stains, it is probable that it was mainly this portion of the epithelial junctional complex that was identified by light microscopists as the terminal bar.

The Macula Adherens or Desmosome. The third component of the typical junctional complex of columnar epithelium is the *macula adherens*, which corresponds to the desmosome of classical histology and is commonly referred to by this name. These appear with the light microscope merely as dense dots or fusiform thickenings of the cell boundaries, but they are resolved in electron micrographs as bipartite structures consisting of plaquelike local differentiations of the opposing membranes. The cell surfaces are 15 to 20 nm apart, and the opposing membranes are of normal dimensions but appear thickened owing to the presence of a thin but very dense layer closely applied to their cytoplasmic surface (Fig. 2–11). Immediately subjacent to this dense plaque is a thicker layer consisting of a feltwork of fine filaments. Tonofilaments in the cytoplasm converge upon the desmosomes and appear to terminate in their inner layer. High-resolution micrographs suggest that many of the tonofilaments form hairpin loops in the matt of filaments associated with the dense plaque and turn back into the cytoplasm. The desmosomes are thus sites of attachment of the cytoskeleton to the cell surface as well as sites of cell-to-cell adhesion. As in the case of the zonula adherens, freeze-cleaved preparations show no distinctive internal differentiation of the cell membrane at desmosomes.

In thin sections, a slender intermediate dense line is often seen in the middle of the intercellular space between the two halves of the desmosome (Fig. 2–11). Occasionally, with intense heavy-metal staining, there is also a suggestion of delicate striations traversing the intercellular space. The integrity of desmosomes is dependent on the presence of calcium. Perfusion of tissue with calcium-free media or immersion in a chelating agent results in separation of the two halves.

In simple cuboidal or columnar epithelia, there is often a circumferential row of desmosomes below the zonula adherens forming the third element of the typical junctional complex, but additional desmosomes may be found scattered at random over the lateral cell surfaces. In stratified squamous epithelia, zonulae occludentes and zonulae adherentes may be absent, but desmosomes are unusually abundant, attaching the ends of the short processes that were erroneously interpreted by light microscopists as intercellular bridges.

The formation of one half of a desmosome evidently induces simultaneous formation of the complementary half by the neighboring cell. Hemidesmosomes are not seen on the boundaries between cells. They are found, however, on the basal surface of stratified squamous epithelia where the cells are exposed to the underlying basal lamina (Fig. 2–12).

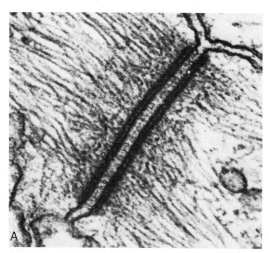

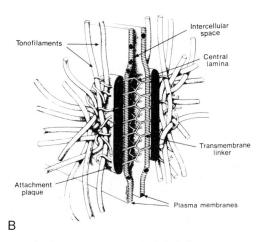

Figure 2–11. *A,* Electron micrograph of a desmosome from amphibian epidermis showing the attachment plaque and tonofilaments forming recurving loops in the adjacent cytoplasm. (Micrograph courtesy of D. Kelly.)

B, Schematic representation of the structure of the desmosome. (Redrawn from Staehelin, L. A., and B. E. Hill. Sci. Am. *238:*146, 1978. Copyright Scientific American, Inc. All rights reserved.)

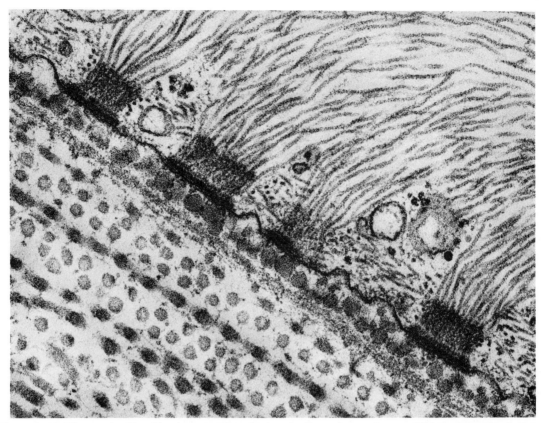

Figure 2–12. Micrograph of hemidesmosomes along the basal cell membrane of an amphibian epidermal cell. Notice the tonofilaments converging on the hemidesmosomes. At lower left are cross sections of collagen fibers in the connective tissue underlying the epithelium. (Micrograph courtesy of D. Kelly.)

The Nexus or Gap Junction. A junctional specialization that went undetected by light microscopy is the *gap junction,* also called the *nexus,* or *communicating junction.* At these sites the intercellular space is reduced to a narrow slit about 2 nm wide. This intercellular gap is of constant width throughout and at no point do the opposing membranes appear to be fused. When epithelial tissues are exposed to an extracellular electron-opaque tracer, such as lanthanum, it penetrates the intercellular space and is visible as a thin dense line about 2 nm wide between the opposing membranes. Where the plane of section passes tangentially to the cell membrane providing an *en face* view of the interspace, a highly ordered pattern is seen in the specialized portions of the opposing membranes. The lanthanum outlines hexagonally packed globular subunits with a center-to-center spacing of 9 nm. With the freeze-fracturing technique, the replica of the outwardly directed inner half-membrane (P-face) shows a high concentration of closely packed particles within the membrane (Fig. 2–13 *B*).

When cells some distance apart in an epithelial sheet are impaled with microelectrodes, they can be shown to be electrically coupled. In replicas of high resolution a minute central depression can be detected in each 8-nm intramembrane particle on the P-face of the junction. This corresponds to a 1.5- to 2-nm central pore seen better in negatively stained isolated gap junctions where the contrast medium penetrates the pore (Fig. 2–13 *C*). The globular particles in such preparations appear to be composed of six subunits arranged radially around the pore. The junctional particles extend through the lipid bilayer and project into the intercellular gap where they attach to corresponding particles in the opposing membrane. The alignment and end-to-end bonding of the junctional particles forms units called *connexons.*

The flow of ions through the hydrophilic channels of the connexons explains the electrical coupling of cells throughout an epithelium. Microinjected fluorescent dyes of low molecular weight can also be shown to pass-

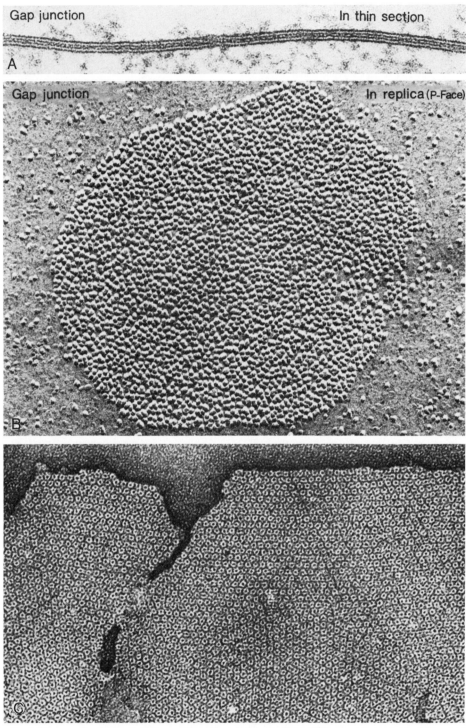

Figure 2–13. *A,* Micrograph of a gap junction as it appears in thin sections. (Micrograph courtesy of Kiyoshi Hama.) *B,* Freeze-fracture replica of the P-face of a gap junction. (Micrograph courtesy of D. Albertini.) *C,* Isolated gap junctions as they appear in negatively stained preparations. The connexons have a central dot representing the central 1.5- to 2-nm channel, filled with the contrast medium. (Micrograph courtesy of B. Gilula.)

from cell to cell via gap junctions. Cyclic AMP and other small molecules can also pass through these communicating junctions and may play an important role in coordinating the responses of groups of epithelial cells to hormonal and neural stimuli. Proteins, nucleic acids, and other macromolecules greater than 1200 M.W. do not pass through the connexons.

Junctional specializations of this type are not confined to epithelia but are also seen at the so-called electrical synapses in the invertebrate central nervous system and between cellular units of smooth and cardiac muscle. There is compelling evidence that in these latter the nexuses or gap junctions are the low-resistance pathways through which excitation passes rapidly from cell to cell, permitting the muscle to function as if it were a syncytium (see Chapter 10).

The Basal Surface of Epithelia

The basal surface of most epithelia is smooth contoured and unspecialized. However, in certain transporting epithelia (especially those of the renal tubules, and the ciliary epithelium of the eye) the cell membrane may be deeply infolded, partitioning the basal cytoplasm into multiple narrow alcoves containing mitochondria. Some of these are open to the cytoplasm above. Others appear to be closed compartments and are in fact undermining processes extending laterally from the base of neighboring cells. The effect of this basal specialization is to create a labyrinthine system of extracellular clefts that greatly increase the area of the cell surface engaged in pumping of solute to generate an extracellular osmotic gradient that moves water and electrolytes across the epithelium.

At the boundary between epithelia and the underlying connective tissue is a supporting structure called the *basal lamina* or *basement membrane.* The latter term commonly used in descriptions based on light microscopy often includes other components of the extracellular matrix and is therefore less specific than the term basal lamina, which describes the continuous layer seen underlying epithelia in electron micrographs. A similar layer surrounds smooth, skeletal, and cardiac muscle cells, Schwann cells, and certain other sessile cells of mesenchymal origin. The term *external lamina* is more appropriate for this circumferential investment than basal lamina or basement membrane.

The basal lamina consists of two zones— one of low density adjacent to the cell membrane called the *lamina rara* or *lamina lucida,* and one of greater density adjacent to the connective tissue matrix called the *lamina densa.* The two are of about equal thickness, 40 to 60 nm, but in a few exceptional examples the lamina densa may be two to three times thicker. Substructure is difficult to resolve in the lamina rara, which generally appears as a clear zone. The lamina densa consists of a dense meshwork of randomly oriented filaments approximately 4 nm in diameter. The basal and external laminae are formed by the cells with which they are associated, and consist largely of Type IV collagen, laminin, and proteoglycan rich in heparan sulfate.

Type IV collagen to date has been found exclusively in basal laminae. It consists of three alpha chains richer in carbohydrate side chains than those of other collagens, and these alpha chains retain the propeptide extensions at the ends of the molecule that are usually cleaved off in the extracellular processing of collagen. Their persistence is thought to prevent assembly of Type IV collagen into cross-banded fibers. Instead, the molecules become cross-linked to form a resilient three-dimensional meshwork.

Laminin is a glycoprotein of 900,000 M.W. with a distinctive crosslike molecular configuration. It seems to be localized exclusively in basal laminae where it is bound to Type IV collagen in the lamina densa and less abundantly in the lamina rara.

The proteoglycans of basal laminae vary in their glycosaminoglycan composition in different tissues. Proteoglycans are commonly rich in heparan sulfate, which gives the basal lamina a strong anionic charge that probably plays a role in cell attachment and in its function as a selective filter.

In addition to these components that are synthesized and secreted by the associated cells, there may be varying small amounts of fibronectin on the connective tissue face of the basal lamina and this may have a role in binding it to the underlying stroma.

The primary function of the basal lamina is to provide a physical support for the epithelium. Its structural framework of Type IV collagen gives it considerable tensile strength, and at the same time it is flexible enough to permit stretching and recoil in epithelia lining hollow organs subject to changes of caliber. The basal lamina also provides for cell attachment possibly by specific binding sites in the cell membrane for its constituent proteins. A third function, best exemplified in the basal lamina of capillary endothelium, is ultrafiltration. This has been most thoroughly investigated in the kidney, where the urine is formed as an ultrafiltrate of the blood circulating through the capillaries of the glomerulus. There the basal lamina acts as a sieve holding back molecules on the basis of their size, shape, and electrostatic charge. During embryonic development the basal laminae act as a substrate for cell migration and influence differentiation of the overlying cells by inductive interaction with the cell membranes. In repair after injury to an epithelium in postnatal life, the persisting basal lamina serves as a substrate guiding the migration of new cells from the margins of the wound to reestablish epithelial continuity.

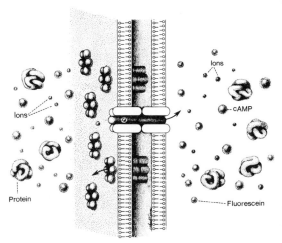

Figure 2–14. Schematic representation of the connexons and their subunits in a portion of a gap junction. The hydrophilic pores through the connexons permit passage of ions and small molecules such as cyclic AMP or the dye fluorescein, but exclude larger molecules. (Redrawn after Tagawa, B., and T. Lowenstein. In Weismann, G., and R. Claiborne, eds.: Cell Membranes: Biochemistry, Cell Biology and Pathology. New York, H. P. Publishing Co., 1975.)

SPECIALIZATIONS OF THE FREE SURFACE

Striated Border

Under the light microscope a number of absorptive columnar epithelia have a refractile border at the free surface that exhibits a fine vertical striation at high magnifications. This *striated* or *brush border* is found in electron micrographs to consist of *microvilli*, slender cylindrical cell processes 80 to 90 nm in diameter and 1 to 2 μm long (Fig. 2–15). The microvilli stand erect and parallel and are closely packed, with approximately 60 per square micrometer of epithelial surface. Each is enclosed in an extension of the plasma membrane and collectively they result in a 15- to 30-fold increase in surface area exposed to the lumen compared with that of a flat apical surface. At the tips of the microvilli, delicate branching filaments 3 to 5 nm in diameter project from the membrane forming a conspicuous surface coat or *glycocalyx* at the luminal surface of the epithelium (Fig. 2–15). The fine filaments making up this layer are terminal oligosaccharides of integral membrane proteins. Staining histological sections with cytochemical methods for carbohydrates renders the glycocalyx visible at the light microscope level.

The cytoplasm in the interior of each microvillus contains a bundle of 25 to 35 actin filaments, which are attached to the membrane at the tip and extend downward into the apical cytoplasm (Fig. 2–16). The filaments are cross-linked into a bundle by a polypeptide called *villin*, and at regular intervals of 33 nm along their length fine cross filaments project laterally, linking the core bundle to the membrane of the microvillus. The actin filaments extending downward from the bases of the microvilli are anchored in a zone of transversely oriented interwoven filaments making up the *terminal web* of the cell. This structure has a number of components and a complex organization that is still being worked out. It contains myosin, tropomyosin, and several smaller polypeptides associated with a dense meshwork of 6-nm actin filaments and 10-nm intermediate filaments. A peripheral band of circumferentially oriented actin filaments is closely bound to the zonula adherens of the junctional complex.

It was formerly thought that interaction of actin filaments of the rootlets with myosin in the terminal web might actively shorten the microvilli. The core filaments are now believed to have a cytoskeletal function, stiffening the microvilli and helping to maintain their parallel array. Contraction of the terminal web can, however, decrease the diameter of the cell apex, making its surface bulge into the lumen and thereby spreading apart the tips of the microvilli and expanding the intervillous spaces.

Microvilli occur on the free surface of most

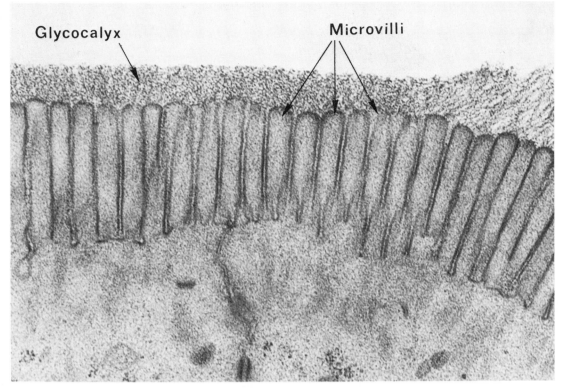

Figure 2–15. Electron micrograph of the brush border of an intestinal epithelial cell showing the closely packed microvilli. The layer on the tips of the microvilli is the glycocalyx, a mat of fine filaments that are terminal oligosaccharides of membrane glycoproteins. (Micrograph courtesy of S. Ito.)

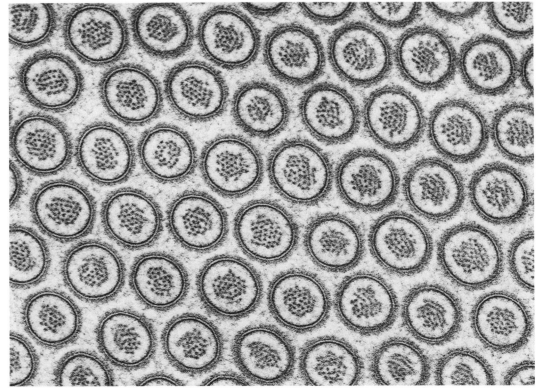

Figure 2–16. Micrograph of transverse sections of the microvilli in the brush border of intestinal epithelium showing the thinner glycocalyx on the sides of the microvilli and the actin filaments in their core. (Micrograph courtesy of A. Ichikawa.)

epithelia, but they form a typical striated border only where they are very numerous and closely packed as they are on the absorptive epithelium of the intestine. Biochemical analysis of brush borders isolated from this epithelium has shown that their membrane is rich in enzymes that carry out the terminal steps in digestion of carbohydrates. Thus, the intestinal brush border is a structural adaptation for increasing the digestive and absorptive efficiency of the epithelium by greatly amplifying the surface area of membrane exposed to nutrients in the intestinal lumen. In epithelia that are not highly specialized for absorption or transport the microvilli are relatively sparse, shorter, and more variable in their orientation. In such cells the terminal web and actin cores of the microvilli are less well developed.

Stereocilia

The pseudostratified columnar epithelium lining the epididymal duct in the male has a unique surface specialization. Under the light microscope a pyriform tuft of cell processes projects from each cell several microns into the lumen (Fig. 2–17). At high magnifications the individual processes within this tuft are resolved as slender, hairlike structures as long as cilia but more slender. Because they were nonmotile they were named *stereocilia* to distinguish them from the motile *kinocilia*.

In electron micrographs they have the appearance of very long, flexible microvilli but somewhat thicker at the base and tapering to a narrower tip. They have a core bundle of actin filaments that extends into and through a moderately well developed terminal web. The stereocilia are parallel at their base but become increasingly sinuous and entwined toward their tips. Their function is not entirely clear but the epididymal epithelium is known to absorb 90 per cent of the original volume of fluid secreted by the testis, and the increased surface provided by the stereocilia no doubt contributes to the efficiency of the epithelium in concentrating the seminal plasma in its passage through the long epididymal duct.

Cilia

Cells specialized for transport of fluid or a film of mucus along the surface of an epithelium have motile, hairlike cell processes called

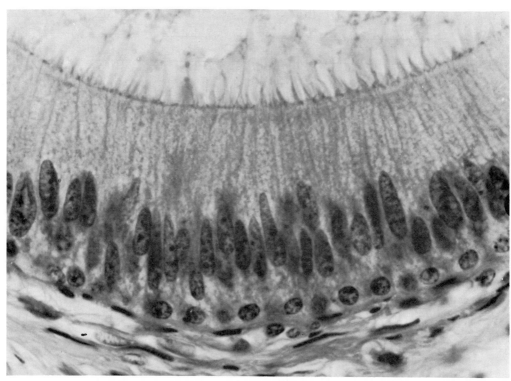

Figure 2–17. Photomicrograph of pseudostratified columnar epithelium of the human epididymis. Notice the tufts of long flexible stereocilia projecting from each cell.

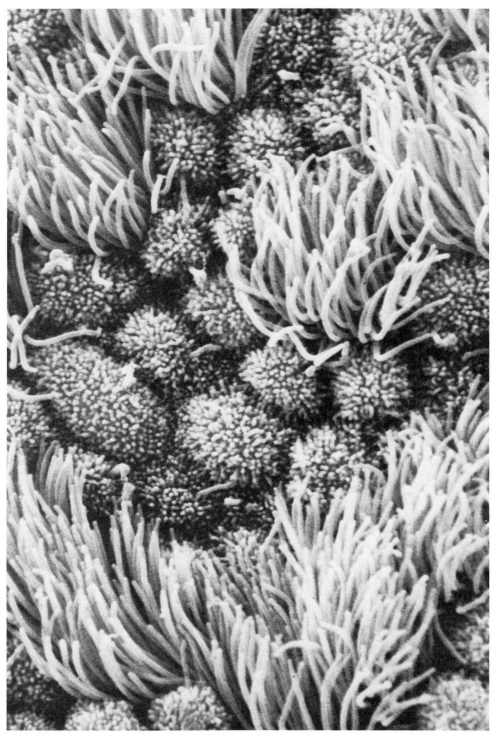

Figure 2–18. Scanning micrograph of the luminal surface of the epithelium of the human oviduct, which contains ciliated and nonciliated cells. The latter bear many short microvilli. (Micrograph from Gaddum-Rosse, P. R. Blandau, and R. Tiersch. Am. J. Anat. *138*:269, 1973.)

cilia. These execute rapid to-and-fro oscillations in the direction of movement of the luminal contents. There are from 50 to 100 or more per cell, arranged in rows with microvilli between the rows. They are 7 to 10 μm long and 0.2 μm in diameter and easily resolved with the light microscope (Fig. 2–5). Their form and arrangement are revealed more dramatically in the three-dimensional images provided by scanning electron microscopy (Fig. 2–18).

On living cells cilia beat rapidly in a consistent direction. If the rate of beat is slowed down in cinematographic analysis, each cilium is observed to stiffen on the more rapid forward or *effective stroke* and to become flexible on the slower *recovery stroke.* Cilia may have an *isochronal rhythm,* in which all cilia beat together, but more commonly those on ciliated epithelia exhibit a *metachronal rhythm,* in which the successive cilia in each row start their beat in sequence so that each is slightly more advanced in its cycle than the preceding one. This sequential activation of the cilia results in the formation of waves that sweep slowly over the surface of the epithelium as a whole. When viewed from above with the microscope, this activity is reminiscent of the waves that run before the wind across a field of grain. The metachronal waves of ciliated epithelia, however, are regular in the periodicity of their occurrence and constant in direction. The effect of this coordinated activity of the cilia is to move a blanket of mucus slowly over the epithelium or to propel fluid and particulate matter through the lumen of a tubular organ.

With the light microscope, no internal structure is discernible in cilia to account for their movement, but under the electron microscope cilia are found to have a core structure called the *axoneme,* consisting of longitudinal microtubules that have a constant number and precise arrangement. In transverse sections, two single microtubules are located in the center of the axoneme, with nine doublet tubules uniformly spaced around them (Figs. 2–19 and 2–20). At the base of each cilium is a cylindrical *basal body* with a structure identical to that of a centriole, with nine triplet microtubules in characteristic pinwheel arrangement making up

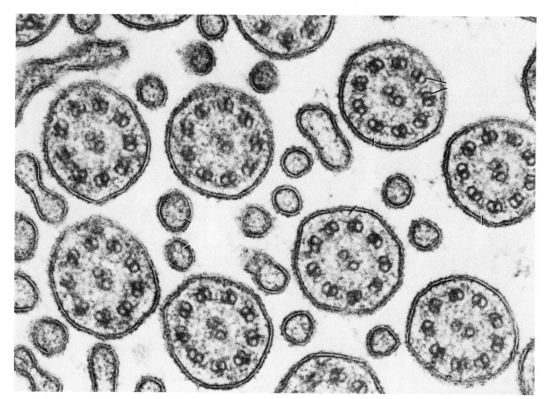

Figure 2–19. Micrograph parallel to the surface of tracheal epithelium, affording a comparison of the cross-sectional appearance of the cilia and the intervening microvilli. (Micrograph from Simionescu, M., and N. Simionescu. Reproduced from The Journal of Cell Biology 70:608, 1976 by copyright permission of The Rockefeller University Press.)

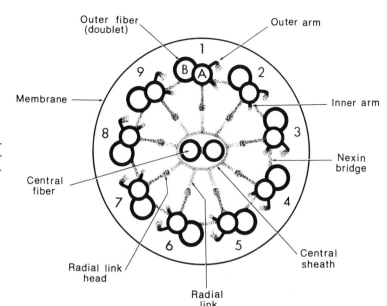

Figure 2–20. Diagram of the cross-sectional appearance of the components in the axoneme of a cilium. (Redrawn after R. Linck.)

the wall of the hollow organelle. The microtubules of the axoneme extend throughout the length of the ciliary shaft. The central pair terminate at the base of the cilium, but the nine peripheral doublets are continuous with the two inner subunits of the nine triplets in the wall of the basal body.

The central pair of microtubules in the axoneme of cilia have much in common with the microtubules found in the cytoplasm of nearly all cells. The doublets are rather different. They are not composed of two similar tubules adherent along one side. Instead, there is one complete tubule with a circular cross section, *subunit A,* and an incomplete tubule, *subunit B,* which has a C-shaped cross section. The latter is fused to subunit A along its edges so that the resulting doublet has a figure-eight cross section with a segment of the wall of tubule A closing the defect in the wall of tubule B (Fig. 2–20). The wall of the microtubules is composed of *tubulin* heterodimers arranged end-to-end to form *protofilaments.* The wall of subunit A of the doublets consists of 13 protofilaments while subunit B has 10 and shares 3 with subunit A. Each doublet has two rows of short *arms* that project from subunit A toward the next doublet in the row. The arms diverge slightly and are directed clockwise from the point of view of an observer looking along the ciliary shaft from base toward tip. Each arm has three subunits and contains the protein *dynein,* which has adenosine triphosphatase activity. Radial *spokes* extend inward from subunit A to a sheath around the central pair of microtubules (Fig. 2–20).

The doublet microtubules of the axoneme are the structures responsible for movement of the cilium. It was originally thought that they were contractile. If they were, those on the concave side during the effective stroke would be expected to shorten. Instead, it has been shown that these doublets actually extend further into the ciliary tip than those on the convex side (Fig. 2–21). Bending therefore occurs without shortening of any of the microtubules. It is now generally accepted that ciliary motion involves a sliding-microtuble mechanism comparable with the sliding-filament mechanism of muscle contraction. The ATPase activity of the dynein arms liberates the energy necessary to generate sliding of the microtubules, and the radial spokes attaching to the central microtubule complex provide the resistance to shear that is needed to convert microtubule sliding into bending.

Convincing evidence for this interpretation has come from the observation that in mutant protozoa that fail to form the radial spokes, the cilia do not execute bending movements. The essential role of dynein in energizing microtubule sliding has found confirmation in a rare congenital anomaly of humans in which the arms on the doublets are lacking and the cilia and sperm flagella are immobile.

Classical cytologists believed that the formation of cilia was preceded by repeated division of an initial pair of centrioles until the required number of basal bodies was produced. These then became arranged in rows beneath the cell surface, and each gave rise to a cilium. More recent studies of cili-

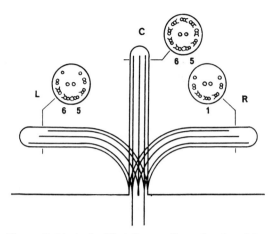

Figure 2–21. A simplified diagram illustrating the sliding microtubule hypothesis of ciliary motility. At center, cilium C is straight and the doublets of the axoneme terminate at the same level. A transverse section near the tip would show all nine peripheral doublets. At left, cilium L is bent toward doublets 5 and 6, which project farthest toward the tip. Doublet 1 terminates first and is missing from cross sections near the tip. Doublets become single near their termination; hence, 9 and 2 are shown as singlets. At right, cilium R is bent toward doublet 1, which now projects farthest. Doublets on the concave side of the cilium are present in transverse sections, while 5 and 6 on the convex side are missing. If the microtubules shortened to produce bending, the relative lengths of those on the convex and concave side would be the reverse of that shown here. The observations therefore favor a sliding mechanism rather than contractile elements. (Figure modified after Sleigh, M. A. Endeavour *30*:11, 1971.)

ogenesis have shown that the basal bodies arise in two ways. (1) They may originate in the same manner in which centrioles are duplicated in the mitotic cycle—a dense, ring-like procentriole arising in end-to-side relationship to a preexisting centriole (Fig. 2–22). The centriole seems to act merely as a site of induction or nucleation for a process of self-assembly in which one or several radially arranged new centrioles form from fibrogranular precursor material. (2) Multiple basal bodies may arise *de novo* without participation of a preexisting centriole. In this case, they develop around dense spherical bodies variously called *procentriole organizers* or *deuterosomes*. Clusters of small, round, fibrous granules (filosomes) appear to be their precursor material. Multiple *procentrioles* develop around the organizer center and grow by accretion at their ends until they attain the appropriate length. The newly formed centrioles move to the cell surface where they function as basal bodies, initiating polymerization of tubulin to form the axonemes of the cilia. Once initiated, the assembly of the ciliary shaft is rapid and self-

perpetuating—the ends of the doublets that polymerize on the ends of the triplets in the wall of the basal body then become sites for deposition of additional subunits until the cilium has attained the normal length (Fig. 2–22).

Flagella

Flagella differ from cilia in their greater length, the character of their movements, and the number per cell—their internal structure is the same as that of cilia. In their most typical form, flagella occur singly or in pairs on free-swimming cells. They are the motor organs of many protozoa reaching lengths of 15 to 30 μm. They are located at the anterior pole and have an undulatory movement in which waves of bending are propagated along the flagellum, pulling the organism through its fluid medium. The spermatozoa of nearly all multicellular animals are propelled by a flagellum that extends posteriorly and moves the cell body forward. In marine invertebrates the internal structure of the sperm flagellum is identical to that of a cilium. In higher forms in which the sperm flagellum may reach a length of several hundred micrometers, there is an additional row of nine dense longitudinal fibers peripheral to the nine doublets of the axonemé. Multiple flagella occur on epithelial cells in certain segments of the nephron in lower vertebrates, but when flagella occur on epithelia in mammals there is only one per cell; it may be no longer than a cilium and probably has a similar pattern of movement. Such vestigial flagella are found on cells of the renal tubules; in the ducts of many glands; in the rete testis; and on the nonciliated cells of uterine epithelium (Fig. 2–23). What their function may be is not apparent unless simple agitation of the fluid in the lumen may have some desirable physiological consequences. Still more puzzling is the observation that single short flagella occur on the cells in some epithelial organs that lack a lumen, such as the anterior lobe of the hypophysis and the islets of Langerhans. Here the flagella simply project into the intercellular spaces or into the connective tissue stroma, where their agitation would seem to serve no useful purpose. Similar abortive flagella have been described occasionally on smooth muscle cells, on the stromal cells of the endometrium, and on mesenchymal derivatives in many other organs. Some of these cilia or flagella have a normal appearing axoneme; others lack the central pair of tu-

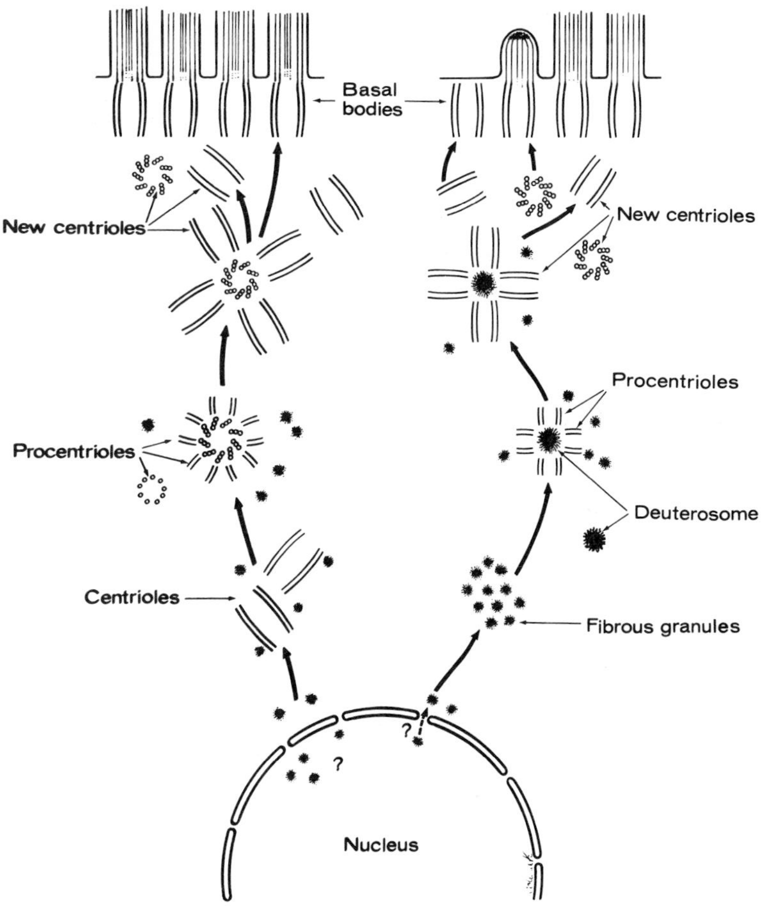

Figure 2–22. Schematic depiction of the alternative origins of basal bodies during ciliogenesis. New basal bodies may form around one or both of the preexisting centrioles, as indicated at left, or they may arise *de novo* from fibrogranular precursors coalescing around centers of organization called procentriole organizers or deuterosomes, as shown at right. The latter mechanism accounts for most of the basal bodies formed. (From Fawcett, D. W. *In* Beatty, R. A., and S. Glueckson-Waelsch, eds.: Genetics of Spermatozoa. Edinburgh, 1972.)

bules. Because some sensory epithelia employ modified cilia or flagella as receptor organelles, it has been speculated that the nonmotile flagella found sporadically on a wide range of cell types may also have a sensory function, but there is no experimental evidence to support this.

It is an interesting example of the unity of nature that the same basic structural organization is found in the axoneme of cilia and flagella throughout the plant and animal kingdoms. Those that enable the protozoa to swim about in a drop of pond water have exactly the same cross-sectional appearance as those that help to remove dust and bacteria from the sinuses and respiratory passages of humans.

BLOOD VESSELS AND NERVES

As a rule, epithelia covering surfaces or lining cavities are not penetrated by blood vessels. The nutritive substances from the blood vessels of the underlying connective tissue reach the epithelial elements after passing through the basal lamina and the narrow intercellular spaces between the epithelial cells. If the epithelium is unusually thick, as in the skin, the underlying connective tissue usually forms vascular *papillae*, which project into the deep surface of the epithelium. These facilitate nutrition by shortening the diffusion distance to the cells in the superficial layers. In a few sites such as the stria vascularis of the cochlea and the maternal layer of some epitheliochorial placentae, loops of blood capillaries may actually penetrate among the cells of the epithelium. Such intraepithelial capillaries are rare in other organs.

In the epidermis, olfactory mucosa, and many other epithelia, numerous terminal branches of sensory nerve fibers pierce the basement lamina and run in the interstices among the epithelial cells. The epithelia of the stomach and the cervix of the uterus, on

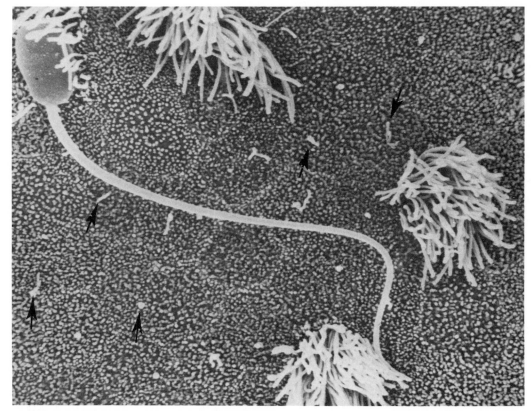

Figure 2–23. Scanning micrograph of a spermatozoan lying on the surface of the uterine epithelium. The illustration permits comparison of the length of the sperm flagellum with that of the cilia on three ciliated cells in this field. Each of the nonciliated cells has a single centrally placed vestigial flagellum *(at arrows).* (From Motta, P., P. Andrews, and K. R. Porter: Microanatomy of Cell and Tissue Surfaces. Philadelphia, Lea & Febiger, 1977, p. 173.)

the other hand, seem to lack sensory nerve endings, and the mucous membranes of these organs can be rubbed or cauterized in the unanesthetized patient without discomfort.

EXTRANEOUS CELLS

Lymphocytes normally invade the epithelium from the connective tissue in some organs. For example, individual lymphocytes are very often found in the epithelium of the intestinal tract. Peyer's patches in the intestinal submucosa are large accumulations of lymphoid cells, and the overlying epithelium is often infiltrated by a multitude of lymphocytes that may push aside and distort the epithelial cells. Similarly, the epithelium overlying the tonsils is extensively infiltrated by lymphocytes. In all these examples the lymphocytes represent a part of the body's immunological defenses against invasion by microorganisms from the environment. At certain phases of the reproductive cycle of rodents, and to a lesser extent in humans, a

great number of leukocytes of various kinds migrate through the vaginal epithelium. It is not surprising that these actively motile cells can insinuate themselves between the sessile epithelial cells, but how they breach the basement lamina and separate the desmosomes and even the occluding junctions of epithelium, and how these latter are restored to their previous relations after the migratory cell has passed, are problems that remain unsolved.

RENEWAL AND REGENERATION OF EPITHELIUM

Epithelia, especially those that cover the outer surface of the body and line the intestinal tract, are subject to constant mechanical and other trauma. Under physiological conditions, their cells continuously perish and are shed. This is especially manifest in the stratified squamous epithelium of the epidermis, where the superficial cells undergo keratinization, a peculiar kind of differentiation that leads to death and desquamation of the superficial cells. In the gastrointestinal tract, cells are continually exfoliated at the tips of the villi. On the other hand, in the respiratory passages and especially in most of the glands, degeneration of the epithelium is rare, and the cells are correspondingly long-lived.

The physiological loss of cells in the epithelium is balanced by a corresponding regeneration. The keratinized cells lost from stratified squamous epithelium are replaced by mitotic proliferation of relatively undifferentiated cells in the deeper layers near the base of the epithelium. These cells differentiate and become keratinized during their ascent to the epithelial surface. The simple columnar epithelia of the stomach and the intestine are regenerated from proliferating undifferentiated cells in the neck of the gastric glands or in the intestinal crypts of Lieberkühn. The rate of normal physiological loss and replacement is so great that the epithelial covering of the intestinal villi is entirely replaced every few days (see Chapter 26).

The epithelial cells are nonmotile as a rule. In healing wounds, however, epithelial cells flatten out into a thin sheet that rapidly spreads to cover large denuded areas of connective tissue. In the initial stages of this repair there is no mitotic activity, but proliferation begins later at the margins of the wound, providing the cells necessary to restore the covering epithelium to its normal thickness.

REFERENCES

JUNCTIONAL SPECIALIZATIONS

Barr, L., W. Berger, and M. M. Barr: Electrical transmission at the nexus between smooth muscle cells. J. Gen. Physiol. *51*:347, 1968.

Brightman, M. W., and T. S. Reese: Junctions between intimately apposed cell membranes in vertebrate brain. J. Cell Biol. *40*:648, 1969.

Farquhar, M. G., and G. E. Palade: Junctional complexes in various epithelia. J. Cell Biol. *17*:375, 1963.

Gilula, N. B., M. L. Epstein, and W. H. Beers: Cell-to-cell communication and ovulation. A study of the cumulus–oocyte complex. J. Cell Biol. *78*:58, 1978.

Gilula, N. B., O. R. Reeves, and A. Steinbach: Metabolic coupling, ionic coupling and cell contracts. Nature *235*:262, 1972.

Kelly, D.: Fine structure of desmosomes, hemidesmosomes and an adepidermal globular layer in developing newt epidermis. J. Cell Biol. *28*:51, 1966.

Leblond, C. P., H. Puchtler, and Y. Clermont: Structures corresponding to terminal bars and terminal web in many types of cells. Nature *786*:764, 1960.

Lowenstein, W. R.: Intercellular communication. Sci. Am. *222*:79, 1970.

Lowenstein, W. R.: Cellular communication through membrane junctions. Arch. Intern. Med. *129*:299, 1972.

Pitts, J. D. and J. W. Simms: Permeability of junctions between animal cells. Intercellular transfer of nucleotides but not macromolecules. Exp. Cell. Res. *104*:153, 1977.

Staehelin, A.: Structure and functions of intercellular junctions. Int. Rev. Cytol. *39*:191, 1974.

BASAL LAMINA

Dodson, J. D., and E. D. Hay: Secretion of collagenous stroma by epithelium grown in vitro. Exp. Cell. Res. *65*:215, 1971.

Hay, E. D., and J. P. Revel: Autoradiographic studies of the origin of the basement lamella in Ambystroma. Dev. Biol. 7:152, 1963.

Kanwar, Y. S., and M. G. Farquhar: Anionic sites in the glomerular basement membrane: *in vivo* and *in vitro* localization in the laminae rarae by cationic probes. J. Cell Biol *81*:137, 1979.

Kanwar, Y. S., and M. G. Farquhar: Presence of heparan sulfate in the glomerular basement membrane. Proc. Natl. Acad. Sci. USA 76:1303, 1979.

Kefalides, N. A., A. Alper, and C. C. Clark: Biochemistry and metabolism of basement membranes. Int. Rev. Cytol. *61*:167, 1979.

Martinez-Hernadez, A., and P. S. Amenta: The basement membrane in pathology. Lab. Invest. *48*:656, 1983.

Pierce, G. B., T. F. Beals, J. Sri Ram, and A. R. Midgley: Basement membranes. IV. Epithelial origin and immunological cross reactions. Am. J. Pathol., *45*:929, 1964.

Pierce, G. B., A. R. Midgley, and J. Sri Ram: Histogenesis of basement membrane. J. Exp. Med. *117*:339, 1963.

SPECIALIZATIONS OF THE FREE SURFACE

Afzelius, B. Q.: A human syndrome caused by immotile cilia. Science *193:317, 1976.*

Bennett, H. S. : Morphological aspects of extracellular polysaccharides. J. Histochem. Chyochem. *11*:2, 1963.

Fawcett, D. W.: Cilia and flagella. *In* Brachet, J., and A. E. Mirsky, eds.: The Cell: Biochemistry, Physiology, Morphology. Vol. II. New York, Academic Press, 1961.

Fawcett, D. W., and K. R. Porter: A study of the fine structure of ciliated epithelia. J. Morphol. *94*:221, 1954.

Gibbons, I. R., and A. J. Rowe: Dynein: a protein with adenosine triphosphatase activity from cilia. Science *149:*424, 1965.

Ito, S.: The surface coat of enteric microvilli. J. Cell Biol. 27:475, 1965.

Pedersen, H., and H. Rebbe: Absence of arms on the axoneme of immobile human spermatozoa. Biol. Reprod. *12*:541, 1975.

Satir, P.: Studies on cilia. III. Further studies on the cilium tip and a "sliding filament" model of ciliary motility. J. Cell Biol. *39*:77, 1968.

Sleigh, M. A.: Cilia. Endeavour 30:11, 1971.

Warner, F. D.., and P. Satir: The structural basis of ciliary bend formation. Radial spoke positional changes accompanying microtubule sliding. J. Cell Biol. *63*:35, 1974.

Witman, G. B., J. Plummer, and G. Sander: Chlamydomonas flagellar mutants lacking radial spokes and central tubules. Structure, composition and function of specific axonemal components. J. Cell Biol. *76*:729, 1978.

REGENERATION AND RENEWAL

Arey, L. B.: Wound healing. Physiol. Rev. *16*:327, 1936.

Bertalanffy, F. D., and K. P. Nagy: Mitotic activity and renewal rate of the epithelial cells of human duodenum. Acta Anat. *45*:362, 1961.

Leblond, C. P., R. C. Greulich, and J. P. M. Pereira: Relationship of cell formation and cell migration in the renewal of stratified squamous epithelia. *In* Montagna, W., and R. E. Billingham, eds.: Advances in Biology of the Skin. Vol. 5. New York, Pergamon Press, 1964.

Leblond, C. P., and B. E. Walker: Renewal of cell populations. Physiol. Rev. *36*:255, 1956.

Lipkin, M., P. Serlock, and B. Bell: Cell proliferation kinetics in the gastrointestinal tract of man. Gastroenterology *45*:721, 1963.

Messier, B., and C. P. Leblond: Cell proliferation and migration as revealed by radioautography after injection of thymidine-H3 into male rats and mice. Am. J. Anat. *106*:247, 1960.

3

GLANDS AND SECRETION

EXOCRINE GLANDS

Secretion is the process by which some cells take up small molecules from the blood and transform them by intracellular biosynthetic mechanisms into a more complex product that is then released from the cell. The chemical transformations involved in secretion are active processes consuming energy in contrast to *excretion* as exemplified by the passive diffusion of carbon dioxide across the epithelium lining the lung, or the filtration of blood in the kidney to form urine.

Cells and associations of cells specialized for secretion are called *glands*. We define three major categories of glands on the basis of the path of release of their products. Those that deliver their product into a system of ducts opening onto an external or internal surface are called *exocrine glands*. Those that release their product into the blood or lymph for transport to target cells in another part of the body are called *endocrine glands*. Those that release their product into the extracellular space for simple diffusion to target cells in the immediate vicinity are called *paracrine glands* or *paraneurones*.

Secretion has traditionally been regarded as a function of epithelial cells because it was in these that accumulation and liberation of the product could be observed directly with the light microscope. However, since indirect autoradiographic methods have become available for tracing uptake of precursors and discharge of product, it has become obvious that the traditional definition must be extended to include many nonepithelial mesenchymal derivatives such as fibroblasts, chondroblasts, and osteoblasts that release substances into the extracellular space to form the fibrous and amorphous components of the connective tissues.

Much has been learned in recent years about the intracellular sites of synthesis and the mechanisms of secretion by correlating electron microscopic and biochemical observations. These primary events at the subcellular level will be reviewed before we proceed to a discussion of the histological organization and classification of glands.

SYNTHESIS AND RELEASE OF PROTEIN SECRETORY PRODUCTS

Glandular cells often contain granules or droplets that represent intracellular accumulation and storage of their secretory products. Just as all cells are continually performing chemical work in maintaining their structural integrity and internal organization, most glandular cells are synthesizing and secreting their products continually at minimal levels. They can often be stimulated to increase the rate of delivery of their product, and much of the information on secretion gained by traditional histologists depended on observation of the cytological changes associated with stimulated or exaggerated activity. It was observed, for example, that when glandular cells were stimulated, the number of secretory granules in their cytoplasm decreased concomitantly with the increase in outflow of secretion from the ducts. After depletion of the granules, the basophilic substance of the cytoplasm seemed to become more prominent, the Golgi apparatus hypertrophied, the nucleus increased slightly in volume, and the nucleolus enlarged. Each of these organelles was therefore thought to be involved in some way in the synthetic activities of the cell. As the secretory granules began to reaccumulate, they first appeared in very close association with the Golgi apparatus and this organelle was therefore thought to be the site of concentration of material synthesized elsewhere in the cytoplasm.

Ultrastructural and biochemical studies have now substantiated these classical observations of light microscopists and have made it possible to define more precisely the respective roles of the various cell organelles in the secretory process. The cell type that has been most thoroughly studied is the pancreatic acinar cell (Fig. 3–1), which secretes several protein enzymes into the digestive juice. The description of the cellular mechanisms of protein synthesis and of the intracellular secretory pathways that follows is based largely on studies of this cell but it applies equally to a great variety of other glandular cells producing secretions rich in protein.

The chemical nature of a cell product is determined in the nucleus. The information or "blueprint" for construction of the protein products of cells is encoded in the sequence of nucleotides in the DNA of the chromosomes. The protein synthesized by a cell depends on which regions of its chromosomes are active at the time—in other words,

which sequences in the DNA molecules (genes) are exposed and available for transcription of information. The cell components that are capable of utilizing this information for synthesis of protein reside in the cytoplasm. There must therefore be intermediaries or messenger molecules to carry the information from the nucleus to the cytoplasm, and there must be avenues of communication between these two compartments of the cell. Three classes of ribonucleic acid (RNA) molecules are essential for the transfer of genetic information and its translation during protein synthesis. These are *messenger RNA* (mRNA), *transfer RNA* (tRNA), and *ribosomal RNA* (rRNA). All three are formed by transcription of specific segments of the chromosomal DNA molecule. A region of one of the chromosomes that is concerned with elaboration of ribosomal RNA is closely associated with the nucleolus. This organelle is the site of union of ribosomal RNA with protein to form nucleoproteins that then pass into the cytoplasm to form ribosomes. The pathway that all three types of RNA take to the cytoplasm is through the pores in the nuclear envelope.

In the cytoplasm, the ribosomes become

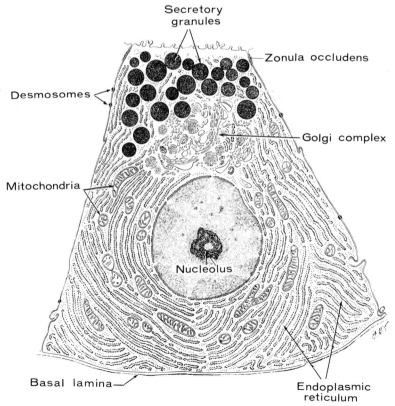

Secretory granules

Zonula occludens

Desmosomes

Golgi complex

Mitochondria

Nucleolus

Basal lamina

Endoplasmic reticulum

Figure 3–1. Drawing of the fine structure of a pancreatic acinar cell, which can be considered typical of exocrine glandular cells secreting a protein product.

associated with the site of initiation of protein synthesis at one end of the long molecules of mRNA and subsequently move along the length of the molecule, "reading" in each successive set of three nucleotides (codons) the instructions that determine the sequence of assembly of amino acids in the protein being synthesized. The appropriate amino acid is brought to the site of assembly on the ribosome by a molecule of tRNA. There are specific tRNAs for each of the 20 amino acids. A molecule of tRNA carrying its specific amino acid recognizes and attaches itself to the appropriate complementary site on the mRNA. Its amino acid is then inserted into the protein molecule being developed on the ribosome. The ribosome moves along the mRNA to the next codon, and the first tRNA molecule is released. Other ribosomes in turn become attached to the vacated initiation site and follow along after the first, reading the same message and synthesizing the same kind of protein molecule. In this way numerous ribosomes become associated with the same mRNA molecule to form a chain of interconnected ribosomes. These assemblages, called *polyribosomes* or *polysomes,* are found in elec-

tron micrographs either free in the cytoplasmic matrix or attached to the outer surface of the limiting membrane of the endoplasmic reticulum (Figs. 3–2, 3–3, 3–4). The free polyribosomes are concerned with synthesis of the integral proteins of the cell, while those attached to the endoplasmic reticulum are involved in synthesis of secretory proteins for export from the cell. The vast majority of ribosomes in glandular cells are associated with the reticulum.

The mRNAs for secretory proteins have a special sequence of nucleotides, the *signal codons,* that is lacking on messengers for integral proteins. When these codons have been read, the resulting *signal peptide* binds in the cytoplasmic matrix to a *signal recognition particle* consisting of polypeptides and a small 7s RNA molecule. This particle serves as an adapter binding the ribosome and the emerging signal peptide to receptor proteins within the membrane of the reticulum. Interaction of the signal receptor particle and signal sequence with the membrane is believed to cause aggregation of *ribosome receptor proteins* in such a way as to form a transmembrane channel through which the lengthen-

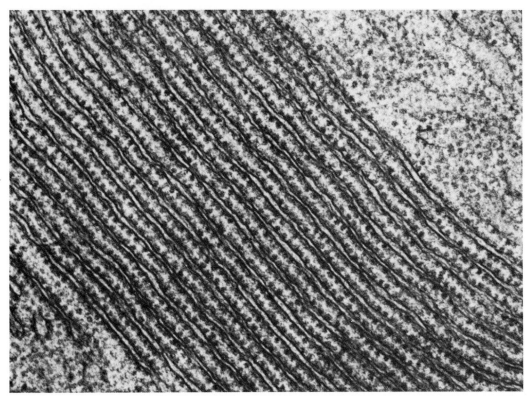

Figure 3–2. An area of cytoplasm from a glandular cell at higher magnification, showing the ribosomes attached to the outer surfaces of several closely spaced cisternae of the endoplasmic reticulum.

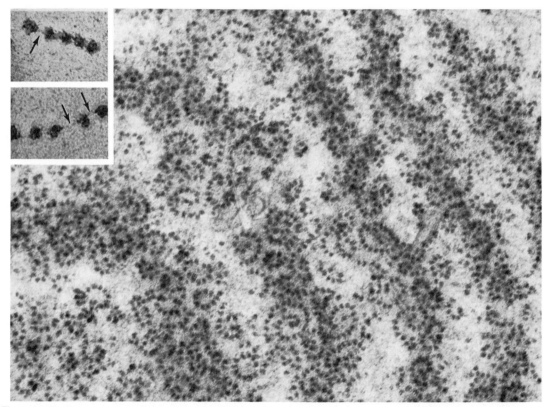

Figure 3–3. Electron micrograph of an oblique section passing tangentially to several parallel cisternae of the endoplasmic reticulum, showing numerous spiral and rosette configurations of polyribosomes. (Courtesy of E. Yamada.) Insets show positively stained, isolated ribosomes connected by a thin strand *(arrows)* representing the messenger RNA. (Courtesy of C. Hall and A. Rich.)

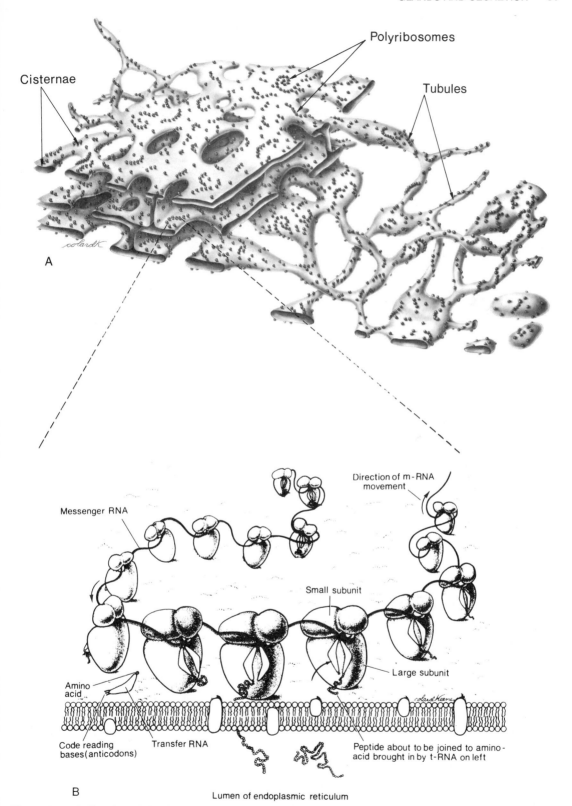

Cisternae

Polyribosomes

Tubules

A

Direction of m-RNA movement

Messenger RNA

Small subunit

Large subunit

Amino acid

Code reading bases (anticodons)

Transfer RNA

Peptide about to be joined to amino-acid brought in by t-RNA on left

B

Lumen of endoplasmic reticulum

Figure 3–4. *A,* Drawing of the three-dimensional configuration of the cisternae and tubules making up the rough endoplasmic reticulum. Ribosomes occur in spirals and rosettes on the outer surface of the membrane.

B, Schematic depiction of a strand of messenger RNA and its associated ribosomes on the membrane of the endoplasmic reticulum. Polypeptide chains of increasing length from the 5′ end *(right)* to the 3′ end *(left)* pass through channels formed by assembly of integral receptor proteins in the underlying membrane. The nascent polypeptides thus are translocated into the lumen. (Redrawn after E. C. Jordan, Oxford/Carolina Biological Reader, 45–9616, Carolina Biological Supply Co., Burlington, North Carolina.)

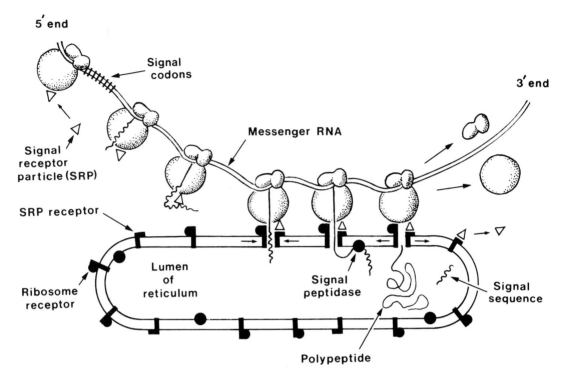

Figure 3–5. Schematic representation of the signal hypothesis and the elements involved in attachment of the polyribosomes to the membrane of the reticulum and translocation of the nascent polypeptide into its lumen. Codons at the 5′ end of the mRNA determine an initial amino acid sequence called the "signal." When the nascent polypeptide chain emerges from the ribosome, its signal sequence binds an 11s *signal recognition protein* (SRP). This in turn binds to an *SRP receptor* in the membrane. Interaction of *ribosome receptor* and *SRP receptor* forms a transmembrane pore through which the lengthening polypeptide chain is translocated into the lumen of the reticulum. The signal segment of the polypeptide is subsequently cleaved off by a *signal peptidase* located on the inner aspect of the limiting membrane of the reticulum. (Redrawn after Blöbel, G. *In* International Cell Biology 1976–1977, p. 320; and Walter, P., and G. Blöbel. J. Cell Biol. *91*:557, 1981. Reproduced from The Journal of Cell Biology by copyright permission of The Rockefeller University Press.)

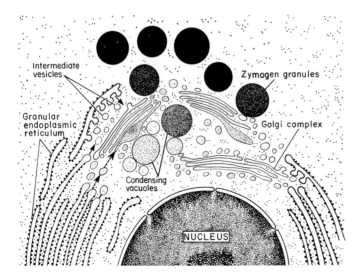

Figure 3–6. Diagram of the Golgi region of a glandular cell, showing smooth-surfaced intermediate vesicles budding from the endoplasmic reticulum. The product carried in these vesicles to the forming face of the Golgi complex emerges from its secretory face in condensing vacuoles. These concentrate the product to form zymogen granules.

ing polypeptide chain extends into the lumen of the reticulum. When elongation of the nascent polypeptide chain has moved the signal sequence into the cistern, a *signal peptidase* on the inner aspect of the membrane cleaves off the signal sequence. After the entire message has been translated and synthesis of the polypeptide chain terminated, the ribosome separates from the reticulum, and it is assumed that the underlying channel in the membrane is obliterated by dissociation of the signal receptor particle and lateral diffusion of the ribosome receptor proteins. The signal sequence coding on mRNA for secretory protein and the occurrence of signal recognition particles in the cytoplasm capable of binding to receptor in the membrane ensures that the translation machinery of the cell is coupled to the translocation machinery in the endoplasmic reticulum. The newly synthesized molecules of secretory protein are thus segregated within the reticulum and transported in its fluid contents to the supranuclear Golgi region of the cell.

On ribosome-free regions of the reticulum in the vicinity of the Golgi complex, small evaginations of its membrane pinch off as free vesicles each containing a small quantity of the newly synthesized protein. These *intermediate* or *transport vesicles* carry the product from the endoplasmic reticulum to the Golgi complex. The site of fusion of the transport vesicles with the membranes of the Golgi complex is debated but it is the prevailing view that the vesicles fuse with one another to form a flattened saccule or cistern at the convex surface of the organelle, commonly referred to as its *forming face*. This cistern with its content of cell product is then thought to progress through the organelle to its concave *secretory face* as successive cisternae are formed behind it. According to this interpretation, all cisternae in the stack constituting the Golgi complex are involved in processing the product. In the outermost cisternae the product is dilute and, owing to extraction during specimen preparation, these cisternae usually appear empty in electron micrographs. However, the protein is progressively concentrated as the cistern moves through the organelle and it is usually preserved in the cisternae at the secretory

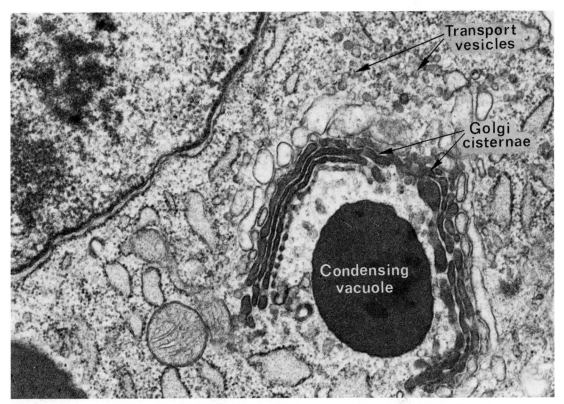

Figure 3–7. Golgi region of an actively secreting glandular cell showing transport vesicles and concentration of the product in the inner cisternae of the Golgi complex and in a condensing vacuole.

face as a moderately dense content (Fig. 3–7). The innermost cistern at the secretory face of the Golgi rounds up into small *condensing vacuoles,* which subsequently coalesce with each other and with contributions from the succeeding cistern to form a single large condensing vacuole. With further concentration of its contents, this vacuole becomes a typical dense *secretory granule* (Fig. 3–8). In its transit through the Golgi complex, the secretory protein not only undergoes a 20 to 25 per cent concentration but is also chemically modified by formation of disulfide bonds and addition of polysaccharide chains. The secretory granules accumulate in the apical cytoplasm for transient storage. When the glandular cell is stimulated to release its product, the granules are moved into contact with plasmalemma. Their limiting membrane fuses with the cell membrane at the point of contact and the contents flow into the lumen (Fig. 3–9). As the granule is evacuated, its membrane is incorporated in the cell surface. Thus, the secretory product leaves the cell without any discontinuity being produced in the plasmalemma. This process of release of material from cells is called *exocytosis.*

The excess membrane added to the plasmalemma during exocytosis is retrieved from the cell surface and recycled through the Golgi complex. Small patches of surface membrane invaginate to form clathrin-coated vesicles that move into the cytoplasm and fuse with the distended peripheral portions of the Golgi cisternae or with condensing vacuoles. Other vesicles fuse with lysosomes and are degraded.

In recapitulation, secretory protein is synthesized on polyribosomes associated with the endoplasmic reticulum. It is sequestered in the lumen of this organelle and transported through it to the Golgi region of the cell. There, transport vesicles transfer it to the Golgi complex, which concentrates and packages the product in granules limited by a membrane capable of fusing with the cell membrane to release the secretion by exocytosis. The mitochondria participate in the process by providing ATP for the energy-requiring steps of synthesis and transport. Incorporated amino acids traverse this intracellular biosynthetic pathway much more rapidly than was previously imagined. The mean transit time of exportable protein in

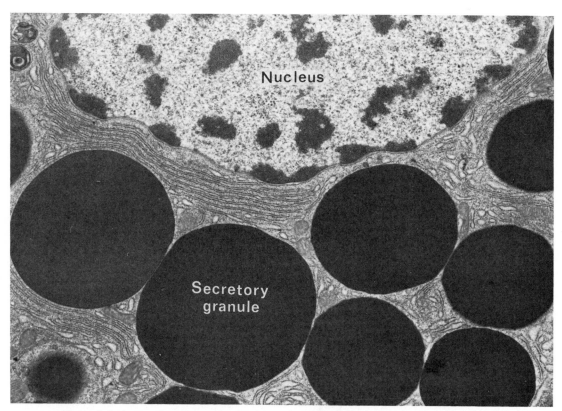

Figure 3–8. Juxtanuclear region of a glandular cell showing fully condensed secretory granules.

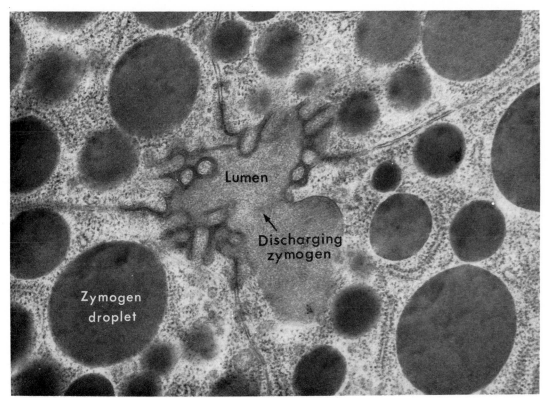

Figure 3–9. Electron micrograph of the lumen of an acinus and the apical portions of four acinar cells. Large dense zymogen droplets or granules are found in the cell apex. The limiting membrane of one of these has fused with the cell membrane and its zymogen is being discharged into the lumen.

the pancreatic acinar cells is now estimated to be about 50 minutes.

In glandular cells whose secretion is rich in carbohydrate as well as protein, the Golgi complex plays an active synthetic role in addition to concentrating and packaging the product. The assembly of the carbohydrate component of such secretions has been shown to depend on glycosyltransferases located in the membranes of the Golgi cisternae. In cells secreting mucus and other glycoproteins, the Golgi complex appears to be the principal site of synthesis of the polysaccharides and their conjugation with protein previously synthesized on the ribosomes of the endoplasmic reticulum.

Much more is known about the transcription and translation of genetic information and the regulation of protein synthesis than has been indicated here. Some of this will already be familiar to students well prepared in cell and molecular biology. Others may wish to consult a modern textbook of biochemistry for additional details.

MECHANISMS FOR RELEASE OF SECRETORY PRODUCTS

Histologists have traditionally distinguished three mechanisms by which cells discharge their secretory products.

1. *Merocrine secretion* was defined as release through the cell membrane with the cell remaining intact. The limited resolution of the light microscope did not reveal how this was accomplished but it was assumed either that the secretory material diffused through an intact membrane or, more likely, that whole granules passed out through transient discontinuities in the membrane. Electron microscopic observations on exocytosis have now shown how a product can be released in bulk without the creation of discontinuities in the membrane. Merocrine secretion is now understood to consist of release by the process of exocytosis, involving fusion of the limiting membrane of the secretory granule with the cell membrane.

2. *Apocrine secretion* was believed to involve loss of part of the apical cytoplasm along with the material secreted. Despite this loss, the cell was believed to be able to restore continuity of its surface and reaccumulate product. This form of secretion is less common and has been less thoroughly studied. Electron microscopic observations on the mammary gland, which is generally accepted as an apocrine gland, substantiate the belief that some of the cell is lost, but this loss involves only a segment of the membrane and a thin rim of cytoplasm around the lipid component of the secretion—certainly a less drastic loss of cell substance than was envisioned by light microscopists.

3. *Holocrine secretion* consists of release of whole cells into the excretory ducts or total discharge of the contents of cells, leading to their complete destruction. In sebaceous glands, the cells break down with an outpouring of their cytoplasm and accumulated lipid. Release of spermatozoa from the seminiferous epithelium of the testis is regarded as a form of holocrine secretion in which living cells are the product.

Although the traditional terms merocrine, apocrine, and holocrine have required some redefinition, they will continue to be used until their mechanisms are better understood and a more precise terminology evolves.

CLASSIFICATION OF EXOCRINE GLANDS

Exocrine glands may be *unicellular* or *multicellular*. The latter are further classified, according to the organization and geometry of their epithelial component, as *tubular, alveolar, tubuloalveolar, saccular,* and so forth.

Unicellular Glands

In mammals, the most common and indeed virtually the only example of a unicellular gland is the *mucous* or *goblet cell* found scattered among the columnar cells of the epithelium on many mucous membranes. It secretes *mucin,* a glycoprotein, which upon hydration forms a lubricating solution called *mucus.* A fully developed cell of this type has an expanded apical end filled with pale droplets of *mucigen,* and a slender basal end containing a compressed nucleus and a small amount of deeply staining basophilic cytoplasm. The term *globlet cell* is descriptive of

the form of the cell, which has an expanded cup-shaped rim of cytoplasm called the *theca* filled with secretory droplets, and a thin base, like the stem of a goblet, extending to the basal lamina of the epithelium (Fig. 3–10).

The mucigen droplets tend to swell and coalesce during specimen preparation and are seldom resolved as separate entities. They are better preserved by freeze-drying and they stain well with the periodic acid–Schiff reaction because of their polysaccharide content.

The finer structure of goblet cells is difficult to study because of the degree to which their organelles are compressed into the basal cytoplasm. The basophilia of the cytoplasm results from the abundance of free and attached ribosomes. The latter are deployed on the surface of the cisternae arranged roughly parallel to the cell surface in the paranuclear and basal cytoplasm. The Golgi complex is well developed and located between the compressed nucleus and the mucigen droplets in the theca. The individual droplets of mucigen are enveloped by extremely delicate membranes that are often broken in preparation of the specimen.

The synthesis of mucigen involves the synthesis of protein in the manner previously

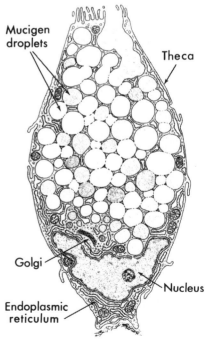

Figure 3–10. Drawing of the fine structure of an intestinal goblet cell. (From Lentz, T. L. Cell Fine Structure. Philadelphia, W. B. Saunders Co., 1971.)

described for protein-secreting cells in general. However, autoradiography after administration of ^{35}S or ^{3}H-glucose shows that the label goes directly to the supranuclear region, thus establishing that the synthesis of the carbohydrate moiety and sulfation of the glycoprotein of the mucigen take place in the Golgi complex. In discharging the secretion, the membrane of individual secretory droplets or of groups of coalesced droplets fuses with and becomes part of the plasma membrane, permitting the mucus to pour out onto the surface.

The secretion of mucus proceeds more or less continuously and the cell retains its goblet form for most of its life span—which is only two to four days in the intestinal mucosa. Although goblet cells normally pass through only one long secretory cycle, they may be made to expel nearly all of their secretion at once. Under these conditions, they soon resume mucosynthesis and refill their theca.

Multicellular Glands

The simplest form of multicellular gland is a sheet of epithelium consisting of a ho-

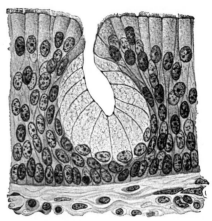

Figure 3–12. Intraepithelial gland from the pseudostratified ciliated epithelium of the laryngeal surface. (After V. Patzelt, from Schaffer.)

mogeneous population of secretory cells (Fig. 3–11). The surface epithelium of the gastric mucosa and of the uterine lining at certain stages belong to this category, sometimes described as a *secretory sheet*.

Intraepithelial glands are intermediate between a secretory sheet and a simple tubular gland. They are small accumulations of glandular cells (usually mucous) that lie wholly within the thickness of the epithelium but are arranged around a small lumen of their own (Fig. 3–12). In man, examples are found in the pseudostratified columnar epithelium of the nasal mucosa and in the ductuli efferentes and urethra of the male reproductive tract.

All other multicellular glands arise as tubular invaginations of an epithelial sheet and extend into the underlying connective tissue (Fig. 3–11). The glandular cells are usually confined to the *terminal* or *secretory* portions of the tubular invagination. Secretion elaborated by the gland cells reaches the surface directly, or through an *excretory* duct consisting of less specialized, nonsecretory cells.

In many glands, the surface available for release of secretion is further increased by development of many extremely fine canals, the *secretory canaliculi*, which extend from the lumen between glandular cells. These slender extracellular passages are often branched, and they end blindly before reaching the basal lamina. They have no walls of their own but are formed by apposition of groovelike excavations in the surface of adjoining cells. They are usually lined by numerous microvilli. The parietal cells of the gastric glands are exceptional in appearing to have an in-

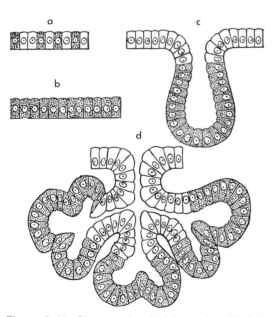

Figure 3–11. Diagram of unicellular and multicellular glands. *a*, Granular; glandular cells are scattered singly among clear, common epithelial cells. *b*, Glandular cells arranged in a continuous sheet—secretory epithelial surface. *c*, Simplest type of multicellular gland; the area lined with glandular cells forms a saclike invagination into the subjacent tissue. *d*, Multicellular gland of greater complexity; the glandular spaces are lined partly with glandular cells (terminal portions), partly with common epithelium (excretory ducts).

tracellular system of canaliculi. Electron microscopy has shown, however, that these so-called *intracellular canaliculi* are not actually within the cytoplasm but are deep invaginations of the cell surface. They are limited by the plasma membrane and their lumen is therefore actually extracellular, like that of the more common *intercellular canaliculi*.

Simple Exocrine Glands. The elaborate scheme of classification of glands may seem to the student unnecessarily complex but it has the advantage of permitting more precise description of the great variety of patterns of association of secretory cells found in the body. Multicellular glands are designated as *simple* or *compound* depending on whether or not their avenue of communication with the surface is branched. A *simple exocrine gland* is one in which the functional unit is connected directly to the surface epithelium via an unbranched duct (Fig. 3–13). Glands fulfilling this criterion are further categorized on the basis of the configuration of their terminal or secretory portion. Thus, they may be described as *simple tubular, simple coiled tubular, simple branched tubular,* and *simple acinar* (or *alveolar*).

In *simple tubular glands,* there is no excretory duct and the terminal portion is a straight tubule that opens directly onto the epithelial surface. The intestinal glands of Lieberkühn are examples (Fig. 3–13a).

In *simple coiled tubular glands,* the terminal portion is a long coiled tubule connected to the surface by an unbranched excretory duct (Fig. 3–13b). The common sweat glands belong to this category. In the larger apocrine sweat glands, the terminal portions do branch.

In *simple branched tubular glands,* the tubules of the terminal portion bifurcate into two or more branches, which may be somewhat coiled near their ends (Fig. 3–13d). An excretory duct may be absent, as in the glands of the stomach and uterus, or there may be a short excretory duct, as in some of the small glands of the oral cavity, the tongue, and the esophagus, and in the glands of Brunner in the duodenum.

In the *simple acinar* (or *simple alveolar*) *glands,* the terminal portion is expanded to form a spherical or elongated sac. If only one acinus is associated with one excretory duct, the gland is a *simple acinar gland* (Fig. 3–13e). This type is thought not to occur in mammals. If the acinus is subdivided by partitions into several smaller compartments, or if several acini are arranged along a duct, it is a *simple branched acinar gland* (Fig. 3–13f, g). Examples are the sebaceous glands of the skin and the meibomian glands of the eyelids.

Compound Exocrine Glands. The duct of a compound exocrine gland branches repeatedly. Such a gland can be thought of as consisting of a variable number of simple glands at the ends of an arborescent system of ducts of progressively diminishing caliber (Fig. 3–14). Thus, there are *compound tubular,* and *compound acinar glands.*

In *compound tubular glands,* the terminal portions of the smallest lobules are more or less coiled tubules, usually branching. To this category belong the pure mucous glands of the oral cavity, glands of the gastric cardia, some of the glands of Brunner (Fig. 3–15), the bulbourethral glands, and the renal tubules. In special cases, the terminal coils anastomose.

In *compound acinar glands* (also called *compound alveolar glands*), the terminal portions have been described as occurring in the form of spherical or pear-shaped units with a small lumen (Fig. 3–14a). As a rule, however, the

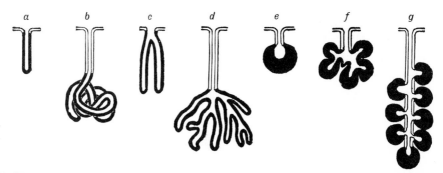

Figure 3–13. Diagrams of simple exocrine glands. *a,* Simple tubular; *b,* simple coiled tubular; *c* and *d,* simple branched tubular; *e,* simple alveolar; *f* and *g,* simple branched acinar. Secretory portions black; ducts double-contoured.

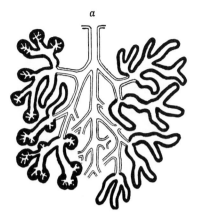
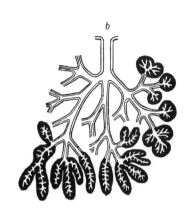

Figure 3–14. Diagram of compound exocrine glands. *a,* Mixed compound tubular and tubuloacinar; *b,* compound acinar. Secretory portions black; ducts double-contoured.

form is that of irregularly branched tubules with numerous acinar lateral outgrowths from the wall and on the blind ends. These glands would be more corrrectly designated *compound tubuloacinar (tubuloalveolar).* To this group belong most of the larger exocrine glands—the salivary glands, glands of the respiratory passages, and the pancreas (Fig. 3–16).

Some authors add another category called *compound saccular glands,* which differ from the compound alveolar type only in their much larger size, and particularly in the larger lumen of their secretory end pieces. The examples commonly cited are the mammary gland and the prostate gland. Other authors, however, include these organs among the compound tubuloacinar glands.

In some cases the excretory ducts do not all join into a single main duct but open independently on a restricted area of a free epithelial surface. Such is the case with the lacrimal, mammary, and prostate glands.

In addition to classification according to

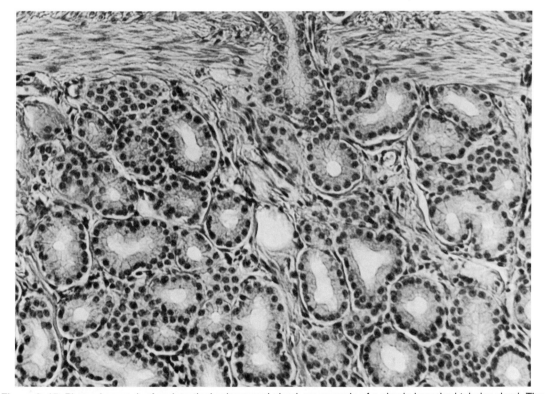

Figure 3–15. Photomicrograph of an intestinal submucosal gland, an example of a simple branched tubular gland. The duct, seen penetrating the muscularis mucosae at the top of the micrograph, is unbranched, but the secretory portion branches repeatedly and presents many cross-sectional profiles when sectioned.

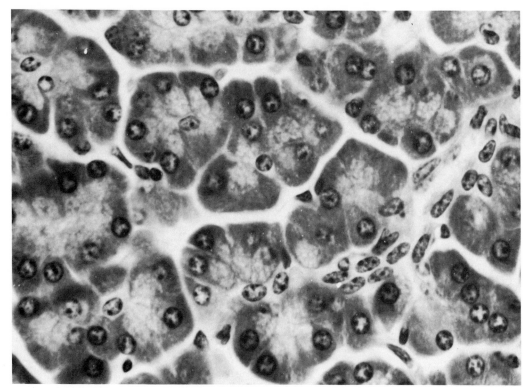

Figure 3–16. Photomicrograph of the pancreas, a compound tubuloacinar gland. A small duct is sectioned longitudinally at right of figure. The duct branches to the several acini that are clustered around it.

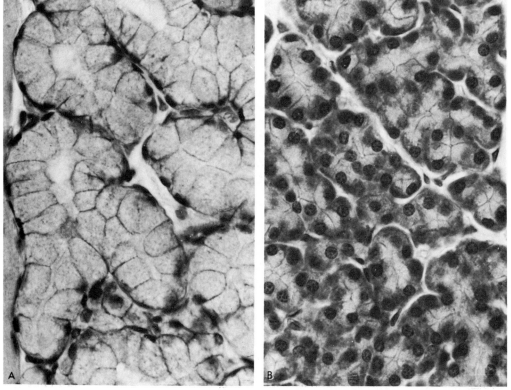

Figure 3–17. Photomicrographs illustrating the contrasting appearance of a mucous gland *(A)* and a serous gland *(B)*, both from the tongue.

histological organization, compound glands are often classified according to the nature of the secretion they produce. Thus, they may be designated as *mucous, serous,* or *mixed.* Mucous glands secrete a viscous material with a lubricating or protective function (Fig. 3–17A); serous glands have a watery secretion often rich in enzymes (Fig. 4–17B).

In mucous glands the major portion of the cell is occupied by mucigen droplets, and appears pale and highly vacuolated in histological sections. The nucleus is displaced far to the base and is often greatly flattened by the accumulated mucigen droplets. In serous glands the cells are generally smaller and their nucleus is spherical and situated in the basal half of the cell surrounded by deeply basophilic cytoplasm. The apex of the cell may be clear, owing to extraction of the secretory material (Fig. 3–17B), or, where the secretory product is preserved, it may stain as discrete granules. The ultrastructure of serous cells is similar to that of the pancreatic acinar cell but with somewhat less extensive development of the endoplasmic reticulum.

Mixed glands contain both mucous and serous cells. Mucous cells often make up the greater part of the gland, with somewhat flattened serous cells forming crescentic caps, called *serous demilunes,* over the ends of the alveoli. The cells of the demilunes are in communication with the lumen via intercellular secretory canaliculi (Figs. 3–18, 3–19).

HISTOLOGICAL ORGANIZATION OF EXOCRINE GLANDS

There are certain common features in the organization of the larger glands. They are usually enclosed in a condensation of connective tissue that forms the capsule of the organ. Septa of connective tissue extending inward from the capsule divide the gland into grossly visible subdivisions called *lobes.* These in turn are partitioned by thinner septa into smaller units called *lobules,* still visible with the naked eye (Fig. 3–20). These are separated to some extent into microscopic *lobules* of glandular units, but as a rule collagenous connective tissue penetrates for only a short distance into the lobule before giving way to a delicate network of reticular fibers surrounding the terminal ducts and secretory acini or tubules. The connective tissue components of a gland are collectively called the *stroma,* and its epithelial portion, the *parenchyma.*

Blood vessels, lymphatics, and nerves of glands usually show a pattern of distribution similar to that of the connective tissue. They

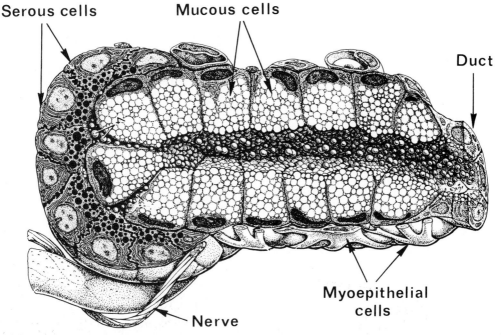

Figure 3–18. Drawing of the end piece of a tubuloalveolar salivary gland showing the mucous cells and the serous demilune. (Modified from Krstić, R. V. Gewebe des Menschen und der Saugetiere. Heidelberg, Springer-Verlag, 1978.)

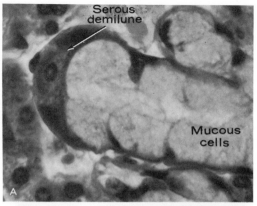

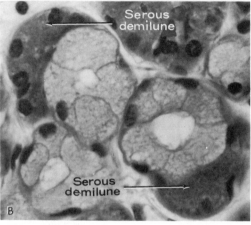

Figure 3–19. Photomicrograph of the terminal portions of the submandibular gland. This is an example of a mixed gland; some of the terminal elements are purely mucous, others have crescentic caps of serous cells called demilunes. The relationship is seen to better advantage in longitudinal section *(A)* than in transverse section *(B)*.

penetrate the capsule and follow the collagenous septa and the thinner partitions between the lobules, and from there send branches to the parenchyma. Within the lobule they are ultimately enclosed by reticular connective tissue. The blood and lymph capillaries form networks around small groups of acini and terminal ducts. The major vascular supply is supplemented in most glands by a collateral circulation mediated through capsular vessels of small caliber. The terminal nerve fibers branch, and their final divisions end on the surfaces of the acini.

The duct system of a complex exocrine gland conducts the product of the gland cells to a free external or internal body surface. The ducts may also modify the secretion during its passage. The *main duct* of the gland divides in the connective tissue to form *lobar ducts.* Their further branchings in the septa between lobules are called *interlobular ducts,*

while the ducts of the microscopic lobules are called *intralobular ducts.* The latter are continuous with the *intercalary ducts,* whose branches communicate with the secretory acini either directly, via intercellular canaliculi, or by a combination of these arrangements. The epithelium of the largest ducts may be simple or stratified columnar. As the duct becomes smaller, the epithelium is first simple columnar, then cuboidal, and finally squamous.

CONTROL OF EXOCRINE SECRETION

Many glands secrete continuously at a low level but are stimulated under certain conditions to secrete more abundantly. The mechanisms for physiological control of secretion vary greatly from gland to gland. In many the stimulation is mediated solely via the autonomic nervous system. In other glands the stimulus is hormonal, and in some there is a dual mechanism. It is well known, for example, that the sight or smell of food will increase the secretion of acid, mucus, and digestive enzymes in the stomach. These psychic stimuli are mediated via the vagus

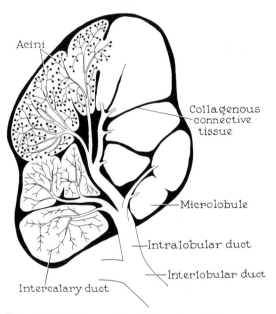

Figure 3–20. Diagram showing branches of duct system and their relationship to secretory portion in a lobule of a compound tubuloacinar gland. Collagenous stroma separates (often incompletely) the microscopic lobules. The main duct shown is a branch of the interlobular duct. The interlobular duct branches into intralobular ducts of several orders. These are continuous with fine terminal intercalary ducts that end in the secretory portion. (Modified from Heidenhain.)

nerves and are abolished if these are cut. On the other hand, food placed in the stomach also initiates gastric and pancreatic secretion even if it has not previously been seen or tasted. Secretion in this case depends on the intrinsic nerves in the organ and upon locally produced hormones. Activation of nerves in the gastric mucosa releases the transmitter *acetylcholine,* which stimulates release of the hormone *gastrin* from endocrine cells in the mucosa, and this in turn activates secretion by the gastric glands. Gastrin-secreting cells may also respond directly to the presence of food as a result of its detection by modified microvilli that are believed to have a chemo-receptor function.

There are no visible morphological criteria that enable the histologist to determine whether a given gland is under control of hormones, but nervous control can be inferred from the observation of nerve endings in close contact with the secretory cells. In the pancreas, nerve endings can be found inside the basal lamina of the acini, in close contact with the base of the exocrine cells. These cells are also known to be responsive to the hormone *gastrin,* produced in the stomach, and *secretin* and *cholecystokinin,* secreted in the duodenum. Thus, multiple factors are involved in the control of pancreatic secretion.

ENDOCRINE GLANDS

Phylogenetically, three main mechanisms have developed in animals to integrate the functions of their different tissues and organs. To some degree these are recapitulated in vertebrate ontogeny. The earliest mechanism to appear involves substances that simply diffuse through the intercellular spaces to influence the behavior or function of other cells at a limited distance from the source (paracrine secretion). Integration by simple diffusion of chemical messengers is slow, poorly controlled, and of limited usefulness in larger metazoa. This primitive humoral mechanism was later supplemented by development of a nervous system consisting of cells that had acquired the capacity to respond to external stimuli and to rapidly conduct a signal over the surface of their long cell processes (axons) to affect other cells. The nervous system increased in complexity and became highly efficient in dealing with elaborate integrated patterns of behavior involving precise and rapid motor events. The

two integrative systems have been supplemented by development of ductless *endocrine glands* whose cells synthesize chemical agents called *hormones* that are carried in the circulating blood to distant parts of the body, where they act upon specific *target organs.* These chemical messengers tend to have a longer latent period because they are distributed by the blood, but they produce more sustained effects than the signals carried by nerves.

Endocrine glands arise in the embryo as tubular evaginations or solid outgrowths from lining epithelia, but later in their development their connection with the surface is lost. They are penetrated by blood vessels, which form a very rich capillary plexus in intimate relationship to the cords, follicles, or acini of the endocrine glands. The close proximity of the cells to a dense vascular bed favors release of secretory product into the blood.

The fully developed endocrine gland is usually completely dissociated from exocrine glandular tissue, but in a few examples there is relatively little morphological separation of the endocrine tissue from an exocrine gland. Thus, the small islets of Langerhans, the endocrine component of the pancreas, are scattered throughout the much greater bulk of the exocrine portion of the gland (see Chapter 28). Similarly, in the testis, the Leydig cells secreting male sex hormone are located in interstitial tissue between the tubules comprising the exocrine portion of the organ (see Chapter 31). Thus, in these *mixed glands,* one group of cells secretes into a duct system while another group delivers its secretion into the blood. In the unique case of the liver, the cells secrete bile into the intercellular terminations of a duct system, but the same cells also release internal secretions into the blood flowing through sinusoids between the sheets of hepatic cells.

The principal endocrine glands are the *hypophysis, thyroid, parathyroid, pancreas, adrenals, pineal, testes,* and *placenta.* These are so diverse in their architecture that they do not lend themselves to classification on the basis of their histological organization. The chemical nature of their hormones is also varied, including modified amino acids, peptides, proteins, glycoproteins, and steroids. It is not surprising, therefore, that one cannot describe cytological features common to all endocrine cells. It is possible, however, to assign them to categories related to the chemical nature of their product.

CYTOLOGY OF POLYPEPTIDE-SECRETING ENDOCRINE GLANDS

As might be expected, endocrine cells secreting peptide and glycoprotein hormones have many ultrastructural features in common with the protein-secreting exocrine cells described previously, but there is a significant difference in the degree of development of the organelles concerned with protein synthesis. The granular endoplasmic reticulum is much less extensive. This is consistent with the great difference in the volume of product produced. The acinar cells of the exocrine pancreas produce over 1 liter of enzyme-rich digestive juice per day, whereas the output of a polypeptide- or glycoprotein- secreting endocrine gland would be measured in milligram or microgram quantities.

The beta cell of the pancreatic islets, which secretes the hormone *insulin,* can be considered representative of this category of endocrine cells. Electron micrographs of these cells show a few meandering profiles of rough endoplasmic reticulum, and clusters of free ribosomes in a cytoplasmic matrix of low density. There is a small Golgi apparatus and numerous membrane-limited granules 200 to 300 nm. in diameter. As in exocrine glandular cells, the granules are formed in the Golgi complex. They tend to be somewhat more numerous at the vascular pole of the cell but occur in considerable numbers throughout the cytoplasm (Fig. 3–21). In humans insulin occurs in the form of pleomorphic crystals within membrane-limited secretory vesicles, but in common laboratory animals the secretory granules are uniformly dense and homogeneous. With minor differences in cytology and granule size, this same description would apply to the alpha cells of the pancreas, which secrete *glucagon;* the somatotrophs, thyrotrophs, gonadotrophs, and corticotrophs of the hypophysis (secreting *growth hormone, thyroid stimulating hormone, gonadotrophic hormone,* and *adrenocorticotrophic hormone*); and the ultimobranchial or C cells of the thyroid (secreting *calcitonin*). In all of these, it is clear that the intracellular secretory pathway involves synthesis on ribosomes, segregation in the reticulum, concentration in the Golgi complex, and storage in membrane limited granules.

The thyroid gland belongs to the category of protein-secreting endocrine glands, but differs from the others in that its product, *thyroglobulin,* is stored extracellularly. The

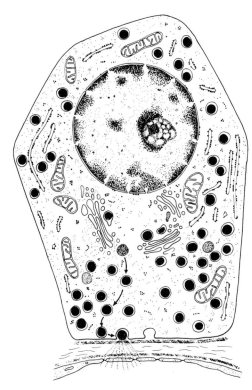

Figure 3–21. Schematic representation of the mechanism of release in endocrine cells producing protein or peptide hormones. Membranes bounding the granules coalesce with the cell membrane. The exteriorized granule disintegrates and the hormone diffuses into the blood through the fenestrated endothelium of an adjacent capillary or sinusoid.

cells are arranged in a simple cuboidal epithelium bounding spherical follicles with a central cavity. The cells have an extensive endoplasmic reticulum in the form of cisternae distended with the proteinaceous precursor of the secretory product (Fig. 3–22). In the Golgi complex, this material is packaged in membrane-limited secretory vesicles that do not accumulate in the cytoplasm but pass directly to the apical surface and discharge their content into the lumen of the follicle by exocytosis.

CYTOLOGY OF STEROID-SECRETING ENDOCRINE CELLS

The steroid-secreting endocrine cells of the ovary, testis, and adrenal gland are all quite similar to their ultrastructure, and are very different from protein and peptide-secreting cells. They have little granular endoplasmic reticulum and relatively few free ribosomes. Their most characteristic feature is a remark-

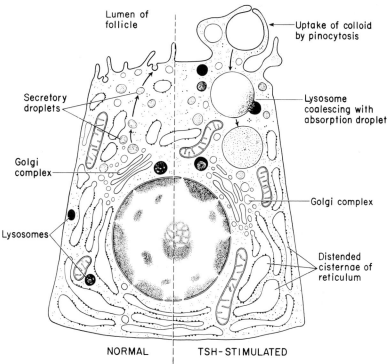

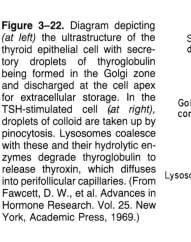

Figure 3–22. Diagram depicting *(at left)* the ultrastructure of the thyroid epithelial cell with secretory droplets of thyroglobulin being formed in the Golgi zone and discharged at the cell apex for extracellular storage. In the TSH-stimulated cell *(at right),* droplets of colloid are taken up by pinocytosis. Lysosomes coalesce with these and their hydrolytic enzymes degrade thyroglobulin to release thyroxin, which diffuses into perifollicular capillaries. (From Fawcett, D. W., et al. Advances in Hormone Research. Vol. 25. New York, Academic Press, 1969.)

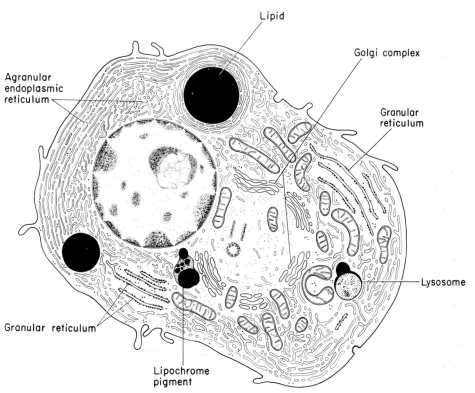

Figure 3–23. Schematic drawing of the characteristic cytologic features of a steroid-secreting cell. Most notable are the large Golgi complex and extensive smooth-surfaced endoplasmic reticulum. (From Fawcett, D. W., et al. Advances in Hormone Research. Vol. 25. New York, Academic Press, 1969.)

ably extensive smooth-surfaced endoplasmic reticulum in the form of a close-meshed network of branching and anastomosing tubules (Figs. 3–23, 3–24). The juxtanuclear Golgi complex is very large but has no associated secretory granules. Lipid droplets are present in the cytoplasm in greater or lesser numbers depending on the organ and the species. Mitochondria are numerous and of variable size and often have an unusual internal structure, with tubular or vesicular amplifications of the internal membrane instead of the usual lamellar or foliate cristae. These cells also contain lysosomes and peroxisomes and have a tendency to accumulate deposits of lipochrome pigment.

Steroid-secreting cells store very little hormone but may store a precursor, cholesterol. The lipid droplets, when present, contain cholesterol esters as well as triglycerides. The steroid-secreting cells in some species depend mainly on cholesterol from the blood, while those of other species synthesize much of the cholesterol they utilize for hormone synthesis. The enzymes for synthesis of cholesterol reside mainly in the membranes of the smooth endoplasmic reticulum. The initial step in conversion of cholesterol to steroid hormones is cleavage of its side chain by an enzyme in the mitochondria. Several subsequent steps in steroidogenesis involve enzymes in the reticulum. In the case of the adrenal steroids, there are additional steps in the synthesis that take place in the mitochondria. Little is known about how cholesterol and the intermediate products in steroidogenesis are moved back and forth between mitochondria and the reticulum to accomplish the successive biosynthetic steps. Since there is no appreciable storage of hormone, these cells must maintain the organelles needed to synthesize steroids on demand. The extensive development of the smooth endoplasmic reticulum thus represents a specialization to ensure the presence of the enzymes necessary for rapid synthesis of steroid hormone. The observation that the lipid content of steroid-secreting cells diminishes on stimulation is interpreted as mobilization and depletion of stored precursors during enhanced hormone production. It is not yet known what role is played by the prominent Golgi complex, but the fact that it increases in size in response to trophic hormone stim-

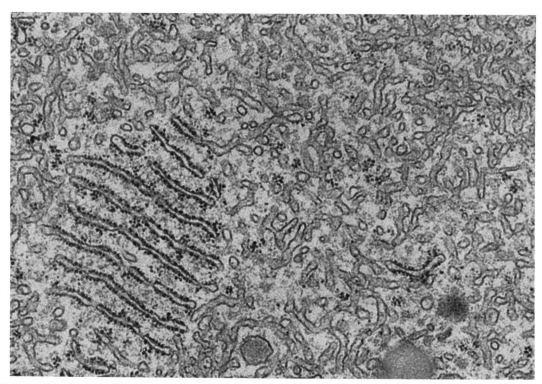

Figure 3–24. Electron micrograph of a small area of cytoplasm from a cell of the human fetal adrenal cortex. A few cisternae of granular endoplasmic reticulum are present, but most of the cytoplasm is occupied by branching tubules of the smooth endoplasmic reticulum. (Micrograph courtesy of N. S. McNutt.)

ulation indicates that it is involved in some way in the secretory process. No consistent morphological changes associated with the release of steroid have been reported, and nothing can be said at present about the mechanism of release or its regulation.

STORAGE AND SECRETION OF HORMONES

Endocrine glands differ greatly in the amount of hormone stored and in the site of storage. As previously noted, the steroid-secreting endocrine glands have no visible secretory granules and they store little or no hormone. They are evidently able to vary their rate of synthesis and release to keep pace with current needs. The thyroid gland, on the other hand, is unique among endocrine glands in that it stores hormone extracellularly in the lumen of the follicles and ordinarily contains enough to meet normal needs for several weeks. The several endocrine glands that secrete protein, glycoprotein, or polypeptide hormones, as well as those that secrete catecholamines, store their product intracellularly in membrane-limited granules in sufficient numbers to represent one to three weeks' supply. This latter category of endocrine glands with intracellular storage has been the most thoroughly studied with respect to the composition of the granules and their mechanism of release.

The neurohypophyseal hormones (*vasopressin* and *oxytocin*) are stored in the neurosecretory granules together with specific soluble proteins called *neurophysins*. These proteins seem to serve as "carriers" for the hormones in the hypothalamo-neurohypophyseal tract. The binding of the hormones to them may prevent diffusion of the biologically active molecules out of the vesicles in which they are stored. Zymogen granules, alpha-cell granules of the pancreas, calcitonin-containing granules, granules of various pituitary cell types, and the granules of the adrenal medulla all appear dense in electron micrographs and have similar histochemical staining reactions. The presumption is that in all of these the hormones are bound to or at least associated with a class of proteins comparable to the neurophysins. All these glands release their secretion by exocytosis entirely comparable with that described above for the exocrine pancreas but less easily observed because the quantities of material released are smaller. It follows from this mode of secretion that the soluble protein and other components of the granules are discharged as well as the hormones. Their fate is poorly understood. The biologically active hormones evidently become dissociated from the other constituents extracellularly and are free to diffuse into the blood vessels.

Active hormone secretion requires a mechanism not only for release of the membrane-limited granules (exocytosis) but also for transport of the granules to the cell surface. In glands, whether the cells are polarized toward the lumen of an acinus or toward a blood vessel, this transport must be selective and directional. Recent studies indicate that microtubules and possibly the microfilaments of the cytoplasm may be involved in this phase of the secretory process. The evidence for this is more pharmacological than morphological, and rests upon the demonstration that colchicine and other alkaloids that are known to prevent polymerization of tubulin to form microtubules also block the release of secretory products. A relation between microtubules and the secretory process was suggested first by the observation that colchicine prevents release of insulin from the pancreatic beta cells. Similar observations have been made for release of catecholamines from the adrenal medulla and for secretion of thyroxin by the thyroid gland.

In the case of the thyroid, there is also evidence for involvement of the microfilaments of the cytoplasm. The fungal metabolite *cytochalasin B* is known to cause the disappearance of microfilaments and to block a number of cellular processes involving protoplasmic movement. When this substance is added to the medium in which mouse thyroid glands are being maintained in vitro, the normal response to hormonal stimulation is blocked. Both colloid droplet uptake from the follicle lumen and release of hormone into the medium are suppressed. The action of cytochalasin B on the secretory process suggests that microfilaments, as well as microtubules, are involved. Since uptake of colloid by macropinocytosis is an initial step in thyroxin release, it may be that the motility of the ectoplasm necessary for formation of the engulfing pseudopods is the process that requires microfilaments. A word of caution may be in order. The conclusions drawn from these observations assume that the action of colchicine and of cytochalasin is specific for microtubules and for microfilaments, respectively. The possibility that either or both may have toxic effects on other components or activities of the cell has not been ruled out.

In the case of the thyroid, which stores its product, *thyroglobulin,* extracellularly, the mechanism for release of hormone into the blood is more complex. Droplets of colloid are taken up by pinocytosis from the lumen of the follicle. Within the cell the droplets fuse with lysosomes, and the thyroglobulin is degraded by hydrolytic enzymes liberating *thyroxin,* which diffuses through the base of the cell into the perifollicular capillaries. Thus, participation of lysosomes is an integral part of the normal secretory process in this particular endocrine gland but occurs in few others (Fig. 3–22).

In a number of endocrine cells, lysosomes do play a role in disposal of unneeded stores of secretion. For example, when the young of a lactating rat are weaned, there is a large excess of secretory granules in the mammotrophic cells of the anterior pituitary. These coalesce with lysosomes and are degraded by autophagy. Endoplasmic reticulum and ribosomes no longer required for minimal rates of hormone secretion suffer a similar fate.

RELATION OF ENDOCRINE CELLS TO BLOOD AND LYMPH VASCULAR SYSTEMS

Despite their histological and cytological diversity, a common feature of endocrine glands is their great vascularity. Nearly every cell is in close relation to one or more thin-walled vessels of a rich vascular bed. In some glands, the vessels are typical capillaries; in others, they are more appropriately described as sinusoids. The latter are generally larger than true capillaries and are more variable in shape—often conforming to the contours of the interstices they occupy among the plates or cords of epithelial cells that constitute the parenchyma of the endocrine gland. In the pituitary and adrenal glands, the endothelium of the sinusoids was formerly believed to be phagocytic to colloidal dyes, and it was traditionally included in the reticuloendothelial system. This interpretation has not been substantiated in ultrastructural studies, which show that the phagocytic potential resides in perivascular cells rather than in the endothelium.

Whether the vessels of endocrine glands are true capillaries or sinusoids, the lining endothelium is extremely thin and fenestrated. The only exception is the interstitial tissue of the testis, which has unfenestrated capillaries. In all cases the diffusion distance between the secretory cells and the blood is short, and the intervening structural components to be traversed are (1) a thin basal lamina around the endocrine cells, (2) a narrow perivascular space, (3) the basal lamina of the capillary endothelium, and (4) the thin diaphragms of the capillary pores. None of these appears to constitute a significant barrier to access of the hormones to the blood.

In addition to the microscopic structure of the vascular bed, a consideration of the pattern of drainage of blood from an endocrine gland, at a somewhat grosser level, may be relevant to an understanding of its function. For example, the hypothalamic releasing hormones are liberated into capillaries of the median eminence of the hypothalamus, which are drained via special hypophyseoportal vessels to responsive target cells immediately downstream in the anterior lobe of the pituitary. Similarly, the mammalian adrenal gland consists of two portions arranged concentrically—an outer *cortex* that secretes steroid hormones and an inner *medulla* composed of cells that synthesize the catecholamines *epinephrine* and *norepinephrine*. No capsule or sharp boundary separates the two zones, and much of the blood supply flows centripetally from the cortex, carrying steroid hormones downstream to the cells of the medulla. It now appears that a relatively high concentration of cortical steroids may be necessary for induction and maintenance of an enzyme in the medulla that is essential for epinephrine synthesis. Thus, the local "downstream" effects of hormones may be as important as their effects exerted at a distance via the general circulation.

In most endocrine organs the hormones are released exclusively into the blood, but recent physiological studies indicate that in a few instances the lymphatics may also be significant pathways for egress of hormones. This is particularly true of the perifollicular lymphatics of the thyroid and the intertubular lymphatics of the rodent testis.

CONTROL MECHANISMS AND INTERRELATIONS WITHIN THE ENDOCRINE SYSTEM

Endocrine glands modify the function of specific target organs. In the course of evolution, some have also developed the capacity to sense changes in the concentration of metabolites or cell products in the body fluid; others have become specifically responsive to the hormones of other endocrine glands, and still others are stimulated by secretory products of the central nervous system. The activity of the brain and of the endocrine glands has become so closely integrated that changes in one are reflected in alterations in function of the other. On the basis of these interactions, a variety of control mechanisms has evolved that ensure the coordinated functioning of organs situated at a distance from one another. These mechanisms serve to maintain the constancy of the internal environment of the organism.

One of the simplest forms of control is the case in which a hormone acts upon a target organ, causing its cells to discharge a substance into the extracellular compartment. The resulting change then acts back upon the endocrine gland to *decrease* its output of hormone. This is commonly referred to as a *negative feedback mechanism*. The release of the hormone insulin from the beta cells of the pancreas drives glucose into cells and lowers blood sugar (Fig. 3–25). The lowered concentration of blood sugar, in turn, acts back upon the beta cells to diminish insulin release. Similarly, parathyroid hormone acts upon bone cells to mobilize calcium, and the elevated blood calcium, by negative feedback, depresses release of parathyroid hormone.

A somewhat greater degree of complexity is encountered when the endocrine gland is

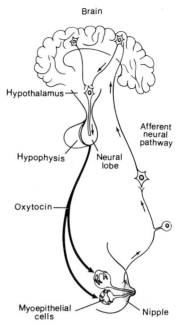

Figure 3–26. Illustration of the neuroendocrine interrelationships involved in the suckling reflex. Stimulation of the nipples generates sensory impulses that pass to the central nervous system via the dorsal root ganglia. In the brain these impulses are relayed to the hypothalamus, where they activate neurosecretory cells whose processes extend into the neural lobe of the hypophysis. Stimulation of these cells results in release of the hormone oxytocin, which is carried in the blood to the breast, where it causes contraction of myoepithelial cells around acini of the mammary gland, expelling milk. No feedback mechanism is involved.

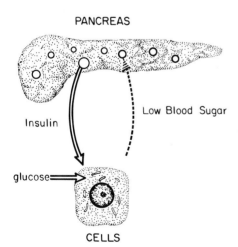

Figure 3–25. Drawing of a simple endocrine feedback mechanism. Insulin, the hormone from the islets of Langerhans in the pancreas, promotes entry of glucose into other cells of the body. The resulting low blood sugar acts back upon the alpha cells in the pancreas to reduce the release of insulin.

under control of the nervous system. The milk ejection reflex is a good example of a simple neuroendocrine mechanism in which the train of integrated events begins with a peripheral sensory stimulus. In this case, the tactile stimulus to the nipple, involved in suckling, is conducted over afferent neural pathways via the dorsal nerve roots and spinal cord to the brain and thence to neurosecretory cell bodies in the hypothalamus (Fig. 3–26). Stimulation of these cells results in release of the hormone *oxytocin* from their terminations in the posterior lobe of the pituitary. This hormone carried back to the breast via the bloodstream causes contraction of myoepithelial cells around the glandular acini, resulting in ejection of milk. Feedback control is not a feature of this neuroendocrine reflex.

The neuroendocrine response to stress is more complex, involving more steps in the sequence of events; it depends on a special vascular pathway from hypothalamus to pituitary and is under negative feedback control. A painful stimulus reaching the hypothalamus over afferent neural pathways stimulates cell bodies whose axons end in close relation to small blood vessels in the median eminence of the hypothalamus (Fig. 3–27). *Adrenocorticotrophic hormone releasing hormone* (ACTH-RH) is liberated at the nerve ending and carried in the blood via the special hypophyseoportal system of blood vessels to the anterior lobe of the hypophysis, where it causes specifically responsive cells to release *adrenocorticotrophic hormone* (ACTH) into the general circulation. When this hormone reaches the adrenal cortex, steroid hormones, called *glucocorticoids,* are released. These reach all the cells in the body and modify their function in various ways that increase the ability of the organism to tolerate prolonged muscular activity, trauma, infection, or intoxications. Adrenal steroids carried back to the brain exert a "negative feedback" on the cells of the hypothalamus, diminishing their output of ACTH-RH.

The complex system of neuroendocrine interrelations that control the female reproductive cycle will be discussed in Chapter 32. The few examples cited here may provide sufficient introduction to the mode of operation of the endocrine system to enable the student to appreciate the correlations of structure and function that appear in later chapters.

The transmitter substances released at the nerve terminals have a very transient existence, being inactivated in a matter of seconds by specific enzymes at the endings. In the slower-acting endocrine integrative system, the hormones are quite variable in their half lives in the circulation, which range from a few minutes to several days. Some hormones are transported in the blood in combination with specific *carrier proteins.* Inactivation or degradation of the hormone may take place at the target organ or in the liver or kidney. Some hormones enter their target cells to exert their effects; others are evidently able to act simply by binding to specific receptor sites on the cell membrane.

RECEPTORS AND MECHANISM OF HORMONE ACTION ON TARGET ORGANS

Hormones circulating in the blood reach all of the tissues. The selectivity of their action on particular organs depends on the presence in the membranes of the target cells of specific *receptors* having a high binding affinity for that hormone. The receptors are integral protein molecules of the cell membrane. Their number varies in different target organs but may be of the order of 10,000 molecules per cell. They are not static components of the plasma membrane but are in a dynamic state of turnover. There is normally a preprogrammed rate of receptor synthesis and insertion into the membrane, but their number may change with the state of cell differentiation and can be influenced by exposure to unphysiological levels of the specific hormone (homospecific regulation). The action of one hormone on a cell may induce the appearance of receptors for a second hormone (heterospecific regulation). The responsiveness of target cells is a function of the number of available receptors. Tissues that do not respond to a given hormone invariably lack receptors for that hormone.

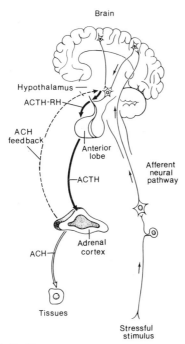

Figure 3–27. More complex neuroendocrine relationships involved in response to stress. A painful peripheral stimulus reaching the brain is relayed to neurosecretory cells in the hypothalamus. These liberate ACTH releasing hormone (ACTH-RH) into the vessels of the hypophyso-portal system. Carried downstream to the anterior lobe, this hormone stimulates corticotrophs to release ACTH. The ACTH borne by the blood to the adrenal cortex causes release of corticosteroids (ACH) that are carried to cells throughout the body, inducing protective metabolic responses. Adrenocortical hormones act back upon the hypothalamus to suppress liberation of ACTH-RH.

The biochemical mechanisms by which hormones elicit a response in their target cells have been a subject of intensive investigation. Two principal mechanisms have emerged. In the case of steroid hormones, the hormone–receptor complex is translocated to the cell nucleus where it becomes associated with acceptor sites on the chromatin. There it activates gene transcription, which in turn directs the appropriate synthetic activities of the responding cell.

The action of other hormones is mediated by a mechanism discovered in studies on the effects of norepinephrine and glucagon on the liver (Fig. 3–28). In binding to receptors, these molecules become associated with an enzyme, *adenyl cyclase,* in the cell membrane. The activated enzyme catalyzes the formation of *cyclic AMP* from adenosine triphosphate (ATP). Intracellular accumulation of cyclic AMP activates *protein kinases,* enzymes that set in motion a train of events leading to the characteristic response of the target cell to the hormone. These findings led to the "second messenger" concept. Briefly stated, a hormone, the "first messenger," is carried in the blood and activates adenyl cyclase in the target cell membrane, resulting in an increase in the "second messenger," cyclic AMP, which induces a specific response. In all instances in which this mechanism is operative, the action of the hormone can be duplicated by application of exogenous cyclic AMP to the target cells.

This mode of coupling a stimulus to its response is involved in the action of the hypophyseal hormones adrenocorticotropin, thyrotropin, and gonadotropins, and in the release of calcitonin from the parafollicular cells of the thyroid. It also mediates those examples of exocrine secretion that are initiated by the neurotransmitter norepinephrine. An explanation of the remarkable diversity in the responses of various target cells to a single second messenger is still being sought. All the effects of cyclic AMP appear to be mediated by controlling the activity of protein kinases that catalyze the transfer of phosphate from ATP to protein. The diversity of the responses of target cells, therefore, seems to depend, not on the control system, but on the distinctive proteins available and on their varied biological activities when phosphorylated.

The second messenger, cyclic AMP, is commonly involved in the category of *nonexcitable tissues* such as liver, other glands, and adipose tissue. Another mechanism by which stimuli evoke cellular responses utilizes an ionic messenger, the divalent cation Ca^{2+}. Calcium is principally involved in coupling stimulus to response in *excitable tissues* such as nerve and muscle, where ion currents lead to action potentials propagated over the cell surface from the site of the initial stimulus. Stimulus-induced fluxes in free intracellular Ca^{2+} are controlled by an ubiquitous regulatory protein, *calmodulin,* which can activate a number of enzymes involved in the physiological responses of cells. Among its other functions, calmodulin plays a role in activation of adenyl cyclase by modulating the local concentration of Ca^{2+}. The validity of the sharp distinction often made between the ionic and cyclic AMP mechanisms of stimulus-response coupling is now in doubt since it has been shown that the two often interact in achieving a cellular response.

Although our understanding of the mechanisms by which binding of hormones to receptors results in propagation of signals to the appropriate synthetic pathways within the cell is still incomplete, enough is known to explain several diseases whose pathogenesis was previously obscure. The congenital disorder *testicular feminization* is now known to be a genetic abnormality of receptor function. Individuals with a male chromosome

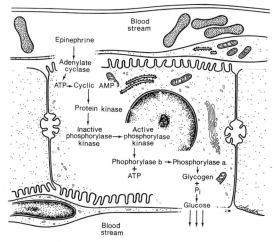

Figure 3–28. Diagram of the mechanism of action of hormones. The hormone epinephrine (first messenger) carried to the liver cell membrane in the blood activates the enzyme adenylate cyclase in the cell membrane, causing it to convert some of the ATP of the cytoplasm into cyclic AMP (second messenger). This then activates a protein kinase, which activates a second kinase. The second kinase initiates a four-step sequence that converts glycogen into glucose, which then passes out into the bloodstream in the hepatic sinusoids.

complement (46 XY) at conception fail to develop testicular function and male external genitalia because of receptor anomalies that result in complete insensitivity of the target tissues to the hormone dihydrotestosterone. In some patients the receptors are completely absent. In others they are present but the hormone–receptor complex lacks the ability to activate gene transcription in the nucleus. Comparable receptor abnormalities are responsible for *familial male pseudohermaphroditism*.

Endocrine disturbances may arise in adults as a consequence of development of auto-antibodies that bind to receptors on specific target organs. Patients with Graves' disease (thyrotoxicosis) have an abnormal immunoglobulin in their serum that binds to the receptor for thyrotropic hormone and activates adenyl cyclase, resulting in continual stimulation of the cells to produce excess thyroid hormone. By competing with thyrotropic hormone for binding sites, the immunoglobulin overrides the endocrine control mechanisms that normally govern thyroid function. Similarly, rare cases of *diabetes* are attributable to an abnormal immunoglobulin that competes with insulin for receptor sites. In this condition, the immunoglobulin is not stimulatory and therefore acts as an insulin antagonist.

NEUROENDOCRINE CELLS, PARANEURONES

As stated earlier in this chapter, two systems for coordinating the activities of cells in the body have long been recognized: (1) the nervous system, providing rapid point-to-point communication and using *chemical neurotransmitters* released at special synaptic sites on long cell processes; and (2) the endocrine system, acting more slowly and using *hormones* transported to distant target cells by the blood. The neurotransmitters are commonly monoamines or amino acids; the hormones are small glycoproteins, polypeptides, or steroids.

The separation of neurones from endocrine cells was narrowed in the 1930s by the description of cells in the nervous system that have the form of neurones but contain secretory granules that are transported along their axonal processes, releasing their contents into perivascular spaces to be carried in the blood to their target cells. The discovery of these neurosecretory cells established an important linkage between the nervous and endocrine system and initiated a new field of research called *neuroendocrinology*.

The traditional distinction between neural and endocrine systems was further clouded by the discovery that the neurotransmitter *norepinephrine* is also a hormone released into the circulation by endocrine cells in the adrenal medulla. Conversely, the peptide hormone *vasopressin*, released in the neurohypophysis, has been found to serve as a neurotransmitter for certain cells in the hypothalamus. A dozen or more peptides have now been found to relay signals between endocrine cells and their targets. Cells releasing these peptides occur singly or in small groups in various regions of the brain, and are widely distributed in the gastrointestinal tract. In contrast to the compact endocrine glands, these dispersed cells collectively make up a *diffuse neuroendocrine system,* which can be regarded as a third system for coordinating cellular activities using chemical messengers commonly referred to as *neuropeptides.* These isolated cells, possessing properties in common with both neurones and endocrine cells, are now the focus of much investigative interest. Twenty or more morphologically similar but functionally distinct cell types have been identified in the epithelium of the gut and its associated glands. These have been called the *entero-endocrine cells* or *gastroenteropancreatic (GEP) endocrine cells* (Chapter 26). But these terms are not sufficiently inclusive, for cells with the same peptide secretory products have also been found widely dispersed in the central nervous system. Some, but not all, of these cells have the capacity for *amine precursor uptake* and *decarboxylation* and have been grouped together by some investigators under the acronym *APUD cells*.

Thus, the traditional view of histologists that neurones were so differentiated in structure and function that they could easily be identified on the basis of shape and possession of certain distinctive organelles has been progressively eroded. The electron microscope showed that some of the structural components believed to be unique to neurones were common to many cell types. "Neurofilaments" and "neurotubules" do not differ significantly from the cytoskeletal filaments and microtubules of cells in general. The "Nissl bodies" are simply parallel arrays of cisternae of the endoplasmic reticulum and associated polyribosomes. And the defining physiological property of membrane depolarization is now known to be shared with several endocrine cells. A consensus has gradually developed that there are overlapping properties and a broad continuity between neurones and endocrine cells.

It has been suggested that the numerous cell types of the diffuse endocrine system should be regarded as closely related to neurones and might appropriately be called *paraneurones.* They all have in common the presence of small secretory granules or vesicles concentrated at the base or vascular pole of the cell. The cytoplasm is usually electron lucent, the endoplasmic reticulum sparse, and the Golgi apparatus relatively small. They secrete substances identical with or closely related to known neurosecretions or neurotransmitters (peptides and sometimes monoamines). They have the morphological characteristics of cells specialized for reception of a stimulus and release of a secretion in response. The products of some are released into the bloodstream for transport to distant target cells. The products of many others simply diffuse to neighboring epithe-

lial cells or adjacent nerve cells. This local action is described as *paracrine secretion* to distinguish it from blood-borne distribution of hormones from the *endocrine glands.* Cytological criteria alone do not permit unambiguous identification of the cells releasing a particular peptide. Such identification must be accomplished immunocytochemically by using fluorescein-labeled antibodies against each of the biologically active peptides.

Included in the paraneurone category are the several endocrine cell types of the gut exemplified by the gastrin cell, which has microvilli serving a chemoreceptor function, and basal granules that release hormone (Fig. 3–29A). Similar in structure and sensory function are the gustatory cells of the lingual taste buds (Fig. 3–29B); the basal granular cells of the bronchial epithelium that sense hypoxia of the respired air (Fig. 3–29C); the principal cells of the carotid body (Fig. 3–29D); and the olfactory cells of the nasal epithelium (Fig. 3–29E). In addition to these cells with a chemoreceptor function, there are mechanoreceptor cells such as the hair

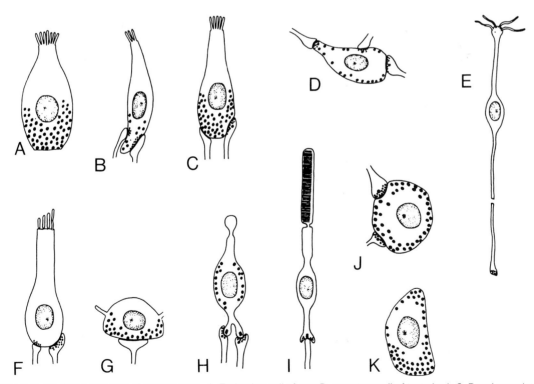

Figure 3–29. Principal types of paraneurons. *A,* Endocrine cell of gut; *B,* gustatory cell of taste bud; *C,* Basal granulated cell of bronchus; *D,* chief cell of the carotid body; *E,* olfactory cell; *F,* hair cell of the inner ear; *G,* Merkel cell of the skin; *H,* avian pinealocyte; *I,* visual cell of retina; *J,* adrenal chromaffin cell; *K,* endocrine cell of adenohypophysis, parafollicular cell of thyroid, or pancreatic islet cell. (Modified after Fujita, T., et al. *In* Farner, D., and K. Lederis, eds.: Neurosecretion: Molecules, Cells, Systems. New York, Plenum Press, 1982.)

cells of the inner ear (Fig. 3–29*F*) and the Merkel cells of the epidermis (Fig. 3–29*G*). Possibly qualifying as paraneurones are the avian pinealocytes that retain some photoreceptor function (Fig. 3–29*H*) and the phylogenetically related visual cells of the mammalian retina (Fig. 3–29*I*). Finally, there are noninnervated endocrine cells such as those of the adenohypophysis, the parafollicular cells of the thyroid, and the pancreatic islet cells (Fig. 3–29*J*).

The paraneurone concept is still evolving, but is a convenient generalization that encompasses several more narrowly defined categories and brings some order out of the terminological chaos that has resulted from the rapid discovery of numerous types of granulated cells secreting a bewildering variety of hormones or transmitters. The finding of isolated cells with a sensory apex and a secretory base in hydroids and other invertebrates suggests that paraneurones and their secretory products have been highly conserved in evolution and may well have antedated development of the neural and endocrine coordinating systems.

REFERENCES

EXOCRINE GLANDS, GENERAL

Bowen, R. H.: The cytology of glandular secretion. Q. Rev. Biol. *4*:299, 484, 1929.

Nassonov, D.: Das Golgische Binnennetz und seine Beziehungen zu Sekretion. Morphologische und experimentelle Untersuchungen an einiger Saugetierdrusen. Arch. Mikr. Anat. *100*:433, 1924.

Scharrer, E., and B. Scharrer: Neurosekretion. *In* von Mollendorff, W., and W. Bargman, eds.: Handbuch der Mikroskopisches Anatomie des Menschen. Vol. 6, Part 5. Berlin, Springer-Verlag, 1954.

PROTEIN SECRETION

Amsterdam, A., I. Ohad, and M. Schramm: Dynamic changes in the ultrastructure of the acinar cell of the rat parotid gland during the secretory cycle. J. Cell Biol. *41*:753, 1969.

Blöbel, G., P. Walter, C. N. Chang, B. M. Goldman, A. H. Erickson, and V. R. Lingappa: Translocation of protein across membranes. The signal hypothesis. *In* Secretory Mechanisms. Symp. Soc. Exp. Biol. Vol. 33. Cambridge, Cambridge University Press, 1979.

Castle, J. D., J. D. Jamieson, and G. E. Palade: Radioautographic analysis of the secretory process in the parotid acinar cell of the rabbit. J. Cell Biol. *53*:290, 1972.

Farquahar, M. D.: Recovery of surface membrane in anterior pituitary cells. Variations in traffic detected with ionic and cationic ferritin. J. Cell Biol. *77*:R35–R42, 1978.

Herzog, V., and H. Reggio: Pathways of endocytosis from luminal plasma membrane in rat exocrine pancreas. Eur. J. Cell Biol. *21*:141, 1980.

Jamieson, J. D., and G. E. Palade: Production of secretory proteins in animal cells. *In* Brinkley, B. B., and K. R. Porter, eds.: International Cell Biology. New York, Rockefeller University Press, 1977.

Leblond, C. P., and G. Bennett: Role of the Golgi apparatus in terminal glycosylation. *In* Brinkley, B. B., and K. R. Porter, eds.: International Cell Biology. New York, Rockefeller University Press, 1977.

Neutra, M., and C. P. Leblond: Synthesis of the carbohydrate of mucus in the Golgi complex as shown by electron microscope radioautography of goblet cells from rats injected with glucose-H3. J. Cell Biol. *30*:119, 1966.

Palade, G. E.: Intracellular aspects of the process of protein secretion. Science *189*:347, 1975.

Walter, P., I. Ibrahimi, and G. Blöbel: Translocation of proteins across the endoplasmic reticulum. J. Cell Biol. *91*:545, 1981.

ENDOCRINE SECRETION

Fawcett, D. W., J. A. Long, and A. L. Jones: The ultrastructure of the endocrine glands. Recent Prog. Hormone Res. *25*:315, 1969.

Grossman, M. I.: Integration of neural and hormonal control of gastric secretion. Physiologist *6*:349, 1963.

O'Malley, B. W., and W. T. Schrader. The receptors of steroid hormones. Sci. Am. *234*:32, 1976.

Schally, A. U., A. J. Kastin, and A. Arimura: Hypothalamic hormones: the link between brain and body. Am. Scientist *65*:712, 1977.

Smith, A. D.: Storage and secretion of hormones. Sci. Basis Med. *74*:102, 1972.

Turner, C. D., and J. T. Bagnara: General Endocrinology. 5th ed. Philadelphia, W. B. Saunders Co., 1971.

CONTROL OF SECRETION

Rasmussen, H.: Cell communication, calcium ion and cyclic adenosine monophosphate. Science *170*:404, 1970.

Sutherland, E. W.: On the biological role of cyclic AMP. J.A.M.A. *214*:1281, 1970.

PARACRINE SECRETION

Feyrter, F.: Uber die peripheren endokrinen (parakrinen) Drüsen des Menschen. 2nd ed. Vienna, Wilhelm Mudrich, 1953.

Fujita, T.: Concept of paraneurons. Arch. Histol. Jpn. *40*(Suppl):1, 1977.

Fujita, T., T. Iwanaga, Y. Kusumato, and S. Yoshie: Paraneurons and neurosecretion. *In* Farner, D. S., and K. Lederis, eds.: Neurosecretion: Molecules, Cells, Systems. New York, Plenum Publishing Corp., 1982.

Pearse, A. G. E.: The diffuse neuroendocrine system and the APUD concept: related endocrine peptides in brain, intestine, pituitary, placenta, and anuran cutaneous glands. Med. Biol. *55*:115, 1977.

4

BLOOD

Blood is a fluid tissue consisting of *erythrocytes* (red blood cells) and *leukocytes* (white blood cells) suspended in *blood plasma*. It circulates in the vascular system, transporting oxygen from the lungs and nutrients from the digestive tract to other tissues throughout the body, and carrying carbon dioxide to the lungs and nitrogenous waste products to the kidneys for excretion. Blood also plays an essential role in the integrative function of the endocrine system by distributing hormones from their sites of production to their distant target organs.

All the connective tissues of the body are composed of cells distributed in an abundant extracellular matrix. Cartilage, for example, consists largely of intercellular material that is a firm gel, and in bone the extracellular matrix is a highly organized scaffolding of mineralized fibers. Blood has traditionally been classified as a connective tissue in which the intercellular substance is fluid. Obviously it is not a "connective tissue" in the sense of binding together and preserving the structural integrity of the organism, but only in the sense that it maintains logistic support and communication between the tissues and organs of the body.

The boundaries of the several kinds of tissues are not always clearly defined. The fibers of connective tissue proper extend into the extracellular matrix of cartilage and bone. Similarly the circulating blood is not functionally separable from the connective tissue around the blood vessels, for fluid constituents of the blood are constantly filtering through the capillary walls to contribute to the fluid phase of the connective tissue matrix. Concurrently, metabolites are diffusing from the tissue fluid back into the bloodstream. This continual exchange of substances between the blood plasma and tissue fluid is essential for survival of the cells in all the organs.

It was formerly thought that all the blood cells carried out their principal functions in the bloodstream, but when it became possible to radiolabel cells and trace their migrations, it soon became evident that only the erythrocytes and platelets function entirely within the confines of the vascular system. The several types of leukocytes are only very transiently in the blood and are constantly migrating through the walls of capillaries and venules to become free cells of the connective tissues. It is there that they carry out their functions, complete their short life span, and degenerate. The blood is simply the vehicle for transport of the leukocytes from the bone marrow, where they are generated, to the tissues to carry out their appointed tasks.

The volume of blood in humans is approximately 5 liters, accounting for 7 per cent of body weight. Erythrocytes make up about 45 per cent of this volume, the leukocytes and platelets make up 1 per cent, and the remainder is blood plasma, the transparent yellow liquid that constitutes the extracellular matrix of this tissue. When blood is drawn from the circulation, it rapidly clots to a deep red, jelly-like mass, but if clotting is prevented by an anticoagulant the cellular elements can be centrifuged to the bottom of the tube, providing a useful measure of the packed cell volume and a clear view of the plasma.

A thorough knowledge of the normal histology of blood is of great importance in medical and veterinary practice, for no tissue is examined more often for diagnostic purposes. Study of stained blood smears under the microscope not only yields information about diseases that primarily affect the blood and blood-forming organs, but also may provide evidence of viral, bacterial, and parasitic infections. It enables the physician to identify the nature of the disease; to follow its course; and to evaluate the effectiveness of his treatment.

ERYTHROCYTES

The *erythrocytes* are the minute corpuscles that impart the red color to the blood. They develop in the bone marrow as true cells but, before entering the circulation, they extrude their nucleus, losing the capacity for DNA-directed protein synthesis. Their mitochondria and other membrane-limited organs are also lost and they are thus reduced to plastids* whose cytoplasm consists mainly of hemoglobin. In this structural simplification the erythrocytes become specialized for the primary function of transporting oxygen from the lungs to the tissues and carbon dioxide from the tissues to the lungs. Anucleate erythrocytes are characteristic of mammals. In birds, reptiles, amphibia, and fish, the erythrocytes retain a nucleus but its chromatin is functionally inert.

The normal number of erythrocytes per cubic millimeter of blood is about 5.4 million in men and 4.8 million in women. These numbers are increased somewhat by residence at high altitude. The mammalian erythrocyte has a highly consistent and characteristic shape (Figs. 4–1B, 4–3). It is a biconcave disc about 7.5 μm in diameter, 1.9 μm in maximal thickness, and has a surface area of approximately 140 square micrometers. The biconcave shape of the erythrocyte

*Since they lack the defining organelles of true cells, the terms "red blood *cell*" and "erythrocyte" are inappropriate. *Erythroplastid* would be a more accurate description, but *erythrocyte* is so widely used it is not likely to be replaced.

is well adapted to its function, for in this form it presents a surface area 20 to 30 per cent greater in relation to its volume than it would if it were spherical. This increased surface favors the immediate saturation of its hemoglobin with oxygen as the erythrocyte passes through the pulmonary capillaries. The total surface area of the erythrocytes in an average human is 3800 square meters—some 2000 times the total body surface. The enormous surface area of the erythrocytes results in great efficiency in oxygen and carbon dioxide transport.

The uniformity of shape of erythrocytes in blood smears is not entirely representative of their form in the peripheral circulation. They are very pliable and may be deformed to bell-like or paraboloid shape when flowing through capillaries. This deformation is dependent on the velocity of blood flow and is a consequence of hydrodynamic force and viscous drag. Since the altered configuration results in a further increase in surface area, this transient shape change may have some significance in gas exchange.

When fresh blood is examined in a thick smear under the microscope, the erythrocytes are often observed to associate in stacks called *rouleaux* (Fig. 4–1A). This phenomenon does not occur when blood is circulating but only when it is still or stagnant. It is often considered a surface tension effect but its physical basis is in fact poorly understood.

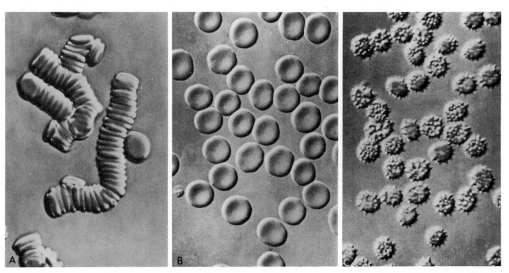

Figure 4–1. Photomicrographs of fresh blood viewed by Nomarski optics. *A,* Erythrocytes in vitro often aggregate like stacked coins; this is called rouleau formation. *B,* Normally, erythrocytes are biconcave discs with an obvious central depression and a thicker rim. *C,* Erythrocytes may assume a spiny configuration with 10 to 30 spicules evenly distributed over the surface and are then referred to as echinocytes. This change in form is often called crenation, and usually occurs during specimen preparation but may occur in pathological conditions in vivo. (Micrographs courtesy of Marcel Bessis.)

The shape of erythrocytes is sensitive to various factors in the surrounding medium. In moderately hypotonic solution they swell and may become uniconcave. In strongly hypotonic solution the membrane is stretched and becomes leaky or ruptures, allowing the hemoglobin to escape, leaving behind an empty membrane called an *erythrocyte ghost.* This disruption is called *hemolysis.* In moderately hypertonic solution erythrocytes become flattened but do not otherwise alter their shape. Under various experimental conditions in vitro, erythrocytes assume a spiny configuration with 10 to 30 spicules regularly distributed over their surface, and are then called *echinocytes* (Fig. 4–1C). This change of form is referred to as *crenation.* It was formerly attributed to hypertonicity of the medium but is now known to be due to other factors. Formation of echinocytes can be induced in vitro by exposure to fatty acids, lysolecithin, anionic compounds, or elevated pH.

Unstained erythrocytes have a pale yellow or tan color due to their content of *hemoglobin,* the respiratory pigment that makes up about 33 per cent of their mass. Hemoglobin is the most essential biochemical component of the erythrocyte. It is a protein with a molecular weight of 65,000 consisting of four polypeptide globin chains. An iron-containing heme group is bound to each chain of the tetramer.

Humans are genetically capable of synthesizing and incorporating into hemoglobin four structurally different polypeptide chains designated alpha (α), beta (β), gamma (γ), and delta (δ). Hemoglobin of the normal adult, called hemoglobin A (HbA), contains two alpha and two beta chains. This form accounts for 96 per cent of the hemoglobin while 2 per cent is of a second type (HbA$_2$), consisting of two alpha and two delta chains, and less than 2 per cent is fetal hemoglobin (HbF), composed of two alpha and two gamma chains. HbF greatly predominates over the others during fetal life but diminishes in amount in the postnatal period. In certain types of anemia (thalassemia), there is a persistence of abnormally high levels of fetal hemoglobin.

A separate genetic locus determines the structure of each of the four globin chains, and a variety of inherited disorders of hemoglobin synthesis have been discovered that involve relatively minor amino acid substitutions in the beta chain but nevertheless have profound physiological effects. These exam-

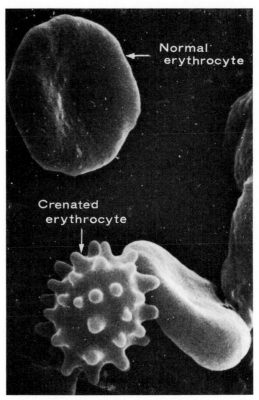

Figure 4–2. Scanning electron micrograph of two normal biconcave erythrocytes and one crenated erythrocyte. (Micrograph courtesy of Marcel Bessis.)

ples of disease involving defects at the molecular level are now of great clinical interest. A classical example is hemoglobin S (HbS) associated with *sickle cell anemia.* It differs from normal only in the substitution of valine for glutamine at one site on the beta chain, but this substitution is enough to make it less soluble than normal in the reduced condition and results in formation of long tactoids that deform the red cells into bizarre sickle forms, which block capillaries and are prone to hemolysis.

Normally, the erythrocytes in a dry smear of peripheral blood stain deep pink or salmon color with Wright's stain (Fig. 4–7). Some of the young red cells that have lost their nucleus shortly before entering the circulation and are not yet completely mature may have a bluish or greenish tinge due to the basophilic staining of small numbers of residual ribosomes. These are called *polychromatophilic erythrocytes* or *reticulocytes.* The latter term refers to the fact that when blood smears are stained with brilliant cresyl blue, the remaining ribonucleoprotein is precipitated by the dye into a delicate basophilic network in the otherwise acidophilic hemoglobin-rich cytoplasm. Within 24 hours after entering the blood from the bone marrow, the reticulocytes mature into adult erythrocytes. Reticulocyte number in adult humans averages about 0.8 per cent of the total erythrocytes of blood. The *reticulocyte count* is used clinically as a rough index of the rate of erythrocyte formation. In patients with anemia, elevation of the count is a valuable sign of response to treatment.

A detailed description of abnormal forms of erythrocytes is more appropriate for textbooks of hematology or pathology, but a few of the descriptive terms may be useful here. Abnormal variation in size of red cells is described as *anisocytosis*. Red cells that are larger than normal are *macrocytes*, and an anemia characterized by such cells is a *macrocytic anemia*. Deviation from the normal shape is described by the term *poikilocytosis*. The concentration of hemoglobin per cell is less than normal when the rate of red cell formation is relatively greater than the rate of hemoglobin synthesis. Under these circumstances, each erythrocyte contains an abnormally small quantity of hemoglobin. It appears paler and is described as *hypochromic*, as opposed to normal or *normochromic* erythrocytes.

Electron micrographs of erythrocytes reveal a homogeneous content of considerable density that at high magnification has a finely granular texture representing molecules of hemoglobin (Fig. 4–3). Microtubules and filaments found in the cytoskeleton of other cells are not observed. Owing to the ready availability of erythrocytes and the ease with which the plasmalemma can be purified after hemolysis, more is known about the erythrocyte membrane than about any other. The biconcave shape and elasticity of the red cell are attributed to a complex of peripheral proteins on the inner aspect of the membrane, which are organized in a deformable reinforcing meshwork. The principal component of this unusual cytoskeleton is *spectrin*, a large asymmetrical molecule composed of two polypeptide subunits of 240,000 and 220,000 M.W. It normally occurs as a tetramer (920,000 M.W.), a long, flexible, rodlike molecule 200 nm long. The erythrocyte cytoskeletal complex is believed to be made up of a meshwork of spectrin rods linked together by *actin* oligomers. This web is attached to the membrane by another protein called *ankyrin*, which binds to both spectrin and one of the integral membrane proteins (Fig. 4–4). Spectrin and ankyrin were thought to occur only in erythrocytes but there is now evidence that they occur in certain other cell types and may play a role in membrane–cytoskeleton linkage.

To students, these ultrastructural details of the erythrocyte cytoskeleton may seem to be esoteric, but they have recently acquired clinical significance insofar as they explain the cellular abnormalities observed in certain hereditary hemolytic anemias of humans, including *hereditary spherocytosis* and *hereditary elliptocytosis*. In these conditions there are varying degrees of membrane instability resulting in deformations in shape of the erythrocytes and excessive fragility. Underlying these abnormalities, patients may have deficiencies of spectrin or of ankyrin or defective binding of spectrin to actin and the integral protein of the erythrocyte membrane. The study of these skeletal protein mutants sheds

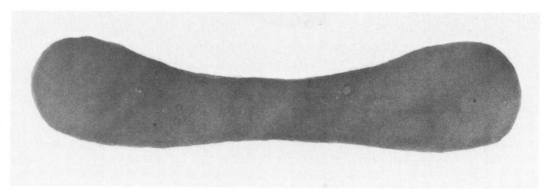

Figure 4–3. In a micrograph of an erythrocyte in thin section, its cytoplasm is devoid of organelles and consists of a homogeneous suspension of hemoglobin molecules that at high magnification give the interior a finely granular texture.

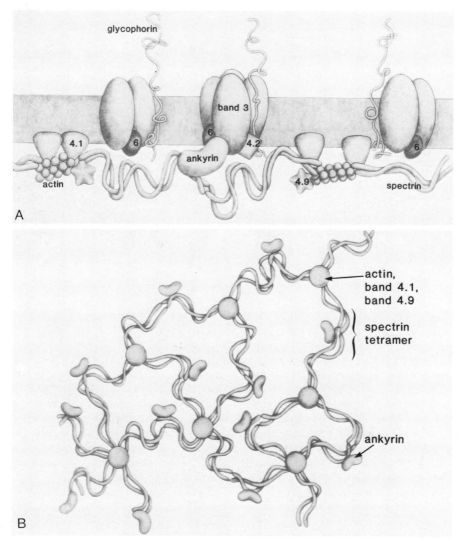

Figure 4–4. *A,* Drawing of the components of the erythrocyte cytoskeleton–a meshwork beneath the plasma membrane. The links of the network consist of dimers of spectrin joined end to end, the nodal points being a complex of spectrin, actin, and protein 4. The cytoskeleton is bound to the integral transmembrane protein 3 by a cross-linking protein, ankyrin. *B,* Drawing depicting the configuration of the cytoskeleton as it would appear in a view of the inner aspect of the erythrocyte membrane. (From C. M. Cohen, Semin. Hematol. *20*:141, 1983 by permission of Grune & Stratton, Inc.)

light upon the relationships of the cytoskeleton to the membrane not only in erythrocytes but in cells generally.

PLATELETS

The *thromboplastids* or *platelets* are minute, colorless, anucleate corpuscles found in the blood of all mammals. They are involved in the clotting of blood at sites of injury to blood vessels and are essential in the protection of the organism against excessive blood loss. Their functional equivalents in lower vertebrates are nucleated cells called *thrombocytes*.

Platelets are flat, biconvex discs 2 to 3 μm in diameter, round or ovoid when viewed on the flat and fusiform in profile when seen on edge. In human blood their number ranges from 150,000 to 350,000 per cubic millimeter. In stained blood smears they exhibit two concentric zones—a thin, pale-blue peripheral zone called the *hyalomere,* and a thicker central region, the *chromomere* or *granulomere* containing small azurophil granules.

In electron micrographs, the granulomere usually contains one or two mitochondria and numerous small clear vesicles (Fig. 4–5). Glycogen is present in the form of scattered particles. Varying numbers of membrane-bounded dense granules, 0.2 μm in diameter,

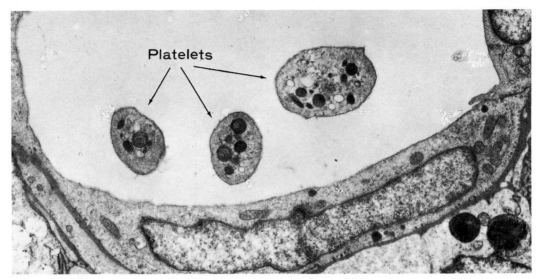

Figure 4–5. Electron micrograph of circulating platelets in the lumen of a capillary.

correspond to the azurophil granules seen with the light microscope. These are commonly called α *granules*. In some species the platelets have a second category of very dense 0.5-μm granules that are believed to contain the vasoactive substance serotonin (5-hydroxytryptamine). A few tubular invaginations extend from the plasmalemma into the interior of the platelet. These are residual elements of the system of cytoplasmic membranes in the megakaryocytes from which the platelets arise (see Chapter 7). They may have no functional significance in the mature platelet.

The hyalomere lacks membranous organelles and is characterized by a finely filamentous electron-lucent cytoplasm similar in texture to the peripheral ectoplasmic zone of leukocytes and other motile cells. Its most conspicuous structural element in equatorial sections is a bundle of 10 to 15 microtubules that run circumferentially near the plasma membrane (Fig. 4–6*B*). When cut transversely, the microtubule bundle is represented by a cluster of small circular profiles at either end of the sectioned platelet (Fig. 4–6*A*). These microtubules are a cytoskeletal specialization serving to maintain the discoid form of the platelet. A similar marginal band is found in the nucleated erythrocytes of fish, reptiles, and birds, which are also flattened biconvex discs.

Platelets contain contractile material with properties similar to those of actomyosin extracted from muscle. Under appropriate physicochemical conditions this material ex-

tracted from platelets will form in vitro thin filaments and thicker filaments identifiable as *actin* and *myosin* respectively. Thus, the mechanism of platelet contraction is believed to have features in common with that of muscle. The contractile material of circulating platelets is present mainly in monomeric form, but platelet activation during blood clotting seems to initiate polymerization of actin and myosin monomers into the filamentous form necessary for contraction.

Determinations of the life span of platelets using the isotopic label Cr^{51} indicate that they survive eight to 11 days in the normal circulation. Despite their small size and lack of a nucleus, they are able to carry out many of the metabolic activities of whole cells. They consume oxygen, are rich in adenosine triphosphate (ATP), and contain 25 or more enzymes and several pharmacologically active compounds.

The principal functions of platelets are to patch small defects in the endothelial lining of blood vessels and to limit hemorrhage by promoting local coagulation of the blood. In the circulation, platelets exhibit no tendency to adhere to each other, to other cells, or to the lining of the blood vessels, but when they encounter surfaces to which they are not normally exposed, they rapidly adhere. This adhesive property is expressed in vitro by sticking to glass, plastic, or other solid substrates. By convention, *platelet adhesion* is defined as the sticking of platelets to solid surfaces, and *platelet aggregation* is the sticking of platelets to each other.

At sites of vascular injury they adhere to damaged endothelium and to exposed collagen, forming a layer of platelets over the denuded area. The adhering platelets are activated by this contact to break down their ATP and release ADP onto their surface and into the surrounding medium. ADP is a potent inducer of platelet aggregation and other platelets stick to those initially deposited. These in turn are activated and induce further aggregation. The mass of platelets on the vessel wall thus continues to enlarge, producing a *platelet thrombus* and finally a hemostatic plug.

Concurrently with platelet aggregation, other complex reactions of blood clotting are set in motion. A substance called *tissue thromboplastin* released from the injured tissue of the vessel wall initiates a series of reactions in blood plasma that convert *prothrombin* to *thrombin*. Thrombin catalyzes the conversion of plasma *fibrinogen* to *fibrin*, which polymerizes as a feltwork of cross-striated fibrils that enmesh erythrocytes and platelets to form a gelatinous *clot*.

In the process of aggregation and activation, the platelets undergo dramatic morphological changes. They extend numerous slender processes, release the content of their granules, and ultimately coalesce into a coherent viscous mass. Associated with their degranulation, phospholipid is released, which reacts with other plasma components to produce *platelet thromboplastin*. This in turn acts to promote progression of the clotting process initiated by tissue thromboplastin.

Within an hour or so after its formation, the blood clot shrinks to about half its original volume. This is attributed to polymerization of actin and myosin filaments during the viscous metamorphosis of the platelets triggered by thrombin, and their interaction to produce contraction of the clot. The hemostasis achieved by occluding the lumen is supplemented by active constriction of the injured vessel. This is in part a direct consequence of mechanical stimulation of the vessel wall at the time of injury, but there is evidence that diffusible substances released from the platelet mass also play a role. The serotonin of the platelets may be involved and proteolytic enzymes activated in the clotting process may result in production of bradykinin and other vasoactive peptides.

The clotting process is essential for limitation of hemorrhage but can also be life-threatening when it is initiated on the walls of coronary arteries—causing *coronary thrombosis,* the basis of the familiar "heart attack." Similarly, when clots that have formed in injured veins of the extremities break loose from the vessel wall, they may be carried to the lungs, resulting in fatal *pulmonary embolism.*

Defects in platelets or in plasma factors participating in the clotting mechanism are responsible for a number of human and animal diseases. Clotting defects attributable to platelets may be due to quantitative deficiency in their production, *thrombocytopenia,* or to qualitative abnormalities of structure and function, *thrombocytopathia.* An example of the latter is the condition called *thrombasthenia,* in which platelet numbers may be normal but there is deficiency of adhesion, poor aggregation, and diminished clot retraction. In some inherited diseases such as *thrombocytopenic purpura,* a defect in platelet production is linked to abnormal fragility of the small vessels, resulting in spontaneous capillary bleeding manifested by multiple "black-and-blue" areas over the surface of the body.

Blood coagulation is an extraordinarily complex process involving the interaction of at least 12 plasma factors in addition to the platelets. Inherited single deficiencies of many of these factors have been described. The best known of these disorders is the bleeding disease *hemophilia.*

LEUKOCYTES

In addition to the red cells, the blood of all mammals contains a number of types of colorless cells, the *leukocytes* or *white blood corpuscles.* They are true cells with a nucleus and cytoplasm and all are spherical in the blood but more or less ameboid in the tissues or on a solid substrate. There are five kinds of leukocytes in the blood (Figs. 4–6, 4–8). They are categorized according to the presence or absence of specific cytoplasmic granules (*granular* and *nongranular*) and according to the shape of their nucleus (*mononuclear** or *polymorphonuclear*). The granular leukocytes are further classified according to the

---

*This misleading term would seem to imply possession of a single nucleus. All the leukocytes have one nucleus. *Mononuclear* (referring to lymphocytes and monocytes) unfortunately has come into general use as a contraction of *monomorphonuclear* (a simple unlobulated nucleus) in contrast to *polymorphonuclear* (a complex lobulated or segmented nucleus).

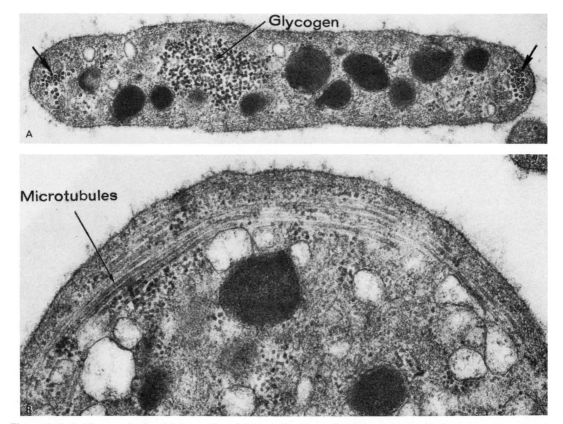

Figure 4–6. *A,* Micrograph of a platelet sectioned through its narrow dimension, showing its dense secretory granules and an aggregation of glycogen particles. At arrows are cross sections of the bundle of microtubules that runs circumferentially in the rim of the platelet. *B,* A platelet sectioned parallel to the broad dimension. Here the bundle of microtubules that helps to maintain the discoid shape of the platelet is seen in longitudinal section. (Micrographs courtesy of O. Behnke.)

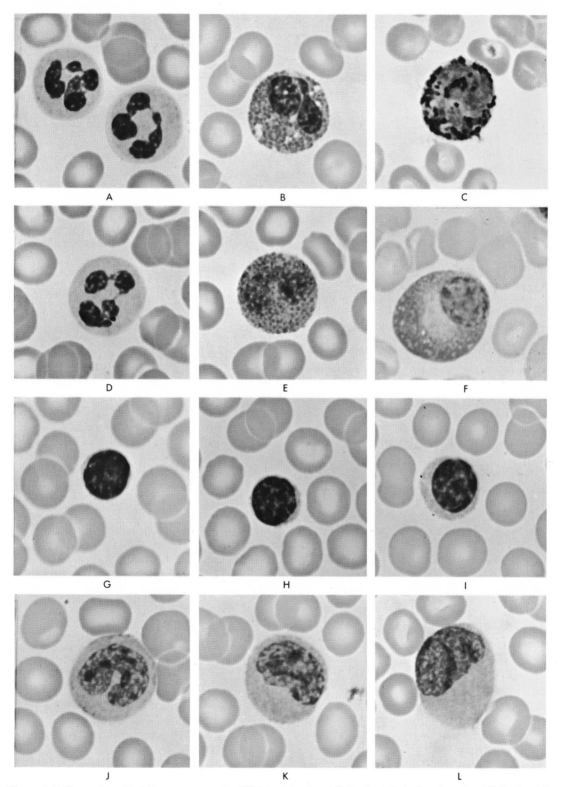

Figure 4–7. Human blood cells form a smear after Wright's stain. *A* and *D,* Neutrophilic leukocytes. *B* and *E,* Eosinophilic leukocytes. *C,* Basophilic leukocyte. *F,* Plasma cell; this is not a normal constituent of the peripheral blood but is included here for comparison with the nongranular leukocytes. *G* and *H,* Small lymphocytes. *I,* Medium lymphocytes. *J, K,* and *L,* Monocytes.

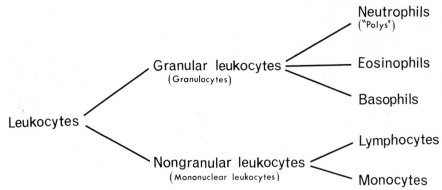

Figure 4–8. Classification of leukocytes. The granular leukocytes, especially the neutrophils, are polymorphonuclear. The nongranular leukocytes are often referred to as "mononuclear" leukocytes, an unfortunate term that implies that the others are multinuclear. The point of contrast is shape, not number of nuclei. Monomorphonuclear would more accurately describe the morphological distinction between the nongranular leukocytes and the polymorphonuclear granulocytes.

staining affinities of their granules (*neutrophils, eosinophils, basophils*).

The number of circulating leukocytes is normally in the range of 5000 to 9000 per mm³ of blood. The number is subject to some variation with age and even at different times of day in the same individual. Thus, minor variations are of little clinical significance, but in the presence of acute infections (appendicitis, pneumonia, and so forth) the *white blood count* may rise to 20,000 or even 40,000 per mm³.

The relative proportions of the various types of leukocytes are normally fairly constant: neutrophils, 55 to 60 per cent; eosinophils, 1 to 3 per cent; basophils, 0 to 0.7 per cent; lymphocytes, 25 to 33 per cent; monocytes, 3 to 7 per cent. Because different disease processes may affect the numbers of one cell type more than others, the *differential leukocyte count* is diagnostically valuable.

NEUTROPHILIC LEUKOCYTES (NEUTROPHILS)

Neutrophils are the most abundant of the leukocytes, constituting 55 to 65 per cent of the total count. In absolute numbers, there are 3000 to 6000 per mm³ or 20 to 30 billion in the circulation at any one time. They are 7 μm in diameter in the circulating blood and 10 to 12 μm in diameter in dry smears, and are easily recognized by their highly characteristic nucleus consisting of two or more lobules connected by narrow strands (Fig. 4–7A). The number of nuclear lobes depends in part on the age of the cell. When they are first released into the blood, the

nucleus has a simple elongate shape. Such cells are often described as *"band forms."* A constriction subsequently develops, resulting in a bilobed nucleus, and the process of elongation and constriction continues with time until, in older neutrophils, there may be five or more segments or lobes. The proportion of band forms or young cells in the differential count is a useful index of the rate of entry of new neutrophils into the circulation. The normal life span of these cells is about eight days, but a major part of this is spent in reserve in the bone marrow. The variability of nuclear shape is the basis for the other name applied to this cell type—*polymorphonuclear leukocyte.* In clinical parlance this is often abbreviated so that neutrophils are also referred to as "polys."

The nuclear chromatin occurs in deeply staining clumps, and a nucleolus cannot be identified. Since these cells are fully differentiated, with no synthetic capacity, they no longer need a nucleolus for assembly of ribosomal RNA. In a small proportion of the neutrophils of women, the chromatin representing the condensed X chromosomes forms a minute separate lobule—often described as the *"drumstick"* because of its characteristic shape (Fig. 4–9). Thus, it is possible to determine from a blood smear the genetic sex of the individual by examining a large number of neutrophils for the presence of this nuclear appendage.

The cytoplasm of the neutrophil, when properly stained, is stippled with very small granules that have little affinity for the dyes. These are the so-called *specific granules* (Fig. 4–7A, D). In addition to these, there are larger, reddish-purple *azurophil granules*. The

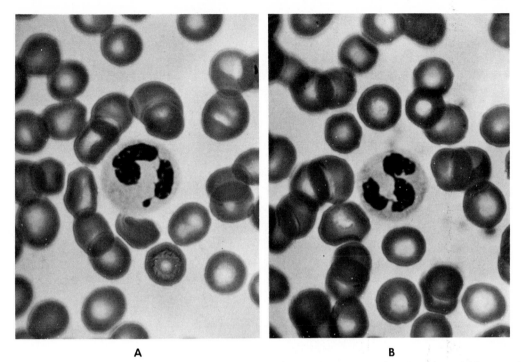

A   B

Figure 4–9. *A,* Erythrocytes and a neutrophilic leukocyte from a woman showing the "drumstick" appendage characteristic of the female. *B,* A comparable field from the blood smear of a man. (Photomicrograph courtesy of M. Barr.)

granules are often quite inconspicuous in routinely stained smears and they are therefore studied to better advantage in living leukocytes viewed by phase-contrast microscopy or in electron micrographs. In the guinea pig and rabbit, the granules are more conspicuous than in the human, and are stainable with either acid or basic dyes but show a predilection for eosin. Therefore, in these species these cells are sometimes called *pseudoeosinophils.*

In electron micrographs of human leukocytes the neutrophil granules may be found almost anywhere in the cell, but they tend to be absent from a thin peripheral zone of cytoplasm, which is rich in fine filaments that seem to be concerned with cell motility (Fig. 4–10). Centrally situated in the cell adjacent to the nucleus is a small Golgi complex and a pair of centrioles. The specific granules are round or elongate like rice grains. In some species the azurophil granules are more spherical and distinctly larger, but in neutrophils of humans it is difficult to distinguish the granule types on morphological criteria alone. However, the enzyme myeloperoxidase is localized exclusively in the azurophil granules (Fig. 4–11) and can be used as a cytochemical marker to identify this granule type. In addition to peroxidase, the azurophil

granules contain histochemically demonstrable acid phosphatase, β-glucuronidase, and a number of other hydrolytic enzymes for which no staining method exists. They are therefore regarded as primary lysosomes. The specific granules, which greatly outnumber the azurophils, lack lysosomal enzymes but contain alkaline phosphatase and a variety of poorly characterized basic proteins, called *phagocytins,* which have significant antibacterial activity.

Neutrophils are in the first line of defense of the body against invasion by pathogenic bacteria. At sites of inflammation, they adhere to the walls of postcapillary venules and their ameboid motility enables them to insinuate themselves between the endothelial cells and into the connective tissues to attack bacteria. The neutrophils are avidly phagocytic; i.e., they have the capacity to extend pseudopods around bacteria, take them into their cytoplasm in membrane-bounded vacuoles (Fig. 4–14), and destroy them with hydrolytic enzymes. In the presence of bacterial infection, a message is somehow transmitted to the bone marrow that stimulates increased production and release of neutrophils. Thus, the number of circulating polymorphonuclear leukocytes increases and the percentage of young band forms is elevated.

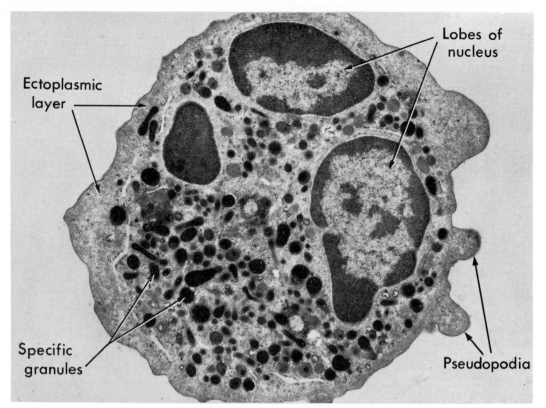

Figure 4–10. Electron micrograph of a guinea pig polymorphonuclear leukocyte. The nucleus has several lobes that appear separate in this plane of section. The cytoplasm is filled with specific granules of varying shape. A thin ectoplasmic zone of cytoplasm rich in actin is important in pseudopod formation and ameboid locomotion of the cell.

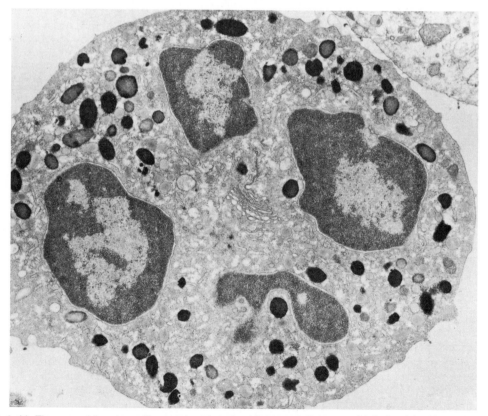

Figure 4–11. The azurophil and specific granules of neutrophils are not always easily distinguished in routine electron micrographs, but in this neutrophil stained by the cytochemical reaction for peroxidase, only the azurophil granules (primary lysosomes) are stained. (From Bainton, D., J. Ullyot, and M. Farquhar. J. Exp. Med. *134*:907, 1971.)

Although neutrophils are able to take in other types of particles by *nonspecific phagocytosis*, they are especially effective against bacteria. Their efficiency in this defensive role is enhanced if the body has developed specific antibodies as a result of previous exposure to the same type of bacteria. Under these circumstances, blood-borne antibody (IgG) binds to the surface antigen of the bacterium and a derivative of the complement system of the plasma (C_3b) binds to the antigen-antibody complex. IgG and C_3b act as ligands binding the bacterium to specific receptors for these molecules present in the plasma membrane of neutrophils. Attachment and interiorization of the bacterium is thereby facilitated. Plasma components such as IgG and C_3b that coat bacteria are collectively called *opsonins*. Phagocytosis of opsonized particles is described as *immune-phagocytosis* to distinguish it from nonspecific uptake of particles that have not been coated with ligands.

The neutrophil responds to attachment of the particle by local invagination and by extension of pseudopods (Fig. 4–12). As the enveloping pseudopods bring more of the cell surface into contact with the surface of the bacterium, the ligand-receptor binding spreads laterally from the point of initial contact, tightly zippering up the cell membrane to the surface of the bacterium around its entire circumference, so that it becomes enclosed in a deep recess in the leukocyte surface. When the enveloping cell processes meet beyond the bacterium, their membranes fuse. The invaginated membrane and its enclosed bacterium separate from the plasmalemma and move into the cytoplasm as a *phagocytic vacuole* (Fig. 4–13). The membrane of one or more lysosomal granules then coalesces with the membrane of the vacuole, discharging into it their hydrolytic enzymes (Fig. 4–14) to digest the bacterium.

Another mechanism associated with phagocytosis by neutrophils is the generation of

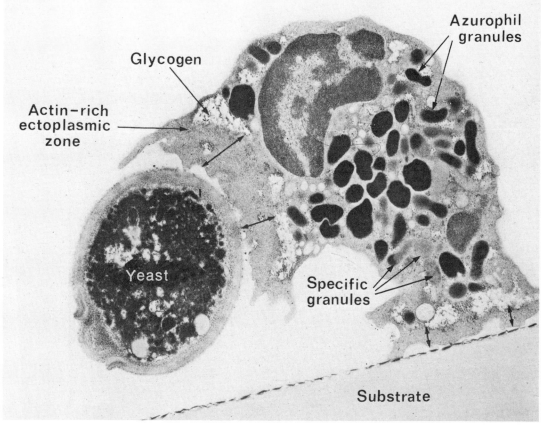

Figure 4–12. The highly motile, avidly phagocytic neutrophils accumulating at sites of inflammation are the first line of defense against invading microorganisms. Shown here is a neutrophil beginning to phagocytize a yeast in vitro. Notice the thickening of the ectoplasmic zone *(double arrows)* and extension of lamellipodia in the region of contact with the organism. (Micrograph courtesy of D. Bainton.)

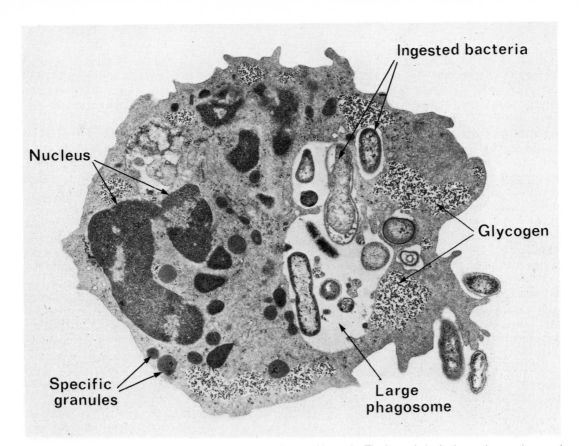

Figure 4–13. Micrograph of a neutrophil that has ingested several bacteria. The bacteria in the large phagocytic vacuole show signs of incipient degeneration resulting from this bacteriostatic and hydrolytic environment. (Micrograph courtesy of D. Bainton.)

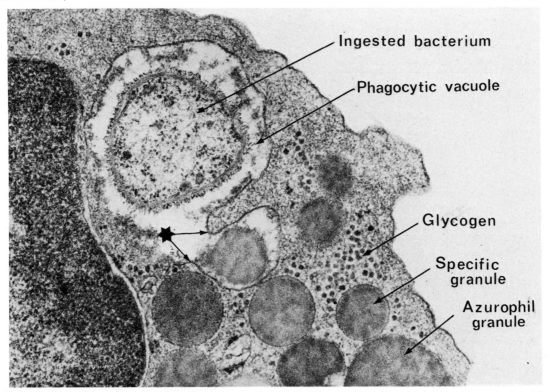

Figure 4–14. Portion of a neutrophil that has recently phagocytized a bacterium. Arrows (⋆) show the continuity of the membrane of the phagosome with that of a granule about to discharge its contents into the phagosome. (Micrograph from D. Bainton. *In* Williams, R. C. and H. H. Fudenberg, eds. Phagocytic Mechanisms in Health and Disease. New York, Intercontinental Medical Book Corporation, 1972, p. 130.)

superoxide anions by an oxidase present on their surface membrane. Some of the superoxide is converted to hydrogen peroxide and both are carried into the phagocytosis vacuoles. There, in the presence of myeloperoxidase contributed by coalescing lysosomes, hydrogen peroxide reacts with chloride ions to form hypochlorite—a potent bactericide.

Much has been learned about the role of the lysosomal azurophil granules, but much less is known about how the specific granules exert their antibacterial effect. However, it is clear that these cells have evolved multiple complementary bactericidal strategies. The pus that accumulates in boils and abscesses consists of millions of dead and dying neutrophilic leukocytes that have carried out their mission.

The azurophil and specific granules of the polymorphonuclear leukocytes function primarily in the intracellular destruction of foreign invaders. These cells are not considered to be secretory in the usual sense. However, under certain circumstances the hydrolytic enzymes that are normally confined within the membranes of granules or within phagocytosis vacuoles may escape into the surrounding tissue. Fusion of lysosomes may occur before closure of the phagocytosis vacuole, resulting in leakage of degradative enzymes into the extracellular space. This is especially apt to occur if the ratio of particles to phagocytes is high or when the foreign particle size is too large to be completely ingested. Among the enzymes escaping are collagenase and elastase, which can break down collagenous and elastic fibers, and other proteases that may attack cellular components of the connective tissue. Thus, the neutrophils may damage, to some extent, the tissues they are defending. Such effects may contribute to the pain and swelling at sites of inflammation.

EOSINOPHILIC LEUKOCYTES (EOSINOPHILS)

Eosinophils arise from precursors in the bone marrow. After three or four days of maturation the eosinophil is released and probably spends only three or four hours in the bloodstream en route to the connective tissues, where it remains for the remainder of its eight- to 12-day life span. Eosinophils represent 1 to 3 per cent of the total population of blood leukocytes, but for every one in the blood there are about 300 in the tissues. They are 9 μm in diameter in suspension and about 12 μm when flattened out in dried blood smears. Eosinophils are easily recognized by their relatively coarse specific granules, which stain pink with Wright's blood stain (Fig. 4–7B, E). The nucleus is less segmented than that of neutrophils and usually appears bilobed. In rats and mice, the nucleus has a ring form. The chromatin pattern is less coarse than it is in neutrophils. There is a granule-free cell center around a pair of centrioles, a small Golgi apparatus, and a few mitochondria. The endoplasmic reticulum is not extensive.

The most conspicuous feature of this cell is its specific granules. These display rather striking interspecific variations in their ultrastructure. In laboratory rodents, each granule contains a single, equatorial, discoid crystal (Fig. 4–15). In humans the crystals may be single or multiple and quite variable in form. In cats, eosinophil granules have a dense cylindrical inclusion with a concentric lamellar substructure. In all species, the crystalline inclusions are embedded in an amorphous or finely granular matrix and enclosed by a membrane.

Upon isolation and analysis, eosinophil granules contain several of the lysosomal enzymes but are unusually rich in peroxidase. Lysozyme and phagocytin, the antibacterial agents present in the specific granules of neutrophils, are lacking in eosinophil granules. In addition to the specific granules, eosinophils contain a few azurophil granules and thus have two classes of primary lysosomes. The eosinophil granules also contain a protein of 11,000 M.W. rich in the amino acid arginine. This *major basic protein* (MBP) present in the crystalloids is thought to be responsible for the strong affinity of eosinophil granules for acid dyes. The granules also contain myeloperoxidase, arylsulfatase, β-glucuronidase, acid phosphatase, ribonuclease, and cathepsin.

The precise role of eosinophils in the body's defense mechanisms is not well defined. They are greatly increased in number in parasitic diseases and various forms of allergy. Repeated injections of foreign protein are attended by local and general increases in eosinophils mobilized from large reserves in the bone marrow. They do not normally phagocytize bacteria, but they do selectively ingest and destroy antigen-antibody complexes. Eosinophils appear to be attracted to sites where basophils and mast cells abound. They are believed to respond

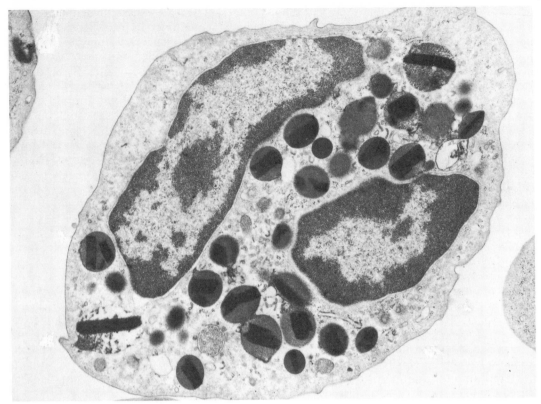

Figure 4–15. Micrograph of a guinea pig eosinophilic leukocyte. The specific granules contain one or more dense polyhedral crystals.

to *eosinophil chemotactic factors* released by basophils and mast cells. Just how they interact with these cells is not known but they may counteract the inflammatory effects produced by the histamine and other mediators that these cells secrete. Although eosinophils are found in connective tissue throughout the body, they are especially numerous beneath the epithelia of the alimentary and respiratory tracts where penetration of foreign antigens is likely to occur.

The factors regulating release of eosinophils from the marrow are poorly understood but there is evidence suggesting that a diffusible substance formed at sites of antigen-antibody interaction in inflamed tissue is carried back to the marrow, causing discharge of more eosinophils into the circulation. Injections of adrenocortical hormone or hydrocortisone result in a marked reduction in circulating eosinophils. It is believed that these hormones exert this effect by interfering with the mobilization of eosinophil reserves from the marrow.

BASOPHILIC LEUKOCYTES (BASOPHILS)

Basophils are the least numerous of the granulocytes, accounting for only 0.5 per cent of the total leukocyte count. They are slightly smaller than neutrophils, measuring about 10 μm in diameter in stained blood smears. The elongated nucleus is often bent into a U or J shape and may appear bilobed, but segmentation is less obvious than in other granulocytes. The specific granules are larger, fewer, and less closely packed than those of eosinophils (Fig. 4–7C). They are metachromatic, staining purple with toluidine blue or alcoholic thionine. They are water soluble in the human and with aqueous stains may be distorted and partially dissolved, but in dried smears, or in tissue sections after alcoholic fixation, they are usually preserved. Their properties vary in different species. The large oval granules of guinea pig basophils are insoluble in water but stain only faintly. In the dog, the granules are quite small and are assembled in a compact group. Basophilic leukocytes seem to be absent from the circulation in cat, rat, and mouse.

In electron micrographs, basophils have a small Golgi apparatus, a few mitochondria, and occasional strands of endoplasmic reticulum. The cytoplasmic matrix contains varying amounts of glycogen. The specific granules are round, oval, or angular and about 1.2 μm in diameter (Fig. 4–16). They have a substructure composed of 12- to 26-nm dense particles embedded in a less dense matrix. In some other mammalian species, the dense subunits of the basophil granules are arranged in a highly ordered lattice. Basophil granules are *peroxidase* positive and contain *histamine* and the sulfated mucopolysaccharide *heparin,* which is responsible for their metachromasia. There is no evidence at present that they contain lysosomal enzymes.

The basophils of the blood have a number of properties in common with the mast cells of connective tissues. Both have metachromatic granules containing histamine and heparin. Both are degranulated by histamine-liberating drugs and when exposed to antigen in sensitized individuals. Many investigators formerly considered the basophil to be a circulating form of the mast cell, but it is now generally agreed that they are from distinct cell lines. The basophils arise in the bone marrow; the mast cells probably originate from precursors in the connective tissue, but this is debated. The basophil is much smaller and has a polymorphous nucleus and fewer granules. It is the current view that although these two cell types have different origins, their functions are very similar. The tissue mast cells are relatively sessile whereas the circulating basophils can be rapidly mobilized at sites where they are needed to supplement the resident population of mast cells.

An important property of basophils and mast cells is the presence in their surface membrane of specific receptors for immunoglobulin E (IgE). IgE is a minor component of normal blood serum but may be increased up to 20-fold in persons suffering from hay fever, asthma, or allergic dermatitis. It is the *reaginic antibody* (i.e., antibody against allergens) that results in *immediate hypersensitivity,* as opposed to delayed, *cell-mediated hypersensitivity* (see Chapter 13). Human basophils carry from 10,000 to 40,000 molecules of IgE bound to their surface receptors. When an allergen is introduced into the tissues, it combines with IgE on the basophils and mast cells. This triggers their rapid degranulation and release of histamine and other mediators. The histamine released is in part responsible for itching and in-

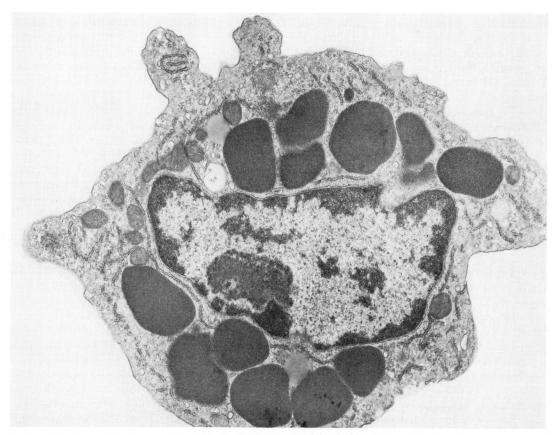

Figure 4–16. Micrograph of a basophil leukocyte. The large granules are somewhat irregular in outline and vary in their density.

creased permeability of postcapillary venules that results in tissue edema and local swelling.

Basophils that have migrated from the blood into the dermis and subcutaneous connective tissue are now recognized as major participants in the form of cell-mediated immunity called *cutaneous basophil hypersensitivity.* Although in the blood there are only 30 to 40 basophils per mm^3, they are found in concentrations of 300 to 600 per linear millimeter in sections of skin from previously sensitized guinea pigs reacting to a challenging dose of parenterally administered antigen.

LYMPHOCYTES

Lymphocytes are the second most numerous class of leukocytes in the blood, constituting 20 to 35 per cent of the circulating white blood cells. In blood smears, they are small spherical cells with an intensely staining, slightly indented nucleus, and a thin rim of clear blue cytoplasm (Fig. 4–7G, H). They are 7 to 9 μm in diameter, which is only slightly larger than the erythrocytes. They contain no specific granules. In electron micrographs they have a small Golgi complex, a pair of centrioles, and a few mitochondria. Endoplasmic reticulum is usually lacking but the cytoplasm is rich in ribosomes. Occasionally observed are small, dense lysosomes that correspond to the azurophil granules reported by hematologists.

Histologists traditionally categorized lymphocytes as large, medium, and small on the basis of their diameter and relative amount of cytoplasm. These were thought to represent successive stages in their evolution from a larger precursor, the lymphoblast. The small lymphocytes were long considered to be an end stage capable of surviving only a few days, after which they were believed to degenerate or to be eliminated from the body by migration into the lumen of the intestine. When methods were developed for radiolabeling cells, following their migrations and measuring their longevity, the traditional interpretation of lymphocytes proved to be erroneous. It is now known that there are two functionally distinct categories of small lymphocytes designated *B lymphocytes* and *T lymphocytes.* These differ in their developmental background, life span, and functions. They are not distinguishable morphologically, but distinctive surface markers can be detected by immunofluorescence.

The lymphocytes are the cells principally involved in the immune responses of the body, and their functions will be discussed in greater detail in a later section on the immune system (Chapter 13). It suffices here to describe briefly what those responses are. When foreign substances in the environment, usually proteins or polysaccharides, get into the body, they stimulate formation of *immune globulins* that circulate in the blood plasma and are capable of combining with and neutralizing the harmful effects of the inducing substance. An animal that has become protected in this way is said to have developed an *immunity.* The substance that induces an immune response is called an *antigen* and the specific globulin molecules that appear in the blood to counteract it are called *antibodies.*

When an antigen is introduced into the body for the first time, there is a conditioning of the antibody-producing cells or their precursors that extends over a number of weeks and may result in low levels of circulating antibody. The events taking place in this latent period are described as the *primary response.* If a second exposure to the same antigen occurs weeks or months afterward, there is a dramatic and rapid rise in synthesis of antibody globulin, resulting in a titer of circulating antibody 10 to 100 times the previous level. This is called the *secondary response.* If a number of injections of antigen are given, the elevated level of circulating antibody may be maintained for years. This component of the bodily defenses, which depends on blood-borne antibodies, is called the *humoral immune response.* The lymphocytes are the cells that recognize an antigen as foreign to the body and respond to an initial encounter by undergoing certain changes that may have no effect upon their appearance but which endow them with a specific "memory" for that antigen, which conditions their behavior when exposed at a later time to the same antigen.

If lymphocytes are placed in tissue culture and stimulated by phytohemagglutinin or other mitogens, they enlarge, acquire increased numbers of ribosomes, and take on the appearance of large lymphoblasts (Fig. 4–18). After this initial period of hypertrophy, they begin to divide. This unexplained stimulation by phytohemagglutinin is of interest because it duplicates in vitro the normal response of lymphocytes upon exposure to antigens in vivo. The repeated division of lymphoblastic cells gives rise to clones of "memory cells," each of which expresses on

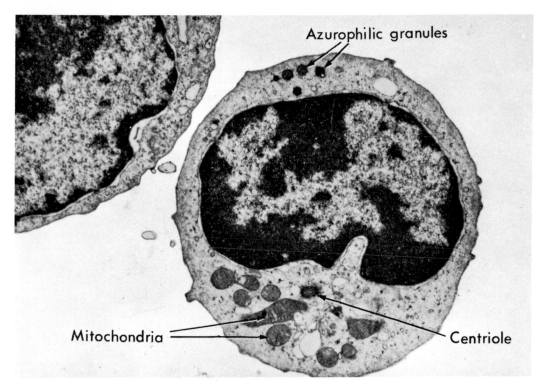

Figure 4–17. Micrograph of a guinea pig lymphocyte. The nucleus is indented and has a coarse pattern of heterochromatin. A centriole and several mitochondria are seen in the cytoplasm. Although it is a nongranular leukocyte, the lymphocyte may contain a few small azurophil granules.

its surface specific combining sites or receptors for the inducing antigen. Some of these lymphocytes go on to differentiate into *plasma cells*, which synthesize specific antibody against that antigen. The proliferative response of lymphocytes in response to antigen thus serves to amplify the production of specific antibody. Although we refer to B lymphocytes as a single class, there are, in an immunological sense, as many kinds of memory lymphocytes as the number of different antigens that have, at one time or another, invaded the body.

The T and B lymphocytes do not function independently in the immune response. For many antigens, subpopulations of T cells are required to provide an additional stimulus to the B cells for the production of antibody to occur. These are designated *"helper" T cells.* Other subpopulations of T cells are capable of depressing production of antibody by B cells. These are called *"suppressor" T cells.* The mechanism of T-cell regulation of B-cell function is unclear. It is not evident whether direct contact between the interacting cells is required in vivo or whether diffusible products of the T cells are involved.

T lymphocytes participate in a number of immunological processes in addition to the regulation of antibody production. They have the capacity to seek out antigenic foreign cells and to interact with macrophages so as to promote destruction of the foreign cells by cytotoxic and phagocytic mechanisms. Protective reactions of this kind are distinguished from the humoral immune response by the term *cell-mediated immunity.*

The mechanisms of the interaction of lymphocytes and macrophages in immunological responses are still poorly understood. In in vitro studies, T-cell functions, such as antigen-dependent proliferation and development of "helper" capacity, have been shown to require a contribution from macrophages. Conversely, several macrophage functions are modified by interaction with immune T cells and appropriate antigen. The biologically active molecules produced by lymphocytes in their immunoregulatory functions are called *lymphokines.* An increasing number of these are being identified. One that has attracted intense interest is *interferon,* which has the capacity to inhibit replication of certain viruses and suppress the multiplication of some intracellular parasites. It also enhances several functions of macrophages including phagocytosis. In addition, interferon is reported to inhibit proliferation of normal

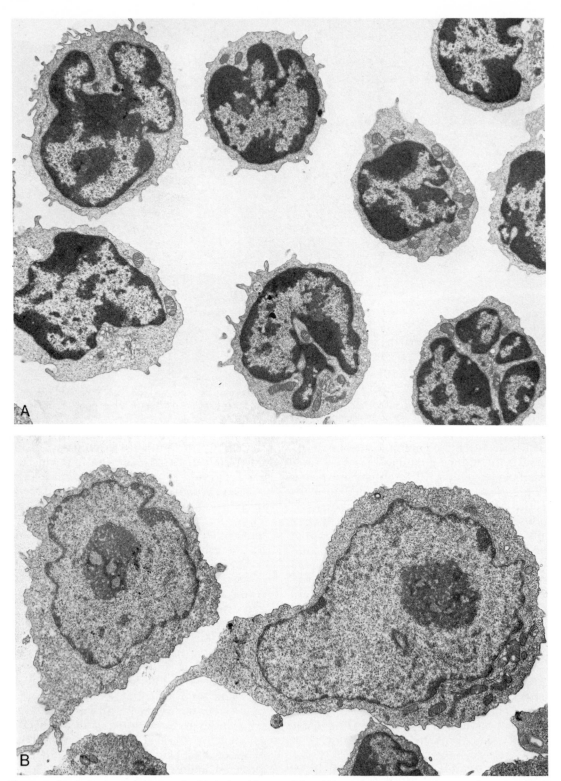

Figure 4–18. *A,* Bovine lymphocytes freshly isolated from peripheral blood and placed in culture medium containing a lectin, concanavalin A. *B,* At the same magnification, after 72 hours in culture many of the lymphocytes have transformed into metabolically active large lymphoblasts with prominent nucleoli and little heterochromatin. This in vitro transformation mimics that occurring in vivo when lymphocytes are exposed to antigen.

and malignant cells in vitro, and its potential for suppressing the growth of cancers is now being explored.

The lymphocytes were formerly believed to arise almost exclusively in the lymph nodes and other lymphoid organs, while other leukocytes were formed in the bone marrow. The principal basis for this assumption was the observation that if the thoracic duct, which drains lymph and lymphocytes from the lymph nodes back to the bloodstream, was severed and exteriorized, the number of lymphocytes in the blood rapidly fell. Since the number entering the blood daily from this source was very large, it seemed reasonable to infer that their life span must be very short, for if a comparable number were not leaving the blood daily, the lymphocyte count would rise rapidly to astronomical numbers. Neither of the conclusions drawn from these observations has proved to be correct.

It is now known that large numbers of B lymphocytes are generated in the bone marrow. Approximately one quarter of all the nucleated marrow cells are lymphocytes. Although some of these no doubt belong to the pool of recirculating long-lived B and T lymphocytes, many of them arise from stem cells in the marrow, and continuously emigrate to the peripheral lymphoid organs as virgin B lymphocytes capable of mediating primary humoral immune responses. Primary B lymphocytes are constantly turning over in the peripheral lymphoid tissues. Labeled young lymphocytes persist in spleen and lymph nodes for only about a week. The large-scale genesis and emigration of B lymphocytes in the marrow suggests that the population of rapidly renewing primary B lymphocytes in the spleen is maintained almost exclusively by the continuous influx of cells from the marrow. Most of these studies have been carried out on mice but it seems likely that the same events occur in humans, although the time course may differ.

The first indication that the lymphocytes in lymphoid organs were transient residents arising elsewhere came from experiments that antedated application of radiolabeling with tritiated thymidine. It was observed that a thoracic duct fistula resulted not only in a decrease in the number of blood lymphocytes, but also in a gradual diminution in the number of lymphocytes emerging from the duct. If this outflow depended solely on new formation of lymphocytes in the lymph nodes, the output from the thoracic duct should have been maintained. Thus, it was shown that the lymphocytes entering the blood from the thoracic duct are not all newly formed in the nodes, as had been thought. A substantial proportion enter the nodes from the blood, remain for a while, and then leave via the lymph. When tritiated thymidine is infused into the afferent lymphatic to a node, it is found that fewer than 5 per cent of the emerging cells are labeled. The vast majority have traversed the node from the blood.

It is now universally accepted that lymphocytes are continually migrating between lymph nodes, spleen, and connective tissues, using the blood as a common path. The lymphocytes found in the blood, despite their uniform appearance, consist of different populations. The majority are part of the recirculating pool of long-lived (months to years) lymphocytes, capable of participating in cell-mediated immunity. A smaller proportion are short-lived (weeks or months) but are capable of transformation to antibody-producing cells on antigenic stimulation (see Chapter 13).

MONOCYTES

The typical *monocyte* measures 9 to 12 μm in diameter, but in blood smears, where monocytes are greatly flattened in the drying process, they may be up to 17 μm in diameter. They constitute 3 to 8 per cent of the leukocytes of the circulating blood. Their enumeration is subject to some error because they cannot always be sharply differentiated from large lymphocytes. The cytoplasm is more abundant than in lymphocytes, and instead of a clear, pale blue, it tends to have a grayish-blue tint with scattered small azurophil granules (Fig. 4–7 *J, K, L*). In older monocytes, the nucleus is eccentric in position and oval or reniform. Its chromatin is more finely granular and more uniformly dispersed in the nucleoplasm, so that the nucleus as a whole appears less intensely stained. One or more nucleoli are present but are seldom seen in routine blood smears.

In electron micrographs the nucleoli are obvious, and the cytoplasm contains a conspicuous Golgi complex, a few cisternal profiles of rough endoplasmic reticulum, a moderate number of free ribosomes, and some glycogen granules. In addition, there are in each section 15 to 20 granules with a dense homogeneous content (Fig. 4–19). These correspond to the azurophil granules seen in stained smears. They exhibit cytochemical staining reactions for acid phosphatase, arylsulfatase, and peroxidase, and hence are considered to be primary lysosomes.

The origin of monocytes and their relation to lymphocytes were long obscured by the contradictory theories of blood formation. More recently, experiments involving radio-labeling of cells of the marrow and lymphoid organs and their transfusion into x-irradiated host animals have now resolved much of this controversy. It has been convincingly demonstrated that monocytes originate in the bone marrow from precursors called *promonocytes.* After a developmental period of one to three days they enter the circulation. Those found in the peripheral blood represent cells in transit from the marrow to their ultimate destination in the tissues. They spend only about a day and a half in the blood, then migrate into the connective tissue of various organs throughout the body, where they differentiate into tissue macrophages. They are capable of mitotic division and of continued enzyme synthesis in the tissues. They seem to perform no function while in the blood but survive for months in the tissues, where they are a mobile reserve of scavengers that play a valuable defensive role by phagocytosis and intracellular digestion of invading microorganisms. They may also be essential for the processing of antigens prior to the development of antibodies by immunocompetent lymphoid cells associated with them in the tissues.

OTHER COMPONENTS OF BLOOD

Since blood is a tissue composed of cells suspended in a fluid extracellular matrix, the *blood plasma,* it may be appropriate to comment briefly on some of the more important constituents of this matrix. There are three major types of plasma proteins—*albumin, globulin,* and *fibrinogen.*

Albumin is the most abundant and smallest of the plasma proteins with M.W. of about 59,000. It is synthesized by the liver and its principal function is to maintain the colloid

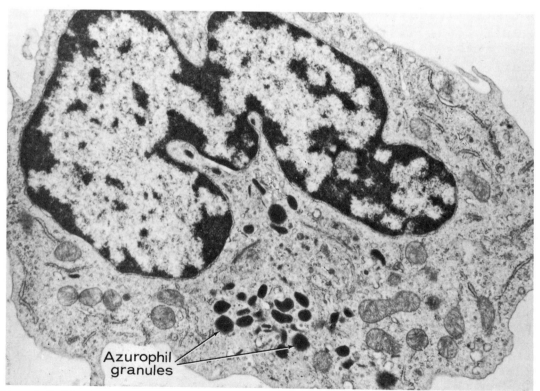

Figure 4–19. Micrograph of a typical rabbit monocyte showing its irregularly shaped nucleus, occasional cisternal profiles of rough endoplasmic reticulum, and a small cluster of azurophil granules (lysosomes) near the Golgi complex. (Micrograph courtesy of D. Bainton.)

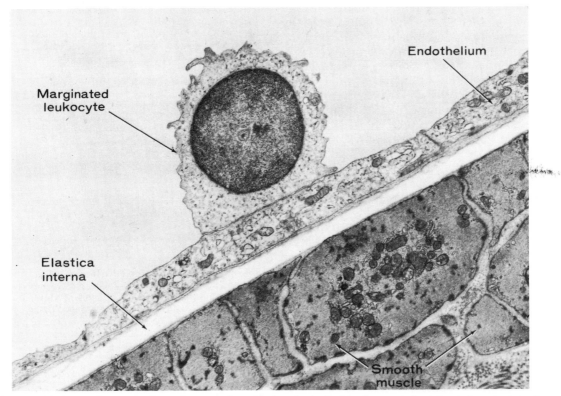

Figure 4–20. At one time or another, a large number of leukocytes in the blood are not circulating but are temporarily adherent to the endothelium of small blood vessels as shown here. This population is referred to as the "marginated pool" of leukocytes.

osmotic pressure within the blood capillaries, which prevents excessive loss of fluid to the tissues. In addition, a variety of substances that are relatively insoluble in water dissolve more readily in the presence of blood proteins. Plasma albumin plays an important part in the transport of these metabolic products.

The globulins include proteins of a wide range of M.W., 80,000 to several million. They are divided into several fractions. The greatest interest is centered on the *gamma globulins* because this fraction includes the *immune globulins* or *antibodies*, which are the basis of the immunological defenses of the body against bacteria, toxins, and other foreign proteins. These important globulins are synthesized in the cells of the lymphoid organs. The *beta globulins* function in the transport of hormones, metal ions, and lipid.

The beta globulin called *transferrin* combines with iron, copper, and zinc. Its principal function is to transport iron. In conditions in which there is increased need for iron for hemoglobin synthesis, as in nutritional deficiency of iron or in pregnancy, there is a compensatory increase in this trans-

port protein in the plasma. In liver disease or pernicious anemia, the concentration of transferrin is reduced. A protein of rather similar function, *ceruloplasmin*, contains nearly all the copper of the blood and is believed to regulate utilization of copper by reversibly binding and releasing it at various sites in the body. In the rare inherited disorder of copper metabolism, Wilson's disease, ceruloplasmin is markedly reduced.

Serum lipoproteins, globulins involved in lipid transport, attain such a large size that they can be visualized electron microscopically as spherical particulates of varying size. They can therefore be included among the microscopic formed elements of the blood. These serum lipoproteins can be separated from plasma by physical techniques of ultracentrifugal flotation or electrophoresis, and are divided into four major groups on the basis of size. (1) The *chylomicrons,* ranging in size from 100 nm to 500 nm are the largest and are detectable by dark-field light microscopy. (2) The *very-low-density lipoproteins* (VLDL) generally fall within a size range of 25 to 70 nm and are not visible by light microscopy. (3) The *low-density* or *beta lipopro-*

teins (LDL) are considerably smaller. In addition to their characteristic sizes, the lipoproteins are distinguishable biochemically by their differing proportions of various classes of lipids associated with specific apoproteins.

In the nutrition of mammals, the lipoproteins are the form in which lipids absorbed in the gastrointestinal tract are transported in the blood to the liver. The chylomicrons formed in the absorptive epithelium of the intestine are transiently increased in the blood after a fat-rich meal. The VLDL are the form in which lipid is transported from the liver to the adipose tissue.

Other classes of lipoproteins are persistently elevated in certain disease conditions. The continued presence of high circulating levels of lipoprotein is thought to predispose to atherosclerosis, or hardening of the arteries. The normal lipoproteins are spherical droplets or particles but, interestingly enough, in diseases involving obstruction of the bile duct, abnormal lipoproteins, which have an unusual discoid shape, may appear in the blood. These easily associate in rouleaux under the usual conditions of isolation and negative staining.

Plasma clotting factors are the major defense of the body against serious blood loss. An essential component of this mechanism is *fibrinogen,* a protein synthesized in the liver and circulating in the blood plasma as long, asymmetrical molecules of 330,000 M.W. When *prothrombin,* also present in plasma, is activated by *thromboplastin* of tissue or platelet origin, enzymatically active *thrombin* is produced, resulting in polymerization of fibrin to form the fibrous meshwork of a clot. Various hemorrhagic disorders may result from impaired synthesis of fibrinogen or deficiency of prothrombin.

REFERENCES

ERYTHROCYTES

Bessis, M., and J. P. Thiéry: Les cellules du sang vues au microscope à interférences (système Nomarski). Rev. d'Hematol. *12*:518, 1957.

Bennett, V., and D. Branton: Selective association of spectrin with the cytoplasmic surface of human erythrocyte plasma membranes. J. Biol. Chem. *252*:2753, 1977.

Bennett, V., and P. J. Stenbuck: Human erythrocyte ankyrin. Purification and properties. J. Biol. Chem. *255*:2540, 1980.

Bishop, C., and D. M. Surgenor, eds.: The Red Blood Cells. New York, Academic Press, 1964.

Branton, D., C. M. Cohen, and J. Tyler: Interaction of cytoskeletal proteins on human erythrocyte membrane. Cell *24*: 24, 1981.

Cohen, C. M.: The molecular organization of the red-cell membrane skeleton. Sem. Hematol. *20*:141, 1983.

Harrison, P. R.: Analysis of erythropoiesis at the molecular level. Nature *262*:353, 1976.

Ingram, V.: The Hemoglobins in Genetics and Evolution. New York, Columbia University Press, 1963.

Patek, J., and S. E. Lux: Red Cell membrane skeletal defects in hereditary and acquired hemolytic anemias. Sem. Hematol. *20*:189, 1983.

Perutz, M. F.: Hemoglobin structure and respiratory transport. Sci. Am. *239*:92, 1978.

PLATELETS

Biggs, R., and R. G. Macfarlane: Human Blood Coagulation and Its Disorders. 3rd ed. Philadelphia, F. A. Davis Co., 1962.

Fox, J. E. B., and D. R. Phillips: Polymerization and organization of actin filaments within platelets. Sem. Hematol. *20*:243, 1983.

Johnson, S. A., R. W. Monto, J. W. Rebuck, and R. C. Horn, Jr., eds.: Blood Platelets (A Symposium). Boston, Little, Brown & Co., 1961.

Marcus, A. J., and M. B. Zucker: The Physiology of Blood Platelets. New York, Grune & Stratton, 1965.

Shattil, S. J., and J. S. Bennett: Platelets and their membranes in hemostasis: physiology and pathophysiology. Ann. Intern. Med. *94*:108, 1981.

Weiss, H. J.: Platelet physiology and abnormalities of platelet function. N. Engl. J. Med. *203*:531, 580, 1975.

White, J. G., and C. C. Clauson: Biostructure of platelets. Ultrastruct. Pathol. *1*:533, 1980.

NEUTROPHILS

Anderson, D. R.: Ultrastructure of normal and leukemic leukocytes in human peripheral blood. J. Ultrastr. Res. (Suppl.):5, 1966.

Athens, J. W.: Granulocyte kinetics in health and disease. Natl. Cancer Inst. Monogr. *30*:135, 1969.

Bainton, D. F.: Primary lysosomes of blood leukocytes. *In* Dingle, J. T., and R. T. Dean, eds.: Lysosomes in Biology and Pathology. Amsterdam, North Holland Publishing Co., 1976.

Cohn, Z. A., and S. I. Morse: Functional and metabolic properties of polymorphonuclear leukocytes. I. Observations on the requirements and consequences of particle ingestion. J. Exp. Med. *111*:667, 1960.

Daems, W.: On the fine structure of human neutrophilic leukocyte granules. J. Ultrastruct. Res. *24*:343, 1968.

Hirsch, J. G., and Z. A. Cohn: Degranulation of polymorphonuclear leukocytes following phagocytosis of microorganisms. J. Exp. Med. *118*:1005, 1960.

Klebanoff, S. J.: Antimicrobial mechanisms in neutrophilic polymorphonuclear leukocytes. Sem. Hematol. *12*:117, 1975.

Lisiewicz, J.: Human Neutrophils. Bowie, MD, Charles Press Publishers, 1980.

Murphy, P.: The Neutrophil. New York, Plenum Publishing Co., 1976.

Spitznagel, J. K., F. G. Dalldorf, and M. S. Liffell: Characterization of azurophil and specific granules purified from human polymorphonuclear leukocytes. Lab. Invest. *30*:774, 1978.

Weissmann, G., R. B. Zurier, P. J. Spieler, and I. M. Goldstein: Mechanisms of lysosomal enzyme release from leukocytes exposed to immune complexes and other particles. J. Exp. Med. *134*:149, 1971.

EOSINOPHILS

Beeson, P. B., and D. A. Bass: The Eosinophil. Philadelphia, W. B. Saunders Co., 1977.

Hudson, G.: Quantitative study of eosinophil granulocytes. Sem. Hematol. *5*:166, 1968.

Litt, M.: Eosinophils and antigen-antibody reactions. Ann. N.Y. Acad. Sci. *116*:964, 1964.

BASOPHILS

Ackerman, G. A.: Cytochemical properties of the blood basophilic granulocyte. Ann. N.Y. Acad. Sci. *103*:376, 1963.

Askenase, P. W.: Role of basophils, mast cells and vasoamines in hypersensitivity reactions with a delayed time course. Prog. Allergy *23*:199, 1977.

Dvorak, H. F., and A. M. Dvorak: Basophilic leucocytes: structure, function and role in disease. Clin. Haematol. *4*:651, 1975.

Dvorak, H. F., and A. M. Dvorak: Basophils, mast cells, and cellular immunity in animals and man. Hum. Pathol. *3*:454, 1972.

Ishizaka, T., and K. Ishizaka: Biology of immunoglobulin E. Molecular basis of reaginic hypersensitivity. Prog. Allergy *19*:60, 1975.

Terry, R. W., D. F. Bainton, and M. G. Farquhar: Formation and structure of specific granules in basophilic leukocytes of the guinea pig. Lab. Invest. *21*:65, 1969.

Wolf-Jürgensen, P.: The basophilic leukocyte. Ser. Haematol. *1*:45, 1968.

Zucker-Franklin, D.: Electron microscopic study of human basophils. Blood *29*:878, 1967.

LYMPHOCYTES

See References, Chapter 7 and 13.

MONOCYTES

See References, Chapter 5.

CONNECTIVE TISSUE PROPER

5

Connective tissue consists of cells and extracellular fibers embedded in a gel-like ground substance or matrix rich in tissue fluid. Traditionally the fibers have been considered to be of three kinds: *collagen fibers, reticular fibers,* and *elastic fibers.* The collagenous and reticular fibers have now been found to be different morphological forms of the same fibrous protein, collagen. Nevertheless, it is useful for descriptive purposes to retain the term reticular fiber for bundles composed of *fibrils* of collagen 50 nm or less in diameter, and the term collagen *fiber* for larger bundles consisting of unit fibrils 50 to 150 nm in diameter.

In recent years, there has been rapid progress in characterizing the macromolecules of the extracellular matrix of connective tissue. These have been found to occur in much greater variety than previously assumed. Many of these molecules belong to a class of compounds called *proteoglycans.* This term describes complex molecules containing a core of protein to which *glycosaminoglycans* are covalently bound. The latter in turn consist of linear polymers of repeating disaccharides. The proteoglycans may involve different core proteins and several classes of glycosaminoglycans linked to the core in varying numbers. This results in great diversity at the molecular level, which endows proteoglycans with considerable versatility in their structural and organizational functions. The time-honored concept of an "amorphous ground substance" has become obsolete as more has been learned about the configuration and interactions of its macromolecular constituents. The general term *extracellular matrix* (ECM), now widely used, embraces the proteoglycans, the collagen, elastin, and the more recently discovered structural proteins *fibronectin, chondronectin,* and *laminin.* Collectively these form the stable material that surrounds connective tissue cells and underlies epithelia.

There are several cell types in connective tissue. These can be categorized as *fixed cells,* a more or less permanent resident population, and *wandering cells,* which are transient emigrants from the bloodstream.

The relative abundance of the various kinds of fibers, cells, and matrix varies greatly in connective tissue from one region of the body to another, depending on the local structural requirements. For convenience in description and communication, histologists have attempted to classify connective tissues. But classification is often difficult and inexact and should not be interpreted too rigidly, since various types grade into one another through transitional forms and one type may be transformed into another if the local conditions change.

Categorical terms are usually assigned according to whether the fibers are loosely interwoven or densely packed. Thus, we distinguish *loose connective tissue* and *dense connective tissue.* Within the latter category, it is useful to add modifiers to indicate whether the fibers have an ordered or a disordered arrangement. Thus, in *dense irregular connective tissue,* the fibers are closely interwoven in random orientation, whereas in *dense regular connective tissue,* the fibers are arranged in parallel bundles as in tendons; or in flat sheets, as in aponeuroses. In addition to these designations, several kinds of specialized connective tissue are named to indicate their predominant component, or identifying feature: e.g., *mucous* connective tissue, *reticular* tissue, *adipose* tissue, *pigment* tissue, and so on. These examples and the *lamina propria* of the gastrointestinal mucosa are all variants of loose connective tissue, which is a common form that can be discussed as the prototype of connective tissues in general.

LOOSE CONNECTIVE TISSUE

Loose connective tissue develops from the mesenchyme that remains after the other tissues of the embryo have been formed. An interlacing fabric of very fine collagenous fibers is deposited in the meshes of the reticulum of stellate mesenchymal cells. These fine fibrils formed early, adsorb metallic silver when treated with alkaline solutions of reducible silver salts, and are blackened. Because of this staining property, they were formerly considered to be distinct from collagen and were called *reticular fibers* and their substance designated *reticulin*. They are now known to be simply one of the several molecular species of collagen. As development progresses, coarser fibers are formed that associate in bundles and have the staining properties of the form of collagen that predominates in the connective tissues of the adult organism. Although "reticulin" is no longer regarded as a distinct chemical entity, the terms *reticulum* and *reticular fibers* continue to be useful to designate fibrous elements whose size is smaller than, and arrangement different from, those of the more prevalent collagenous fibers in the adult.

As development progresses the mesenchymal cells gradually change their character, elongating and stretching out along the surface of the collagen fiber bundles to become *fibroblasts*, the principal cells of connective tissue. Other cell types, either differentiating from mesenchymal cells or emigrating from the blood, take up residence in the interstices of the fabric of interwoven fibers. Like a collapsed sponge, this tissue contains innumerable potential spaces, normally occupied by a small amount of matrix but capable of becoming enlarged and distended with fluid. These extracellular interstitial spaces are the minute chambers or compartments seen by the early histologists, who are responsible for the term *areolar tissue* (from *areola*, a small space), a common synonym for loose connective tissue.

EXTRACELLULAR MATRIX

The supportive functions of the connective tissue depend largely on the properties of its extracellular matrix. The fibers are responsible for its tensile strength and resilience and form a scaffolding on which its fixed cells are deployed. The aqueous phase of the matrix is the medium through which all nutrients and waste products must pass in transit between the blood and the cells of the body. The consistency, composition, and state of hydration of the matrix can exert an important influence upon this vital exchange.

Collagen Fibers

Collagen fibers are present in varying abundance in all types of connective tissues. In unstained preparations of loose connective tissue, they appear as colorless strands 0.5 to 20 μm in diameter and of indefinite length. They run in all directions and if not under tension they tend to have a slightly wavy course (Fig. 5–1). At high magnification, a longitudinal striation can be detected in the larger collagen bundles, indicating that these consist of smaller parallel fibers. With polarization microscopy, even the smallest collagen fibers visible with the light microscope exhibit form birefringence attesting to the presence of elongated submicroscopic units oriented in the direction of the fiber axis. Seen in stained histological sections, collagen fibers are acidophilic, staining pink with eosin, blue with Mallory's trichrome, and green with Masson's trichrome stain.

When examination of collagen is pursued down to the electron microscopic level, the smaller fibers detectable by light microscopy are found to be composed of parallel fibrils 20 to 100 nm in diameter. These are the oriented subunits responsible for the form birefringence observed when collagen is examined in polarized light. In electron micrographs, these *unit fibrils* are cross-striated with transverse bands repeating every 64 to 67 nm along their length. When stained with phosphotungstic acid and viewed at high magnification, several additional bands can be resolved within each 67-nm period (Fig. 5–2). In addition to the typical fibrils with 67-nm cross-banding, collagen fibrils with a periodicity of about 240 nm occur rarely in certain tissues.

Collagen fibers are flexible but offer great resistance to a pulling force. The breaking point of collagen fibers in human tendon is reached with a force of several hundred kilograms per square centimeter, and at this tension they have elongated only a few percent of their original length. When collagen is denatured by boiling, it yields the familiar substance *gelatin*. With more gentle treatment, it is possible to extract from rapidly developing or repairing connective tissues

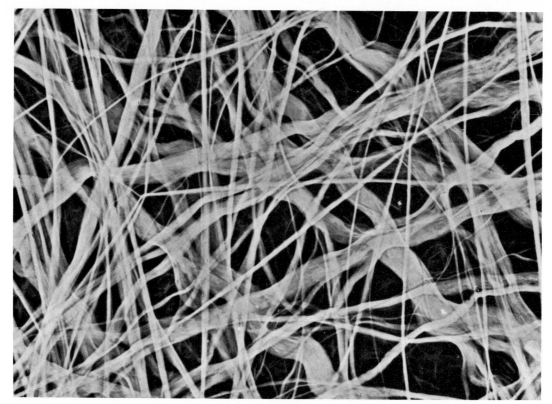

Figure 5–1. Photomicrograph of collagenous fibers in a thin spread of rat mesentery. Notice the variation in fiber diameter and the wavy course of the larger fibers. The preparation was stained by a silver method and the photograph printed as a negative to simulate more closely the appearance of the fibers in fresh material. (From Fawcett, D. W. *In* Greep, R. O., ed.: Histology. Philadelphia, Blakeston Co., 1953. Reproduced by permission of McGraw-Hill Book Co.)

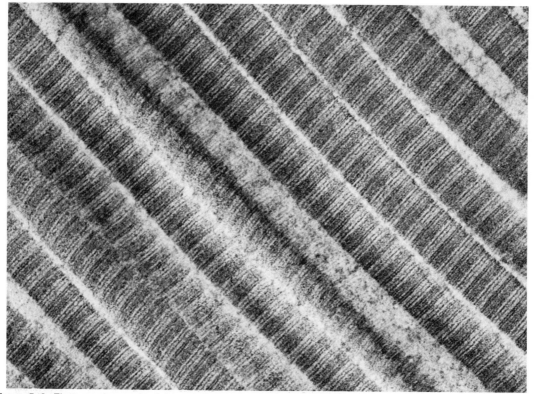

Figure 5–2. Electron micrograph of the unit fibrils of collagen showing their characteristic pattern of cross striations. (Micrograph courtesy of D. Friend.)

several collagen fractions with different solubility properties. Extracting at neutral pH yields a solution containing the tropocollagen molecules, which had not yet polymerized or had just begun to form protofilaments. This is the *neutral-soluble fraction*. If the tissue is further extracted with citrate at pH 3, the *acid-soluble fraction* is obtained. The remaining collagen, which can only be extracted with very drastic procedures, is designated the *insoluble fraction*. These three fractions are believed to represent successive stages in the extracellular polymerization of collagen molecules to form fibers.

The tropocollagen molecule is about 300 nm in length and 1.4 nm in diameter, and is made up of three polypeptide chains, called α chains, each having a M.W. of approximately 100,000. These have a left-handed helical configuration and are entwined and cross-linked to form a right-handed triple helix with each complete turn spanning a distance of 8.6 nm (Fig. 5–3).

When the cold neutral-soluble fraction of collagen is warmed to body temperature, the tropocollagen molecules spontaneously polymerize to form cross-striated fibrils with the 67-nm periodicity of native collagen. In this process, the 300-nm molecules are oriented parallel, overlapping one another by about one quarter of their length, and leaving a short empty space or lacuna between the NH_2 terminal of one molecule and the COOH terminal of the next (Fig. 5–4). The staggered array of molecular and hole zones is responsible for the cross striation of the fibers seen in negatively stained preparations. The accumulation of the contrast medium in the hole zones results in dark bands. The light bands where no stain penetrates are the regions in which molecular overlapping is complete.

Banding patterns that do not normally occur in nature can be produced in vitro by varying the conditions under which the collagen is reconstituted. When a solution of collagen and serum α-glycoprotein is dialyzed against water, the fibers that are formed have a periodicity of 240 nm instead of the 67 nm characteristic of native collagen. This is called *fibrous long-spacing (FLS) collagen* (Fig. 5–5). Precipitation of collagen from acid solution by addition of adenosine triphosphate yields short segments about 300 nm long instead of fibers. This form is called *segment long-spacing (SLS) collagen*. In both of the long-spacing forms, the molecules come together side to side and in register with no overlap. The length of the period or segment is therefore approximately the same as the length of the collagen molecule. Both of these, as well as the native collagen fibers, can be redissolved and polymerized in either of the other forms by controlling the physiochemical conditions. Knowledge of these unnatural forms of collagen is of limited value to students of histology or pathology, but it has contributed significantly to our understanding of the molecular organization of collagen and the mechanisms involved in fiber formation.

Collagen was formerly considered to be a unique protein whose size, helical structure, and amino acid composition had been highly conserved in the course of evolution. In recent years, however, improved analytical methods have led to the discovery of differences in amino acid sequence in α chains of collagen extracted from different tissues in the body. Instead of a single protein, collagen is now regarded as a family of closely related but genetically distinct molecules. At least seven types of collagen have been described to date.

The most ubiquitous is *Type I collagen* found in abundance in skin, bone, tendon, and cornea. It occurs in striated fibrils 20 to 100 nm in diameter that aggregate to form larger collagen fibers. Its molecular subunits are made up of α chains of two kinds differing slightly in amino acid composition and

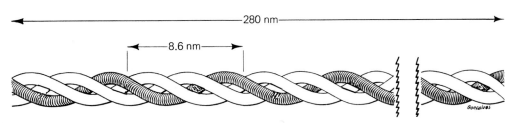

Figure 5–3. In Type I collagen each molecule (tropocollagen) is composed of two alpha-1 chains (shown here unshaded) and one alpha-2 (shaded) polypeptide chains entwined in a helical configuration. Each gyre of the helix spans a distance of 8.6 nm. (From Junqueira, L. C., and J. Carneiro. Basic Histology. 3rd ed. Los Altos, CA, Lange Medical Publications, 1980.)

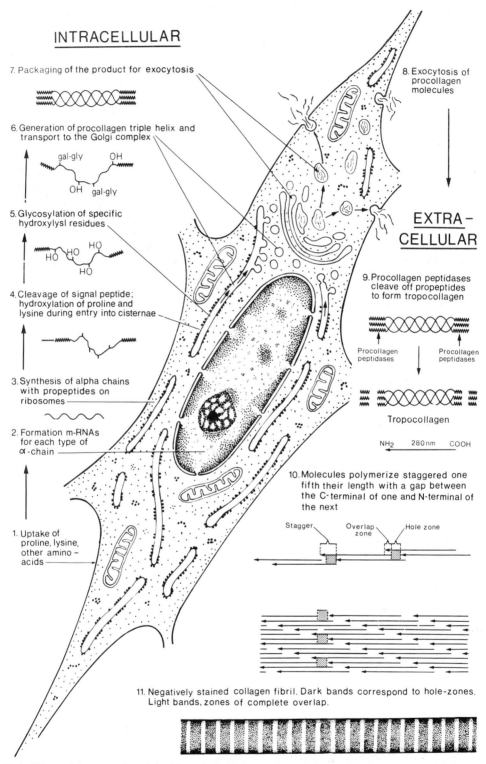

INTRACELLULAR

7. Packaging of the product for exocytosis

6. Generation of procollagen triple helix and transport to the Golgi complex

gal-gly   OH

OH   gal-gly

5. Glycosylation of specific hydroxylysl residues

HO   HO

HO   HO

HO

4. Cleavage of signal peptide; hydroxylation of proline and lysine during entry into cisternae

3. Synthesis of alpha chains with propeptides on ribosomes

2. Formation m-RNAs for each type of α-chain

1. Uptake of proline, lysine, other amino-acids

8. Exocytosis of procollagen molecules

EXTRA-CELLULAR

9. Procollagen peptidases cleave off propeptides to form tropocollagen

Procollagen peptidases   Procollagen peptidases

Tropocollagen

NH_2 280 nm   COOH

10. Molecules polymerize staggered one fifth their length with a gap between the C-terminal of one and N-terminal of the next

Stagger   Overlap zone   Hole zone

11. Negatively stained collagen fibril. Dark bands correspond to hole-zones. Light bands, zones of complete overlap.

Figure 5–4. Schematic presentation of the biosynthetic events and organelle participation in the formation of collagen. On left, successive intracellular events are defined; on right, the steps leading to extracellular assembly of cross-striated collagen fibrils. (Modified after Junqueira, L. C., and J. Carneiro. Basic Histology. 3rd ed. Los Altos, CA, Lange Medical Publications, 1980.)

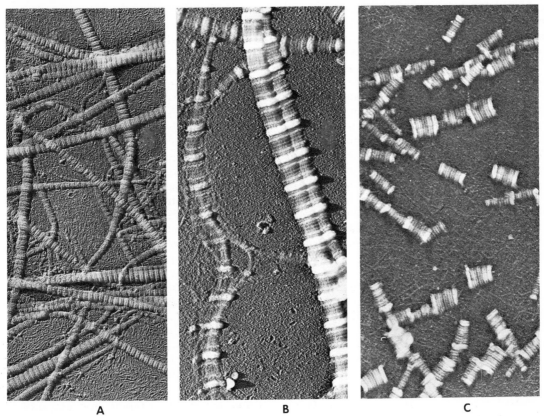

A   B   C

Figure 5–5. Electron micrograph of the different forms that can be produced upon reconstitution of collagen in vitro. *A,* Fibrils with the 64-nm period of native collagen—precipitated from solution by dialysis against 1 per cent NaCl. *B,* Fibrous long-spacing (FLS) collagen produced from a mixture of α_1 acid glycoprotein of serum and collagen solution dialysed against water. *C,* Segment long-spacing (SLS) collagen precipitated from acid solution of collagen by addition of ATP. (Micrographs courtesy of Gross, J., F. O. Schmitt, and J. H. Highberger.)

sequence, one being designated the $\alpha1(I)$ and the other the $\alpha2(I)$ chain. In the complex nomenclature that has evolved, the complete molecule of Type I collagen is abbreviated $[\alpha1(I)_2\alpha_2(I)]$.

Type II collagen is characteristic of cartilage but also occurs in embryonic cornea and notochord, the nucleus pulposus, the vitreous body of the eye, and elsewhere. In cartilage, it forms thin 10- to 20-nm fibrils, but in other microenvironments it may form larger fibrils morphologically indistinguishable from those of Type I collagen. It consists of α chains of a single kind, designated $\alpha1(II)$, and since there are three of these, the molecule is described $[\alpha1(II)]_3$.

Type III collagen is abundant in loose connective tissue, blood vessel walls, dermis of the skin, and stroma of various glands. It appears to be a major constituent of the slender 50-nm fibers that have traditionally been called reticular fibers (see below). It is composed of a single kind of α chain, $\alpha1(III)$, and the molecule is abbreviated $[\alpha1(III)]_3$.

Collagen Types I, II, and III, which form connective tissue fibers, are referred to as *interstitial collagen.* The basal lamina underlying epithelia contains collagen that does not polymerize into fibrils but instead forms a mat of randomly oriented molecules in association with proteoglycans and the structural proteins laminin and fibronectin. The collagens of the basal lamina are difficult to extract in pure form and have been less thoroughly studied than the interstitial collagens. The best characterized is *Type IV collagen,* which consists of three identical α chains—$\alpha1(IV)$—and the molecule is designated $[\alpha1(IV)]_3$. Chains distinctly different from other known α chains have been extracted from basal laminae and are collectively referred to as *Type V collagen,* but their association ratio remains to be clarified.

The functional significance of the molecular heterogeneity and differing distribution of collagen types is still obscure. Statements as to distribution of the several molecular types of collagen are based largely on biochemical extraction from various organs and tissues. The types specified in Table 5–1 predominate in the locations given but it would be misleading to suggest that those are the only collagens present. In most locations the connective tissues include more than one type of collagen. Biochemical identification of the predominant type in a given organ does not provide information on the range of fiber sizes, their orientation, their degree of aggregation into fiber bundles, or their relationship to the proteoglycan constituents of the extracellular matrix. Information of this kind must be obtained by microscopic methods such as immunohistochemical localization with type-specific antibodies, and visual analysis at high resolution with the electron microscope.

When the several molecular types of collagen were discovered, it was tempting to speculate that each might polymerize in a characteristic fibril size and that the different categories of fibrils were deployed in distinctive patterns. However, evidence to date indicates that fiber diameter is not closely correlated with collagen type. When examined with the electron microscope, connective tissues that are relatively rich in Types I, II, or III collagen by biochemical analysis all contain varying proportions of microfibrils (~4

nm in diameter); slender nonstriated fibrils (~10 nm); intermediate-sized striated fibrils (~25 nm); and larger striated fibrils (~50 nm). Only Type I collagen, such as occurs in tendons, appears to form very large fibrils up to 190 nm in diameter, but in this tissue, too, fibrils in the 50-nm range mingle with the large fibrils (Fig. 5–28). It seems clear that the widely distributed 50-nm striated fibrils with 67-nm periods may be composed of Types I, II, or III collagen and fibrils of this size are not confined to reticular connective tissue, as has been widely assumed. The size and architectural pattern of the fibrils formed in different organs does not appear to depend solely on genetically determined differences in collagen molecules, but is influenced by their post-translational modification; by their relationship to glycosaminoglycans in the matrix; and by other factors in the regional microenvironment. Apart from their intrinsic interest, analysis of all these factors is relevant to human and veterinary medicine since, as discussed in a later section, a number of collagen diseases can be explained by failures at specific steps in the complex process of synthesis, secretion, post-translational modification, and extracellular assembly of collagen molecules.

Although the electron microscope is the

Table 5–1. CHARACTERISTICS OF DIFFERENT COLLAGEN TYPES

Collagen Type	Molecular Formula	Tissue Distribution	Optical Microscopy	Ultrastructure	Site of Synthesis	Interaction with Glycosaminoglycans	Function
I	$[\alpha 1(I)]_2\alpha_2$	Dermis, bone, tendon, dentin, fascias, sclera, organ capsules, fibrous cartilage	Closely packed, thick, non-argyrophilic, strongly birefringent yellow or red fibers. Collagen fibers.	Densely packed, thick fibrils with marked variation in diameter	Fibroblast, osteoblast, odontoblast, chondroblast	Low level of interaction, mainly with dermatan sulfate	Resistance to tension
II	$[\alpha 1(II)]_3$	Hyaline and elastic cartilages	Loose, collagenous network visible only with picrosirius stain and polarization microscopy	No fibers; very thin fibrils embedded in abundant ground substance	Chondroblast	High level of interaction, mainly with chondroitin sulfates	Resistance to intermittent pressure
III	$[\alpha 1(III)]_3$	Smooth muscle, endoneurium, arteries, uterus, liver, spleen, kidney, lung	Loose network of thin, argyrophilic, weakly birefringent greenish fibers. Reticular fibers.	Loosely packed thin fibrils with more uniform diameters	Smooth muscle, fibroblast, reticular cells, Schwann cells, hepatocyte	Intermediate level of interaction, mainly with heparan sulfate	Structural maintenance in expansible organs
IV	$[\alpha 1(IV)]_3$	Epithelial and endothelial basal laminae and basement membranes	Thin, amorphous, weakly birefringent membrane	Neither fibers nor fibrils are detected	Endothelial and epithelial cells	Insufficient data	Support and filtration

Modified from Junqueira, L. C., and Carneiro, J. Basic Histology. 4th ed. Los Altos, CA, Lange Medical Publishers, 1983.

instrument of choice for identification of the subunit structure of collagen fiber bundles, it does not lend itself to study of the orientation and pattern of fibers with respect to whole organs and their functional subunits. For this purpose the light microscope is more suitable because of its larger field and the greater thickness of the sections that can be examined. Its usefulness is enhanced if the tissue is stained with the picrosirius method and viewed with polarization optics. In reacting with the basic groups of collagen, the long molecules of the dye, Sirius red, orient parallel to the molecules of collagen, enhancing the form birefringence of the fibers. Under the polarizing microscope, one can take advantage of differential coloration and relative enhancement of birefringence to assess the distribution of collagen Types I and III. Thus, in dermis, tendon, fibrous cartilage, bone, dentin, sclera, and cornea where Type I is abundant, the collagen appears as strongly birefringent yellow or red fibers. In uterine smooth muscle, in the walls of arteries, in liver, spleen, and the investment of nerves—tissues all rich in Type III collagen—one finds thin, green, birefringent fibers corresponding in pattern to the silver-impregnated reticular fibers of classical histology. Type II collagen, which is characteristic of cartilage, is poorly or inconsistently stained with this method. Immunofluorescent localization of collagen types using sensitive specific antibodies is in general agreement with the distribution observed in preparations stained with the picrosirius method.

Reticular Fibers

Reticular fibers were identified as a component of connective tissue over a century ago and were long regarded as a fibrous element distinct from collagen. These very slender fibrils (0.5 to 2.0 μm) tend to form delicate networks rather than coarse bundles (Fig. 5–6). They are not apparent in ordinary histological sections but can be selectively stained by reason of their property of adsorbing metallic silver when treated with alkaline solutions of reducible silver salts (Fig. 5–7). Fibers of this nature are the first to appear in the differentiation of embryonic mesenchyme into loose connective tissue, but they gradually give way to increasing numbers of typical collagen fibers in the connective tissue of adults. Reticular fibers persist,

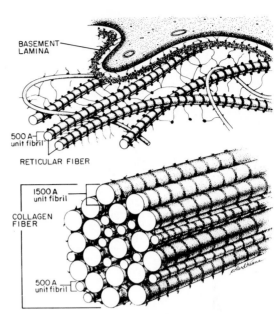

Figure 5–6. Drawing comparing Type IV collagen (basement lamina), Type III (reticular fibers) and Type I (tendon). Fibers characteristic of tendon are a mixture of fibrils 30 to 150 nm in diameter, whereas in reticular fibers the fibrils average 50 to 55 nm in diameter. The small dots associated with these fibrils represent granules of protoglyan. (From Hay, E. D., et al. *In* Gästpar, H., K. Kühn, and R. Marx, eds.: Collagen-Platelet Interactions. Stuttgart, Schattauer, 1978, pp. 129–151.)

however, in delicate networks surrounding adipose cells; smooth muscle cells; the sarcolemma of striated muscle; the endoneurium of nerves; and the stroma of many glandular organs. They are also found in close association with the basal lamina of most epithelia and they form the supporting tissue of lymphoid and blood-forming organs.

With the introduction of the electron microscope, reticular fibers were found to be made up of unit fibrils having the 67-nm periodicity typical of collagen. It is now thought that the difference in argyrophilia of reticular and collagen fibers is not due to a chemical difference in their fibrous proteins, but depends on the size of the fibrils and their relationship to interfibrillar proteoglycans that bind them together. It is now generally accepted that collagenous and reticular fibers are essentially identical biochemically. However, the terms "reticulum" and "reticular fibers," are still widely used to designate small fibrous elements of connective tissue whose size and pattern are different from those of more typical collagen fibers. Recent studies indicate that the collagenous component of reticular fibers is principally Type III collagen.

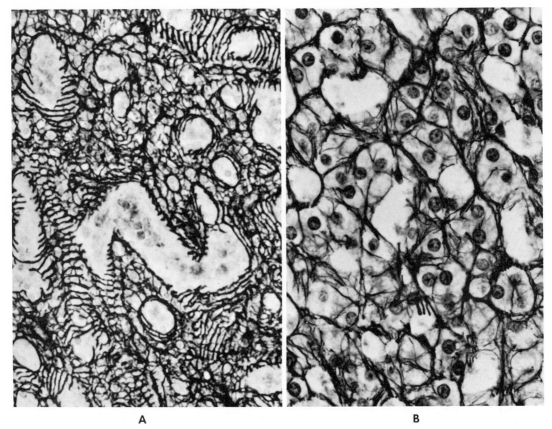

A   B

Figure 5–7. Reticular fibers are distinguished from other collagenous fibers by their smaller size, their reticular pattern, and the fact that they blacken with silver stains. The pattern of reticular fibers in different examples is presented here. A, Reticulum of the spleen. B, Reticular fibers of the adrenal cortex.

Elastic Fibers

Some organs, in their normal function, must yield transiently to externally or internally applied force. Their connective tissue therefore must have sufficient resilience to restore the original state. For example, the aorta, the large vessel conducting blood from the heart, is distended by the outflow from each contraction of the ventricle. Its elastic recoil to resting diameter between beats is essential for maintenance of continuous flow from the intermittent pumping action of the heart. Similarly, the lungs are expanded during inspiration and return passively to initial volume during expiration. The aorta and lungs are especially rich in *elastic fibers*, but connective tissues throughout the body contain similar fibers that have the ability to be stretched by a small force and to return to their original dimensions when the force is removed. Elastic fibers can be stretched to their breaking point at about 150 per cent of their original length with a force of only 20 to 30 kg/cm². When a fiber breaks, its ends quickly retract and coil up.

In unstained spreads of loose connective tissue, the slender, refractile elastic fibers 0.2 to 1.0 μm in diameter are not plentiful, but they can be distinguished from the more abundant collagen fibers by their small diameter and their tendency to branch and anastomose to form loose networks (Fig. 5–8). They usually are not identifiable in histological sections stained with hematoxylin and eosin, but can be clearly demonstrated when selectively stained by Verhoeff's stain, Weigert's resorcin-fuchsin, or Halmi's aldehyde-fuchsin method.

When present in sufficient numbers, elastic fibers impart a yellowish color to the fresh tissue. Certain elastic ligaments, such as the ligamenta flava of the human vertebral column and the ligamentum nuchae of ruminants, are distinctly yellow. The latter is composed of exceptionally coarse parallel elastic fibers up to 4 or 5 μm in diameter. Elastin is not always in the form of fibers. It takes the form of fenestrated sheets or lamellae in the *elastica interna* and *elastica externa* in the walls of arteries.

Elastic fibers are not made up of fibrillar

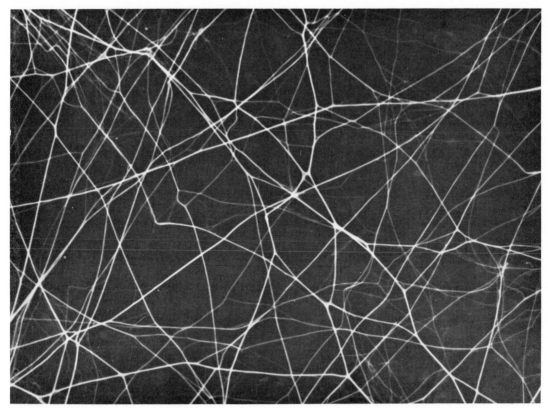

Figure 5–8. Elastic fibers in a spread of rat mesentery, stained with resorcin-fuchsin; the photograph is printed as a negative image. Notice that the fibers are more slender than the collagen fibers in Figure 5–1, and they branch and anastomose to form a network. (From Fawcett, D. W. *In* Greep, R. O., ed. Histology. Philadelphia, Blakiston Co., 1953. Reproduced by permission of McGraw-Hill Book Co.)

subunits that are visible with the light microscope and therefore appear homogeneous. Under polarizing optics, they exhibit a weak birefringence that increases when the fibers are stretched. In electron micrographs, elastic fibers have two components: *microfibrils* approximately 10 nm in diameter aggregated in small bundles that are associated with, or embedded in, a seemingly amorphous component, *elastin* (Fig. 5–9).

Although elastin is usually described as amorphous, a fibrillar substructure has recently been reported in electron micrographs of purified elastin after prolonged extraction with osmium tetroxide or periodate. It is speculated that these treatments may dissove sugar moieties of elastin, unmasking its fibrillar structure. The fibrils are reported to have a diameter of 2 to 4 nm and to be closely packed in parallel array.

Elastin is resistant to boiling and to hydrolysis by dilute acid or alkali under conditions that destroy other connective tissue constituents. It resists digestion by trypsin but when treated with the enzyme *elastase*, prepared from pancreas, it is selectively digested from tissue sections, leaving cells and collagen intact. About 30 per cent of the amino acid residues of elastin are glycine and about 11 per cent are proline. Unlike collagen, elastin is composed mainly of nonpolar hydrophobic amino acids and contains little hydroxyproline and no hydroxylysine. It is relatively rich in valine and contains two unique amino acids, *desmosine* and *isodesmosine*, which serve to cross-link the polypeptide chains.

The microfibrillar component of elastic fibers differs greatly from elastin in amino acid composition. It contains less glycine; contains no hydroxyproline, desmosine, or isodesmosine; and is composed mainly of hydrophilic amino acids. About 5 per cent of the weight of microfibrillar protein consists of neutral sugars.

The role of the microfibrils in fibrogenesis is not clear, but it is thought that they may impose a fibrous form on the polymerizing elastin. During development, the bundles of microfibrils are laid down first in close proximity to the surface of fibroblasts, smooth muscle cells, or other mesenchymal derivatives. The elastin appears later and ultimately makes up the bulk of the fiber, with the

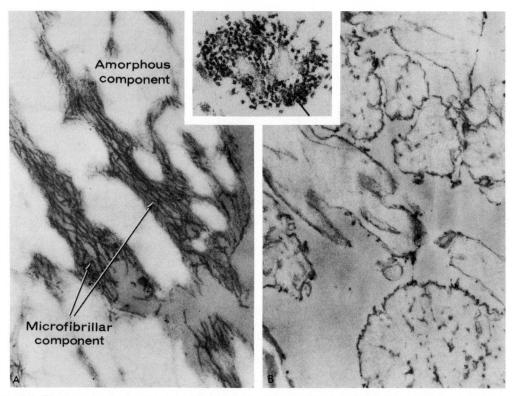

Figure 5–9. Electron micrograph of a preparation of elastic fibers purified from ligamentum nuchae of a fetal calf. *A,* Stained microfibrils are visible around and between the pale amorphous appearing areas of elastin. *B,* The microfibrils have been extracted by chemical treatment that breaks disulfide bonds of protein, leaving behind only the amorphous component of elastic fibers. Inset shows an early stage of elastic fiber formation in cross section. 11-nm microfibrils are seen around a pale core of newly formed elastin. (Micrographs from Ross, R., and P. Bornstein. Sci Am *224:*44, 1971.)

microfibrils forming a layer around its periphery and occurring in small fascicles in its interior. A precursor molecule, *proelastin* or *tropoelastin,* is believed to be synthesized and released at the cell surface. Extracellularly the enzyme lysyl oxidase catalyzes the formation of aldehyde groups on certain lysines. Three of these aldehydic residues condense with a fourth lysine to form the ring structure of the desmosines that cross-link the elastin chains.

In the disease *lathyrism,* which occurs in animals that eat the plant *Lathyrus odoratus,* and in a comparable condition induced experimentally by administration of β-amino-propionitrile, the action of lysyl oxidase is inhibited and both collagen and elastin are incompletely cross-linked.

Other Structural Proteins

In addition to the collagenous and elastic fibers long recognized by light microscopists, there are at least two structural glycoproteins—*fibronectin* and *laminin.* Glycoproteins are distinguished from the proteoglycans of the extracellular matrix by their higher proportion of protein and by characteristic differences in the nature of their polysaccharide side chains. They usually contain hexosamine, galactose, or other sugars with sialic acid in a terminal position on the heterosaccharide chain.

Fibronectin. The term *fibronectin* describes a group of structurally and immunologically related glycoproteins found in connective tissue, in basal laminae of epithelia, and on the surfaces of many cells. As the name implies (*fibra,* fiber; *nectere,* to bind), this protein binds to other fibrous proteins such as collagen and fibrin. It seems to be involved in adhesion of fibroblasts and other cell types to their natural substrates in the tissues, and in the adhesion, spreading, and locomotion of cells on artificial substrates in vitro. The protein has a M.W. of about 440,000 and is composed of two 220,000-dalton polypeptide chains. It is not confined to the tissues but occurs also in the blood plasma where it was first detected and called *cold-insoluble globulin,* a term that has now been discarded in favor of *plasma fibronectin.* The circulating fibronectin is believed to be synthesized by the endothelium lining the vascular system. The fibronectin of the peripheral tissues is reported to be synthesized by fibroblasts, myoblasts, chondrocytes, Schwann cells, astroglial cells, and by a number of epithelia, and the list is increasing. It is not visible in routine histological preparations, and what is known of its distribution is based mainly on immunocytochemical localization with fluorescent antibody.

Fibronectin is an important component of the connective tissue matrix and is present in the basal lamina of epithelia, and in the external lamina around smooth and striated muscle cells. In tissue cultures, where it has been most extensively studied, it appears as a fine fibrillar matrix situated on cells, between cells, and between them and the glass or plastic substrate. There is some evidence suggesting transmembrane association of intracellular actin with extracellular fibronectin, which would account for the observed effects of added fibronectin on cell shape and improved adhesion to substrate.

Fibronectin is found in the α granules of blood platelets, and is released onto their surface and into the environment when platelets are activated by thrombin or by contact with collagen. It has been suggested that surface fibronectin may play a role in platelet aggregation and adhesion to fibrin and collagen in the formation of blood clots.

The fibronectin molecule has along its length a set of highly specific binding domains for macromolecules that occur on cell surfaces and in the extracellular matrix. These binding sites enable fibronectin to mediate adhesion of cells to other cells, to collagen, and to hyaluronic acid and other glycosaminoglycans of the extracellular matrix. Thus, it may play a role in organizing extracellular macromolecules as well as in binding cells to their substrate.

Laminin. Laminin is more restricted in its distribution than fibronectin. It is a large glycoprotein composed of at least two polypeptide chains of M.W. 220,000 and 440,000 joined by disulfide bonds. Laminin is localized mainly in basal laminae and seems to be involved in attachment of epithelia to their supporting layer of Type IV collagen.

Ground Substance

The cells and fibers of connective tissue are surrounded by a translucent matrix that exhibits no structural organization visible with the light microscope. It is commonly referred to, therefore, as the *amorphous ground substance*. It has the physical properties of a viscous solution or thin gel. It is extracted by the aqueous fixatives commonly used and is not visible in histological sections. It can be preserved to some extent if frozen sections of fresh tissue are fixed in ether-formol vapor. In such preparations, it stains with the periodic acid–Schiff reaction for carbohydrates and stains metachromatically with toluidine blue. These tinctorial properties are attributable to the presence of several types of *proteoglycans*—complex macromolecules consisting of a core protein of varying length to which *glycosaminoglycan* (GAG) chains are covalently linked. Glycosaminoglycans are linear polymers of repeating disaccharide units of which one is always a hexosamine. The GAG chains are linked to the core protein at one end and radiate from it in a bottle-brush configuration (Fig. 5–10). The principal glycosaminoglycans of the extracellular matrix are *hyaluronic acid, chondroitin sulfates, dermatan sulfate, keratan sulfate,* and *heparan sulfate* (Table 5–2). These differ in molecular weight, length of chain, and the nature of their disaccharide units. With the possible exception of hyaluronic acid, these glycosaminoglycans do not exist in tissues in the free state, but are always bound to core proteins as components of proteoglycans.

Hyaluronic acid is a major constituent of vitreous humor and synovial fluid but occurs widely in extracellular matrices elsewhere. It is a very long molecule of high molecular weight, which if straightened out would be up to 2.5 μm in length. One of its most important properties is its very high viscosity in aqueous solution, which is largely responsible for the consistency of the ground substance. If fluid is injected into connective tissue, it does not immediately diffuse away from the site but remains localized for a while in a discrete bleb, as though walled off by the viscous interstitial substance. This property of the matrix is believed to serve as a barrier to the spread of bacteria that may gain access to the tissues. It is of interest that the most invasive pathogenic bacteria produce an enzyme *hyaluronidase,* which enables them to depolymerize the hyaluronidase in the extracellular matrix. The viscosity of hyaluronic acid in the synovial fluid of joints makes it well suited for its lubricating function in this site.

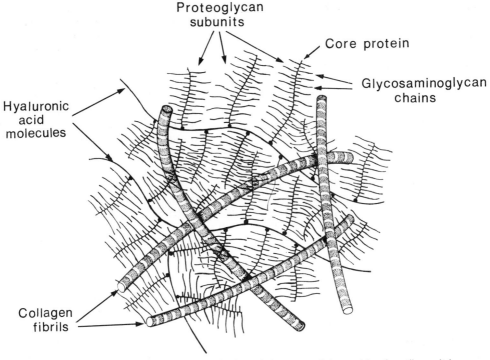

Figure 5–10. Schematic representation of the organization of the extracellular matrix of cartilage. It is composed of collagen fibrils with intertwining proteoglycan aggregates occupying the interstices. The extracellular matrix of connective tissues in general is believed to be similar but with differences in proportions of the several glycosaminoglycans.

Chondroitin sulfate is the predominant glycosaminoglycan in the proteoglycans of cartilage, bone, and large blood vessels but is found in other tissues as well. Dermatan sulfate is most abundant in skin but also occurs in lung, tendon, and elsewhere. Ker-

atan sulfate is found in cornea, cartilage, and nucleus pulposus. Heparan sulfate occurs in liver, aorta, and lung and will no doubt be detected elsewhere as more connective tissues are analyzed.

The proteoglycans of cartilage matrix have

Table 5–2. CONSTITUTION AND DISTRIBUTION OF GLYCOSAMINOGLYCANS IN CONNECTIVE TISSUE AND THEIR INTERACTION WITH COLLAGEN FIBERS

Glycosamino-glycan	Disaccharide Unit	Distribution	Electrostatic Interaction with Collagen
Hyaluronic acid	D-glucuronic acid + N-acetyl-O-glucosamine	Umbilical cord, synovial fluid, vitreous, cartilage	. . .
Dermatan sulfate (chondroitin sulfate B)	L-iduronic acid + N-acetyl-D-galactosamine-6-sulfate	Structures formed by collagen fibers: e.g., dermis, tendon, ligaments, heart valves, organ capsules, sclera, fibrous cartilage, arteries (adventitial layer), nerves (epineurium)	Low levels of interaction, mainly with collagen Type I
Chondroitin 4- or 6-sulfate* (chondroitin sulfate A or C)	D-glucuronic acid + N-acetyl-D-galactosamine 4- or 6-sulfate	Hyaline and elastic cartilage, arterial medial layer, nucleus pulposus of intervertebral discs	High levels of interaction, mainly with collagen Type II
Heparan sulfate	D-glucuronic acid + iduronic acid + N-acetyl-D-glucosamine + glucosamine	Structures rich in reticular fibers: e.g., smooth muscle, liver, spleen, nerves, endoneurium	Intermediate levels of interaction, mainly with collagen Type III

*Chondroitin sulfate can present its sulfate groups in positions 4 or 6. Both of these compounds exist in cartilage and in smaller amounts in other tissues. The biological significance of sulfation in position 4 or 6 is unknown.
From Junqueira, L. C., and Carneiro, J. Basic Histology. 4th ed. Los Altos, CA, Lange Medical Publishers, 1983.

been most extensively studied and can be regarded as representative of the structure of this class of macromolecules. The typical cartilage proteoglycan has about 80 side chains of chondroitin sulfate, each with a M.W. of 20,000, attached to a core protein together with a smaller number of chains of keratan sulfate. At one end of the core protein is a region with few or no attached GAG chains but having instead a number of covalently bound oligosaccharides. This segment of the polypeptide, which is referred to as the HA-binding region, includes an active site that binds with high specificity to hyaluronic acid. The binding of proteoglycan monomers to hyaluronic acid results in formation of *proteoglycan aggregates* of very large size. The sulfate and carboxyl groups on the repeating disaccharide units of the GAG chains result in a high concentration of anionic charges. Thus, the proteoglycans are polyanions and can be stained in tissue sections with cationic substances such as colloidal iron or Alcian blue, which have a high affinity for the anionic groups on the macromolecule.

In their native state, the long straight polysaccharide chains are extended and occupy a large volume in relation to their molecular weight. It is likely that in the connective tissue the extended proteoglycan molecules occupy essentially all the interstitial space in the matrix, and the proteoglycan aggregates are intertwined among the collagen and elastic fibers (Fig. 5–10).

As tissues are routinely prepared for electron microscopy, the polysaccharides are seldom well preserved. Better results are obtained when the polycationic dye ruthenium red is included in the fixative. This appears to preserve the GAG by interaction with its anionic groups, but during dehydration the chains collapse onto the protein core. Thus, in electron micrographs the proteoglycans are represented only by dense matrix granules 10 to 20 nm in diameter. These regrettably provide little information as to the configuration of proteoglycans in their native state, or the relationships of the extended molecules to each other and to the fibrous constituents of the extracellular matrix. In some tissues, there is a suggestion of a highly ordered interaction between the proteoglycans and specific sites along the cross-banded collagen fibrils. A row of proteoglycan granules forming a regular array with a spacing of about 60 nm can be demonstrated along the basal laminae of many epithelia (Fig. 5–6). Their ordered arrangement suggests that

the proteoglycans may play a role in maintaining the structural organization of the basal lamina.

Origin of Connective Tissue Fibers

The sequence of morphological events in formation of collagen is similar whether studied in the embryo, in young scar tissue, or in tissue cultures. Delicate networks of branching and anastomosing argyrophilic fibrils appear among the fibroblasts (Fig. 5–11). The fibrils may follow the outlines of the cells and their processes but they also extend far into the intercellular substance. When studied in electron micrographs, the finest of the developing fibrils are extracellular and have cross striations. As the fibrils increase in number, they rearrange into parallel wavy bundles of appreciable thickness. These lose their ability to be blackened with silver and instead accept stains for collagen.

The constant association of fibroblasts with developing collagenous fibers both in vivo and in vitro early suggested that these cells were involved in fibrogenesis, but their exact role remained a subject of debate. The area of controversy has been narrowed in recent years. It is now widely accepted that collagenous fibers arise extracellularly by polymerization of molecular collagen secreted into the extracellular matrix by fibroblasts. Consistent with this view is the electron microscopic observation that fibroblasts of growing connective tissue have the extensive endoplasmic reticulum and well-developed Golgi complex that we have come to expect of cells actively engaged in protein synthesis. Moreover, if ^{14}C-labeled proline is given to animals in which formation of connective tissue has been induced, labeled collagen can be detected in the microsome fraction isolated from connective tissue cells. Incorporation of labeled amino acid in fibroblasts can also be followed autoradiographically in animals with healing wounds. At early time intervals after administration of tritiated proline, the silver grains, betraying the location of the labeled precursor, are over the endoplasmic reticulum; later they are seen over the Golgi region and still later outside the cell, over newly formed collagen fibers.

The evidence thus points to a synthetic pathway for collagen, similar to that described for other proteins (Fig. 5–4). On the ribosomes of the endoplasmic reticulum, activated amino acids are assembled into polypeptide alpha chains, each composed of

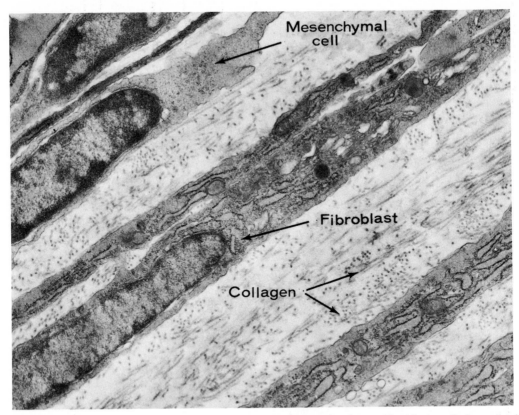

Figure 5–11. Electron micrograph of fibroblasts in developing connective tissue. Fibroblasts actively synthesizing collagen have a well-developed rough endoplasmic reticulum, often with distended cisternae. The relatively undifferentiated cell at upper left has more heterochromatin and little differentiation of its cytoplasm. The newly formed collagen fibrils are slender and randomly oriented.

about 1000 amino acids. Hydroxylation of the prolyl and lysyl residues takes place while the nascent alpha chains are still being synthesized. While the alpha chains are still associated with the ribosomes or immediately after their release into the lumen of the endoplasmic reticulum, they associate in helical configuration to form procollagen molecules with a M.W. of 336,000. The exact location of the other post-translational events is uncertain, but the procollagen molecules appear to be transported through the lumen of the endoplasmic reticulum, and packaged in the Golgi complex. Molecular collagen segregated in Golgi vacuoles is released from the fibroblast when these vacuoles move to the cell surface and discharge their contents into the surrounding ground substance (Fig. 5–4).

A relatively recent development in our understanding of collagen synthesis has been the identification of *procollagen,* an antecedent of the definitive collagen molecule. Procollagen subunits corresponding to α_1 and α_2 chains have a M.W. of 112,000—distinctly larger than the alpha chains of collagen. Their greater length and higher M.W. is

attributed to the presence of an additional sequence of amino acids on the N-terminal end of the molecule. This is the original form in which collagen is synthesized in the cell. Procollagen molecules are unable to polymerize into collagen fibers. However, an enzyme, *procollagen peptidase,* has been identified, which is believed to be located in the cell or at its surface. This cleaves off the telopeptide converting procollagen to collagen at the time of its release from the cell. The resulting collagen molecules are then free to polymerize extracellularly into cross-striated fibrils.

A remaining point of uncertainty concerns the possible role of the cells in determining the arrangement of the fibers. Most histologists assume that the cells simply maintain the appropriate physicochemical conditions in the surrounding ground substance to permit collagen fibers to form extracellularly by a process of spontaneous polymerization similar to that observed in vitro. Such a process could presumably take place at some distance from the fibroblast. The subsequent orientation of the fibrils would be in response to mechanical stresses in the tissue and would not be influenced by the cells. A few investigators believe that new fibrils arise only in very close relation to the cell surface, and that the cells exercise a direct control over their orientation in the connective tissue. It is contended that the orthogonal patterns and other precisely ordered arrangements of collagen fibers in the body are difficult to explain if collagen deposition is a completely independent extracellular phenomenon, whereas, if collagen is deposited in protofibrils that are oriented by fibroblasts, a mechanism is provided for ordering of collagen fibrils by the cells rather than by purely mechanical forces. Further study is needed to resolve this problem.

CELLS OF CONNECTIVE TISSUE

It is convenient to think of the cells of loose connective tissue in two categories: (1) a relatively stable population of *fixed cells*—the fibroblasts (responsible for production and maintenance of the extracellular components) and adipose cells (for storage of reserve fuel); and (2) a population of mobile *wandering cells*—macrophages, eosinophils, mast cells, lymphocytes, and plasma cells (cells concerned mainly with the shorter-term events involved in tissue reaction to injury).

Fibroblast or Fibrocyte

These are the principal cells of the connective tissue that elaborate the precursors of the extracellular matrix components.* Their shape depends to some extent on their physical substrate. They are usually deployed

---

*The student should be aware of troublesome inconsistency in terminology with respect to this cell type. The suffix *-blast* (Greek *blastos,* germ) is often used in naming the formative stages of various cell types. Thus, an *erythroblast* is an early developmental stage of the fully differentiated cell called an *erythrocyte.* Some authors, therefore, use the term *fibroblast* to designate a relatively immature cell actively proliferating and producing components of the extracellular substance, and they apply *fibrocyte* to the relatively quiescent cells of adult connective tissue. This interpretation loses sight of the fact that the term "fibroblast" was originally intended to describe a "fiber-forming cell" and not to name an immature form of a cell called a fibrocyte. Moreover, because most histologists recognize *mesenchymal cells,* persisting in postnatal life, as the undifferentiated progenitors of the connective tissue cells, the use of "fibroblast" in this sense makes an unnecessary distinction and introduces a redundant term. The term *fibroblast,* therefore, is properly used to describe the differentiated cell of adult connective tissue, and it can be considered synonymous with *fibrocyte* (as used by other authors).

along bundles of collagen fibers and appear in sections as fusiform elements with long tapering processes. In other situations they may be flattened, stellate cells with several slender processes. Their cytoplasm is usually eosinophilic like the neighboring collagen. The outlines of the cell bodies are therefore difficult to make out. They are more easily visualized after staining with iron-hematoxylin.

These cells have been extensively studied in tissue culture, where they can be better observed isolated from the interlacing fabric of fibers in which they reside in vivo. In this environment the cells migrate out from the explant into the surrounding medium, with their processes adhering to form a cellular network (Fig. 5–12). It is likely that the fibroblasts in the body also maintain tenuous contacts with one another, but for technical reasons this is difficult to demonstrate.

The elliptical nucleus is usually smoothly contoured but may sometimes be slightly folded. There are one or two nucleoli, and the chromatin is sparse and distributed in small karyosomes. A pair of centrioles and a small Golgi apparatus are situated near the nucleus. Long, slender mitochondria are found mainly in the perinuclear cytoplasm, but may also occur in the processes. Under conditions of stimulation, as in wound healing, when fibroblasts are dividing and actively synthesizing extracellular components, they enlarge and their cytoplasm becomes moderately basophilic. In electron micrographs, quiescent fibroblasts contain a small Golgi complex and only a few cisternal profiles of granular endoplasmic reticulum, but in growing or repairing connective tissue, the Golgi complex becomes very prominent and the endoplasmic reticulum is much more extensive. The cytoplasm usually contains few inclusions except for occasional small fat droplets. Granules staining with the periodic acid–Schiff reaction become numerous under some conditions and may represent intracellular precursors of the glycosaminoglycans of the ground substance.

Majority opinion holds that fibroblasts are fully differentiated cells that ordinarily do not give rise to other types of cells in the connective tissue. There is suggestive evidence, however, that in pathological states and under certain experimental conditions, they can transform into bone cells. It is also widely accepted that fibroblasts may accumulate lipid and become adipose cells, but in both these instances it is difficult to establish with certainty whether it is actually the fibro-

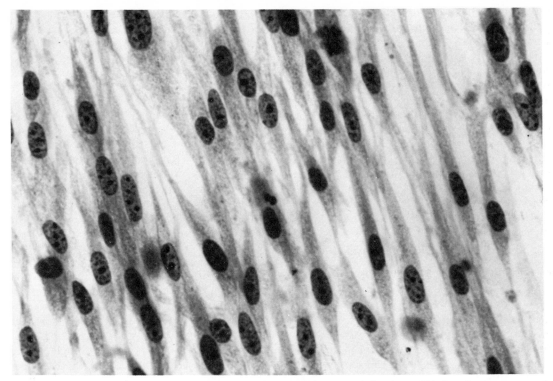

Figure 5–12. Photomicrograph of fibroblasts in cell culture illustrating their spindle shape. This form is also common in vivo but the processes may be branched, resulting in more stellate forms.

blasts or their undifferentiated mesenchymal progenitors that undergo these transformations.

Mesenchymal Cells

It is widely accepted that a population of cells that retain the developmental potentialities of embryonic mesenchymal cells persists in the adult organism. They are somewhat smaller than fibroblasts, but otherwise have much the same appearance and cannot easily be distinguished from them in ordinary histological sections. In loose connective tissue they are usually deployed along the blood vessels, especially along capillaries. In electron micrographs (Fig. 5–11), these small cells have a somewhat coarser chromatin pattern, few mitochondria, and little or no rough endoplasmic reticulum. These characteristics serve to distinguish them from synthetically active fibroblasts.

Many investigators regard these cells, rather than fibroblasts, as the precursors of adipose cells. When capillaries are obliged to grow and change the character of their walls in response to altered hemodynamic conditions, the smooth muscle cells required seem to be recruited by differentiation of these pluripotential cells in the perivascular connective tissue.

Adipose Cells

Among the sessile cells in loose connective tissue are some that are specialized for the synthesis and storage of lipid. These *adipose cells* or *fat cells* accumulate lipid to such an extent that the nucleus is flattened and displaced to one side, and the cytoplasm becomes so thinned out that it is resolved only as a thin line around the rim of the single large lipid droplet (Figs. 5–13, 5–14). So inconspicuous are the nucleus and cytoplasm that the fat cells in fresh connective tissue have the appearance of large glistening drops of oil. They may occur singly in the connective tissue but are more often found in groups. There is a marked tendency for them to be located along the course of small blood vessels. When they accumulate in such large numbers that they become the predominant component, crowding out other cell types, the resulting tissue is called *adipose tissue* or *fat* (see Chapter 6). All intermediate grades between loose connective tissue and typical adipose tissue can be found.

In the preparation of the usual histological

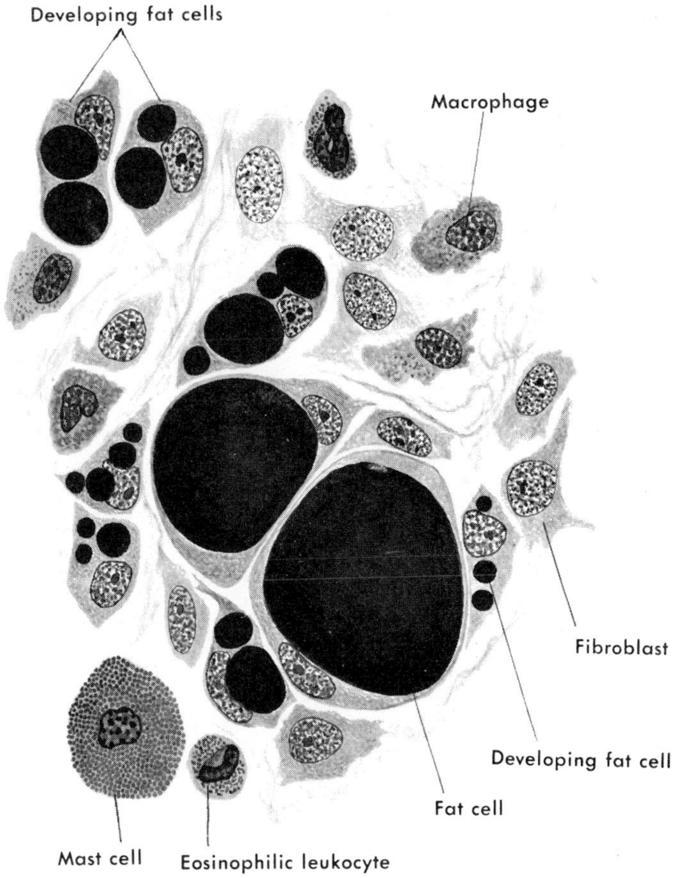

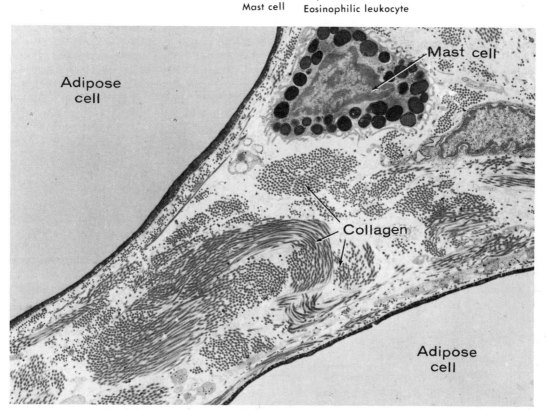

Figure 5–13. Drawing of cells in subcutaneous loose connective tissue of a rat. The osmium tetroxide of the fixative preserved and blackened the lipid droplets in several adipose cells in different stages of development. (After A. A. Maximov.)

Developing fat cells

Macrophage

Fibroblast

Developing fat cell

Fat cell

Mast cell   Eosinophilic leukocyte

Mast cell

Adipose cell

Collagen

Adipose cell

Figure 5–14. Electron micrograph of portions of two adipose cells and the intervening collagenous fibers. Relative to the mast cell and the fibroblast at upper right, the adipose cells are enormous. Only a small portion of each is included in this field, but enough to show their thin peripheral layer of cytoplasm and the homogeneous lipid content, which usually is not stained black by osmium after primary glutaraldehyde fixation.

section the lipid droplets of the adipose cells are dissolved out during dehydration, and there remains only the thin layer of cytoplasm, slightly thickened in one area to accommodate the nucleus. Despite the extreme thinness of the rim of cytoplasm, a juxtanuclear Golgi apparatus can be demonstrated, and filamentous mitochondria are distributed around the entire circumference of the lipid droplet. The individual fat cells are surrounded by a delicate network of reticular fibers.

Adipose cells develop from fusiform cells that resemble fibroblasts, but, as indicated above, these are generally believed to be mesenchymal cells that persist into postnatal life in the adventitia of the small blood vessels of the connective tissue. During their early development they may contain multiple small lipid droplets, but these ultimately coalesce into a single drop (Fig. 5–13). The fully formed fat cell is incapable of mitotic division. Any new areas of adipose cells that develop in adult life must therefore arise from undifferentiated precursors.

Macrophages

The connective tissues contain mononuclear cells of varying appearance that have in common the ability to take particulate material into their cytoplasm and to degrade the ingested substances with hydrolytic enzymes. This activity is called *phagocytosis* (see Chapter 1) and any cells that exhibit it are described as *phagocytes*. The principal phagocytes in normal connective tissue are the *macrophages*. Because of their remarkable capacity to destroy bacteria, dead cells, and debris resulting from injury, such cells are important in maintenance and repair of tissues and in the body's defense against invading microorganisms.

Traditionally, histologists were obliged to rely exclusively upon the shapes of cells, their staining properties, and their relationship to other tissue components for their identification. Using these morphological criteria, two main categories of phagocytes were distinguished—*free macrophages* and *fixed macrophages;* one motile and wandering through the ground substance of the connective tissue, the other sessile and stretched out along the bundles of collagen fibers. These two forms of tissue phagocytes were considered to be distinct in their origins and, to some extent, in their functions. The former were

believed to stem from monocytes emigrating from the blood. The latter were thought to originate in the connective tissue by differentiation from persisting mesenchymal cells.

The development of methods for tracing cell lineages by labeling with radioisotopes; the use of chromosome markers; and immunological techniques for detecting specific receptors on the surface of cells have all provided compelling evidence that the mononuclear phagocytes all originate from precursors in the bone marrow; are transported in the blood as monocytes; migrate through the endothelium of postcapillary venules; and take up residence in the tissues. To some extent, their morphology is dependent on the organ in which they are found and on the degree of their activity. It is now widely accepted that the free and fixed macrophages of the connective tissue are different functional phases in the life history of cells of the same lineage.

The circulating monocytes of the blood are a reserve of potential phagocytes that can be rapidly mobilized at sites where they are needed. In inflammatory reactions, additions are made to the resident population of phagocytes by emigration of monocytes from the blood and their transformation to free macrophages. A monocyte that has recently arrived in the tissues is a spherical cell 10 to 14 μm in diameter with an eccentric, reniform nucleus and a faintly basophilic cytoplasm. In electron micrographs it has a relatively smooth surface, a sparse endoplasmic reticulum, and few cytoplasmic inclusions. After its activation and transformation to a macrophage, the surface is highly irregular with many microvilli and lamellipodia, and the cytoplasm contains numerous phagocytic vacuoles, secondary lysosomes, and residual bodies (Fig. 5–15). These cells have an ameboid locomotion. Therefore, the shape they present in sections depends on their configuration at the moment of their immobilization by the fixative.

A large proportion of the macrophages in normal connective tissue are relatively inactive and are deployed along fibrous components of the tissue as stellate or fusiform cells that are difficult to distinguish from fibroblasts. Their nucleus is somewhat smaller and more deeply stained. The cytoplasm is more heterogeneous, often containing granules and vacuoles of varying size. In this configuration, the cells correspond to the fixed macrophages or *histiocytes* of the classical lit-

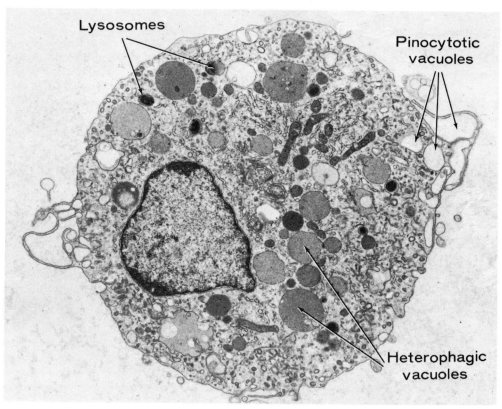

Figure 5–15. Micrograph of a free macrophage in edematous loose connective tissue showing the typical heterogeneity of the cytoplasm containing numerous lysosomes, vesicles, and heterophagic vacuoles. Thin ruffles or lamellipodia were fixed in various phases of their pinocytotic activity.

erature on histology and histopathology. When appropriately stimulated, these sessile macrophages detach from the fibers, withdraw their processes, and migrate as free macrophages to sites of tissue injury or bacterial invasion. After the acute inflammatory reaction subsides, the survivors presumably disperse and revert to their sessile, resting form.

In certain forms of chronic inflammation, aggregated macrophages may take on a polygonal shape due to close packing and mutual deformation. In this form, they are described as *epithelioid cells.* Around splinters or other foreign bodies in the tissues that are too large to be engulfed and destroyed by intracellular digestion, macrophages may coalesce to form huge multinucleate masses called *foreign-body giant cells.* The morphological transformations of mononuclear phagocytes that occur in inflamed connective tissue in vivo can also be observed when leukocytes from blood are cultivated in vitro. In such cultures, the only leukocytes capable of survival are the monocytes. These rapidly

transform to macrophages that eliminate by phagocytosis the dead and dying leukocytes of other types. Thus, in a few days, pure cultures of macrophages are obtained (Fig. 5–16). The cells flatten out uniformly spaced on the glass substrate or, if sufficiently crowded, may assume an epithelioid appearance. The culture vessel acts as a foreign body and, after prolonged cultivation, multinucleate giant cells are formed.

Monocytes and their derivatives have the unique property of rapid adherence to glass or plastic surfaces. When mixed populations of cells from blood, peritoneal exudates, or spleen are introduced in suspension into a culture flask, monocytes and mature macrophages settle onto the floor and soon become firmly adherent. Other cell types remain unattached and after a few hours can be washed away. By this device, pure cultures can be obtained for experimental purposes without waiting for the contaminating cell types to be eliminated by phagocytosis. Thus, adherence to glass has become one of the defining characteristics of mononuclear phagocytes.

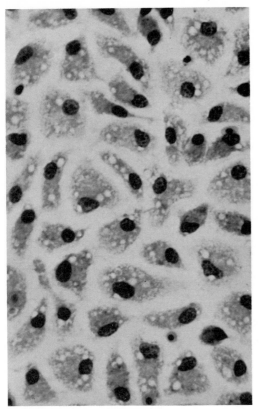

Figure 5–16. Photomicrograph of a culture of macrophages that have differentiated in vitro from peripheral blood monocytes.

The ability to follow in vitro the same sequence of cellular transformation that occurs in inflamed tissues has made it possible to study in considerable detail the cytological and cytochemical changes associated with the transition of monocytes to macrophages and epithelioid and giant cells. Accompanying the acquisition of phagocytic properties, there is an increase in cell volume and a striking enlargement of the Golgi apparatus, which becomes the site of active formation of numerous lysosomes. During the intracellular digestion of ingested material, the lysosomes discharge their content of hydrolytic enzymes into the phagocytotic vacuoles. Thus, the number of lysosomes diminishes during active phagocytosis. They accumulate again in abundance in the epithelioid and giant cells that develop after cellular debris and other material available for phagocytosis has been eliminated.

In their defensive role against pathogenic bacteria, macrophages do not function independently. They are assisted by antibodies (*immunoglobulins*) and *complement* present in blood serum. If specific antibody is present,

it binds to antigen on the surface of bacteria. A component of *complement* (C_3) in turn binds to the antigen-antibody complex and serves as a ligand promoting phagocytosis by facilitating attachment of the bacterium to specific receptors (Fc) in the membrane of the macrophage. The phagocytic and cytotoxic capabilities of macrophages are also enhanced by products of other cells in the connective tissue, notably the lymphocytes.

Conversely, products of macrophages influence lymphocytes. Their role in immunity will be discussed in more appropriate context in Chapter 13. It will suffice here to note that the interaction of macrophages with lymphocytes is an essential step in the initiation and regulation of an immune response. Antibody production, both in vivo and in vitro, is greatly impaired in the absence of macrophages. It is postulated that they process antigen to make it more immunogenic, but to date the exact mechanisms by which macrophages participate in antibody production have not been clearly defined. They are also required to generate cytotoxic cells in cell-mediated immune responses.

FREE CELLS OF CONNECTIVE TISSUE

In addition to the fixed or sessile cell types of connective tissue, there are several types of migratory cells that are emigrants from the blood—*lymphocytes, monocytes, eosinophils, basophils,* and *neutrophils.* Because of their capacity for ameboid locomotion and their tendency to congregate at sites where their services are needed, their numbers in the connective tissue are highly variable, depending on the local conditions. They were formerly regarded as blood cells carrying out essential functions in the circulation and only secondarily leaving the blood to take up residence in the connective tissue. The development of ingenious methods for tagging these cells, determining their life span, and following their movements in the body has brought about a fundamental change in our interpretation of their mission. It is now known that the primary functions of these cells are performed extravascularly in the connective tissue.

Monocytes and the Mononuclear Phagocyte System

The structure of monocytes was described and illustrated in Chapter 4, and their capacity to transform into macrophages, giant cells, and epithelioid cells has been discussed in the foregoing section. It remains to consider them in the context of a broader spectrum of phagocytic cell types that are widely distributed in the body. In addition to those already mentioned, the alveolar phagocytes of the lung, the microglia of the brain, the Kupffer cells of the liver, and certain stromal cells of the bone marrow and lymphoid organs all share the property of avid phagocytosis. Although these were formerly believed to arise from different precursors, histologists early recognized the desirability of grouping them together on the basis of their shared structural and behavioral features. Metchnikoff (1892) considered them as a diffuse cell system, which he termed the *macrophage system*. Relying on the uptake and storage of vital dyes as a measure of phagocytic capacity, Aschoff (1924) broadened the concept to include the specialized endothelium lining the sinusoids of spleen and bone marrow and proposed the inclusive term *reticuloendothelial system* (Fig. 5–17), which is still widely used and strongly defended by its proponents.

The term and its definition are now criticized on several grounds. The vital dye trypan blue not only accumulates in highly phagocytic cells, but when used in high concentration may be taken up in smaller amount by fluid-phase pinocytosis in unspecialized endothelium, in fibroblasts, and even in adipose cells—cells not truly phagocytic. The uptake of vital dyes is therefore a necessary but an insufficient criterion for inclusion in the system.

The development of methods for marking cells with radioisotopes and for recognizing stable surface antigens made it possible to trace cell lineages and to carry out cytokinetic studies that have significantly changed our concept of this system. Van Furth (1969) proposed the term *mononuclear phagocyte system* to include all highly phagocytic cells and their precursors. This includes a number of the cell types previously assigned to the reticuloendothelial system and several additional ones (Fig. 5–18). It excludes fibroblasts, endothelial cells, reticulum cells, dendritic cells, and others that ingest vital dyes at very low rates. The great appeal of the unifying concept of a mononuclear phagocyte system is that labeling and cytokinetic studies show that all of its members belong to the same cell lineage, originating in the bone marrow and being transported in the blood to their functional sites in the tissues. Wherever found they exhibit a positive histochemical reaction for esterase, contain peroxidase-positive granules, and have receptors for IgG and complement on their surface.

Since the cells of the mononuclear phagocyte system pass through several developmental stages and express different degrees of functional activity, there is need for descriptive terms for these states. Macrophages that are present at any given site in the absence of an exogenous stimulus are called *resident macrophages*. Those that have acquired enhanced functional activity in response to

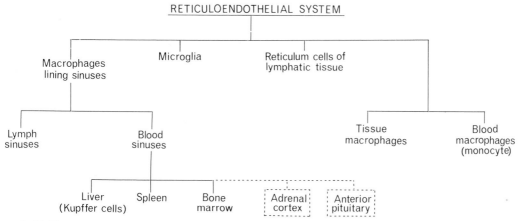

Figure 5–17. The reticuloendothelial system as traditionally defined—a diffuse system of macrophages and phagocytic endothelial cells lining blood sinuses in various organs. Although widely separated, they were grouped together because they shared similar phagocytic properties. The sinusoids of the pituitary and adrenal were originally included but are shown here in interrupted lines because electron microscopy has revealed that it is not the endothelium, but perivascular macrophages, that are phagocytic in these organs. The alleged phagocytic activity of splenic sinusoids is now seriously questioned, and in the liver these properties reside in the Kupffer cells and not in the endothelium proper. Thus, the endothelial component of the system has been largely eliminated by application of modern research methods.

Mononuclear Phagocyte System

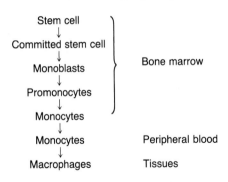

Stem cell
↓
Committed stem cell
↓
Monoblasts   } Bone marrow
↓
Promonocytes
↓
Monocytes
↓
Monocytes   Peripheral blood
↓
Macrophages   Tissues

Normal State
connective tissue (histiocyte)
liver (Kupffer cell)
lung (alveolar macrophage)
lymph nodes (free and fixed macrophages;
    interdigitating cell?)
spleen (free and fixed macrophages)
bone marrow (fixed macrophage)
serous cavities (pleural and peritoneal
    macrophages)
bone (osteoclasts)
central nervous system (CSF macrophages; brain
    macrophages)
skin (histiocyte; Langerhans cell?)
synovia (type A cell)
other organs (tissue macrophage)

Inflammation
exudate macrophage
exudate-resident macrophage
epithelioid cell
multinucleated giant cell (Langhans type
    and foreign-body type)

Figure 5–18. The concept of a mononuclear phagocyte system has replaced the reticuloendothelial system. This is a group of widely disseminated cell types that not only share similar morphology and phagocytic potential but also have a common origin from the monocytes of the blood. Included in this system are all the cell types specified in parenthesis after the organ or tissue in which they are located. (After von Furth, R. Immunobiology *161*:178, 1982.)

an environmental stimulus are called *activated macrophages*. Macrophages of varying degrees of activity attracted to the same site by a given substance are referred to as *elicited macrophages*. These terms find their greatest use in studies on the inflammatory response of tissues.

Lymphocytes

The smallest of the free cells of the connective tissue are lymphocytes that have emigrated from the blood. Their structural and functional role in immune responses have been discussed in Chapter 4. They may be found in small numbers in normal connective tissue throughout the body but are greatly increased at sites of chronic inflammation. They are normally abundant in the lamina propria of the respiratory tract and are especially concentrated in the loose connective tissue that underlies the epithelium of the gastrointestinal tract, where they are involved in protective immunosurveillance against the bacterial flora and antigenic foreign substances present in the gut lumen.

Plasma Cells

Plasma cells are ovoid cells with an eccentric nucleus and an intensely basophilic cytoplasm. They vary in size but usually fall within the range of 10 to 20 μm. The nucleus is spherical, and its abundant heterochromatin occurs in unusually coarse clumps that tend to be evenly spaced around the periphery in a radial pattern that is a useful identifying characteristic of this cell type. A prominent, lightly staining area adjacent to the

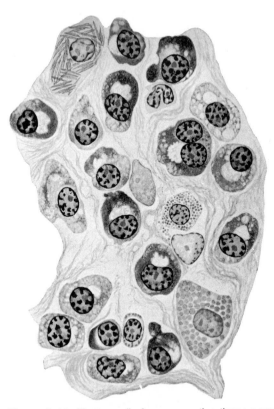

Figure 5–19. Plasma cells from connective tissue near the human tonsil. Several transitional forms between lymphocytes and plasma cells are drawn. The mature plasma cells are intensely basophilic, and a conspicuous paler region adjacent to the nucleus is the site of the large Golgi complex. (After A. A. Maximov.)

nucleus is the site of its large Golgi apparatus. The remainder of the cytoplasm is strongly basophilic.

In electron micrographs the coarse chromatin pattern is equally striking. There is a well-developed juxtanuclear Golgi complex and a pair of centrioles. The most conspicuous ultrastructural feature of the cytoplasm is an extensive system of cisternae of the rough endoplasmic reticulum (Fig. 5–20). The cisternae are usually narrow and in close parallel array, but in some cells they may be less highly ordered and their lumen may be distended with a flocculent material of low electron density. The plasma cell thus has the ultrastructural features of a highly active protein-secreting cell. The varying appearance of its endoplasmic reticulum probably reflects differing degrees of activity and accumulation of secretory product.

Plasma cells are the principal producers of antibodies, the immunoglobulins that participate in the humoral immune responses of the body (Fig. 5–21). These cells arise extravascularly by further differentiation of B lymphocytes that have migrated into the tissues from the blood. They are most numerous in the lymph nodes and spleen but may be found anywhere in the connective tissue where lymphocytes abound. Thus, they are common among the population of free cells in the lamina propria of the intestinal tract.

The B lymphocytes that are the immediate precursors of plasma cells make up only a small percentage of the circulating lymphocytes. They carry in their surface membrane molecules of immunoglobulin that they have produced in response to an initial encounter with an antigen earlier in their relatively long life span. These serve as specific receptors for that antigen in a subsequent exposure anywhere in the body. When antigen binds to these surface receptors, the antigen-antibody complexes aggregate and are taken into the cell by endocytosis. These events trigger transformation of the lymphocyte into a lymphoblast that divides repeatedly, giving rise to a clone of B lymphocytes all bearing the same antigenic specificity. Some members of this clone differentiate into plasma cells that synthesize and release large amounts of specific antibody. The remainder are added to the population of recirculating B lymphocytes with specificity for that particular antigen. This enables the individual to mount a more vigorous and sustained immune re-

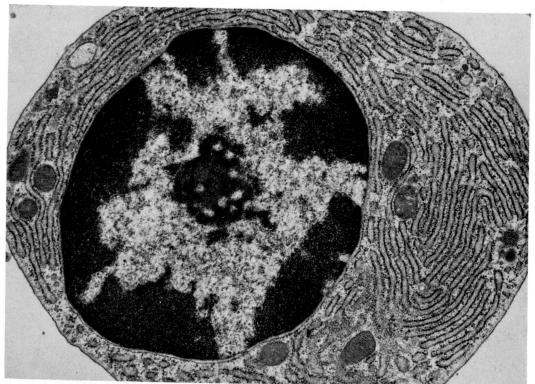

Figure 5–20. Electron micrograph of a plasma cell illustrating the coarse pattern of heterochromatin and the extensive rough endoplasmic reticulum. The large Golgi complex is not included in this plane of section.

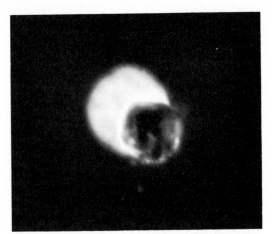

Figure 5–21. Fluorescence photomicrograph of a human plasma cell reacted with fluorescein-conjugated antibody against gamma globulin. The strong fluorescence of the cytoplasm identifies the cell as a site of immunoglobulin synthesis. (From Mellors, R., and L. Korngold. J. Exp. Med. *118*:387, 1963.)

sponse to reintroduction of the antigen to the body at a later time. The plasma cells formed have a limited life span in the lymphoid organs and connective tissue, and degenerate after a few weeks of active antibody synthesis.

Plasma cells are unusual among protein-secreting cells in that their product is not normally packaged and stored in conspicuous cytoplasmic granules. Instead, it appears to be transported from the Golgi complex to the cell surface in small vesicles and is released at the same rate as it is produced.

Occasional plasma cells contain spherical inclusions called *Russell bodies*. These stain with histochemical reactions for both protein and carbohydrate and also to some degree with fluorescein-conjugated antibody against immunoglobulin. In electron micrographs they are found within distended cisternae of the endoplasmic reticulum. Although the glycoprotein Russell bodies contain immunoglobulin, they are not regarded as normal secretory product but probably represent an aberrant state of the cell. Whether their presence is indicative of a defect in synthesis or transport is not known. It is speculated that they may be accumulations of light chains not used in the assembly of complete immunoglobulin molecules.

The train of evidence implicating plasma cells in antibody production extends back over 30 years and includes contributions from several disciplines. It was first observed that intensive immunization of animals was attended by a marked increase in the number of their plasma cells. It was later found that humans with *hyperglobulinemia*, an excess of circulating antibodies, had a high concentration of these cells in their tissues, whereas persons with congenital *agammaglobulinemia* developed no plasma cells at sites of antigenic stimulation and had a complete failure of antibody synthesis. Compelling direct evidence finally resulted from the demonstration of antibody production in vitro by individual plasma cells isolated from the tissues by microsurgery. Immunocytochemical methods localized antibody by light microscopy within plasma cells (Fig. 5–21) and electron microscopy localized antibody within the cisternae of the endoplasmic reticulum.

Eosinophils

The structure and functions of eosinophils have been presented in Chapter 4 and need not be reviewed here. Their function in the normal connective tissue is yet to be elucidated. What little is known has been deduced from observations of their behavior at sites of inflammation or parasitic invasion.

Eosinophils are often found in close proximity to basophils and mast cells, and it is possible that they inactivate histamine and other mediators released by these cells in inflammation. The most dramatic eosinophil responses are seen in parasitic diseases such as schistosomiasis, trichinosis, and ascariasis in which circulating eosinophils may rise to 90 per cent of the leukocyte count. In humans or experimental animals that have previously mounted an immune response to the parasite, a second invasion is rapidly followed by accumulation of very large numbers of eosinophils around the parasite larvae. Degranulation and release of MBP and other substances not yet identified results in killing and destruction of the larvae. This killing effect of the eosinophils is dependent on the presence of antiparasite antibody. In animals lacking such antibodies, this rapid mobilization and degranulation of eosinophils does not take place, and dissemination of parasites and severe disease may occur before immunity develops.

Mast Cells

The mast cells of connective tissue have several of the cytological and functional characteristics previously described for basophilic leukocytes (Chapter 4), but they are a distinct cell type. The basophils develop in the marrow, circulate in the blood, and migrate through the endothelium of small venules into the connective tissue. The mast cells originate in the connective tissue. They are especially abundant near the small blood vessels and have long been thought to develop from persisting perivascular mesenchymal cells. However, recent experimental evidence indicates that they differentiate from hemopoietic stem cells. Thus, it now seems likely that circulating stem cells enter the connective tissues from the blood and there differentiate into mast cells. Mast cells can also arise from preexisting mast cells by mitotic division.

Mast cells have a round or oval nucleus and their cytoplasm is filled with several hundred granules (Fig. 5–22), which stain metachromatically with toluidine blue or thionine. This property of changing the color of blue dyes to purple is due to their content of *heparin*, a sulfated acid mucopolysaccharide.

In electron micrographs, mast cells are observed to have numerous villous projections and undulant surface folds (Fig. 5–23).

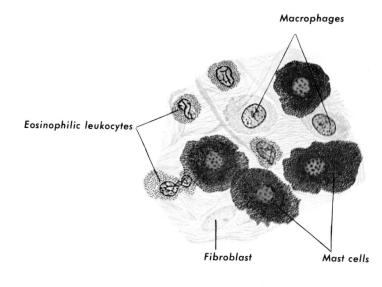

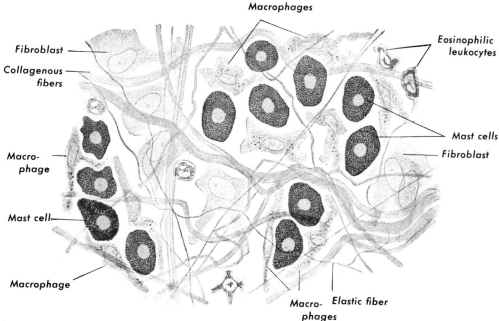

Figure 5–22. Mast cells in loose connective tissue of the rat. Upper figure was drawn from a preparation fixed and stained with hematoxylin-eosin-azure II. Lower figure depicts a fresh preparation stained supravitally with neutral red. The mast cell granules have bound the dye. Other elements of the tissue are largely unstained. (After A. A. Maximov.)

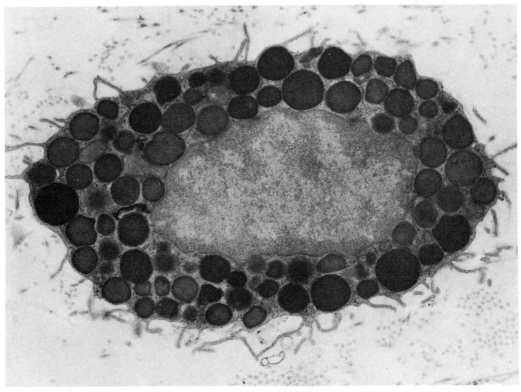

Figure 5–23. Electron micrograph of a mast cell from loose connective tissue of the rat.

The Golgi complex is well developed; the endoplasmic reticulum is sparse and the mitochondria relatively few. The dense granules are bounded by a membrane and display considerable variability in their substructure from species to species. Their content is finely granular in rodents, but they are quite heterogeneous in humans, with coarse subunits consisting of scrolls of thin lamellae of differing size and orientation. In some species the granules are soluble in aqueous fixatives.

It has long been known that mast cell granules contain *heparin*, an anticoagulant; *histamine*, which increases vascular permeability; and *serotonin*, which causes contraction of smooth muscle. The conditions under which these substances are released and the way in which they function in the connective tissues have become better understood in recent years. Mast cells are now recognized as sensitive sentinels detecting foreign substances and initiating a local inflammatory response in the tissues. Located near mucosal surfaces and along blood vessels, they are strategically situated to detect a variety of threats to the host. Their activation results in prompt release of the preformed chemical mediators stored in their granules and in slower generation of other biologically active

substances that serve to recruit other cell types to participate in local defense mechanisms.

Degranulation of mast cells can be experimentally induced by a number of nonspecific stimuli such as compound 48/80, polylysine, polymyxin B, certain snake venoms, and by lowering of the pH or osmolarity of the surrounding fluid. However, the stimulus most commonly invoking this response in vivo is invasion of the tissues by any foreign substance (antigen) to which the individual is sensitive (allergic). Thus, the activation and degranulation of mast cells is intimately related to the body's immune system (Chapter 13).

In addition to the major class of antibodies (IgG) involved in humoral immunity, the blood serum contains a minor immunoglobulin component, designated IgE, which is implicated in pathogenesis of allergies. The mast cell membrane contains from 50,000 to 300,000 receptors that bind IgE molecules to the cell surface (Fig. 5–24). When exposed to specific antigen, the antigen molecules form complexes with the surface IgE that alter the permeability of the mast cell membrane, permitting influx of calcium. The membrane of the mast cell granules then fuses with the plasmalemma, and the granule contents are discharged into the surrounding connective tissue matrix. This whole process of degranulation or explosive secretion is completed in two to three minutes. The histamine released causes transudation of fluid from dilated small venules, resulting in edema and local swelling. If the antigen is inhaled, histamine released by mast cells on the surface of the airways and in the submucosal connective tissue activates smooth muscle, constricting bronchi and bronchioles, thereby precipitating an asthma attack in susceptible individuals. The actions of histamine are supplemented by similar effects of another mediator generated after granule release called *slow-reacting substance of anaphylaxis* (SRS-A). In addition to these *vasoactive* and *bronchoconstrictive* mediators, discharge of mast cell granules is attended by liberation of *chemotactic mediators*—substances that attract leukocytes. The best characterized of these is *eosinophil chemotactic factor of anaphylaxis* (ECF-A), which induces emigration of eosinophils from the blood and their aggregation in the vicinity of activated mast cells.

Mast cell granules also contain the enzymes β-*glucuronidase hexosaminidase*, *arylsulfatase*, and *chymase*. These too are released by immunologically activated mast cells. Their effects in the extracellular environment are poorly understood, but they may degrade the glycosaminoglycans of the connective tissue ground substance.

Much remains to be learned about the functions of mast cells. It is well established that in allergic individuals their immunologically induced degranulation is responsible for an important train of events in the pathogenesis of both immediate and more persistent inflammatory processes. Recent investigations have focused on these dramatically rapid responses in sensitized animals and allergic humans, but it is likely that under normal conditions they secrete more or less continuously, at a slower rate. The possible significance of this activity for the homeostasis of the connective tissues is largely unknown.

The secretory activity of mast cells in inflammatory reactions is widely accepted but it is possible that they possess other nonse-

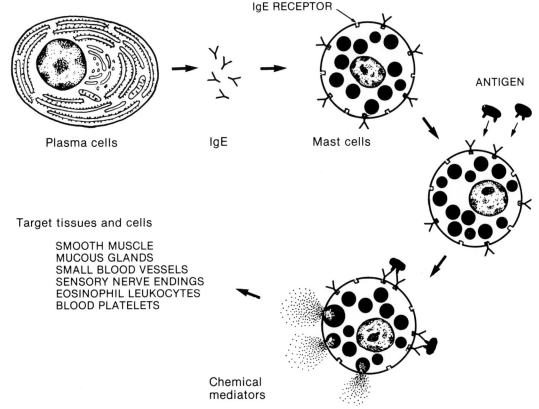

IgE RECEPTOR

ANTIGEN

Plasma cells   IgE   Mast cells

Target tissues and cells

SMOOTH MUSCLE
MUCOUS GLANDS
SMALL BLOOD VESSELS
SENSORY NERVE ENDINGS
EOSINOPHIL LEUKOCYTES
BLOOD PLATELETS

Chemical mediators

Figure 5–24. Schematic representation of the role of mast cells in allergic reactions. IgE produced by mast cells binds to IgE receptors in the mast cell membrane. On a second exposure, antigen binds to IgE and this event triggers mast cell degranulation with release of histamine and other chemical mediators that affect various target tissues and organs.

cretory functions in normal connective tissue. They take up thorium dioxide, used as an undigestible cell marker, and incorporate it in the granules. Marked cells are still detectable in rats after ten months indicating, that under normal conditions mast cells are very long-lived, and there is less turnover of their granules than would be expected if they were continuously secreting by degranulation.

SEROUS MEMBRANES

The serous membranes, *peritoneum, pleura,* and *pericardium*, are thin layers of loose connective tissue covered by a layer of mesothelium. When the membranes are folded, forming the omentum or the mesentery, both free surfaces are covered with mesothelium. The cavities lined by serous membranes always contain a small amount of liquid, the *peritoneal fluid* or *pleural fluid*. The cells in this exudate originate from the serous membrane.

All the elements of the loose connective tissue previously described are found in serous membranes, such as the mesentery. Because they are very thin and require no sectioning, the mesenteries have been favorite sites for the microscopic study of loose connective tissue. A mesentery contains a loose network of collagenous and elastic fibers, scattered fibroblasts, macrophages, mast cells, and a varying number of fat cells.

Physiologically the most important and histologically the most interesting of the serous membranes in mammals is the *omentum*. The membrane is pierced by innumerable holes and is thus reduced to a fine lacelike net formed by collagenous bundles covered by mesothelial cells. Such thin, fenestrated areas have few or no vessels. In the thicker areas where the omentum is a continuous sheet, macrophages are numerous. There are also many small lymphocytes and plasma cells and, occasionally, esoinophils and mast cells (Fig. 5–25). The number of lymphocytes and plasma cells varies considerably in different animal species.

In certain areas, the macrophages and other free cells accumulate in especially dense masses. Such macroscopically visible areas are often arranged along the blood vessels as round or oval patches called *milky spots*. These are sometimes found in the thin netlike part of the omentum. They are especially characteristic of the omentum of the rabbit.

The omentum in man extends downward from the greater curvature of the stomach like a loose curtain or veil over the intestines and is of great clinical importance in the limitation of disease processes in the abdominal cavity. When patients with a recently perforated ulcer are operated upon, it is usually found that the highly mobile omentum has already become locally adherent to the wall of the gut in an effort of nature to close the opening. Similarly, the omentum adheres at sites of inflammation and tends to wall off the process so that a local abscess will form instead of a generalized and often fatal peritonitis. In addition to the protection afforded by the adhesion of the omentum, the free cells of its connective tissue constitute an important mobile reserve to combat infections in the peritoneal cavity.

Free Cells of the Serous Exudate

Normally, the amount of serous exudate in the body cavities is small, but in pathological conditions it may increase enormously. It contains a variety of freely floating cells, including (1) macrophages that originate in the milky spots of the omentum and migrate into the cavity; (2) desquamated mesothelial cells that keep their squamous form or round up; (3) small lymphocytes, the vast majority of which have migrated from the blood vessels of the omentum; (4) eosinophilic leukocytes of hematogenous origin; (5) free mast cells, which are especially abundant in serous exudates of rats and mice; and (6) in pathological inflammatory exudates, enormous numbers of neutrophilic leukocytes.

DENSE CONNECTIVE TISSUE

Dense connective tissue differs from the loose form mainly in the great preponderance of the fibers over the cellular and matrix components. Where the fiber bundles are randomly oriented, the tissue is described as *dense irregular connective tissue*. Where the fibers are oriented parallel to one another or in some other consistent pattern, it is called *dense regular connective tissue*.

Dense Irregular Connective Tissue

This tissue is found in the dermis; in the capsules of many organs; sheaths of tendons

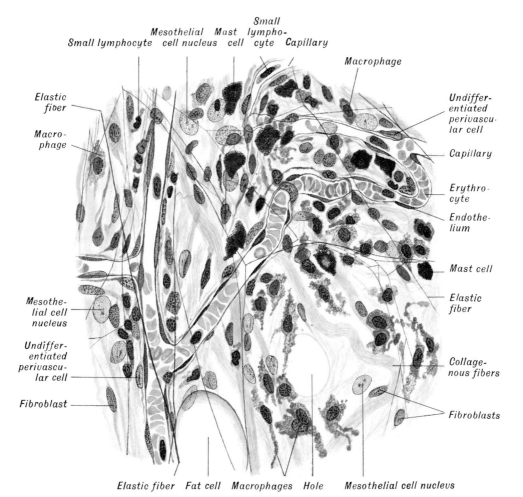

Figure 5–25. Drawing of a spread preparation of human omentum stained with hematoxylin-eosin-azure II. (After A. A. Maximov.)

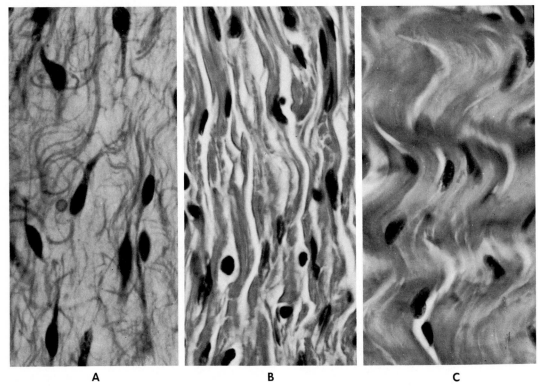

Figure 5–26. Photomicrographs illustrating connective tissues with differing amounts of collagen. *A,* Loose connective tissue from an 8-month-old fetus, showing relatively sparse, slender collagen fibers. *B,* Moderately dense irregular connective tissue with coarse, irregularly oriented bundles of collagen. *C,* Dense connective tissue with very abundant collagen in parallel wavy bundles.

and nerves; beneath the epithelium in parts of the urinary tract; and in many other sites in the body. Its structure in the dermis of the skin can be taken as typical. The elements are the same as in the loose connective tissue but the collagenous bundles are thicker and are woven into a compact feltwork. They are accompanied by extensive elastic networks. The fibers from the dermis continue directly into those of the subcutaneous tissue, but there the fiber bundles are thinner and their arrangement is correspondingly looser. There is less ground substance in the dense connective tissue. Among the densely packed collagenous and elastic fibers are the cells, but these are much more difficult to identify than in the loose tissue. The macrophages are recognizable only by vital staining. Along the small vessels there are always many inconspicuous fusiform cells, which are undifferentiated mesenchymal cells.

Dense Regular Connective Tissue

The collagen bundles of regular connective tissue are arranged according to a precise plan, and the specific arrangement reflects the mechanical requirements of the particular tissue. Macroscopically, the tissue has a distinctly fibrous structure and a characteristic shining white appearance.

Tendon consists predominantly of Type I collagen. It is composed of thick, closely packed bundles of collagen fibrils oriented parallel to the long axis of the tendon. Delicate networks of elastin have been described between the bundles of collagen fibrils, but these are inconspicuous and detectable only after specific staining of elastin.

In transverse sections examined with the electron microscope, the collagen fibrils are of two sizes, one population averaging 60 nm in diameter and the other 175 nm (Fig. 5–28A). The relative numbers of the larger and smaller fibrils vary from tendon to tendon and in different areas of the same tendon. Delicate cross-bridging strands of unknown nature extend laterally from fibril to fibril (Fig. 5–28B).

The fibroblasts, which are the only cells present, are arranged in long parallel rows in the spaces between the parallel collagenous bundles. The cell bodies are rectangular, triangular, or trapezoidal when seen in surface view, and rod-shaped when seen in profile. Their cytoplasm stains darkly with basic dyes and contains a clear centrosome adjacent to the single flattened nucleus. Although the limits between the successive cells in a row are distinct, the lateral limits of the cells are indistinct. In a stained cross section of a tendon, the cells appear as dark star-shaped figures between the collagenous bundles. A tendon consists of a varying number of small tendon bundles bound by loose connective tissue into larger bundles (Fig. 5–27).

In the tendon the fibers form a tissue that is flexible but offers great resistance to pulling force. In certain forms of locomotion, the tendons of limb muscles are stretched when the foot strikes the ground, acting like a tension spring. The subsequent recoil of the tendons to their original length helps push the foot off the ground in the next stride. This mechanical or elastic energy requires no metabolic input such as that involved in muscle contraction. Human sprint-

ers may derive as much as 50 per cent of their locomotor energy from this source. Animals, such as the kangaroo, that have evolved a hopping gait make maximal use of this property of tendons. A kangaroo changing from walking to running actually decreases its oxygen consumption and at 30 miles per hour utilizes no more than an animal half its size running on all four feet at the same speed. The tendons are thus an important source of "free" energy for locomotion.

Ligaments are similar to tendons, except that the elements are somewhat less regularly arranged. In other examples of dense regular connective tissue, such as the *fasciae* and *aponeuroses*, the collagenous bundles and fibroblasts are arranged regularly in multiple sheets or lamellae. In each layer the fibers follow a parallel and often slightly wavy course. In the different layers the direction may be the same or it may change. The fibers often pass from one layer into another. Therefore, a clear isolation of the sheets is seldom possible. The cells that correspond to the tendon cells adapt their shape to the spaces between the collagenous bundles.

In dense connective tissue layers with somewhat less regularly arranged elements, such as the periosteum, sclera, and the like, a section perpendicular to the surface shows successive layers of collagenous bundles cut in the longitudinal, oblique, or transverse direction, and cells that are irregular, flat, or fusiform. In these tissues there are always gradual transitions to neighboring areas, where the elements have a quite irregular, dense arrangement. There is also no sharp distinction between them and the surrounding loose connective tissue.

The substantia propria of the cornea provides an example of dense regular connective tissue made up of successive layers of collagen with the fibrils of one layer oriented at approximately 90 degrees to those in the next layer (Fig. 5–29).

CONNECTIVE TISSUE WITH SPECIAL PROPERTIES

Mucous Connective Tissue

This tissue is found in many parts of the embryo and is a form of loose connective tissue. The classic example of this type of connective tissue is *Wharton's jelly* of the um-

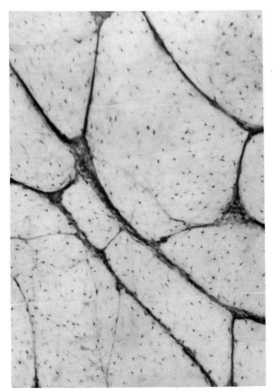

Figure 5–27. Cross section of human tendon. Massive bundles of collagen are separated by darker-staining loose connective tissue. Dots in the paler areas of collagen are nuclei of modified fibroblasts in narrow clefts among the collagen fibers.

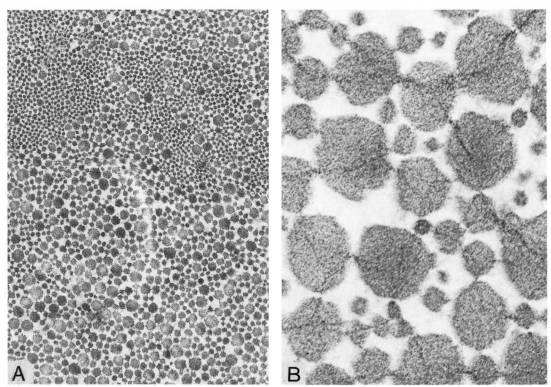

Figure 5–28. Electron micrographs of human tendon. *A,* Transverse section of Achilles tendon showing variations in the distribution and ratio of larger 175-nm fibrils to smaller 60-nm fibrils. *B,* High magnification of a small area of plantaris tendon illustrating linear densities extending from fibril to fibril. (Micrographs from Dyer, R. F. Cell Tissue Res. *168*:247, 1976.)

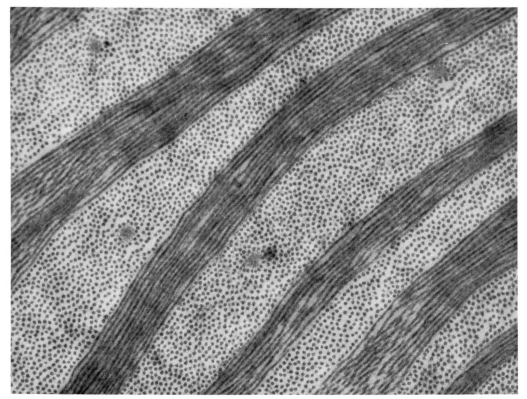

Figure 5–29. Electron micrograph of dense regular connective tissue of the cornea. The collagen is arranged in lamellae with the fibrils in alternate layers oriented at right angles to those in adjacent lamellae. (Micrograph courtesy of M. Jakus.)

bilical cord. The cells are large, stellate fibroblasts whose processes often are in contact with those of neighboring cells. A few macrophages and lymphoid wandering cells are also present. The intercellular substance is very abundant, soft, jelly-like, and homogeneous in the fresh condition. When fixed, much of it is extracted, and the residue contains granular and fibrillar precipitates. It has the staining reactions of mucin and contains thin, collagenous fibers that increase in number with the age of the fetus.

Examples of mucous connective tissue in adult animals are limited to the cockscomb and the dermis and hypodermis of the sex skin of monkeys. In both of these the ground substance is extraordinarily abundant, is of firm consistency, and is influenced by the sex hormones.

Elastic Connective Tissue

In the dense connective tissue of a few stuctures in the body, elastic fibers predominate, and the tissue has a yellow color on inspection with the naked eye. It may appear in the form of strands or sheets of coarse parallel fibers, as in the ligamenta flava of the vertebral column, in the vocal cords, in the ligamentum stylohyoideum, and in the ligamentum suspensorium penis. In these situations, the elastic fibers are thick and either round or flattened in cross section. They branch frequently and rejoin with one another at acute angles, as in a stretched fishing net. In cross section the angular or round areas representing the fibers form small groups. The spaces between the elastic fibers are filled with a delicate feltwork of collagenous fibrils and a few fibroblasts.

The classical example of *dense regular elastic connective tissue* is found in the massive ligamentum nuchae of ruminants. It consists of coarse elastic fibers 10 to 15 μm in diameter, closely associated in parallel bundles. Its stretch and elastic recoil permits grazing animals to cut off grass with their lower incisors with relatively little expenditure of energy.

Scarpa's fascia of the human anterior abdominal wall, which aids in the support of the viscera, also consists largely of elastic fibers. The corresponding layer in the large quadrupeds, called the tunica abdominalis, is a thick yellow sheet of dense elastic tissue several millimeters in thickness, which plays an important role in supporting the viscera while permitting some degree of abdominal distention.

Elastic tissue forms layers in the walls of hollow organs upon which a changing pressure acts from within, as in the largest arteries and in the trachea and bronchi. In the large elastic arteries, the elastic tissue takes the form of a *fenestrated membrane*, a sheet of elastin of variable thickness provided with many irregular openings. The fenestrated membranes are arranged in multiple layers concentric with the lumen of the vessel and are connected with one another by oblique ribbon-like branches. The spaces between the lamellae contain a mucoid ground substance and smooth muscle cells of irregular outline. Fibrous elastic networks, as well as fenestrated elastic membranes, exist in the walls of these vessels and it is difficult to distinguish clearly between the two in sections.

Reticular Connective Tissue

Most of the fibrous elements around the sinusoids of the liver and in the stroma of lymphatic organs, hemopoietic tissue, and the spleen are blackened by silver stains and are thus identified as reticular fibers. The patterns of the fibers in these examples of *reticular connective tissue* are also distinctive. Small bundles of thin collagenous fibrils form complex three-dimensional networks, whose interstices are occupied by large numbers of free cells. Stellate cells of mesenchymal origin are also associated with the argyrophilic reticulum in these organs.

HISTOPHYSIOLOGY OF CONNECTIVE TISSUE

Normal Functions

Connective tissue functions in *mechanical support, exchange of metabolites* between blood and the tissues, *storage* of energy reserves in adipose cells, *protection* against infection, and *repair* after injury.

For its mechanical role the fibrous components are most important, and their abundance and distribution are adapted to the local structural requirements. Delicate networks of reticular fibers support the basement lamina of epithelia, surround the capillaries and sinusoids, and envelop individual muscle fibers and the groups of parenchymal cells that form the functional units of organs. The coarser collagenous fibers abound where greater tensile strength is required. They form the tendons and the aponeuroses, the septa and fibrous capsules of organs. Elastic fibers give the tissues their suppleness and their ability to spring back to their normal relations after stretching. They are especially abundant in hollow organs subject to periodic distention. Loose connective tissue, with its abundant, highly hydrated ground substance, is commonly found beneath the integument, between muscles, and in other sites where mobility of the parts is advantageous. On the other hand, where strength is more important than mobility, dense connective tissue is formed, and its bundles of collagen fibers tend to be oriented so as to resist most efficiently the local mechanical stresses.

Connective tissue plays a significant role in nutrition of the other tissues that it surrounds and permeates. It is evident that all substances reaching the cells of these other tissues from the blood, and all the waste products of their metabolism that are returned to the blood and lymph, must pass through a layer of connective tissue. These metabolites are believed to diffuse through the aqueous phase of the gelatinous ground substance or along thin films of fluid coating the fibers. The exchange of materials is probably influenced by the viscous properties of the ground substance. The polyelectrolyte properties of its glycosaminoglycans suggest that the connective tissue extracellular matrix may also participate in maintaining water and electrolyte balance. In addition to the storage of energy in adipose cells, it is noteworthy that approximately half of the circulating proteins of the body are in the interstitial spaces and, because the proportions of albumin and globulin there differ from those in plasma, it is speculated that the connective tissue may exercise some selectivity in its depot function.

Inflammation

Of great importance in the defense against disease is the reaction of the connective tissue, called *inflammation*. A detailed consideration of this process falls into the sphere of general pathology, but some awareness of its mechanisms is essential to an understanding of the functions of the cellular elements of the blood and connective tissues.

Bacteria or other injurious agents breaching the mechanical barrier provided by epithelia induce an intense reaction in the connective tissue, resulting in local redness, swelling, heat, and pain. Tissue damage causes release of histamine from mast cells, which increases the caliber and rate of flow through the small vessels, resulting in redness and local elevation of tissue temperature. Increased permeability of the walls of postcapillary venules results in escape of fluid, fibrinogen, and immunoglobulins into the extravascular compartment, causing edema and associated swelling.

Other chemical mediators induce selective margination of blood leukocytes, diapedesis, and attraction to the site of injury. The polymorphonuclear leukocytes are the earliest and most abundant emigrants, followed after a day or so by monocytes that transform into macrophages, which phagocytose bacteria and tissue debris and eliminate them by intracellular digestion. If the invading bacteria are of species resistant to destruction, *chronic inflammation* ensues with a change in the nature of the cellular infiltration, with macrophages, lymphocytes, and plasma cells predominating. If the tissue invasion is not successfully controlled by the mobilization of phagocytic cells, the process is contained by proliferation of fibroblasts and formation of a dense wall of collagenous fibers.

The mobilization of neutrophils and monocytes at the site of injury is the result of *chemotaxis*—a vectorial motility of these cells toward substances that are generated by certain bacteria; by activation of serum complement; and by activation of Factor XII of the blood clotting system, which leads to formation of the chemotactic agents *kallikrein* and *plasminogen activator*. The bacteria are rendered more susceptible to phagocytosis by being coated with serum complement and specific antibody that gain access to them as a consequence of the increased permeability of the blood vessels. This enhancement of phagocytosis is called *opsonization*. Some encapsulated bacteria are resistant to destruction by phagocytes because they appear to have the capacity to inhibit fusion of lysosomes with the phagocytic vacuoles.

Repair

The regenerative capacity of fibroblasts and the fact that they respond so readily to injury by proliferation and fibrogenesis make them the principal agents of repair. They are involved in the healing of defects, not only in connective tissue proper, but also in other tissues that have little or no regenerative capacity of their own. For example, the heart muscle that degenerates following a heart attack is replaced by a connective tissue scar.

Although much has been learned about the production of collagen in the histiogenesis and repair of connective tissue, it must be realized that there are also mechanisms for the removal of collagen. This is of great importance in the growth and remodeling of bone and involves local production and release of the enzyme *collagenase.* Collagenase is also detected in mammalian tissues subject to cyclic regression, such as the uterine endometrium.

Hormonal Effects

The adrenocorticotropic hormone of the pituitary and cortisone of the adrenal cortex both tend to lower the glycosaminoglycan content of the ground substance. They also diminish the intensity of the cellular response in inflammation. The response of connective tissues to sex hormones varies greatly with the species, the sex, and the site in the body. The most dramatic effects are on the sex skin of monkeys, where estrogens greatly increase the glycosaminoglycans of the extracellular matrix and in the cockscomb, where testosterone stimulates accumulation of hyaluronic acid and formation of collagen. Less dramatic hormonal effects are detected in the human female in the periodic increase in hydration of the tissues during certain phases of the menstrual cycle.

Disturbances of Collagen Metabolism

Collagen metabolism is affected by age and nutrition and may be rather specifically disturbed in a number of disease states. In some of these specific disorders, recently acquired knowledge of the mechanisms of fibrogenesis has provided a partial explanation of the defect or has made it possible to identify the step in the process where the normal biosynthetic mechanism fails. It has long been known that *scurvy,* the disease resulting from deficiency of vitamin C (ascorbic acid), is attended by an inability to form collagen fibers in normal abundance. It has now been found that addition of ascorbic acid in vitro to suspensions of fibroblasts from scorbutic animals enhances their conversion of proline to hydroxyproline in collagen. This suggests that the basic defect of collagen metabolism in scorbutic animals may be impaired synthesis of hydroxyproline, one of the amino acids peculiar to collagen.

A disease of domestic animals character-ized by bone deformities has been traced to the ingestion of the sweet pea *Lathyrus odoratus.* All the abnormalities of this disease, called *lathyrism,* can be reproduced by administration of β-aminopropionitrile, the toxic agent extracted from the sweet pea plant. Tropocollagen appears to be synthesized normally in such animals but is defective in its ability to form stable collagen fibrils. When tropocollagen is extracted at 0° C from *normal* animals and induced to form fibers by an increase in the temperature to 37° C, the longer it is held at that temperature the less soluble it becomes at 0° C. This time-dependent loss of solubility is believed to be due to formation of increased numbers of bonds between the tropocollagen units. In *lathyritic* animals there is a marked increase in the extractability of tropocollagen from connective tissue at 0° C, and although the extracted tropocollagen is capable of forming typical cross-striated fibers on warming, these fibers retain the ability to redissolve upon cooling even after prolonged periods at 37° C. This and other evidence suggests that ingestion of lathyritic agents results in synthesis of abnormal chains that are not able to cross-link adequately.

A rare inherited disease of humans, *Ehlers-Danlos syndrome,* is characterized by short stature, unusually stretchable skin, hypermobility of joints, and a tendency for joint dislocations. There is a related disease of cattle and sheep called *dermatosparaxis* in which the skin is fragile and very easily torn. Recent evidence indicates that the defect may reside in an abnormally low activity of the enzyme *procollagen peptidase,* which normally converts procollagen to collagen by cleaving off a peptide from the amino-terminal ends of the α_1 and α_2 chains of procollagen.

REFERENCES

GENERAL

Asboe-hanse, G., ed.: Connective Tissue in Health and Disease. Copenhagen, G. Munksgaard, 1954.

Hay, E. D., ed.: Cell Biology of Extracellular Matrix. New York, Plenum Press, 1981.

Kulonen, E., and J. Pikkarainen, eds.: Biology of the Fibroblast. New York, Academic Press, 1973.

Ramachadran, G. N., and A. H. Reddi, eds.: Biochemistry of Collagen. New York, Plenum Press, 1976.

Sandberg, L. B., W. R. Gray, and C. Franzbau, eds.: Elastin and Elastic Tissue. Advances in Experimental Medicine and Biology. Vol. 79. New York, Plenum Press, 1977.

COLLAGEN

Bornstein, P.: The biosynthesis of collagen. Annu. Rev. Biochem. *43*:567, 1974.

Hay, E. D., D. L. Hasty, and K. L. Kiehnan: Morphological investigation of fibers derived from various types. *In* Gastpar, H., K. Kühn, and R. Marx, eds.: Collagen—Platelet Interaction. Stuttgart, York, Schattauer, 1978.

Junqueira, L. C. U., W. Cossermelli, and R. R. Brentani: Differential staining of collagens types I, II and III by sirius red and polarization microscopy. Arch. Histol. Jpn. *41*:267, 1978.

Kivirikko, K. I., and L. Risteli: Biosynthesis of collagen and its alterations in pathological states. Med. Biol. *54*:159, 1976.

LeRoy, E. C.: Collagens and human disease. Bull. Rheum. Dis. *25*:778, 1975.

Mimmi, M. E.: Collagen: its structure and function in normal and pathological connective tissues. Semin. Arthritis Rheum. *4*:95, 1974.

Prokop, D. J., K. I. Kivirikko, L. Tuderman, and N. A. Guzman: Biosynthesis of collagen and its disorders. N. Engl. J. Med. *301*:77, 1979.

ELASTIN

Franzbau, C., and B. Faris: Elastin. *In* Hay, E. D., ed.: Cell Biology of Extracellular Matrix. New York, Plenum Press, 1981.

Gotte, L., M. G. Giro, D. Volpin, and R. W. Horne: The ultrastructural organization of elastin. J. Ultrastruct. Res. *46*:23, 1974.

Gray, W. R., L. B. Sandburg, and J. A. Foster: Molecular model for elastin structure and function. Nature (Lond.) *246*:461, 1973.

Ross, R., and P. Bornstein: Elastic fibers in the body. Sci. Am. *224*:44, 1971.

Ross, R., and P. Bornstein: The elastic fiber. J. Cell Biol. *40*:366, 1969.

Sandberg, L. B., N. T. Soskel, and J. G. Leslie: Elastin structure, biosynthesis and relation to disease states. N. Engl. J. Med. *304*:566, 1981.

GROUND SUBSTANCE

Balacz, E. D.: Glycosaminoglycans and proteoglycans. *In* Chemistry and Molecular Biology of the Intercellular Matrix. Vol. 2. New York, Academic Press, 1970.

Compar, W. D., and T. C. Laurent: Physiological function of connective tissue polysaccharides. Physiol. Rev. *58*:255, 1978.

Hascall, V. C., and G. K. Hascall: Proteoglycans. *In* Hay, E. D., ed.: Cell Biology of the Extracellular Matrix. New York, Plenum Press, 1981.

Lindahl, U., and M. Hook: Glycosaminoglycans and their binding to biological macromolecules. Annu. Rev. Biochem. *47*:385, 1978.

Rosenberg, L., W. Hellman, and A. K. Kleinschmidt: Electron microscopic studies of proteoglycan aggregates from bovine articular cartilage. J. Biol. Chem. *250*:83, 1975.

Ruoslahti, E., E. Engvall, and E. G. Hayman: Fibronectin: current concepts of its structure and function. Collagen Rel. Res., *1*:95, 1981.

Timpl, R., R. Rohde, P. G. Robey, S. I. Rennard, J. M. Foidart, and G. R. Martin.: Laminin—a glycoprotein from basement membranes. J. Biol. Chem. *254*:9933, 1979.

Trelstad, R. L., K. Hayashi, and B. P. Toole: Epithelial collagens and glycosaminoglycans in the embryonic cornea: macromolecular order and morphogenesis in the basement membrane. J. Cell Biol. *62*:815, 1974.

MONONUCLEAR PHAGOCYTE SYSTEM

Aschoff, L.: Das reticulo-endotheliale System. Ergeb. Inn. Med. Kinderheilk. *26*:1, 1924.

van Furth, R.: Current view on the mononuclear phagocyte system. Immunobiology *161*:178, 1982.

van Furth, R., Z. A. Cohn, J. G. Hirsch, J. H. Humphrey, W. G. Spector, and H. L. Langevoort: The mononuclear phagocyte system. A new classification of macrophages, monocytes, and their precursor cells. Bull. W.H.O. *46*:845, 1972.

MACROPHAGES

Cohn, Z. A.: Structure and function of monocytes and macrophages. Adv. Immunol. *9*:163, 1968.

Cohn, Z. A., and B. Benson: The differentiation of mononuclear phagocytes. Morphology, cytochemistry, and biochemistry. J. Exp. Med. *121*:153, 1965.

Gordon, S., and Z. A. Cohn: The macrophage. Int. Rev. Cytol. *36*:171, 1973.

Griffin, F. M., C. Bianco, and S. C. Silverstein: Characterization of the macrophage receptor for complement and demonstration of its functional independence from the receptor for the F_c portion of immunoglobulin G. J. Exp. Med. *141*:1269, 1975.

Griffin, F. M., J. A. Griffin, J. E. Leider, and S. C. Silverstein: Studies on the mechanism of phagocytosis. I. Requirements for circumferential attachment of particle-bound ligands to specific receptors on the plasma membrane. J. Exp. Med. *142*:1263, 1975.

Uananue, R. R., and J. Cerotti: The function of macrophages in the immune response. Semin. Hematol. *7*:225, 1970.

Weiss, L. P., and D. W. Fawcett: Cytochemical observations on chicken monocytes, macrophages and giant cells in tissue culture. J. Histochem. Cytochem. *1*:47, 1953.

MAST CELLS

Dvorak, H. F., and A. M. Dvorak: Basophils, mast cells and cellular immunity in animals and man. Hum. Pathol. *3*:454, 1972.

Fawcett, D. W.: An experimental study of mast cell degranulation and regeneration. Anat. Rec. *121*:29, 1955.

Ishizaka, H., H. Tomioka, and T. Ishizaka: Mechanism of passive sensitization. I. Presence of IgE and IgG molecules on human leukocytes. J. Immunol. *105*:1459, 1970.

Ishizaka, T.: Functions and development of cell receptors for IgE. *In* Johannsen, Strandberg, and Uvnäs, eds.: Molecular and Biological Aspects of Acute Allergic Reactions. New York, Plenum Publishing Co., 1976.

Kitamura, Y., M. Yokoyama, H. Matsudo, and T. Ohno: Spleen colony-forming cell as common precursor for tissue mast cells and granulocytes. Nature *291*:159, 1981.

Lagunoff, O.: Mast cell secretion: membrane events. J. Invest. Dermatol. *71*:81, 1978.

Metzger, H.: The IgE-mast cell system as a paradigm for the study of antibody mechanisms. Immunol. Res. *41*:186, 1978.

Padawer, J., ed.: Mast cells and basophils. Ann. N.Y. Acad. Sci. *103*:1, 1963.

Padawer, J.: Mast cells: extended life span and lack of granule turnover during normal *in vivo* conditions. Exp. Mol. Pathol. *20*:269, 1974.

Uvnäs, B.: Chemistry and storage function of mast cell granules. J. Invest. Dermatol. *71*:76, 1978.

Wasserman, S. I.: The lung mast-cell: its physology and potential relevance to defense of the lung. Environ. Health Perspect. *35*:153, 1980.

EOSINOPHILS

Archer, R. K.: On the functions of eosinophils in the antigen-antibody reaction. Br. J. Haematol. *11*:123, 1965.

Beeson, P. B., and D. A. Bass: The Eosinophil. Philadelphia, W. B. Saunders Co., 1977.

Hirsch, J. G.: The eosinophil leucocyte. *In* Zweifack, B. W., L. Grant, and R. T. McCluskey, eds.: The Inflammatory Process. New York, Academic Press, 1965.

Hudson, G.: Quantitative study of eosinophil granulocytes. Semin. Hematol. *5*:166, 1968.

Litt, M.: Eosinophils and antigen-antibody reaction. Ann. N.Y. Acad. Sci. *116*:964, 1964.

TENDON

Cooper, R. R., and S. Misol: Tendon and ligament insertion—a light and electron microscopic study. J. Bone Joint Surg. [Br.] *52*:1, 1970.

Dyer, R. F., and C. D. Enna: Ultrastructural features of adult human tendon. Cell Tissue Res. *168*:247, 1976.

Elliott, D. H.: Structure and function of tendon. Biol. Rev. *40*:392, 1965.

Field, P. L.: Tendon fibre arrangement and blood supply. Aust. N.Z. J. Surg. *40*:298, 1971.

6

ADIPOSE TISSUE

Adipose tissue was long considered to be a metabolically inert tissue that passively stored fat, provided insulation against heat loss, and functioned in mechanical support in certain regions of the body. The allocation of a separate chapter to it in recent textbooks of histology is a consequence of its belated recognition as a diffuse organ of primary metabolic importance.

Most animals feed intermittently but consume energy continuously; there must therefore be provision for temporary storage of fuel. Lipid is the most favorable substance for this purpose because it weighs less and occupies less volume per calorie of stored chemical energy than either carbohydrate or protein. Although many tissues contain small amounts of carbohydrate and fat, the adipose tissue serves as the body's most capacious reservoir of energy. About 10 per cent of the total body weight of an average human is fat, representing approximately a 40-day reserve of energy. In obese individuals this may increase to the equivalent of a year or more of normal metabolism. By accumulating lipid in periods of excess food intake and releasing fatty acids in periods of fasting, adipose tissue plays an important role in maintaining a stable supply of fuel. Far from being inert, the cells of this tissue are capable of actively synthesizing fat from carbohydrate and are highly responsive to hormonal and nervous stimulation.

HISTOLOGICAL CHARACTERISTICS OF THE ADIPOSE TISSUES

In most mammals there are two distinct types of adipose tissue, which differ in their color, distribution, vascularity, and metabolic activity. One is the familiar yellow or *white adipose tissue,* which composes the bulk of body fat. The other, called *brown adipose tissue,* is less abundant and occurs only in certain specific areas. There are marked species differences in the relative amounts of the two types of fat. Brown adipose tissue is most abundant in hibernating species. Although it is present in primates, including man, it is relatively inconspicuous and probably does not assume great importance in the economy of these species.

The peripheral parts of lobules of brown adipose tissue often have an appearance strongly suggestive of a transition from one form of fat to the other. This has fostered the widespread belief that brown fat is simply an immature or transitional form of ordinary adipose tissue. For this reason it is sometimes referred to in the literature of pathology as *fetal fat.* The term is not appropriate however, for in those species in which it is best developed, brown fat persists throughout adult life and is morphologically and metabolically sufficiently different to warrant its designation as a distinct type of adipose tissue. We will return to this point in discussing the histogenesis of the adipose tissues.

Unilocular Adipose Tissue

Fat varies in color from white to deep yellow, depending in part on the abundance of carotinoids in the diet. The color resides mainly in the stored lipid. The cells are very large, ranging up to 120 μm in diameter. They are typically spherical but may assume polyhedral shapes because of mutual deformation (Fig. 6–1). A single droplet of lipid occupies most of the volume of the cell. Therefore, adipose cells of this kind are described as *unilocular* to distinguish them from brown fat cells, which contain multiple small droplets and are described as *multilocular.* The nucleus is displaced to one side by the accumulated lipid and the cytoplasm is reduced to a thin rim constituting only about one fortieth of the total volume of the cell. The lipid is usually extracted during prepaof endoplasmic reticulum, and a moderate number of free ribosomes. The thin layer of cytoplasm surrounding the lipid droplet also contains a few mitochondria, 10-nm filaments, and minute vesicles, which may represent the agranular reticulum. Not infrequently there also are small droplets of newly formed lipid that has not yet coalesced with the principal lipid drop (Figs. 6–3 and 6–4). The lipid droplet is not bounded by a membrane but its interface with the cytoplasm may stain more intensely, giving a specious appearance of a limiting membrane. A regular network of orthogonally arranged 6-nm filaments is often observed around the lipid droplet (Fig. 6–6). Similar filaments occurring singly or in small bundles are found randomly oriented elsewhere in the cytoplasm. Each adipose cell is invested by a layer of glycoprotein resembling the basal lamina of epithelia. The plasma membrane shows numerous minute invaginations of the kind that are usually interpreted as evidence for a

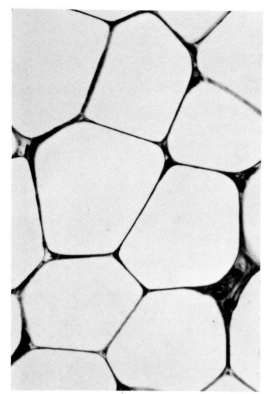

Figure 6–1. Common unilocular adipose tissue prepared by routine methods. The lipid droplet of the cells has been extracted during dehydration and only a thin rim of cytoplasm remains.

ration of histological sections, so that only the plasmalemma and a thin shell of cytoplasm remain. With silver stains each cell is found to be surrounded by delicate reticular fibers. In the angular spaces between the cells are cross sections of capillaries that form a loose plexus throughout the tissue. If well preserved, adipose tissue appears in section as a delicate network with large polygonal meshes (Figs. 6–1 and 6–2), but the cell rims often collapse to varying degrees during preparation, giving the cells an irregular outline.

Adipose tissue is often subdivided into small lobules by connective tissue septa. This compartmentation, visible with the naked eye, is most obvious in regions where the fat is subjected to pressure and has a cushioning or shock-absorbing effect. In other regions, the connective tissue septa are thinner and the lobular organization of the tissue is less apparent.

Examined with the electron microscope, the cytoplasm near the nucleus is found to contain a small Golgi complex, a few filamentous mitochondria, occasional short profiles

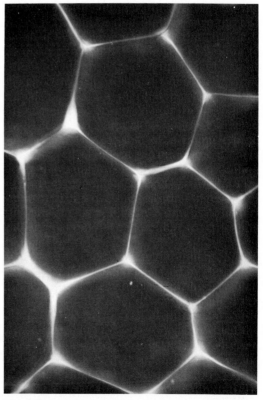

Figure 6–2. A thin spread of adipose tissue of mesentery stained with Sudan black without previous dehydration. Here the lipid droplet has been retained and is stained by the fat-soluble dye, while the surrounding rim of cytoplasm is unstained. (From Fawcett, D. W. *In* Greep, R. O., ed.: Histology. Philadelphia, Blakiston Co., 1953. Reproduced by permission of McGraw-Hill Book Co.)

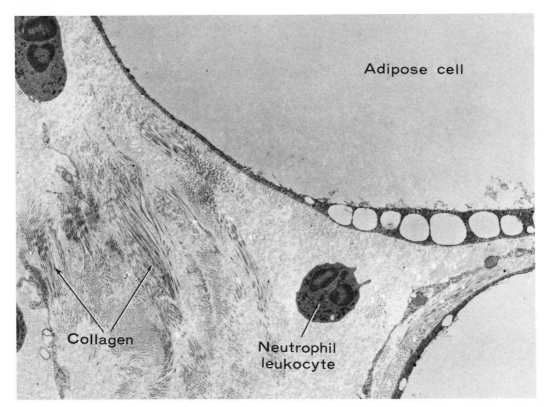

Figure 6–3. Electron micrograph of portions of two unilocular adipose cells from the epididymal fat pad of the rat. Notice the relative sizes of the neutrophil leukocyte and the very large fat cell. The cell at upper right has several small lipid droplets that have not yet coalesced with the large lipid droplets.

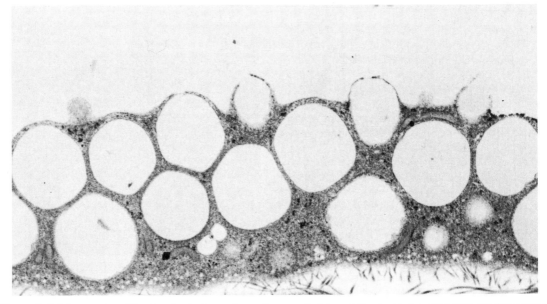

Figure 6–4. Micrographs of the rim of cytoplasm of an adipose cell. A few of the numerous small lipid droplets appear to be discharging their contents into the main lipid droplet at the top of the figure.

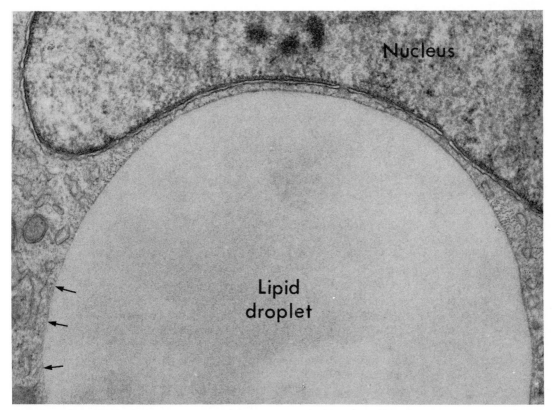

Figure 6–5. Micrograph of a portion of a developing adipose cell. After glutaraldehyde fixation the lipid often is only slightly stained by osmium, and the interface between the lipid and the cytoplasm *(at arrows)* can be seen more clearly. Notice the absence of a membrane around the lipid. (Micrograph courtesy of E. Wood.)

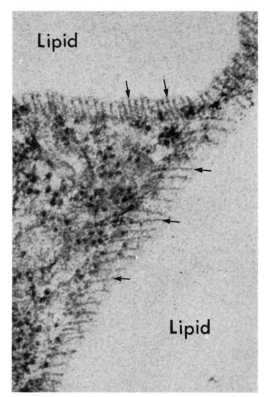

Figure 6–6. Micrograph of portions of two lipid droplets and the intervening cytoplasm in a developing adipose cell. The lipid-cytoplasm interface is sectioned obliquely, revealing *(at arrows)* an ordered array of 10-nm filaments at the boundary. (Micrograph courtesy of E. Wood.)

submicroscopic form of pinocytosis. The significance of these vesicles has been the subject of considerable debate. It has been suggested that they may be involved in uptake of materials used by the cell in lipid synthesis. However, their number is reported to increase greatly during prolonged starvation and after norepinephrine administration. This has led to the speculation that fatty acid and glycerol formed during lipolysis may be transported in vesicles to the cell surface for release. Since it is not easy to determine from fixed images the direction of vesicular transport, the role of these vesicles in the economy of the adipose cell remains unresolved.

In prolonged fasting or in the emaciation associated with chronic illness, adipose tissue may give up much of its stored lipid and revert to a highly vascular tissue containing aggregations of ovoid or polygonal cells with multiple small lipid droplets. In electron micrographs of fat cells decreasing in size during fasting, the cell surface becomes highly irregular in outline with numerous pseudopod-like processes, and the redundant exter-

nal lamina no longer conforms to the cell surface but becomes folded. The cells never revert to simple fusiform elements resembling fibroblasts.

Distribution of Unilocular Adipose Tissue (White Fat)

This type of fat is widely distributed in the subcutaneous tissue but exhibits regional differences, which are influenced by age and sex. In infants and young children there is a continuous subcutaneous layer of fat, the *panniculus adiposus,* over the whole body. In adults it thins out in some regions but persists and grows thicker in certain sites of predilection. These sites differ in the two sexes and are largely responsible for the characteristic differences in body form of males and females. In the male, the principal areas are the nape of the neck, the subcutaneous area overlying the deltoid and triceps muscles, the lumbosacral region, and the buttocks. In the female, subcutaneous fat is most abundant in the breasts, the buttocks, the epitrochanteric region, and the lateral and anterior aspects of the thighs.

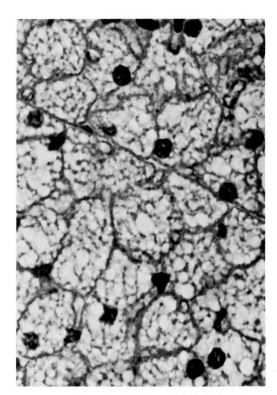

Figure 6–7. Photomicrograph of typical multilocular adipose tissue (brown fat). The polygonal cells contain more cytoplasm than in white fat and have multiple lipid droplets of varying size.

In addition to these superficial fat deposits, there are extensive accumulations in both sexes in the omentum, mesenteries, and retroperitoneal areas. All these areas readily give up their stored lipid during fasting. There are other areas of adipose tissue, however, that do not give up their stored fuel so readily. For example, the adipose tissue in the orbit, in the major joints, and on the palms of the hands and soles of the feet does not seem to be grist for the metabolic mill but instead has the mechanical function of support. These areas diminish in size only after very prolonged starvation.

Multilocular Adipose Tissue (Brown Fat)

The color of this form of adipose tissue ranges from tan to a rich reddish brown. Its cells are smaller than those of white fat and are polygonal in section. The cytoplasm is more abundant and there are multiple lipid droplets of varying size (Fig. 6–7). The spherical nucleus is somewhat eccentric in position but is seldom displaced to the periphery of the cell. A small Golgi apparatus is present, as well as numerous large spherical mitochondria. In electron micrographs the mitochondria occupy a large part of the cytoplasm and have numerous cristae that may extend across the full width of the organelle (Fig. 6–8). The endoplasmic reticulum is not well developed, and only a few profiles of the smooth-surfaced form can be found. The lipid droplets do not appear to develop within the reticulum but are free in the cytoplasm. Scattered ribosomes and variable amounts of glycogen are also present in the cytoplasmic matrix.

The connective tissue stroma of brown adipose tissue is very sparse and the blood supply exceedingly rich (Fig. 6–9). The cells are therefore in more intimate association with one another and with the capillaries than is the case in unilocular fat. Numerous small unmyelinated nerve fibers can be demonstrated among the brown fat cells by silver staining methods and in electron micrographs. Naked axons are frequently encountered in close apposition to the surface of the adipose cells.

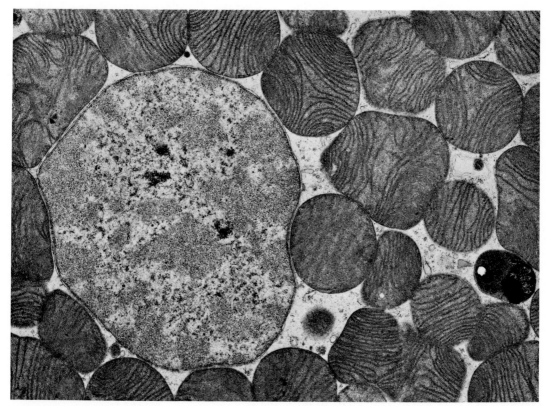

Figure 6–8. Electron micrograph of the nucleus and adjacent cytoplasm of a brown adipose cell from a bat recently aroused from hibernation. Typical of this tissue is a great abundance of very large mitochondria with cristae traversing the entire width of the organelle.

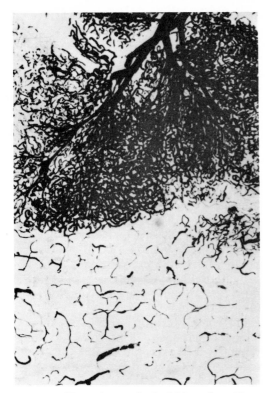

Figure 6–9. Photomicrograph of a thick section of brown and white adipose tissue in which the blood vessels have been injected with India ink. The vascular network of the brown adipose tissue *(above)* is extraordinarily rich and has a glandlike pattern, while that of the white fat *(below)* is relatively sparse. (From Fawcett, D. W. J. Morphol. *90*:363, 1952.)

The histological organization of brown fat is always distinctly lobular, and the pattern of distribution of the blood vessels within lobes and lobules resembles that found in glands. In animals subjected to prolonged fasting the brown fat gradually becomes more deeply colored and reverts to a compact, glandlike mass of epithelioid cells bearing no resemblance to a connective tissue (Fig. 6–10). The depletion of lipid in brown adipose tissue is more rapid in animals subjected to a cold environment.

The brown color of the tissue is in large part attributable to the high concentration of cytochromes in its extraordinarily abundant mitochondria. The relative oxidative capacity of brown adipose tissue, based on cytochrome oxidase, is greater than that of cardiac muscle.

Distribution of Multilocular Adipose Tissue

Brown or multilocular adipose tissue arises in embryonic life in certain specific sites, and

no new areas develop after birth. This is in contrast to ordinary fat cells, which may develop in almost any area of loose connective tissue, and new adipose cells may appear at any time in postnatal life. Brown adipose tissue may not occur in all mammals, but its presence has been established in representatives of at least seven of the orders, including primates. It is prominent in the newborn of all the species in which it occurs and is a distinct and conspicuous tissue in the adults of hibernating species. In some nonhibernating species, including man, the multilocular condition of the lipid in its cells gradually diminishes postnatally by coalescence of the droplets, so that the cells may gradually come to resemble those of unilocular adipose tissue. For this reason, there has been some debate as to whether or not there are two physiologically distinct types of adipose tissue in well-nourished human adults. The bulk of the evidence now indicates that two types do exist, even though they may be difficult to distinguish morphologically in well-nourished adults. Brown fat is well differentiated

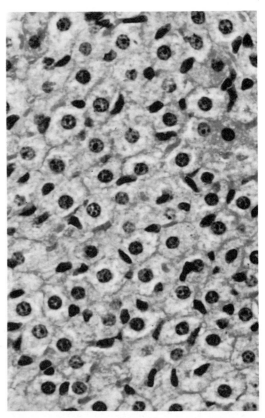

Figure 6–10. Brown adipose tissue that has been depleted of lipid after prolonged fasting, or after hypophysectomy, takes on the appearance of a compact glandular epithelium. Its cells bear no resemblance to fibroblasts.

as early as the twenty-eighth week in the human fetus, and in the newborn constitutes about 2 to 5 per cent of total body weight. In adults, all the fat may appear to be of the unilocular variety, but in the elderly, in persons with chronic wasting diseases, or in starvation, glandlike masses of multilocular fat cells reappear in the same regions where they are found in the newborn. Moreover, two types of *lipomas* (fatty tumors) occur in man—one resembling unilocular adipose tissue and the other resembling brown adipose tissue. These observations lend support to the view that both types of adipose tissue are represented in man throughout life.

In the common laboratory rodents, brown fat occurs in two symmetrical interscapular fat bodies, in thin lobules between muscles around the shoulder girdle, and in the axillae. It fills the costovertebral angle and forms long slender lobules on either side of the thoracic aorta. Smaller lobules are also found in the anterior mediastinum, along the great vessels in the neck, and in the hilus of the kidney. Brown adipose tissue is less extensive in primates, but in young macaques and in newborn humans, sizable masses can be found in the axillae and in the posterior triangles of the neck. Smaller lobules are found near the thyroid, along the carotid sheath, and in the hilus of the kidney.

HISTOGENESIS OF ADIPOSE TISSUE

Histogenesis of adipose tissue has long been controversial and unanimity has yet to be achieved. Histologists of the last century considered adipose tissue to be merely loose connective tissue in which lipid had accumulated in many of the fibroblasts. According to this interpretation, any and all connective tissue could become adipose tissue when dietary intake exceeded energy expenditure. Connective tissue is ubiquitous; however, in obesity, adipose cells do not become universally and evenly distributed but develop preferentially in certain sites while others remain unchanged. For example, the eyelids, nose, ears, scrotum and genitalia, and the back of the hands and feet rarely accumulate fat. This would be hard to explain if adipose cells could arise from fibroblasts wherever they occurred.

Later histologists maintained that unilocu-lar adipose cells differentiate from special formative cells, called *lipoblasts*, that arise from mesenchymal cells in late fetal and early postnatal life. According to this interpretation, the characteristic pattern of fat deposits in the adult would reflect the distribution and relative abundance of the lipoblasts formed in the fetal and neonatal period. These hypothetical lipoblasts are fusiform or stellate cells with no cytological features that clearly distinguish them from other relatively undifferentiated connective tissue cells. Some histologists therefore consider it unnecessary to postulate a separate category of committed stem cells but prefer to interpret the immediate precursors of adipose cells as persisting pluripotential mesenchymal cells.

The view prevailing now is that there are two processes of adipose tissue formation in mammals (Fig. 6–11). In one taking place in fetal life and called *primary fat formation,* special epithelioid precursor cells are laid down in lobular, glandlike arrangements. These accumulate multiple lipid droplets and become the multilocular adipose tissue found in most mammalian species. In addition, adipose cells can arise in late fetal and early postnatal life by accumulation of lipid in relatively undifferentiated cells of connective tissue without these cells becoming organized into epithelioid glandlike lobules. This *secondary fat formation* results in the disseminated unilocular adipose tissue of the adult.

These two distinct modes of histogenesis of fat are identifiable in the human. In postnatal life, however, the multiple lipid droplets in cells of areas of primary fat formation tend to coalesce, resulting in a tissue closely resembling unilocular adipose tissue. Thus, in the well-nourished adult there appears to be only one morphological type of adipose tissue, but there are in fact two, differing in their ontogeny and physiology.

In affluent developed countries, obesity is a major health problem. Excess adipose tissue puts an added strain on the circulatory system and increases the risk for those predisposed to myocardial infarction and hypertension. Obesity developing in adult life commonly results from accumulation of excess lipid in a normal number of unilocular adipose cells *(hypertrophic obesity).* In severe obesity, however, there may also be a greater than normal number of adipose cells *(hypercellular obesity).* The precursor cells are formed in the early postnatal period and adipose cells are incapable of proliferation later in life. There

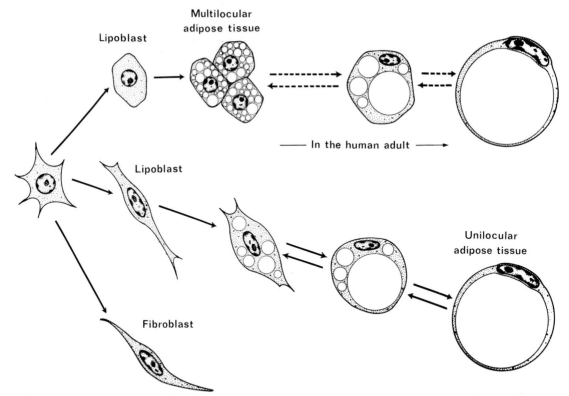

Figure 6–11. Schematic representation of histogenesis of the adipose tissues. Mesenchymal cells differentiate into fibroblasts and two kinds of lipoblasts. One forms glandlike aggregations of epithelioid cells that accumulate multiple lipid droplets and develop into multilocular adipose tissue. In primates, including humans, the lipid droplets may coalesce to varying degrees in well-nourished adults, so that the tissue comes to resemble unilocular adipose tissue. The other kind of lipoblast, which is fusiform and more widely dispersed in the embryonic connective tissues accumulates lipid that coalesces into a single large droplet, forming typical unilocular adipose tissue. In prolonged fasting, when the lipid is depleted, the two types of adipose tissue revert to tissues of different appearance. Neither reverts to a spindle-shaped cell that could be mistaken for a fibroblast.

is now experimental and clinical evidence that overfeeding in the early weeks of life can induce formation of greater numbers of adipose cell precursors, resulting in a greater risk of hypercellular obesity in adult life. Infants achieving an early body weight over the 97th percentile are reported to be three times as likely to become obese adults as are other infants. Conversely, infants who were born in a period of famine in Europe near the end of World War II had roughly one third the incidence of adult obesity compared with a similar group born in a period of plenty in the first summer of peace.

Thus, it seems clear that the level of nutrition in the early weeks of life can influence the number of adipose cell precursors. While adult hypertrophic obesity may occur from dietary excess in anyone, severe hypercellular obesity is more likely to occur in those who were overnourished as infants.

HISTOPHYSIOLOGY OF ADIPOSE TISSUE

Since the introduction of isotopic tracers for use in studying metabolism, it has been clearly shown that the lipid in fat depots is not an inert energy reserve drawn upon only in periods of inanition. On the contrary, the lipid is continuously being mobilized and renewed even in an individual in caloric balance. The half life of depot lipid in the rat is about eight days, which means that almost 10 per cent of the fatty acid stored in adipose cells is replaced each day by new fatty acid. The same kind of continual renewal occurs in man, but the quantities and time course of these events are not known with the same precision as in laboratory animals.

The histophysiology of adipose tissue can best be understood by analogy to deposits and withdrawals from a metabolic reserve bank or revolving fund. The "deposits" may be in the form of (1) fatty acids from the chylomicrons formed from dietary lipid, (2) fatty acids synthesized from glucose in the liver and transported to the adipose tissue in the form of serum lipoprotein, or (3) triglyceride synthesized from carbohydrate in the adipose cells themselves. "Withdrawals" are made by enzymatic hydrolysis of triglyceride and release of free fatty acids into the blood. With a continuous supply of glucose, lipolysis and release of free fatty acids are negligible. With alternations of fasting and feeding, which is the usual feeding pattern, lipolysis is increased severalfold during periods of fasting. The normal balance is greatly affected by hormones and by the action of the nervous system.

In the deposition of fat from circulating chylomicrons and very-low-density lipoproteins, the triglycerides of these blood-borne particles are hydrolyzed in the adipose tissue capillaries by an enzyme, lipoprotein lipase, which is believed to be synthesized by adipose cells and subsequently localized in membrane at the luminal surface of the endothelium in the neighboring capillaries. The fatty acid resulting from lipoprotein hydrolysis traverses the endothelium, diffuses across the narrow extracellular space, and enters the adipose cells. The role of micropinocytotic vesicles in fatty acid transport and uptake is moot. In the thin rim of cytoplasm, fatty acids are combined with α glycerophosphate, an intermediate product of glucose metabolism, to form triglyceride (neutral fat), which is added to the lipid droplet. The smooth endoplasmic reticulum is the organelle principally involved in the reesterification of the fatty acids to form the triglycerides.

Much has been learned in recent years about the morphological and biochemical differentiation of adipose cells by studying a cell line, designated 3T3, which originated from disaggregated cells of a mouse fetus at the stage when adipose cell precursors were first appearing. When growth is arrested in cultures of these 3T3 preadipose cells, they exhibit in vitro the same morphological and biochemical changes that occur in adipose tissue development in vivo. Lipid droplets accumulate and the cells progressively assume the spherical shape of fat cells. Accompanying triglyceride accumulation, the rate of their endogenous fatty acid synthesis, measured by incorporation of labeled acetate,

increases up to 100-fold. Comparable increases are measured by incorporation of exogenous fatty acid into triglyceride. The activity of lipoprotein lipase also increases two orders of magnitude during in vitro adipose conversion.

Hormonal Influences

In many tissues under endocrine control, the hormones act by stimulating the enzyme adenyl cyclase in the cell membrane, which generates from ATP, the intracellular "second-messenger" cyclic AMP. The differing responses of various target organs to this common messenger depend on its activation of organ-specific protein kinases. Several hormones affect the release of fatty acid from adipose tissue—the hypophyseal hormones adrenocorticotropin (ACTH), thyrotropin (TSH), and luteinizing hormone (LH) and the adrenomedullary hormone epinephrine. The fat cell membrane contains specific receptors for each of these. The receptors regulate access of the hormones to adenyl cyclase. The cyclic AMP generated within the adipose cell activates lipase that degrades stored triglyceride to fatty acids and glycerol, which are released into the bloodstream. The importance of this process is evident when one considers that in humans, it results in release of nearly 200 g of free fatty acid a day, the oxidation of which in other tissues accounts for about 80 per cent of the basal oxygen consumption.

The characteristic differences in adipose tissue distribution in males and females has already been alluded to. Because hormones circulate freely in the blood and presumably reach all tissues in approximately equal concentrations, these differences in fatty distribution imply either that there are genetically determined differences in distribution of cells having the capacity to develop into fat cells, or that there are regional differences in sensitivity of the cells to circulating sex hormones. This regional difference in sensitivity does not seem to be restricted to the effects of sex hormones, for an excess of *adrenocortical hormone* results in a characteristic distribution of fat, of which a prominent feature is an accumulation of fat over the lower cervical region, producing a deformity referred to as "buffalo hump."

The hormone *insulin* is the main physiological factor controlling the uptake of glucose by adipose tissue and the synthesis of fat from carbohydrate. Whether given in vivo or added to the medium of adipose tissue incubated in vitro, it appears to stimulate the transport of glucose into the cell and to accelerate its metabolism along all of the paths open to it. It has an effect on the rate at which glucose is converted to glycogen and also acts on fatty acid synthetase. Oxygen consumption is stimulated because of the accelerated conversion of glucose to fatty acid. The effects of insulin in promoting glycogen deposition can be demonstrated morphologically and are very much more pronounced in brown than in white fat (Figs. 6–12, 6–13).

In the absence of insulin, as in diabetes, there is a rise in blood glucose, a diminished utilization of glucose, an increase in unesterified fatty acids in the plasma, and an increase in blood lipoproteins. Carbohydrates are normally used preferentially as an energy source, but in the diabetic, in whom carbohydrates cannot be utilized because of the deficiency

of insulin, the required energy is derived principally from fat.

Influence of the Autonomic Nervous System

Adipose tissue is rather richly innervated, especially the brown fat. The function of the nerves can be demonstrated experimentally by cutting the nerves of the interscapular fat body on one side of the midline, leaving the nerve supply to the other side intact. Within the first few postoperative days it becomes apparent that the fat cells on the denervated side are larger than those on the normal side. The differences in the two sides are more dramatic if the animal is then deprived of food and placed in a cold environment. These environmental conditions ordinarily lead to a rapid mobilization of lipid from the fat depots. In animals unilaterally denervated, the fat cells on the side with the nerves intact are rapidly depleted of lipid, while the

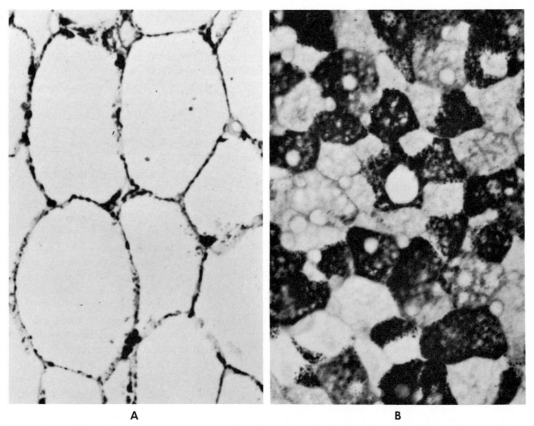

A   B

Figure 6–12. *A,* White adipose tissue of a rat refeeding after a period of fasting. The dark granular deposits in the rim of cytoplasm are glycogen, which subsequently disappears as the carbohydrate is used in synthesis of triglycerides. *B,* Under the same experimental conditions, considerably more glycogen is deposited in multilocular adipose tissue, but not all cells accumulate carbohydrate to the same degree. Some, therefore, stain relatively little with the periodic acid–Schiff reaction used here. A similar deposition of glycogen can be induced in unfasted animals by administration of excess insulin. (From Fawcett, D. W. J. Morphol. *90:*363, 1952.)

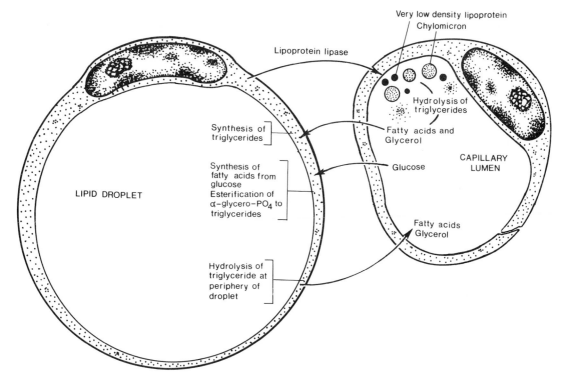

Figure 6–13. Schematic representation of lipid transport between the blood and adipose cells. An enzyme, lipoprotein lipase, probably synthesized by adipose cells, is localized in the endothelium of the adjacent capillaries. Lipid is carried in the bloodstream to the adipose cells in the form of chylomicrons from the intestine and very-low-density lipoproteins from the liver. In the capillaries, these are hydrolyzed by lipoprotein lipase to fatty acids and glycerol, which diffuse to the cytoplasm of the adipose cells where they are reesterified to triglyceride, which is added to the stored lipid. Glucose diffusing to the fat cells may also be used in the synthesis of triglycerides from carbohydrate. Upon neural or hormonal stimulation, elevated cyclic AMP activates a cytoplasmic lipase, which hydrolyzes triglyceride from the periphery of the droplet, and the resulting fatty acids and glycerol diffuse back to the capillaries and are carried in the blood to tissues throughout the body.

fat cells on the denervated side retain an almost normal content of lipid. It is thus demonstrated that the presence of nerves is necessary for normal mobilization of lipid from adipose tissue.

The chemical mediator norepinephrine is present in abundance in innervated adipose tissue but is low or absent after denervation. It is through release of norepinephrine from the nerve endings that the nerves control the mobilization of fatty acids from adipose tissue. Injection of small amounts of exogenous norepinephrine inhibits the action of insulin on fat cells and approximately doubles the amount of free fatty acid in the blood plasma. The norepinephrine brings about the activation of adipose tissue lipase, increasing the rate of hydrolysis of triglycerides. In patients who have an adrenomedullary tumor (pheochromocytoma) that secretes excessive amounts of norepinephrine, the plasma concentration of fatty acids may be several hundred times the normal level.

Brown Adipose Tissue as a Heat Generator

It has long been noted that brown adipose tissue is more abundant in animal species that hibernate, and it was assumed to have a function related to winter dormancy. There is now evidence that one of its functions is to serve as a "chemical furnace"—an oil burner to heat the animal during arousal from hibernation.

Homeothermic animals maintain their body temperature within a rather narrow range. When exposed to an unfavorable cold environment, they decrease their heat loss by constricting peripheral blood flow and increase their metabolism to generate more heat. The *basal metabolic rate* is the heat production or oxygen consumption in a resting, fasting animal in a thermoneutral environment. In a cold environment, extra heat can be produced by shivering— a form of involuntary isometric exercise. In addition to *shiv-*

ering thermogenesis, many species are capable of *nonshivering thermogenesis*—an increase in heat production that occurs without any increase in electrical activity in skeletal muscle. Brown adipose tissue has been found to be the most important site of nonshivering thermogenesis. Upon stimulation, it is capable of the highest oxygen consumption recorded for any organ. Its maximal consumption may represent a rate of heat production hundreds of times the average heat production of other organs, and the blood flow through this tissue can increase to seven times its own volume per minute.

When a hibernating animal begins to arouse, there is a marked increase in oxygen consumption and generation of heat without shivering. Nerve impulses to the brown adipose tissue release norepinephrine at the nerve endings, which leads to activation of lipase in the fat cells and breakdown of triglyceride to fatty acid and glycerol. Oxidation of fatty acid and reesterification of some of the fatty acid then occurs, with consumption of oxygen and generation of heat that serves to warm the blood flowing through the fat, secondarily raising the temperature of the animal as a whole.

Correlated with this function are some unusual features of the mitochondria. Oxidative phosphorylation is difficult to demonstrate in mitochondrial fractions from brown adipose tissue. The elementary particles or inner membrane subunits that are usually present on the mitochondrial cristae are thought to be the sites of phosphorylation enzymes. These have not been demonstrated in normal numbers in negatively stained mitochondria from brown adipose tissue. A deficiency of oxidative phosphorylation in mitochondria would be a surprising finding in any other normal tissue, but it is consistent with the needs of a system concerned mainly with heat production.

The heat generation by brown fat can be demonstrated visually by the new technique of thermography (Fig. 6–14). The thermograph scans across the body, detecting the infrared radiation from surfaces, and registers the temperature-dependent intensity of radiation on a photographic plate. When a bat arousing from hibernation is scanned, the thin wing membranes rapidly equilibrate with the ambient temperature, and most of the body is still relatively cool. However, a sharply delineated "hot area" is found on the thermograph, coinciding with the location of the interscapular brown fat. Thus, in hibernating species brown adipose tissue performs two important roles during arousal from dormancy: oxidation of lipid to produce heat within the brown fat, and release into the circulation of oxidizable substrates for utilization by other tissues.

When newborns of nonhibernating species such as the rat and rabbit are exposed to the cold or when they are infused with physiological amounts of norepinephrine, there is a substantial increase in oxygen consumption, and thermocouples embedded in their interscapular brown fat register a local production of heat.

It has now been shown that the human infant makes use of the same mechanism for heat generation. An infant placed in an environment at 23°C immediately after birth

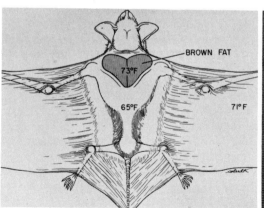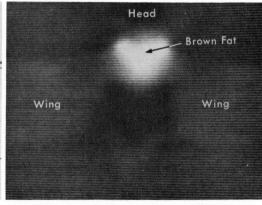

Figure 6–14. Thermograph of a bat during arousal from hibernation. Scanning the animal for detection of infrared radiation reveals a "hot spot" in the area corresponding to the interscapular brown adipose tissue. During arousal this tissue acts as a chemical "furnace," producing heat carried in the bloodstream to warm the rest of the body. (Thermograph courtesy of J. Hayward.)

will have approximately double the metabolic rate of an infant at 33°C and will accomplish this without shivering. There is an associated increase in the level of glycerol in the blood, resulting from lipolysis of triglycerides. Under these conditions, thermography reveals areas of elevated skin temperature over the sites of brown adipose tissue at the nape of the neck and in the axillae. It is possible that this adipose tissue may also have some slight thermogenic function in adults, but this is yet to be demonstrated.

REFERENCES

UNILOCULAR ADIPOSE TISSUE

Cushman, S. W.: Structure-function relationships in the adipose cell. I. Ultrastructure of the isolated adipose cell. II. Pinocytosis and factors influencing its activity in the isolated adipose cell. J. Cell Biol. 46:326, 342, 1970.

Green, H.: The adipose conversion of 3T3 cells. In Ahmad, F., T. R. Russell, J. Schultz, and R. Werner, eds.: Miami Winter Symp. Differentiation and Development. Vol. 15. New York, Academic Press, 1978.

Greenwood, M. R. C., and J. Hirsch: Postnatal development of adipocyte cellularity in the normal rat. J. Lipid Res. 15:474, 1979.

Heindel, J. J., L. Orci, and B. Jeanrenaud: Fat mobilization and its regulation by hormones and drugs in white adipose tissue. In Peters, C. (ed.): International Encyclopedia of Pharmacology and Therapy. Oxford, Pergamon Press, 1:175–373, 1975.

Hirsch, J., and B. Batchelor: Adipose tissue cellularity in human obesity. Clin. Endocrinol. Metab. 5:299, 1976.

Jeanrenaud, B.: Dynamic aspects of adipose tissue metabolism. A review. Metab. Clin. Exp. 10:535, 1961.

Napolitano, L.: The differentiation of white adipose cells: an electron microscope study. J. Cell Biol. 18:663, 1963.

Napolitano, L., and H. T. Gagne: Lipid depleted white adipose cells. Anat. Rec. 147:273, 1963.

Renold, A. E., and G. F. Cahill, eds.: Adipose Tissue Handbook of Physiology. Sec. 5. Washington, D.C., American Physiological Society, 1965.

Sheldon, H.: The fine structure of the fat cell. In Rodahl, K., and B. Issekutz, eds.: Fat As A Tissue. Baltimore, McGraw-Hill Book Co., 1964.

Slavin, B. G.: The cytophysiology of mammalian adipose tissue. Int. Rev. Cytol. 33:297, 1972.

MULTILOCULAR ADIPOSE TISSUE

Cannon, B., and B. W. Johansson: Non-shivering thermogenesis in the newborn. Mol. Aspects Med. 3:119, 1980.

Fawcett, D. W.: A comparison of the histological organization and histochemical reactions of brown fat and ordinary adipose tissue. J. Morphol. 90:363, 1952.

Foster, D. O., and M. L. Frydman: Tissue distribution of cold-induced thermogenesis in conscious warm- or cold-acclimated rats reevaluated from changes in tissue blood flow: the dominant role of brown adipose tissue in the replacement of shivering by non-shivering thermogenesis. Can. J. Physiol. Pharmacol. 57:257, 1979.

Himms-Hagen, J.: Cellular thermogenesis. Annu. Rev. Physiol. 38:315, 1976.

Lindberg, O., ed.: Brown Adipose Tissue. New York, American Elsevier Publishing Co., 1970.

Lindberg, O., J. de Pierre, E. Rylander, et al.: Studies of the mitochondrial energy-transfer system of brown adipose tissue. J. Cell Biol. 34:293, 1967.

Merklin, R. J.: Growth and distribution of human fetal brown fat. Anat. Rec. 178:637, 1974.

Nedergaard, J., and O. Lindberg: The brown fat cell. Int. Rev. Cytol. 74:310, 1982.

Nicholls, D. G.: Brown adipose tissue mitochondria. Biochim. Biophys. Acta 549:1, 1979.

Sidman, R. L., and D. W. Fawcett: The effect of peripheral nerve section on some metabolic responses of brown adipose tissue. Anat. Rec. 118:487, 1954.

Sidman, R. L., M. Perkins, and N. Weiner: Noradrenaline and adrenaline content of adipose tissues. Nature 193:36, 1962.

Smith, R. E., and B. A. Horwitz: Brown fat and thermogenesis. Physiol. Rev. 49:330, 1969.

7

CARTILAGE

Cartilage is a specialized form of connective tissue consisting of cells, called *chondrocytes,* and extracellular fibers embedded in a gel-like *matrix.* The intercellular components predominate over the cells, which are isolated in small cavities within the matrix. Unlike other connective tissues, cartilage has no nerves or blood vessels of its own. The colloidal properties of its matrix are therefore important to the nutrition of its cells and are in large measure responsible for its firmness and resilience. The capacity of cartilage for rapid growth while maintaining a considerable degree of stiffness makes it a particularly favorable skeletal material for the embryo. Most of the axial and appendicular skeleton is first formed in cartilage models, which are later replaced by bone.

Cartilage is of more restricted occurrence in postnatal life, but it continues to play an indispensable role as the long bones grow in length in the immature individual, and it persists in the adult on the articular surfaces of the long bones. Except where it is exposed to the synovial fluid in joints, cartilage is invariably enclosed in a dense fibrous connective tissue called the *perichondrium.*

Three kinds of cartilage, *hyaline, elastic,* and *fibrocartilage,* are distinguished on the basis of the amount of extracellular matrix and the relative abundance of the collagenous and elastic fibers embedded in it. Hyaline cartilage is the most common and most characteristic type, and the others can be regarded as modifications of it (Fig. 7–1).

HYALINE CARTILAGE

In the adult, hyaline cartilage is found on the ventral ends of the ribs, in the tracheal rings and larynx, and on the joint surfaces of bones. It is a somewhat elastic, semitransparent tissue with an opalescent bluish gray tint. Its histological appearance is most easily understood from a consideration of its mode of development.

Histogenesis of Cartilage

At sites of future cartilage formation in the embryo, the mesenchymal cells first withdraw their processes and become crowded together in dense aggregations called *protochondral tissue* or *centers of chondrification.* The nuclei of the cells are very close together and the cell boundaries are indistinct (Fig. 7–2A,B). As the cells enlarge and differentiate, they secrete around themselves a metachromatic extracellular matrix (Fig. 7–2C). Tropocollagen is secreted at the same time, but the fibrils that form extracellularly tend to be masked by the hyaline matrix in which they are embedded. As the amount of interstitial material increases, the cells become isolated in separate compartments or *lacunae* and gradually take on the cytological characteristics of mature cartilage cells or *chondrocytes* (Fig. 7–3).

The continuing growth of cartilage takes place by two different mechanisms. Mitosis is observed among the cells for a rather long period. After the constriction of the cytoplasm in such a division, a new partition of interstitial substance quickly develops and separates the two daughter cells. These in turn may divide, giving rise to clusters of four, and so on. The mitotic division of the chondrocytes and the secretion of new matrix between the daughter cells lead to an expansion of the cartilage from within, which is referred to as *interstitial growth.*

The mesenchyme surrounding the cartilage primordium condenses to form a special layer, the perichondrium, which merges with the cartilage on one side and with the adjacent connective tissue on the other (Fig. 7–4). Throughout embryonic life the cells on the inner or *chondrogenic layer* of the perichondrium constantly differentiate into chondrocytes, secrete matrix around themselves, and

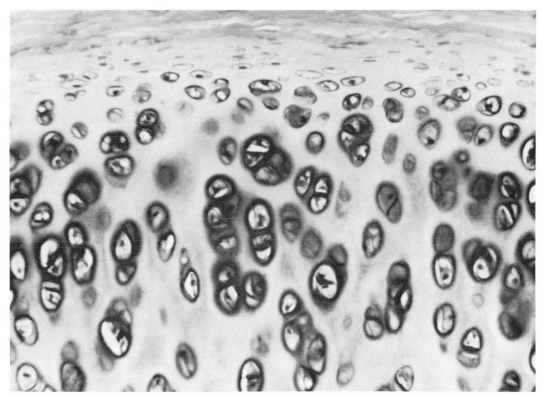

Figure 7–1. Hyaline cartilage from the trachea of a guinea pig. Notice the more intense staining of the capsular or territorial matrix immediately surrounding the groups of isogenous cells. The cells immediately beneath the perichondrium *(top)* recently added in appositional growth are single and elongated.

in this way contribute new cells and matrix to the surface of the mass of cartilage. This process is called *appositional growth.* The ability of the perichondrium to form cartilage persists but remains latent in the adult.

The Chondrocytes

In the layers of cartilage immediately beneath the perichondrium or under the free surface of articular cartilage, the lacunae are elliptical in section, with the long axis parallel to the surface, while deeper in the cartilage they are semicircular or angular. The cells in living cartilage usually conform to the shape of the lacunae that they occupy, but fixation and dehydration may result in their retraction from the wall of the lacuna, so that they may appear stellate. Mature cartilage cells in higher vertebrates rarely if ever have processes visible with the light microscope, but in electron micrographs their surface is quite irregular. The cells tend to be clustered in small groups (Fig. 7–1). Each group is said to be *isogenous* because it represents the prog-

eny of a single chondrocyte that underwent a few mitotic divisions in the course of the interstitial growth of the cartilage. In the cartilage of the epiphyseal plates of long bones, cell division in a consistent plane results in an arrangement of the cartilage cells in long columns that are later invaded by advancing bone (Fig. 7–6).

The nucleus of the chondrocyte is round or oval and contains from one to several nucleoli, depending on the species. There is a juxtanuclear cell center with a pair of centrioles and a well-developed Golgi apparatus. The surrounding cytoplasm contains elongated mitchondria, occasional lipid droplets, and variable amounts of glycogen. When new matrix is being formed in growing or regenerating cartilage, the cytoplasm becomes more basophilic and the Golgi region becomes unusually large. Under these conditions of active growth, electron micrographs show a well-developed granular endoplasmic reticulum with moderately distended cisternae. The saccules of the Golgi complex tend to be dilated, and there are numerous asso-

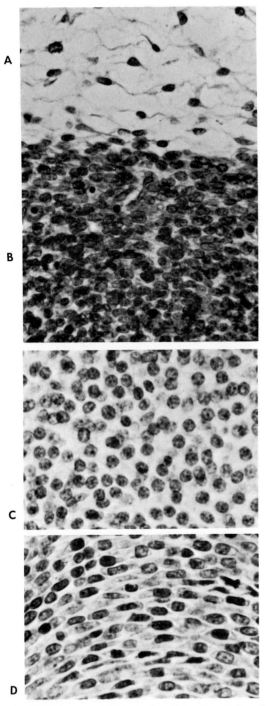

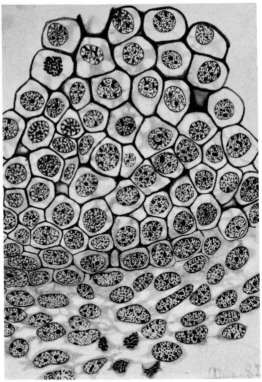

Figure 7–3. Development of cartilage from mesenchyme in a 15-mm guinea pig embryo. The mesenchyme *(below)* gradually merges into the protochondral tissue with interstitial substance *(above)*. (After A. A. Maximow.)

Figure 7–2. In the histogenesis of cartilage, mesenchymal cells *(A)* withdraw their processes and become crowded together to form an area of precartilage *(B)*. In newly formed embryonic cartilage *(C)*, the densely aggregated cells of the precartilaginous stage have been moved apart by deposition of clear hyaline matrix between them. The cells then become angular *(D)* and isolated in clearly demarcated lacunae.

ciated vacuoles of varying size that sometimes contain filaments or granules. Similar vacuoles are also seen at the cell surface, where they appear to be discharging their contents into the surrounding matrix. In cartilage that is not actively growing, the endoplasmic reticulum is less extensive and the Golgi complex not as prominent.

Cartilage Matrix

In fresh hyaline cartilage the matrix appears homogeneous. This is due in part to the fact that the ground substance and the collagen embedded within it have approximately the same refractive index and in part to the small size of the collagen fibrils. The matrix is deeply colored with the periodic acid–Schiff reaction for carbohydrates. It also has a marked affinity for basic dyes and stains metachromatically with toluidine blue. The principal constituents of the extracellu-

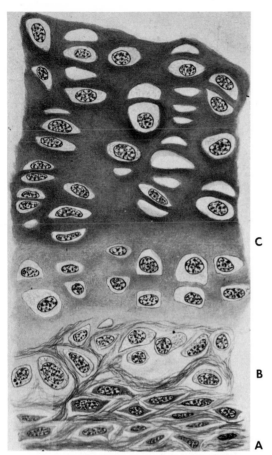

C

B

A

Figure 7–4. Hyaline cartilage from xiphoid process of rat. *A,* Transition layer adjacent to perichondrium. *B,* Continuation of collagenous fibers from perichondrium into interstitial substance of cartilage. *C,* Columns of isogenous groups of cartilage cells, some of which have fallen out of the lacunae in processing. (After A. A. Maximow.)

plex carbohydrates called glycosaminoglycans. These radiate from the core protein in a bottle-brush configuration. The principal glycosaminoglycans of cartilage matrix are *chondroitin sulfate* and *keratan sulfate.* There are typically about 80 chondroitin sulfate chains and about 100 keratan sulfate chains associated with each core protein molecule. At one end of the core protein is a polypeptide segment relatively free of glycosaminoglycan side chains, the so-called hyaluronic acid–binding region. The proteoglycan molecules are bound at this end, via a link protein, to very long *hyaluronic acid* molecules spaced at intervals of about 30 nm. The *proteoglycan aggregates* so formed occupy the interstices of the meshwork of collagen fibrils. In the hydrated state in vivo the extended proteoglycan molecules occupy very large volumes relative to their molecular weight. The entwining of the proteoglycan aggregates with the collagen fibrils is depicted schematically in Figure 5–10, Chapter 5. These relationships cannot be directly visualized by routine methods, for when tissues are processed for electron microscopy, the glycosaminoglycan chains collapse onto the core protein during dehydration. The proteoglycan monomers thus appear in sections of ruthenium red–stained cartilage as dense granules of irregular shape dispersed in the meshes of the collagenous framework. The molecular organization of the extracellular matrix in the hydrated state is ideally suited to its function on the weight-bearing articular surfaces of bones. The fibrillar scaffolding of collagen determines and maintains tissue shape and resists tensile forces, while the proteoglycan aggregates occupying its interstices provide a hydrated viscous gel that absorbs compressive forces.

The matrix immediately surrounding each group of isogenous cells usually stains more deeply than elsewhere (Fig. 7–1). This deeply basophilic rim is called the *capsular* or *territorial matrix,* while the less basophilic areas between cell groups are called the *intercapsular* or *interterritorial matrix.* The deeper staining of the territorial matrix suggests that the concentration of chondroitin sulfate is higher in the immediate vicinity of the cells.

Secretion of Matrix Components

The chondrocytes synthesize and secrete the collagen and proteoglycans of the sur-

lar matrix of hyaline cartilage are *Type II collagen* and *proteoglycans.* The collagen fibrils are generally quite thin (10–20 nm) and unlike other collagens they usually lack a distinct cross-banding. They are assembled from molecules composed of a single type of α chain designated α1(II). The fibrils are not organized in bundles but form a loose meshwork throughout the matrix.

The proteoglycans of cartilage have been thoroughly studied and have a more complicated structure than many other members of this class of macromolecules. The core protein forming the backbone of the proteoglycan is about 300 nm in length and has a molecular weight of about 250,000. The remainder of the molecule consists of the com-

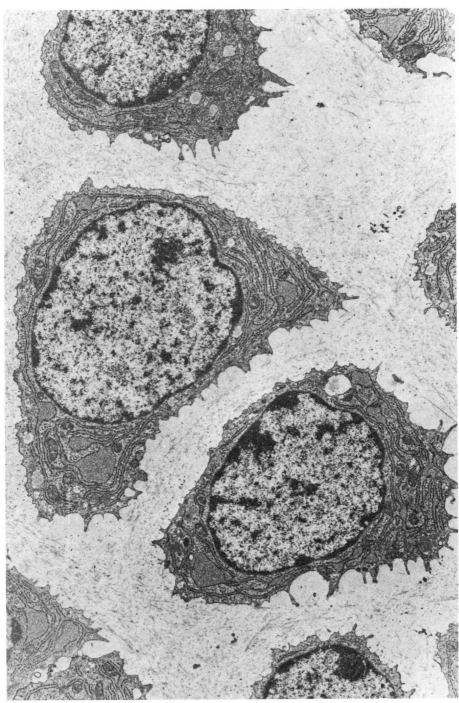

Figure 7–5. Electron micrograph of chondrocytes and matrix of mouse trachea illustrating the irregular outlines of the cells, their well-developed granular endoplasmic reticulum, and other organelles. (Micrograph from Seegmiller, R., C. Ferguson, and H. Sheldon. J. Ultrastruct. Res. *38*:288, 1972.)

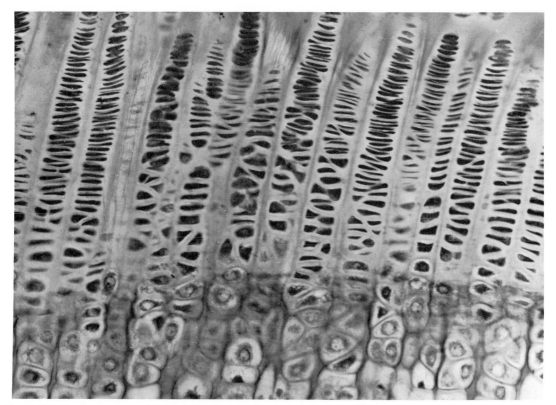

Figure 7–6. Hyaline cartilage of the epiphyseal plate of rabbit tibia. Here the cartilage cells are arranged in long parallel columns. From above downward, zones of cartilage cell proliferation, maturation, hypertrophy, and degeneration can be recognized.

rounding matrix. After injection of tritiated proline into experimental animals that are actively forming cartilage, this amino acid precursor of collagen can be localized by radioautography over the endoplasmic reticulum of the chondrocytes in 10 minutes; over the Golgi complex in 30 minutes; over secretory vacuoles at the cell periphery at three hours; and at longer time intervals over the extracellular matrix. Thus, the synthesis of collagen follows the same intracellular path as the secretion of protein by glandular cells.

The same train of events can be demonstrated in the elaboration of matrix proteoglycans. The synthesis of the core protein and the initial steps of oligosaccharide addition occur on the ribosomes of the endoplasmic reticulum. After accumulation of the initial product in the cisternae and transport to the Golgi, chondroitin sulfate chains are rapidly added to complete assembly of proteoglycans. The completed molecules, packaged in secretory vacuoles, are moved to the cell surface and released by exocytosis. In electron micrographs both filamentous and

granular material can be found in the same vacuole, suggesting that collagen and proteoglycans are synthesized concurrently and packaged together for exocytosis. Secretion of hyaluronic acid and linking proteins probably take place similarly. However, the proteoglycans are secreted as monomers, and their assembly into aggregates occurs extracellularly.

In hyaline cartilage of adults the collagen network in the matrix does not seem to be renewed, but the proteoglycans slowly turn over and are replaced by molecules newly synthesized by the chondrocytes. These cells are thus involved in maintenance of the normal structure of the matrix, and are capable of responding to altered conditions of weight bearing and attrition by altering the rate of turnover of the proteoglycans. Some of the structural changes observed in the cartilage of aging osteoarthritic individuals are probably a consequence of a declining ability of chondrocytes to replace proteoglycans at a rate sufficient to keep pace with wear and tear. In the inflammatory reaction associated

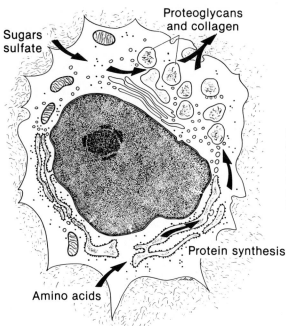

Figure 7–7. Diagram of the intracellular pathway for synthesis of matrix components. Amino acids are incorporated into protein at the ribosomes. Sugar and sulfates are believed to be incorporated into polysaccharide in the Golgi region and combined to form the protein-polysaccharide mucopolysaccharide released into the surrounding matrix. (Courtesy of E. Hay and J. P. Revel.)

with rheumatoid arthritic disorders, proteases released may rapidly degrade the core proteins of proteoglycans and impair their normal function in the matrix.

ELASTIC CARTILAGE

In mammals this variety of cartilage is found in the external ear, the walls of the external auditory and eustachian canals, the epiglottis, and in parts of the corniculate and cuneiform cartilages. It differs from hyaline cartilage macroscopically in its yellowish color and its greater opacity and elasticity.

Its cells are similar to those of hyaline cartilage; they are of the same rounded shape, are also surrounded by capsules, and are scattered singly or in isogenous groups of two or four cells. The interstitial substance differs from that of hyaline cartilage by being permeated by frequently branching fibers, which are positive in all staining methods for elastin (Fig. 7–8). They form a network that is often so dense that the ground substance is obscured. In the layers beneath the perichondrium, the feltwork of the elastic fibers is looser. The elastic fibers of the cartilage continue into the perichondrium.

In the histogenesis of elastic cartilage in the embryo, a primitive connective tissue develops, containing fibroblasts and fibrillar bundles that do not give reactions characteristic of either collagen or elastin. These indifferent fibers later acquire typical staining properties for elastin. The cells secrete matrix around themselves and become recognizable as chondrocytes. As in hyaline cartilage, a perichondrium is formed and initiates appositional growth.

FIBROCARTILAGE

Fibrocartilage occurs in a few regions of dense connective tissue in the body. In small areas with poorly defined limits, typical cartilage cells and a small amount of matrix are found among the abundant fibrous elements. It occurs in the intervertebral discs; in certain articular cartilages; in the symphysis pubis; in the ligamentum teres femoris; and in the sites of attachment of certain tendons to bones. The encapsulated cartilage cells lie singly or in pairs, or are sometimes aligned in rows between bundles of collagen fibers (Fig. 7–9). The matrix is quite inconspicuous except in the immediate vicinity of the cells, where its presence can be inferred from the characteristic form of the lacunae.

Fibrocartilage is closely associated with the connective tissue of the capsules and liga-

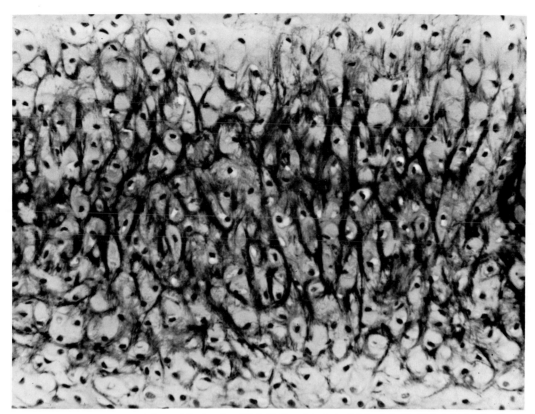

Figure 7–8. Elastic cartilage of the epiglottis of a child. Notice the dark-staining elastic fiber bundles in the matrix between cell groups. (From Fawcett, D. W., *In* Greep, R. O., ed.: Histology. Philadelphia, Blakiston Co., 1953. Reproduced by permission of McGraw-Hill Book Co.)

ments of joints. It is a transitional form between cartilage and dense connective tissue, and the gradual transition from one to the other can be observed in the adult, as well as during histogenesis in the embryo. In the intervertebral discs, for example, the hyaline cartilage connected with the vertebrae shows distinct collagenous fibers in its matrix. These then become associated into thick bundles, which almost entirely displace the ground substance while the cartilage cells retain their typical form and their capsular matrix. Finally, this typical fibrocartilage merges into connective tissue, the fusiform cells of which have tapering processes and are not enclosed in lacunae.

Fibrocartilage develops in much the same way as ordinary connective tissue. In the beginning there are typical fibroblasts separated by a large amount of collagen. Then these cells become rounded, are transformed into cartilage cells, and surround themselves with a thin layer of capsular matrix. The abundant fibrous interstitial substance becomes infiltrated only slightly, with cartilaginous ground substance.

OTHER VARIETIES OF CARTILAGE AND CHONDROID TISSUE

There is a transitory phase in the embryonic development of hyaline cartilage when it is composed of closely packed cells having thin capsules and collagen fibers in its intercellular substance. In this underdeveloped condition the cartilage may remain throughout life in certain sites in the bodies of higher organisms. It occurs often in lower vertebrates (fishes and amphibians) and is still more common in invertebrates. Such tissue has been variously called *pseudocartilage, fibrohyaline tissue, vesicular supporting tissue,* and *chondroid tissue.* This tissue serves as a local mechanical support for the surrounding tissue.

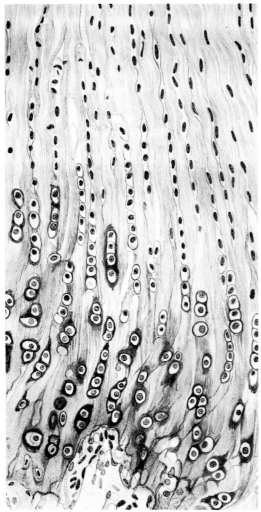

Figure 7–9. Low-power drawing of fibrocartilage at insertion of tendon into the tibia of a rat. Note the direct transformation of rows of tendon cells *(top)* into cartilage cells surrounded by deeply staining matrix. (Drawn by Miss A. Nixon.)

The tissue composing the *notochord* of vertebrate embryos has a similar structure. Here there is a cylindrical shaft of variable thickness, which consists of large, closely packed cells distended with fluid. The notochordal tissue has a different embryologic origin from that of the cartilage and of the other connective tissues.

REGENERATION OF CARTILAGE

In amphibians, cartilage is regenerated in a manner resembling histogenesis of cartilage in the embryo. After a wound or excision of a portion of cartilage in adult mammals, no such independent regeneration takes place. Instead, one sees at first in the injured area only necrotic and atrophic changes. The defect is then filled by connective tissue, which grows in from the perichondrium or from fascia in the vicinity of the injured area. The fibroblasts of this ingrowing granulation tissue may then round up, produce capsules around themselves, and become transformed into new cartilage cells. Thus, if cartilage is replaced in the adult mammal, this takes place mainly by metaplasia of loose connective tissue.

Such cartilaginous metaplasia sometimes takes place in connective tissue under the influence of simple mechanical forces acting from the outside, such as pressure, particularly when combined with friction. It is claimed that the presence of cartilage on the joint surfaces of bones is related to the constant mechanical influences to which a normal joint is subjected while functioning. When these mechanical conditions disappear, as happens in dislocation of bones, the cartilage often undergoes dedifferentiation. On the other hand, cartilage is laid down in the primordia of the joint surfaces in the embryo at a time when there are probably no mechanical forces acting on the joint.

Although cartilage has only limited regenerative capacity, it has been shown that components of the matrix can be rapidly reformed if the cells remain intact. Injection of a crude preparation of papain into young rabbits results in a collapse of their ears. This is attended by a loss of basophilia of the cartilage matrix and by a loss of its proteoglycans and elastic components, demonstrable in electron micrographs. After 48 hours the regeneration of matrix components is already far advanced and the ears are largely restored to their normal erect position.

REGRESSIVE CHANGES IN CARTILAGE

The most important regressive change in cartilage, *calcification,* normally precedes the type of bone formation called *endochondral ossification* (Fig. 7–10). The cartilage cells in a center of ossification undergo a regular sequence of cytological changes accompanied by characteristic changes in the neighboring

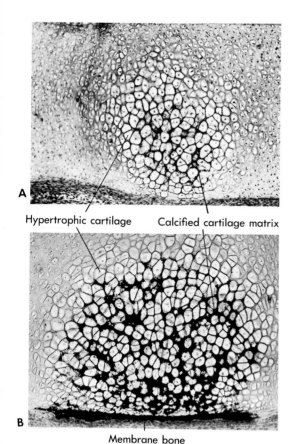

Hypertrophic cartilage   Calcified cartilage matrix

Membrane bone

Figure 7–10. Two stages in calcification of the cartilage model of the calcaneus in rats. *A,* Two days after birth; *B,* four days after birth. The calcium salts appear black because of the silver nitrate stain. Undecalcified preparations stained with von Kóssa's method. (After W. Bloom and M. A. Bloom.)

matrix. In the epiphyseal plate of long bones where the cells become arranged in parallel columns, these changes are observed in successive zones along the length of the column. Distinct zones of *proliferation, maturation, cartilage cell hypertrophy,* and *cell degeneration* can be recognized (Fig. 7–6). In the zone of hypertrophic cartilage cells, the matrix undergoes calcification.

At sites where cartilage matrix undergoes calcification, small membrane-limited structures are found, called *matrix vesicles.* Because they are limited by a typical unit membrane and sometimes contain ribosomes or other recognizable cytoplasmic components, it is assumed that they arise by being budded off from the chondrocytes. The vesicles have been isolated in centrifugal fractions and found to contain acid phosphatase and ATPase activity. They are found at all levels in the epiphyseal plate but are concentrated in the zone of hypertrophic cartilage cells. In the early stages of calcification of the hyaline matrix, minute crystals of hydroxyapatite are seen within and at the surface of the matrix vesicles. It is believed that the vesicles may have the capacity to bind and concentrate calcium, resulting in precipitation of hydroxyapatite in their immediate vicinity. As the nests of apatite crystals enlarge and merge, the cartilage becomes opaque, hard, and brittle. Because of these changes in the matrix, the zone of cartilage cell hypertrophy is also known as the *zone of provisional calcification.* The relation of these events to the process of ossification will be discussed in greater detail in Chapter 8.

In man, ossification of certain cartilages also occurs as a normal age change and may take place in some parts of the larynx as early as 20 years of age.

HISTOPHYSIOLOGY OF CARTILAGE

Cartilage in joints has the remarkable property of sustaining great weight and at the same time allowing the bones, which carry this weight, to move easily and smoothly against one another. In other places, such as the ear and the respiratory passages, cartilage serves as a pliable yet resistant framework that prevents the collapse of the tubular organ it surrounds. Finally, cartilage in many bones makes possible their growth in length and is important in determining their size and shape.

Far from being an inert tissue, cartilage, through its participation in the growth of bones, is a fairly delicate indicator of certain metabolic disturbances. It reflects *nutritional deficiencies,* especially of protein, minerals, or vitamins. For example, the thickness of the epiphyseal cartilage plate diminishes rapidly when a young rat is placed on a protein-deficient diet or on one lacking in vitamin A. When vitamin C is withheld from guinea pigs, producing *scurvy,* cessation of matrix formation may be accompanied by changes in the cells and by distortion of their columnar arrangement. Absence of vitamin D is attended by a deficient absorption of calcium and phosphorus from the diet and leads to *rickets,* in which the epiphyseal cartilages continue to proliferate but fail to calcify, and the growing bones become deformed by weight bearing.

The participation of cartilage in the growth in length of bones is in part under control of several hormones, of which the most important is the pituitary *growth hormone*. Hypophysectomy in young rats leads to a thinning of the epiphyseal plate of long bones, with cessation of mitosis and a decrease in the number and especially in the size of its cells. After a short time the cartilage fails to be eroded and growth of the bone ceases. When growth hormone is injected into such animals, the cartilage undergoes a striking metamorphosis and within a few days resembles that of a normal young growing animal, and the bone resumes its growth. The response of the cartilage varies with the dose level and has been used to assay extracts containing the hormone. Long-continued administration of the hormone produces giant rats, this being made possible in part by growth of cartilage after it would normally have ceased growing. Further, the injection of the hormone into older rats, in which cartilage proliferation has stopped, can to some extent reactivate its growth, with subsequent increase in the size of its bones.

REFERENCES

Ali, S. Y., S. W. Sajdera, and H. C. Anderson: Isolation and characterization of calcifying matrix vesicles from epiphyseal cartilage. Proc. Natl. Acad. Sci USA 67:1513, 1970.

Anderson, H. C.: Vesicles associated with calcification of the matrix of epiphyseal cartilage. J. Cell Biol. 41:59, 1969.

Anderson, D. R.: The ultrastructure of elastic and hyaline cartilage in the rat. Am. J. Anat. 114:403, 1964.

Anderson, H. C., T. Matsuzwa, S. W. Sajdera, and S. Y. Ali: Membranous particles in calcifying matrix. Trans. N.Y. Acad. Sci. 32:619, 1970.

Anderson, H. C. and S. W. Sajdera, 1971. The fine structure of bovine nasal cartilage. Extraction as a technique to study proteoglycans and collagen in cartilage matrix. J. Cell Biol. 49:650

Becks, H., C. W. Asling, M. E. Simpson, C. H. Li, and H. M. Evans: The growth of hypophysectomized female rats following chronic treatment with pure pituitary growth hormone. III. Skeletal changes—tibia, metacarpal, costochondral junction and caudal vertebrae. Growth 13:175, 1949.

Bonucci, E.: Fine structure of early cartilage calcification. J. Ultrastr. Res. 20:33, 1967.

Bonucci, E.: Fine structure and histochemistry of calcifying globules in epiphyseal cartilage. Zeitschr. f. Mikroskop. Anat. 103:192, 1970.

Cameron, D. A., and R. A. Robinson: Electron microscopy of epiphyseal and articular cartilage matrix in the femur of the newborn infant. J. Bone Joint Surg. 40:163, 1958.

Christner, J. E., M. L. Brown, and D. D. Dziewiatkowski: Interactions of cartilage proteoglycans with hyaluronate. J. Biol. Chem. 254:4624, 1979.

Comper, W. D., and T. C. Laurent: Physiological function of connective tissue polysaccharides. Physiol. Rev. 58:255, 1978.

Glücksmann, A.: Studies on bone mechanics in vitro. II. The role of tension and pressure in chondrogenesis. Anat. Rec. 73:39, 1939.

Goldman, G. C., and N. Lane: On the site of sulfation in the chondrocyte. J. Cell Biol. 21:353, 1964.

Goldman, G. C., and K. R. Porter: Chondrogenesis, studies with the electron microscope. J. Biophys. Biochem. Cytol. 8:719, 1960.

Hascall, G. K.: Cartilage proteoglycans: comparison of sectioned and spread whole molecules. J. Ultrastruct. Res. 70:369, 1980.

Hascall, V. C.: Interaction of cartilage proteoglycans with hyaluronic acid. J. Supramol. Struct. 7:101, 1977.

Lane, J. M., and C. Weiss: Review of articular cartilage collagen research. Arthritis Rheum. 18:553, 1975.

McCluskey, R. T., and L. Thomas: The removal of cartilage matrix *in vivo* by papain. J. Exp. Med. 108:371, 1958.

Minns, R. J., and F. S. Stevens: The collagen fibril organization in human articular cartilage. J. Anat. 123:437, 1977.

Revel, J. P., and E. D. Hay: An autoradiographic and electron microscopic study of collagen synthesis in differentiating cartilage. Zeitschr. f. Zellforsch. 61:110, 1963.

Seegmiller, R., C. C. Ferguson, and H. Sheldon: Studies on cartilage. VI. A genetically determined defect in tracheal cartilage. J. Ultrastruct. Res. 38:288, 1972.

Seegmiller, R., E. C. Fraser, and H. Sheldon: A new chondrodystrophic mutant in mice. Electron microscopy of normal and abnormal chondrogenesis. J. Cell Biol. 48:580, 1971.

Sheldon, H., and F. B. Kimball: Studies on cartilage. III. The occurrence of collagen within vacuoles of the Golgi apparatus. J. Cell Biol. 12:599, 1962.

Sheldon, H., and R. A. Robinson: Studies on cartilage. I. Electron microscope observations on normal rabbit ear cartilage. II. Electron microscopic observations on rabbit ear cartilage following the administration of papain. J. Biophys. Biochem. Cytol. 4:401, 1958; 8:151, 1960.

Silberberg, R., M. Hasler, and M. Silberberg: Submicroscopic response of articular cartilage of mice treated with estrogenic hormone. Am. J. Pathol. 46:289, 1965.

Silberberg, R., M. Silberberg, and D. Feir: Life cycle of articular cartilage cells: an electron microscope study of the hip joint of the mouse. Am. J. Anat. 114:17, 1964.

Thomas, L.: Reversible collapse of rabbit ears after intravenous papain and prevention of recovery by cortisone. J. Exp. Med. 104:245, 1956.

Wolbach, S. B., and C. L. Maddock: Vitamin-A acceleration of bone growth sequences in hypophysectomized rats. Arch. Pathol. 53:273, 1952.

Zambrano, N. Z., Montes, G. S., Shigihara, K. M., Sanchez, E. M., and Junqueira, L. C.: Collagen arrangement in cartilages. Acta Anat. (Basel) 113:26, 1982.

8

BONE

Bone, in common with other connective tissues, consists of cells, fibers, and ground substance, but unlike the others its extracellular components are calcified, making it a hard, unyielding substance ideally suited for its supportive and protective function in the skeleton. It provides for the internal support of the body and for the attachment of the muscles and tendons essential for locomotion. It protects the vital organs of the cranial and thoracic cavities, and it encloses the bloodforming elements of the bone marrow. In addition to these mechanical functions, it plays an important metabolic role as a mobilizable store of calcium, which can be drawn upon as needed in the homeostatic regulation of the concentration of calcium in the blood and other fluids of the body.

Bone has a remarkable combination of physical properties—high tensile and compressive strength while at the same time having some elasticity and being a relatively lightweight material. At all levels of the organization of bones, from their gross form to their submicroscopic structure, their construction ensures the greatest strength with great economy of material and minimal weight. Despite its strength and hardness, bone is a dynamic living material, constantly being renewed and reconstructed throughout the lifetime of the individual. Owing to its continual internal reconstruction and its responsiveness to external mechanical stimuli, it can be modified by the surgical procedures and appliances of the orthopedic surgeon or the orthodontist. It is also surprisingly responsive to metabolic, nutritional, and endocrine influences. Disuse is followed by *atrophy* with loss of substance; increased use is accompanied by *hypertrophy*, with an increase in the mass of bone.

MACROSCOPIC STRUCTURE OF BONES

Upon inspection with the naked eye or hand lens, two forms of bone are distinguishable, *compact* (substantia compacta) and *spongy* (substantia spongiosa), also called *cancellous bone*. The latter consists of a three-dimensional lattice of branching bony spicules or *trabeculae* delimiting a labyrinthine system of intercommunicating spaces that are occupied by *bone marrow*. Compact bone appears as a solid continuous mass in which spaces can be seen only with the aid of the microscope. The two forms of bone grade into one another without a sharp boundary (Fig. 8–3).

In typical long bones, such as the femur or the humerus, the *diaphysis* (shaft) consists of a thick-walled hollow cylinder of compact bone with a voluminous central *medullary cavity* (marrow cavity) occupied by the bone marrow. The ends of long bones consist mainly of spongy bone covered by a thin peripheral cortex of compact bone (Figs. 8–2, 8–3). The intercommunicating spaces among the trabeculae of this spongy bone, in the adult, are directly continuous with the marrow cavity of the shaft. In the growing animal the ends of long bones, called the *epiphyses*, arise from separate centers of ossification and are separated from the diaphysis by a cartilaginous *epiphyseal plate* (Fig. 8–1), which is united to the diaphysis by columns of spongy bone in a transitional region called the *metaphysis*. The epiphyseal cartilage and the adjacent spongy bone of the metaphysis constitute a growth zone, in which all increment in length of the growing bone occurs. On the articular surfaces at the ends of long bones, the thin cortical layer of compact bone is covered by a layer of hyaline cartilage, the *articular cartilage*.

With few exceptions, bones are invested by *periosteum*, a layer of specialized connective tissue, which is endowed with *osteogenic potency*. That is to say, it has the ability to form bone. A covering of periosteum is lacking on those areas at the ends of long bones that are covered with articular cartilage. It is also absent at the sites where tendons and ligaments are inserted and on the surfaces of the patella and other sesamoid bones that are formed within tendons. It is also lacking on

199

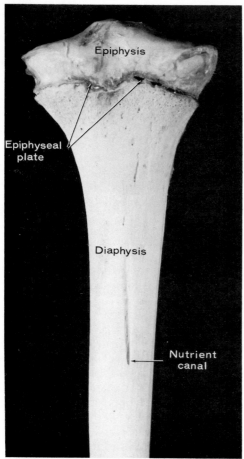

Figure 8–1. Photograph of the upper half of the tibia of a young girl showing the proximal bony epiphysis, the cartilaginous epiphyseal plate, and the shaft or diaphysis.

(Labels in figure: Epiphysis, Epiphyseal plate, Diaphysis, Nutrient canal)

the subcapsular areas of the neck of the femur and of the astragalus. Where functional periosteum is absent, the connective tissue in contact with the surfaces of bone lacks osteogenic potency and does not contribute to the healing of fractures. The marrow cavity of the diaphysis and the cavities of spongy bone are lined by the *endosteum*, a thin cellular layer that also possesses osteogenic properties.

In the flat bones of the skull, the substantia compacta forms, on both surfaces, relatively thick layers that are often referred to as the *outer* and *inner tables*. Between them is a layer of spongy bone of varying thickness called the *diploë*. The periosteum on the outer surface of the skull is called the *pericranium*, while the inner surface is lined by the *dura mater*. Although different terms are applied to these connective tissue coverings of the flat bones, they do not differ significantly in

their structure or osteogenic potency from the periosteum and endosteum of long bones. However, defects in the calvaria resulting from injury often do not heal completely in adults.

MICROSCOPIC STRUCTURE OF BONES

If a thin ground section of the shaft of a long bone is examined with the microscope, it is apparent that the contribution of the cellular elements of bone to its total mass is small. Compact bone is largely composed of the mineralized interstitial substance, *bone matrix*, deposited in layers or *lamellae* 3 to 7 μm thick (Figs. 8–4, 8–5). Rather uniformly spaced throughout the interstitial substance of bone are lenticular cavities, called *lacunae*, each completely filled by a bone cell or *osteocyte*. Radiating in all directions from each lacuna are exceedingly slender, branching tubular passages, the *canaliculi*, that penetrate the interstitial substance of the lamellae, anastomosing with the canaliculi of neighboring lacunae (Figs. 8–6, 8–7). Thus, although the lacunae are spaced some distance apart, they form a continuous system of cavities interconnected by an extensive network of minute canals. These slender passages are believed to be essential to the nutrition of the bone cells. Whereas cartilage can be sustained by diffusion through the aqueous phase of the gel-like hyaline matrix, the deposition of calcium salts in the interstitial substance of bone evidently reduces its permeability. However, the maintenance of a system of intercommunicating canaliculi provides avenues for exchange of metabolites between the cells and the nearest perivascular space.

The lamellae of compact bone are disposed in three common patterns. (1) The great majority are arranged concentrically around longitudinal vascular channels within the bone to form cylindrical units of structure called *haversian systems* or *osteons*. These vary in size, being made up of four to 20 lamellae. In cross section, the haversian systems appear as concentric rings around a circular opening (Figs. 8–6, 8–8*A*). In longitudinal section, they are seen as closely spaced bands parallel to the vascular channels (Figs. 8–5, 8–9). (2) Between the haversian systems are angular fragments of lamellar bone of varying size and irregular shape. These are the *interstitial systems* (Fig. 8–4). The limits of the haversian

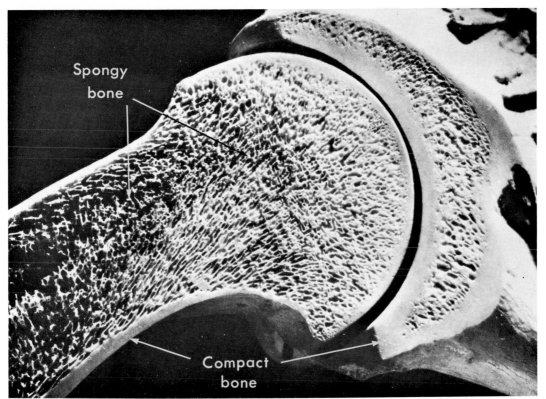

Figure 8–2. Photograph of a sagittal section of the proximal end of the humerus in relation to the glenoid fossa of the scapula at the shoulder joint. These are dry bones, and the cartilaginous articular surfaces of the joint are not present. The figure is presented here to illustrate the appearance and distribution of spongy and compact bone. (After A. Feininger, from *Anatomy of Nature.* Crown Publishers. With permission of Time, Inc.)

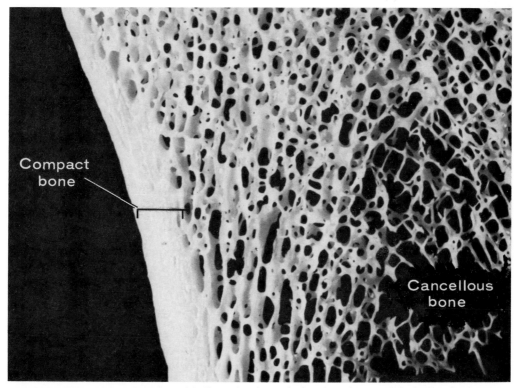

Figure 8–3. A thick ground section of the tibia illustrating the cortical compact bone and the lattice of trabeculae of the cancellous bone.

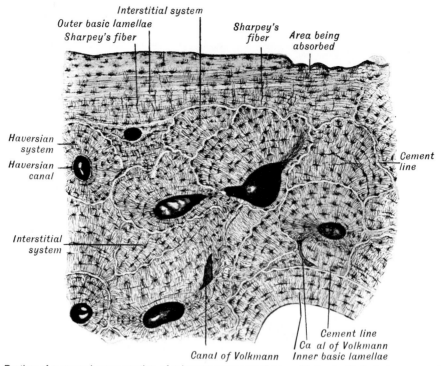

Figure 8–4. Portion of a ground cross section of a human metacarpal bone. Stained with fuchsin, mounted in Canada balsam. (After Schaffer.)

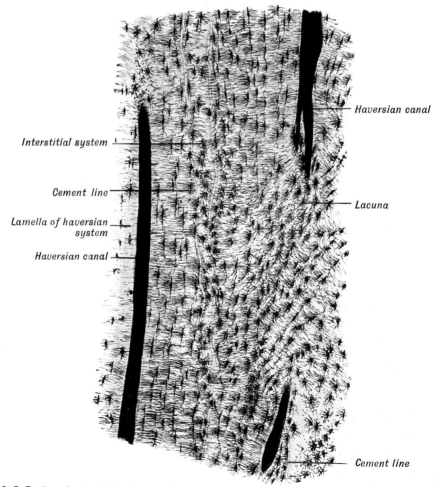

Figure 8–5. Portion of a longitudinal, ground section of the ulna of man; stained with fuchsin. (After Schaffer.)

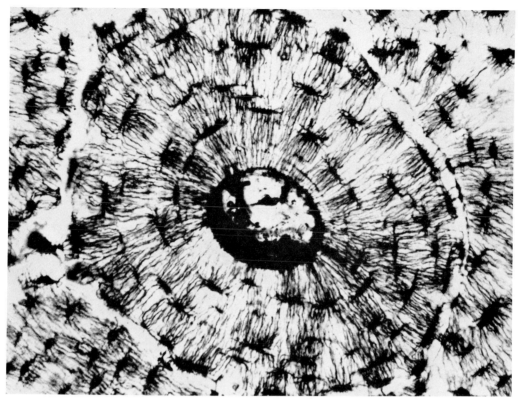

Figure 8–6. Ground section of human femur, showing a typical haversian system and the lacunae and canaliculi. (After Fawcett, D. W. *In* Greep, R. O., ed.: Histology. Philadelphia, Blakiston Co., 1953. Reproduced by permission of McGraw-Hill Book Co.)

systems and interstitial systems are sharply demarcated by refractile lines called *cement lines*. In cross section, the interior of compact bone thus appears as a mosaic of round and angular pieces cemented together (Fig. 8–8A). (3) At the external surface of the cortical bone, immediately beneath the periosteum, and on the internal surface, subjacent to the endosteum, there may be several lamellae that extend uninterruptedly around much of the circumference of the shaft. These are the *outer* and *inner circumferential lamellae* (Fig. 8–9).

Two categories of vascular channels are distinguished in compact bone on the basis of their orientation and their relation to the lamellar structure of the surrounding bone. The longitudinal channels in the centers of the haversian systems are called *haversian canals*. They are 22 to 110 μm in diameter and contain one or two blood vessels ensheathed in loose connective tissue. The vessels are, for the most part, capillaries and postcapillary venules, but occasional arterioles may also be found. The haversian canals are connected with one another, and

communicate with the free surface and with the marrow cavity via transverse and oblique channels called *Volkmann's canals*. These can be distinguished from the haversian canals in sections by the fact that they are not surrounded by concentrically arranged lamellae but traverse the bone in a direction perpendicular or oblique to the lamellae. The blood vessels from the endosteum and, to a lesser extent, from the periosteum communicate with those of the haversian systems via Volkmann's canals. The vessels are often larger than those in the osteons.

Although it is generally correct, the traditional description of haversian canals as being longitudinal and Volkmann's canals as being oblique or transverse is an oversimplification. Reconstruction of osteons from serial sections has shown that they are not always simple cylindrical units but may branch and anastomose and have a rather complex three-dimensional configuration. Thus, obliquely oriented vascular channels surrounded by concentric lamellae may be encountered. Despite their atypical orientation, these are clearly cross-connecting haversian canals.

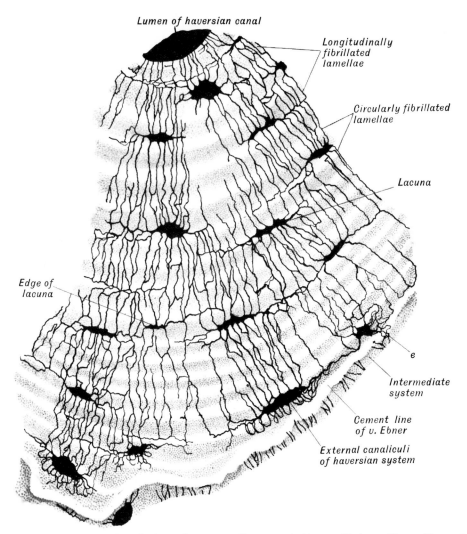

Lumen of haversian canal

Longitudinally
fibrillated
lamellae

Circularly fibrillated
lamellae

Lacuna

Edge of
lacuna

e

Intermediate
system

Cement line
of v. Ebner

External canaliculi
of haversian system

Figure 8–7. Sector of a cross section of a haversian system of a macerated human hip bone. The cavities and canaliculi are filled with a dye: *e,* connection of canaliculi of the haversian system with those of an intermediate system. (After A. A. Maximow.)

Figure 8–8. Section of bone from the midshaft of the human fibula as revealed by four different optical methods. *A,* Ground section photographed through the ordinary bright field microscope. The lacunae, haversian systems, and interstitial lamellae are clearly shown. *B,* The same section photographed through the polarizing microscope shows the alternating bright and dark concentric layers in the haversian systems that result from the differing orientation of collagen fibers in the successive lamellae. *C,* In a historadiogram of the same section, the differing shades of gray in the scale from nearly white to nearly black reflect the differing concentrations of calcium. In the haversian canals, there has been no absorption of the x-rays and the film is therefore black. The most recently deposited haversian systems are incompletely calcified and appear dark gray, whereas older ones containing higher concentrations of calcium are lighter. The old interstitial lamellae, being fully calcified, are most highly absorptive and therefore appear white. *D,* The 14-year-old girl from whom this specimen was taken had been given a daily dose of the antibiotic Achromycin (tetracycline) for 15 consecutive days at one period of her illness. Amputation of the leg was carried out 230 days later. Achromycin is incorporated into the matrix of bone being deposited at the time of its administration and imparts a fluorescence to the newly formed bone. In the section shown here, transilluminated with ultraviolet light in a fluorescence microscope, the white areas represent areas of bone laid down during the 15-day Achromycin treatment. The nonfluorescent central portions of the same haversian systems represent bone deposited after cessation of the treatment. (Courtesy of R. Amprino.)

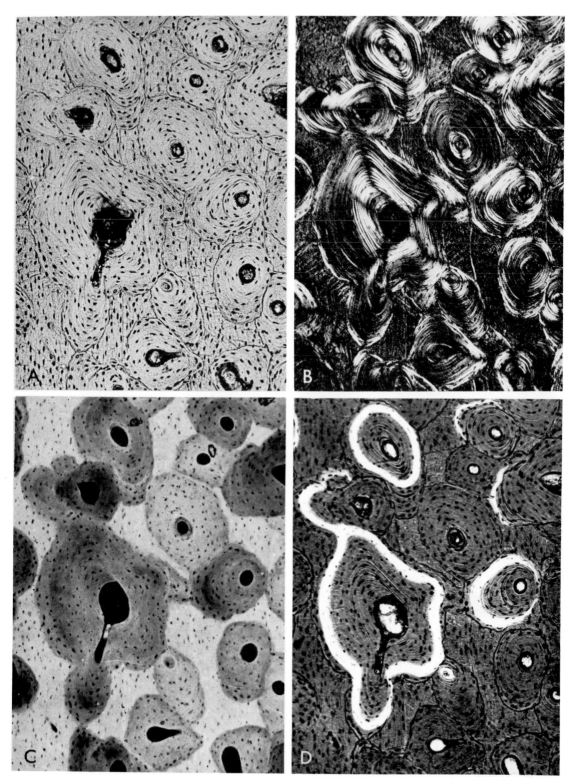

Figure 8–8. *See opposite page for legend.*

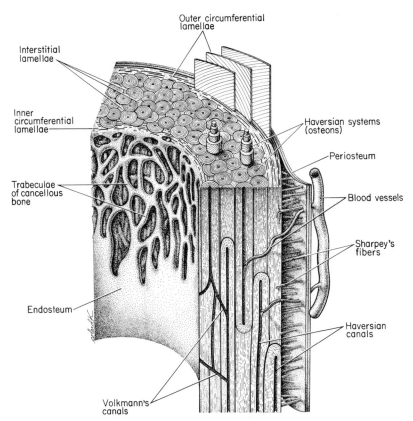

Figure 8–9. Diagram of a sector of the shaft of a long bone, illustrating the disposition of the lamellae in the osteons or haversian systems, the interstitial lamellae, and the outer and inner circumferential lamellae. (After A. Benninghoff. Lehrbuch der Anatomie des Menschen. Berlin, Urban & Schwarzenberg, 1949.)

Cancellous bone is also composed of lamellae, but its trabeculae are relatively thin and usually are not penetrated by blood vessels. Therefore, there generally are no haversian systems but merely a mosaic of angular pieces of lamellar bone. The bone cells are nourished by diffusion from the endosteal surface via the minute canaliculi that interconnect lacunae and extend to the surface.

The periosteum is subject to considerable variation in its microscopic appearance, depending on its functional state. During embryonic and postnatal growth there is an inner layer of bone-forming cells, *osteoblasts*, in direct contact with the bone. In the adult, the osteoblasts revert to a resting form (*osteoprogenitor cells*) and are indistinguishable from other spindle-shaped connective tissue cells. If a bone is injured, however, the bone forming potentiality of these cells is reactivated; they take on the appearance of typical osteoblasts and participate in the formation of new bone. The outer layer of the periosteum is a relatively acellular dense connective tissue containing blood vessels. Branches of these vessels traverse the deeper layer and enter Volkmann's canals, through which they communicate with the vessels of the haversian canals. These numerous small vessels entering Volkmann's canals from the periosteum may contribute to maintaining its attachment to the underlying bone. In addition, coarse bundles of collagenous fibers from the outer layer of the periosteum turn inward, penetrating the outer circumferential lamellae and interstitial systems of the bone. These are called *Sharpey's fibers* or *perforating fibers* (Figs. 8–9, 8–10). They arise during growth of the bone when thick collagenous bundles become incarcerated in the bone matrix deposited during the subperiosteal formation of new lamellae. When the perforating fibers are uncalcified, they occupy irregular canals penetrating the compact bone from the periosteal surface in a direction perpendicular or oblique to the lamellae. When calcified, they appear as irregular radial streaks in the outer portion of the cortical bone. They serve to anchor the periosteum firmly to the underlying bone. They vary greatly in number in

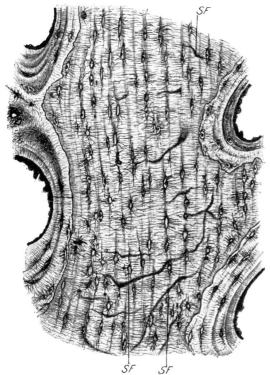

Figure 8–10. Portion of a cross section of a human fibula. *SF,* Sharpey's fibers. (After Schaffer.)

different regions, being particularly numerous in some bones of the skull and at sites of attachment of muscles and tendons to the periosteum of long bones. In addition to Sharpey's fibers, some elastic fibers penetrate the cortical bone from the periosteum, either together with or independent of the collagenous bundles.

The endosteum is a thin layer of squamous cells lining the walls of those cavities in the bone that house the bone marrow. It is the peripheral layer of the stroma of the bone marrow where it is in contact with bone, and it resembles the periosteum in its osteogenic potencies, but is much thinner—usually a single layer of cells without associated connective tissue fibers. All the cavities of bone, including the haversian canals and the marrow spaces within spongy bone, are lined by endosteum.

BONE MATRIX

The interstitial substance of bone is composed of two major components, an organic matrix and inorganic salts, each comprising about 50 per cent of its dry weight. The organic matrix consists of collagenous fibers embedded in a ground substance. In adult mammals, about 95 per cent of the organic matrix is collagen.

Ground Substance

The chemical composition of the extracellular substance of bone has not been studied as thoroughly as that of cartilage, owing in part to the fact that it represents a relatively small fraction of the organic matrix of bone. The positive periodic acid–Schiff reaction, the faint metachromasia of some areas of bone matrix, and the autoradiographic demonstration of incorporation of ^{35}S all provide indirect histochemical evidence for the presence of glycosaminoglycans. Analyses of extracts of whole bones have identified at least three such amino sugar–containing macromolecular components—chondroitin sulfate, keratan sulfate, and hyaluronic acid. However, it is evident that the concentration of sulfated glycosaminoglycans in the ground substance of bone is much less than in cartilage, for bone matrix is usually acidophilic in its staining properties.

Collagen

The collagen of bone, like that of common connective tissue, occurs in the form of cross-striated fibers 50 to 70 nm in diameter, with a 67 nm repeating period. Collagen of bone is predominantly Type I, but differs in some of its physical properties. It fails to swell in dilute acid and is insoluble in solvents used successfully to extract collagens from other tissues. Thus, it seems to have a greater degree of intermolecular bonding.

In mature lamellar bone, the collagen fibers are highly ordered in their arrangement. Those within each lamella of a haversian system are parallel in their orientation, but the direction of the fibers in the successive lamellae changes. This change in orientation of the fibers is responsible for the alternation of bright and dark layers in haversian systems viewed with polarizing optics (Fig. 8–8B). Some disagreement persists as to the precise arrangement of the fibers. In decalcified preparations viewed at high magnification, refractile lamellae with a fine circumferential striation alternate with less refractile layers having a stippled or punctate aspect. This appearance was originally interpreted as indicating a regular alternation of lamellae with circularly and with longitudinally oriented fibrils. This was apparently an oversimplification. Some investigators have insisted that collagen-rich lamellae alternate with collagen-poor lamellae and that this difference is as important as the direction of the fibers in accounting for the microscopic appearance of the haversian systems. Others have suggested that the fibers within a given collagen-rich lamella are not parallel but form two sets of fibers intersecting in a lattice-like pattern. Most histologists, however, seem to believe that the fibrils in all the lamellae run helically with respect to the axis of the haversian canal, but that the pitch of the helix changes sufficiently from one lamella to the next to account for the differences observed under bright-field and polarization microscopes.

Bone Mineral

The inorganic matter of bone consists of submicroscopic deposits of a form of calcium phosphate, very similar, but not identical, to the mineral hydroxyapatite (Ca_{10} [PO_4]$_6$ [OH]$_2$). Bone mineral is probably deposited initially as amorphous calcium phosphate and subsequently reordered to form crystalline hydroxyapatite. In its final phase, the calcium phosphate is present as thin plates or slender rodlike crystals 1.5 to 3 nm in thickness and about 40 nm long. These are situated on and within the substance of collagen fibers in the matrix. The crystals are not randomly distributed but recur regularly at intervals of 60 to 70 nm along the length of the fibers.

Bone mineral contains significant amounts of the citrate ion $C_6H_5O_7^{\equiv}$ and the carbonate ion $CO_3^=$. Citrate is considered to be in a separate phase, located on the surfaces of crystals. The site of carbonate is still a matter of debate; it may be located on the surface of crystals, or it may substitute for $PO_4^{\equiv}$ in the crystal structure, or both. Substitution of the fluoride ion F^- for OH^- in the apatite crystal is common; its amount depends mainly on the fluoride content of the drinking water. Magnesium and sodium, which are normal constituents of body fluids, are also present in bone mineral, which to some extent serves as a storage depot for these elements. The isotopes ^{45}Ca and ^{32}P can, of course, substitute for the stable ^{40}Ca and ^{31}P in the hydroxyapatite crystal. Foreign cations, such as Pb^{++}, Sr^{++}, and Ra^{++} (^{226}Ra), if ingested, may also substitute for Ca^{++}. In the fission of uranium in nuclear reactors or of uranium or plutonium in the detonation of nuclear weapons, a large number of radioactive elements are liberated. Some of these, on gaining access to the body, are incorporated in bone. The most hazardous of these *bone-seeking isotopes* is ^{90}Sr. As a result of their radioactivity, isotopes may cause severe damage to bone and to the blood-forming cells in the marrow. A few of these bone-seeking isotopes, including ^{239}Pu, do not enter the bone mineral but have instead a special affinity for the organic constituents of bone. Studies of the rate of turnover of the inorganic substances in bone have been greatly aided by the use of bone-seeking isotopes.

During development and growth, the amount of organic material per unit volume remains relatively constant, but the amount of water decreases and the proportion of bone mineral increases, attaining a maximum of about 65 per cent of the fat-free dry weight of the tissue in the adults. In the poorly calcified bone of individuals suffering from *rickets* or *osteomalacia*, the mineral content may be as low as 35 per cent.

If bone is exposed to a weak acid or a chelating agent, the inorganic salts are removed. The bone thus demineralized loses most of its hardness but is still very tough and flexible. It retains its gross form and a nearly normal microscopic appearance. On the other hand, if the organic constituents are extracted from a bone, the remaining inorganic constituents retain the gross form of the bone and, to a certain extent, its microscopic topography, but the bone has lost much of its tensile strength and is as brittle as porcelain. Thus, it is clear that the hardness of bone depends on its inorganic constituents, while its great toughness and resilience reside in its organic matrix, particularly the collagen. Without either one, bone would be a poor skeletal material, but with both, it is a highly ordered, remarkably resistant tissue, superbly adapted, at all levels of its organization, for its chemical and mechanical functions.

THE CELLS OF BONE

In actively growing bones four kinds of bone cells are distinguishable: *osteoprogenitor cells, osteoblasts, osteocytes,* and *osteoclasts.* Although the first three are usually described as distinct cell types, there is clear evidence of transformation from one to the other, and it is evidently more reasonable to regard them as different functional states of the same cell type. Such reversible changes in appearance are examples of cell *modulation*, in contrast to *differentiation*, which is the term reserved for progressive and apparently irreversible specialization in structure and function. The osteoclasts have a separate origin from monocytes formed in the bone marrow and circulating in the blood.

Osteoprogenitor Cells

Like other connective tissues, bone develops from embryonic mesenchyme. It retains in postnatal life a population of relatively undifferentiated cells that have the capacity for mitosis and for further structural and functional specialization. These *osteoprogenitor cells* have pale-staining, oval or elongate nuclei and inconspicuous acidophilic or faintly basophilic cytoplasm. They are found on or near all the free surfaces of bone: in the endosteum; in the innermost layer of the periosteum; lining the haversian canals; and on the trabeculae of cartilage matrix at the metaphysis of growing bones.

The osteoprogenitor cells are active during the normal growth of bones and may be activated in adult life during internal reorganization of bone or in the healing of fractures and repair of other forms of injury. Under any of these conditions, they undergo division and transform into the bone-forming osteoblasts.

After administration of tritiated thymidine, the osteoprogenitor cells are the only cells found to be labeled in autoradiographs at early time intervals. At later times, silver grains can also be found over the nuclei of osteoblasts, indicating that some of the osteoprogenitor cells have become transformed into bone-forming cells. The osteoblasts can also revert to osteoprogenitor cells when osteogenesis subsides.

Many authors refer to these potentially osteogenic cells as mesenchymal cells, but this term implies that they have a broader range of latent developmental potentialities than has been demonstrated. It may yet be shown that these cells can also develop into adipose cells, into fibroblasts, and into hemopoietic cells of the bone marrow. If this should be true, "mesenchymal cell" would indeed be the more appropriate designation. In the meantime, a majority of contemporary investigators of bone prefer the more limited implications of the term osteoprogenitor cell.

Osteoblasts

The *osteoblasts* are responsible for formation of bone matrix and are invariably found on the advancing surfaces of developing or growing bone. During active deposition of new matrix, they are arranged in an epithelioid layer of cuboidal or low columnar cells connected to one another by short slender processes. The nucleus with its single prominent nucleolus is often at the end of the cell farthest from the bony surface. The cells are clearly polarized toward the underlying bone, with a well-developed Golgi apparatus situated between the nucleus and the cell base. The mitochondria are elongated and fairly numerous. The cytoplasm is intensely basophilic, owing to its large content of rough endoplasmic reticulum.

The osteoblasts give a strong histochemical reaction for alkaline phosphatase, and the periodic acid–Schiff reaction reveals in cytoplasmic vacuoles small pink-staining granules that are believed to represent precursors of the bone matrix. When active new formation of bone ceases and the osteoblasts revert to spindle form, these granules disappear from the cytoplasm, and the phosphatase reaction of the cells rapidly declines.

In electron micrographs, osteoblasts are seen to have the structure expected of cells actively engaged in protein synthesis (Fig. 8–11). The endoplasmic reticulum is extensive and its cisternae are often in parallel array. Their membranes are studded with ribosomes, and these are also present in great numbers in the cytoplasmic matrix. The Golgi membranes are well developed and have numerous associated vacuoles. Sizable vesicles containing an amorphous or flocculent material of appreciable density apparently correspond to the PAS-staining granules observed with the light microscope. Small lipid droplets and membrane-limited dense bodies, interpreted as lysosomes, are also encountered occasionally.

Osteocytes

The principal cells of fully formed bone are the *osteocytes*, which reside in lacunae within the calcified interstitial substance. The cell body is flattened, conforming to the

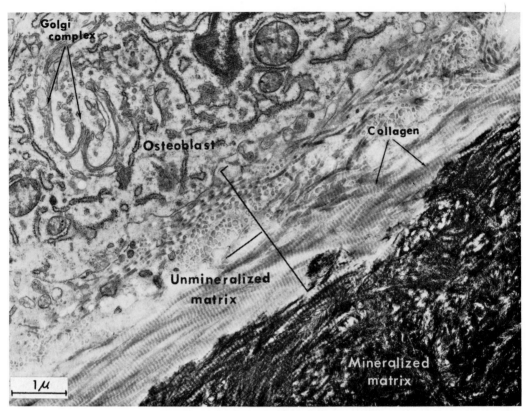

Figure 8–11. Edge of a resorption canal being filled in by lamellar bone. At upper left is a portion of an osteoblast containing a prominent Golgi zone and abundant granular reticulum. Subjacent to it are the collagen fibrils of two unmineralized lamellae, and at lower right is the dense mineralized bone. (From Cooper, et al. J. Bone Joint Surg. 48A:1239, 1966.)

shape of the lenticular cavity that it occupies, but there are numerous slender processes that extend for some distance into canaliculi in the surrounding matrix. How far they penetrate into the canaliculi of adult mammalian bone could not be ascertained by light microscopy. However, electron microscopic studies have shown that the processes of neighboring osteocytes are in contact at their ends. Moreover, their apposed membranes are specialized to form gap junctions or nexuses at their sites of contact (Fig. 8–12). Thus, the bone cells are not completely isolated in their lacunae but appear to be in communication with one another and ultimately with the cells at the surface via a series of cell-to-cell junctions of low electrical resistance, permitting flow of ions and possibly of small molecules. This finding may explain how cells deep within the calcified matrix of bone can respond to hormonal stimuli that would seem to have direct access only to cells in the immediate vicinity of blood vessels.

The nuclear and cytoplasmic characteristics of osteocytes at the light microscopic level are similar to those of osteoblasts except that the Golgi region is less conspicuous and the cytoplasm exhibits less affinity for basic dyes. In electron micrographs of osteocytes that have only recently been incorporated into bone, the Golgi apparatus is still rather large and the endoplasmic reticulum is quite extensive (Fig. 8–13). In osteocytes situated deeper in bone matrix, these organelles have undergone some regression (Fig. 8–14). Although these cells appear less active in protein synthesis, they are by no means metabolically inert.

In its development, an osteocyte is essentially an osteoblast that has become surrounded by bone matrix. Isolated within its lacuna, it undergoes some cytological dedifferentiation, but remains active. Considerable indirect evidence has accumulated indicating that the osteocyte exerts an important influence on the surrounding osseous matrix. The

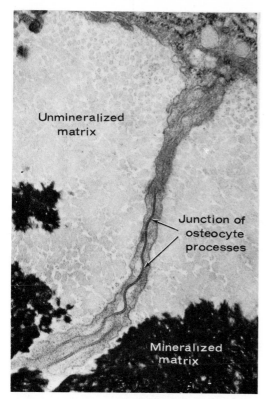

Figure 8–12. Electron micrograph of portions of cell processes from two neighboring osteocytes traversing the zone of unmineralized matrix lining a lacuna. Note the nexus or gap junction where the processes overlap. (From Holtrop, M. E., and M. J. Weinger. Proc. Fourth Parathyroid Conference, Internat. Congress Series No. 243. Amsterdam, Excerpta Medica, 1971.)

phenomenon of *osteolysis* is an active physiological process whereby the bone matrix immediately surrounding osteocytes is modified and bone salt is resorbed. It is the current belief that the osteocytes play an active role in the release of calcium from bone to blood, and hence participate in the homeostatic regulation of its concentration in the fluids of the body.

Parathyroid hormone is the principal regulator of the blood calcium level. Its administration has a microscopically visible effect on the osteocytes and on the staining reactions of the adjacent bone matrix. Because the response of the blood calcium level to parathyroid hormone is too rapid to be accounted for by osteoclastic erosion of bone, the primary action of the hormone may be to stimulate osteocytic osteolysis.

The osteocyte is believed to be capable of modulation to other cell types. When released from its lacuna during bone resorption, it may revert to a quiescent osteoprogenitor cell.

Osteoclasts

Closely associated with areas of bone resorption are the *osteoclasts*—giant cells 20 to 100 μm in diameter and containing as many as 50 nuclei. They were first described a century ago and believed to be the active agents in bone resorption. Although this view has been a subject of continuing debate, the great bulk of recent evidence supports this interpretation. Osteoclasts are frequently found in shallow concavities in the surface of bone, called *Howship's lacunae*. It was this relationship that first suggested to early investigators of the histology of bone that these lacunae were formed by an erosive action of osteoclasts. In the turnover and remodeling of bones that occurs in growing animals, osteoclasts are always most abundant in those areas known to be undergoing resorption. No one questioned the close topographical relation of these cells to sites of resorption, but some argued that the osteoclasts arose by coalescence of osteocytes liberated from surrounding matrix in the course of bone resorption, and that they therefore should be regarded as products rather than as agents of bone resorption. This interpretation now has few adherents, as the evidence for an active role of osteoclasts in bone resorption has become compelling. Osteoclasts actively engaged in bone resorption show an obvious polarity. The nuclei tend to congregate near the outer surface, which is smooth contoured, while the side adjacent to the bone exhibits a radial striation that was long interpreted as a "brush border" but which has now been shown by electron microscopy to have an infolded structure that makes the term "ruffled border" more appropriate. There are deep infoldings of the plasma membrane, which delimit a large number of closely packed clavate or foliate processes of highly variable size and shape, separated by narrow extracellular clefts (Fig. 8–16). Small crystals of bone mineral liberated from the bone matrix may be found deep in these clefts.

The plasma membrane itself is specialized in the region of the ruffled border. It bears on its inner or cytoplasmic surface a nap of exceedingly small, bristle-like appendages 15 to 20 nm in length and spaced about 20 nm apart. This bristle coat makes the membrane in this elaborately infolded region appear

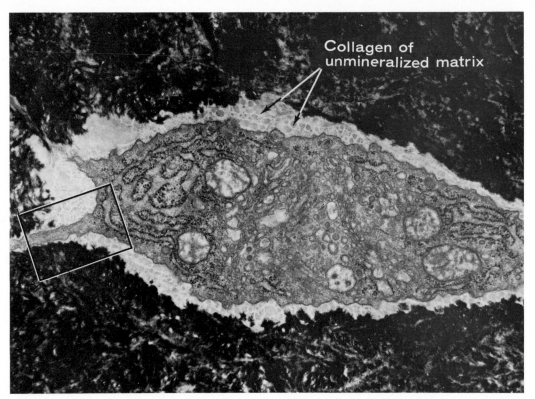

Figure 8–13. Electron micrograph of an osteocyte. The plane of section does not include the nucleus. Notice that the Golgi complex is still quite well developed, and numerous cisternal profiles of endoplasmic reticulum are present. At the left, a cell process is seen extending into a canaliculus. An area similar to that in the rectangle is seen at higher magnification in Figure 8–15. (Micrograph courtesy of M. Holtrop.)

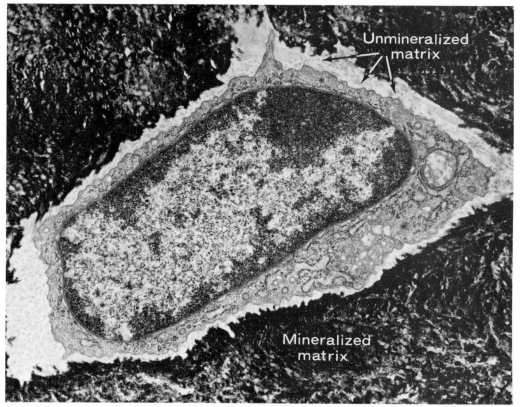

Figure 8–14. Electron micrograph of an osteocyte. Notice that it completely fills its lacuna. The clear area around the cell is in fact occupied by unmineralized matrix in which the collagen fibers are faintly visible. The mineralized matrix is black owing to the electron scattering of the apatite crystals. (Micrograph courtesy of M. Holtrop.)

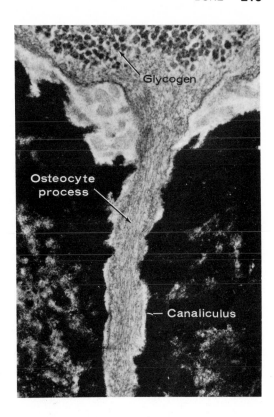

Figure 8–15. Osteocyte process extending from cell body *(above)* into a canaliculus *(below)*. Notice the high concentration of cytoplasmic filaments in the cell process. (Micrograph courtesy of M. Holtrop.)

thicker than the unspecialized unit membrane elsewhere on the cell surface. In contrast to a typical brush border, which is a very well-ordered and stable differentiation, the ruffled border of the osteoclast seems to be highly active and constantly changing its configuration. Cinematographic studies of these cells in vitro have shown that processes are continually being extended and retracted and changing their position.

The nuclei of osteoclasts resemble those of osteoblasts and are in no way unusual. The cytoplasm is slightly basophilic when stained with basic dyes at controlled pH, but in routine histological sections it is usually eosinophilic and highly vacuolated. There are multiple Golgi complexes distributed among the nuclei, and a number of centriole pairs corresponding to the number of nuclei. The centrioles may gather together in a centrosome region. The rod-shaped or short filamentous mitochondria of osteoclasts are very numerous and tend to congregate near the ruffled border. In contrast to other bone cells, the cytoplasmic vacuoles of osteoclasts stain supravitally with neutral red—a property that can be used to advantage in locating these multinucleate cells in fresh bone for experimental manipulation. Many of the vacuoles and granules also give a positive histochemical reaction for acid phosphatase, in-

dicative of their lysosomal nature. In electron micrographs, the granules are for the most part dense, spherical, 0.2 to 0.5 μm in diameter, and membrane limited, but larger vesicular structures 0.5 to 3 μm in diameter may also be secondary lysosomes.

Despite the evidence of activity of the osteoclast surface where it is in contact with bone, there is little evidence that these cells are mechanically erosive or even highly phagocytic. The exact mechanisms by which they accomplish the simultaneous degradation of the organic matrix and the dissolution of bone mineral still elude us, but there are rather clear indications that they secrete hydrolytic enzymes, including collagenase, which are responsible for digestion of matrix components.

The experiments upon which this conclusion is based depend on the fact that maintenance of normal levels of blood calcium in the intact animal depend on the actions of two hormones that act antagonistically on bone. Administration of *parathyroid hormone* causes mobilization of calcium by promoting bone resorption, while *calcitonin* acts to suppress mobilization of calcium from bone. Both hormones are also effective when applied to isolated bone fragments maintained in vitro. Thus, addition of parathyroid hormone to organ cultures results in appearance

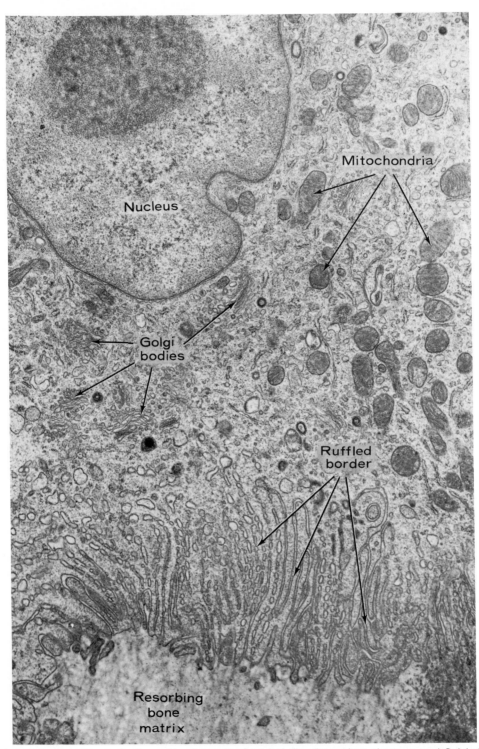

Figure 8–16. Electron micrograph of a portion of an osteoclast, including the nucleus above, several Golgi elements, and the ruffled border closely applied to an area of resorbing bone matrix at bottom of figure. (Micrograph courtesy of P. Garrant.)

of resorption cavities in the bone and markedly accelerated release of calcium and phosphate into the medium as a result of solubilization of bone mineral. There is also an increase in liberation of hydroxyproline from degradation of collagen of the bone matrix. Concomitant with these evidences of bone resorption, appreciable quantities of several lysosomal acid hydrolases are also released into the medium, whereas there is no detectable release of nonlysosomal enzymes from the cells of the culture. It is suggested, therefore, that the lysosomal enzymes are secreted by osteoclasts. Parathyroid hormone also greatly increases the rate of production of lactate and citrate by the bone explants, causing them to acidify their medium much more rapidly than other cells in culture. From consideration of such experiments, it is pro-

posed that lysosomal acid hydrolases of osteoblasts are active in resorption of the organic matrix of bone and that the stimulated local acid production solubilizes bone mineral and at the same time creates a pH favorable to the action of acid hydrolases.

The surface membrane of osteoclasts around the periphery of the active ruffled border is very smooth and closely applied to the underlying bone (Fig. 8–17). This observation has led to the speculation that the close application of the cell to its substrate in the clear zone around the periphery of the ruffled area might help to seal off the active portion of the cell and enable it to maintain a microenvironment conducive to solubilization of mineral and to optimal activity of hydrolytic enzymes.

There is additional physiological evidence

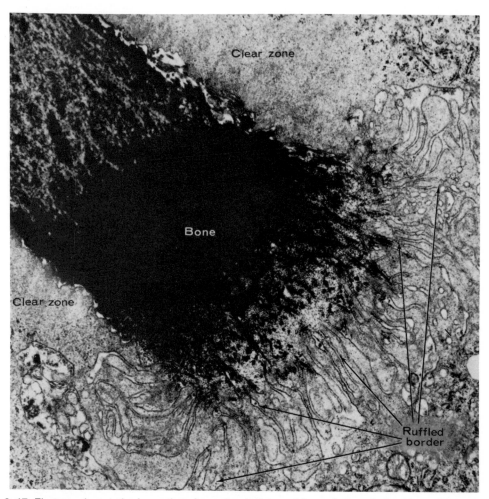

Figure 8–17. Electron micrograph of a portion of an osteoclast around the end of a spicule of bone. Notice the ruffled border at the end of the bone, where it is undergoing resorption. A smooth contoured portion of the osteoclast surface with a subjacent clear zone of ectoplasm is closely applied to the bone around the periphery of the ruffled border. (Micrograph courtesy of M. Holtrop.)

for a direct action of hormones on the osteoclast. Administration of parathyroid hormone is reported to cause depolarization of the osteoclast membrane and an increase in the rate of RNA synthesis, while calcitonin polarizes the cell membrane and inhibits the effect of parathyroid hormone on RNA synthesis. Calcitonin also causes disappearance of the ruffled border, a change in the character of the membrane, and separation of osteoclasts from the bone surface.

It is generally accepted that the multinucleate osteoclasts arise by coalescence of uninucleate cells, but a consensus as to the identity of the precursor cell has been reached only recently. Osteoprogenitor cells, osteoblasts, and osteocytes liberated from the matrix have all been proposed and strongly defended. However, some 30 years ago, in experiments that involved labeling of hemopoietic cells with tritiated thymidine, it was observed in radioautographs that some osteoclasts contained labeled nuclei. Since the nuclei of such cells do not divide and hence would not have incorporated thymidine during DNA replication, it was concluded that the labeled osteoclasts arose by fusion of mononuclear cells of bone marrow origin. Although this interpretation was slow to gain acceptance, confirmatory observations with labeling experiments of other design have accumulated. Perhaps the most compelling evidence for the origin of osteoclasts from cells circulating in the blood has been provided by ingenious experiments with mice of a mutant strain that have *osteopetrosis*—an excessive accumulation of spongiosa in their long bones due to impaired osteoclastic resorption of bone during development. When such osteopetrotic mice are surgically joined to normal littermates in parabiosis, the excess spongiosa disappears from their bones within six weeks, and they remain cured even after separation from their normal parabiont. The conclusion is inescapable that the mononuclear progenitors of the osteoclasts originated from the blood of the normal mouse while their circulatory systems were in continuity. Osteoclasts are now believed to arise by fusion of monocytes, and although they are not phagocytic in the usual sense, osteoclasts are considered members of the diffuse mononuclear phagocyte system.

HISTOGENESIS OF BONE

Bone always develops by replacement of a preexisting connective tissue. Two different modes of osteogenesis are recognized in embryos. When bone formation occurs directly in primitive connective tissue, it is called *intramembranous ossification*. When it takes place in preexisting cartilage, it is called intracartilaginous or *endochondral ossification*. In endochondral ossification the bulk of the cartilage must be removed before bone deposition begins, and the distinctive features of this mode of ossification are more concerned with the resorption of cartilage than with deposition of bone. The actual deposition of bony tissue is essentially the same in the two modes of ossification. Bone is first laid down as a network of trabeculae, the *primary spongiosa*, which is subsequently converted to more compact bone by a filling in of the interstices between trabeculae. Occasionally, under pathological conditions, bone may arise in tissues not belonging to the osseous system, and in connective tissues not ordinarily manifesting osteogenic properties. This is called *ectopic bone formation*.

Intramembranous Ossification

Certain flat bones of the skull—the frontal, parietal, occipital, and temporal bones and part of the mandible—develop by intramembranous ossification and are referred to as *membrane bones*. The mesenchyme condenses into a richly vascularized layer of connective tissue, in which the cells are in contact with one another by long tapering processes, and the intercellular spaces are occupied by randomly oriented delicate bundles of collagen fibrils embedded in a thin, gel-like extracellular matrix. The first sign of bone formation is the appearance of thin strands or bars of a denser eosinophilic matrix (Fig. 8–18). These strands of bone matrix tend to be deposited approximately equidistantly from neighboring blood vessels, and since the vessels form a network, the earliest trabeculae of bone matrix also develop in a branching and anastomosing pattern (Fig. 8–19). Simultaneously with the appearance of those first strands of eosinophilic extracellular matrix, there are changes in the neighboring primitive connective tissue cells. They enlarge and gather in increasing numbers on the surface of the trabeculae, assuming a cuboidal or columnar form while still remaining adherent to one another via shortened processes. Concurrently with the changes in their size and shape, the cells become intensely basophilic and are thereafter identified as osteoblasts. Through their synthetic and secretory activity, additional bone matrix

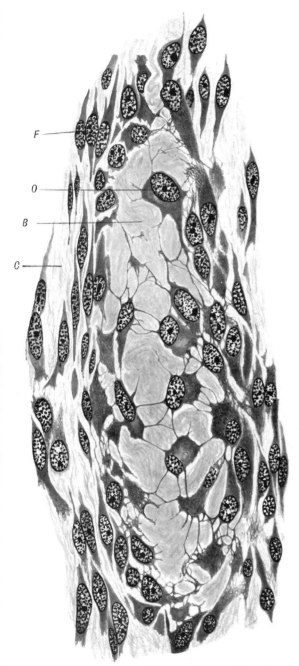

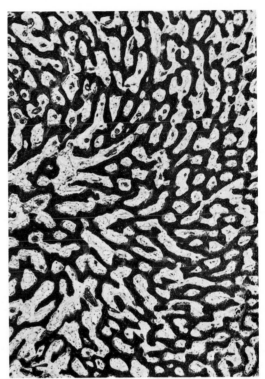

Figure 8–19. Photomicrograph of the pattern of trabeculae in the primary spongiosa of intramembranous bone formation.

Figure 8–18. Beginning of intramembranous bone formation in the skull of a 5.5-cm cat embryo. *B,* Homogeneous thickened collagenous fibers, which become the interstitial bone substance. *C,* Collagenous interstitial substance. *F,* Connective tissue cells. *O,* Connective tissue cells, with processes, which become osteoblasts and later bone cells. Eosin-azure stain. (After A. A. Maximow.)

(osteoid) is deposited, and the trabeculae become longer and thicker.

Collagen molecules are secreted together with the proteoglycans of the matrix, and they polymerize extracellularly to form great numbers of randomly interwoven fibrils of collagen throughout the trabeculae of osseous matrix. This early intramembranous bone in which the collagen fibers run in all directions is often called *woven bone,* to distinguish it from the *lamellar bone* formed in subsequent remodeling, which contains collagen in highly ordered parallel arrays. Woven bone is permeated by relatively large tortuous channels occupied by blood vessels and connective tissue. The osteocytes are distributed uniformly but oriented at random. In lamellar bone, on the other hand, the osteocytes are arranged in regular concentric order around relatively straight vessels in slender haversian canals (Fig. 8–20).

At a very early stage in the replacement of the interstitial substances of primitive connective tissue by bone matrix, the latter becomes a site of deposition of calcium phosphate. All of the matrix subsequently secreted by the osteoblasts calcifies after a very short lag. Thus, in electron micrographs, there is only a narrow zone of osteoid between the bases of the osteoblasts and the heavily mineralized matrix of the underlying trabeculae (Fig. 8–11). As the trabeculae thicken by accretion, some of the osteoblasts at their surface become incarcerated in the newly deposited matrix, and one by one they are buried within its substance to become bone cells—osteocytes. The osteocytes thus sequestered in lacunae within the newly de-

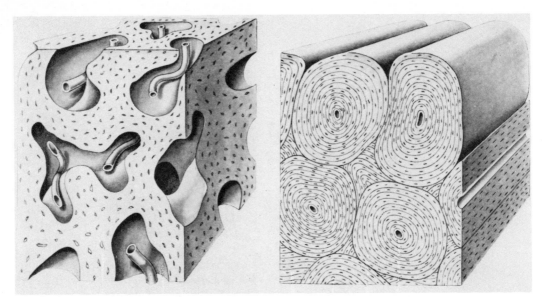

Figure 8–20. Three-dimensional diagrammatic representation of the differences in architecture of woven bone *(A)* and lamellar bone *(B)*. (From Hancox, N. M. *Biology of Bone*. Cambridge, England, Cambridge University Press, 1972.)

posited matrix nevertheless remain connected to osteoblasts at the surface by slender processes. The canaliculi of bone are formed by deposition of matrix around these cell processes. As rapidly as the ranks of osteoblasts on the surface of the trabeculae are depleted by their incorporation into the bone, their numbers are restored by differentiation of new osteoblasts from primitive cells of the surrounding connective tissue. Mitotic division is frequent in these progenitor cells but is rarely if ever observed in osteoblasts.

In areas of the primary spongiosa that are destined to become compact bone, the trabeculae continue to thicken at the expense of the intervening connective tissue until the spaces around the blood vessels are largely obliterated. The collagen fibrils in the layers of bone that are deposited on the trabeculae in this progressive encroachment upon the perivascular spaces gradually become more regularly arranged and come to resemble lamellar bone. Although the irregularly concentric layers formed may bear a superficial resemblance to haversian systems, they are not true lamellar bone because their collagen is randomly oriented.

In those areas where spongy bone will persist, the thickening of the trabeculae ceases and the intervening vascular connective tissue is gradually transformed into hemopoietic tissue. The connective tissue surrounding the growing mass of bone persists and condenses to form the periosteum. The

osteoblasts that have remained on the surface of the bone during its development revert to the fibroblast-like appearance as growth ceases and persist as the quiescent osteoprogenitor cells of the endosteum or of the periosteum. If they are again called upon to form bone, their osteogenic potentialities are reactivated and they again take on the morphological characteristics of osteoblasts.

Endochondral Ossification

Bones at the base of the skull, in the vertebral column, in the pelvis, and in the extremities are called *cartilage bones* because they are first formed of hyaline cartilage, which is then replaced with bone in the process called *endochondral ossification*. This can best be studied in one of the long bones of an extremity. The first indication of the establishment of a *center of ossification* is a striking enlargement of the chondrocytes at the middle of the shaft of the hyaline cartilage model (Fig. 8–21). The cells in this region hypertrophy, glycogen accumulates within them, and their cytoplasm becomes highly vacuolated. As the chondrocytes hypertrophy there is an enlargement of their lacunae at the expense of the intervening cartilage matrix, which is gradually reduced to thin fenestrated septa and irregularly shaped spicules. The remaining hyaline matrix in the region of hypertrophic cartilage cells becomes calcifiable, and small granular

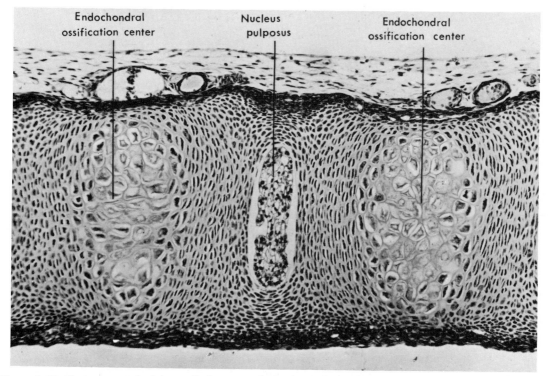

Endochondral   Nucleus   Endochondral
ossification center   pulposus   ossification center

Figure 8–21. Photomicrograph of the cartilaginous vertebral column of a mouse embryo, showing in the center of each vertebra an area of hypertrophied cartilage cells that represents an early stage in the establishment of a center of endochondral ossification.

aggregations and nests of crystals of calcium phosphate are deposited within it (Fig. 8–25C). Regressive changes in the hypertrophied cartilage cells, including swelling of their nuclei and loss of chromatin, are followed by their death and degeneration.

Concurrently with these hypertrophic and regressive changes in the chondrocytes in the interior of the cartilage model, the osteogenic potencies of cells in the *perichondrium* are activated, and a thin layer of bone, the *periosteal band* or *collar,* is deposited around the midportion of the shaft (Figs. 8–22B, 8–25A). At the same time, blood vessels from the investing layer of connective tissue (now called the periosteum) grow into the diaphysis, invading the irregular cavities in the cartilage matrix created by the enlargement of the chondrocytes and confluence of their lacunae (Figs. 8–22E,F, 8–23, 8–24). The thin-walled vessels branch and grow toward either end of the cartilage model, forming capillary loops that extend into the blind ends of the cavities in the calcified cartilage. Primitive pluripotential cells are carried into the interior of the cartilage in the perivascular tissue of the invading blood vessels. Some of these cells differentiate into hemopoietic elements of the bone marrow. Others differen-

tiate into osteoblasts, which congregate in an epithelioid layer on the irregular surfaces of spicules of calcified cartilage matrix and begin to deposit bone matrix upon them. The earliest bony trabeculae formed in the interior of the cartilage model thus have a core of calcified cartilage and an outer layer of bone of varying thickness. Owing to the different staining affinities of calcified cartilage and bone, these trabeculae have a mottled heterogeneous appearance and are easily distinguished from the homogeneous trabeculae of woven bone formed under the periosteum by intramembranous ossification.

It is common practice to include in the term *primary center of ossification* all the early morphological changes described above, whether they occur in the interior of the cartilage model or under the perichondrium. This usage is intended only to distinguish the diaphyseal center, which appears first, from *secondary centers of ossification,* which develop much later in the epiphyses. Some investigators, however, reserve the term primary center of ossification for the subperiosteal collar on the grounds that this is the first true bone formed, even though its formation is heralded by earlier changes in the chondrocytes in the interior of the model.

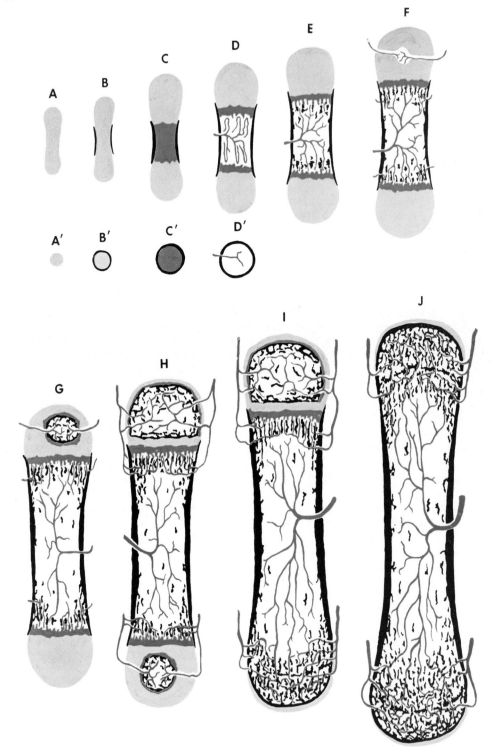

Figure 8–22. Diagram of the development of a typical long bone as shown in longitudinal sections *(A to J)* and in cross sections *A', B', C',* and *D'* through the centers of *A, B, C, and D.* Pale blue, cartilage; purple, calcified cartilage; black, bone; red, arteries. *A,* Cartilage model. *B,* Periosteal bone collar appears before any calcification of cartilage. *C,* Cartilage begins to calcify. *D,* Vascular mesenchyme enters the calcified cartilage matrix and divides it into two zones of ossification *(E). F,* Blood vessels and mesenchyme enter upper epiphyseal cartilage and the epiphyseal ossification center develops in it *(G).* A similar ossification center develops in the lower epiphyseal cartilage *(H).* As the bone ceases to grow in length, the lower epiphyseal plate disappears first *(I)* and then the upper epiphyseal plate *(J).* The bone marrow cavity then becomes continuous throughout the length of the bone, and the blood vessels of the diaphysis, metaphyses, and epiphyses intercommunicate.

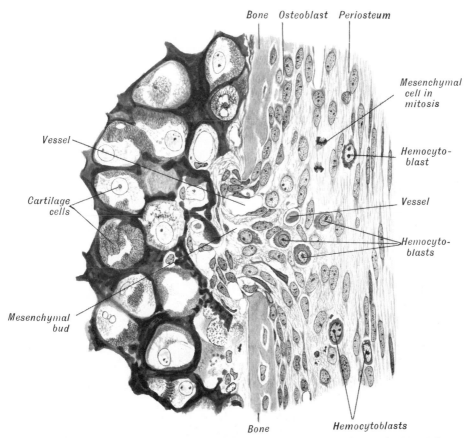

Figure 8–23. Part of longitudinal section through the middle of the diaphysis of the femur of a 25-mm human embryo. Mesenchyme with vessels entering calcified cartilage through an opening in the periosteal bone collar. Eosin-azure stain. (After A. A. Maximow.)

Mechanism of Calcification

The mechanism by which mineral is deposited in the organic matrix of cartilage and bone has been a subject of much debate and numerous hypotheses. One of the most widely accepted of these holds that the initiation of mineralization in bone is analogous to the familiar induction of crystallization from metastable solutions in vitro by adding a seed crystal or by scratching the wall of the beaker—a process called *heterogeneous nucleation*. The foreign matter disturbs the equilibrium in the solution and causes a clustering of molecules that results in formation of small nuclei capable of growing to form crystals. In the case of bone, it is believed to be the highly ordered "crystalline" collagen fibers of the matrix that act as the nucleation catalyst for transformation of calcium and phosphate in solution in the tissue fluids into the solid-phase mineral deposits. In support of this theory, it has been shown that reconstituted pure collagen fibers and demineralized bone are able to induce formation of apatite crystals when introduced into metastable solutions of inorganic calcium and phosphate. The fact that fibers of the native type, with 67-nm periodicity, are the only form of collagen capable of inducing this change led to speculation that nucleation of bone mineral is dependent on, or is at least facilitated by, the particular arrangement of molecules in these fibers. This interpretation derives added support from the observation that in electron micrographs of early stages of mineralization, the deposits of calcium phosphate are localized on specific regions of the cross-banded fibers.

During their formation of linear polymers, the collagen molecules overlap a short distance (Fig. 8–27). When these linear polymers associate laterally to form fibrils, they pack in such a way that discontinuities or "holes" exist within the fibers between the tails and heads of successive molecules. In negatively stained collagen, the contrast medium penetrates the fiber and fills these holes, producing the broad, dark bands that are characteristic of such preparations. The

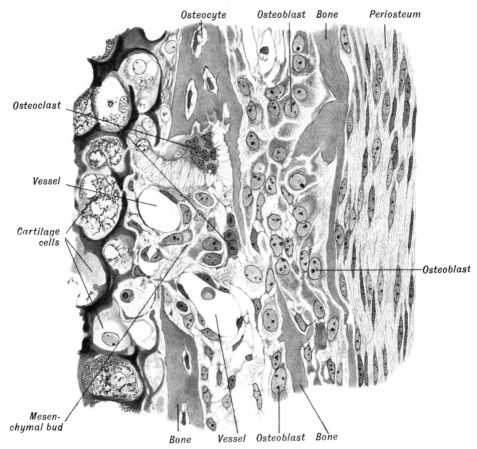

Figure 8–24. Part of longitudinal section through the middle of the diaphysis of the humerus of a human embryo of eight weeks. The process of ossification has advanced slightly farther than in Figure 8–23. Eosin stain. (After A. A. Maximow.)

earliest deposits of bone mineral produce a similar pattern of dense bands and therefore are believed to be localized in the holes within the collagen fibers (Fig. 8–27).

Persuasive as the evidence is for this attractive theory, it does not fully explain the localization of the process or the absence of calcification in many other collagen-rich tissues. It is evident too that collagen cannot be the only initiator of calcification. The organic matrix of the developing enamel of teeth, for example, is composed of a very different protein, but it is rapidly and heavily mineralized. A number of investigators insist that collagen does not act alone in vivo but that its interaction with chondroitin sulfate or some other glycosaminoglycan in the matrix may result in a particular stereochemical configuration that promotes apatite crystal formation. Evidence for this hypothesis is fragmentary, but it would seem to be in better accord with morphological observations on early stages of mineralization that show an

irregular pattern of crystal deposits on and between collagen fibers. It may also have an advantage over the collagen-centered nucleation theory in helping to explain those instances of mineralization, such as in epiphyseal cartilage, in which the initial deposits are localized without obvious topographical relation to typical 67-nm collagen fibers.

Clearly, this chapter in the story of bone development is not closed. Many details of the calcification process and its regulation remain to be worked out.

Growth in Length of Long Bones

In the continuing growth in length of the cartilage model after the appearance of the diaphyseal center of ossification, the chondrocytes in the adjacent regions of the epiphyses become arranged in longitudinal columns instead of in the small groups usually found in hyaline cartilage (Fig. 7–6). The cells within the columns are separated by thin

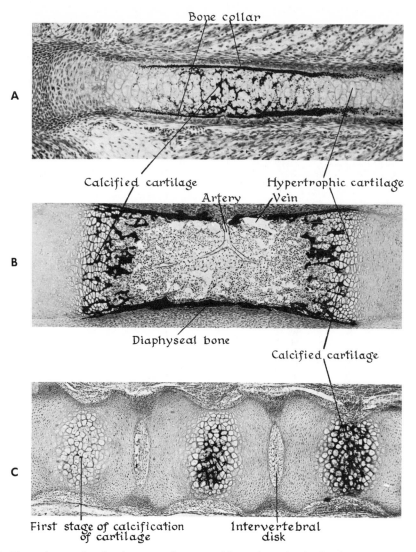

Bone collar

A

Calcified cartilage   Hypertrophic cartilage
              Artery   Vein

B

Diaphyseal bone

Calcified cartilage

C

First stage of calcification   Intervertebral
        of cartilage   disk

Figure 8–25. Photomicrographs showing several stages of bone formation in developing rats. From formalin-fixed, undecalcified sections stained with silver nitrate to show bone salt (black). *A,* Longitudinal section through second rib of 18-day rat embryo; calcification of the periosteal bone collar is further advanced than that of the cartilage. *B,* Section of metatarsal of 4-day rat, in which ossification is proceeding toward the epiphyses; the hypertrophic cartilage is not completely calcified. *C,* Three stages in calcification of vertebrae in 20-day rat embryo. (Courtesy of W. Bloom and M. A. Bloom.)

transverse septa, while adjacent columns are separated by wider longitudinal bars of hyaline matrix. As endochondral ossification progresses from the center of the shaft toward either end of the cartilage model, the chondrocytes undergo the same sequence of changes as described for the establishment of the diaphyseal center, but the process is now more orderly. Along the length of the epiphyseal cell columns are several recognizable zones, corresponding to various stages in the cytomorphosis of the cartilage cells. At some distance from the diaphyseo-epiphyseal junction is a *zone of proliferation,* where frequent

division of the small flattened cells provides for continual elongation of the columns. Next comes a *zone of maturation,* in which the cells that are no longer dividing gradually enlarge. This is followed by a *zone of hypertrophy,* with very large vacuolated cells. Since the matrix in this latter region becomes the site of calcium deposition, this may also be called the *zone of provisional calcification.* And finally, at the diaphyseal end of the columns is a zone wherein the chondrocytes are degenerating and the open ends of their enlarged lacunae are being invaded by capillary loops and osteoprogenitor cells from the marrow spaces

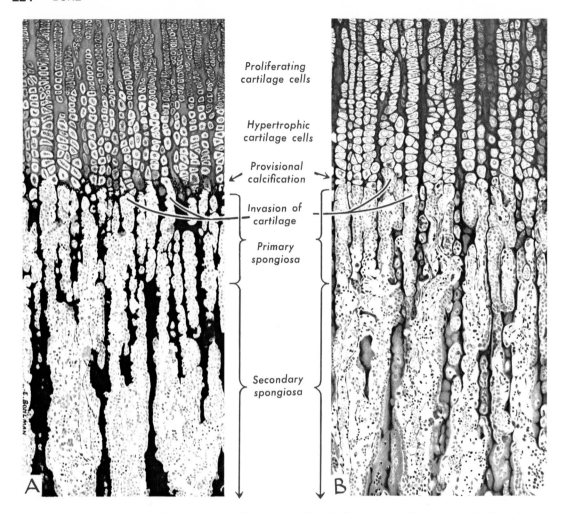

Proliferating
cartilage cells

Hypertrophic
cartilage cells

Provisional
calcification

Invasion of
cartilage

Primary
spongiosa

Secondary
spongiosa

Figure 8–26. Endochondral ossification in longitudinal sections through the zone of epiphyseal growth of the distal end of the radius of a puppy. *A,* Neutral formalin fixation; no decalcification. Von Kóssa and hematoxylin-eosin stain. All deposits of bone salt are stained black; thus, bone and calcified cartilage matrix stain alike. *B,* Zenker-formol fixation; decalcified. Hematoxylin-eosin-azure II stain. Persisting cores of cartilage matrix in trabeculae of bone take a deep blue or purple stain, whereas bone stains red. It is impossible to tell where calcium deposits had been.

of the diaphysis (Fig. 8–26). As the spaces at the lower ends of the columns are invaded, osteoblasts differentiate and congregate on the surfaces of the irregularly shaped longitudinal bars of calcified cartilage that persist between them. A thin new layer of bone matrix is then deposited on the surface of the cartilage. Under favorable conditions it begins to calcify nearly as rapidly as it is laid down, and thus it becomes bone. Electron microscopy has shown, however, that a superficial layer of uncalcified *preosseous tissue* or *osteoid,* 1 μm or less in thickness, is always present on forming bony surfaces (Fig. 8–11). There may be further lag in calcification under conditions of local failure in the supply of calcium or phosphate. When such a failure becomes general and osteoid accumulates in excess, the condition is known as

rickets in growing children or as *osteomalacia* in adults.

The distribution of calcified cartilage and new bone is best demonstrated in undecalcified sections in which the bone mineral has been stained black with silver by the von Kóssa method (Fig 8–26A). The transitional zone where the cartilage is being replaced by advancing bone is called the *metaphysis.* The primary spongy bone in this zone undergoes extensive reorganization as the growth processes pass it by. As the bone grows longer, the diaphyseal ends of the trabeculae are continually being eroded by osteoclasts at about the same rate that additions are made at the epiphyseal end, with the result that the spongiosa of the metaphysis tends to remain relatively constant in length.

Centers of ossification have appeared in

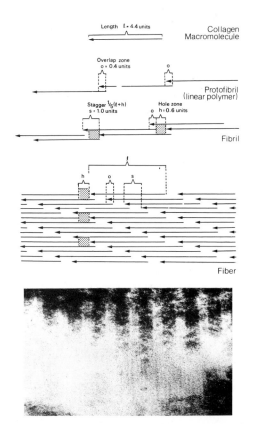

Length ℓ = 4.4 units

Collagen Macromolecule

Overlap zone
o = 0.4 units

Protofibril (linear polymer)

Stagger ⅕(ℓ + h)
s = 1.0 units

Hole zone
h = 0.6 units

Fibril

Fiber

Figure 8–27. Diagram of the overlapping staggered arrangement of molecules in a collagen fiber, showing the small discontinuities or holes that are thought to be sites of nucleation of apatite crystals in the mineralization of bone. (Modified from Glimcher, M. J., and S. M. Krane. *In* Gould, B. S., and G. N. Ramachandran, eds.: A Treatise on Collagen. Vol. II. New York, Academic Press, 1968.)

the diaphysis of each of the principal long bones of the skeleton by the third month of fetal life. Much later, usually after birth, the epiphyses show in their interior the characteristic chondrocyte hypertrophy that heralds the onset of endochondral ossification, and they in turn are invaded by blood vessels and osteogenic tissue from the perichondrium to establish *secondary centers of ossification* at either end of the developing long bones (Fig. 8–22C,H) These differ from the diaphyseal centers in that there is no associated deposition of subperichondral bone. The expansion of these secondary centers gradually replaces all of the epiphyseal cartilage except that which persists as the *articular cartilage* and a transverse disc between the epiphysis and diaphysis called the *epiphyseal plate* (Fig. 8–22J). The latter contains the cartilage columns whose proliferative zone is responsible for all subsequent growth in length of long bones. Under normal conditions the rate of multiplication of cartilage cells in this zone is

in balance with the rate of their degeneration and removal at the diaphyseal end of the columns. The epiphyseal plate therefore retains approximately the same thickness. Growth in length is the result of the cartilage cells continually growing away from the shaft and being replaced by bone as they recede. The net effect is an increase in the length of the shaft.

At the end of the growing period, proliferation of cartilage cells slows and finally ceases. Continued replacement of the cartilage by bone at the diaphyseal end of the columns then results in complete removal of the epiphyseal cartilage, and the bony trabeculae of the metaphysis then become continuous with the spongiosa of the bony epiphysis. This process of elimination of the epiphyseal plate is referred to as *closure of the epiphysis*. When this has taken place, no further longitudinal growth of the bone is possible. The times of closure and the relative contribution of each of the two epiphyses of a long bone to its overall growth may differ markedly. Growth in length of the femur, for example, takes place mainly at the distal epiphysis; growth of the tibia, mainly at the proximal epiphysis. Such information is of clinical value in radiology and orthopedic surgery.

Because all increment in length of a bone is limited to its epiphyseal plates, injury to this region may result in serious impairment of growth. In cases of retarded growth of one leg attributable to general neurovascular disturbances, such as may occur in the limb of a child who has had poliomyelitis, the orthopedic surgeon can take advantage of existing knowledge of the normal rates of growth at the various epiphyseal plates and of the times of their normal closure, to select the appropriate time and site for a surgical obliteration of an epiphysis in the normal leg. Such a procedure, if appropriately timed, may retard growth of the normal leg just enough to permit the slower growing leg to catch up and thus achieve an equalization of leg length by the time that growth in stature of the individual ceases.

Growth in Diameter of Long Bones

The long bones of the extremities are first laid down in cartilage models, and, as indicated in the foregoing section, their growth in length depends on endochondral ossification. The growth in diameter of the shaft, however, is the result of deposition of new membrane bone beneath the periosteum. The compact bone forming the shaft of a fully developed long bone is almost entirely the product of subperiosteal intramembranous ossification.

After establishment of the primary ossification center, the ends of the cartilage model continue to elongate and broaden by proliferation of chondrocytes and elaboration of new matrix, but such interstitial growth is no longer possible in the center of the diaphysis, where the cartilage is regressing and being replaced by bone. The diameter of the endochondral component in the middle of the diaphysis, therefore, cannot be appreciably greater than the diameter of the cartilage model in the early embryo at the time of establishment of the primary center of ossification. To keep pace with the rapid interstitial growth of the cartilage at the ends, increase in thickness of the shaft is accomplished by a progressive thickening of the *periosteal band* or *collar* formed around the middle of the cartilaginous diaphysis at the onset of ossification. This results in deposition of a lattice of trabeculae of intramembranous woven bone, forming the wall of the diaphysis.

Bone resorption is as important to the growth of bones as is bone deposition, and the deposition of new bone on the outside of the shaft is accompanied by the appearance of osteoclasts that erode the inner aspect of the subperiosteal trabeculae to enlarge the marrow cavity. The rates of external apposition of new bone and internal resorption are so adjusted that the cylindrical shaft expands rapidly while the thickness of its wall increases more slowly.

Because of the continual internal resorption and reorganization of bone during development, the record of the topographical distribution of endochondral and intramembranous ossification in earlier stages of development is continually erased. Therefore, the extent of the contribution of the periosteum to the fully formed long bone is seldom fully appreciated. It is informative in this regard to examine developing long bones of the manatee, an aquatic mammal in which resorption of bone to form the secondary marrow cavity does not take place. In fetal bones of this species (Figs. 8–28, 8–29), the primary spongiosa of endochondral bone has a characteristic hourglass distribution. The two conical regions, with their apices meeting at the site of the original ossification center, result from uniform growth in length and breadth of the ends of the cartilage model. The area between the diverging sides of the two cones is filled in by a thick collar of trabeculae of periosteal origin. Such bones, lacking the capacity for the resorption that occurs in the histogenesis of long bones in other species, provide an instructive view of the basic topography of the cartilaginous and membranous components of all long bones (Fig. 8–29).

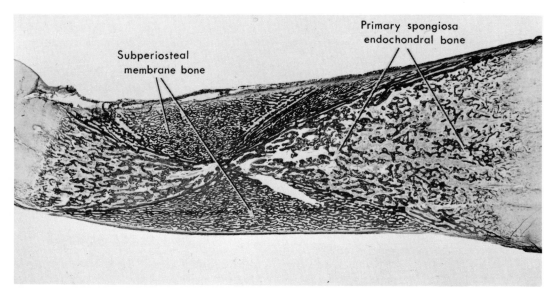

Figure 8–28. Photomicrograph of the humerus in a fetal manatee in longitudinal section. In this species, whose bones lack a secondary marrow cavity, the respective contributions of subperiosteal and endochondral bone to the formation of the shaft of a long bone are more evident than in bones of other species. (After Fawcett, D. W. Am. J. Anat. 71:271, 1942.)

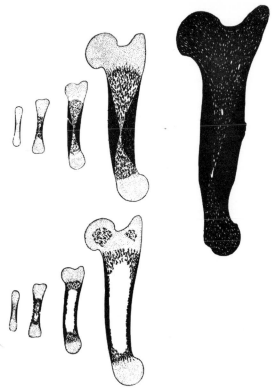

Figure 8–29. Diagrammatic representation of the development of a manatee bone *(above)* compared with that of a typical mammal *(below)*. (After Fawcett, D. W. Am. J. Anat. *71*:271, 1942.)

Surface Remodeling of Bones

Although growing bones are constantly changing their internal organization, they retain approximately the same external form from an early fetal stage into adult life. It is apparent that this would not be so if new bone were deposited at a uniform rate at all points beneath the periosteum. Instead, the shape of a bone is maintained during growth by a continual remodeling or sculpturing of its surface, which involves bone deposition in some areas of the periosteum and bone absorption in other areas. That this is true was demonstrated in the middle of the eighteenth century by madder feeding experiments. With this method of vital staining, the bone deposited during a period of feeding on madder root was stained red, while areas that were stable or were undergoing resorption remained unstained. It was clearly shown that some areas of the surface of long bones stained while others did not. The general features of these early experiments have now been confirmed and extended by means of newer techniques employing bone-seeking

isotopes or the antibiotic tetracycline, both of which are deposited preferentially in newly forming bone.

Typical of such experiments are those localizing the sites of osteogenesis in the growing rat tibia. This bone supports a large articular surface, and the epiphysis is considerably broader than the shaft. Thus, it is possible to distinguish a cylindrical region in the middle of the shaft and a conical region toward the end, where it expands to the width of the epiphysis. If a bone-seeking isotope is given to a growing rat and autoradiographs are then made of longitudinal sections of the tibia, the sites of new bone formation are disclosed by the distribution of silver grains in the overlying emulsion. In the conical region of the bone, the silver grains are aligned immediately subjacent to the endosteum, whereas in the cylindrical portion of the shaft they are found beneath the periosteum (Fig. 8–31). Study of parallel histological sections reveals numerous osteoclasts beneath the periosteum of the conical region and beneath the endosteum of the cylindrical segment. Thus, it is clear that in the surface remodeling of this bone, the periosteum plays opposite roles in neighboring regions on the surface of the same bone. Subperiosteal bone deposition is occurring in the cylindrical portion of the shaft while subperiosteal bone absorption is taking place in the conical region. Similarly, bone is being

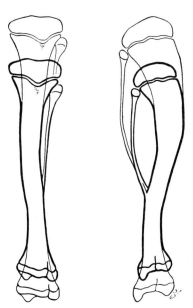

Figure 8–30. Diagram to illustrate remodeling during growth of tibia and fibula of rat, viewed from anterior aspect and in profile. (After Wolbach.)

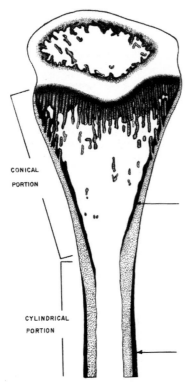

CONICAL
PORTION

CYLINDRICAL
PORTION

Figure 8–31. Diagram based on an autoradiograph of the head of the tibia of a growing rat killed a few hours after receiving an injection of ^{32}P. The localization of high concentrations of silver grains in the autoradiograph is depicted here in black. In addition to the new bone in the epiphysis and at the metaphysis, bone is being deposited under the endosteum in the conical portion and beneath the periosteum in the cylindrical portion of the shaft *(arrows).* (Drawing based on studies of Leblond et al. Am. J. Anat. *86*:289, 1950. After Fawcett, D. W. *In* Greep, R. O., ed.: Histology. Philadelphia, Blakiston Co., 1954. Reproduced by permission of McGraw-Hill Book Co.)

formed at the endosteal surface of the cone and absorbed on the inner aspect of the cylinder. As a consequence of these activities, the midportion of the shaft is expanding radially and its marrow cavity is being enlarged. While the bone as a whole is elongating by growth at the epiphyseal plate, the diverging wall of the conical region of the shaft is being straightened and is contributing, at its lower end, to the lengthening of the cylindrical region of the shaft.

Similarly, in the skull vault, the assumption that growth of the flat bones at the sutures could account for enlargement of the cranial cavity to accommodate the growing brain is not sufficient as an explanation. As the radius of curvature of the growing skull vault increases, the bones become less convex. Therefore, not only must bone resorption take place on the inside of the calvarium concurrently with bone deposition on the outer surface, but also the rates of deposition and absorption must differ from the center to the periphery of each cranial bone in order to account for its flattening as the radius of curvature of the skull vault increases. How these local variations in function of endosteum and periosteum are controlled in space and time to mold and shape the bone constantly during its growth is a fascinating unsolved problem in morphogenesis.

Internal Reorganization of Bone

The conversion of the primary lattice of trabeculae laid down in intramembranous ossification into compact bone is attributed to thickening of the trabeculae and a progressive encroachment of bone upon the perivascular spaces until these are largely obliterated. As the process advances, bone is deposited in ill-defined layers with randomly oriented collagen fibers but since these are disposed more or less concentrically around vascular channels, they come to bear a superficial resemblance to haversian systems. They are sometimes called *primitive haversian systems*, but they should be clearly distinguished from the more precisely ordered lamellar systems comprising the *definitive haversian systems* of adult bone. The latter arise only in the course of the internal reorganization of primary compact bone that is referred to as *secondary bone formation*.

At scattered points in the compacta, usually in those areas laid down earliest, cavities appear as a result of osteoclastic erosion of primary bone. Such *absorption cavities* enlarge to form long cylindrical cavities occupied by blood vessels and embryonic bone marrow. When they reach a considerable length, destruction of bone ceases; the osteoclasts give way to osteoblasts, and concentric lamellae of bone are laid down on the walls of the cavity until it is filled in to form a typical haversian system of lamellar bone. The lamellae of this and subsequent generations of haversian systems have the ordered arrangement of collagen and the change in its orientation in successive layers that are characteristic of osteons in adult bone. In man from about the age of 1 year onward, only lamellar bone of this character is deposited within the shafts of long bones. This secondary bone eventually replaces all the primitive haversian systems.

The outer limits of secondary haversian systems are defined by distinct *cement lines.*

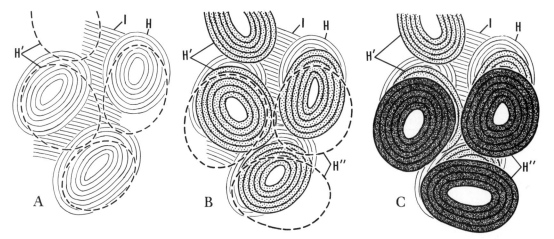

Figure 8–32. Diagram of stages in formation of three generations of haversian system, *H*, *H'*, and *H"*. *I*, Interstitial lamellae. (Modified from Prenant.)

These are layers of bone matrix formed whenever a period of resorption is followed by new bone formation. They are collagen poor, have staining properties different from other layers of matrix, and are not traversed by canaliculi.

The internal bone destruction and reconstruction do not end with the replacement of primary by secondary bone, but continue actively throughout life. Resorption cavities continue to appear and to be filled in by third, fourth, and higher orders of haversian systems (Fig. 8–32). The interstitial lamellae of adult bone represent persisting fragments of earlier generations of haversian systems largely removed in the continuing internal reorganization. At any one time there may

be seen in a cross section (1) mature osteons, in which all rebuilding activity has come to an end and which form the great mass of structural bone upon which the weight-bearing function of the skeleton depends; (2) actively forming new osteons, in which concentric layers of preosseous tissue are being laid down and progressively calcified; and (3) absorption cavities being hollowed out in preparation for formation of new osteons.

The rate of lamellar bone formation can be determined by administration of tetracycline at two different times and measurement of the thickness of bone between the two resulting bands of labeled bone (Fig. 8–33). Such studies show that 1 μm per day is a fair average for the human and for any given

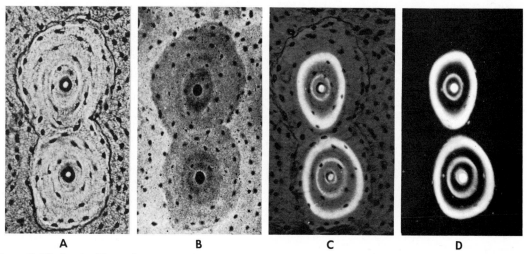

Figure 8–33. A pair of haversian systems from the midshaft of the tibia of a 9-month-old dog given two 5-day courses of treatment with a tetracycline separated by an interval of 19 days. *A*, Ordinary microscopy. *B*, Historadiogram. *C* and *D*, Fluorescence microscopy. The bone deposited during Ledermycin (demeclocycline) treatment fluoresces, and the design of this experiment permits one to visualize the amount of bone deposited in each 5-day period. Of particular interest is the fact that the inner band, corresponding to the second period of administration, is narrower than the first, demonstrating that in this instance there is slowing down in the rate of concentric bone deposition as the formation of the haversian system progresses. (Courtesy of R. Amprino.)

haversian system the rate of deposition slows as the osteon nears completion. The formation time for a haversian system in the adult is four to five weeks. Different values are found in young growing bone and in pathological states. The newly deposited lamellar bone continues to calcify over a considerable period of time. A historadiogram therefore reveals a mixture of haversian systems of varying age, displaying all degrees of mineralization (Fig. 8–8C). By this continuous turnover, the organism is assured a continuing supply of new bone to carry out its skeletal and metabolic functions. It also provides the plasticity that enables bone to alter its internal architecture to adapt to new mechanical conditions.

Repair of Bone

After a fracture the usual reactions of any tissue to severe injury are seen, including hemorrhage and organization of the clot by ordinary granulation tissue. The granulation tissue becomes denser connective tissue. Car-tilage and fibrocartilage then develop within it, forming a *fibrocartilaginous callus* that fills the gap between the ends of the fragments. The new bone, which will ultimately unite the fragments, begins to form at some distance from the fracture line, by activation of osteoprogenitor cells of the deeper layers of the periosteum and endosteum. A meshwork of subperiosteal trabeculae, the *bony callus*, is formed, and a similar formation of new bone of endosteal origin occurs in the medullary cavity around the cartilaginous callus. As healing progresses, the latter is gradually eroded, with only enough cartilage matrix remaining to provide a framework for deposition of new bone in the area. As in endochondral bone formation, ossification of the fibrocartilaginous callus is accomplished by its gradual replacement with bone. *Bony union* of the fracture is complete when the new spongy bone from the two fragments meets and becomes continuous across the fracture line. After this there is compaction and reorganization, with resorption of excess bone and internal reconstruction, resulting

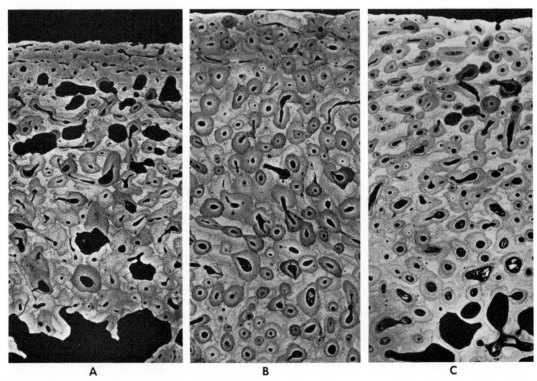

A   B   C

Figure 8–34. Cross section of the anteromedial sector of the midshaft of the femur as revealed by negative historadiography. *A*, At age 7. *B*, At age 20. *C*, At age 65. Notice in the child *(A)* there are large resorption cavities *(black)* and large, irregularly shaped haversian systems. At the surface of the compacta, the thick zone of periosteal bone is invaded by resorption cavity. Large remnants of periosteal primary bone are found in the interstices between the secondary osteons in the middle zone of the compacta. These remnants are fewer and smaller in the older perimedullary zone at the bottom of the figure. In the 20-year-old man *(B)*, the compacta is much thicker. Secondary haversian systems and remnants of primary bone persist in the subperiosteal zone. Elsewhere, the osteons are fairly regular in outline and are separated by remnants of preexisting osteons. (Courtesy of R. Amprino.)

finally in a bridging of the gap with compact bone.

In certain locations, where the connective tissue surrounding the bone lacks osteogenic potency, such as the subcapsular areas of the neck of the femur and of the astragalus, and the surfaces of the *sesamoid bones* formed within tendons (e.g., patella, pisiform), healing of fractures occurs without a periosteal reaction and without a fibrocartilaginous callus. If there is good apposition of the fragments, the cancellous bone of the marrow cavity unites, without any callus formation. If apposition is poor or nonexistent, repair may occur only as a relatively weak, fibrous union.

Ectopic Bone Formation

As already stated, intramembranous bone forms from a connective tissue, with the transformation of mesenchymal cells into osteoprogenitor cells, osteoblasts and osteocytes. The return of these cells to fibroblast-like osteoprogenitor cells has also been described. The influences under which ordinary connective tissue gives rise to bone in the embryo are poorly understood, but it is clear that previously undifferentiated cellular elements of primitive connective tissue are capable of transformation to the cells characteristic of bone.

It would appear that, once cells have exhibited osteogenic potencies, these can be readily evoked again for an indeterminate period after the cells have returned to an indifferent morphological state. Thus, in the healing of fractures, cells in the deepest layers of the periosteum and endosteum, under the stimulus of trauma, reassume the form of osteoblasts and once again are actively engaged in osteogenesis. Moreover, cells grown from bone in tissue culture, and having lost the morphological characteristics of osteoblasts, once again form bone when implanted into the anterior chamber of the eye.

Furthermore, under certain conditions, bone may be formed spontaneously from connective tissue that is not in association with the skeleton. This *ectopic ossification* has been described in such diverse locations as the pelvis of the kidney, the walls of arteries, the eyes, muscles, and tendons. In the long tendons of the legs of turkeys, bone formation is a normal event. From these observations it may be inferred that many types of connective tissue have latent osteogenic potencies that are exhibited only rarely. This conclusion is supported by experimental production of bone in connective tissue after ligation of the renal artery and vein and after a variety of experimental manipulations, such as transplantation of bladder epithelium to the fascia of the anterior wall of the abdomen, or after injection of alcoholic extracts of bone into muscle.

Many attempts have been made to utilize the osteogenic potencies of periosteum and bone by transplanting these tissues to areas in which it is desired that new bone be formed. The modern "bone bank," which supplies fragments of bone preserved by freezing or by other means, is the fruit of these efforts. Transplants of fresh autogenous bone ordinarily survive and proliferate. Homografts are antigenic and give rise to an immune response that leads ultimately to death of the transplanted tissue. Heterografts usually do not survive, but if calf bone is refrigerated and stored, it loses some of its antigenicity and may therefore be suitable for use in bone banks. Grafts of such tissue favor induction of new bone formation by the cells of the host.

Primitive connective tissue cells within the orbit of advancing bone, as in the formation of medullary bone in birds, assume the form of osteoblasts before they actually participate in osteogenesis. This observation, together with those upon the behavior of bone grafts just cited, suggests that the presence of bone itself may be an important factor in activating osteogenic potencies. There is thus histological evidence in favor of *induction* of bone formation, although attempts to isolate a specific inductor substance have so far given equivocal results.

HISTOPHYSIOLOGY OF BONE

As the principal tissue making up the skeletal system, bone functions in support of the soft tissues; it carries the articulations and provides attachment for the muscles involved in locomotion; and it forms a rigid covering for protection of the nervous system and of the hemopoietic tissue. In addition to these mechanical functions, it plays an important role as a large store of calcium and phosphorus that can be drawn upon to maintain the normal levels of these elements in the blood and to provide for the mineral requirements of other tissues.

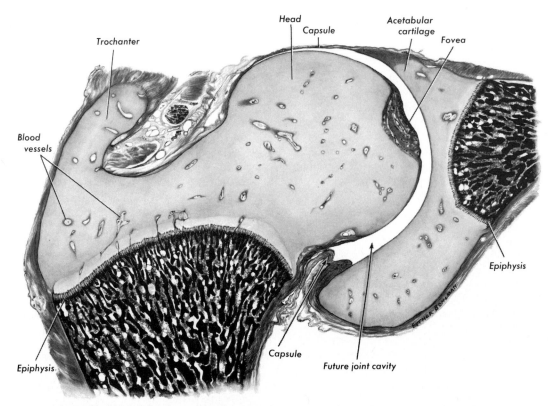

Figure 8–35. Section through head of the femur of a 26-cm human fetus. (From a preparation of H. Hatcher.)

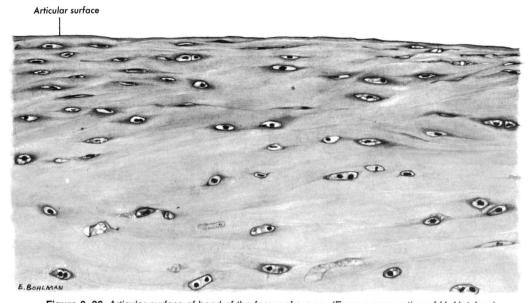

Figure 8–36. Articular surface of head of the femur of a man. (From a preparation of H. Hatcher.)

Bone as a Store of Mobilizable Calcium

It is impossible to overemphasize the importance of calcium in the vital functions of the body. It is essential for the activity of many enzymes. It is indispensable for maintenance of cell cohesion and of the normal permeability of cell membranes. It is required for contraction of muscles and for coagulation of the blood. It is not surprising, therefore, that the homeostatic mechanisms of the body regulate the concentration of plasma calcium with remarkable constancy, the normal range being between 9 and 11 mg per 100 ml. Most of the calcium in the body (99 per cent) is, of course, in the bones. There is a constant interchange of calcium between bone and the blood, which results in maintenance of the relatively constant calcium ion concentration in the plasma. The minute hydroxyapatite crystals present a surface area for exchange with the extracellular fluids that is of the order of 100 to 300 square meters per gram. It has been estimated that during each minute in the life of an adult man, one of every four calcium ions present in the blood exchanges with similar ions in the bones.

A dual mechanism for homeostatic regulation of the blood calcium level has been postulated. One part, acting by diffusion and simple equilibrium between blood and the labile fraction of bone mineral, is adequate to maintain a constant but low calcium level of approximately 7 mg per 100 ml of blood plasma. Not all of the bone contributes equally to this function. The most labile calcium apparently is located in the younger and incompletely calcified osteons. It is these that are most sensitive to ionic variations in the internal environment. Therefore, the continued remodeling of the adult skeleton has metabolic as well as mechanical significance. It provides a pool of young osteons, which can rapidly respond in homeostatic regulation by taking up or releasing calcium. As these osteons mature and become more heavily mineralized, they become progressively less available to the extracellular fluids, and these older osteons probably contribute more to the mechanical function of the skeleton. They are ultimately replaced in their physiological function by a new generation of osteons. These two categories are sometimes referred to as *metabolic* and *structural bone*. The second part of the dual mechanism required to elevate and maintain the plasma calcium at the normal level of 10 mg per 100 ml is mediated by *parathyroid hormone*, and involves resorption of bone mineral and organic matrix through the action of osteoclasts.

The responsiveness of the skeleton to the metabolic needs of other organ systems is best illustrated in those species in which there are unusual periodic demands for calcium. Perhaps the most striking example is found in birds in the laying cycle, during which considerable amounts of calcium are required in the oviduct for deposition of the eggshell. To meet this need, many trabeculae in the marrow cavities of the long bones are resorbed, only to be restored after the egg is laid and again removed to provide the shell for the next egg in the clutch. Less dramatic examples of mobilization of calcium from the skeleton are also observed in mammals. While the antlers of deer are growing, there is a mild rarefaction of bone throughout the skeleton, and in dairy cows producing large amounts of milk there may be a detectable osteoporosis associated with the considerable calcium loss in the milk. Human reproduction does not involve such unusual demands for calcium. There is no doubt, however, that during pregnancy the maternal skeleton is drawn upon to some extent for calcification of the fetal skeleton, and during prolonged lactation it is the source of some of the calcium lost in milk. In normal individuals there is no detectable radiological change in the skeleton, but when pregnancy or lactation is superimposed upon severe nutritional deficiency or impaired absorption of calcium, *osteomalacia* results, and may become so severe as to result in pathological fractures.

Endocrine Effects Upon Bone

The skeletal system is affected by several hormones. The most important of these is *parathyroid hormone*. Its participation in maintenance of the normal levels of circulating calcium was referred to earlier. The activity of the parathyroid glands appears to be regulated by a *negative feedback* mechanism, in which the blood Ca^{++} level itself exerts a direct effect upon parathyroid activity. Parathyroid hormone has multiple sites of action. One of the earliest detectable effects after its administration is on the kidney, where it causes a rapid increase in excretion of phosphate in the urine. This in turn affects the plasma calcium levels. The hormone appears to have a dual effect upon bone. Its initial effect is believed to be on osteocytes, stimulating osteocytic osteolysis. A long-continued increase in circulating parathyroid hormone results in induction of osteoclast formation and accelerated bone remodeling. Since bone resorption under the influence of parathyroid hormone results in destruction of stable crystals of hydroxyapatite, as well as of the organic matrix, this mechanism makes available, for homeostatic regulation, an otherwise inaccessible source of calcium.

Grafts of parathyroid to bone in vivo and confronted cultures in vitro have demonstrated that the gland causes resorption by direct action on bone. In clinical *hyperparathyroidism*, bone is extensively absorbed and is replaced by fibrous tissue containing large numbers of osteoclasts. This results in the pathological condition described as *osteitis fibrosa* (von Recklinghausen's disease).

Opposing the action of parathyroid hormone is the polypeptide hormone *calcitonin* or *thyrocalcitonin*, which originates from special cells in the thyroid gland. This hormone inhibits bone resorption and thus tends to lower blood calcium. It is currently hypothesized that parathyroid hormone and calcitonin act together to prevent or counteract any significant perturbation of the homeostatic regulation of plasma calcium concentration. A fall in plasma calcium below a certain level would presumably result in increased release of parathyroid hormone and suppression of calcitonin release. The effect of this would be an increased rate of bone resorption and movement of calcium from bone to blood, thereby returning the plasma calcium to normal. Conversely, a supranormal blood calcium concentration would stimulate release of calcitonin and suppress release of parathyroid hormone. These effects would tend to return the elevated plasma calcium to normal.

The effects of the gonadal hormones upon bone vary greatly with the species. In the example of the laying bird cited previously, an entire new system of trabeculae of medullary bone is produced by stimulation of the endosteal lining in the estrogenic phase of the egg-laying cycle. These trabeculae serve to accumulate calcium for later use in formation of the eggshell. The same changes can be induced by administration of exogenous *estrogens*. Concurrently with the storage of calcium in medullary bone, the liver forms a phosphoprotein that appears in the blood and is transported to the ovarian follicle, where it is stored in the egg yolk as *phosphovitellin*, the major source of phosphate for growth and development of the chick embryo.

Mice react to administration of estrogens in a manner qualitatively similar to that of birds. Endosteal bone formation is enhanced, but in this case does not seem to serve any physiological function. Endosteal bone formation has not been reported in rats. In this species, estrogens inhibit normal resorption of the spongiosa during endochondral ossification, resulting in a greatly elongated and dense spongiosa in the metaphysis. The osteoporosis occasionally seen in women after the menopause is attributed by some to the decline in ovarian function, but it does not respond favorably to treatment with estrogens.

The gonadal hormones in some way play an important part in determining the rate of skeletal maturation. In normal human development the time of appearance of the various ossification centers and the time of fusion of the epiphyses with their diaphyses is remarkably constant. The progress of these events at any given time during development is intimately related to the developmental state of the reproductive system. Thus, in precocious sexual development, skeletal maturation is accelerated and growth is stunted, owing to premature epiphyseal closure. On the other hand, in testicular hypoplasia or prepubertal castration, epiphyseal union in the long bones is delayed, and the arms and legs become disproportionately long.

The growth of bone is also markedly influenced by the *growth hormone* (somatotropin) of the anterior hypophysis. Hypophysectomy results in cessation of growth at the epiphyseal plate; upon administration of growth hormone, growth recommences. Growth hormone injected into rats that have been both thyroidectomized and hypophysectomized produces skeletal growth, whereas thyroxine produces maturation but only moderate growth. Coordination between growth and maturation may be restored by administration of both hormones.

Nutritional Effects Upon Bone

Growth of the skeleton is quite dependent upon nutritional factors. Deficiencies of minerals or of essential vitamins are often detected more easily in bone than in other tissues. A gross dietary deficiency of either calcium or phosphorus leads to rarefaction of bone and increased liability to fractures. Even if the intake of these elements is adequate, a deficiency of *vitamin D* may interfere with their intestinal absorption and lead to *rickets*. In this condition, ossification of the epiphyseal cartilages is disturbed, the regular columnar arrangement of the cartilage cells disappears, and the metaphysis becomes a disordered mixture of uncalcified cartilage and poorly calcified bone matrix. Such bones are easily deformed by weight bearing.

In long-standing deficiency of calcium and of vitamin D, especially when aggravated by pregnancy, the bones of adults come to contain much uncalcified osteoid tissue, a condition known as *adult rickets* or *osteomalacia*. Although the condition is aggravated by the increased demands of pregnancy, the diminution in calcium content in this condition is due mainly to failure of calcification of new bone formed in the turnover of this tissue, rather than to decalcification of previously calcified bone.

Deficiency of *vitamin C* leads to profound changes in tissues of mesenchymal origin, producing the condition known as *scurvy* or *scorbutus*, in which the primary defect is an inability to produce and maintain the intercellular substance of connective tissues. In the case of bone, it results in deficient production of collagen and bone matrix, with consequent retardation of growth and delayed healing of fractures.

Deficiency of *vitamin A* results in a diminution in the rate of growth of the skeleton. The vitamin controls the activity, distribution, and coordination of osteoblasts and osteoclasts during development. Among other things, resorption and remodeling fail to enlarge the cranial cavity and spinal canal at a rate sufficient to accommodate growth of the brain and spinal cord. Serious damage therefore results to the central nervous system. In hypervitaminosis A, erosion of the cartilage columns accelerates without a compensating increase in the rate of multiplication of cells in the proliferative zone. The epiphyseal plates may therefore be completely obliterated, and growth may cease prematurely.

JOINTS AND SYNOVIAL MEMBRANES

Bones are joined to one another by connective tissue structures that permit varying degrees of movement between the adjoining bones. Such structures are called joints or articulations. These present extreme variations in character, which depend primarily on the type of bones that are joined and the varying degrees of motion permitted by the articulation. Thus, in some cases, as in the skull, the joints are immovable, and the connected bones are separated only by a thin connective tissue layer, the sutural ligament. Other joints are slightly movable, such as the intervertebral articulations. Here the succeeding vertebrae are joined by dense fibrous tissue and cartilage. Still other bones are freely movable upon one another, and here the ends of the bones are completely covered by cartilage, and the articular surfaces are surrounded by fibrous capsules.

Joints in which there is little or no movement are called *synarthroses*. There are three types of these: if the connection between the bones is of bone, it is a *synostosis;* if it consists of cartilage, a *synchondrosis;* and if of connective tissue, a *syndesmosis*. Joints that permit free movement of the bones are called *diarthroses*.

The articular surface of the bones in diarthroses is covered with hyaline cartilage. Although the opposing cartilages are not covered by connective tissue, a small area of perichondrium at their margins is reflected backward into the lining of the joint capsule. At this point, there are many cartilage cells extending into the synovial membrane.

The joint capsules are composed of an external layer consisting of dense fibrous tissue called the *fibrous layer* and an inner *synovial layer,* which is more cellular and is thought to secrete the viscid, colorless liquid of the joint cavity. However, joint membranes exhibit many variations in structure. The synovial layer is sometimes thrown into folds, which may project for surprising distances into the cavity. The larger of these folds frequently contain vessels. In other cases the two layers appear fused, or the synovial layer may rest directly on muscle, fatty tissue, or periosteum. It has been suggested that the synovia be classified according to the tissues on which they lie: that is, loose connective, dense fibrous, or adipose, tissue.

Synovial membranes that rest on loose connective tissue usually cover those parts of the joints not subjected to strain or pressure. As a rule, they have a definite surface layer, separated from the underlying tissue of the joint by loose connective tissue. The surface layer consists of collagenous fibers inter-

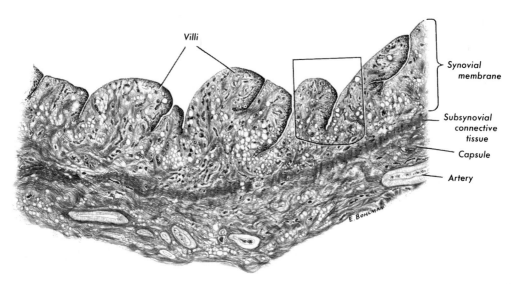

Figure 8–37. Section through capsule of the knee joint of a young man, showing the villi and connective tissue components. The area outlined is shown at higher magnification in Figure 8–38. (From a preparation of H. Hatcher.)

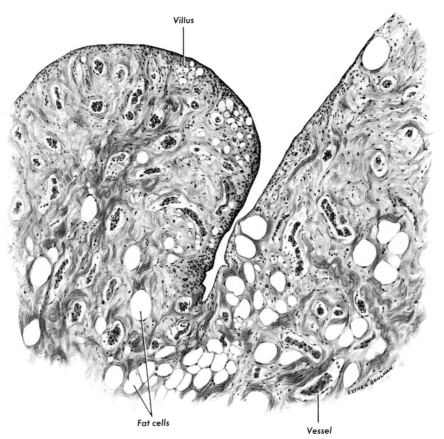

Figure 8–38. Synovial membrane of a young adult. (Higher magnification of the area outlined in Fig. 8–37.) Note the irregularity in concentration of cells toward the free surface of the villus and the irregular distribution of fat cells. (From a preparation of H. Hatcher.)

spersed with fibroblasts. The collagenous fibers either are irregularly arranged or may be oriented along the main lines of stress. In addition to the fibroblasts, there are a few macrophages, leukocytes, and lymphoid wandering cells. In addition to blood vessels, the loose connective tissue contains many lymphatics.

The fibrous type of synovial membrane covers the interarticular ligaments and tendons and lines those parts of the joints that are subject to strain. The adipose type of synovial membrane covers the fat pads that project into some joint cavities. The synovial membrane in this case usually consists of a single layer of cells resting on a thin layer of connective tissue.

Folds of the synovial membrane either may be transient formations, which depend on the position of the joint, or permanent villi, which project into the joint cavity. Some of these villi are short and have a broad base (Fig. 8–37), while others may be thin and long. The larger folds contain blood vessels, lymphatics, and occasionally lobules of adipose tissue (Fig. 8–38). There is an increase in the size and number of the villi with age. New islets of cartilage are formed in them by metaplasia of the synovial fibroblasts.

There are two plexuses of lymphatics, as a rule, within the synovial membranes—a superficial and a deep plexus. The nerves that accompany the blood vessels end beneath the surface in terminal arborizations or end bulbs. Pacinian corpuscles are always present in synovial membranes.

When injured, the synovial membrane reacts, like any other connective tissue, by forming granulation tissue, and after some weeks may be completely regenerated. The synovial fluid is normally small in amount and seems to be a dialysate of blood, to which have been added small amounts of hyaluronic acid and a very few lymphocytes, monocytes, and macrophages.

REFERENCES

Amprino, R., and A. Engstrom: Studies on x-ray absorption and diffraction of bone tissue. Acta Anat. *15*:1, 1952.

Barland, P., A. B. Novikoff, and D. Hamerman: Electron microscopy of the human synovial membrane. J. Cell Biol. *14*:207, 1962.

Barnicot, N. A.: The local action of the parathyroid and other tissues on bone in intracerebral grafts. J. Anat. *82*:233, 1948.

Bélanger, L. F.: Osteocytic osteolysis. Calcif. Tissue Res. *4*:1, 1969.

Bélanger, L. F., J. Robichon, B. B. Migicovsky, D. H. Copp, and J. Vincent: Resorption without osteoclasts (osteolysis.) *In* Sognnaes, R. F., ed.: Mechanisms of Hard Tissue Destruction. Washington, DC, American Association for the Advancement of Science, 1963.

Bernard, G. W., and D. C. Pease: An electron microscopic study of initial intramembranous osteogenesis. Am. J. Anat., *125*:271, 1969.

Bloom, W., M. A. Bloom, and F. C. McLean: Calcification and ossification: medullary bone changes in the reproductive cycle of female pigeons. Anat. Rec. *81*:443, 1941.

Bonucci, E.: The locus of initial calcification in cartilage and bone. Clin. Orthop. *78*:108, 1971.

Cohen, J., and W. H. Harris: The three dimensional anatomy of haversian systems. J. Bone Joint Surg. *40A*:419, 1958.

Cooper, R. R., J. W. Milgram, and R. A. Robinson: Morphology of the osteon. An electron microscopic study. J. Bone Joint Surg. *48A*:1239, 1966.

Fawcett, D. W.: The amedullary bones of the Florida manatee. Am. J. Anat. *71*:271, 1942.

Fishman, D. A., and E. D. Hay: Origin of osteoclasts from mononuclear leucocytes in regenerating new limbs. Anat. Rec. *143*:329, 1962.

Gaillard, P. J.: Parathyroid gland and bone in vitro. VI. Dev. Biol. *1*:152, 1959.

Glimcher, M. J.: Molecular biology of mineralized tissues with particular reference to bone. *In* Oncley, J. L., et al., eds.: Biophysical Science—A Study Program. New York, John Wiley & Sons, 1959.

Glimcher, M. J., A. J. Hodge, and F. O. Schmitt: Macromolecular aggregation states in relation to mineralization: the collagen-hydroxyapatite system as studied in vitro. Proc. Natl. Acad. Sci. USA *43*:860, 1957.

Glimcher, M. J., and S. M. Krane: The organization and structure of bone and the mechanism of calcification. *In* Ramachandran, G. N., and B. S. Gould, eds.: Treatise on Collagen. IIB: Biology of Collagen. London, Academic Press, 1968.

Goldhaber, P.: Oxygen dependent bone resorption in tissue culture. *In* Greep, R. O., and R. V. Talmage, eds.: The Parathyroids. Springfield, IL, Charles C Thomas, 1961.

Hancox, N. M., and B. Boothroyd: The osteoclast in resorption. *In* Sognnaes, R. F., ed.: Mechanisms of Hard Tissue Destruction. Washington, DC, American Association for the Advancement of Science, 1963.

Harris, W. H., and R. P. Heaney: Skeletal renewal and metabolic diseases of bone. N. Engl. J. Med. *28*:253, 1969.

Heinen, J. H., G. H. Dabbs, and H. A. Mason: The experimental production of ectopic cartilage and bone in the muscles of rabbits. J. Bone Joint Surg. *31*:765, 1949.

Heller, M.: Bone. *In* Bloom, W., ed.: Histopathology of Irradiation from External and Internal Sources. National Nuclear Energy Series. New York, McGraw-Hill Book Co., 1948.

Heller, M., F. C. McLean, and W. Bloom: Cellular transformations in mammalian bones induced by parathyroid extract. Am. J. Anat. *87*:315, 1950.

Holtrop, M. E.: The ultrastructure of osteoclasts during stimulation and inhibition of bone resorption. IV

International Congress of Endocrinology, Washington, DC, 1972.

Holtrop. M. E.: The ultrastructure of bone. Am. Clin. Lab. Sci. *5*:264, 1975.

Jackson, S. F.: The fine structure of developing bone in the embryonic fowl. Proc. R. Soc. Lond. *B146*:370, 1957.

Jones, S. J., and A. Boyde: Some morphologic observations on osteoclasts. Cell Tissue Res. *185*:387, 1977.

Jowsey, J.: Studies of the haversian systems in man and some animals. J. Anat. *100*:857, 1966.

Kallio, D. M., P. R. Garant, and C. Minkin: Evidence of coated membranes in the ruffled border of the osteoclast. J. Ultrastruct. Res. *37*:169, 1971.

Lacroix, P.: Bone and cartilage. *In* Brachet, J., and A. E. Mirsky, eds.: The Cell: Biochemistry, Physiology, Morphology. Vol. V. New York, Academic Press, 1961.

Lacroix, P., and A. Budy, eds.: Radioisotopes and bone: a symposium. Oxford, Blackwell Scientific Publications, 1962.

Leblond, C. P., G. W. Wilkinson, L. F. Belanger, and J. Robichon: Radioautographic visualization of bone formation in the rat. Am. J. Anat. *86*:289, 1950.

McLean, F. C., and W. Bloom: Calcification and ossification; calcification in normal growing bone. Anat. Rec. *78*:333, 1940.

McLean, F. C., and A. M. Budy: Radiation, Isotopes, and Bone. New York, Academic Press, 1964.

McLean, F. C., and R. E. Rowland: Internal remodeling of compact bone. *In* Sognnaes, R. F., ed.: Mechanisms of Hard Tissue Destruction. Washington, DC, American Association for the Advancement of Science, 1963.

Maximow. A. A.: Untersuchungen über Blut und Bindegewebe. III. Die embryonale Histogenese des Knochenmarks der Säugetiere. Arch. f. Mikr. Anat. *76*:1, 1910.

Mears, D. C.: Effects of parathyroid hormone and thyrocalcitonin on the membrane potential of osteoclasts. Endocrinology *88*:1021, 1971.

Miller, E. J., and G. R. Martin: The collagen of bone. Clin. Orthop. *59*:195, 1968.

Neuman, W. F., and M. W. Neuman: The Chemical Dynamics of Bone Mineral. Chicago, University of Chicago Press, 1958.

Owen, M.: Histogenesis of bone cells. Calcif. Tissue Res. *25*:205, 1978.

Roberts, E. D., F. K. Ramsey, W. P. Switzer, et al.: Electron microscopy of porcine synovial cell layer. J. Comp. Pathol. *79*:41, 1969.

Robinson, R. A., and D. A. Cameron: Bone. *In* Electron Microscopic Anatomy. New York, Academic Press, 1964.

Schenk, R. K., D. Spiro, and J. Wiener: Cartilage resorption in the tibial epiphyseal plate of growing rats. J. Cell Biol. *34*:275, 1967.

Scott, B. L.: Thymidine-³H electron microscopic radioautography of osteogenic cells in the fetal rat. J. Cell Biol. *35*:115, 1967.

Sledge, C. B.: Some morphologic and experimental aspects of limb development. Clin. Orthop. *44*:241, 1966.

Vaes, G.: On the mechanism of bone resorption: the action of parathyroid hormone on the excretion and synthesis of lysosomal enzymes and on the extracellular release of acid by bone cells. J. Cell Biol. *39*:676, 1968.

Vincent, J.: Microscopic aspects of mineral metabolism in bone tissue with special reference to calcium, lead, and zinc. Clin. Orthop. *26*:161, 1963.

Walker, D. G.: Osteopetrosis cured by temporary parabiosis. Science *180*:875, 1973.

Walker, D. G.: Control of bone resorption by hemopoietic tissue. J. Exp. Med. *142*:651, 1975.

Whitson, S. W.: Tight junction formation in the osteon. Clin. Orthop. *86*:206, 1972.

Young, R. W.: Cell proliferation and specialization during endochondral osteogenesis in young rats. J. Cell Biol. *14*:357, 1962.

Young, R. W.: Specialization of bone cells, *In* Frost, H., ed.: Bone Biodynamics. Boston, Little, Brown, & Co., 1964.

Zichner, D.: The effects of calcitonin on bone cells in young rats: an electron microscope study. Isr. J. Med. Sci. *7*:359, 1971.

9

BONE MARROW AND BLOOD CELL FORMATION

The cells of the blood are short-lived and are continuously replaced from sources outside of the circulation. The process of blood cell formation is called *hemopoiesis* and the sites where it takes place are termed *hemopoietic organs*. The principal hemopoietic organs in adult mammals are the bone marrow, spleen, lymph nodes, and thymus. This chapter is devoted to the bone marrow, which is by far the most important site of hemopoiesis. The role of the spleen, lymph nodes, and thymus in the formation and maturation of blood cells will be discussed in later chapters.

Marrow occupies the cylindrical cavities of the long bones and the interstices of the spongiosa in vertebral bodies, ribs, sternum, and the flat bones of the cranium and pelvis. It accounts for 4 to 6 per cent of body weight and has a total volume nearly equal to that of the liver. It is a soft, highly cellular tissue consisting of precursors of the blood cells, macrophages, adipose cells, reticular cells, and reticular fibers. The relative proportions of these several cell types undergo changes with age, and vary in different regions of the skeleton. At birth, all the bones contain deep red hemopoietically active marrow. The red color is largely attributable to the enormous numbers of developing erythrocytes it contains. At 4 to 5 years of age, the number of blood-forming cells begins to diminish and the number of adipose cells increases. With this shift in relative abundance of hemopoietic and adipose cells, the color of the marrow gradually changes from deep red to yellow. The transformation of hemopoietically active red marrow to relatively inactive yellow marrow occurs earlier and progresses further in the distal portions of the long bones. In adults, red marrow persists only in the proximal ends of the humerus and femur, and in vertebrae, ribs, sternum, and ilia. Fatty transformation of the marrow in the peripheral segments of the appendicular skeleton is believed to be related to the slightly lower temperature of these parts. Yellow marrow can revert to red in response to elevated temperature or unusual demands for blood cells.

PRENATAL HEMOPOIESIS

During prenatal life, there are three successive phases in which the principal site of hemopoiesis shifts from one region of the embryo to another. Formation of blood is first detectable in the mesenchyme of the body stalk and in neighboring areas of the yolk sac in the second week of life when the embryo is only a few millimeters long. Clusters of mesenchymal cells in these areas round up and differentiate into large basophilic cells that assemble in aggregations called *blood islands*. In this *mesoblastic phase of hemopoiesis*, nearly all of the cells formed are erythrocytes. The earliest basophilic cells of the blood islands differentiate into *primitive erythroblasts*. These synthesize hemoglobin and develop into erythrocytes, which differ from those of postnatal life in the nature of their hemoglobin and in the fact that they have a nucleus (Figs. 9–1, 9–2).

After establishment of blood islands in the yolk sac, accumulations of round basophilic cells also appear, at about six weeks of gestation, in the primordium of the liver, initiating the *hepatic phase of hemopoiesis*. These cells resemble the erythroblasts of postnatal hemopoiesis and are called *definitive erythroblasts*. They ultimately give rise to anucleate

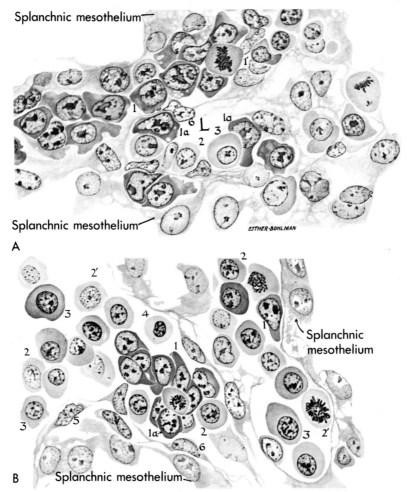

Splanchnic mesothelium

Splanchnic mesothelium

Splanchnic mesothelium

Splanchnic mesothelium

A

B

Figure 9–1. Two sections through folds of the wall of the yolk sac of a 24-day human embryo (H1516 Univ. Chicago Emb. Coll.). *A*, Early stage of hemopoiesis, consisting of proliferating extravascular hemocytoblasts *(1, 1')*; *L*, lumen of a small vessel containing a few primitive polychromatophilic erythroblasts. *B*, Later stage of hemopoiesis showing transformation of hemocytoblasts *(1)* into primitive basophilic erythroblasts *(1a)*, primitive polychromatophilic erythroblasts *(2, 3)*, and primitive erythrocytes *(4)*; *5*, mesenchymal cells; *6*, endothelium. Hematoxylin-eosin-azure II stain. (From Bloom, W., and F. W. Bartelmez. Am. J. Anat. 67:21, 1940.)

erythrocytes unlike those arising from primitive erythroblasts, which retain their nucleus. In the second month, granular leukocytes and megakaryocytes appear in small numbers in the sinusoids of the liver. Somewhat later the spleen, as well as the liver, becomes a site of hemopoiesis.

In the early embryo, the skeleton consists entirely of hyaline cartilage that is subsequently replaced by bone. In the fourth month, blood vessels begin to penetrate into cavities created by programmed degeneration of chondrocytes in the cartilage models of the bones. The blood vessels carry with them mesenchymal cells that differentiate into bone-forming osteoblasts and reticulum cells destined to form the stroma of the bone marrow. Concurrently with establishment of these ossification centers in the cartilaginous skeleton, blood formation begins in the prim-

itive bone marrow, initiating the *myeloid phase of hemopoiesis.* Hemopoiesis in the liver and spleen then declines, and thenceforth the bone marrow is the major blood-forming organ.

In the transition from mesoblastic to hepatic, to myeloid hemopoiesis, it was formerly believed that mesenchymal cells in each of these successive sites gave rise independently to primitive blood-forming cells. It has now been demonstrated that various blood-cell types in the adult, including pluripotential stem cells, can migrate in the bloodstream from organ to organ. Therefore, it is now thought that, in the embryo, successive sites of hemopoiesis are probably seeded by migration of stem cells from the preexisting sites of blood formation.

The liver and spleen in the adult do not normally participate in blood formation, but

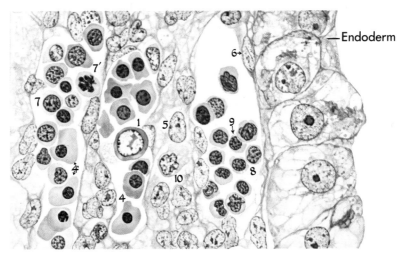

—Endoderm

Figure 9–2. Section through yolk sac of a 20-mm human embryo. In addition to circulating primitive erythrocytes, there are two foci developing polychromatophilic definitive erythroblasts. *1,* Hemocytoblast; *4,* primitive erythrocytes; *5,* mesenchymal cells; *7 and 8,* early and late definitive polychromatophilic erythroblasts with one in mitosis at *7';* *9,* normoblast; *10,* lymphoid wandering cell. Hematoxylin-eosin-azure II stain. (From Bloom, W., and F. W. Bartelmez. Am. J. Anat. *67:*21, 1940.)

in diseases attended by marrow failure, *extra-medullary hemopoiesis* may be resumed in these organs.

STRUCTURAL ORGANIZATION OF BONE MARROW

The bone marrow consists of closely packed hemopoietic cells, reticular cells, and adipose cells occupying all the extravascular spaces around an extensive system of thin-walled venous sinuses. The blood cells develop extravascularly and must pass through the walls of the sinuses to enter the circulation. Some familiarity with the unusual vascular architecture of bones is essential to an understanding of marrow histology.

The arterial blood supply comes from two sources. The cortical osseous tissue is penetrated from outside by branches of a network of small vessels in the surrounding periosteum. Some of the capillaries within the cortex are continuous at the corticomedullary boundary with an elaborate network of anastomosing thin-walled venous sinuses within the marrow. These sinuses, in turn, converge upon wider *collecting sinuses* radially arranged around a large, longitudinally oriented *central sinus.* The major arterial supply to long bones is from a *nutrient artery,* which enters the marrow cavity through the nutrient canal and bifurcates into ascending and descending branches. The great majority of the fine branches resulting from their ramification

within the medullary cavity enter Volkmann's canals and join the vascular network within the cortex. Very few intramedullary branches communicate directly with the sinuses of the marrow. Thus, most of the blood reaching the sinuses has first entered the osseous tissue either from periosteal vessels or from endosteal branches of the nutrient artery, and has secondarily entered the medullary sinuses at the corticomedullary junction. The significance of this indirect transosteal routing of the blood is not known, but it may be necessary in order to maintain the optimal physicochemical environment for hemopoiesis.

The vascular sinuses of the marrow are 50 to 75 μm in diameter with a thin endothelial lining. Histologists had long assumed that the endothelium was discontinuous to allow passage of newly formed blood cells into the circulation. This view was sustained by early electron microscopic studies, which reported sizable openings in the sinus wall. It is now agreed that these were artifacts, for in scanning and transmission electron microscopic studies in which care has been taken to preserve the marrow *in situ* and avoid mechanical damage, the sinuses have been shown to have no permanent apertures that would permit passage of blood cells. The endothelium is composed of flattened cells joined together by junctional complexes as in other epithelia. In the extremely attenuated peripheral portions of the cells, clusters of endothelial pores may be found. A typical basal lamina is absent but there may be scattered extravascular deposits of flocculent material of similar nature.

Reticular cells are deployed in a discontinuous adventitial layer over the abluminal surface of the sinuses with their long branching processes extending into the surrounding myeloid tissue in intimate association with the differentiating blood cells. They are strategically situated to participate in inductive or regulatory interactions with the hemopoietic stem cells, but if they have such a function it has yet to be convincingly demonstrated. Their principal function seems to be mechanically supportive. They synthesize and maintain the delicate framework of reticular fibers that form the sparse stroma of the marrow.

The adventitial reticular cells in normal marrow are estimated to cover 40 to 60 per cent of the abluminal surface of the sinuses, leaving the remainder accessible to mature blood cells for transmural migration into the bloodstream. In response to circulating toxins and possibly to hemopoietic hormones, the reticular cells may change their shape, exposing more endothelial surface for egress of cells. In experimentally induced active transmural cell transport, the adventitial cover may be reduced to less than 20 per cent of the sinus surface.

The passage of mature blood cells into the circulation does not take place by separating endothelial cells at their junctions, but is transcellular. The migrating cell presses the abluminal membrane of the endothelial cell into contact with the adluminal membrane, and the two fuse to form a transient *migration pore* (Fig. 9–3). This opening may be somewhat enlarged by the cell in transit but does not exceed 4 μm in diameter, and continuity of the endothelium is rapidly restored after the blood cell has become free in the lumen of the sinus. The endothelium is the major barrier in the path of the exiting mature blood cells. It appears to be actively involved in the process and there is suggestive evidence that it may exercise some selectivity in control of the transcellular traffic.

The organization of the extravascular hemopoietic compartment of the marrow is difficult to study with the light microscope owing to the crowding and superimposition of cells in histological sections, and the difficulty of obtaining adequately fixed preparations

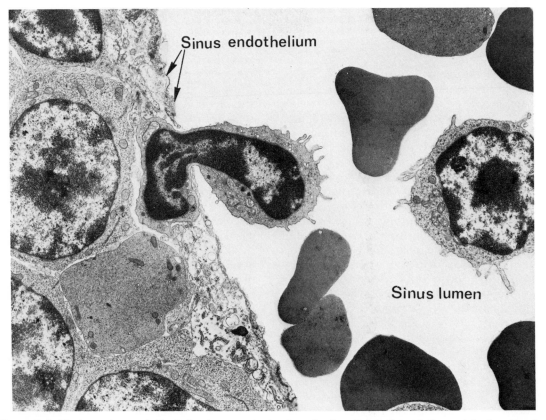

Figure 9–3. Electron micrograph illustrating transmural migration of a lymphocyte through the endothelium into the sinus lumen.

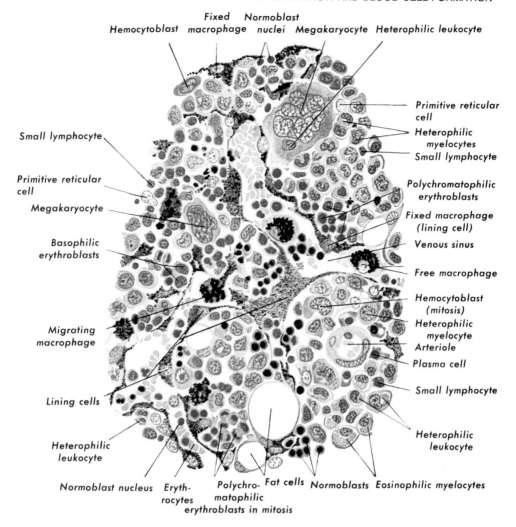

Fixed — Normoblast
Hemocytoblast — macrophage — nuclei — Megakaryocyte — Heterophilic leukocyte

Primitive reticular
cell

Heterophilic
myelocytes

Small lymphocyte

Small lymphocyte

Polychromatophilic
erythroblasts

Primitive reticular
cell

Fixed macrophage
(lining cell)

Megakaryocyte

Venous sinus

Basophilic
erythroblasts

Free macrophage

Hemocytoblast
(mitosis)

Heterophilic
myelocyte

Migrating
macrophage

Arteriole

Plasma cell

Lining cells

Small lymphocyte

Heterophilic
leukocyte

Heterophilic
leukocyte

Normoblast nucleus — Eryth-rocytes — Polychro-matophilic erythroblasts in mitosis — Fat cells — Normoblasts — Eosinophilic myelocytes

Figure 9–4. Section of bone marrow of rabbit that had injections of lithium carmine and India ink. Hematoxylin-eosin-azure II stain. (After A. A. Maximow.)

without mechanical damage (Fig. 9–4). However, some patterns of cell association have emerged. Erythropoiesis tends to occur in clusters near the sinuses, while granulocytes develop near the center of the hemopoietic spaces. Megakaryocytes are typically situated adjacent to the sinus wall with processes projecting through apertures into the lumen. Macrophages and lymphocytes are scattered throughout the marrow. Adipose cells arise by accumulation of lipid in adventitial reticular cells and hence are usually in close proximity to sinuses. The spatial and functional relationships of cell types are considered further below.

HEMOPOIETIC STEM CELLS

In the bone marrow, as in other organs where the cell population is continually re-newed, a small number of cells have the capacity for both self-duplication and differentiation. Such cells are called *stem cells*. If their progeny are able to differentiate into several different types of mature blood cells, they are described as *pluripotential hemopoietic stem cells* (PHSC). The differentiation of such a cell involves first, a loss in the ability to develop along multiple alternative paths and later, gradual acquisition of distinctive new morphological features and functional properties typical of more mature blood cells. The immediate progeny of a pluripotential stem cell that retain the capacity for self-renewal, but are able to differentiate only into a single end-cell type, are termed *unipotential stem cells* or *committed stem cells*.

Recognition of hemopoietic stem cells poses an insuperable problem for the microscopist. For visual identification of different cell types, he is obliged to rely on size, shape, staining properties, nuclear configu-

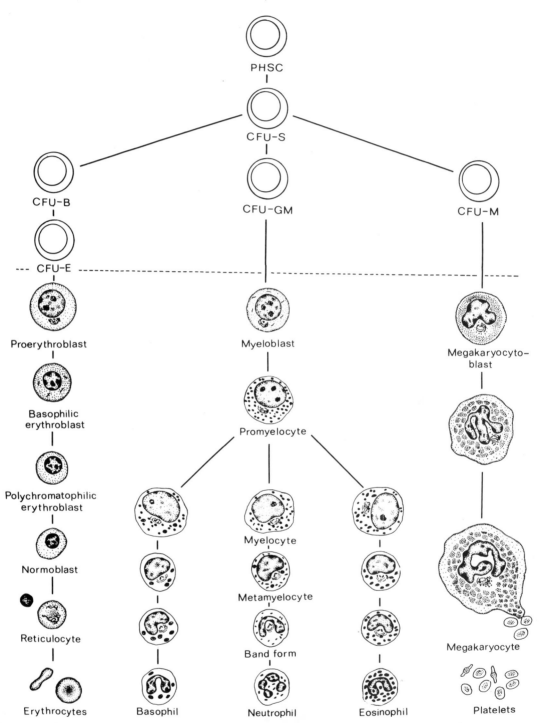

Figure 9–5. Diagram of the principal myelopoietic cell lineages. Above the dotted line are the stem cells, which are not microscopically distinguishable but are identified by spleen assay—pluripotential hemopoietic stem cell (PHSC); colony-forming unit–spleen (CFU-S); colony-forming unit–burst (CFU-B); colony-forming unit–erythrocyte (CFU-E); colony-forming unit–granulomonocyte (CFU-GM); and colony-forming unit–megakaryocyte (CFU-M). Below the dotted line are the morphologically recognizable cell lines that differentiate from these stem cells.

ration or chromatin pattern, and presence or absence of specific granules. The distinctive features required for identification are acquired late in the course of differentiation and are largely lacking in the early stages of the several blood-forming cell lines. Thus, although histologists and hematologists can agree upon a functional definition of a stem cell, they cannot identify it with any degree of confidence at the light or electron microscope level. It is safe to assume that it is a small spherical cell with a rim of basophilic cytoplasm around a nucleus relatively poor in condensed chromatin. Thus, it cannot be dependably distinguished from one of the several kinds of lymphocytes. Therefore, stem cells are commonly dealt with as hypothetical or statistical entities rather than recognized cell types.

Stem cells are detected and their several categories are distinguished by testing their developmental potential in an in vivo or in vitro assay system. The most widely used experimental procedure consists of injecting suspensions of hemopoietic cells into the bloodstream of mice that have been X-irradiated with a dosage sufficient to destroy the proliferative capacity of their own cells. The injected cells "home" into the spleen and marrow of the recipient mouse. After several days, the spleen contains grossly visible small colonies, each having developed by proliferation of a single stem cell and differentiation of its progeny. This assay detects a broad class of stem cells designated *colony-forming units–spleen* (CFU-S). The stem cells giving rise to the individual colonies can be more narrowly defined by examining the nature of their differentiated progeny. If these include two or more blood cell types, the cell of origin was a *pluripotential* stem cell (PHSC). If the progeny are all of the erythrocyte lineage, they arose from a *unipotential* stem cell, designated a *colony-forming unit–erythroid* (CFU-E). Similarly, if they all belong to the megakaryocyte line, they arose from a *colony-forming unit—megakaryocyte* (CFU-M). Other colonies contain both granulocytes and monocytes and arise from a bipotential stem cell referred to as a *colony-forming unit–granulo-monocyte* (CFU-GM).

Kinetic studies indicate that there are in the mouse as few as one pluripotential stem cell per 10,000 nucleated marrow cells—a total of about 40,000. The spleen contains about one twentieth this number. They have also been detected in small numbers in peripheral blood and are therefore capable of being transported from the marrow to other sites. This may account for the occurrence of extramedullary hemopoiesis in certain diseases. The pluripotential stem cells are *slowly* proliferating but give rise to more *rapidly* proliferating unipotential stem cells (CFU-E or CFU-M), limited to production of granulocytes and/or cells of the monocyte-macrophage lineage.

Much of our understanding of the kinetics and cell lineages in the early stages of hemopoiesis has been based on spleen colony assays in irradiated mice, but there is every reason to believe that the same principles apply to the human. Culture systems have now been developed in which progenitor cells from human marrow are stimulated with hemopoietic growth factors and give rise to clonal colonies in a semisolid matrix of agar, fibrin, or methyl cellulose. These in vitro systems promise to permit studies of kinetics and control mechanisms of human hemopoiesis comparable with those carried out in the mouse.

ERYTHROPOIESIS

The erythrocytes have a life span of about 120 days and are then removed from the blood and destroyed in the spleen. The maintenance of normal numbers in the circulation requires their continuous formation in the bone marrow. Each day some 2×10^{10} new erythrocytes enter the circulation.

Although blood cell development is a continuous process, it is customary to consider it as occurring in three phases: hemopoietic *stem cells*, committed *progenitor cells*, and morphologically recognizable *maturation stages*. Through lack of criteria for its visual identification, the pluripotential stem cell giving rise to all blood cells is designated the colony-forming unit (CFU). Some of the progeny of this slowly replicating cell lose their pluripotentiality and become irreversibly committed to production of erythrocytes. Hematologists studying the characteristics of these unipotential progenitor cells in cultures have distinguished two successive stages: *erythroid burst-forming units* (E-BFU or CFU-B) and *erythroid colony-forming units* (E-CFU or CFU-E). The former have a higher proliferation rate and require a relatively high concentration of the stimulating factor *erythropoietin*. The latter proliferate more slowly and are responsive to erythropoietin in low concentration. With further differentiation, the erythroid progenitor cells (E-CFU or

CFU-E) become morphologically identifiable as *proerythroblasts*. These are round cells 14 to 19 μm in diameter, with a thin rim of basophilic cytoplasm and a large nucleus, which has a rather uniformly dispersed chromatin pattern and two or more nucleoli.

Each proerythroblast undergoes a series of divisions to produce several smaller *basophilic erythroblasts*. These have a deeply basophilic cytoplasm, a more coarsely clumped chromatin pattern, and no visible nucleoli (Fig. 9–6). The disappearance of nucleoli is asso-

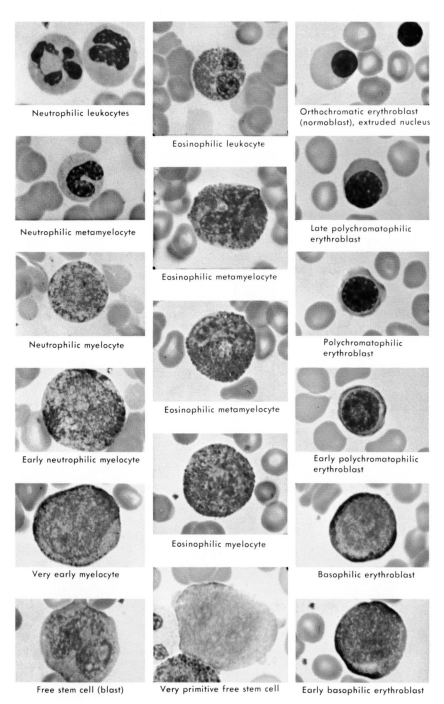

Neutrophilic leukocytes	Eosinophilic leukocyte	Orthochromatic erythroblast (normoblast), extruded nucleus
Neutrophilic metamyelocyte		Late polychromatophilic erythroblast
Neutrophilic myelocyte	Eosinophilic metamyelocyte	Polychromatophilic erythroblast
Early neutrophilic myelocyte	Eosinophilic metamyelocyte	Early polychromatophilic erythroblast
Very early myelocyte	Eosinophilic myelocyte	Basophilic erythroblast
Free stem cell (blast)	Very primitive free stem cell	Early basophilic erythroblast

Figure 9–6. Photomicrographs of developing blood cells in human bone marrow, showing steps in the transformation of stem cells into neutrophilic and eosinophilic leukocytes and into erythrocytes, as seen in dry smears stained with Wright's blood stain.

ciated with cessation of nuclear synthesis of new ribosomal protein. In electron micrographs, the cytoplasm contains a profusion of free polyribosomes but few or no profiles of endoplasmic reticulum. Synthesis of hemoglobin is already in progress at this stage. It is recognizable in electron micrographs as fine cytoplasmic particles of relatively low density. In stained marrow smears observed with the light microscope, its presence is obscured by the intense blue staining of the ribonucleoprotein of the cytoplasm.

The progeny of the division of basophilic erythroblasts are *polychromatophilic erythroblasts*, recognizable by their smaller overall size, their smaller nucleus with more condensed chromatin, and the characteristic staining reaction of their cytoplasm, which ranges from bluish-gray through gray-greens of diminishing intensity (Fig. 9–6). Since no new ribosomes are formed after disappearance of the nucleoli, there is a progressive decrease in their concentration as a consequence of the succeeding divisions. At the same time, the hemoglobin synthesized on the polyribosomes steadily accumulates (Fig. 9–7). The range of tinctorial affinities exhibited by the polychromatophilic erythroblasts reflects the progressively changing proportions of ribosomes (which bind the blue components of the dye mixture) and of hemoglobin (which has an affinity for the eosin).

When the cells have acquired nearly their full complement of hemoglobin, their cytoplasm is distinctly eosinophilic with only a slight tinge of residual blue. The nucleus is now small, eccentric, and deeply stained. Such cells (7 to 14 µm) are called *orthochromatic erythroblasts* (also called *normoblasts*). In electron micrographs, their heterochromatin is in coarse blocks with little intervening nucleoplasm. The cytoplasm is devoid of organelles except for an occasional mitochondrion (Figs. 9–8, 9–9C). The cytoplasmic matrix presents a rather uniform fine gray granularity, owing to the high concentration of hemoglobin. Widely scattered clusters of ribosomes are still present (Fig. 9–9C).

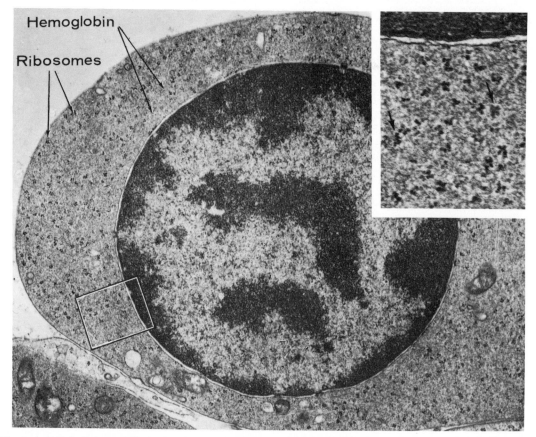

Hemoglobin

Ribosomes

Figure 9–7. Polychromatophilic erythroblasts from guinea pig marrow showing coarse blocks of heterochromatin in the nucleus, and cytoplasm consisting mainly of hemoglobin and polyribosomes. In inset, polyribosomes *(at arrows)* can be distinguished from the smaller, less dense granular background of hemoglobin.

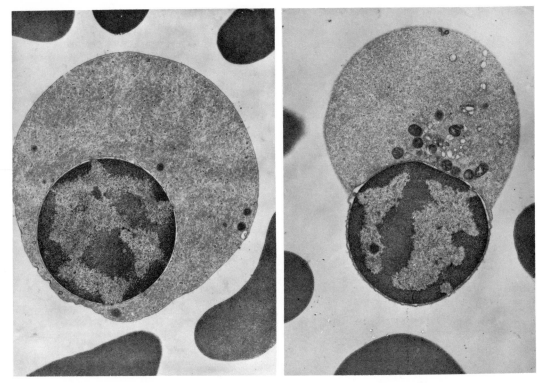

Figure 9–8. Electron micrographs of human orthochromatic erythroblasts (normoblasts). The cell at right is extruding its nucleus. Notice that the nucleus is pinched off, enclosed in a portion of the cell membrane and a thin layer of cytoplasm, and does not pass through a break in the membrane as was previously believed.

The eccentric nucleus is then extruded and pinched off, with a very thin film of cytoplasm enclosed by a portion of the plasma membrane (Fig. 9–8). The extruded nuclei are ingested and destroyed by macrophages. The anucleate portion, an erythrocyte, is ultimately released into the bloodstream. Newly formed erythrocytes contain small amounts of basophilic material dispersed in the hemoglobin, and consequently have a slightly greenish tint instead of the clear salmon pink of more mature forms. These are described as *polychromatophilic erythrocytes*. However, if fresh blood smears are stained with cresyl blue, the residual ribosomes are clumped and the aggregates formed appear as a bluish skein or network in the otherwise pink cytoplasm. Under these conditions of staining, the recently formed erythrocytes are called *reticulocytes*.

The percentage of reticulocytes in a blood smear is a dependable index of the rate of formation of new red blood cells and is widely used in following the recovery of patients from blood loss or their response to treatment for anemia. In man, the erythrocyte generation time from stem cell to circulating blood cell is about a week.

There is a reserve of reticulocytes in the marrow somewhat greater than the number in the circulation. In the continual turnover of erythrocytes, about 1.9×10^{10} erythrocytes are destroyed each day and the same number of new ones are produced in the marrow. Old or damaged erythrocytes undergo changes in their surface membrane, notably a loss of sialic acid residues, and are selectively removed from the circulation in the spleen and phagocytized by macrophages. Iron released in the degradation of their hemoglobin is transported by plasma transferrin back to the marrow for reutilization in hemoglobin synthesis. The remainder of the degraded hemoglobin is transformed into the bile pigment *bilirubin* and excreted.

GRANULOPOIESIS

In common with all other blood cells, the granulocytes originate from the morphologically undefined pluripotential stem cell now referred to as the colony-forming unit (CFU-S). These cells having a high capacity for self-renewal give rise to several types of progenitor stem cells including one committed to

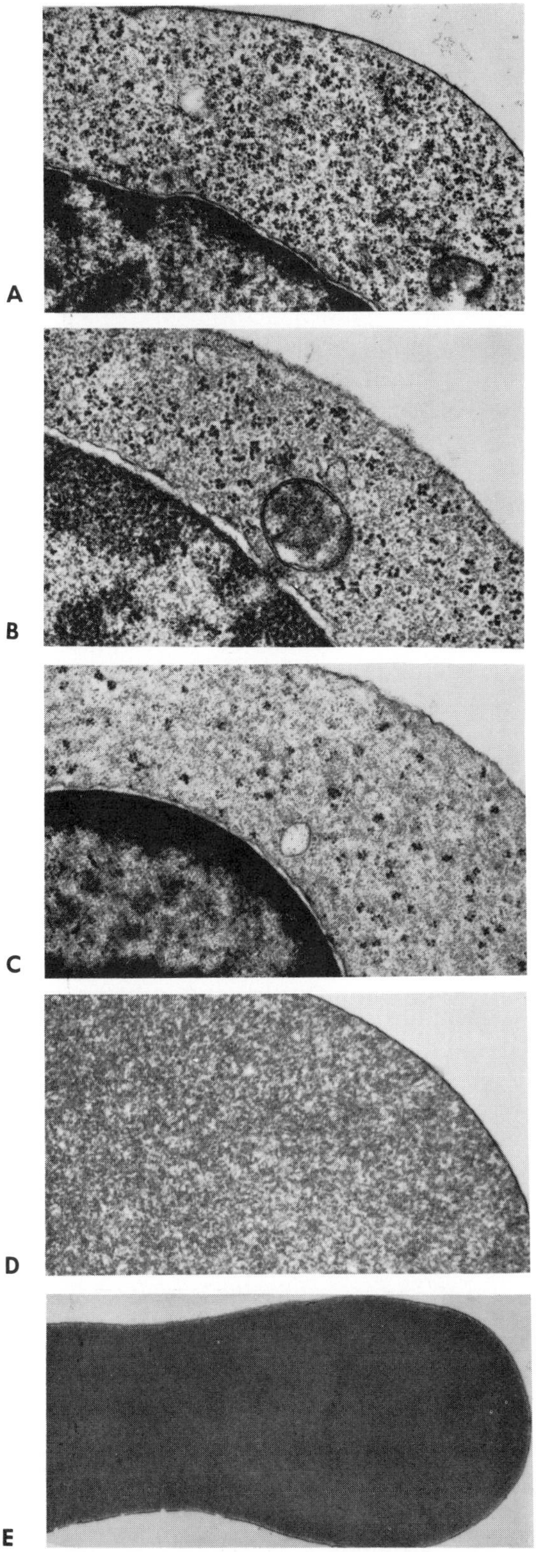

Figure 9–9. A series of electron micrographs illustrating the decline in number of ribosomes and progressive increase in hemoglobin in the cytoplasm during the differentiation of the guinea pig erythrocyte. *A,* Basophilic erythroblast; *B,* polychromatophilic erythroblasts; *C,* orthochromatic erythroblast (normoblast); *D,* reticulocyte; *E,* erythrocyte.

formation of granulocytes and monocytes (GM-CFU). These differentiate into *myeloblasts,* the earliest morphologically recognizable cell of the granulocyte series.

The myeloblast is a relatively small cell with a large nucleus containing three or more nucleoli. The cytoplasm is basophilic and devoid of granules. In its further development, the cell enlarges and acquires small, metachromatic *azurophil granules.* It is then called a *promyelocyte.*

The promyelocyte has a reniform nucleus, multiple nucleoli, and a dispersed chromatin pattern. Early in its development, a small number of azurophil granules are clustered near the cell center (Fig. 9–6). In electron micrographs, these are dense, somewhat irregular in outline, 0.1 to 0.25 μm in diameter, and membrane bounded. A few cisternal profiles of rough endoplasmic reticulum are present, and abundant free ribosomes. The Golgi complex is situated in an indentation of the nucleus, and numerous transitional vesicles are observed between the cisternae of the reticulum and the convex outer face of the Golgi. Condensing vacuoles containing dense cores arise at the inner concave face of the Golgi. These dense-cored vacuoles fuse, forming larger ones containing multiple dense bodies that coalesce to form azurophil granules. In the human, the content of the condensing vacuoles is a flocculent precipitate instead of dense cores and morula forms characteristic of these cells in the rabbit. Otherwise, the mechanism of azurophil granule formation is not significantly different.

More advanced promyelocytes exhibit a striking increase in size from about 16 to about 24 μm in diameter (Figs. 9–10, 9–11, 9–12). There is a concomitant increase in number of azurophil granules, which are now dispersed throughout the cytoplasm. The chromatin is more condensed and clumped along the nuclear envelope and around the nucleoli. The endoplasmic reticulum is more extensive and is often somewhat distended during this phase of rapid synthesis of granule protein.

After one or more mitotic divisions, the resulting late promyelocytes are considerably smaller, the chromatin is more condensed, and nucleoli are inconspicuous. Although azurophil granules still occupy much of the cytoplasm, the peak period of their formation has passed and there is a notable decrease in the size of the Golgi and the extent of the reticulum.

From stem cell through the late promyelocyte stage, the development of all types of

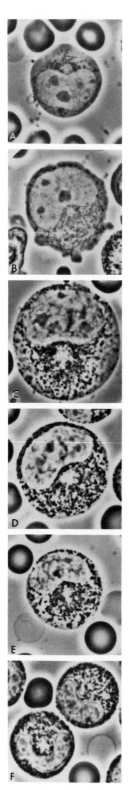

Figure 9-10. Phase-contrast photomicrographs of pro-myelocytes *(A, B)*, neutrophilic myelocytes *(C, D, E)*, and metamyelocytes *(F)* from human bone marrow. (Photographs from Ackerman, A. Zeitschr. f. Zellforsch. *121*:153, 1972.)

granulocytes is essentially the same. The granulocyte lineage then diverges along three separate paths of differentiation with the appearance in the *myelocytes* of *specific granules* with differing tinctorial properties and distinctive ultrastructure.

Neutrophilic Myelocytes

The *neutrophilic myelocyte* is distinguished from the promyelocyte by its smaller size; by the more variable shape of the nucleus and greater condensation of its chromatin; by the smaller size of its Golgi complex; and especially by the presence in its cytoplasm of a second type of granule that has little affinity for stains in routine marrow smears. In electron micrographs these are less dense than azurophil granules and often elongated, resembling rice grains. The formative stages of the specific granules are said to be associated with the convex surface of the Golgi complex. Thus, in the development of neutrophils, two populations of granules are formed at different times. The azurophil granules arise in the promyelocyte stage at the concave face of the Golgi apparatus, and the specific granules are formed in the myelocyte stage at its convex face. The azurophil granules contain histochemically demonstrable peroxidase, acid phosphatase, arylsulfatase, β-galactosidase, β-glucuronidase, esterase, and 5′-nucleotidase and therefore are considered to be primary lysosomes (Fig. 9–13). The specific granules contain alkaline phosphatase and poorly characterized bacteriostatic proteins.

From the progenitor cell through the myelocyte stage, four to seven divisions occur. Mitotic divisions then cease and subsequent differentiation involves changes in nuclear form, diminution in number of mitochondria and other organelles, slight condensation of the cytoplasm, and the appearance in it of small amounts of glycogen.

The next stage, the *metamyelocyte*, is distinguishable from the myelocyte mainly by the shape of its nucleus, which is deeply indented (Fig. 9–14). Two granule types are still present, but specific granules now make up over 80 per cent of the granule population. Nuclear modeling continues, resulting in a cell with a slender, straight, or curved nucleus, referred to as a *band-form*. During final maturation of the neutrophil, the nucleus becomes constricted into multiple small lobules connected by extremely thin regions.

The entire transit time from stem cell to mature granulocyte is about ten days. The

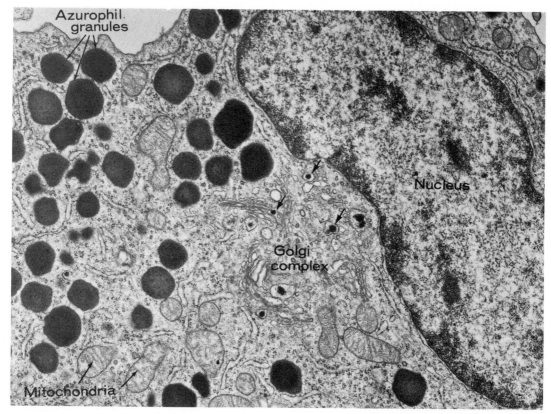

Figure 9–11. Electron micrograph of promyelocyte from rabbit marrow. Dense-cored vacuoles associated with the Golgi complex represent formative stages of azurophil granules. Enlargement and coalescence of these gives rise to the large dense mature granules seen elsewhere in the cytoplasm. (Electron micrograph from Bainton, D., and M. Farquhar. J. Cell Biol. *28*:277, 1966.)

production rate in the human is estimated to be about 1.6×10^4/kg/day, of which the great majority are neutrophils. A large reserve of metamyelocytes, band-forms, and mature neutrophils is maintained in the marrow, perhaps as great as ten times the daily production. These can be mobilized to meet unusual demands. Mature neutrophils are preferentially released, but in infections many band-forms and even metamyelocytes enter the circulation.

Eosinophilic Myelocytes

These are less numerous than neutrophilic myelocytes. The nucleus has a rather coarse pattern of peripheral clumps of chromatin. The cytoplasm is slightly basophilic and the specific granules are distinctly larger and eosinophilic. In electron micrographs there are many cisternal profiles of endoplasmic reticulum and abundant free ribosomes. Two populations of granules are discernible— dense azurophil granules and somewhat less dense specific granules. The eosinophil granules are rich in peroxidase, and cytochemical staining for this enzyme is useful in revealing the intracellular pathway for synthesis, segregation, and packaging of the enzyme into specific granules. In eosinophilic myelocytes, peroxidase reaction product can be demonstrated in the perinuclear cistern, throughout the endoplasmic reticulum, and in the Golgi saccules and forming granules (Fig. 9–16). In later stages after granule formation has ceased, the enzyme is found only in the specific granules. A similar distribution is reported for acid phosphatase and arylsulfatase. Thus, the myelocytes appear to be capable of synthesizing and concentrating several proteins simultaneously.

The nucleus of eosinophil metamyelocytes is indented, and in mature eosinophils it is usually bilobed. No band-form occurs and the nucleus never acquires the degree of lobulation seen in neutrophils. In late myelocytes and metamyelocytes, the contents of the specific granules begin to crystallize, and one finds in micrographs a heterogeneous population of granules, some remaining

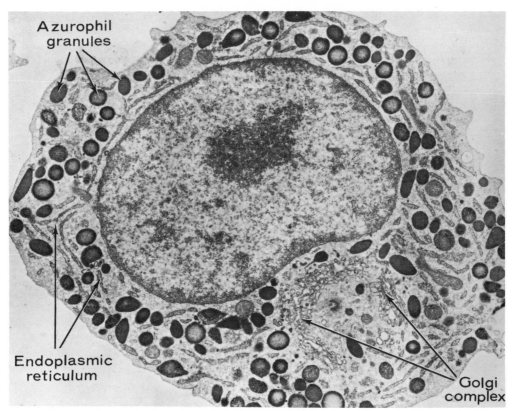

Figure 9–12. Electron micrograph of a polymorphonuclear promyelocyte, the largest cell of the neutrophilic series, treated for peroxidase. The cytoplasm is packed with peroxidase-positive azurophil granules, and a positive reaction is seen throughout the reticulum. Specific granules are not yet present. (From Bainton, D., J. Ullyot, and M. Farquhar. J. Exp. Med. *134*:907, 1971.)

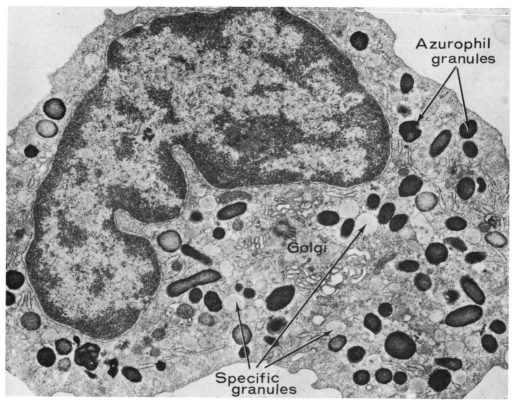

Figure 9–13. Electron micrograph of polymorphonuclear neutrophilic myelocyte stained with the peroxidase reaction. The azurophil granules are strongly reactive but the specific granules are unstained. (From Bainton, D., J. Ullyot, and M. Farquhar. J. Exp. Med. *134*:907, 1971.)

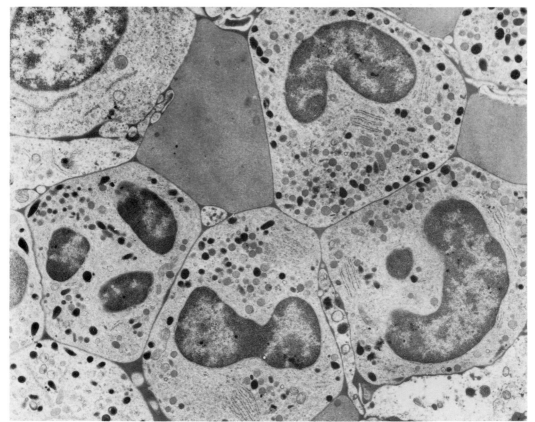

Figure 9–14. Micrograph of a group of neutrophilic metamyelocytes and band forms from baboon bone marrow. The dense azurophil granules are few relative to the specific granules.

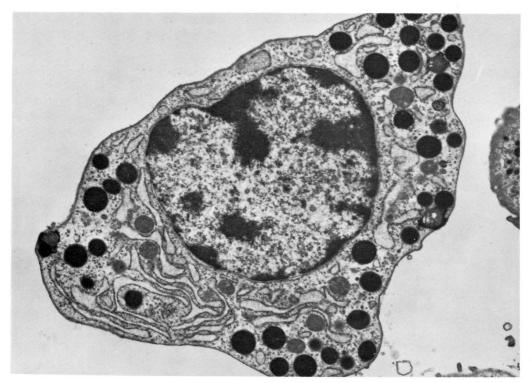

Figure 9–15. Eosinophilic myelocyte from guinea pig bone marrow. There is a well-developed endoplasmic reticulum and the specific granules are distinctly larger than those of neutrophilic myelocytes. The crystals in the granules have not yet developed.

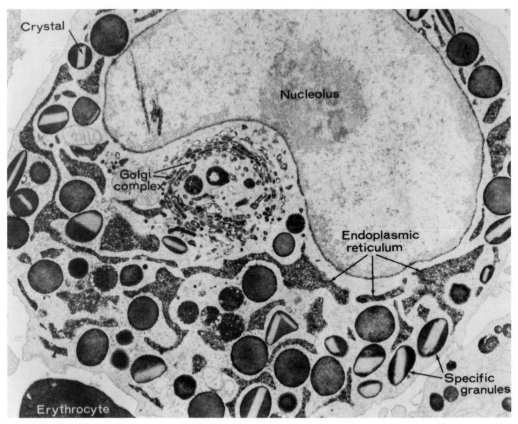

Figure 9–16. Eosinophilic myelocyte of rat, stained by the cytochemical reaction for peroxidase. Formation of specific granules is continuing and reaction product is found in the perinuclear cisterna and throughout the endoplasmic reticulum–also in the Golgi complex and specific granules. (Micrograph from Bainton, D., and M. Farquhar. J. Cell Biol. 45:54, 1970.)

dense and homogeneous, others having crystals of varying form surrounded by a matrix of low density (Fig. 9–17).

Basophilic Myelocytes

These are rarely observed in preparations of human marrow owing to their small numbers and the difficulty of preserving their granules, which are soluble in aqueous media and are partially or completely extracted during fixation and staining. They have a paler-staining nucleus than other myelocytes. The cytoplasm contains relatively few specific granules, which are metachromatic and vary considerably in size. The nucleus of meta-myelocytes is deeply indented, and that of mature basophils is constricted into two and occasionally three lobes.

MONOPOIESIS

Experimental studies of spleen colonies has revealed that the monocyte-macrophage cell line shares with the granulocytes a common committed stem cell, the colony-forming unit–granulocyte/macrophage (CFU-GM). A *monoblast* is described from colonies in cell culture but is identified with difficulty in the marrow. Its division gives rise to *promonocytes*. About half of the promonocytes of the marrow are rapidly proliferating to generate nonproliferating *monocytes*. The remainder constitute a reserve of very slowly renewing progenitor cells that can be activated to meet unusual demands for tissue macrophages.

The pool of promonocytes in human marrow is estimated to be about 6×10^8/kg body weight and the monocyte production rate about 7×10^6/kg body weight per hour. The stem cell to monocyte transit time is about 55 hours and they probably remain in the circulation no more than 16 hours before emigrating to the tissues, where they differentiate into macrophages—the functional phase of this cell line. Maintenance of the macrophage population in the tissues depends mainly on the continuous influx of monocytes from the blood. Macrophages are capable of cell division, but under normal conditions

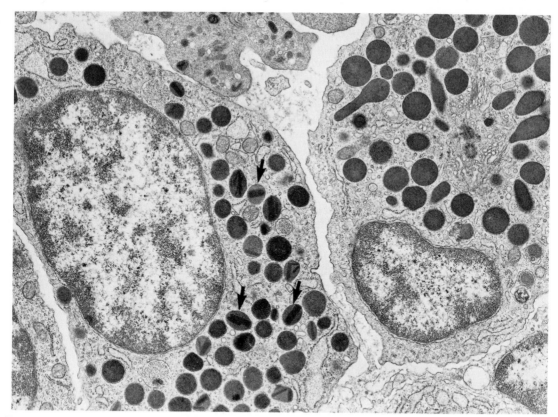

Figure 9–17. Micrograph of a pair of late eosinophilic myelocytes from rat bone marrow. Endoplasmic reticulum is less extensive and crystals are forming in the specific granules *(at arrows).*

their proliferation does not contribute substantially to renewal of the population in the tissues.

THROMBOPOIESIS

Thrombocytes and platelets are cellular elements in the blood of vertebrates concerned with protection against blood loss by promoting clotting at sites of tissue injury.

The term *thrombopoiesis* refers to the developmental events in hemopoietic organs leading to formation of thrombocytes and platelets. The thrombocytes in lower vertebrates are nucleated cells that develop by successive division and differentiation of precursor cells called thromboblasts in a manner similar to the derivation of erythrocytes from erythroblasts. The anucleate platelets of mammals, which are the functional equivalent of the thrombocytes of amphibia, reptiles, and birds, are formed by fragmentation of the

Figure 9–18. Summary diagram of the timing of events in differentiation of polymorphonuclear neutrophils. (From Boggs, D., and M. Chernack. J. Reprod. Fertil., Suppl. *10*:32, 1970.)

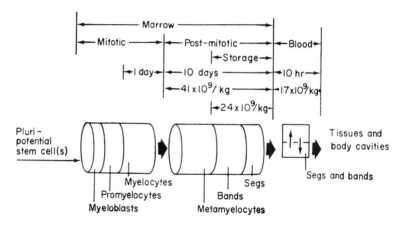

cytoplasm of huge polymorphonuclear cells called *megakaryocytes,* found among the other hemopoietic cells in the bone marrow. The nucleus of these giant polyploid cells contains from eight to 16 sets of chromosomes and occasionally as many as 64. Thus, if platelets arose by nuclear and cytoplasmic division as do thrombocytes in lower vertebrates, 64 cells at most would result. But megakaryocytes will produce 4000 to 8000 platelets. Therefore, in mammals a significant increase in productive capacity has been gained by the unique device of cytoplasmic fragmentation.

The very large size of the megakaryocytes, 50 to 70 μm, makes them the most conspicuous blood-forming cell in the marrow. The cell body is roughly spherical but may have blunt cytoplasmic processes projecting from its surface (Fig. 9–19). The nucleus is remarkably elaborate, with multiple lobes of varying size interconnected by constricted regions. The nucleoplasm has a moderately coarse chromatin pattern and contains numerous indistinct nucleoli. The cytoplasm appears rather homogeneous in routine marrow smears, but after appropriate fixation and special staining a concentric zonation is apparent. A narrow perinuclear zone is surrounded by a broad region stippled with numerous fine azurophil granules, which may be either uniformly distributed or gathered in small clusters, depending on the stage of development of the megakaryocyte. Groups of centrioles are found in bays among the lobules of the complex nucleus. Mitochondria are numerous and quite small. A single compact Golgi apparatus is demonstrable in a juxtanuclear location in young megakaryocytes, but in mature forms multiple small Golgi bodies are widely dispersed in the cytoplasm. At the periphery is a rim of clear cytoplasm of irregular outline and varying thickness, which is devoid of granules.

Megakaryocyte Development

The committed stem cell of mammalian thrombopoiesis, designated *colony-forming unit–megakaryocyte* (CFU-M), gives rise to the earliest morphologically identifiable cell of this lineage, the *megakaryoblast.* This is a large cell with round or indented nucleus, loose chromatin pattern, and inconspicuous nucleoli. The cytoplasm is basophilic and largely free of specific granules. In electron micrographs, it contains moderate numbers of polysomes, a few cisternae of endoplasmic reticulum, a juxtanuclear Golgi complex, and large mitochondria. If two nuclei are present, these fuse at the next nuclear division and the cell (2n) subsequently increases rapidly in size while undergoing a series of atypical nuclear divisions that are not accompanied by division of the cytoplasm. In each of these divisions, the centrioles replicate and a complex multipolar spindle is formed. At metaphase, the chromosomes become arranged in several equatorial planes and give rise at anaphase to several chromosome groups that then reconstitute a single lobulated nucleus of larger size. After a short interval, another similar episode of division occurs with daughter groups of chromosomes again reconstituting a single large nucleus at telophase. Thus, cells with 4n, 8n, 16n, and higher orders of polyploidy are formed without division of the cytoplasm. The successive doubling of DNA content in cells of this series has been verified by microspectrophotometry. Frequencies of 4n, 8n, 16n, 32n, and 64n are respectively 1.6, 10, 71.2, 17.1, and 0.1 per cent.

Although there is a concurrent increase in volume of the megakaryocyte, there is little differentiation of its cytoplasm until it has synthesized all of the DNA it will ultimately possess. Since the volume attained by a cell is a function of its ploidy, and not all progress to the same degree of polyploidy, megakaryocytes vary considerably in size and in the number of platelets they can form.

In the *promegakaryocyte* stage (30–45 μm in diameter), a prominent cell center develops containing a number of centriole pairs corresponding to the degree of polyploidy. In the subsequent increase in cytoplasmic volume, its basophilia diminishes and newly formed azurophilic granules become dispersed throughout.

The fully formed reserve *megakaryocyte,* not yet active in platelet formation, is 50 to 70 μm in diameter and possesses a very large, highly lobulated nucleus. Fine azurophil granules are widely disseminated in the central region of the cytoplasm, but generally absent from a narrow peripheral zone of pale blue ectoplasm. This rim of clear ectoplasm becomes less conspicuous in mature *platelet-forming megakaryocytes,* and the azurophil granules become clustered in small groups separated by narrow aisles of agranular cytoplasm.

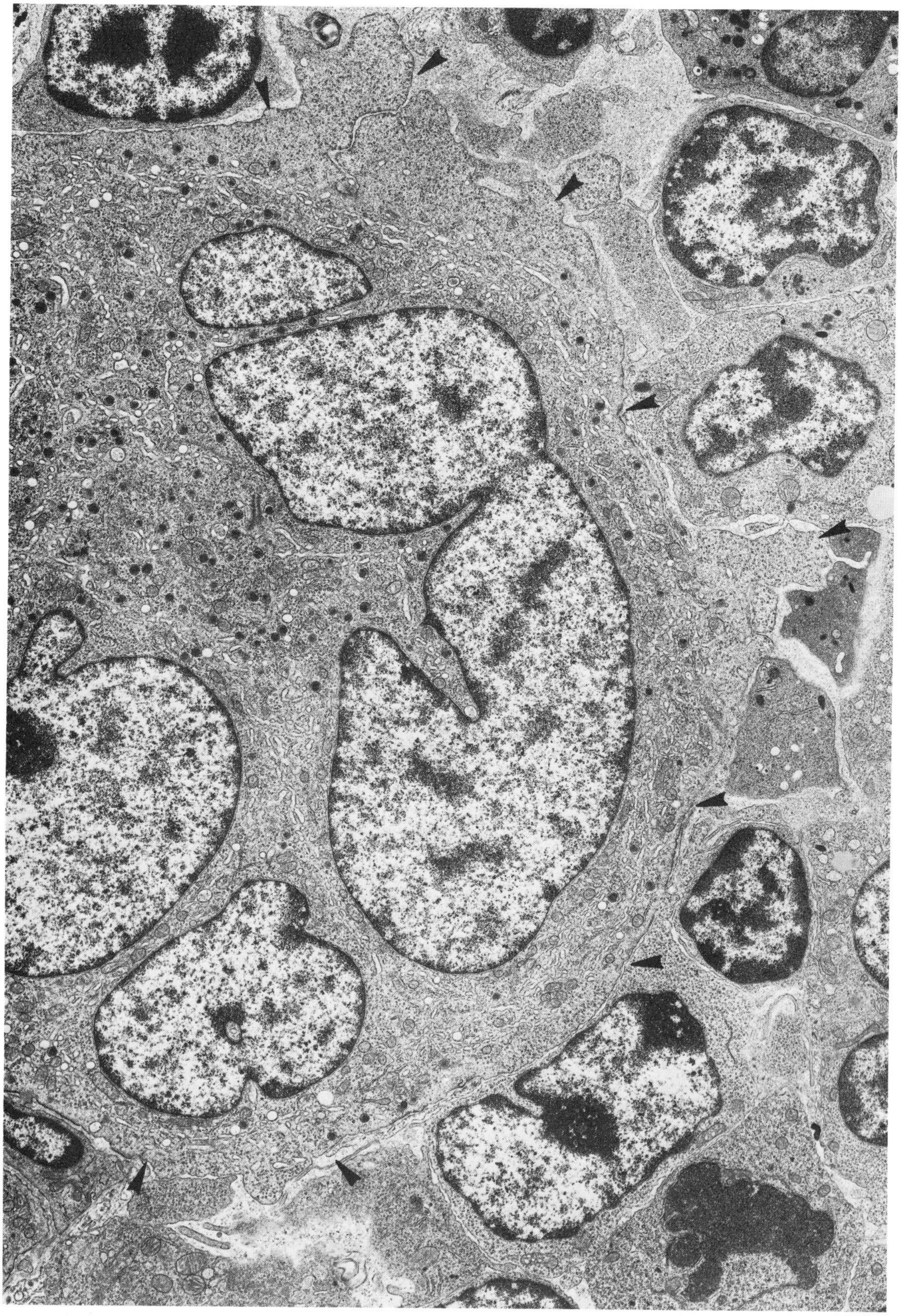

Figure 9–19. Micrograph of rat bone marrow including a portion of a megakaryocyte. The limits of the cell are outlined by arrowheads. Its very large size and multilobulate nucleus can be compared with the smaller hemopoietic cells at right of figure.

Ultrastructural Basis of Platelet Formation

The fragmentation of the megakaryocyte cytoplasm to form platelets was quite accurately described by Wright in 1906 using the light microscope, but the nature of the cytoplasmic differentiation that makes this possible had to await electron microscopic examination. Concurrently with the aggregation of azurophil granules into clusters, small vesicles appear in the cytoplasm and become aligned in rows that pursue a meandering course between the groups of granules. Electron micrographs in various planes of section suggest that the "vesicles" originally described may, in fact, be parallel tubular structures that appear to be vesicles when cut transversely. If it were possible to visualize these linear arrays of tubules in three dimensions, it would be obvious that they are actually arranged in intersecting planes that partition the cytoplasm into units 1 to 3 μm in diameter, each containing a cluster of granules and representing a future platelet. The limiting membranes of the aligned tubular profiles seen in micrographs of matur-ing megakaryocytes ultimately fuse side-to-side and their coalescence results in a three-dimensional lattice of paired *platelet demarcation membranes* that bound a continuous system of narrow clefts or cisternae that outline the nascent platelets (Fig. 9–20).

Since its discovery, the platelet demarcation system has been variously interpreted as an unusual configuration of smooth endoplasmic reticulum; a derivative of the Golgi complex; a unique organelle arising from membranogenic centers in the cytoplasm; or a product of invasion of the megakaryocyte cytoplasm by the surface membrane. There is now little reason to believe that the demarcation system originates from any of the membranous organelles of the cytoplasm. When these cells are exposed to solutions of ferritin or horseradish peroxidase, which do not penetrate biomembranes, these extracellular tracers readily enter the cisternae of the demarcation system. Such experiments clearly demonstrate communication with the extracellular space and strongly support derivation of the system from the surface membrane. The alternative possibility that the system develops from cytomembranes and

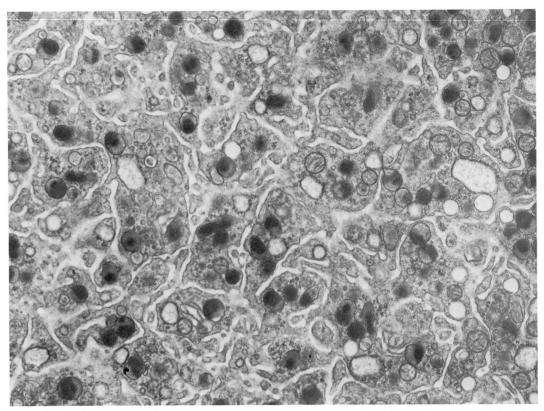

Figure 9–20. Micrograph of a small area of megakaryocyte cytoplasm, showing the platelet demarcation channels outlining future platelets.

secondarily establishes open communication with the cell surface is rendered unlikely by the cytochemical demonstration that the demarcation membranes possess enzymatic activity that is characteristic of the cell surface and not found in membranes of the cytoplasm. It is now widely accepted that the tubules found in the cytoplasm arise by invagination of the plasmalemma. These become oriented with their long axes parallel and, by side-to-side fusion of their membranes, the tubules are reorganized into flat sheets limiting an extensive system of cisternae. The two sheets of membrane bounding any one segment of the system will form the membranes of adjacent nascent platelets.

Release of Platelets

Megakaryocytes are located in subendothelial relationship to the vascular sinuses of the marrow. From this position, processes of mature megakaryocytes penetrate through the endothelium, and large segments of their cytoplasm come to project into the lumen. These structures, sometimes called *proplatelets*, may contain as many as 1200 platelet subunits and it is estimated that a single megakaryocyte may produce and cast off about six proplatelets, ultimately giving rise to 8000 platelets. The discharge of the proplatelets leaves behind around the polymorphous nucleus a thin residual layer of cytoplasm bounded by an intact cell membrane. The possibility that these *residual megakaryocytes* might reconstitute their cytoplasm and produce another set of platelets has not been excluded. It is generally assumed, however, that they degenerate and are replaced by differentiation of new megakaryocytes from stem cells. About 10 per cent of megakaryocytes observed in bone marrow appear to be degenerating cells that have lost nearly all of their cytoplasm in platelet production.

Fragmentation of the proplatelets probably takes place mainly in the vascular sinuses of the marrow, but some enter the general circulation and are carried to the lungs where they break up into individual platelets. Entire megakaryocytes may also enter the circulation. Their presence in the blood has been abundantly documented. They are also found occasionally in spleen, liver, and kidney, but are most abundant in the vascular channels of the lung. These pulmonary megakaryocytes originate in the bone marrow and are carried in the blood to the lung.

Their large size results in their entrapment at sites where the narrowing of the pulmonary vessels prevents their passage. Tens of thousands of megakaryocytes are believed to reach the lungs every minute. Their significant contribution to platelet production is made evident by the observation that the platelet count in blood taken from the pulmonary veins is higher than in that from the pulmonary artery.

Kinetics of Thrombopoiesis

Considerable information has accumulated on the kinetics of thrombopoiesis. The generation time from stem cell to platelet-producing megakaryocyte is estimated to be about ten days in humans. A humoral regulatory mechanism seems to ensure that production is responsive to the need for circulating platelets. Bleeding or performance of exchange transfusions producing low levels of platelets (*thrombocytopenia)* is followed, in several days, by a three- to fourfold increase in megakaryocyte numbers in the marrow and a rebound in circulating platelets to 150 to 200 per cent of the initial level. A hypothetical humoral agent, *thrombopoietin*, is believed to be responsible for this positive feedback, but efforts to isolate a thrombopoiesis stimulating factor from plasma and urine have not been notably successful to date.

LYMPHOPOIESIS

Blood cells were traditionally divided into two categories according to their presumed sites of origin. The lymphocytes and monocytes were referred to as the "lymphoid" elements of the blood reflecting the belief that they arose in the lymphoid organs (lymph nodes, spleen, and thymus). The granulocytes, erythrocytes, and platelets formed in the bone marrow were referred to as the "myeloid" elements and their development was collectively termed *myelopoiesis*. This terminological distinction persists in common usage although some of the assumptions upon which it was based are no longer valid. Monocytes have now been shown to arise in the marrow from a progenitor cell that is also capable of giving rise to granulocytes, It is therefore no longer appropriate to consider it a lymphoid cell.

Although considerable proliferation of

stimulated lymphocytes occurs in the peripheral lymphoid organs throughout life, the lymphopoietic stem cells originate in the bone marrow. Those destined to become T lymphocytes leave the marrow and are carried in the blood to the cortex of the thymus where they proliferate and acquire their characteristic surface markers as they move into the medulla, whence they are transported to the spleen and there undergo further maturation before becoming members of the long-lived recirculating population of small lymphocytes.

The genesis of B lymphocytes has been more clearly defined in birds than in mammals. The stem cells migrate from the bone marrow to an appendage of the avian cloaca called the *bursa of Fabricius* in much the same way that T-cell precursors populate the thymus. In the bursa, they differentiate into mature B cells and then enter the recirculating pool of small lymphocytes. The location of the functional equivalent of the bursa of Fabricius in mammals has been a subject of controversy. The genesis of B lymphocytes appears to take place in multiple sites including gut-associated lymphoid tissue, spleen, and bone marrow. It has become apparent, however, that the bone marrow is probably the major primary site of lymphopoiesis in mammals. In laboratory rodents in which it can be studied with radiolabeled tracers, the marrow has a high continuous rate of lymphocyte production throughout fetal and postnatal life. Lymphocytes constitute 30 per cent of all nucleated marrow cells and at all ages exceed the number of erythroblasts. The dividing precursors of small lymphocytes are somewhat larger cells with a leptochromatic nuclear pattern, a very thin rim of cytoplasm with few organelles. These so-called *transitional cells* are actively proliferating and constitute about one fifth of all marrow lymphocytes. Production rate of small lymphocytes in mouse marrow is calculated to be of the order of 10^8 cells per day. Although ethical considerations exclude quantitation by similar methods in the human, proportionally high rates of marrow lymphocytes are assumed. The resulting lymphocytes progressively acquire the IgG surface markers typical of B lymphocytes and continuously emigrate in very large numbers to the peripheral lymphoid tissues.

REGULATION OF HEMOPOIESIS

Much research has been done to discover how hemopoiesis is regulated to maintain the normal numbers of each cell type in the circulation. We still know little about what determines which of several alternative pathways of differentiation will be taken by the progeny of pluripotential stem cells; however, it is becoming apparent that multiple factors are involved. Some originate locally as components of the *hemopoietic microenvironment*. Others are *humoral agents* that originate elsewhere in the body and are blood-borne to the marrow to stimulate the proliferation of particular cell lineages.

Hemopoietic Microenvironment

Although stem cells may be carried in the blood throughout the body, hemopoiesis is confined to certain tissues and organs that provide a favorable environment for their proliferation. Appropriate local conditions may be acquired by some organs and lost by others, as exemplified in the changing location of the principal site of hemopoiesis during embryonic life from yolk sac to liver and spleen, and then to the marrow. The stem-cell assay based on colony formation in the spleen of irradiated mice depends on the existence in that organ of an environment capable of attracting and supporting proliferation of pluripotential cells transported in the blood. Creation of such an environment is a function of radio-resistant cellular elements of the stroma. Ectopic sites of hemopoiesis can be established in experimental animals by transplantation of marrow stroma. After some initial degenerative changes, the tissue becomes revascularized and ultimately is repopulated with hemopoietic cells. The mechanism by which migratory stem cells recognize and lodge in tissues that will support their growth is not known. The next step of *commitment* to a particular path of differentiation seems to require interaction with cells of the stroma. Local factors provided by the stroma are also necessary to sustain *proliferation* and *maturation* of the hemopoietic cells. Whether stem cell commitment and proliferation are accomplished by cell contact or production of diffusible stimulatory substances is not known, but the most likely candidate for carrying out these functions is believed to be the dendritic reticular cell, although other cells may be involved.

The stroma of different organs or in different regions of the same organ favor development of different cell lineages. Stem cells lodging in the spleen of irradiated mice give rise to colonies that are predominantly erythroid, while those settling in depleted marrow produce a preponderance of granulocyte/monocyte colonies. Stem cells rarely form lymphoid colonies in the spleen but those lodging in thymus or lymph nodes do so regularly.

The study of long-term cultures of bone marrow has provided equally persuasive evidence of the influence of microenvironment. In such cultures the cells produced are granulocytes, largely neutrophils. In addition, there is an extensive growth of stromal elements including endothelial cells, reticular cells, adipose cells, and macrophages. A dominant feature of cultures active in granulopoiesis is the presence of clusters of adipose cells. The differentiating granulocytes are invariably found in very close relationship to fat cells or the processes of reticular cells.

Granulopoietic mouse marrow cultures can be switched to erythropoiesis by addition of serum from anemic mice to the medium. The changeover is accompanied by a regression of the population of adipose cells and emergence of a new pattern of cell association. All stages of the erythroid series are found clustered around large mononuclear phagocytes in a configuration closely resembling the "erythroblastic islets" commonly observed in marrow in vivo.

Thus, it is evident from experimental studies both in vivo and in vitro that the microenvironment plays a very important role in the regulation of hemopoiesis. The stromal cells are intimately involved, and the specific cell associations favoring granulopoiesis differ from those favoring erythropoiesis.

Humoral Regulation of Hemopoiesis

Because blood cells are short-lived and may spend only a small portion of their life span in the circulation, they must be continually replaced by formation of large numbers of new cells. In this process of continual renewal, the relative numbers of the several cell types remain remarkably constant. This implies a need for some mechanism of monitoring the numbers in the circulation, and the existence of specific humoral growth regulators acting back upon the hemopoietic tissue to control the rate of formation and release of new cells of each type. While in most cases the means of sensing changes in the circulating population remains obscure, considerable progress has been made in detecting and characterizing the molecules involved in humoral regulation of specific hemopoietic cell lineages.

The control of erythropoiesis was the first to be studied and is best understood. Blood loss stimulates the marrow to increase its production and release of erythrocytes. Transfusion of excess erythrocytes is followed by suppression of erythropoiesis. With no change in blood volume, an enhanced need for oxygen transport also stimulates the marrow. It was observed nearly a century ago that in the physiological adaptation to high altitude, the body responds to hypoxia by increasing the number of circulating erythrocytes. It was initially concluded that the marrow was *directly* responsive to the oxygen content of the blood. However, this reasonable interpretation was later shown to be incorrect in ingenious experiments on parabiotic rats that share a common circulation. When only one member of the pair was exposed to hypoxia, both members showed enhanced erythropoiesis. This and other experiments clearly demonstrated that the hypoxic stimulus to the marrow was mediated by a blood-borne humoral agent. This was initially named *erythropoiesis stimulating factor* but is now called *erythropoietin*. Erythropoietin is a glycoprotein of 70,000 molecular weight. It can be detected in plasma and urine of hypoxic animals and in humans with diseases attended by oxygen deficiency. Erythropoietin synthesis is inversely related to the oxygen tension prevailing in the tissues. The site of its synthesis is mainly in the kidney.

Maintenance of normal numbers of circulating erythrocytes depends on (1) continuing stimulation of the marrow by erythropoietin, (2) a marrow capable of responding, and (3) an adequate supply of iron to meet the needs of the marrow for synthesis of hemoglobin. A normal marrow not only provides for continual replacement of erythrocytes, but is also capable of rapid increase in output to four or five times the basal rate. The body contains only limited reserves of iron in the form of *ferritin,* a protein capable of accumulating 2000 or more atoms of iron. It is found in various cells throughout the body but notably in the liver. Iron is transported in the plasma by an iron-binding globulin, *transferrin,* and is taken up by specific transferrin receptors on the surface of erythropoietic cells and interiorized for use in hemoglobin synthesis. The amount of available iron may limit the response of the marrow to erythropoietic stimulation, resulting in *iron deficiency anemia.*

To account for the regulation of circulating granulocytes, hematologists have long postulated a specific humoral factor comparable with erythropoietin. Validation of the existence of such a substance requires demonstration that it is capable of stimulating new granulocyte production in vivo. This has been difficult to achieve because factors other than formation of new cells influence the granulocyte count. In the presence of a bacterial infection, there is a rapid and large increase in the number of circulating neutrophils. The rapidity of this response suggests that it is due to mobilization of reserves rather than to the production of new cells. The population of neutrophils within the vascular system customarily falls into two categories: (1) those that are flowing with the blood—the *circulating pool of leukocytes* and (2) those that are temporarily adherent to the vascular endothelium in various parts of the circulatory system—the *marginated pool of leukocytes.* Normally the neutrophils are about equally divided between these two pools, but in response to exercise, epinephrine administration, and other stimuli there may be a massive movement of marginated cells into the bloodstream, doubling the number in the circulating pool without increased granulopoiesis in the marrow.

Under normal circumstances, eight to ten days elapse after the last myelocyte division before the myelocytes complete their maturation and enter the blood. Thus, the greater part of the life span of these cells is spent in the marrow where there are very large reserves of band-forms and mature neutrophils capable of entering the circulation on demand—approximately 15 times as many as there are in the blood. Very marked increases in circulating neutrophils can thus be achieved by their release without an immediate change in production rate. Neverthe-

less, as infection continues, there is an acceleration of granulopoiesis. A humoral agent, variously termed *leukopoietin* or *granulopoietin,* is believed responsible for carrying to the marrow the signal to produce more neutrophils. Convincing experimental evidence for such a substance has been difficult to obtain in vivo, but systems have now been developed for cloning populations of hemopoietic cells in semisolid culture medium in vitro. This has made it possible to detect specific macromolecules that control proliferation and maturation of the progeny of single colony-forming cells, which are the earliest committed progenitors of the various hemopoietic cell lines. Cell proliferation within each colony is dependent on the presence in the medium of a specific *colony-stimulating factor* (CSF). Committed cells that give rise to granulocytes are bipotential. The colonies formed may contain only granulocytes, only monocyte-macrophages, or mixtures of the two. These cells are therefore called *granulocyte-macrophage colony-forming cells* (GM-CFC). The colony-stimulating factor controlling development of these cell types is designated GM-CSF. It is a glycoprotein with a molecular weight of about 45,000 and biochemical properties resembling those of erythropoietin. It can be found in various tissues but its major source seems to be the mononuclear phagocyte system. Bacterial endotoxins increase the release of this colony-stimulating factor by macrophages in vitro, suggesting a mechanism whereby the presence of bacterial products in infections can increase granulocyte production by bone marrow. For this colony-stimulating factor to qualify as a true granulopoietin, it will have to be demonstrated that its repetitive or continuous administration will result in a sustained increase in new circulating granulocytes in vivo. This is yet to be accomplished.

Perturbations of the numbers of circulating platelets are followed by compensatory adjustments in thrombopoiesis. Blood plasma from thrombocytopenic patients is reported to stimulate platelet production when injected into laboratory animals. The stimulatory effect of thrombocytopenic plasma can be detected not only by platelet counts, but by measuring increased incorporation of radioisotope into platelets after administration of ^{75}Se-selenomethionine or ^{35}C-sodium sulfate. Thus, there is strong indirect evidence for feedback regulation of platelet numbers by a thrombopoietin, but little is known about the sensing mechanism responsible for activating its synthesis and release.

There is no persuasive evidence for a feedback control of B-lymphocyte production comparable with the poietins that regulate production of other blood cells. By analogy with effects of bleeding or hemolysis on erythropoiesis, one might expect a marrow response to deletion of circulating lymphocytes. Immunological suppression of circulating lymphocytes has no significant effect upon lymphocyte production in the marrow. On the other hand, mice raised under germ-free conditions have a markedly reduced rate of lymphocyte production. It is concluded that a normal basal level of marrow lymphopoiesis is regulated by local microenvironmental factors, but may be augmented by exogenous antigenic stimulation.

REFERENCES

GENERAL

Tavassoli, M., and J. M. Yoffey: Bone Marrow Structure and Function. New York, Alan Liss, 1983.
Wickramasinghe, S. N.: Human Bone Marrow. Oxford, Blackwell Scientific Publications, 1975.

PRENATAL HEMOPOIESIS

Bloom, W., and F. W. Bartelmez: Hematopoiesis in young human embryos. Am. J. Anat. 67:21, 1940.
Johnson, F. R., and M. A. G. Moore: Role of stem cell migration in initiation of mouse foetal liver haemopoiesis. Nature (Lond.) 258:726, 1975.
Moore, M. A. G., and D. Metcalf: Ontogeny of the haemopoietic system: yolk sac origin of in vivo and in vitro colony forming cells in developing mouse embryo. Br. J. Haematol. 18:279, 1970.

ORGANIZATION OF THE BONE MARROW

Becher, R. P., and De Bruyn, P. P. H.: The transmural passage of blood cells into myeloid sinuses and the entry of platelets into the sinusoidal circulation. A scanning electron microscopic investigation. Am. J. Anat. 145:183, 1976.
De Bruyn, P. P. H., P. C. Breen, and T. B. Thomas: The microcirculation of the bone marrow. Anat. Rec. 168:55, 1970.
De Bruyn, P. P. H., S. Michelson, and T. B. Thomas: Migration of blood cells of the marrow through the sinusoidal wall. J. Morphol. 144:417, 1971.
Hudson, F., and J. M. Yoffey: Ultrastructure of the reticuloendothelial elements of guinea pig bone marrow. J. Anat. 103:515, 1968.
Weiss, L.: The hemopoietic microenvironment of the bone marrow: an ultrastructural study of the stroma in rats. Anat. Rec. 186:161, 1976.
Weiss, L., and L. T. Chen: The organization of hemopoietic cords and vascular sinuses in bone marrow. Blood Cells 1:617, 1975.

HEMOPOIETIC STEM CELLS

Dexter, T. M.: Hemopoiesis in long-term bone marrow cultures. A review. Acta Haematol. 62:299, 1979.

Dexter, T. M., T. D. Allen, L. G. Lajtha, L. G. Krizra, N. Testa, and M. A. S. Moore: In vitro analysis of self-renewal and commitment of hemopoietic stem cells. In Hematopoietic Mechanisms. Cold Spring Harbor Symp. Quant. Biol. 42:63, 1978.
Lajtha, L. G.: Haemopoietic stem cells: Concepts and definitions. Blood Cells 5:447, 1979.
Quesenberry, P., and L. Levitt: Haematopoietic stem cells. N. Engl. J. Med. 30:755, 819, 1979.
Till, J. E., and E. A. McCulloch: Hemopoietic stem cell differentiation. Biochim. Biophys. Acta 605:431, 1980.

ERYTHROPOIESIS

Bessis, M.: Life Cycle of the Erythrocyte. Sandoz Monographs. Basle, Sondoz Ltd., 1966.
Campbell, F. R.: Nuclear elimination from the normoblast of fetal guina pig liver as studied with electron microscopy and serial section techniques. Anat. Rec. 160:539, 1968.
Harrison, P. R.: Analysis of erythropoiesis at the molecular level. Review article. Nature (Lond.) 262:353, 1976.
Hillman, R. S., and C. A. Finch: Erythropoiesis normal and abnormal. Semin. Hematol. 4:427, 1967.

GRANULOPOIESIS

Ackerman, G. A.: Ultrastructure and cytochemistry of the developing neutrophil. Lab. Invest. 19:290, 1968.
Ackerman, G. A.: The human neutrophil myelocyte. A correlated phase and electron microscopic study. Z. Zellforsch. Mikrosk. Anat. 121:153, 1971.
Bainton, D. F., and M. G. Farquhar: Origin of granules in the polymorphonuclear leukocytes. Two types derived from opposite faces of the Golgi complex in development. J. Cell Biol. 28:277, 1966.
Bainton, D. F., and M. G. Farquhar: Differences in enzyme content of azurophil and specific granules of polymorphonuclear leukocytes. II. Cytochemistry and electron microscopy of bone marrow cells. J. Cell Biol. 39:299, 1968.
Bainton, D. F., and M. G. Farquhar: Segregation and packaging of granule enzymes in eosinophilic leukocytes. J. Cell Biol. 45:54, 1970.
Boggs, D. R.: The kinetics of neutrophilic leukocytes in health and disease. Semin. Hematol. 4:1, 1967.
Scott, R. E., and R. G. Horn: Ultrastructural aspects of neutrophil granulocyte development in humans. Lab. Invest. 23:202, 1970.

MONOPOIESIS

Meuret, G.: Origin, ontogeny and kinetics of mononuclear phagocytes. Adv. Exp. Med. Biol. 73:Pt.A:71, 1976.
Nichols, B. A., D. F. Bainton, and M. G. Farquhar: Differentiation of monocytes: origin, nature, and fate of their azuropohil granules. J. Cell Biol. 50:498, 1971.
van Furth, R., and Z. A. Cohn: The origin and kinetics of mononuclear phagocytes. J. Exp. Med. 128:415, 1968.
van Furth, R.: Current view on the mononuclear phagocyte system. Immunobiology 161:178, 1982.
Whitlaw, D. M., M. F. Bell, and H. F. Batho: Monocyte kinetics. Observations after pulse labelling. J. Cell Physiol. 72:65, 1968.

THROMBOPOIESIS

Becher, R. P., and P. P. H. DeBruyn: The transmural passage of blood cells into myeloid sinusoids and entry of platelets into the sinusoidal circulation: a scanning microscope investigation. Am. J. Anat. *145*:183, 1976.

Behnke, O.: An electron microscope study of the megakaryocyte of rat bone marrow. I. The development of the demarcation membrane system and the platelet surface coat. J. Ultrastruct. Res. *24*:412, 1968.

Ebbe, S.: Biology of megakaryocytes. Prog. Hemost. Thromb. *3*:211, 1976.

Hansen, M., and N. T. Pedersen: Circulating megakaryocytes in blood from antecubital vein in healthy adult humans. Scand. J. Haematol. *20*:371, 1978.

Metcalf, D., H. R. MacDonald, N. Odartchenki, and B. Sordat: Growth of mouse megakaryocyte colonies *in vitro.* Proc. Natl. Acad. Sci. USA. *72*:1744, 1975.

Pedersen, N. T.: The pulmonary vessels as a filter for circulating megakaryocytes in rats. Scand. J. Haematol. *13*:225, 1974.

Pedersen, N. T.: Occurrence of megakaryocytes in various vessels and their retention in the pulmonary capillaries in man. Scand. J. Haematol. *21*:369, 1978.

Penington, D. G.: The cellular biology of megakaryocytes. Blood Cells *5*:5, 1979.

Shaklai, M., and M. Tavassoli: Demarcation membrane system in rat megakaryocyte and the mechanism of platelet formation. J. Ultrastruct. Res. *62*:270, 1978.

Tavassoli, M.: Megakaryocyte-platelet axis and the process of platelet formation and release. Blood *55*:537, 1980.

LYMPHOPOIESIS

Osmond, D. G.: Formation and maturation of bone marrow lymphocytes. J. Reticuloendothel. Soc. *17*:99, 1975.

Osmond, D. G., M. T. E. Fahlman, G. M. Fulop, and D. M. Rahal: Regulation and localization of lymphocyte production in the bone marrow. *In* Microenvironments in Haemopoietic and Lymphoid Differentiation. Ciba Foundation Symposium 84. London, Pitman Medical, 1981.

Rosse, C.: Small lymphocyte and transitional cell populations of the bone marrow. Their role in the mediation of immune and hemopoietic progenitor cell functions. Int. Rev. Cytol. *45*:155, 1976.

Yoffey, J. M.: Transitional cells of haemopoietic tissues: origin, structure, and developmental potential. Int. Rev Cytol. *62*:311, 1980.

REGULATION OF HEMOPOIESIS

Allen, T. D.: Haemopoietic microenvironments in vitro: ultrastructural aspects. *In* Microenvironments in Haemopoietic and Lymphoid Differentiation. Ciba Foundation Symposium 84. London, Pitman Medical, 1981.

Burgess, A. W., J. Camakaris, and D. Metcalf: Purification and properties of colony stimulating factor from mouse lung conditioned medium. J. Biol. Chem. *252*:1998, 1977.

Golde, D. W., and M. J. Cline: Regulation of granulopoiesis. N. Engl. J. Med. *231*:1388, 1974.

Gordon, A. S., and E. D. Zanjani: Some aspects of erythropoietin physiology. *In* Gordon, A. S., ed.: Regulation of Hematopoiesis. New York, Appleton-Century-Crofts, 1971.

Jacobson, L. O., E. Goldwasser, W. Fried, and L. Pizak: Role of the kidney in erythropoiesis. Nature (Lond.) *179*:633, 1957.

Metcalf, D.: Regulation of hemopoiesis. Nouv. Rev. Fr. Hematol. *20*:521, 1978.

Miyake, T., C. K. H. Kung, and E. Goldwasser: Purification of human erythropoietin. J. Biol. Chem. *252*:5558, 1977.

Reissman, K. R.: Studies on the mechanism of erythropoietic stimulation in parabiotic rats during hypoxia. Blood *5*:372; *16*:1411, 1960.

Rifkind, R. A., and P. A. Marks: The regulation of erythropoiesis. Blood Cells *1*:417, 1975.

Robinson, W. A., and A. Magalik: The kinetics and regulation of granulopoiesis. Semin. Hematol. *12*:7, 1975.

Trentin, J. J.: Hemopoietic inductive microenvironments. *In* Cairnie, A. B., et al., eds. Stem Cells of Renewing Cell Populations. New York, Academic Press, 1976.

Wolf, N. S.: The haemopoietic microenvironment. Clin. Haematol. *8*:469, 1979.

10

MUSCULAR TISSUE

Contractility is one of the fundamental properties of protoplasm and is exhibited in varying degree by nearly all cell types. In muscular tissue the ability of the cells to convert chemical energy into mechanical work through contraction has become highly developed.

Two broad categories of muscle are distinguished—*smooth muscle* and *striated muscle*. Smooth muscle is composed of fusiform, uninucleate cells. It contracts in response to stimulation by the autonomic nervous system and thus is not subject to voluntary control. Striated muscle associated with the skeleton is responsible for locomotion and other *voluntary movements* of vertebrates and is innervated by the cerebrospinal nervous system. It consists of very long cylindrical units, which are multinucleate syncytia containing large numbers of closely packed cytoplasmic filaments in a highly ordered arrangement that results in a distinctive pattern of cross striations along the length of the cellular elements, traditionally called *muscle fibers*.

The muscular wall of the heart is a unique form of striated muscle whose rhythmic contraction is involuntary. *Cardiac muscle* differs from *skeletal muscle* in that its branching fibers are not syncytial but are formed of individual cellular units joined end to end.

SMOOTH MUSCLE

Smooth muscle forms the contractile portion of the wall of the digestive tract from the middle of the esophagus to the internal sphincter of the anus. It provides the motive power for mixing the ingested food with digestive juices and for its propulsion through the absorptive and excretory portions of the tract. Smooth muscle is also found in the walls of the ducts in the glands associated with the alimentary tract, in the walls of the respiratory passages from the trachea to the alveolar ducts, and in the urinary and genital ducts. The walls of the arteries, veins, and larger lymphatic trunks contain smooth muscle. In the skin it forms minute muscles called arrectores pilorum, responsible for elevation of hairs. In the areola of the mammary gland it participates in the erection of the nipple, and in the subcutaneous tissue of the scrotum it causes the wrinkling of the skin that accompanies elevation of the testes. In the eye it forms the musculature of the iris and of the ciliary body, which is concerned with accommodation and with constriction and dilation of the pupil.

The Smooth Muscle Fibers

Smooth muscle fibers are long, spindle-shaped cells. Where they are closely associated in bundles or sheets, their boundaries are difficult to resolve with the light microscope, but by special maceration techniques the fibers can be isolated, and their long fusiform shape is then evident. They vary greatly in length in different organs. In the pregnant human uterus, they may reach 0.5 mm in length. Their average length in the musculature of the human intestine is about 0.2 mm. The smallest smooth muscle cells in the walls of small blood vessels may be only 20 μm long.

In longitudinal sections, a single elongated nucleus is found to occupy the thickest part of the fiber, about midway along its length. The long nuclear profile is rounded at the ends (Fig. 10–1). The chromatin usually forms a delicate pattern uniformly dispersed in the nucleoplasm, but in the smooth muscle of some organs it tends to be aggregated along the inner surface of the nuclear envelope. There are two or more nucleoli, depending on the species. In smooth muscle fixed in contraction, the passively distorted nuclei may be deeply indented along their margins or may take on a helical form.

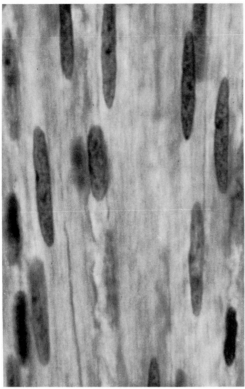 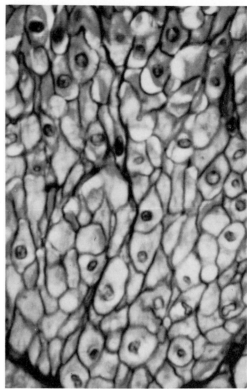

Figure 10–1   **Figure 10–2**

Figure 10–1. Photomicrograph of a longitudinal section of smooth muscle from the tunica muscularis of intestine.

Figure 10–2. Photomicrograph of a transverse section of smooth muscle from the tunica muscularis of the human stomach. The section was stained with the periodic acid–Schiff reaction, which stains the glycoprotein external lamina of the muscle cells, accentuating their outline.

The cells of smooth muscle are offset with respect to one another, so that the thick middle portion of one is juxtaposed to the thin ends of adjacent cells. In transverse sections, smooth muscle therefore presents a mosaic of rounded or irregularly polygonal profiles varying from less than 1 μm to several micrometers across (Fig. 10–2). Only the largest profiles, those representing sections through the thick middle portion of the fibers, contain a centrally placed cross section of the nucleus. No nucleus is found in the smaller profiles, which represent sections at various levels in the tapering ends of the fusiform cells.

The cytoplasm of muscle cells is called *sarcoplasm.* In smooth muscle it appears quite homogeneous in the living state and is almost equally devoid of structure after routine fixation and staining. However, after use of special stains, or after gentle maceration in acid, fine longitudinal striations can be demonstrated, running the full length of the cell. These are the *myofibrils,* the contractile material of smooth muscle. They are birefringent under the polarizing microscope, but show no sign of the alternating isotropic and anisotropic transverse bands that are characteristic of the myofibrils of striated muscle.

After appropriate cytological staining methods, mitochondria can be seen throughout the sarcoplasm, but they tend to congregate near the poles of the elongated nucleus. A pair of centrioles and a small Golgi apparatus can also be demonstrated. In some organs the sarcoplasm of smooth muscle may contain glycogen.

In the development of mammary and sweat glands, certain cells of ectodermal origin become specialized for contraction. The cell body of these *myoepithelial cells* has some of the characteristics of epithelial cells, but their base is drawn out into several radiating processes that contain myofilaments. These portions of the cell have an appearance closely resembling the sarcoplasm of smooth muscle cells.

Mode of Association of Smooth Muscle Fibers

Smooth muscle cells may occur singly or in small groups in ordinary connective tissue, as in the lamina propria of the intestinal villi, where their contraction shortens the villi and helps expel lymph from the lacteals. In the walls of blood vessels, where smooth muscle fibers serve only to change the caliber of the lumen, they are oriented circumferentially, occurring as isolated fibers in the smallest arterioles and as a continuous layer in vessels of larger size. In the wall of the intestine, smooth muscle is arranged in separate longitudinal and circumferential layers. The coordinated action of these layers forms constrictions that move along the intestine as peristaltic waves, propelling the contents through the lumen. In other hollow organs, such as the bladder or uterus, the smooth muscle forms poorly defined layers of elaborately interlacing coarse bundles oriented in different directions. The connective tissue fibers outside the muscle layer continue into the spaces between the cells and bind them into bundles. Between the thicker bundles or layers of smooth muscle cells is a small amount of loose connective tissue containing fibroblasts, collagenous and elastic fibers, and a network of capillaries and nerves. Connective tissue cells are seldom found within smooth muscle bundles, but the clefts between muscle cells are nevertheless occupied by thin reticular fibers, which branch irregularly and form a delicate network investing the individual smooth muscle cells. This reticulum can be stained with Mallory's aniline blue method and still more distinctly with the Bielschowsky silver impregnation method. The reticular fibers are embedded in a layer of intercellular material that appears in sections stained with the periodic acid–Schiff (PAS) reaction as a continuous pattern of magenta lines outlining every muscle cell (Fig. 10–2).

The pull of each contracting cell in smooth muscle is transmitted to the surrounding sheath of reticular fibers, which are continuous with those of neighboring cells and ultimately with those of the surrounding connective tissue. This arrangement permits the force of contraction of the entire layer of the smooth muscle to be uniformly transmitted to the surrounding parts.

The Fine Structure of Smooth Muscle

In electron micrographs the elongated nucleus of the extended smooth muscle cell is smoothly contoured and rounded at the ends. The juxtanuclear sarcoplasm contains long slender mitochondria, a few tubular elements of granular endoplasmic reticulum, and numerous polyribosomes. A small Golgi complex is located near one pole of the nucleus. The bulk of the sarcoplasm is occupied by exceedingly thin, parallel myofilaments associated in bundles that correspond to the myofibrils seen with the light microscope. These are oriented, for the most part, parallel to the long axis of the muscle cell. Interspersed among the bundles of myofilaments are mitochondria, occurring singly or in small clusters, and having a prevailing longitudinal orientation. Scattered through the contractile substance of the cell are oval or fusiform dense areas (Figs. 10–3 and 10–4). At high magnification these appear to be traversed by myofilaments embedded in a dense amorphous matrix. Similar densities are distributed at intervals along the inner aspect of the plasmalemma. The exact nature of these dense areas in the sarcoplasm is not known. Their fine structural resemblance to the dense regions found at desmosomes, at zonulae adherentes of epithelia, and the Z bands of striated muscle suggests that the dense component of all of these may be similar and may have a cohesive function. The occurrence of dense bodies in smooth muscle at nodal points where myofilaments seem to be bonded together laterally, and also where they are attached to the cell surface, is consistent with this speculation. The plasmalemma between the specialized sites of myofilament attachment is characteristically studded with small vesicular inpocketings or caveoli like those seen in endothelial cells and commonly interpreted as evidence of micropinocytosis (Fig. 10–6). However, these vesicles do not appear to dissociate from the membrane and move into the sarcoplasm as one would expect if they were involved in endocytosis. It has been suggested that they may sequester and release calcium and may thus play a role in control of contraction and relaxation comparable with that of the sarcoplasmic reticulum of striated muscle. But the exact physiological significance of these membrane invaginations remains unclear.

In the early electron microscopic studies all vertebrate striated muscles and many unstriated muscles of invertebrates were found to contain two distinct sets of parallel filaments. This led to the expectation that all muscle cells would be found to have a contractile apparatus consisting of two kinds of sarcoplasmic filaments. This expectation was not immediately borne out in studies of mammalian smooth muscle. The filaments were thinner and less well ordered than in striated

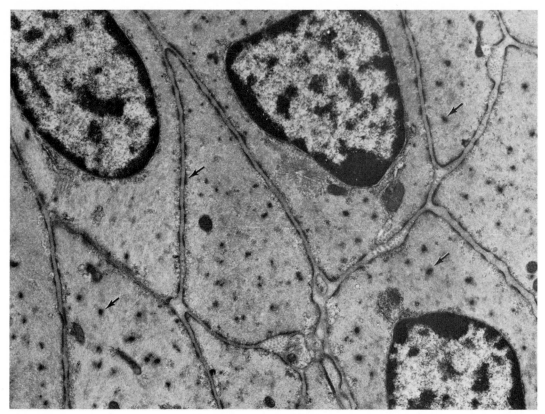

Figure 10–3. Electron micrograph of smooth muscle in transverse section. The cells are separated by wide intercellular clefts occupied by glycoprotein cell coats and small bundles of collagen fibrils. Scattered through the cytoplasm and at the periphery of the cell *(at arrows)* are densities that are sites of lateral bonding of filaments of the cytoskeleton and sites of attachment of myofibrils to the cell membrane.

muscle, and thicker filaments were only rarely seen. The inconsistency in results of electron microscopy of smooth muscle proved to be a technical problem. The routine procedure of postfixation with osmium solutions distorts or depolymerizes actin filaments and is probably destructive to myosin filaments in this tissue. The corresponding filaments in striated muscle are much more stable. In more recent studies using improved methods of preservation, it has been possible to distinguish punctate profiles of two sizes that are interpreted as cross sections of two kinds of filaments comparable with the myosin and actin filaments of striated muscle (Fig. 10–5). The existence of a two-filament contractile system in smooth muscle is now generally accepted, and the morphological evidence is strongly supported by biochemical isolation of both actin and myosin and their interaction in vitro to form a complex capable of contraction upon addition of adenosine triphosphate.

Actin is relatively much more abundant than in striated muscle and the filaments are grouped together in bundles associated with myosin filaments in a ratio of 12:1 or higher, compared with 6:1 in striated muscle. Information on the three-dimensional arrangement of the filaments is still incomplete, but they appear to be grouped together in contractile units attached at each end to the cell membrane. The organization of the myosin molecules and the structural polarity of the filaments formed differs from that of myosin in striated muscle. Thick filaments isolated from smooth muscle are quite variable in length (3–8 μm) and they possess projecting cross bridges at regular intervals along their entire length. Thus, the molecules do not have the antiparallel arrangement that results in a central bare area on myosin filaments of striated muscle (Fig. 10–25B). The molecular organization of the thin filament is very similar to filamentous actin of striated muscle. How the shearing action between the thick and thin filaments takes place during contraction is still poorly understood. The integrity of the contractile system is strongly dependent on the extracellular calcium con-

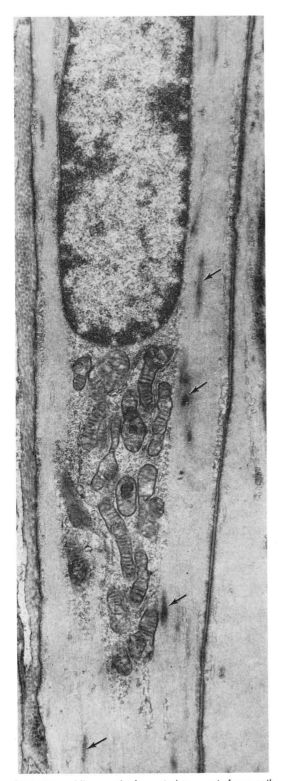

Figure 10–4. Micrograph of a central segment of a smooth muscle cell in longitudinal section. The uniform gray region at the periphery is occupied by myofilaments that are not resolved at this magnification. A conical region of sarcoplasm extending from the pole of the elongate nucleus contains numerous mitochondria and a few profiles of rough endoplasmic reticulum.

centration. If smooth muscle is perfused with mammalian Krebs-Ringer solution containing a physiological concentration of calcium ions, the myofilaments are present in normal abundance and distribution in electron micrographs (Fig. 10–6A). If it is then perfused with the same solution containing the chelating agent EDTA, myofilaments are largely absent (Fig. 10–6B). The filaments are restored and contractility regained upon subsequent perfusion with the original solution.

In addition to the contractile filaments, smooth muscle cells contain a well-developed cytoskeleton consisting of 10-nm filaments, which form structural attachments with the sarcoplasmic dense bodies and the plasma membrane. The cytoskeletal elements are not easily identified in routine micrographs, but the filaments and their association with the dense bodies are clearly visualized in preparations in which the myosin and actin filaments have been extracted (Fig. 10–6B). Opinion is divided as to whether the dense bodies are at nodal points in the cytoskeletal network of 10-nm filaments or whether they are also sites of attachment of the actin filaments.

Cell-to-Cell Relations in Smooth Muscle

In electron micrographs the surface of each smooth muscle cell is invested by a thick extracellular coating that corresponds in its fine structure to the basal lamina of epithelia and to the *external lamina* of other mesenchymal derivatives. This is clearly the component responsible for the PAS reaction of the intercellular spaces of smooth muscle (Fig. 10–2). Small bundles of collagen fibrils, which correspond to the argyrophilic reticulum, are lodged in clefts between or within the glycoprotein surface coatings of adjacent smooth muscle cells.

Owing to the presence of this thick extracellular layer, adjacent smooth muscle cells are separated by a distance of 40 to 80 nm. Typical desmosomes are not found. However, the specialized dense areas in which the myofilaments terminate at the surface of adjacent cells are too often opposite one another for their distribution to be entirely random. An intermediate dense line may be found in the intercellular material between two such opposing dense regions. Thus, in spite of the considerable distance that separates the cells, there is a complementarity to the specialized areas of their surfaces that

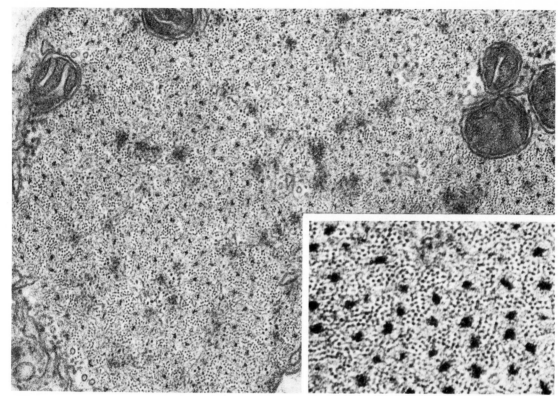

Figure 10–5. Micrograph of a vascular smooth muscle cell in cross section, clearly showing thick and thin filaments. Inset shows the same at higher magnification. (Micrograph from Somlyo, A. P., C. E. Devine, and A. V. Somlyo. *In* Vascular Smooth Muscle. Heidelberg, Springer-Verlag, 1972.)

suggests cell-to-cell cohesion at these sites, as at the desmosomes of epithelia. Contraction results in force applied at many points of insertion of myofilaments on the periphery of the cell. The contracted cell becomes ellipsoid and may exhibit numerous invaginations of its surface at points of attachment of myofilament bundles. The force is probably transmitted to neighboring cells, mainly through the reticular connective tissue sheath, but long-range forces of attraction acting at multiple dense areas of specialization on the opposing cell surfaces may also be involved.

In certain limited areas of the surface of visceral smooth muscle, the intercellular substance is lacking and the membranes of neighboring cells come into very close association. At these sites, the intercellular space is narrowed to 2 nm or less, and the opposing plasmalemmae, in freeze-cleaved preparations, exhibit closely packed 9-nm particles in hexagonal array within the plane of the membrane. These junctional specializations are therefore typical *gap junctions* or *nexuses*, and are believed to be sites of low electrical resis-

tance, permitting free movement of ions and spread of excitation from one cellular unit to another throughout the muscle mass.

Although smooth muscle cells are specialized for their primary contractile function, they also synthesize and release components of the extracellular matrix. Cultures of smooth muscle cells have been shown to produce collagen and elastin. Thus, they are not dependent on fibroblasts for formation of their extracellular matrix.

Physiological Properties and Contractile Mechanism of Smooth Muscle

Smooth muscle is distinguished from striated muscle not only by its histological and cytological appearance but also by its physiological and pharmacological properties. Its contractions are slower than those of other types of muscle, but it is able to sustain forceful contraction for long periods with relatively little expenditure of energy. Depending on the site, contraction may be initiated by nerve impulses, hormonal stimula-

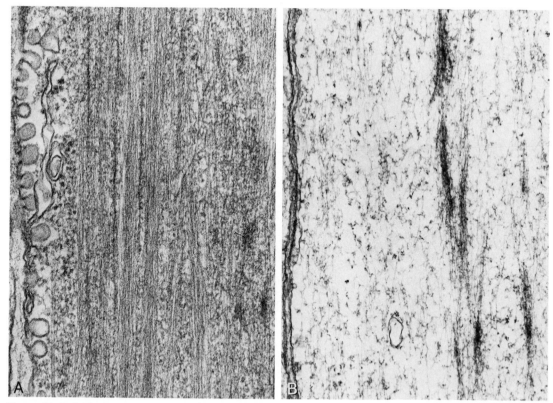

Figure 10–6. *A,* Micrograph of smooth muscle cell perfused with Krebs-Ringer solution, showing bundles of longitudinal filaments. *B,* Muscle perfused with Krebs-Ringer solution containing the calcium chelating agent EDTA. The myofilaments are no longer present. The 10-nm cytoskeletal filaments and dense bodies remain. Upon reperfusion with the original solution the filaments reappear and contractility is restored. (Micrographs from Cooke, P. Eur. J. Cell Biol. 27:55, 1982.)

tion, or local changes arising within the muscle itself. One of the more important local stimuli initiating contraction is stretching of the muscle fibers, which can change the membrane potential and initiate a wave of contraction. The ability of smooth muscle to respond to stretch is particularly important in the physiology of the bladder, gastrointestinal tract, and other hollow viscera, whose contents are evacuated by contractions.

Although usually treated by morphologists as a single type of muscle, smooth muscle is adapted to a variety of functions and differs markedly in its physiological properties in different organs. *Vascular smooth muscle,* in the blood vessels, behaves rather like skeletal muscle in that its activity is usually initiated by nerve fibers (vasomotor nerves), and there is little evidence of conduction between cellular units. *Visceral smooth muscle,* on the other hand, bears certain functional resemblances to cardiac muscle in that it has a myogenic autorhythmicity; the entire cell mass behaves as though it were a single unit with impulses

being conducted from cell to cell via the gap junctions.

Two forms of contraction are recognized in visceral smooth muscle: *rhythmic contraction* and *tonic contraction.* In the former, periodic spontaneous impulses are generated and spread through the muscle, accompanied by a wave of contraction. In addition, smooth muscle maintains a continuous state of partial contraction called *muscle tone* or *tonus.* The cause of the tonic contraction is no better understood than the genesis of the rhythmic contractions. The degree of *tonic contraction* may change greatly, without any change in the frequency of the *rhythmic contraction,* and vice versa. The two forms of contraction thus appear to be independent.

There are several other physiological and pharmacological differences in smooth muscle of different organs. For example, the amounts of *actin* and *myosin* in smooth muscle of the uterus are under endocrine control. Its cells hypertrophy during pregnancy, and show a striking increase in the size of the

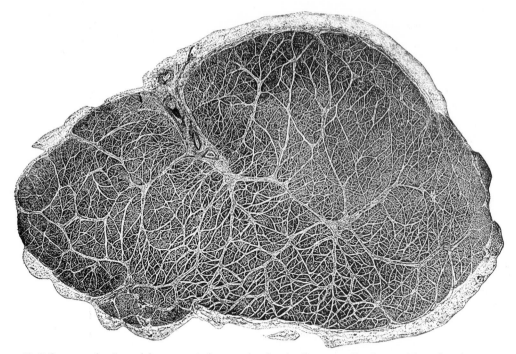

Figure 10–7. Cross section through human sartorius muscle, showing the connective tissue of the epimysium surrounding the entire muscle, and the perimysium enclosing muscle fiber bundles of varying size. (Photograph by Müller, from Heidenhain.)

Golgi apparatus and the extent of the granular endoplasmic reticulum. Physiological changes also occur during the normal estrus cycle. Ribonucleic acid synthesis is one of the early responses of the uterus to estrogen stimulation, and the organelles concerned with protein synthesis become more prominent during estrus than at other times. Uterine musculature in the terminal stages of pregnancy is also responsive to the hormone *oxytocin*, elaborated by the posterior lobe of the hypophysis. Smooth muscle in other parts of the body is relatively unresponsive to hormones other than epinephrine.

SKELETAL MUSCLE

Histological Organization

The unit of histological organization of skeletal muscle is the *fiber,* a long cylindrical multinucleate cell visible with the light microscope. Large numbers of parallel muscle fibers are grouped into *fascicles*, which are visible to the naked eye in fresh muscle. The fascicles are associated in various patterns to form the several types of *muscles* recognized by the anatomist—unipennate, bipennate,

and so on. The individual muscle fibers, the fascicles, and the muscle as a whole are each invested by connective tissue that forms a continuous stroma, but its different parts are designated by separate terms for convenience of description. The entire muscle is enclosed by a connective tissue layer called the *epimysium* (Fig. 10–7). Thin collagenous septa that extend inward from the epimysium, surrounding each and all of the fascicles, collectively make up the *perimysium,* and the exceedingly delicate reticulum that invests the individual muscle fibers constitutes the *endomysium.* The connective tissue serves to bind together the contractile units and groups of units and to integrate their action; it also allows a certain degree of freedom of motion between them. Thus, although the muscle fibers are very closely packed together, each is somewhat independent of adjacent fibers, and each fascicle can move independently of neighboring fascicles.

The blood vessels supplying skeletal muscle course in the connective tissue septa and ramify to form a rich capillary bed around the individual muscle fibers (Fig. 10–9). The capillaries are sufficiently tortuous to permit their accommodation to changes in length of the fibers, by straightening during elongation and contorting during contraction.

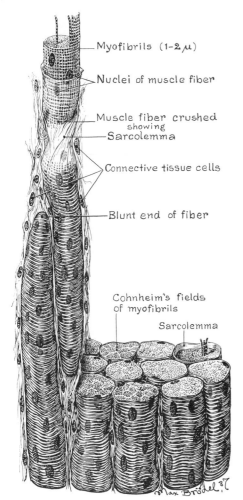

Myofibrils (1-2μ)

Nuclei of muscle fiber

Muscle fiber crushed showing Sarcolemma

Connective tissue cells

Blunt end of fiber

Cohnheim's fields of myofibrils

Sarcolemma

Figure 10–8. Drawing of the relationships of skeletal muscle fibers. (From Brödel, M. Bull. Johns Hopkins Hosp. *61*:295, 1937.)

In muscles that do not taper at the ends, such as the sartorius, the fibers apparently continue without interruption through the entire length of the muscle. It is generally believed, however, that in most muscles the fibers are shorter than the muscle as a whole, seldom extending from its origin to its insertion, but being connected at one end to connective tissue septa within the muscle and at the other to the tendon.

The thickness of the muscle fibers ranges from 10 to 100 μm or more, depending on the species and the particular muscle examined. Fibers within the same muscle may vary considerably in their caliber. During the growth of the organism, the diameter of the fibers increases with age, and in the grown individual it may undergo further increase in response to strenuous muscular activity—a phenomenon referred to as *hypertrophy of use*

and exemplified in the bulging biceps of the boxer and the leg muscles of the ballerina. Conversely, the fibers may become thinner in muscle immobilized for long periods as in the treatment of fracture, a change called *atrophy of disuse.*

Cytology of the Muscle Fiber

The individual fibers can be separated by teasing fresh muscle apart under a dissecting microscope. In addition to the obvious transverse striations that give this type of muscle its name, a more delicate longitudinal striation is also discernible within the muscle fiber. The structural basis of this longitudinal striation becomes apparent when samples of muscle are treated with dilute nitric acid. In such macerated specimens, the *sarcolemma*, the limiting membrane of the fiber, is destroyed; the cytoplasmic matrix, called the *sarcoplasm*, is extracted; and the contractile substance of the muscle fiber separates into a large number of thin, parallel, cross-striated *myofibrils.* The fine longitudinal striation detectable within the fresh muscle fiber is thus attributable to the parallel arrangement of myriad myofibrils within its sarcoplasm. The transverse striation comes about because each myofibril is made up of cylindrical segments or bands of different refractility that alternate regularly along its length. The corresponding segments of the closely packed parallel myofibrils are usually in register, so that the striations appear to extend across the whole width of the fiber (Figs. 10–11, 10–12).

Each muscle fiber is invested by a delicate membrane just visible with the compound microscope. In teased fresh preparations, where the fiber has been torn or crushed, it appears as a thin, transparent film (Fig. 10–8). This investment has traditionally been called the sarcolemma. It has recently become apparent from electron microscopic studies that this film, visible with the light microscope, is not a single component but consists of the plasmalemma of the muscle fiber, its glycoprotein external coating, and a delicate network of associated reticular fibers. In current usage, the term *sarcolemma* is reserved for the plasmalemma of the muscle fiber, and the other components of the traditional sarcolemma are separately designated. The sarcolemma differs in no essential respect from the limiting membrane of any other cell. It should be realized that this membrane alone is not resolved by the ordinary microscope under the usual conditions of observation,

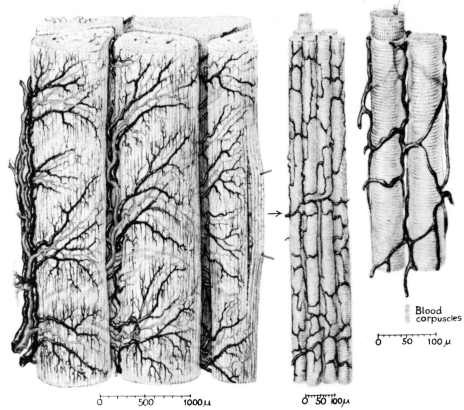

Figure 10–9. *A,* Drawing of the blood supply of muscle bundles in the human rectus abdominis muscle. *B,* The capillary network of the muscle fibers. *C,* The same at higher magnification. (From Brödel, M. Bull. Johns Hopkins Hosp. *61*:295, 1937.)

but with the added thickness of its associated amorphous and fibrous investments, a limiting layer is visible.

The nuclei of the striated muscle fiber are numerous. No actual number can be specified, for this depends on the length of the muscle, but in a fiber several centimeters long there would be several hundred nuclei. They are elongated in the direction of the fiber. Their position varies according to the type of muscle and the animal species, but in the great majority of skeletal muscles of mammals the nuclei are located at the periphery of the fiber, immediately beneath the sarcolemma. This is especially apparent in transverse sections (Fig. 10–10). This characteristic position is a helpful criterion for distinguishing skeletal from cardiac muscle, in which the nuclei are centrally located.

The nuclei of the muscle cells usually have one or two nucleoli and moderately abundant chromatin distributed along the inner aspect of the nuclear envelope. A small number of other nuclei, of similar elongated form but with a coarser chromatin pattern, are closely associated with the surface of the muscle fibers. These belong to elongated *satellite cells,* which are flattened against the muscle fiber or occupy shallow depressions in its surface and are enclosed within the same investing layer of glycoprotein and reticular fibers. The cytoplasm of the satellite cell is scanty and its boundary with the muscle fiber usually cannot be resolved with the light microscope. Skeletal muscle fibers have a limited capacity for regeneration. After minor injury muscle fibers often regenerate. The satellite cells within the intact external lamina serve as stem cells that proliferate and differentiate into myoblasts, which fuse to form myotubes and ultimately new muscle fibers. If the injury has resulted in disruption of the external lamina, regeneration does not occur; the area is invaded by fibroblasts and fibrous scar tissue is formed.

The sarcoplasm of a muscle fiber corre-

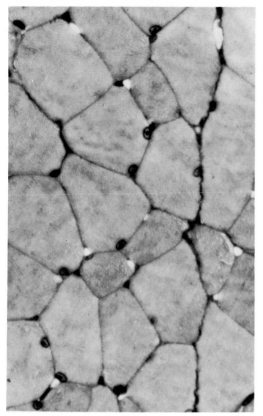

Figure 10–10. Photomicrograph of skeletal muscle fibers in cross section, illustrating their polygonal outline and the peripheral position of their nuclei.

This network appeared to surround all of the myofibrils and was called the *sarcoplasmic reticulum.* It was demonstrated with difficulty by the light microscope, and many observers doubted its reality, but the presence of this organelle has now been verified in electron micrographs and will be described later in this chapter.

Lipid droplets are found in varying numbers in the muscles of some species. They may be situated between the myofibrils or among the clusters of mitochondria at the poles of the nuclei and at the periphery of the fiber. In appropriately stained preparations, small amounts of glycogen can be demonstrated throughout the sarcoplasmic matrix. In addition to these microscopically visible inclusions, the sarcoplasm of the living muscle contains the oxygen-binding protein *myoglobin.* In muscle at rest, oxygen probably remains bound to myoglobin, but when demand for oxygen increases, it dissociates from myoglobin and is available for oxidations. In man, myoglobin is of relatively little significance in skeletal muscle, but in diving mammals and in birds, it is especially abundant and probably of great physiological importance.

Most of the interior of the muscle fiber is occupied by myofibrils 1 to 2 μm in diameter. In transverse sections they are resolved as fine dots either uniformly distributed or grouped in polygonal areas called the *fields of Cohnheim.* Whether this polygonal pattern represents the true distribution of myofibrils or is a consequence of shrinkage was long debated. The weight of evidence now favors its interpretation as a shrinkage artifact, and no functional significance is now attached to Cohnheim's fields.

In longitudinal sections of muscle the feature of greatest interest is the cross striation of the myofibrils. The cylindrical segments of the myofibrils, which are markedly refractile and dark in fresh muscle, stain intensely with iron-hematoxylin in histological sections, while the less refractile, alternate segments remain essentially unstained (Fig. 10–11). When muscle is examined with the polarizing microscope, the contrast of the bands is reversed. The dark-staining bands are now birefringent or anisotropic *(A bands)* and therefore appear bright, whereas the *light* staining bands are isotropic *(I bands)* or only very weakly anisotropic and thus appear *dark.* In the most commonly used terminology, the

sponds to the cytoplasm of other types and can be defined as the contents of the sarcolemma exclusive of the nuclei. It consists, therefore, of a typical cytoplasmic matrix and the usual cell organelles and inclusions as well as the myofibrils peculiar to muscle. Although not visible in routine preparations, the Golgi apparatus can be demonstrated by special staining methods. As might be expected in a multinucleate syncytium, there are multiple small Golgi bodies, which are located near one pole of each nucleus throughout the muscle fiber. The mitochondria (formerly called *sarcosomes*) are most abundant near the poles of the nuclei and immediately beneath the sarcolemma, but they also occur in the interior of the fiber, where they are distributed in longitudinal rows between the myofibrils.

Several early cytologists examining preparations of muscle that were impregnated with heavy metals described a lacelike network of dark strands in the interfibrillar sarcoplasm.

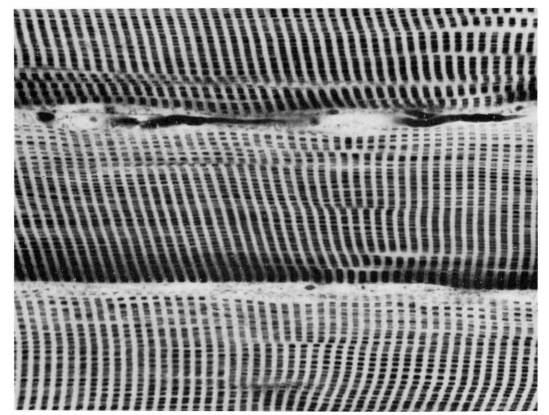

Figure 10–11. Photomicrograph of three muscle fibers in longitudinal section. The transverse dark A bands and light I bands are clearly shown. Preparation stained with iron-hematoxylin.

principal bands are named A band and I band, according to their appearance in polarized light. The relative lengths of the bands vary, depending on whether the muscle is examined at resting length, during contraction, or when passively stretched. The length of the A band remains constant in all phases of contraction, but the I band is most prominent in stretched muscle, is shorter at resting length, and is extremely short in contraction. Both in stained preparations and in living muscle viewed with phase contrast, a dark transverse line, the Z *line*, bisects each I band. The repeating structural unit, to which all the morphological events of the contractile cycle are referred, is the *sarcomere*, which is defined as the segment between two successive Z lines and therefore includes an A band and half of the two contiguous I bands. In histological sections of skeletal muscle, the A bands, I bands, and Z lines are usually the only cross striations discernible, but in exceptional preparations a paler zone, called the *H band*, may be seen traversing the center of

the A band. In its center is a narrow dark line, the *M band* or M line, located precisely in the middle of the A band. Although all these features of the cross-banded pattern of striated muscle can be seen with the light microscope, they can be demonstrated and interpreted more clearly in electron micrographs, and will be discussed in greater detail below in the section on the ultrastructure of the sarcoplasm.

Cytological Heterogeneity of Skeletal Muscle Fibers

When muscles are examined in the fresh condition by the naked eye, they differ somewhat in color. It has also been recognized since the late 1800s that the fibers making up a single muscle are not uniform in their size or cytological characteristics. In *red muscles,* small dark fibers with a granular appearance predominate, whereas in *white muscles,* paler fibers of larger diameter predominate. Differences among the fibers were not con-

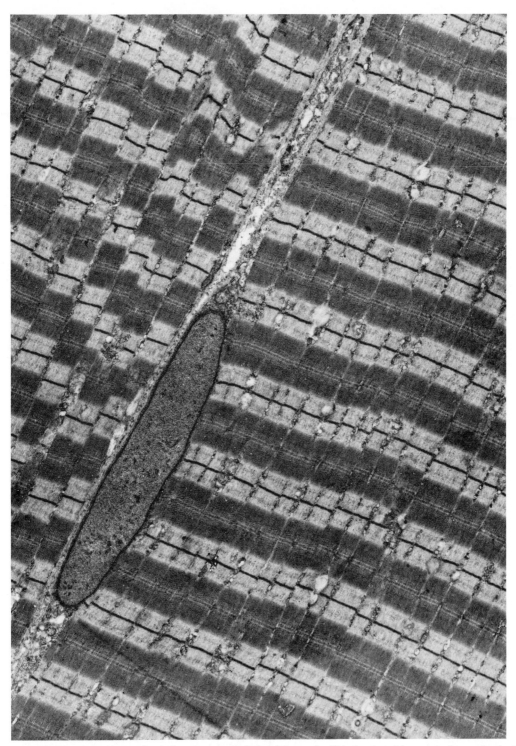

Figure 10–12. Electron micrograph of glycerin-extracted skeletal muscle. This treatment improves the contrast of the myofibrils. Observe the uniform diameter of the myofibrils and the peripheral location of the nucleus. Corresponding bands of adjacent myofibrils are usually in register across the muscle fiber. Where they are out of register, as at upper left, this is usually an artifact of specimen preparation.

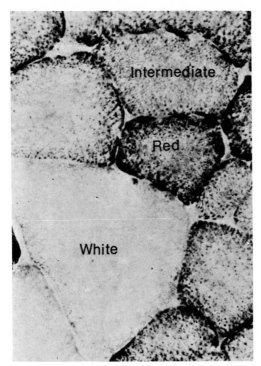

Figure 10–13. Photomicrograph of skeletal muscle in cross section stained for the enzyme succinic dehydrogenase. Three categories of fibers are distinguished: small red fibers rich in peripheral mitochondria; large white fibers with relatively few mitochondria; and fibers with intermediate characteristics. (Photomicrograph courtesy of G. Gautier.)

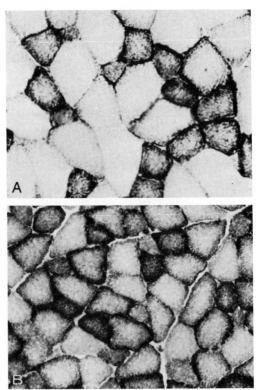

Figure 10–14. Succinic dehydrogenase reaction in skeletal muscle. *A,* Plantaris muscle of a control guinea pig. *B,* Same muscle of an animal after 8 weeks of running on a treadmill. The fiber population of the exercised muscle is more homogeneous—nearly all fibers are small and rich in mitochondria. (Photomicrographs from Faulkner, J. A. *In* Podolsky, R. J., ed.: Contractility of Muscle Cells and Related Processes. Englewood Cliffs, NJ, Prentice-Hall, 1944.)

spicuous in routine histological preparations, but when histochemical methods for localizing enzymatic activity became available, the distinctions between fiber types could be clearly demonstrated and defined more accurately. Staining for the enzyme succinic dehydrogenase clearly identifies the smaller red fibers because of their great abundance of mitochondria. Differences in myoglobin concentration and in myofibrillar adenosine triphosphatase and phosphorylase activity can also be demonstrated.

The multiplicity of fiber types recognizable by these methods has led to some terminological confusion. In the interests of simplicity and continuity with tradition, we adopt here the terms *red, intermediate,* and *white* fibers. The red fibers are small in diameter, rich in myoglobin (Figs. 10–13, 10–14, 10–15,) and have a richer blood supply. In electron micrographs, the Z lines are thicker; profiles of sarcoplasmic reticulum are more complex in the region of the H band; and the mitochondria located in the periphery of the fibers and in rows between the myofibrils are nu-

merous, large, and provided with many cristae. Such fibers, also called *slow fibers,* are easily stimulated but have a slow conduction rate (50–80 m/sec) and are innervated by small axons. On the other hand, white fibers, also called *fast fibers,* are larger in diameter; their Z lines are relatively narrow; the pattern of sarcoplasmic reticulum is simpler and the mitochondria are sparse, with subsarcolemmal and interfibrillar accumulations generally absent. They have a rapid conduction rate (70–110 m/sec); are less easily stimulated; are innervated by larger axons; and have a less rich blood supply. There are also differences in the neuromuscular junctions.

The variations in color of different muscles are a reflection of the differing proportion of the three fiber types. The proportions are usually fairly constant for a given muscle, and it was formerly thought that the mechanical and metabolic properties of muscle fibers

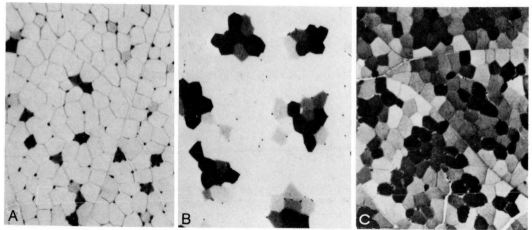

Figure 10–15. Sections of the longissimus muscle of rabbit *(A)*, pig *(B)*, and ox *(C)*, reacted for myoglobin. The species differences in the number of distribution of myoglobin-positive cells is obvious. (Photomicrograph from Cassens, R. G. J. Histochem. Cytochem. *18*:364, 1970.)

were immutable. It is now known that, under appropriate conditions, a fast muscle fiber can be changed into a slow one and vice versa. If the innervations of a postural and a locomotor muscle are cross-transplanted, there is a gradual change in the mechanical and chemical properties of the muscles. Forced exercise training can also increase capillary number, mitochondrial density, and activity of oxidative enzymes (Fig. 10–14).

The Ultrastructure of the Sarcoplasm

The common organelles observed in the sarcoplasm do not depart significantly in fine structure from those in other cell types. The small Golgi complex found near many of the nuclei does not appear especially active. The mitochondria are abundant at the poles of the nuclei and beneath the sarcolemma. In addition, a considerable number are lodged in narrow clefts between the myofibrils. In keeping with the high energy requirements for muscle contraction, the mitochondria have very numerous, closely spaced cristae. Their intimate association with the contractile elements brings the source of chemical energy (ATP) close to the sites of its utilization in the myofibrils.

An important organelle that cannot profitably be studied with the light microscope is the *sarcoplasmic reticulum*, a continuous system of membrane-limited *sarcotubules* that extend throughout the sarcoplasm and form a close-meshed canalicular network around each myofibril (Figs. 10–16, 10–17). This organelle corresponds to the endoplasmic reticulum of

other cell types, but in muscle it is largely devoid of associated ribosomes and exhibits a highly specialized repeating pattern of local differentiations that bear a constant relationship to particular bands of the striated myofibrils. The tubules of the reticulum overlying the A bands have a prevailing longitudinal orientation but anastomose freely in the region of the H band (Fig. 10–17). At regular intervals along the length of the myofibrils, the longitudinal *sarcotubules* are confluent with transversely oriented channels of larger caliber called *terminal cisternae*. Pairs of parallel terminal cisternae run transversely across the myofibrils in close apposition to a slender intermediate element, the transverse tubule, commonly called the *T tubule*. These three associated transverse structures constitute the so-called *triads* of skeletal muscle (Figs. 10–16, 10–17). In amphibian muscle, the triads are found encircling each I band at the level of the Z line (Fig. 10–17). In mammalian muscle there are two triads to each sarcomere, situated at the junctions of each A band with the adjacent I bands. The lumen of the slender T tubule does not open into the adjacent cisternae and, strictly speaking, is not a part of the sarcoplasmic reticulum. Its limiting membrane is continuous with the sarcolemma and its lumen communicates with the extracellular space at the cell surface. It is therefore to be regarded as a slender tubular invagination of the sarcolemma penetrating deep into the interior of the muscle fiber. To emphasize their separate identity and to distinguish the T tubules from elements of the sarcoplasmic reticulum, they

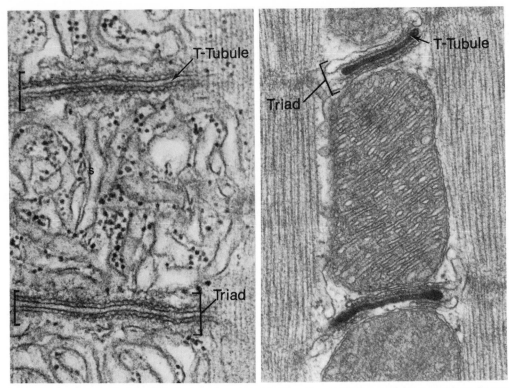

Figure 10–16. *A,* Micrograph of a longitudinal section of skeletal muscle, passing tangential to a myofibril. Observe the longitudinal tubules of the sarcoplasmic reticulum and two transversely oriented triads at the level of the A-I junctions. Glycogen particles are present among the sarcotubules. *B,* Longitudinal section of muscle that has been immersed in peroxidase. The dense-reaction product of the peroxidase is present in the lumen of the tubules, demonstrating continuity of the lumen with the extracellular space. (Micrograph courtesy of D. Friend.)

are referred to collectively as the *T system* of the muscle fiber.

The longitudinal tubules and terminal cisternae of the sarcoplasmic reticulum are now known to regulate the concentration of calcium ions in the microenvironment of the myofibrils. The limiting membrane of the reticulum possesses an active calcium transport mechanism, and calcium is stored within this organelle. Neurally induced depolarization of the sarcolemma is conducted into the muscle fiber by the T tubules. An ATP-dependent mechanism at the junctions of the T tubules with the terminal cisternae of the triads results in release of calcium from the sarcoplasmic reticulum, triggering contraction of the myofibrils. When depolarization of the sarcolemma by nerve impulses ends, calcium is actively transported back into the sarcoplasmic reticulum. The lowering of the calcium concentration around the myofibrils brings about cessation of their contraction.

The Substructure of the Myofibrils. The myofibrils, the smallest units of the contrac-

tile material visible with the light microscope (Fig. 10–18*C,D*), are found in electron micrographs to be composed of smaller units, the *myofilaments* (Fig. 10–18*E*). These are of two kinds, differing in dimensions and chemical composition. The cross-banded pattern of striated muscle reflects the arrangement of these two sets of submicroscopic filaments. The thicker *myosin* filaments, 15 nm in diameter and 1.5 μm long, are parallel and about 45 nm apart. The parallel arrays of myosin filaments are the principal constituent of the A band and determine its length (Fig. 10–18*E*). The filaments are slightly thicker in the middle and taper toward both ends. They are held in register by slender cross connections that are aligned at the midpoint of the A band, giving rise to the transverse density recognized as the M line. In cross sections at the level of the H band, the filaments are disposed in an extremely regular array (Fig. 10–18*G*). The thinner *actin* filaments, 5 nm in diameter, extend about 1 μm in either direction from the Z line and

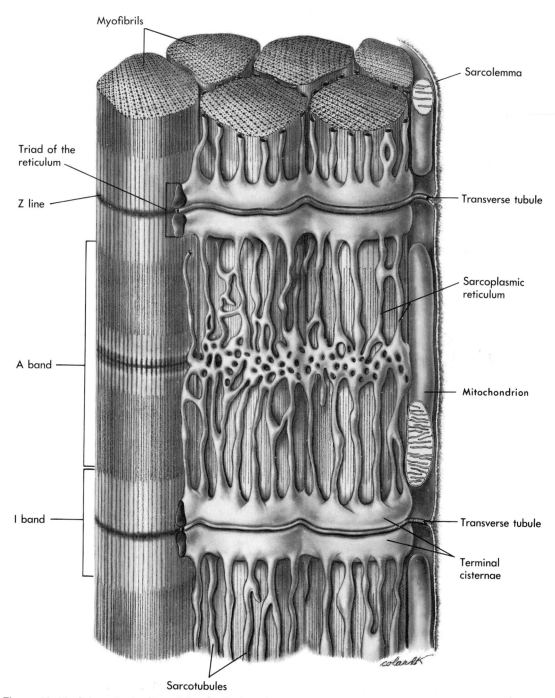

Myofibrils

Sarcolemma

Triad of the
reticulum

Z line

Transverse tubule

A band

Sarcoplasmic
reticulum

Mitochondrion

I band

Transverse tubule

Terminal
cisternae

Sarcotubules

Figure 10–17. Schematic drawing of the distribution of the sarcoplasmic reticulum around myofibrils of amphibian skeletal muscle. The longitudinal sarcotubules are confluent with transverse terminal cisternae. A slender transverse T tubule extending inward from the sarcolemma is flanked by two terminal cisternae to form the "triads" of the reticulum. In amphibian muscle *(depicted here)* the triads are at the Z lines. In mammalian muscle, there are two to each sarcomere, located at the A-I junctions. (Modified from Peachey, L. J. Cell Biol. *25*:209, 1965; from McNutt, S., and D. W. Fawcett. J. Cell Biol. *42*:46, 1969.)

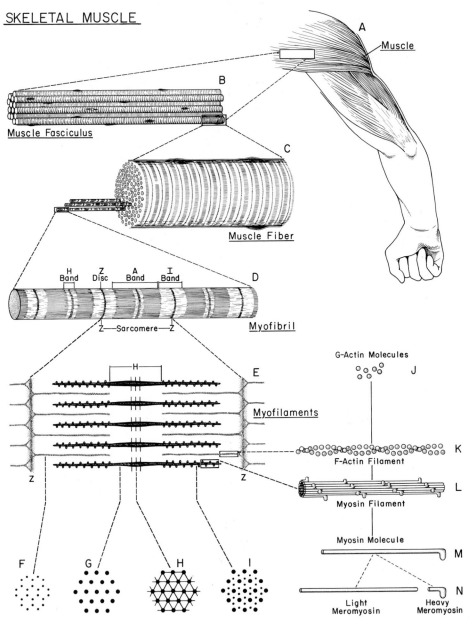

Figure 10–18. Diagram of the organization of skeletal muscle from the gross to the molecular level. *F, G, H,* and *I* show the arrangement of filaments in cross section at the levels indicated. (Drawing by Sylvia Colard Keene.)

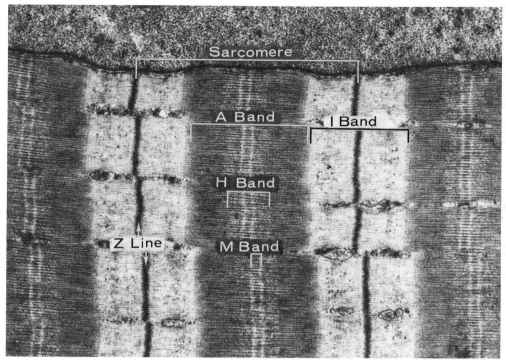

Figure 10–19. Micrograph of several juxtanuclear myofibrils labeled to indicate the various bands in the normal pattern of cross striations in relaxed skeletal muscle.

thus constitute the I band. They are not limited to this band, however, but extend some distance into the adjacent A band, where they occupy the interstices between the hexagonally packed thick filaments. Thus, in cross sections near the ends of the A band, the punctate profiles of six thin actin filaments are evenly spaced around each

myosin filament (Figs. 10–18*I*, 10–22). The depth to which the ends of the actin filaments penetrate into the A band varies with the degree of contraction (Fig. 10–20). In the relaxed condition, the thin filaments that extend into the A band from opposite ends do not meet. The distance between their ends determines the width of the H band, which

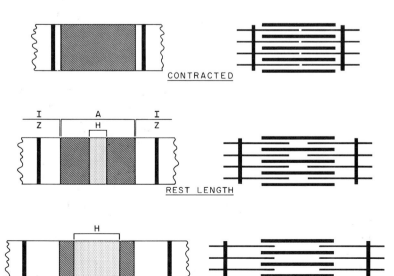

Figure 10–20. *Left,* a schematic representation of the changing appearance of the cross striations in different phases of contraction. *Right,* the differing degrees of interdigitation of the thick and thin filaments corresponding to the different patterns of striation.

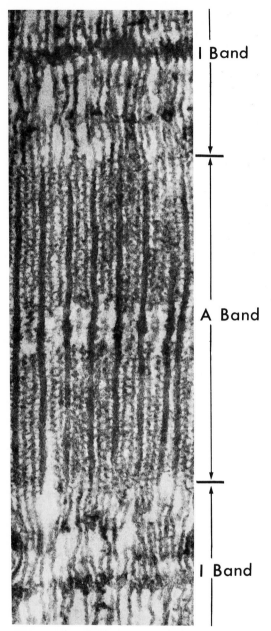

I Band

A Band

I Band

Figure 10–21. Electron micrograph of a sarcomere of rabbit psoas muscle. In the I band, only thin actin filaments are present. In the A band *(central portion of figure),* the thin filaments interdigitate with a set of thicker myosin filaments. Cross bridges between the myosin and actin filaments recur at regular intervals in the region of overlap. (Micrograph courtesy of H. Huxley.)

and this narrow interval is traversed by regularly spaced cross bridges that extend radially from each myosin filament toward the neighboring actin filaments (Figs. 10–18, 10–21, 10–24).

The details of the interrelation of filaments of successive sarcomeres at the Z disc are still a subject of debate, but certain points seem to be adequately established. Each actin filament approaching the Z line appears to be continuous with four diverging thin strands called Z filaments. Each of these runs obliquely through the Z disc to one of the actin filaments on the other side. The actin filaments approaching the Z line from opposite sides are offset, so that in longitudinal sections the cross-connecting Z filaments produce a characteristic zigzag pattern. In addition to the Z filaments, there appears to be a dense amorphous component simply referred to as "Z disc material" or "Z disc matrix." This component varies in abundance in different skeletal muscles and is more easily extractable than the filaments. Its association with the Z disc seems quite selective for when the matrix material is added back to extracted glycerinated muscle, it accumulates around the Z filaments and restores the Z band density. The exact chemical nature of the Z filaments is not yet clear. In addition to the complex of actin filaments, the Z band contains the protein α-*actinin,* which contributes to its electron density and probably plays a role in binding the actin filaments together.

At the level of the Z bands, each myofibril is surrounded by a honeycomb-like network of *desmin* filaments and *vimentin* filaments. It is believed that the networks of 10-nm filaments extending across the muscle fiber serve to link adjacent myofibrils together and thus maintain the lateral register of the sarcomeres.

Although no further detail can be observed in electron micrographs of thin sections of muscle, the analysis of the contractile material has been carried further by mechanical disintegration of myofibrils under conditions that permit the release of the individual myofilaments. These have been studied with the electron microscope after metal shadowing and with negative staining procedures.

The isolated thick filaments are 1.5 μm long. They have a smooth central region, but toward either end they bear short lateral projections corresponding to the cross bridges seen between the thick and thin filaments in intact myofibrils. When further dis-

is defined as the central region of the A band that is not penetrated by the actin filaments. In stretched myofibrils the H band is therefore broad, whereas in the contracted state it is very narrow or entirely absent (Fig. 10–20). In the region of their interdigitation at the ends of the A band, the parallel thick and thin filaments are only 10 to 20 nm apart,

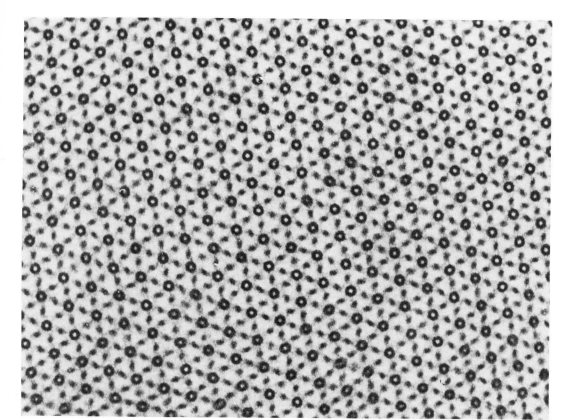

Figure 10–22. Micrograph of a cross section through the A band of insect flight muscle at high magnification, showing the orderly arrangement of actin filaments around the larger myosin filaments. The general pattern is similar in vertebrate muscle but usually does not exhibit such a highly ordered "crystalline" lattice. (Micrograph courtesy of H. Ris.)

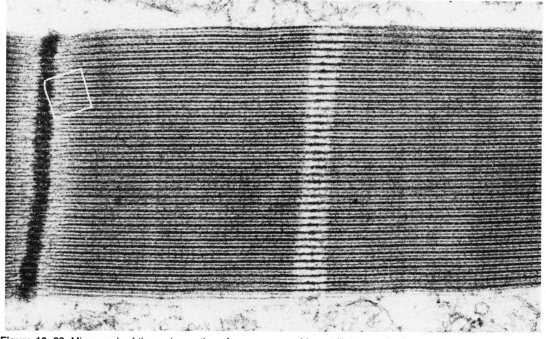

Figure 10–23. Micrograph of the major portion of a sarcomere of insect flight muscle. Cross bridges between the thick and thin filaments are barely detectable, but are more apparent if an area of mammalian muscle comparable with that in the square is examined in replica after rapid freezing, cleaving, and deep-etching (see Fig. 10–24). (High-voltage micrograph courtesy of H. Ris.)

← —— I band —————→ Z line←—— I band —————→/←— A band ——→

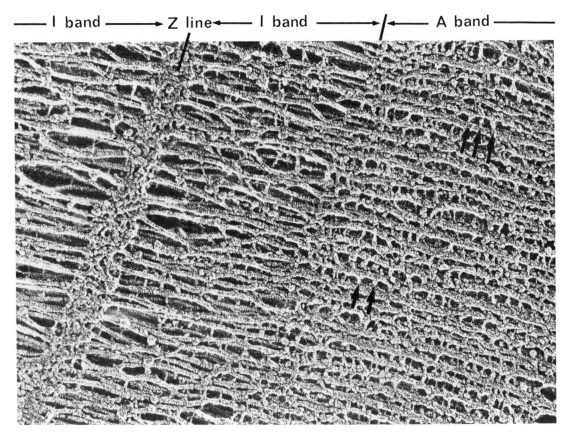

Figure 10–24. Micrograph of a region of skeletal muscle (comparable with that indicated in the square in Fig. 10–23) prepared by rapid freezing in liquid helium, deep-etching, and rotary shadowing. The cross bridges between the myosin and actin filaments are evident. (Micrograph courtesy of N. Hirokawa and J. Heuser.)

sociation of the filaments is carried out, myosin molecules are obtained. These are rodlike structures about 200 nm long and 2 to 3 nm in diameter, consisting of two helically entwined polypeptides each terminating in a globular head that diverges laterally from the backbone of the molecule (Fig. 10–25A). The heads of the molecule form the cross bridges of the myosin filament and are the site of ATP binding and myosin-ATPase activity. Upon enzymatic proteolysis the myosin molecule is cleaved into two fragments—a straight fragment of 150,000 M.W. representing the greater part of the length of the molecule and called *light meromyosin (LMM)*, and a shorter fragment called *heavy meromyosin* (HMM), which includes the heads and a short portion of the rodlike backbone of the molecule. Upon further proteolysis, heavy meromyosin yields two subfragments—HMM-S2 (60,000 M.W.), a terminal portion of rod, and HMM S-1, consisting of the two heads that extend at an angle from the rod (Fig. 10–25A). Because of its actin-

binding property, the S-1 fragment is useful in detecting actin filaments by binding to them in morphologically distinctive arrowhead configuration.

Under appropriate physicochemical conditions, myosin molecules will self-assemble in vitro to reconstitute myosin filaments. In so doing they become arranged parallel with the rod portions oriented toward the center of the nascent filament and heads toward the ends (Fig. 10–25B). The overlapping molecules are staggered so that the projecting heads recur at intervals of 14.3 nm, and each pair is rotated 120 degrees with respect to its neighbors to give them a spiral course along the filament. The bare central segment, corresponding to the H band, is a region consisting only of the overlapping antiparallel rod portions of the molecules (Fig. 10–25B).

Isolated thin filaments are about 1 μm in length and are identified biochemically as filamentous actin *(F-actin)*. At very high magnifications they have a beaded appearance, and have been shown to consist of globular

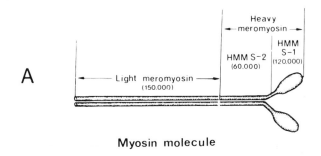

Myosin molecule

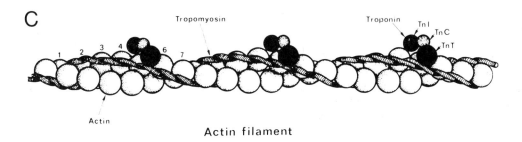

Myosin filament

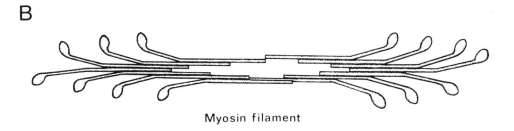

Actin filament

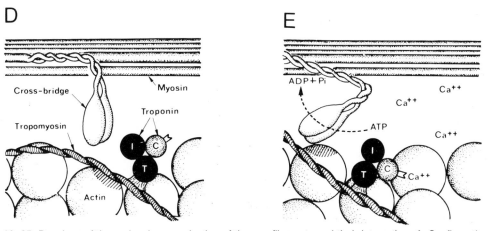

Figure 10–25. Drawings of the molecular organization of the myofilaments and their interaction. *A,* Configuration of an isolated myosin molecule and the fragments obtained when the molecule is cleaved by controlled proteolysis. *B,* Schematic representation of the antiparallel arrangement of myosin molecules in the thick filament. The filament is greatly foreshortened here for illustrative convenience. *C,* The double helical configuration of the actin filament and its associated tropomyosin and troponin. (Redrawn after Junqueira, L. C., and J. Carniero. Basic Histology. Los Altos, CA, Lange Medical Publishers, 1983.) *D* and *E,* Current interpretation of the mechanism of translocation of the actin filament. Calcium binding causes a change in configuration of the troponin-tropomyosin complex, exposing the myosin binding site on actin. The myosin heads energized by ATP then change their angle, moving the actin filament. (Modified after Ganong, W. F. In Review of Medical Physiology, 11th ed. Los Altos, CA, Lange Medical Publishers, 1983.)

subunits 5.6 nm in diameter polymerized to form two strands entwined in a helix with each gyre about 36 nm in length (Fig. 10–25C). The filaments can be dissociated into the globular monomeric subunits (G-actin). When reassembled in vitro, the monomers are consistently oriented to give the filament a definite polarity. In the intact myofibril the actin filaments on either side of the Z line have opposite polarity.

Associated with the double helix of actin is a filament of *tropomyosin* that courses along the groove between the two entwined strands of actin (Fig. 10–25C). The tropomyosin molecule is about 40 nm in length and consists of two polypeptide chains in alpha helical configuration. The molecules are arranged end to end to form the tropomyosin filament.

At regular intervals of about 40 nm along the actin filament, a molecular complex called *troponin* is bound to each molecule of tropomyosin (Fig. 10–25C). It consists of three subunits: one (TnT) that attaches it to tropomyosin; another (TnC) that has a binding site for calcium; and a third (TnI) that inhibits interaction of actin and myosin. When the calcium concentration of the sarcoplasm is low, the tropomyosin filament is so situated that it blocks the myosin binding site on the G-actin monomers. When the calcium concentration rises, calcium is bound to the TnC subunit of troponin, resulting in a configurational change in the complex that changes the position of tropomyosin, exposing the underlying binding site, permitting interaction of the myosin heads with the G-actin subunits of the thin filament, and triggering the movement of the cross bridges that results in displacement of the actin filaments toward the center of the A band (Fig. 10–25D,E).

Sliding Filament Mechanism of Contraction

Although classical cytologists described the changes in the relative lengths of the bands during muscle shortening, these observations suggested no satisfactory explanation of the contractile mechanism. The most common speculation envisioned a process of shortening due to reversible folding and cross-linking of long molecules. In the past two decades, however, detailed analysis of the submicroscopic organization of muscle by electron microscopy and x-ray diffraction has not only revealed the structural relationships responsible for the cross striations but also led to an entirely new concept of the mechanism of contraction. Basic to the new theory was the observation that the length of the A band remains constant during contraction, while the lengths of the H band and the I band both decrease. A possible explanation for these changes in the pattern of cross-banding became apparent when the electron microscope revealed two interdigitating sets of filaments. According to the *sliding filament hypothesis*, when a muscle contracts, the thick and thin filaments maintain the same length but slide past each other, so that the ends of the actin filaments extend farther into the A band, narrowing and ultimately obliterating the H band. As a consequnce of the deeper penetration of the A band by the I filaments, the Z disc is drawn closer to the ends of the adjacent A bands, and there is an overall shortening of the myofibril (Fig. 10–20).

Because the heads of the myosin molecules forming the cross bridges are the only visible structures by which a force could be developed between the thick and thin filaments, it is assumed that this is their function.

Contraction may involve displacement of as much as 300 nm in each half of the sarcomere, while displacement of the distal ends of the bridges from the perpendicular is no more than 10 nm. Therefore, during a single contraction hundreds of bridge-forming and bridge-breaking cycles must take place to produce the observed displacement. For a time some doubt was cast upon the involvement of the bridges in translocation of the actin filaments by the observation in electron micrographs that the interfibrillar distance in some phases of contraction appeared to be greater than the length of the bridging heads of the myosin molecules. This paradox was resolved by the discovery of flexible regions at the base of the heads and at the junction of the heavy meromyosin subunit with the linear backbone of the molecule (Fig. 10–25B). These two flexible couplings permit the heads to attach to the actin filaments over a range of different interfilament distances and still preserve the same orientation relative to the actin. What part of the molecule is the site of development of the force that results in filament movement remains uncertain. But since it is unlikely that it could reside in the flexible region of the molecule, it is speculated that it is in the head, and it is postulated that there is a force generating *active* change in the effective angle of the attachment of the heads to the actin filament.

In the sliding filament mechanism of muscle contraction, the conversion of chemical energy to mechanical work seems to involve the following train of events. In the resting muscle, ATP binds to the ATPase sites on the heads of the myosin molecules (Fig. 10–25D). However, actin is required as a cofactor in the breakdown of ATP to release energy, and interaction of myosin with actin is prevented in the resting muscle by the troponin-tropomyosin blockade of the binding sites on the actin filament. Release of calcium into the surrounding sarcoplasm in response to a nerve impulse is followed by binding of calcium ions to the TnC subunit of troponin (Fig. 10–25E). This results in a change in configuration of the complex that moves the tropomyosin deeper into the groove in the actin helix, exposing the myosin binding sites on the actin filament. Binding activates the myosin ATPase with release of energy from ATP. Active bending or shape change induced in the myosin heads displaces the actin filaments a short distance toward the center of the A bands. This permits alignment of other ATPase-prepared myosin heads with another set of actin subunits for binding in a new cycle of bridge-making and breaking. Contraction continues until calcium ions are taken up and sequestered in the sarcoplasmic reticulum. Troponin-tropomyosin complexes again cover the binding sites on the actin filaments, restoring the resting state (Fig. 10–25D).

Coupling of Excitation to Contraction

The attention of physiologists has long been focused upon the problem of explaining how the myofibrils throughout the muscle fiber are activated simultaneously and almost instantaneously after arrival of a nerve impulse at the sarcolemma. These events take place too rapidly to be explained by inward diffusion of an activating substance liberated from an excitable surface membrane. In a new approach to this problem, a microelectrode was applied to the surface of an isolated muscle fiber and it was found that a local reduction in membrane potential was not equally effective at all points on the surface. It resulted in inward spread of an impulse, leading to contraction only if the tip of the microelectrode was over certain sensitive spots. In frog muscle, these sensitive points

were located only over the I band. There appeared, therefore, to be a structural component at the center of each I band that is responsible for inward conduction.

The discovery of the sarcoplasmic reticulum and the finding of transversely oriented triads at the level of each Z line led to the suggestion that these might be the submicroscopic structures involved in the inward spread of activation. The demonstration that the membranes of the T tubules are continuous with the sarcolemma and that their lumen is open to the extracellular space provided the necessary final link in the evidence for the participation of the T tubules in excitation-contraction coupling. In muscle fibers of amphibians the T tubules are found at the level of the Z disc, while in the skeletal muscle of mammals they are found at the boundary between the A and I bands. Thus, in mammals there are two T tubules to each sarcomere.

The Myoneural Junction

The specialized junctional region at the termination of a motor nerve on skeletal muscle fibers is called the *motor end plate*. It is recognized with the light microscope as a slightly elevated plaque on the muscle fiber, marked by a local accumulation of nuclei (Fig. 10–26A,B). The nuclei are of at least two morphologically distinguishable types. The so-called "arborization nuclei" belong to the terminal sheath cells (Schwann cells) associated with the motor nerve endings. These cells are collectively referred to as the *teloglia*. The second category of nuclei, usually larger and less intensely stained, were called "sole nuclei" in the classical literature. These are simply the nuclei of the underlying muscle fiber that congregate in the region of the myoneural junction. With special methods of impregnation, it can be shown that the axon of the motor nerve, after losing its myelin sheath, forms a terminal arborization over the clustered nuclei of the end plate. The terminal branches of the axons occupy recesses in the surface of the muscle fiber called *synaptic troughs* or *primary synaptic clefts*. When selectively stained, the surface of the underlying muscle fiber is found to be highly differentiated, forming what appear to be evenly spaced, ribbon-like lamellae attached to the sarcolemma by their edges and projecting from the myoneural interface into the underlying sarcoplasm. This specialization of

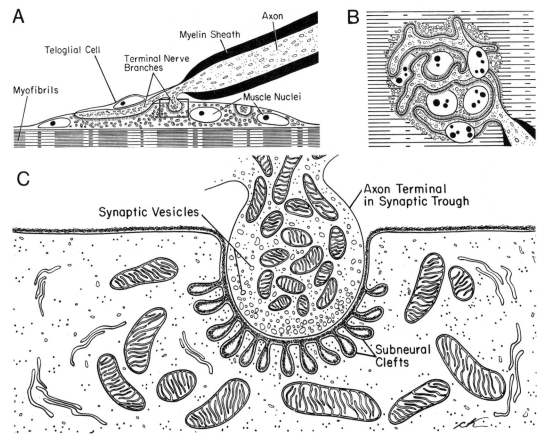

Figure 10–26. Schematic representation of the motor end plate. *A*, End plate as seen in histological sections in the long axis of the muscle fiber; *B*, as seen in surface view with the light microscope; *C*, as seen in an electron micrograph of an area such as that in the rectangle on *A*. (Modified after R. Couteaux.)

the muscle fiber surface is called the *subneural apparatus.*

Electron microscopy has greatly clarified the relationships at the myoneural junction. The teloglial cells cover the outer surface of the axon terminal but never penetrate into the synaptic clefts. Here the nerve and muscle are directly exposed to one another. The so-called "lamellae" of the subneural apparatus are found instead to be narrow *secondary synaptic clefts* formed by infolding of the sarcolemma lining the primary synaptic trough (Fig. 10–26C). These relationships are elegantly displayed in scanning electron micrographs after enzymatic digestion of obscuring connective tissue components. The terminal arborization of the axon in the motor end plate is clearly shown (Fig. 10–27), and if the nerve ending is pulled away the primary and secondary synaptic clefts in the underlying muscle fiber are revealed (Fig. 10–28).

In transmission micrographs the axolemma and the sarcolemma are separated at all points by a glycoprotein boundary layer

similar to that investing the rest of the surface of the muscle fiber. The axoplasm in the nerve terminals contains mitochondria and a very large number of small vesicles (40–60 nm), identical to the *synaptic vesicles* seen at axodendritic synapses in the nervous system (Fig. 10–29). These vesicles are the sites of storage of the neurotransmitter *acetylcholine.* It is estimated that each vesicle may contain 10,000 molecules of acetylcholine. In neural transmission the contents of the synaptic vesicles are released by exocytosis. This takes place at specialized sites in the presynaptic membrane, referred to as *active zones* (Fig. 10–30). When myoneural junctions are studied by the freeze-fracture method the active zones are seen as linear specialization of the membrane running parallel to the ridges and furrows of the subneural specialization of the muscle fiber. The synaptic vesicles cluster in the axoplasm along these active zones (Fig. 10–30B), and in preparations of endings frozen with liquid helium within milliseconds of nerve stimulation, discharging synaptic vesi-

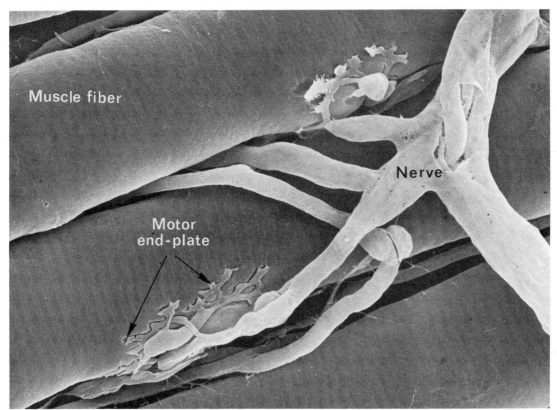

Figure 10–27. Scanning micrograph of motor nerve and two end plates on adjacent muscle fibers. (Micrograph from Desaki, J., and Y. Uehara, J. Neurocytol. *10*:101, 1981.)

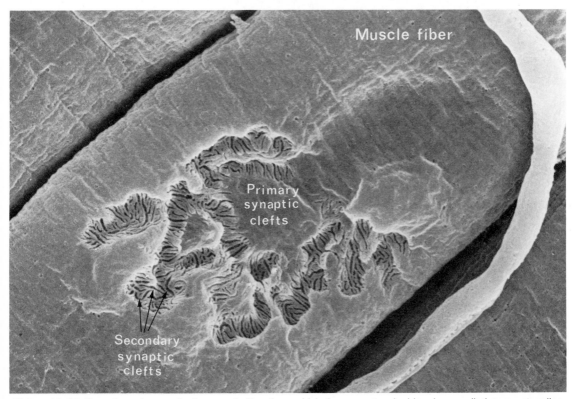

Figure 10–28. Scanning micrograph of a muscle fiber from which the nerve terminal has been pulled away, revealing the underlying primary and secondary synaptic clefts. (Micrograph from Desaki, J., and Y. Uehara, Biomed. Res. 2:Suppl. 139, 1981.)

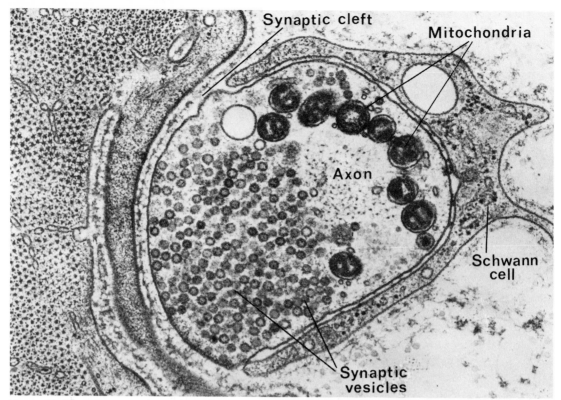

Figure 10–29. Electron micrograph of the nerve ending at the myoneural junction, showing an accumulation of mitochondria and large number of synaptic vesicles in the axoplasm. (Micrograph courtesy of T. Reese.)

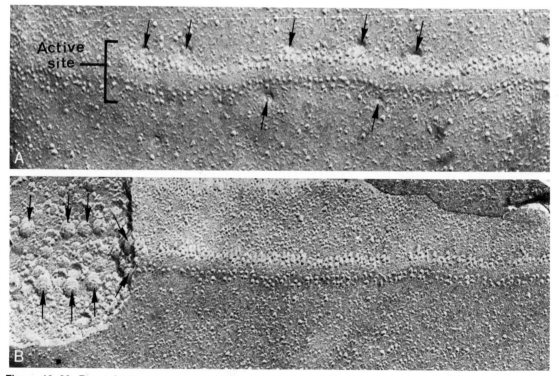

Figure 10–30. Freeze-fracture preparation of the presynaptic membrane at a frog myoneural junction, showing the linear active site. *A,* The nerve was electrically stimulated and the junction frozen within milliseconds; exocytosis of several synaptic vesicles can be seen along the active site *(at arrows)*. *B,* Similar preparation of an unstimulated nerve ending. The fracture plane has broken into the axoplasm showing synaptic vesicles *(at arrows)* clustered near the active site. (Micrograph courtesy of T. Reese.)

cles can be seen along these active zones (Fig. 10–30*A*).

The membrane covering the ridges and clefts of the underlying muscle cell contains a high concentration of *acetylcholine receptors*. In preparations rapidly frozen, deep-etched, and rotary-shadowed these can be seen as closely packed intramembrane particles (Fig. 10–31). When acetylcholine is released into the synaptic cleft, it combines with the receptors and results in a transient increase in the permeability of the membrane to sodium ions. Influx of sodium depolarizes the membrane, generating an *action potential* that is propagated over the sarcolemma and into the T tubules, activating the intracellular release of calcium, which triggers contraction.

The subneural sarcoplasm is unremarkable except for the abundance of its mitochondria. Histochemical studies demonstrate cholinesterase activity in the subneural apparatus of the motor end plate. The major part of this activity is specifically acetylcholinesterase, localized in basal lamina lining the secondary clefts. The acetylcholine released at the motor end plate is rapidly broken down by acetylcholine esterase in the synaptic cleft, thereby limiting the duration of the response to the neurotransmitter.

A reduction in the number of available acetylcholine receptors in myoneural junctions is the basic defect in the human disease *myasthenia gravis,* which is characterized by weakness and fatigability of skeletal muscle. There are normally 30 to 40 million receptors per neuromuscular junction. In myasthenic muscle there is a 70 to 90% reduction in their number.

Neuromuscular Spindles

Skeletal muscle contains complex sensory organs called *muscle spindles.* These fusiform, encapsulated structures consist of several modified striated muscle fibers and their associated nerve endings enclosed in a common sheath. The specialized muscle fibers in the interior of the organ, referred to as *intrafusal fibers,* number from a few to as many as 20, but there are usually about six (Figs. 10–32, 10–33). The fibers are 1 to 5 mm long and attached at their ends to tendon or endomysium. Two distinct types of fibers are present: the *nuclear bag* and *nuclear chain* fibers. Nuclear bag fibers are subdivided into a central or *equatorial segment* and two long tapering *polar segments.* The equatorial segment can be further subdivided on the basis of its struc-

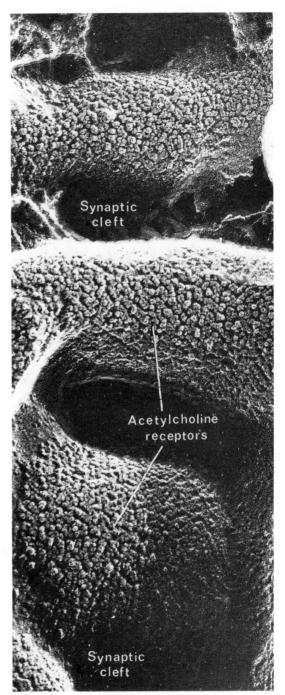

Figure 10–31. Synaptic ridges and clefts of the subneural portion of a motor end plate prepared by rapid freezing, deep-etching, and rotary shadowing. The etching exposes large intramembrane particles in the postsynaptic membrane that are believed to be the acetylcholine receptors. (Micrograph courtesy of N. Hirokawa and J. Heuser.)

tural organization into three regions. The central portion is usually devoid of obvious cross striations and contains an accumulation of 40 to 50 spherical nuclei, which completely

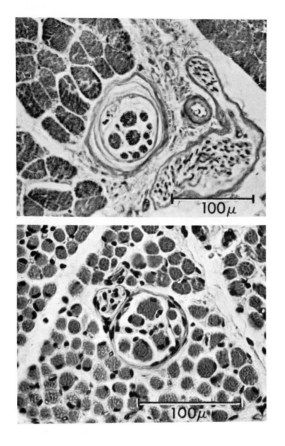

Figure 10–32. *A,* Photomicrograph of a muscle spindle in the lumbrical muscle of a human hand. The equator of the spindle is seen with its laminated capsule and large periaxial space. There are nine intrafusal muscle fibers; three of these are nuclear bag fibers. The other six small muscle fibers, lying in a group, are nuclear chain fibers. A blood vessel and several nerves are also seen. Transverse section. Holmes' silver method. *B,* Muscle spindle in human extrinsic eye muscle. Seven of the muscle fibers are surrounded by a thin capsule and there is a small nerve trunk attached. The muscle spindles are usually smaller than those in the limb muscles and have no nuclear bag fibers in man. Transverse section. Hematoxylin and eosin. (Both photomicrographs courtesy of S. Cooper.)

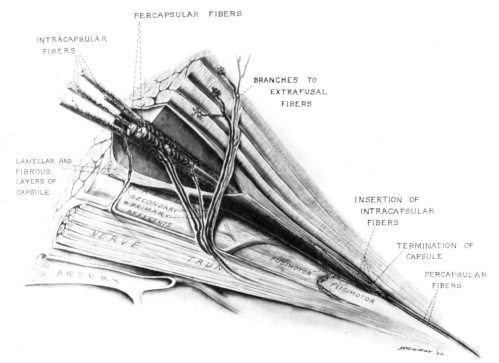

Figure 10–33. Drawing of a muscle spindle and its innervation. The capsule has been cut open to show the periaxial space and the sensory endings of the primary afferent nerves around the central portion of the intrafusal fibers. Near the end of the spindle, fusimotor nerves penetrate, to terminate on the intrafusal fibers in typical motor end plates. (Drawing courtesy of C. F. Bridgman.)

fill and often slightly distend the fiber. This region is referred to as the *nuclear bag*. Extending from it toward either pole is a myotube region, in which oval nuclei are aligned in a row in an axial core of sarcoplasm surrounded by a peripheral layer of cross-striated myofibrils. In the slender polar segments the nuclei are scattered at irregular intervals along the axis of the fiber. In nuclear chain fibers, the nuclei form a single longitudinal row in the central region. The capsule closely invests the poles of the intrafusal fiber but diverges from its surface in the equatorial segment to enclose the *periaxial space*, a fluid filled cavity up to 200 μm in diameter that surrounds the nuclear bag and myotube regions. It has been reported that this space is continuous with the lymphatic system, but this does not seem to have been confirmed, and the space is usually regarded as a closed cavity.

Special kinds of nerve endings are associated with each of the three regions of the intrafusal fiber. The sensory endings supplied by large myelinated afferent fibers are confined to the equatorial segment. The primary sensory or *annulospiral ending* is associated mainly with the nuclear bag or nuclear chain region but may extend into the adjacent myotube region. The endings consist of a complex system of half rings and spirals around the fibers (Figs. 10–33, 10–34). The secondary or *flower-spray* endings are primarily confined to the nuclear chain fibers and localized on either side of the annulospiral endings. Three types of motor terminals are associated with the spindles: fine *fusimotor*, or γ-*efferents* form both motor end plates near the poles of the fibers and unspecialized trail endings near the equatorial region. At the very end of the nuclear bag fibers, collaterals of the motor axons for the extrafusal, slow muscle fibers form "en grappe" terminals, so named because they resemble a bunch of grapes. It must be noted, however, that the details of innervation vary greatly from species to species.

The spindles scattered through skeletal muscles appear to function like miniature strain gauges, sensing the degree of tension in the muscle. The motor innervation of the polar regions of the intrafusal fibers maintains the nuclear bag region under sufficient tension for its stretch receptor endings to be close to their threshold. A further stretch of the equatorial region results in discharge of the spindle afferent fiber, and the frequency of its discharge is proportional to the tension exerted on the intrafusal fiber.

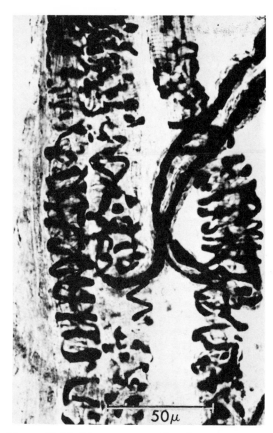

Figure 10–34. Primary nerve ending of a muscle spindle in a cat's plantaris muscle. Two branches of an afferent nerve fiber supply the ending, consisting of two large spirals around the muscle fibers at their nuclear bag regions. Teased gold chloride preparation. (Courtesy of S. Cooper.)

Sensory Nerve Endings in Tendons

There appears to be more than one kind of nerve ending in tendons. In the simplest, unmyelinated nerve fibers ramify over the surface of the collagen bundles. These may possibly give rise to pain sensation on excessive stretch. Of greater interest are the encapsulated *tendon organs*. These are believed to sense tensional stresses produced by muscle pull, and to act as sources of inhibition when muscle contraction becomes excessive. From reconstructions of tendon organs from serial cross sections, it appears that they are composed of specialized, encapsulated fascicles of dense collagen that are subdivisions or branches of the primary tendon of origin or insertion of a muscle. Within this encapsulated region, branches of the entering sensory nerve are entwined among fine bundles of collagen coursing through delicate septa that subdivide the main fascicle of collagen into smaller subunits. Toward the muscle end of the organ, these finer bundles reorganize again into thicker bundles before they interdigitate with the ends of the extrafusal muscle fibers. It is speculated that the spaces between the fine collagen bundles in the relaxed state of the muscle spread open slightly, reducing pressure on the nerve endings lying between them. During muscular contraction, these bundles would straighten and be drawn together, compressing the nerve endings. The compression of the nerve terminals would generate electrochemical events in sensory axons, resulting in transmission of tension information to the central nervous system.

CARDIAC MUSCLE

The heart consists of striated muscle fibers that differ in several respects from those of skeletal muscle. (1) The fibers are not syncytial but are made up of separate cellular units joined end to end by special surface specializations, *intercalated discs,* that run transversely across the fiber (Fig. 10–35). (2) The fibers are not simple cylindrical units but they bifurcate and connect with adjacent fibers to form a complex three-dimensional network.

(3) The elongated nuclei of the cellular units are usually situated deep in the interior of the fiber instead of immediately beneath the sarcolemma (Fig. 10–36). The principal physiological differences between cardiac and skeletal muscle are the spontaneous nature of the beat of cardiac muscle and its rhythmical contraction, which ordinarily is not subject to voluntary control.

The Cytology of Cardiac Muscle

The thin sarcolemma of cardiac muscle is similar to that of skeletal muscle, but the sarcoplasm is relatively more abundant and the mitochondria are much more numerous. The longitudinal striation of the fibers is quite obvious with the light microscope, owing to the subdivision of the contractile material by rows of mitochondria in the interfibrillar sarcoplasm. The pattern of cross striation of the contractile material and the designation of the A, I, M, H, and Z bands is identical to that of skeletal muscle (Fig. 10–37). The myofibrils diverge around the centrally placed nucleus to outline a fusiform axial region of sarcoplasm rich in mitochondria. Near one pole of the nucleus is a small Golgi complex. In the conical regions of sarcoplasm extending in either direction

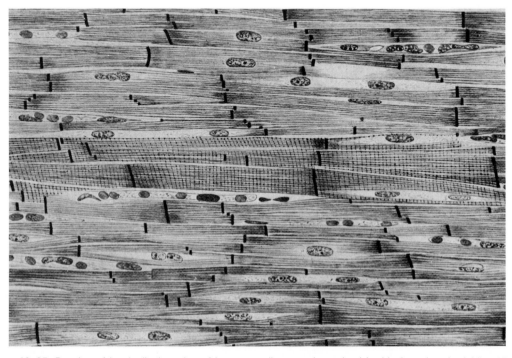

Figure 10–35. Drawing of longitudinal section of human cardiac muscle, stained in thiazin red and toluidine blue to show the intercalated discs. (From H. Heidenhain.)

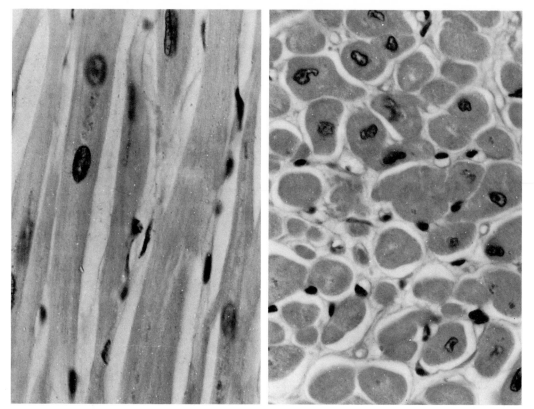

Figure 10–36. *A,* Longitudinal section of human left ventricular muscle, illustrating the variable diameter and branching of the fibers, as well as the central position of the nuclei. In routine hematoxylin and eosin preparations, intercalated discs are not evident. *B,* Cross section of human cardiac muscle.

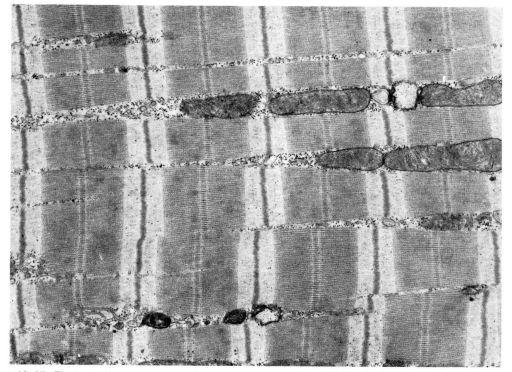

Figure 10–37. Electron micrograph of a portion of a cardiac muscle cell in longitudinal section. The cross-banded pattern of the contractile material is similar to that of skeletal muscle. The numerous mitochondria occupy clefts or fusiform spaces that appear in longitudinal section to subdivide the myofilaments in units comparable with the discrete myofibrils of skeletal muscle. They are, however, much more variable in their width.

from the poles of the nucleus there are often a few droplets of lipid and, in older animals, deposits of lipofuscin pigment. In aged humans this pigment may come to constitute as much as 20 per cent of the dry weight of the myocardium. In small animal species, lipid droplets are plentiful and occur in the interfibrillar sarcoplasm throughout the fiber, often located between the ends of the mitochondria. The sarcoplasm of cardiac muscle is richer in glycogen than is that of skeletal muscle.

At fairly regular intervals along the length of the fibers, the intercalated discs appear as heavy transverse lines. These are relatively inconspicuous in hematoxylin and eosin stains but are clearly revealed in iron-hematoxylin or phosphotungstic acid–hematoxylin preparations. The disc may extend uninterruptedly across the full width of the fiber, but more often it is divided into segments that are offset longitudinally so as to give the disc a steplike configuration. In the repeating pattern of cross striations, the intercalated discs invariably occur at the level of the I bands. They were formerly interpreted as local contraction bands or specializations for intracellular conduction, but they are now known to be devices for maintaining firm

cohesion of the successive cellular units of the myocardium and for transmitting the tension of myofibrils along the axis of the fiber from one cellular unit to the next.

The Submicroscopic Structure of the Sarcoplasm

In electron micrographs, cardiac muscle bears a superficial resemblance to skeletal muscle. Its contractile substance is composed of two sets of myofilaments, thick and thin, in the same interdigitating relationship. In longitudinal section, the tubules of the sarcoplasmic reticulum and rows of mitochondria appear to subdivide the contractile material into myofibrils of variable width (Fig. 10–37). However, upon close examination of transverse sections (Figs. 10–38, 10–39), it becomes evident that the myofilaments are not organized in discrete myofibrils as they are in skeletal muscle. In cross sections the circular profiles of the sarcotubules are aligned in rows that partially demarcate polygonal or irregular areas of myofilaments, but these are usually confluent with adjacent areas of myofilaments over some fraction of their perimeter. Mitochondria often appear completely surrounded by myofilaments (Fig.

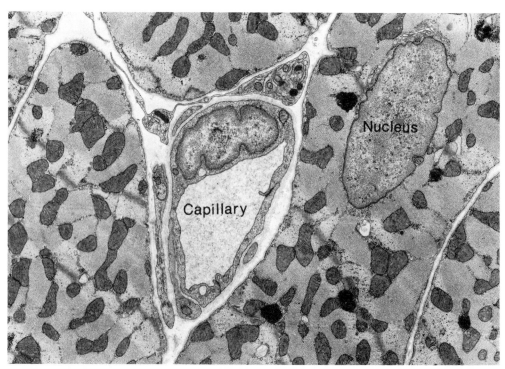

Figure 10–38. A low-power electron micrograph of portions of several cardiac muscle fibers in cross section, illustrating the abundance of large mitochondria, the central location of the nucleus, and the intimate relation of the muscle fibers to the capillaries. Cat papillary muscle.

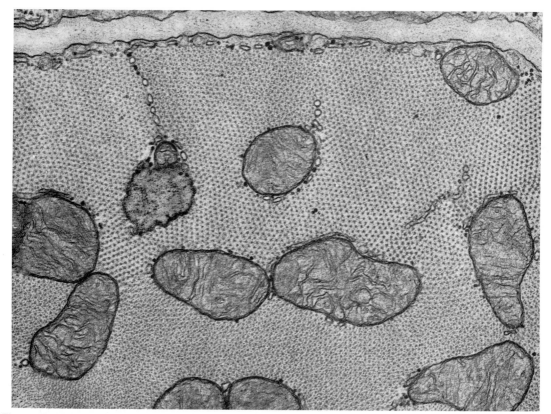

Figure 10–39. Electron micrograph of a small peripheral area of a cardiac muscle fiber in cross section. The myofilaments are not associated in discrete myofibrils with clearly defined limits, but instead form a more or less continuous field interrupted by mitochondria.

10–39). Thus, the contractile substance of cardiac muscle forms a continuum that can be thought of as a large cylindrical mass of parallel myofilaments incompletely subdivided into irregular fascicles by deep incisures and by fusiform or lenticular clefts of sarcoplasm that are occupied by mitochondria and the other organelles essential to the contractile mechanism.

The continuous nature of the contractile mass is not peculiar to cardiac muscle but is also found in certain relatively slow, *tonic* skeletal muscles, particularly in amphibia. The German term *Feldstruktur* has been adopted to describe this pattern of organization of the myofilaments, and the term *Fibrillenstruktur* is applied to the pattern of separate myofibrils that is typical of fast, *twitch* muscles.

The large mitochondria of cardiac muscle have very numerous, closely spaced cristae that often exhibit a periodic angulation of their membranes, giving them a zigzag configuration. As a rule, the mitochondria are about the length of one sarcomere (2.5 μm)

but may occasionally be 7 or 8 μm long. Spherical lipid droplets are often located between the ends of the mitochondria. Glycogen occurs in the form of 30 to 40-nm dense granules crowded into the interstices among the mitochondria. The bulk of the glycogen is located in the interfibrillar sarcoplasm, but particles may also be found aligned in rows between the myofilaments (Fig. 10–41B). They are particularly numerous in the I band and occur more sparsely in the H band. Both the glycogen and the lipid may be used as energy sources for the contractile activity of the myocardium.

The T System and the Sarcoplasmic Reticulum

The tubular invaginations of the sarcolemma that comprise the T system of cardiac muscle are larger than the corresponding intermediate elements of the triads in skeletal muscle. These tubules, representing inward extensions of the extracellular space, are located at the level of the Z lines instead of at

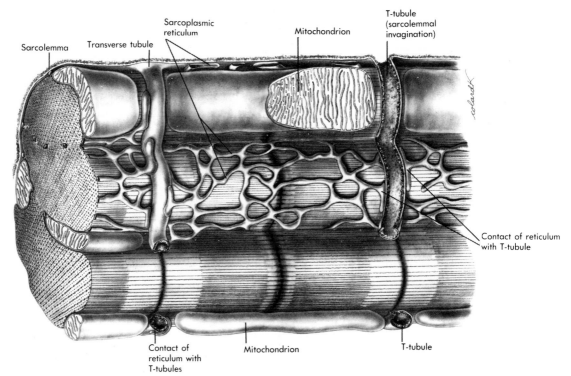

Figure 10–40. Schematic representation of the disposition of the T system and sarcoplasmic reticulum in mammalian cardiac muscle. The transverse tubules are much larger than those of skeletal muscle. The relatively simple sarcoplasmic reticulum has no terminal cisternae and therefore there are no triads. Instead, small expansions to its tubules end in close apposition to the sarcolemma, either at the surface of the fiber or at its inward extension in the T tubules. (From Fawcett, D. W., and N. S. McNutt. J. Cell Biol. *42*:1, 1969.)

the A-I junction and penetrate to the center of the muscle fiber. They are lined by a glycoprotein layer continuous with the external lamina that coats the sarcolemma (Fig. 10–42). Apparently no point in a cardiac muscle fiber is more than 2 to 3 μm from the extracellular space, either at the outer surface of the fiber or in one of the transverse tubules. In addition to playing a role in the coupling of excitation to contraction, these channels no doubt provide important additional surface for the exchange of metabolites between cardiac muscle and the extracellular space.

The sarcoplasmic reticulum is not as highly developed as in skeletal muscle. It consists of a simple plexiform arrangement of tubular elements occupying slender clefts within the mass of myofilaments (Fig. 10–41A). There are no continuous transverse elements of the reticulum comparable with the terminal cisternae of the triads in skeletal muscle. Instead, small terminal expansions of the reticulum here and there are closely applied to the membrane of the T tubes (Fig. 10–42).

Similar contacts are made between small flattened expansions of the reticulum and the sarcolemma at the outer surface of the fiber. The total surface area of the many small sites of apposition of the reticulum to the sarcolemma of cardiac muscle is quite great, but would seem to be considerably smaller than the area of contact between the terminal cisternae and intermediate elements of the triads in skeletal muscle. It is noteworthy, too, that the T tubules in cardiac muscle occur only over the Z lines at the ends of the sarcomeres, whereas in mammalian skeletal muscle there are two triads located at the A-I junctions of each sarcomere. The functional significance of this difference in location of the T system is not fully understood.

The Intercalated Disc

On the transverse portions of the intercalated discs, the opposing ends of the cardiac muscle cells have a deeply sculptured surface. A complex pattern of ridges and papillary projections on each cell fit into corresponding

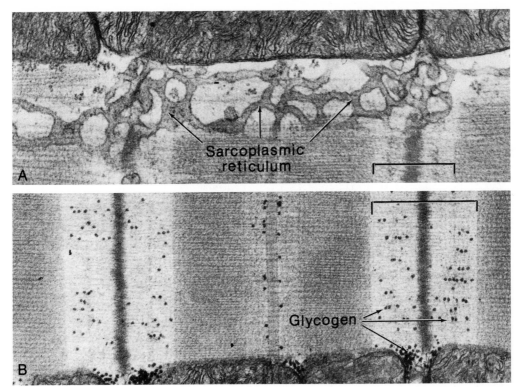

Figure 10–41. Longitudinal sections of cardiac muscle. *A,* The section passes tangentially to an internal surface of the mass of myofilaments and reveals the sarcoplasmic reticulum forming a loose network that continues across the level of the Z lines without any terminal cisternae. *B,* Glycogen particles are seen around mitochondria and between filaments in the I and H bands. The relaxed muscle in these two figures is stretched to different degree. Notice the constancy in length of the I bands, indicated by brackets at right. (From Fawcett, D. W. and N. S. McNutt. J. Cell Biol. *42:*1, 1969.)

grooves and pits in the other cell to form an elaborately interdigitated junction (Figs. 10–43, 10–44). The entire junctional surface of both cells is specialized in various ways for maintaining cell-to-cell cohesion, and one can distinguish areas that are similar in their fine structure to the desmosomes and the zonula adherens of epithelial junctions. However, in the mosaic of different types of surface specialization that constitute the intercalated disc, only the desmosomes are typical with respect to their shape.

The fine structural counterpart of the zonula adherens actually is not beltlike, as is implied by the term *zonula.* Instead there are multiple, moderately extensive but discontinuous areas having irregular and variable outlines. A descriptive term that has been suggested for these is *fascia adherens.*

In longitudinal sections, the opposing cell membranes at the intercalated disc can be identified as two parallel dense lines that follow a sinuous course separated, for the most part, by a 15 to 20-mm intercellular cleft. Over the greater part of the intercalated

disc, the opposing cell surfaces are specialized as fasciae adherentes, with a mat of dense material occurring immediately subjacent to an otherwise unspecialized membrane. The thin filaments of the adjacent I bands terminate in this mat of dense material, which evidently serves to bind the ends of myofilaments to the plasmalemma. At desmosomes along the transverse portions of the disc, the inner leaf of each of the opposing unit membranes is thickened and especially dense. A small condensation of sarcoplasm may be associated with this dense plaque, but the myofilaments usually diverge and do not terminate directly on desmosomes (Fig. 10–44).

At irregular intervals along the disc, the opposing membranes approach to within 2 nm of one another and run parallel for a short distance. These sites of closer apposition were formerly interpreted as "tight junctions" and were termed *maculae occludentes.* Further study of these by the freeze-fracture method has revealed that these correspond instead to the gap junctions of epithelia. There is no fibrous layer or condensation of

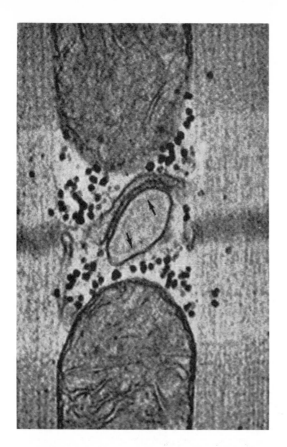

Figure 10–42. Longitudinal section of a small area of a cardiac muscle fiber, illustrating a T tubule cut transversely and a tubule of the reticulum in close apposition to it. The T tubule is lined with a layer of protein-polysaccharide *(at arrows)* like that coating the sarcolemma at the surface of the fiber. The dense granules in the neighboring sarcoplasma are glycogen.

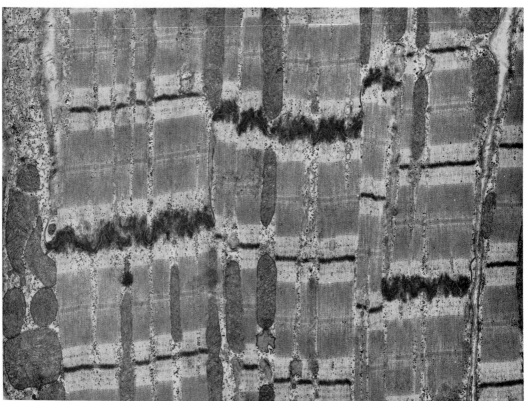

Figure 10–43. Low-power electron micrograph of cardiac muscle in longitudinal section, showing a typical steplike intercalated disc. The transverse portions are highly interdigitated and characterized by an abundance of dense material at the insertions of the myofilaments into the end of the cell. The longitudinal portions of the cell boundary are smooth, unspecialized, and difficult to see at this magnification.

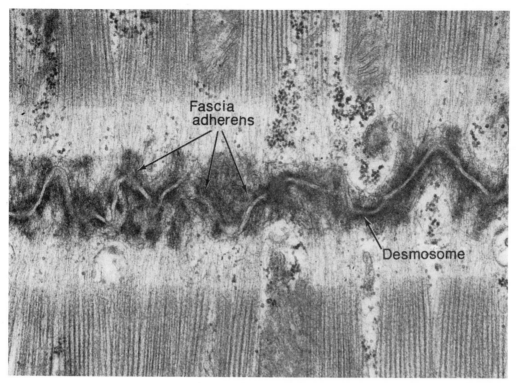

Figure 10–44. Electron micrograph of a transverse segment of an intercalated disc. The portion of the cell junction in which the myofilaments terminate resembles the zonulae adherentes of epithelia, but is here called a fascia adherens. Between sites of myofibril attachment are typical desmosomes. (From Fawcett, D. W., and N. S. McNutt. J. Cell Biol. 42:1, 1969.)

the adjacent sarcoplasm associated with these regions of close apposition.

In addition to the small gap junctions that occur here and there in the transverse portions of the intercalated discs, there are more extensive areas of close membrane apposition on the longitudinal portions of the steplike cell-to-cell junctions, where overlapping processes of successive cells are joined side to side. Considerable emphasis is placed upon these gap junctions because they are areas of low electrical resistance that permit the rapid spread of excitation from cell to cell throughout the heart. Thus, they enable the myocardium to behave as though it were a syncytium. The other specializations of the transverse portions of the intercalated discs, where the surfaces do not have hexagonal arrays of intramembranous particles and are not in such close apposition, evidently have a mechanical significance, being mainly concerned with maintaining cell-to-cell cohesion and transmitting the pull of one contractile unit to the next along the axis of the muscle fibers.

Our understanding of the nature of the forces that bind cells together is still very incomplete, but it is known that calcium ions play an important role. If the beating, isolated heart of an experimental animal is perfused for some time with a calcium-free medium, the heart will soon cease beating. If it is then fixed and examined in thin sections, the individual cells of the muscle fibers are found to have come apart at the intercalated discs. At high magnification it can be ascertained that the membranes, for the most part, are intact but separation has taken place by opening up of the intercellular space. However, at the gap junctions where the membranes are in intimate apposition, the two elements are unable to separate in calcium-free medium, and one or the other of the cells is denuded of its membrane when the ends of the cells are pulled apart in the agonal contractions of the muscle.

Cytological Differences Between Atrial and Ventricular Cardiac Muscle

The fibers of atrial myocardium are basically similar to those of the ventricle described above, but they have a smaller average diameter and the T tubules are few or absent. When found, they tend to be in the larger fibers. It is possible that the smaller fiber diameter may make unnecessary a well-developed system of transverse tubules for inward conduction of the impulse to contract. Despite their smaller diameter, conduction of the action potential over the surface of atrial muscle fibers is said to be more rapid than over ventricular fibers.

Another noteworthy difference is the presence of *specific atrial granules* in these cells. These are membrane-bounded spherical granules 0.3 to 0.4 μm in diameter with a dense homogeneous interior (Fig. 10–45). They are concentrated in the core of sarcoplasm extending in either direction from the poles of the nucleus, usually near the Golgi complex. They have the appearance of secretory granules but until recently their functional significance was a mystery. Two polypeptide hormones have now been extracted from atrial muscle: one, called *cardionatrin*, has potent diuretic and natriuretic effects, and the other, *cardiodilatin*, acts upon vascular smooth muscle, causing relaxation and vasodilation. These polypeptides have been localized immunohistochemically in the granule-containing cells, which are most abundant in the right atrium but also occur in the left atrium. In the light of these unexpected

findings, the right atrium must now be considered an endocrine organ in addition to its contractile and pacemaker functions, and may have a hitherto unsuspected role in the regulation of blood pressure and fluid and electrolyte balance. Its "myoendocrine" cells clearly possess certain morphological and physiological properties in common with the peptide-secreting cells of the gastrointestinal and respiratory tracts.

Cardiodilatin is a polypeptide of 126 amino acids and has a M.W. of about 7500. Cardionatrin is a peptide of 28 amino acids having a sequence similar to a segment of the cardiodilatin molecule. Other small peptides have also been found in extracts of atrium. It is not yet clear whether the myoendocrine cells synthesize a large prohormone that is enzymatically cleaved to form multiple peptide hormones that are stored in the granules, or whether the smaller peptides are fragments produced by the isolation procedure.

Specialized Conducting Tissue of the Heart

In addition to those cells of the myocardium whose primary function is contraction, there is a specialized system made up of

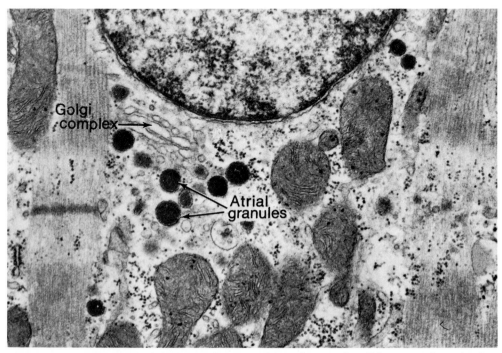

Figure 10–45. Electron micrograph of the juxtanuclear area of a cardiac muscle cell from cat atrium, showing dense spherical atrial granules in the Golgi region. These are now known to contain peptide hormones involved in control of sodium excretion and blood pressure. (From McNutt, N. S., and D. W. Fawcett. J. Cell Biol. *42*:45, 1969.)

modified muscle cells whose function is to generate the stimulus for the heart beat and to conduct the impulse to the various parts of the myocardium in such a way as to ensure the contraction of the atria and ventricles in the proper succession, so that the heart acts as an effective pump. This system consists of the *sinoatrial node* (node of Keith and Flack), the *atrioventricular node* (node of Tawara), and the *atrioventricular bundle* (bundle of His). The sinoatrial node is located beneath the epicardium at the junction of the superior vena cava and the right atrium. The atrioventricular node is found beneath the endocardium in the lower part of the interatrial septum between the attachment of the septal leaf of the tricuspid valve and the opening of the coronary sinus. The atrioventricular bundle originates from the anterior portion of the node and enters the fibrous portion of the interventricular septum, where it soon divides into right and left bundles that are ultimately distributed to the right and left ventricles. Each of these bundles ramifies beneath the endocardium of its respective chamber to form an extensive plexus, from which fine fibers penetrate the myocardium to come into intimate contact with the ordinary contractile fibers.

The specialized cells of the nodal tissue are distinctly smaller than ordinary cardiac muscle fibers and are arranged in a network embedded in an abundant and rather dense connective tissue. In sections, the slender fusiform nodal cells coursing in various directions among the collagen bundles may be difficult to distinguish from the associated fibroblasts, but careful examination reveals their cross striations. In the mammal no connection between the sinoatrial node and the atrioventricular node via specialized conduction tissue has yet been convincingly demonstrated. The nodal fibers appear to be continuous with ordinary atrial muscle fibers. The node is richly innervated by both the sympathetic and parasympathetic divisions of the autonomic nervous system. In addition there are numerous nerve fibers closely associated with the sinoatrial and atrioventricular nodes that are immunoreactive for the peptides *neurotensin* and *substance-P*. The rate and forcefulness of contraction of the heart are affected by these substances as well as by the usual transmitters of the sympathetic and parasympathetic innervation.

In cardiac muscle, which beats rhythmically without nervous or other external stimuli, the cells with the most rapid inherent rhythm

establish the rate of beating of the rest of the myocardium. In warm-blooded animals, the fibers of the sinoatrial node have the most rapid rhythm, and this node is therefore referred to as the "pacemaker" of the heart. The evidence for this resides in the fact that the electrical events associated with each beat begin at the sinoatrial node and travel from there over the atria. Warming or cooling the node increases or decreases, respectively, the rate of the heart beat. Although the heart will normally beat at a rate determined by the inherent rhythm of its pacemaker, this rate can be modified by the autonomic nervous system. Parasympathetic (vagal nerve) stimulation brings about a slowing of the heart and sympathetic stimulation accelerates it.

The fibers of the atrioventricular node are small, like those of the sinoatrial node. The fibers of the atrioventricular bundle are similar at their origin, but more distally in the right and left bundle branches they become larger than ordinary cardiac muscle fibers and take on a highly distinctive appearance. These are the so-called *Purkinje fibers* (Figs. 10–46, 10–47). They have one or two nuclei situated in a clear central mass of sarcoplasm that is rich in mitochondria and glycogen. The myofibrils are relatively sparse and displaced to the periphery, and they are less consistent in their orientation than are those of ordinary cardiac muscle fibers.

The Purkinje fibers of ungulates reach very large size, and for this reason these have been more extensively studied than those of other mammals, but they do not seem to differ in any other important respect. Typical intercalated discs are seldom seen in the conducting tissue. At their ends the Purkinje fibers are said to lose their specific cytological features and to become continuous with the ordinary muscle fibers of the myocardium.

In electron micrographs, the cytoplasmic matrix of the Purkinje cells is of relatively low density and contains numerous randomly oriented mitochondria (Figs. 10–48, 10–49). The myofilaments do not form a continuous contractile mass but are arranged in separate myofibrils that are relatively few in number. Although their prevailing orientation is parallel to the long axis of the cell, they are very poorly ordered compared with those of ordinary cardiac muscle.

The cells have variable and unusual shapes, one often partially surrounding another or sending a large process into a deep recess in the adjoining cell (Fig. 10–49). As a conse-

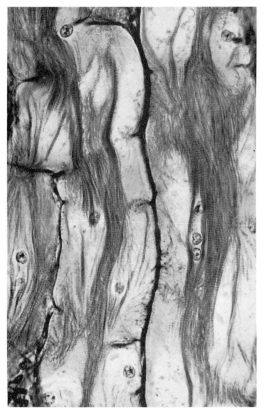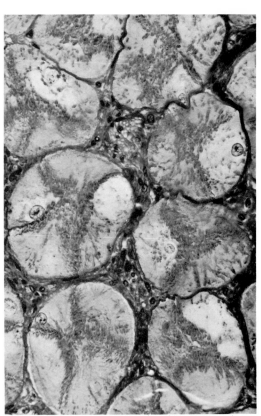

Figure 10–46. Photomicrographs of the very large Purkinje fibers in the moderator band of the bovine heart. In *A* the fibers are cut longitudinally; in *B* they are cut transversely. In both, it is evident that the myofibrils occupy only a small part of the sarcoplasm. The large clear areas are rich in glycogen.

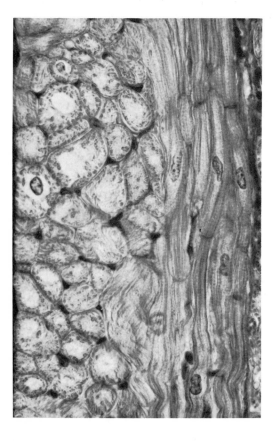

Figure 10–47. Photomicrograph of the specialized conduction tissue of the human atrioventricular bundle. The large Purkinje fibers seen in cross section at left of figure can be compared with the smaller unspecialized heart muscle cut longitudinally at right side of figure.

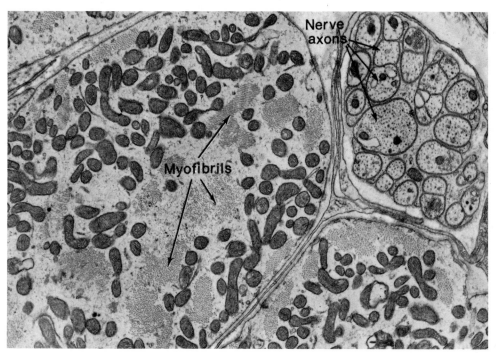

Figure 10–48. Electron micrograph of adjacent areas of two Purkinje fibers and an accompanying nerve in the atrioventricular bundle of the cat heart. The mitochondria are abundant and pleomorphic, and the loosely organized myofilaments occur only in scattered bundles.

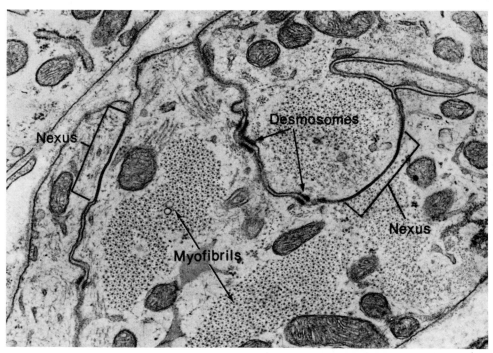

Figure 10–49. Electron micrograph of the cell junctions in the atrioventricular bundle. The cells of the conduction tissue are irregular in shape and have an extensive area of cell-to-cell apposition, on which are numerous desmosomes and nexuses. (Courtesy of D. Feldman.)

quence of their irregular shape, the cells are in extensive contact with one another. Although no typical intercalated discs are found, numerous desmosomes are distributed at irregular intervals along the cell boundaries. There are also areas of close membrane apposition corresponding to gap junctions of ordinary cardiac muscle. Surprisingly, these do not appear to be as numerous or as extensive as in the unspecialized fibers of the myocardium, and the morphological basis for the more rapid conduction in the atrioventricular bundle is not evident. Disease of the conduction system results in asynchrony in the beating of the ventricles or disorders in the timing of the contraction of the atria and ventricles that result in impaired efficiency of the heart.

Nerves to the Myocardium

Although the initiation of the heartbeat is not dependent on the nervous system, the heart is richly innervated. The parasympathetic (vagus) and sympathetic divisions of the autonomic nervous system form extensive plexuses at the base of the heart. Ganglion cells and numerous nerve fibers have been described in the wall of the right atrium, particularly in the region of the sinoatrial and atrioventricular nodes. Stimulation of the vagus nerve slows the heart, and release of norepinephrine from sympathetic nerve endings accelerates it. It is commonly assumed that the autonomic nervous system acts indirectly upon the myocardium by modifying the inherent rhythm of the pacemaker. This view is supported by physiological experiment and by light and electron microscopic observations establishing the presence of large numbers of unmyelinated nerve fibers close to the specialized cells of the nodal and conduction systems (Fig. 10–48). In addition, however, a surprising number of unmyelinated fibers are found in close relation to the ordinary cardiac fibers of the atrium and ventricles. Although it is difficult to determine to which division of the autonomic nervous system these belong, some at least contain granulated vesicles and therefore appear to be sympathetic. Release of catecholamine from these endings apparently exerts a direct effect upon the cardiac muscle.

Neither in ordinary cardiac muscle nor in the conduction tissue do the nerve fibers form specialized endings comparable with the myoneural junctions of skeletal muscle.

Slender axons merely pass near the surface of the cardiac muscle cells. That these are functional endings and not merely passing axons may be inferred from the fact that their axoplasm often contains large numbers of small vesicles identical to those found at other nerve endings and at synapses in the central nervous system.

REFERENCES

SMOOTH MUSCLE

Bozler, E.: Smooth muscle. *In* Rodahl, K., and S. M. Horvath, eds.: Muscle as a Tissue. New York, McGraw-Hill Book Co., 1962.

Bülbring, E., and T. B. Bolton, eds.: Smooth muscle. Br. Med. Bull. 55:27, 1979.

Cooke, P.: A filamentous cytoskeleton in vertebrate smooth muscle fibers. J. Cell Biol. 68:539, 1976.

Cooke, P.: A reversible change in functional organization of the filaments in smooth muscle fibers. Eur. J. Cell Biol. 27:55, 1982.

Devine, C. E., and A. P. Somlyo: Thick filaments in vascular smooth musscle. J. Cell Biol. 49:636, 1971.

Devine, C. E., A. V. Somlyo, and A. P. Somlyo: Sarcoplasmic reticulum and mitochondria as calcium accumulation sites in smooth muscle. Philos. Trans. R. Soc. Lond. [Biol.] 265:17, 1973.

Dewey, M. M., and L. Barr: Intercellular connection between smooth muscle cells: the nexus. Science 137:670, 1962.

Gabella, G., and D. Blundell: Nexuses between smooth muscle cells of the guinea-pig ileum. J. Cell Biol. 82:239, 1979.

Garamvölgyi, N., E. S. Uizi, and J. Knoll: The regular occurrence of thick filaments in stretched mammalian smooth muscle. J. Ultrastruct. Res. 34:135, 1971.

Harman, J. W., M. T. O'Hegarty, and C. K. Byrnes: The ultrastructure of human smooth msucle. I. Studies of cell surface and connections in normal and achalasic esophageal smooth muscle. Exp. Mol. Pathol. 1:204, 1962.

Jones, P. A., T. Scott-Burden, and W. Gevers: Glycoprotein, elastin and collagen secretion by rat smooth muscle cells. Proc. Natl. Acad. Sci. U.S.A. 76:353, 1979.

Kelly, R. E., and R. V. Rice: Localization of myosin filaments in smooth muscle. J. Cell Biol. 37:105, 1968.

Lane, B. P., and J. A. G. Rhodin: Cellular interrelationships and electrical activity in two types of smooth muscle. J. Ultrastruct. Res. 10:470, 1964.

Nonomura, Y., and S. Ebashi: Calcium regulatory mechanism in vertebrate smooth muscle. Biomed. Res. 1:1, 1980.

Rhodin, J. A. G.: Fine structure of vascular walls in mammals with special reference to smooth muscle component. Physiol. Rev. 42:49, 1962.

Ross, R.: The smooth muscle cell. II. Growth of smooth muscle in culture and formation of elastic fibers. J. Cell Biol. 50:172, 1971.

Schoenberg, C. F., and D. M. Needham: A study of the mechanism of contraction in vertebrate smooth muscle. Biol. Rev. 51:53, 1976.

Small, J. V.: Studies on isolated smooth muscle cells: the contractile apparatus. J. Cell Sci. 24:327, 1977.

Small, J. V., and A. Sobiezek: The contractile apparatus of smooth muscle. Int. Rev. Cytol. *64*:241, 1980.

Somlyo, A. P., and A. V. Somlyo: Vascular smooth muscle. I. Normal structure, pathology, biochemistry and biophysics. Pharmacol. Rev. *22*:249, 1970.

SKELETAL MUSCLE

Allbrook, D.: Skeletal muscle regeneration. Muscle and Nerve *4*:234, 1981.

Bennett, H. S.: The structure of striated muscle as seen by the electron microscope. *In* Bourne, G. H., ed.: Structure and Function of Muscle. Vol. I. New York, Academic Press, 1960.

Bourne, G. H., ed.: The Structure and Function of Muscle. 3 Vols. New York, Academic Press, 1960.

Bridgman, C. F., E. E. Shumpert, and E. Eldred.: Insertions of intrafusal fibers in muscle spindles of the cat and other mammals. Anat. Rec *164*:391, 1969.

Cohen, C.: The protein switch of muscle contraction. Sci. Am. *238*:36, 1975.

Cooper, S.: Muscle spindles and other muscle receptors. *In* Bourne, G. H., ed.: Structure and Function of Muscle. Vol. I. New York, Academic Press, 1960.

Couteaux, R.: Motor end plate structure. *In* Bourne, G. H., ed.: Structure and Function of Muscle. Vol. I. New York, Academic Press, 1960.

Desaki, J., and Y. Uehara: The overall morphology of neuromuscular junctions as revealed by scanning electron microscopy. J. Neurocytol. *10*:101, 1981.

Ebashi, S.: Regulatory mechanism of muscle contraction with special reference to the Ca-troponin-tropomyosin system. Essays Biochem. *10*:1, 1974.

Endo, M.: Entry of a dye into the sarcotubular system of muscle. Nature. *202*:1115, 1964.

Franzini-Armstrong, C., and L. D. Peachey: Striated muscle: contractile and control mechanisms. J. Cell Biol. *88*:166, 1981.

Gautier, G. F.: The ultrastructure of three fiber types in mammalian skeletal muscle. *In* Briskey, E. J., R. G. Cassens, and B. B. Marsh, eds.: The Physiology and Biochemistry of Muscle as a Food. Madison, WI, University of Wisconsin Press, 1940.

Gautier, G. F.: The structural and cytochemical heterogeneity of mammalian skeletal muscle fibers. *In* Podolsky, R. J., ed.: Contractility of Muscle Cells and Related Processes. New York, Prentice-Hall, 1971.

Hanson, J., and L. Lowy: The structure of actin filaments and the origin of the axial periodicity in the I-substance of vertebrate striated muscle. Proc. R. Soc. Lond. *B160*:449, 1964.

Hanson, J., and L. Lowy: Molecular basis of contractility in muscle. Br. Med. Bull. *21*:264, 1965.

Heuser, J.: Morphology of synaptic vesicle discharge and reformation at frog neuromuscular junction. *In* Thesleff, S., ed.: The Motor Innervation of Muscle. London, Academic Press, 1976.

Heuser, J. E., T. S. Reese, M. J. Dennis, J. L. Jan, and L. Evans: Synaptic vesicle exocytosis by quick-freezing and correlated with quantal transmitter release. J. Cell Biol. *81*:275, 1979.

Huxley, A. F.: The activation of striated muscle and its mechanical response. Proc. R. Soc. Lond. *B178*:1, 1971.

Huxley, H. E.: Muscle cells. *In* Brachet, J., and A. E. Mirsky, eds.: The Cell; Biochemistry, Physiology, Morphology. Vol. 4. New York, Academic Press, 1960.

Huxley, H. E.: Electron microscopic studies on the structure of natural and synthetic protein filaments from striated muscle. J. Mol. Biol. *7*:281, 1963.

Huxley, H. E.: Evidence for continuity between the central elements of the triads and extracellular space in frog sartorius muscle. Nature *202*:1067, 1964.

Huxley, H. E.: The mechanism of muscle contraction. Science *164*:1356, 1969.

Kelly, D. E., and M. A. Cahill: Filamentous and matrix components of skeletal muscle Z-discs. Anat. Rec. *172*:623, 1972.

Merrillees, N. C. R.: The fine structure of muscle spindles in the lumbrical muscles of the rat. J. Biophys. Biochem. Cytol. *7*:725, 1960.

Morita, S., R. G. Cassens, and E. J. Briskey: Histochemical localization of myoglobin in skeletal muscle of rabbit, pig, and ox. J. Histochem. Cytochem. *18*:346, 1970.

Nonomura, Y., W. Drabikowski, and S. Ebashi: The localization of troponin in tropomyosin paracrystals. J. Biochem. *64*:419, 1968.

Page, S.: Structure of the sarcoplasmic reticulum in vertebrate muscle. Br. Med. Bull. *24*:170, 1968.

Peachey, L. D.: The sarcoplasmic reticulum and transverse tubules of the frog's sartorius. J. Cell Biol. *25*:209, 1965.

Pepe, F. A.: Some aspects of the structural organization of the myofibril as revealed by antibody staining. J. Cell Biol. *28*:505, 1966.

Porter, K. R.: The sarcoplasmic reticulum, its recent history and present status. J. Biophys. Biochem. Cytol. *10*:(Suppl.):219, 1961.

Porter, K. R., and G. E. Palade: Studies on the endoplasmic reticulum. III. Its form and distribution in striated muscle cells. J. Biophys. Biochem. Cytol. *3*:269, 1957.

Uihara, Y., and K. Hama: Some observations on the fine structure of the frog muscle spindle. I. On the sensory terminals and motor endings of the muscle spindle. J. Electron Microsc. *14*:34, 1965.

Zacks, S. I.: The Motor Endplate. Philadelphia, W. B. Saunders Co., 1964.

CARDIAC MUSCLE

de Bold, A. J., and T. G. Flynn: Cardionatrin I—a novel heart peptide with potent diuretic and natriuretic properties. Life Sci *33*:297, 1983.

Fawcett, D. W., and N. S. McNutt: The ultrastructure of the cat myocardium. I. Ventricular papillary muscle. J. Cell Biol. *42*:1, 1969.

Forssmann, W. G., D. Hock, F. Lottspeich, A. Henschen, K. Kreye, M. Christmann, M. Reinecke, J. Metz, M. Carlquist, and V. Mutt: The right auricle is an endocrine organ. Anat. Embryol. *168*:307, 1983.

Jamieson, J. D., and G. E. Palade: Specific granules in atrial muscle cells. J. Cell Biol. *23*:151, 1964.

McNutt, N. S., and D. W. Fawcett: The ultrastructure of the cat myocardium. II. Atrial muscle. J. Cell Biol. *42*:46, 1969.

McNutt, N. S., and D. W. Fawcett: Myocardial ultrastructure. *In* Mammalian Myocardium. New York, John Wiley Sons, 1974.

Metz, J., V. Mutt, and G. Forssmann: Immunohistochemical localization of cardiodilatin in myoendocrine cells of cardiac atria. Anat. Embryol. *170*:123, 1984.

Muir, A. R.: Electron microscope study of the embryology of the intercalated disc in the heart of the rabbit. J. Biophys. Biochem. Cytol. *3*:193, 1975.

Reineke, M. E., E. Weihe, R. E. Carraway, S. E. Leeman, and W. G. Forssmann: Localization of neurotensin immunoreactive fibers in the guinea pig heart: evidence derived by immunohistochemistry, radioimmunoassay, and chromatography. Neuroscience 7:1785, 1982.

Rhodin, J. A., P. Missier, and L. C. Reid: The structure of the specialized impulse-conducting system of the steer heart. Circulation 24:349, 1961.

Simpson, F. O., and S. J. Oertelis: Relationship of the sarcoplasmic reticulum to the sarcolemma in sheep cardiac muscle. Nature 189:758, 1961.

Truex, R. C., and W. M. Copenhaver: Histology of the moderator band in man and other mammals, with special reference to the conduction system. Am. J. Anat. 80:173, 1947.

Truex, R. C., and M. A. Smythe: Recent observations on the human cardiac conduction system with special considerations of the atrioventricular node and bundle. In Electrophysiology of the Heart. New York, Pergamon Press, 1964.

Truex, R. D.: Comparative anatomy and functional considerations of the cardiac conduction system. In de Carvalho, A. P., W. C. de Mello, and B. F. Hoffman, eds.: The Specialized Tissues of the Heart. Amsterdam, Elsevier Publishing Co., 1961.

11

THE NERVOUS TISSUE

JAY B. ANGEVINE

The nervous system comprises the entire mass of nervous tissue in the body. The essential function of nervous tissue is *communication,* which depends upon special signaling properties of the nerve cells and their long processes. These properties express two fundamental attributes of protoplasm: the capacity to react to various physical and chemical agents *(irritability)* and the ability to transmit the resulting excitation from one locality to another *(conductivity).*

Upon reception of a stimulus from the external or internal environment, various forms of energy are transduced to electrical energy by specialized cellular structures, the receptors. Patterns of electrical messages, or nerve impulses, are transmitted from receptors to nervous centers, where they evoke in other nerve cells additional patterns of signals that result in appropriate sensations or responses. By these means, the organism reacts to the events in the world in which it lives and coordinates the functions of its organs. In addition, the nervous system provides the structural and chemical basis of conscious experience. It provides mechanisms for behavior and the regulation of behavior and for maintenance of the unity of the personality.

The *central nervous system* (CNS) consists of the brain and spinal cord and contains the *nerve cells* or *neurons* and a variety of supportive cells, called collectively the *neuroglia.* Nerve impulses conveyed from all parts of the body over the long processes of the nerve cells, called *axons,* come together in the CNS. The *peripheral nervous system* comprises all nervous tissue outside of the brain and spinal cord and functions to keep the other tissues of the body in communication with the CNS. The function of all parts of the organism are thus integrated by a central "clearing house" that controls the activity of the individual as a whole.

The sensory, integrative, and motor functions of nerve cells depend mainly upon irritability and conductivity. In addition, however, some nerve cells possess secretory capabilities similar to those of the endocrine system, which carries out its integrative function by means of blood-borne hormones. The secretory products of such nerve cells are released from axon terminals into a perivascular space, transported somehow into the lumen of the vessel, and carried by the blood to the particular target organ. A neurosecretory system regulating the activity of the adenohypophysis has been thoroughly studied and in recent years great attention has been devoted to functional interaction between the nervous and endocrine systems.

In the evolution of the nervous systems of higher organisms, it is believed that certain cells of primitive Metazoa developed to a high degree the properties of irritability and conductivity, and as a result of their more efficient response and signaling gradually evolved into a rudimentary nervous system. By further specialization, some nerve cells developed the capacity to react to special kinds of exogenous stimuli. These cells, with the corresponding accessory structures distributed throughout the body or near its surface, gave rise to three systems of *sensory receptors:* the *exteroceptive system,* receiving stimuli from the body surface; the *interoceptive system,* receiving stimuli from the internal organs; and the *proprioceptive system,* receiving stimuli from the muscles, tendons, and joints.

Other nerve cells became connected with the peripheral *effector organs,* principally the muscles, forming *neuromotor* systems. Still other nerve cells, collected into a large central mass, assumed the tasks of correlation and integration. These cells receive and modify the impulses arising from the receptors and in turn appropriately influence the effector organs.

311

The cells of the nervous system primarily involved in its special function are the *neurons*. Each neuron has a cell body consisting of a *nucleus* and the surrounding cytoplasm, which is called the *perikaryon*. Typically the cytoplasm is drawn out into several short radiating processes called *dendrites* and into a single long process called the *axon* (Fig. 11–1). The axon, which may attain great length, often emits branches or *axon collaterals* along its course and at its end may exhibit additional fine ramifications.

The size, shape, and other peculiarities of the nerve cell body and the number and mode of branching of its processes are all subject to variation, which results in many morphologically distinguishable kinds of nerve cells (Fig. 11–2). Functional specializations correlate with the morphological diversity. The neurons are anatomically and functionally related by their processes to other nerve cells, or to epithelial, muscular, or glandular cells. At *synapses,* specialized sites of contact between neurons, chemical or electrical signals pass from cell to cell. Transmission is usually in one direction but mixed modes and reciprocal synapses do exist. The countless neurons are morphologically and trophically independent but functionally interrelated at synapses. This fundamental generalization is the *neuron doctrine,* essentially a restatement of the cell theory for the nervous system. The neuron doctrine implies that the nervous system is entirely cellular; that its cells are distinctive in structure and function; and that its cells are not in protoplasmic continuity but are juxtaposed without a significant amount of intervening extracellular substance. Observations with the electron microscope corroborate these basic assumptions of the doctrine and show that the nervous system is a highly specialized epithelium. The nervous system thus reflects its phylogenetic and ontogenetic origin from the ectodermal epithelial layer of the body. Like other epithelia, nervous tissue exhibits junctional complexes, local specializations of the surfaces of adjacent cells that serve to maintain the position of the nerve cells and to stabilize those spatial relations of their processes that are essential to the signaling function of the nervous system.

THE NEURON

The nerve cell, or neuron, is usually large and complex in shape. The volume of cytoplasm in its processes is usually greater—often much greater—than in its perikaryon. The nerve cell body in the CNS generally has several processes. The outline of the perikaryon is typically angular or polygonal,

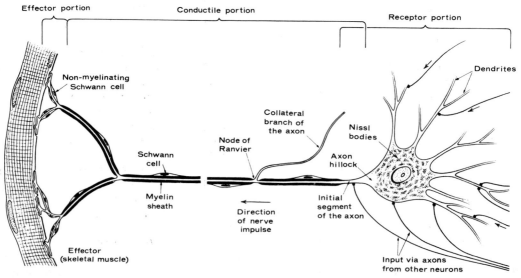

Figure 11–1. Diagrammatic representation of the effector, conductile, and receptor portions of a typical large neuron. The effector endings on skeletal muscle identify this as a somatic motor neuron. The effector endings of many neurons may terminate on the receptor portions of a single neuron. The myelin sheath on the conductile portion of the neuron acts as "insulation" and serves to increase its conduction velocity. The discontinuity in the axon indicates that it is much longer than can be illustrated; sometimes a motor neuron to a limb is 2 or 3 feet long. (Drawing after Bunge in Bailey's Textbook of Histology. 16th ed.)

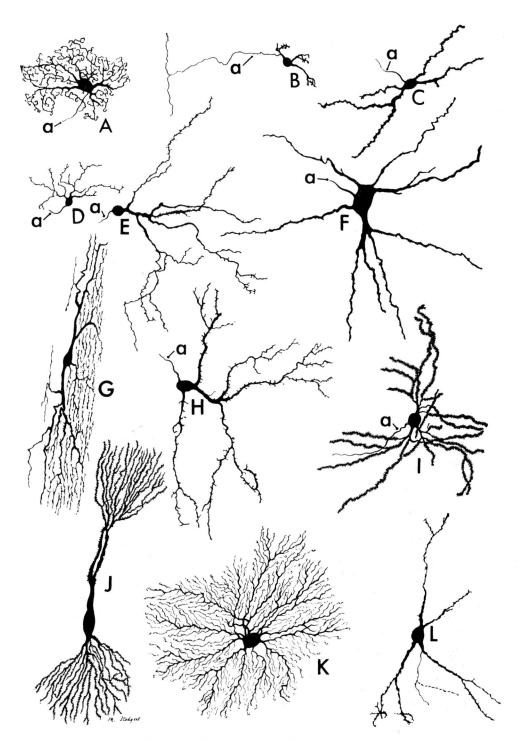

Figure 11–2. Drawing of some characteristic types of neurons whose axons *(a)* and dendrites remain within the central nervous system, illustrating some of the remarkable diversity of cell form exhibited by neurons. *A,* Neuron of inferior olivary nucleus. *B,* Granule cell of cerebellar cortex. *C,* Small cell of the reticular formation. *D,* Small gelatinosa cell of the spinal trigeminal nucleus. *E,* Ovoid cell, nucleus of tractus solitarius. *F,* Large cell of reticular formation. *G,* Spindle-shaped cell, substantia gelatinosa of spinal cord. *H,* Large cell of spinal trigeminal nucleus. *I,* Neuron, putamen of lenticular nucleus. *J,* Double pyramidal cell, Ammon's horn of hippocampal cortex. *K,* Cell from thalamic nucleus. *L,* Cell from globus pallidus of lenticular nucleus. Golgi preparations, monkey brain. (Courtesy of Clement Fox, from Truex, R. C., and M. B. Carpenter. Human Neuroanatomy. 6th ed. Baltimore, Williams and Wilkins, 1969.)

the surfaces between the processes being slightly concave (Figs. 11–3, 11–4). Motor neurons in general and the pyramidal cells of the cerebral cortex (Fig. 11–5) are two of many examples of angular nerve cell bodies. Cell bodies in the dorsal root ganglia, on the other hand, are rounded, and only one process projects from the perikaryon (Fig. 11–6). Regardless of shape, the neuron has a number of distinctive cytological characteristics.

Nucleus

The nucleus is large, pale, spherical, or slightly ovoid, and usually centrally placed within the perikaryon. In most cases there is a single conspicuous nucleolus as well as very fine chromatin particles (Fig. 11–4). Because of uniform dispersion of the chromatin, the nuclei of nerve cells, stained with basic dyes, appear empty and pale and are often described as "vesicular." In smaller nerve cells, the concentration of chromatin may be greater and the vesicular character of the nucleus less obvious. In man, but not in all mammals, the sex chromatin of females is

prominent and is located either near the nucleolus or at the periphery of the nucleus. Although neurons usually contain only one nucleus, binucleate cells are sometimes encountered in autonomic ganglia. In electron micrographs, the nuclear envelope and its pores and the fine structure of the nucleolus and karyoplasm (Fig. 11–8) are not significantly different from the corresponding features in other cells.

Perikaryon

The cytoplasm of the nerve cell is crowded with filamentous, membranous, and granular organelles arranged more or less concentrically around the nucleus. These organelles include the neuronal cytoskeleton, Nissl bodies, Golgi apparatus, mitochondria, centrioles, and various inclusions.

Cytoskeleton. At the electron microscope, the chief components of the neuronal cytoskeleton are neurofilaments and microtubules (Fig. 11–12). Neurofilaments are about 10 nm in diameter and of indefinite length. Unlike other cytoplasmic filaments of com-

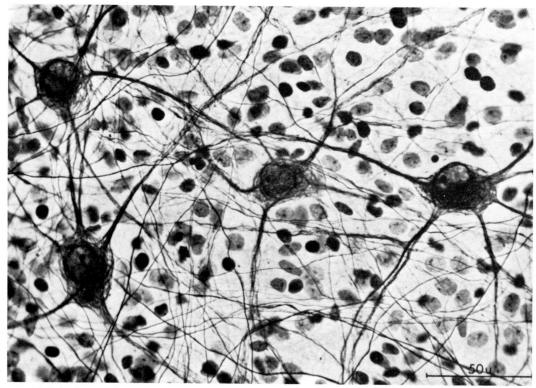

Figure 11–3. In tissue cultures of the nervous system, the three-dimensional configuration of the intact neuron can be seen to better advantage than in sections. Shown here are multipolar neurons from the deep nuclei of the rat cerebellum in a 12-day culture. Notice the neurofibrils in the cell bodies. Holmes stain. (From Hild, W.: Zeitschr. f. Zellforsch. 69:155, 1966.)

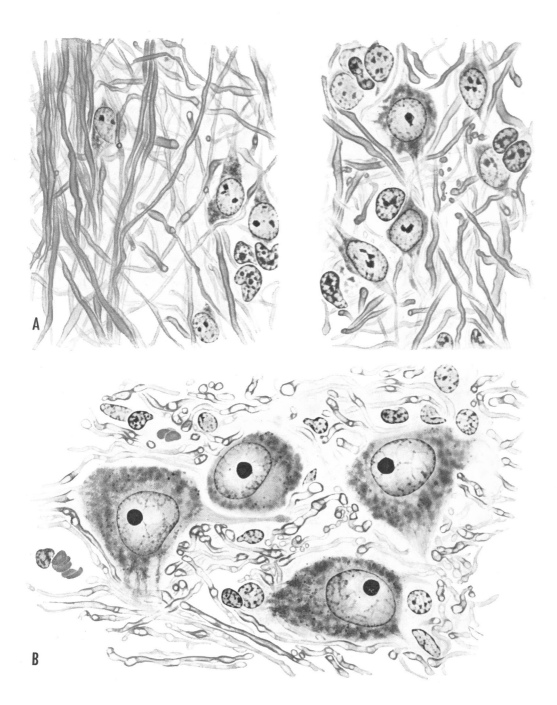

Figure 11–4. *A,* Two areas of section through the optic tectum of a leopard frog, showing blue-stained myelin sheaths and the nerve cell bodies. The small dark nuclei are supporting cells. *B,* Section from pons of man, showing myelin sheaths, nerve cell bodies, and glial cells. *A,* From a frozen section fixed in formalin; *B,* Paraffin section after postmortem formalin fixation. Klüver and Barrera staining methods for cells and myelin sheaths. (Drawn by Esther Bohlman.)

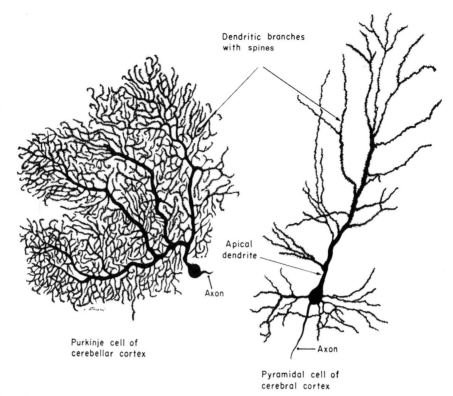

Dendritic branches
with spines

Apical
dendrite

Axon

Purkinje cell of
cerebellar cortex

Axon

Pyramidal cell of
cerebral cortex

Figure 11–5. Drawings of two principal cell types in cerebellar and cerebral cortex. Dendritic branches may provide a very extensive area for attachment of synaptic terminals of many other cortical and subcortical neurons. Golgi preparations, monkey brain. (Courtesy of Clement Fox, from Truex, R. C., and M. B. Carpenter. Human Neuroanatomy. 5th ed. Baltimore, Williams and Wilkins, 1966.)

parable dimensions, they appear at high magnification as minute tubules with a dense wall 3 nm thick and a clear center. They consist of a triplet of proteins of molecular weights 200,000, 150,000 and 70,000 daltons, which

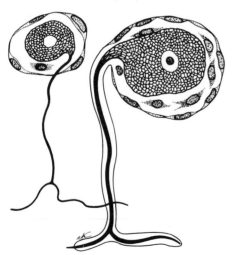

Figure 11–6. Drawing of cells from the nodose ganglion of the vagus nerve. Like neurons in the dorsal root ganglia, their cell bodies are rounded and only one process projects from the perikaryon, which is surrounded by satellite cells. (Redrawn from Ramón y Cajal.)

are different from the constituents of glial filaments and intermediate filaments of other tissues. There is evidence that the 70,000-dalton protein forms the core of the neurofilament, and the other two proteins are helically wound around this core. Microtubules (neurotubules) are long, straight protein tubes with an outer diameter of about 25 nm and a central, pale core of about 10 nm. Their organization and protein composition are the same as in non-neural cells. In the perikaryon, both neurofilaments and microtubules are arranged in tracts that occupy the spaces among Nissl bodies and Golgi complexes and can be followed into the dendrites and axon.

Silver impregnation methods for the light microscope stain a network of fine fibrils in the perikaryon, which continue into the dendrites and axon, where they can be followed to their finest ramifications (Fig. 11–7). These *neurofibrils* arise from a deposition of silver along bundles of neurofilaments. The neurofibrils are much less stable than the neurofilaments and would not be preserved in routine specimen preparation for light microscopy.

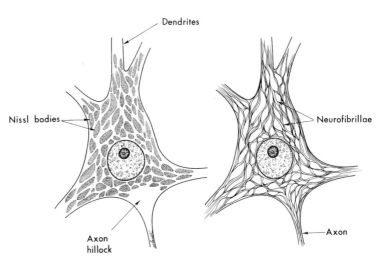

Figure 11–7. Drawings of a motor neuron from the gray matter of the ventral horn of the cat spinal cord stained for Nissl substance (A) and stained by the silver method for demonstrating neurofibrillae (B). The two images are complementary, the network of neurofibrillae running between the areas occupied by Nissl bodies and continuing into the processes. The Nissl bodies are largely confined to the perikaryon but may extend into the dentrites. They usually are not found in the axon hillock.

Nissl Bodies. The Nissl bodies, or chromophilic substance (Figs. 11–4, 11–7), stand out clearly in the cytoplasm of neurons stained with basic dyes and show important changes in some pathological conditions. They are visible in living neurons with phase-contrast microscopy, but are best demonstrated by staining fixed cells with basic aniline dyes—toluidine blue, thionine, or cresyl violet. Thus stained, the bodies appear as deeply basophilic masses or blocks in the perikaryon. The study of Nissl substance in living cells with phase-contrast microscopy or by the freeze-drying method establishes the fact that its clumped pattern in histological sections accurately reflects its distribution in life.

In electron micrographs, Nissl bodies are seen to consist of cisternae of rough-surfaced endoplasmic reticulum in ordered parallel arrays (Figs. 11–8, 11–9). Ribosomes, arranged in loops, rows, and spirals, are attached to the outer surface of the membranes, as in the basophilic bodies of other cell types. They also occur in clusters or rosettes in the cytoplasm between cisternae. Nissl bodies, like the basophilic substance of pancreatic and hepatic cells, represent sites of protein synthesis.

Nissl substance is abundant throughout the cytoplasm, including the dendrites. In the latter it appears under the electron microscope as anastomosing slender tubules and short cisternae. Sites of dendritic branching are frequently occupied by small Nissl bodies. They are usually absent from the most peripheral region of the perikaryon and from the area of the perikaryon in which the axon originates (the *axon hillock*), as well as from the axon itself (Fig. 11–7).

In form, size, and distribution, Nissl bodies vary considerably in different types of neurons. As a rule, they are coarser and more abundant in large neurons, especially motor neurons, and small and few in small neurons. Obvious exceptions are encountered, however. The ganglion cells of the dorsal roots of spinal nerves may attain large size yet typically display a uniform distribution of very fine Nissl bodies. Under differing physiological conditions, and in certain pathological states, Nissl bodies change their appearance.

Golgi Apparatus. A Golgi complex is present in all nerve cells, and when stained selectively with osmium or silver for light microscopy appears as a network of irregular, wavy strands, coarser than the neurofibrillar network. With the electron microscope, the Golgi network appears as clusters of closely apposed, flattened cisternae arranged in stacks and surrounded by myriad small vesicles. The ends of the cisternae are frequently dilated. Areas of typical Golgi cisternae are interconnected by smooth-surfaced tubular elements, often interpreted as *agranular endoplasmic reticulum*. These latter in turn are often continuous with tubules or cisternae of the *granular reticulum*. The Golgi complex is arranged in an arc or a complete circle around the nucleus approximately halfway between it and the surface membrane of the perikaryon (Fig. 11–8). A cytochemical reaction for the enzyme thiamine pyrophosphatase yields a reaction product concentrated in the cisternae on the maturing face of each stack, and the resulting staining is coextensive with the Golgi apparatus as classically delineated by silver or osmium impregnation methods.

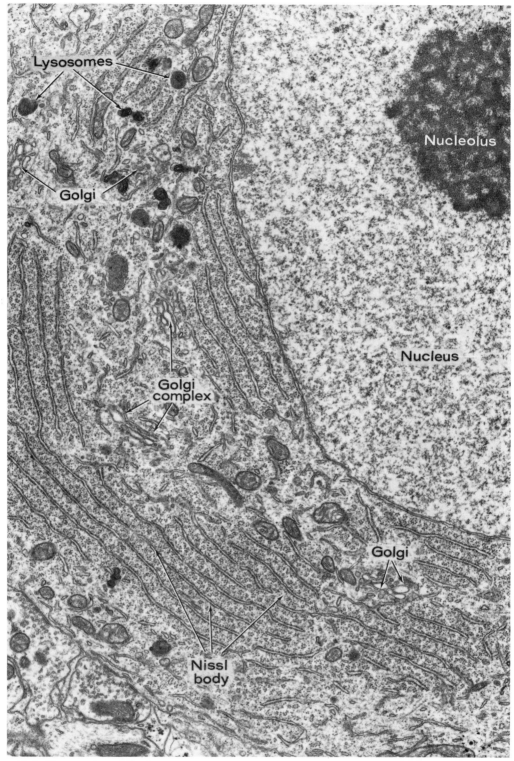

Figure 11–8. Electron micrograph of a portion of the perikaryon of a typical neuron, illustrating the principal organelles. The Golgi complex of the neurons is highly developed and forms a continuous network in the perinuclear cytoplasm; therefore, in a thin section such as this, it is transected at multiple sites. (Micrograph courtesy of Sanford Palay.)

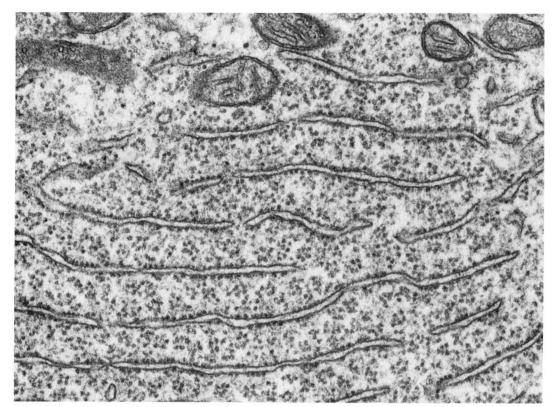

Figure 11–9. Electron micrograph of a Nissl body at higher magnification. It consists of flattened cisternae of the endoplasmic reticulum oriented parallel to each other. In addition to the ribosomes associated with the membranes, there are many clusters of ribosomes in the cytoplasmic matrix between cisternae. (Micrograph courtesy of Sanford Palay.)

Mitochondria. Rodlike or filamentous mitochondria are scattered everywhere, intermingling with Nissl bodies and neurofibrils. They are generally smaller than those of nonnervous tissues, varying from 0.1 to 0.8 μm in diameter, with a preponderance of slender forms that generally measure close to the smaller dimension. They can be demonstrated in fresh nerve cells by supravital staining. Their number varies from cell to cell and in different parts of the same cell; they are especially numerous in axon endings. Their fine structure resembles that of mitochondria in other cells but displays two peculiarities of unknown significance; the cristae are not consistently transversely oriented but often run parallel to the long axis of the mitochondrion, and the dense matrix granules usually present in the inner mitochondrial chamber are either absent or infrequent.

Centrioles. A pair of centrioles is characteristic of preneuronal multiplying cells during embryonic development. In adult neurons of vertebrates, centrioles are only occasionally encountered. Since neurons do not proliferate, the role of this organelle in the adult nerve cell is unknown.

Inclusions. In addition to the organelles already described, there are inclusions in nerve cells that are of more restricted occurrence. Catecholamine-synthesizing neurons contain dense-core vesicles 80 to 120 nm in diameter, filled with neurotransmitter and enzymes involved in their synthesis. Neurosecretory neurons of the hypothalamus are characterized by granules 10 to 30 nm in diameter, which contain the hormones vasopressin and oxytocin and their carrier peptides neurophysins. These granules are transported via the axon to the neurohypophysis, where their hormonal contents are discharged and diffuse into the bloodstream.

In recent years, isolated granule-containing cells of several kinds have been found widely dispersed in the CNS. The granules are immunoreactive for a number of peptides that are also found in the gastrointestinal tract. The physiological significance of these cells is now a subject of intensive investigation.

Pigment granules are frequently encountered in the neuronal perikaryon. The coarse, dark brown or black granules found in neurons in the substantia nigra of the midbrain, the locus ceruleus near the fourth ventricle, the dorsal motor nucleus of the vagus nerve, and the spinal and sympathetic ganglia are undoubtedly *melanin.* The physiological significance of melanin in these sites is unknown. Of more general occurrence, especially in man, are golden brown pigment granules termed *lipofuscin.* They are probably a harmless by-product of normal lysosomal activity that accumulates within the cytoplasm. Gradual increase in amount of lipofuscin with advancing age may displace the nucleus and organelles far to one side of the neuron. Iron-containing granular deposits are found in neurons of the substantia nigra, the globus pallidus, and elsewhere. Their number increases as the individual grows older.

Lipid, encountered as droplets in the cytoplasm, may represent either normal metabolic reserve material or a product of pathological metabolism. Glycogen is found in embryonic neurons, in embryonic neuroglial cells, and in embryonic cells of the ependyma and choroid plexus, but is not present in a histochemically demonstrable quantity in adult nervous tissue.

Processes of Neurons. The cytoplasmic processes of nerve cells are their most remarkable features. In almost all neurons there are two kinds: the dendrites and the axon.

The dendrites provide most of the receptive surface of the neuron, although the cell body, the initial segment of the axon, and axon terminals also may receive afferent fibers from other neurons. Dendrites may be direct extensions of the perikaryon or remote arborizations, as in the peripheral branches of a sensory ganglion cell, in which case a length of typical axon is interposed between perikaryon and dendritic arborization. A neuron usually has several main dendrites; rarely there is only one. Where the dendrites emerge from the cell body they are thick, tapering gradually along their length toward the ends. In most neurons the dendrites are relatively short and confined to the immediate vicinity of the cell body. Each dendrite may divide into primary, secondary, tertiary, and higher orders of branches, of variable shapes and sizes and distributed in diverse patterns (Fig. 11–11). The number and length of the dendrites bear little relation to

the size of the perikaryon, but their pattern of branching is typical for each variety of neuron. The surface of many dendrites is covered with innumerable minute projections or *spines,* which serve as sites of synaptic contact (Fig. 11–5).

In their initial portion, dendrites contain small Nissl bodies, free ribosomes, and mitochondria. In addition, they possess long, straight, parallel microtubules and neurofilaments (Figs. 11–11 and 11–12). With increasing distance from the cell body, microtubules and neurofilaments become the dominant feature of the dendritic cytoplasm. The tubules of the endoplasmic reticulum decrease in number and the ribosomes become sparse, whereas mitochondria remain more or less constant in number per unit length and may actually appear relatively increased in the finer dendritic ramifications.

Through their synapses with axon terminals, the dendrites receive nerve impulses from other functionally related neurons. The numbers of sources from which they are received may be very great. In a Purkinje cell of the cerebellar cortex (Figs. 11–10, 11–11), the terminals upon the dendritic tree number in the hundreds of thousands. The dendrites play a crucial role in the ability of the neuron to integrate information received from its many inputs. The arriving nerve impulses excite or inhibit electrical activity in localized regions of dendritic membrane and thus continuously shift the neuron toward or away from its threshold for signaling a nerve impulse of its own. Although the impulse carried by the axon behaves in an "all-or-nothing" fashion, the integrative capacity of the dendrites depends on graded changes in electrical potential. In certain instances dendrites may transmit, as well as receive, exerting influences upon adjacent dendrites through specialized, reciprocal dendrodendritic synapses. They may also exhibit propagated all-or-nothing signaling within long dendritic shafts (see below). Such findings call for flexibility in the functional characterization of dendrites, or for that matter, any part of the nerve cell, whose parts show great adaptability to special requirements in particular situations.

The *axon* differs considerably from the dendrites. Whereas there are usually several dendrites, there is only one axon to each neuron or, in rare instances, no axon at all (e.g., the amacrine cells of the retina). This cell process often arises from a small conical elevation on the perikaryon devoid of Nissl

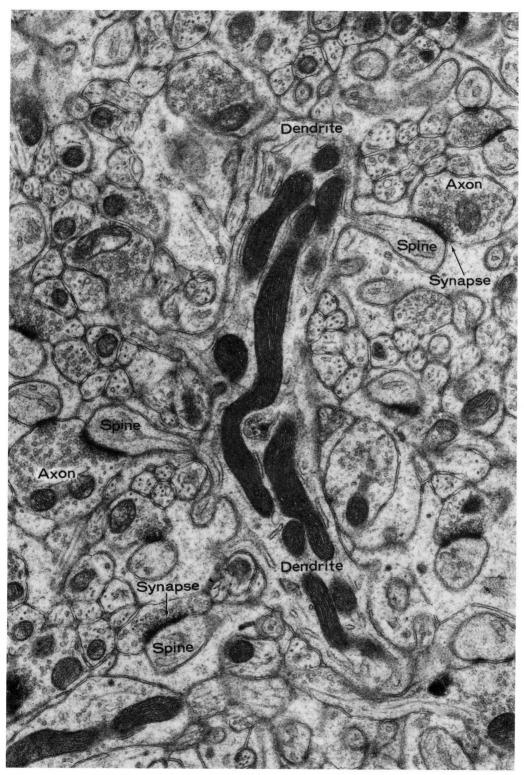

Figure 11–10. Electron micrograph of a small area of cerebellum. A small branch of the dendritic tree of a Purkinje cell running vertically through the field contains several conspicuous mitochondria. Projecting laterally from the dendrite are "spines" or "thorns" with bulbous tips and narrow stalks. Axons of granule cells form synapses with the Purkinje cell dendrite. (From Palay, S. L., and V. C. Palay. Cerebellar Cortex. Berlin, Springer-Verlag, 1974.)

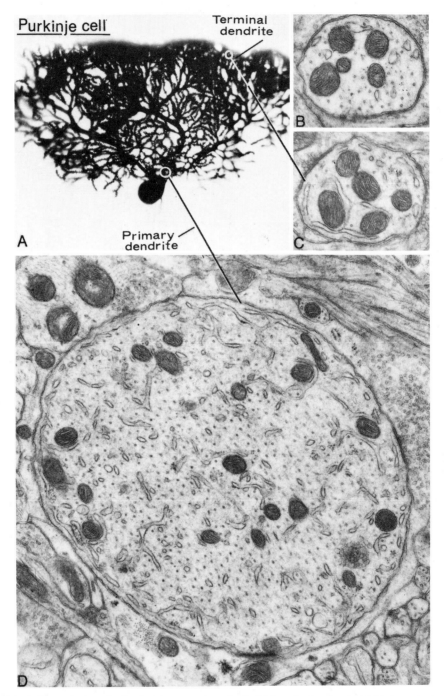

Figure 11–11. *A,* Photomicrograph of a Golgi preparation of a Purkinje cell, showing its highly branched dendritic tree. *B, C,* Electron micrographs of small terminal dendrites of the Purkinje cell located in the molecular layer of the cerebellum. *D,* Cross section of the primary dendrite of a Purkinje cell. Mitochondria, tubular elements of endoplasmic reticulum, and punctate profiles of microtubules are found throughout the dendritic tree, but microtubules are more numerous and more uniformly arranged in the primary dendrite. (Micrograph from Wuerker and Kirkpatrick. *In* Bourne, G. H., and J. F. Danielli, eds.: International Review of Cytology. Vol. 33. New York, Academic Press, 1972.)

bodies, called the *axon hillock*. The axon may arise, however, from the stem of a principal dendrite. The portion of the axon intervening between axon hillock and the beginning of the myelin sheath is called the *initial segment*. In this region, the plasma membrane bears an undercoating of dense material and the microtubules become bundled together into parallel fascicles. Within each fascicle, each microtubule is connected to its neighbors by cross bridges resembling the rungs of a ladder. The axon carries the response of the neuron in the form of a propagated *action potential;* the axon hillock and initial segment of the axon, from which this potential arises, are sometimes called the "trigger zone." The axon does not contain Nissl bodies and usually is thinner and much longer than the dendrites of the same neuron. The axoplasm contains longitudinally oriented tubules of the endoplasmic reticulum, long and extremely slender mitochondria, microtubules, and many neurofilaments.

The axons of many nerve cells have a prominent sheath of material called *myelin,* highly refractile in the fresh condition and appearing black in tissue fixed in osmium tetroxide. The *myelin sheath* of the axon is not part of the neuron but rather a part of an ensheathing cell (see discussion later in this chapter). Its presence or absence exerts an important influence on the physiological properties of the neuron. Because it is associated only with axons, it provides a criterion for recognizing them. There are, however, axons that are devoid of a myelin sheath (*unmyelinated axons*). In electron micrographs, unmyelinated axons and dendrites of large caliber can usually be distinguished by the fact that there is a much greater number of neurofilaments in the axon. The smaller processes are more difficult to distinguish, because the neurofilaments upon which the identification largely depends are less numerous in small axons.

Along its course, the axon may or may not emit collaterals. Unlike the branches of dendrites, which diverge at an acute angle, axonal branches tend to depart at right angles. In certain instances, a neuron may display an extensive system of axon collaterals, which individually ramify into ever finer branches. In such cases, the total length of axon may approach or even exceed that of the dendrites and can extend the sphere of influence of the neuron to a greater number of other neurons. Axon collaterals from many neu-

rons of this kind may combine to form a fibrous plexus of great complexity, enveloping the perikarya of other nerve cells.

The terminal arborization of the axon is composed of primary, secondary, and higher orders of branching, varying greatly in number, shape, and distribution. Often its branches assemble into networks that surround the body of the postsynaptic neuron in the form of a basket, or twist around the dendrites like a clinging vine. In simpler cases, the tips of one or two twigs make very local contact with the surface of a dendrite or the body of another neuron.

The perikaryon, like the dendrites, offers electrically excitable membrane upon which excitatory or inhibitory influences from axon terminals of other neurons can be received and integrated. The axon hillock, or subsequent initial segment, may provide a critically placed receptive zone for inhibitory signals. The pseudounipolar neuron of the craniospinal ganglia transmits a nerve impulse directly from the peripheral to the central branch of its long, single, T-shaped process (Fig. 11–6). Its perikaryon has no synaptic contacts from other neurons and is chiefly of trophic significance, even though its membrane may reflect passage of the action potential in the adjacent process.

Through its ending, the axon transmits nerve impulses to other neurons or to muscle fibers and gland cells. The response of the effector cells is always activity, but the response of neurons may be a varying degree of either excitation or inhibition. There are many types of axon endings, and the same axon may terminate in several different ways and synapse with several different neurons.

In general, dendrites display local changes in membrane potential in response to impulses received. Certain neurons with very long dendrites, however, exhibit propagated dendritic electrical potentials, similar to the action potential characteristic of axons, which appear to summate and convey to the perikaryon weak excitations from remote regions of the dendritic tree.

Neurons are unusual cells, because most of their synthesizing machinery is located in the cell body, but they possess long processes whose maintenance depends on the activity of the perikaryon. Material must therefore pass continuously from the cell body to the dendrites and axon or be returned from the periphery to the cell body. The axon with its terminal arborization largely depends on this

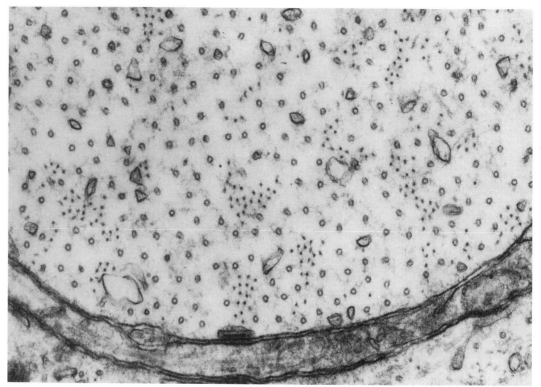

Figure 11–12. Higher magnification of a dendrite from a ventral horn neuron of the spinal cord, showing microtubules and clusters of neurofilaments. (Micrograph courtesy of Raymond Wuerker.)

traffic, whereas dendrites are more independent, because they contain cytoplasmic organelles, especially ribosomes, at least in their portion that is close to the cell body.

Axonal transport is the process by which materials are transferred to or returned from the axon and its terminal arborization; a dendritic transport also takes place but has been studied in less detail. Two forms of transport exist, an *anterograde transport* from the perikaryon to the axon terminal and a *retrograde transport* in the opposite direction. Two components have been identified in the anterograde transport, a fast and a slow one.

The velocity of the fast transport varies from 20 to 400 mm per day. The bulk of the material transported is represented by membrane-bounded organelles, such as tubules of the smooth endoplasmic reticulum, vesicles of various kinds, and some of the mitochondria. In addition, materials of low molecular weight are ferried by the fast transport: these include sugars, amino acids, nucleotides, and calcium. The slow anterograde transport has a velocity of 0.2 to 4 mm per day and carries microtubule and neurofilament proteins of

the axonal cytoskeleton, and numerous proteins of the cytomatrix including actin, clathrin, calmodulin, and various metabolic enzymes. For descriptive purposes the substances transported are now divided into two groups: *slow component a* (SCa), comprising the cytoskeletal proteins, and *slow component b* (SCb), including the cytomatrix proteins. In radiolabeling experiments, both are localized throughout the cross section of the axons but the SCb proteins are found in highest concentration in the subaxolemmal region.

Many of the constituents carried by retrograde transport are the same as those that move in anterograde direction; in addition, retrograde transport conveys to the perikaryon proteins and small molecules that have been picked up by the axonal endings. Some of these proteins travel in tubules, multivesicular bodies, and vesicles that fuse with the lysosomes when they reach the cell body. Retrograde transport is also the pathway followed by toxins, such as tetanus toxin, and neurotropic viruses, such as those of herpes and rabies, to penetrate and invade the central nervous system. The velocity of retrograde transport varies in different axons and is in general slower, about half the rate of the fast anterograde component.

The mechanisms of axonal transport are still poorly understood. The axonal cytoskeleton, especially microtubules, plays an important role in the fast component. For the slow component, one hypothesis holds that the entire cytoskeleton is slowly propelled down along the length of the axon.

One important function of axonal transport is the delivery to the axonal endings of synaptic vesicles and enzymes involved in transmitter metabolism. Synaptic vesicles can travel along the axon as large dense-core vesicles in the neurons that use biogenic amines as neurotransmitters; in other neurons, they probably derive from the tubules of the smooth endoplasmic reticulum. In addition to the enzymes necessary for their synthesis, neurotransmitters themselves can also be transported along the axon, but their quantity is small compared with the amounts synthesized in the endings. An exception to this rule may be represented by neuropeptides and neurosecretory granules produced in the cell body.

DISTRIBUTION AND DIVERSITY OF NEURONS

The core of the central nervous system, the *gray matter* (Fig. 11–13), contains the cell bodies of the neurons, their dendrites, and proximal portions of the axons. Clusters of nerve cell bodies in the gray matter are called *nuclei* (not to be confused with cellular nuclei) and represent functional aggregates of neurons. Surrounding the gray matter more or less concentrically is a zone, devoid of nerve cell bodies, which contains axons of neurons whose cell bodies are located either in the gray matter or in ganglia outside the CNS. This zone is the *white matter,* so-called because the axons here are invested by *myelin,* which is glistening white in the fresh state. Bundles of myelinated fibers in the white matter, which are cable-like functional groupings of nerve fibers, are called *tracts.* In the cerebral hemispheres and cerebellum, additional gray matter with nerve cell bodies arranged in distinct layers forms the cortex surrounding the white matter (Figs. 11–14, 11–15).

A very great variety of neurons can be distinguished in the CNS (Fig. 11–2) on the basis of the number, length, thickness, and mode of branching of the processes, and on the basis of the shape, size, and position of the cell body, as well as of the synaptic relationships. Neurons may have long axons that leave the gray matter, traverse the white matter, and terminate at some distance in another part of the gray matter. Alternatively, axons may leave the CNS and end in the periphery. Such cells with long axons are termed *Golgi Type I* neurons; this type includes the neurons that contribute to formation of the peripheral nerves and those whose axons form long fiber tracts of the brain and spinal cord. In other neurons, the axon is relatively short and does not leave the region of the gray matter where its cell body lies. These cells with short axons, which are especially numerous in the cerebral and cerebellar cortices and in the retina, are *Golgi Type II* neurons.

The shape of the perikaryon varies; it may be spherical, ovoid, pyriform, fusiform, or polyhedral. The absolute size of the cell body also varies between extreme limits, from dwarf neurons of 4-μm diameter (smaller than an erythrocyte) to giants approaching 150 μm. The pyramidal cells of Betz in the mammalian cerebral cortex and the paired Mauthner neurons in the medulla oblongata of certain fishes and amphibians are examples of exceptionally large neurons. Could they be isolated, they would be visible to the naked eye.

True *unipolar neurons* are rare except in early embryonic stages. In *bipolar neurons,* a process projects from each end of the fusiform cell body. Typical bipolar neurons are found in the vestibular and cochlear ganglia, and in the olfactory nasal epithelium. In vertebrate embryos, all neurons of the craniospinal ganglia are first bipolar, but during development the opposing processes shift around the perikaryon and combine into a single process.These neurons are thus called *pseudounipolar.* During embryonic stages, the perikaryon of such neurons is progressively set apart from the region of fusion of the two initial processes. The adult cell body is globular or pear-shaped; a single process arises and divides like the letter T. One branch is directed to the periphery and the other courses in a posterior nerve root to the CNS. The stem process may be relatively short, as illustrated in Figure 11–6, or may run a considerable distance before bifurcating, sometimes enveloping the cell body of origin in a complex tangle. Except in the smallest examples, the initial single process

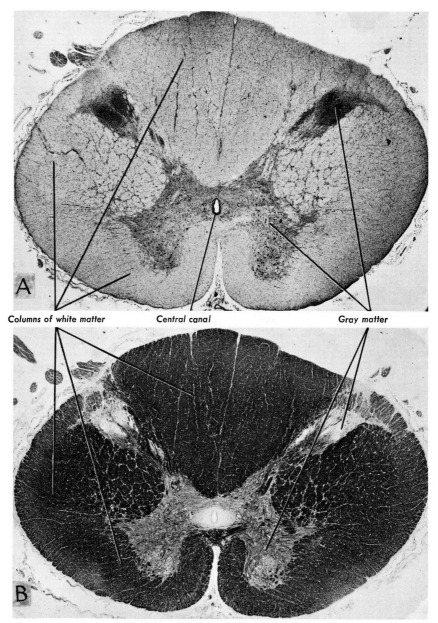

Columns of white matter Central canal Gray matter

Figure 11–13. Sections through human upper cervical spinal cord stained with thionine *(A)* to show cells, and with the Weigert-Weil method *(B)* to show myelinated fibers. Note the external arrangement of the fibers (white matter) and the central, cruciate area containing the cell bodies (gray matter). The ventral surface is below. A portion of the dorsal root is seen in upper left. (Courtesy of P. Bailey.)

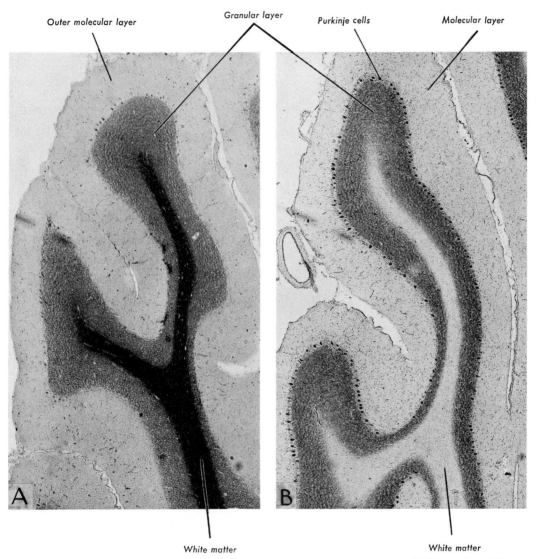

Outer molecular layer   Granular layer   Purkinje cells   Molecular layer

A   B

White matter   White matter

Figure 11–14. Sections of human cerebellar folia stained with the Weigert-Weil method *(A)* for myelinated fibers and with thionine *(B)* for cells. Note the central disposition of the white matter with its myelinated fibers, which stain black with Weigert-Weil and pale with thionine; the outer molecular layer (pale gray), with scattered neurons and the large Purkinje cells; and the intermediate, or granular, layer, composed of cells and fibers. (Courtesy of P. Bailey.)

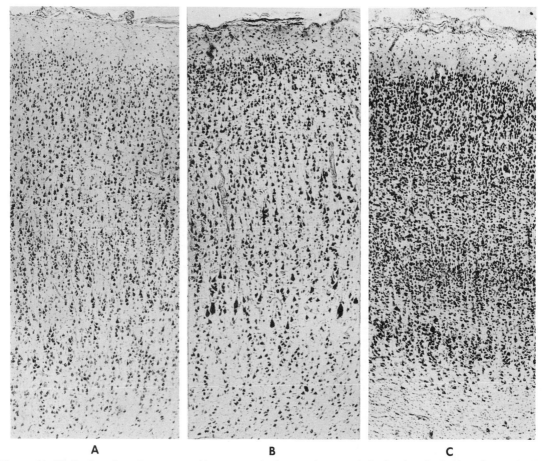

Figure 11–15. Sections from three areas of human cerebral cortex (gray matter), showing distribution of nerve bodies *(A)* in the temporal eulaminate (associational) cortex, *(B)* in the precentral agranular cortex (motor area), and *(C)* in the occipital koniocortex (striate visual cortex). Much stress has been laid on minute differences in lamination of the nerve cells and fibers in these and other areas of the cortex, but there is now a tendency to minimize some of these differences. (Courtesy of P. Bailey.)

and the peripheral and central branches are myelinated. The perikaryon of a pseudouni-polar neuron is ensheathed by two cellular capsules. The inner is made up of small, flat, epithelium-like *satellite cells* that are continu-ous with similar *Schwann cells* enveloping the peripheral process. The satellite cells have a relationship to the ganglion cells that is sim-ilar to that of neuroglial cells (oligodendro-cytes) to neurons in the CNS. Satellite cells, however, differ in structure and embryonic origin from neuroglial cells. The outer cap-sule of pseudounipolar neurons is vascular connective tissue, which extends along the cellular process and continues as the endo-neurium of the nerve fiber.

In the majority of neurons, shape is deter-mined by the number and arrangement of the dendrites (Fig. 11–2). *Stellate* or *star-*

shaped neurons include the motor nerve cells of the ventral gray matter of the spinal cord and of the motor nuclei of the brain stem. Pyramidal neurons are characteristic ele-ments of the cerebral cortex.

Of remarkable shape are the graceful *Pur-kinje cells* of the cerebellar cortex (Figs. 11–5, 11–11*A*) One or two thick dendrites covered with innumerable tiny spines arise from the upper end of the cell body. These branch repeatedly to form a large dendritic arbori-zation, oriented in one plane and shaped like a fan turned at right angles to the long axis of the surrounding cerebellar convolution. The axon enters the white matter beneath the cortex; hence, the Purkinje cell is a Golgi Type I neuron. Synaptic terminals upon the dendrites and body of the Purkinje cell num-ber hundreds of thousands per cell and exhibit, according to their source, specific places and modes of ending upon the postsynaptic surface.

Many more varieties of neurons are found in the cerebral and cerebellar cortices. In diminutive *granule cells*, a few short dendrites radiate in all directions, while the axon and its collaterals remain either in the immediate neighborhood of the cell or at least within the cortical gray matter. Such neurons qualify as Golgi Type II. Neurons in the reticular formation of the brain stem have large, variously shaped perikarya and extensive but poorly branched dendrites. Great attention has been accorded these neurons in recent years because their morphology and synaptic relationships suggest important integrative functions. The multitude of dendrites frequently overlap in complex fashion and receive an input of axons and axon collaterals derived from many sources. The typically long axon may distribute impulses through ascending and descending branches to a considerable portion of the length of the neuraxis and ramify into rich collateral plexuses at different levels. At first glance, these sprawling neurons convey an impression of disorder in the extreme, yet they are encountered in the core of the brain stem, an area upon which the delicate and exquisite control of homeostatic mechanisms depends.

The few examples described give an incomplete picture of the wealth of different kinds of neurons. Many more have been described by numerous investigators. Recent studies, in which the electron microscope and chrome-silver method of Golgi have played complementary roles, have further refined the knowledge of neuronal types. It is apparent that each ganglion, nucleus, or cortical area is composed of (1) a characteristic variety of neurons in differing proportions, each type of cell designed to meet its special functional requirements, and (2) a complex and highly ordered meshwork of dendritic, axonal, and glial processes whose fine structure and relationships are adapted to provide a framework for a particular form of organized activity. The term used to designate this feltwork of processes is *neuropil*. The details of its dense entanglements cannot be resolved in silver preparations and have only begun to be appreciated with the advent of the electron microscope. The neuropil is of great importance in the communications function of nervous tissue; it provides an enormous area for synaptic contact and functional interaction between the processes of nerve cells.

It has been estimated that well over half the cytoplasm of neurons is contained in the neuropil. The great variety of types of neurons and neuropils results in a striking degree of regional heterogeneity in nervous tissue.

The number of nerve cells in the entire nervous system is astronomical, being estimated at 14 billion in man. The tremendous increase in this number in the course of evolution has involved chiefly the integrator cells or *interneurons* of the CNS. The number of *sensory neurons* and associated receptors has also increased, especially in the retina, but to a much lesser extent. The number of *motor neurons* has remained relatively small and in man probably does not exceed two million. The term *final common pathway* is employed to designate the motor neurons by which nerve impulses from many central sources pass to a muscle or gland in the periphery.

THE NERVE FIBER

The *nerve fiber* is composed of an axon and certain sheaths of ectodermal origin. All peripheral axons are enclosed by a sheath of *Schwann cells*, which invest the axon almost from its beginning to near its peripheral termination. The larger peripheral axons are also enveloped in a *myelin sheath*, within the *sheath of Schwann*. The smallest axons of peripheral nerves lack a myelin sheath. It is necessary, therefore, to designate axons as *myelinated* or *unmyelinated*. Fresh myelinated fibers appear as homogeneous, glistening tubes. This refractile property of myelin accounts, as noted earlier, for the white color of fiber tracts of the brain and spinal cord and of numerous peripheral nerves. In stained preparations, the appearance of various constituents of the nerve fiber differs according to the technique applied. With methylene blue vital staining the axon is stained blue, and with silver methods, brown or black, the myelin remaining unstained. Unmyelinated fibers, often difficult to observe by routine histological methods, are well demonstrated by these special techniques. Weigert's method and osmium tetroxide darken the myelin, leaving the axon colorless or light gray (Fig. 11–16). Myelin sheaths are stained blue-green by the Klüver-Barrera method (Fig. 11–4).

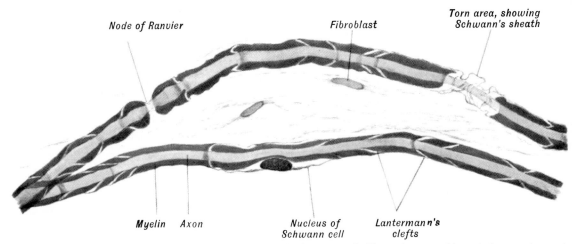

Node of Ranvier   *Fibroblast*   *Torn area, showing Schwann's sheath*

Myelin   Axon   *Nucleus of Schwann cell*   *Lantermann's clefts*

Figure 11–16. Two myelinated fibers of the sciatic nerve of a frog, treated with osmium tetroxide and picrocarmine and teased. (After A. A. Maximow.)

The Sheath of Schwann

This sheath of flattened cells, sometimes called the *neurilemmal sheath*, forms a thin sleeve around the myelin, which surrounds the axon. The Schwann cells, like the neurons, are of ectodermal origin and represent elements similar to neuroglial cells of the CNS, but they are adapted to the special conditions of the peripheral nervous system. In embryonic life, Schwann cells accompany outgrowing axons and migrate from branch to branch until they form complete neurilemmal sheaths. In the adult their nuclei are flattened; a small Golgi apparatus and a few mitochondria can be demonstrated in their attenuated cytoplasm. The myelin and the Schwann sheaths appear distinct with the light microscope and were formerly considered separate structures. The electron microscope, however, shows that myelin is actually part of the Schwann cell, consisting of spirally wrapped layers of its surface membrane (discussed in more detail later). The outer membrane of the Schwann cell and the glycoprotein boundary layer on its outer aspect were resolved with the light microscope as a single layer, traditionally called the *neurilemma*.*

---

*Originally the word *neurilemma*, as employed by European workers early in the twentieth century, meant the connective tissue tunic, continuous with the pia mater, known today as the endoneurium. English-speaking authors, however, used the term to designate the clear layer of Schwann membranes defined above in the text. A related term, *axolemma*, originally referred to the inner membrane of the Schwann cell but is now commonly used to signify the plasmalemma of the axon.

The sheath of Schwann and the myelin sheath are interrupted at regular intervals by *nodes of Ranvier* (Fig. 11–17), which are points of discontinuity between successive Schwann cells along the length of the axon. Here the axon is partially uncovered, being only incompletely enclosed by a complex arrangement of Schwann cell processes. Myelinated axons thus have individual neurilemmal sheaths, divided into segments. Each internodal segment of the sheath between two consecutive nodes of Ranvier is composed of a Schwann cell with its myelin lamellae.

The internodal segments are shorter in the terminal portion of the fiber. The length varies in different nerve fibers and in different species from about 200 to over 1000 μm; the longer and thicker the fibers, the longer the segments. If an axon gives off collateral branches, this takes place at a node of Ranvier.

In fixed preparations of peripheral nerves, the myelin of each segment appears to be interrupted by oblique, cone-shaped discontinuities, the *incisures* or *clefts of Schmidt-Lantermann*, several to each Schwann segment (Figs. 11–16, 11–17). These clefts, seen also in teased fresh or osmicated nerves, represent areas of loosening or local separation of the spirally wrapped myelin lamellae, which are nevertheless continuous across the incisures. The regions between the separated lamellae consist of Schwann cell cytoplasm continuous with that forming the outer sleeve of the nerve fiber on the one hand, and with a thin, inconstant layer of cytoplasm next to the axon on the other.

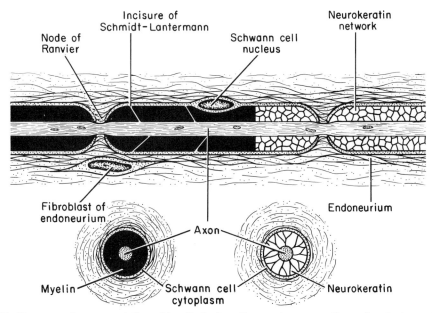

Figure 11–17. Diagrammatic representation of longitudinal sections and cross sections of a single myelinated nerve fiber and its endoneurial sheath. Left half of drawing represents what would be seen after fixation with osmium tetroxide, which preserves the lipid of myelin. Right half represents the appearance after ordinary methods of histological preparation, which extract the myelin and leave behind an artifactitious network of residual protein described as "neurokeratin." (Redrawn from Ham, A. W. Histology, 5th ed. Philadelphia, J. B. Lippincott Co., 1965.)

The exact relationship of the Schwann sheath to unmyelinated axons cannot be visualized with the light microscope, but in electron micrographs it is evident that multiple axons, up to a dozen or more, may occupy deep recesses in the surface of the same Schwann cell (Fig. 11–18). The plasmalemma of the Schwann cell is closely applied to the axon and, as a rule, completely surrounds it. At some point around the periphery of each axon, however, the Schwann cell membrane turns back to form the *mesaxon*, a pair of parallel membranes marking the line of edge-to-edge contact of the encircling sheath cell (Fig. 11–21).

Schwann cells are indispensable for the life and function of the axons of peripheral nerve fibers. In regeneration, the new axon grows out of the proximal stump and follows the path formed by Schwann cells.

The Myelin Sheath

Before the advent of biological electron microscopy, x-ray diffraction analysis suggested that the myelin sheath was composed of concentrically wrapped layers of mixed lipids alternating with thin layers of neurokeratinogenic protein material. Within the layers, the lipid molecules were thought to be oriented with hydrocarbon chains extending radially and with polar groups aligned at the aqueous interfaces, loosely bonded to the proteins. In general electron microscopic studies have supported this interpretation of the molecular organization of myelin and have shown that the alternating layers of mixed lipids and proteins are in fact successive layers of the plasma membrane of the Schwann cell wrapped spirally about the axon.

In electron micrographs at high magnification, compact myelin presents as a series of light and dark lines in a repeating pattern of about 12 nm (Fig. 11–19). The dark line bounding the repeating unit is called the *major dense line* and is about 3 nm thick; it represents the apposition of the inner (cytoplasmic) surfaces of the unit membrane of the Schwann cell. Between major dense lines is a less dense *intraperiod line*. This has been interpreted as representing the union of the outer leaflets of the Schwann cell membrane. However, in recent studies based on high-resolution micrographs of optimally fixed myelin sheaths in spinal roots, a narrow open cleft is resolved between the membranes (Fig. 11–20). If this observation can be generalized, there exists between the outer leaves of the opposing Schwann cell membranes an

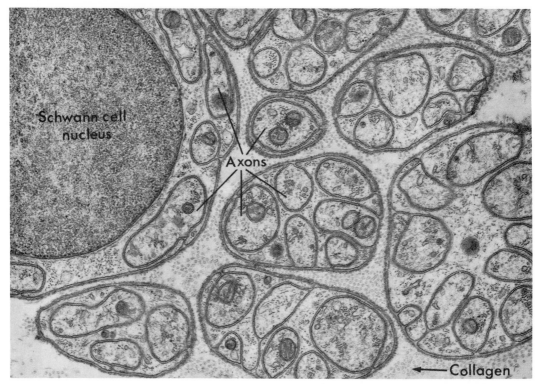

Figure 11–18. Electron micrograph of a small area of unmyelinated nerve from the rat mesentery, showing multiple axons associated with the cross-sectional profile of each Schwann cell. Between these fascicles of unmyelinated axons are unit fibrils of collagen of the endoneurium.

intraperiod gap or channel that is continuous through the myelin sheath from the periaxonal to the endoneurial extracellular spaces.

Where the laminated myelin sheath is interrupted at each node of Ranvier, the axon is surrounded loosely by a collar of minute finger-like processes of the two adjoining Schwann cells. A distinct gap, however, is found between all the membranes in this unmyelinated part of the node (Fig. 11–22). This gap probably is of significance in relation to current flow between axoplasm and the exterior during propagation of the action potential.

In electron micrographs of myelinating peripheral nerves, successive stages can be found in the development of the sheath from a double-layered infolding of the Schwann cell membrane (Fig. 11–21). The mechanism of formation of the spiral, consisting of a few to 50 or more turns around the axon, is still unsettled. It has been suggested that during myelinization the spiral disposition of the myelin lamellae is established by rotation of the sheath cells with respect to the axon. It is difficult, however, to imagine how such

movements could be initiated or controlled so as to result in formation of the precisely uniform laminated structure observed. Studies indicate that the myelin spiral does not develop because of any sort of corkscrew rotation of the axon during growth. If this were the mechanism, the direction of spiral for a particular axon would probably be the same in all its myelin segments, and such is not the case. Apparently the Schwann cell alone actively produces the spiral, and no interaction occurs between individual Schwann cells so far as the direction of spiral is concerned. Formation of new membrane at the free edge of the original infolding of the satellite cell membrane probably extends the fold spirally around the axon without significant change in the relative position of the neuron and its satellite cells. Much remains to be learned concerning the morphogenesis of myelin, but whatever the morphogenetic process, the result is that the axon becomes surrounded by a many-layered sheath.

In myelinated fibers of the central nervous system, certain neuroglial cells (oligoden-

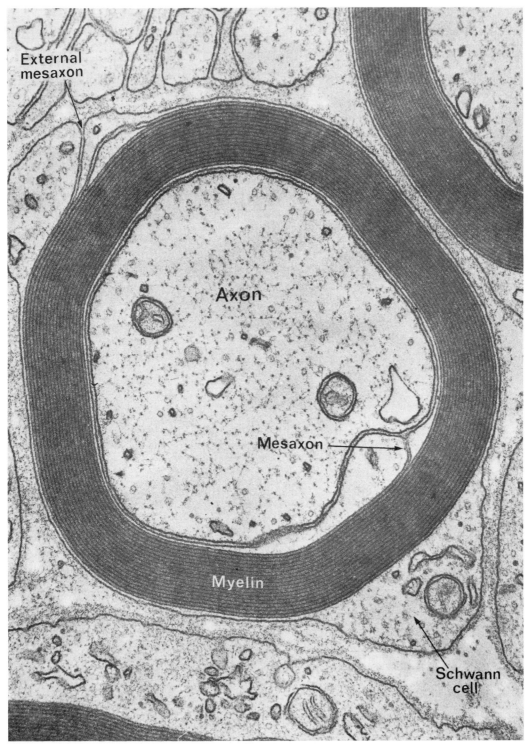

Figure 11–19. Electron micrograph of a large myelinated nerve in a rat spinal root. The myelin sheath consists of a multilayered spiral wrapping of Schwann cell membrane. Two apposed portions of Schwann cell membrane from the **internal mesaxon** extend from the periaxonal space to the innermost layer of myelin. Similarly the two membranes extending from the outermost turn of myelin to the endoneurial space are called the **external mesaxon.** (Micrograph from Coggeshall, R. Anat. Rec. *194*:201, 1979.)

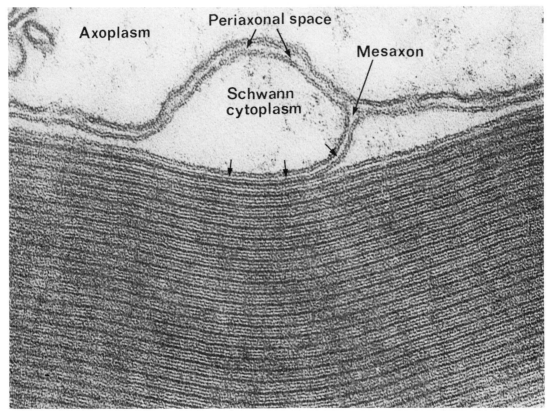

Figure 11–20. At high magnification it can be seen that the periaxonal space continues into the cleft between the opposing external leaflets of the membranes forming the internal mesaxon. This cleft in turn is continuous with a narrow intraperiod gap in the innermost turn of the myelin sheath *(see at arrows)*. (Micrograph from Coggeshall, R. Anat. Rec. *194*:201, 1979.)

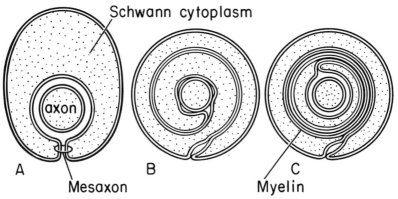

Figure 11–21. Diagrams illustrating the development of nerve myelin. *A,* Earliest stage: axon enveloped by a relatively large Schwann cell. *B,* Intermediate stage: unit membranes of mesaxon and to some extent of axon have come together, line of contact representing future *intraperiod* line of myelin. *C,* Later stage: a few layers of compact myelin have formed by contact of cytoplasmic surfaces of mesaxon loops to make *major dense line* of myelin. (Redrawn from Robertson, J. D. Prog. Biophys. *10*:349, 1960.)

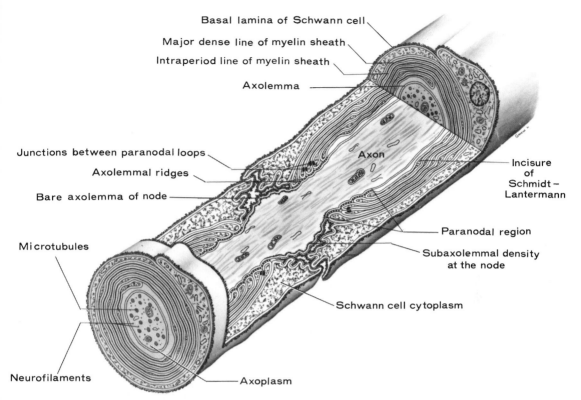

Basal lamina of Schwann cell
Major dense line of myelin sheath
Intraperiod line of myelin sheath
Axolemma

Junctions between paranodal loops
Axolemmal ridges
Bare axolemma of node

Microtubules

Neurofilaments

Axon

Incisure of Schmidt– Lantermann

Paranodal region

Subaxolemmal density at the node

Schwann cell cytoplasm

Axoplasm

Figure 11–22. Diagrammatic representation of the myelin sheath, node of Ranvier, and incisures of Schmidt-Lantermann in a peripheral nerve. (Courtesy of D. Kent Morest.)

droglia) play a role corresponding to that of the Schwann cells in the peripheral nervous system. Nodes of Ranvier occur in the central nervous system, but Schmidt-Lantermann clefts have not been seen.

In ontogenesis, myelin appears relatively late, and the process of myelinization ends some time after birth. Different fiber systems or tracts of the brain and spinal cord become myelinated at different times.

PERIPHERAL NERVES

In their course outside the central nervous system, nerve fibers of varying thickness (from 2 to up to 30 μm) are associated in fascicles and held together by connective tissue to form peripheral nerves. The outer layer of the nerve, the *epineurium*, is made up of connective tissue cells and collagenous fibers, mainly arranged longitudinally (Fig. 11–23). Fat cells may also be found here. Each of the smaller fascicles of a nerve is enclosed in concentric layers of connective tissue forming the *perineurium*. Fine, longi-

tudinally arranged strands of collagenous fibers and fibroblasts pass into the spaces between the individual nerve fibers constituting the *endoneurium*. Where the nerve branches, the connective tissue sheaths become thinner. The smaller branches lack epineurium, and the perineurium cannot be distinguished from the endoneurium, being reduced to a thin, fibrillar layer covered with flat connective tissue cells resembling endothelial cells. Delicate reticular fibrils around each nerve fiber form the tenuous endoneurium. Blood vessels are embedded in the epineurium and perineurium and more rarely in the thicker layers of endoneurium.

It has become customary to classify nerve fibers according to their diameter, because the speed conduction of the action potential varies with the diameter of the fiber. Diameters cover a wide and continuous range from large myelinated to small unmyelinated fibers. In peripheral nerves the fibers fall into three distinct groups. The large fibers, group A, conduct at 15 to 100 meters per second and include motor and some sensory fibers. Group B fibers conduct at 3 to 14 meters per

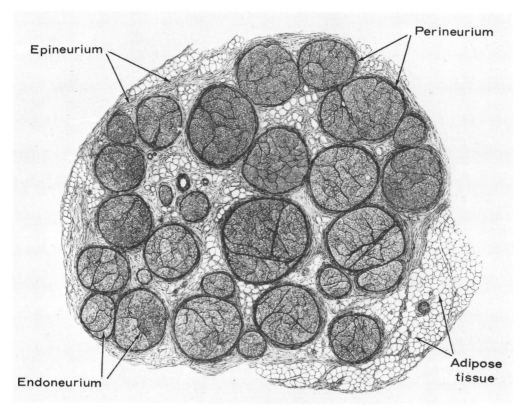

Figure 11–23. Drawing of a histological cross section of a human ulnar nerve at very low magnification, illustrating the perineural adipose tissue, epineurium, perineurium, and endoneurium. (From Bargmann, W. Histologie und mikroskopische Anatomie des Menschen. Stuttgart, Georg Thieme, 1959.)

second and include mainly visceral sensory fibers. The C group, small unmyelinated fibers conducting at 0.5 to 2 meters per second, carry autonomic and some sensory impulses. Other systems of classification besides this one are used in physiological studies.

Motor nerve fibers of the skeletal muscles are thick and heavily myelinated; those of visceral smooth muscle are thin, lightly myelinated, or without myelin. Tactile fibers are medium-sized and moderately myelinated; pain and taste fibers are thinner, with less myelin or none at all, and olfactory nerve filaments are always unmyelinated. Such histologically defined fiber aggregates constitute distinct functional systems: *somatic motor, visceral motor, tactile, gustatory, olfactory,* and so forth.

Clear segregation of functionally different nerve fibers is found in the *spinal roots*. In the ventral root are motor fibers of several types: (1) coarse and heavily myelinated, innervating ordinary skeletal muscle fibers; (2) small and myelinated, terminating on intrafusal muscle fibers; and (3) fine and lightly myelinated, belonging to the autonomic ner-

vous system. The dorsal root contains sensory fibers from superficial and deep cutaneous regions, sensory fibers from muscles and tendons, and afferent fibers from viscera. More than half of the dorsal root fibers are very small axons; most of these distribute with the cutaneous rami. The relative numbers of myelinated and unmyelinated fibers vary widely in different spinal segments and in the same segment in different mammalian species. In the mixed nerve trunks peripheral to the spinal ganglia, the fibers of motor and sensory roots mingle, together with sympathetic fibers from the communicating rami. In mixed trunks stained with hematoxylin and eosin or by another routine method, the lipid constituents of myelin are dissolved out, leaving a loosely arranged protein network called *neurokeratin* (Figs. 11–17, 11–24). A faintly stained axon can usually be seen in the center of this network. In such preparations, myelinated fibers of various sizes are readily identified by the clear zones of extracted myelin surrounding the darkly stained axons. In tissues that have been fixed with glutaraldehyde and osmium tetroxide,

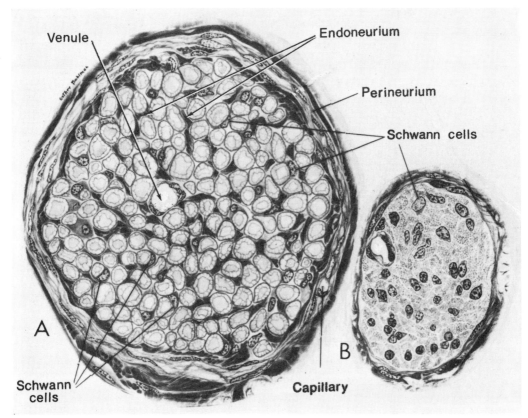

Figure 11–24. Drawing of myelinated *(A)* and unmyelinated nerve *(B)* as they appear in cross section in routine histological preparations. The lipid of the myelin sheaths in *(A)* has been extracted in specimen preparation.

the lipid of the myelin is preserved as a dark rim around the axon (Fig. 11–25).

In the brain and spinal cord, nerve fibers also segregate into functional systems, the *afferent* (incoming) and *efferent* (outgoing) pathways (spinocerebellar, spinothalamic, corticobulbar, corticospinal, and other fiber tracts whose origins and terminations are indicated by binomial nomenclature). Each has a special function.

NERVE ENDINGS

Each peripheral nerve fiber, sensory, motor, or secretory, sooner or later ends in some peripheral organ with one or several terminal arborizations. Some nerve fibers ramify as free endings among the non-nervous tissue cells; others attach to tissue cells by means of specialized terminations. The fibers ending in sensory *receptors* are dendrites; those with *motor* or *secretory* endings are axons, their terminations being called *axon endings*. In general, the structure of the ending is adapted to increase the surface of contact between the neuron and its related non-nervous element. The physicochemical changes that mediate the transfer of the various stimuli from, or the nerve impulses to, a peripheral non-nervous structure have been intensively studied. Three groups of nerve terminations can be distinguished: (1) endings in muscle, (2) endings in epithelium, and (3) endings in connective tissue.

Nerve Endings in Smooth and Cardiac Muscle

From complicated plexuses, thin unmyelinated nerve fibers depart and eventually contact or approach the surface of the muscle cells. *Visceral motor axons* give rise to terminal branches that carry numerous *boutons en passant* filled with synaptic vesicles. These endings remain at a variable distance from the surface of the smooth and cardiac muscle cells and do not form specialized junctions with their membrane. *Visceral sensory fibers* ramify in the connective tissue between smooth muscle bundles or contact the muscle fibers themselves. In cardiac muscle the tissue

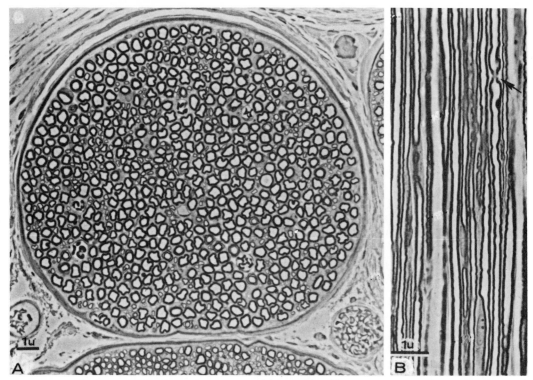

Figure 11–25. A, Cross section of guinea pig sciatic nerve after glutaraldehyde and osmium fixation and embedding in Epon-araldite. The myelin sheaths have been well preserved and appear as black rims around the axons. B, Longitudinal section similarly prepared. Arrow indicates a node of Ranvier. (From Webster, H. In Hubbard, J., ed.: The Vertebrate Peripheral Nervous System. New York, Plenum Press, 1974.)

is permeated by a multitude of thin fibers passing between muscle trabeculae. They appear to end near the surface of the muscle fibers but form no specialized contacts with them.

Motor Nerve Endings in Striated Muscles

The terminations of somatic motor nerves have a more complex structure than those of smooth and cardiac muscle. The motor end plate has already been described in Chapter 10 and need only be reviewed here briefly.

Each motor nerve fiber branches to supply many muscle fibers. The motor neuron together with the muscle fibers it innervates is called a *motor unit*. The myelin sheath ends as a terminal branch of the nerve fiber nears the muscle fiber. The enveloping sheath of Schwann cell cytoplasm continues beyond the termination of the myelin and covers the surfaces of the axonal branch. At the junction of the nerve and muscle fiber there is a local accumulation of sarcoplasm rich in mitochondria and muscle nuclei, the *motor end plate*

(Fig. 11–26). The terminal branches of the nerve fiber ramify and occupy grooves or troughs in the surface of the muscle fiber. Within the expanded axon terminal are numerous mitochondria and *synaptic vesicles*, 40 to 60 nm in diameter. The neurofilaments and microtubules found within the axon usually do not continue into the terminal. The apposed membranes of the axon and of the muscle fiber do not touch but are separated everywhere by a glycoprotein layer continuous with the boundary layer investing the Schwann cell and the sarcolemma. This layer extends into the trough and the narrow gutters formed by infolding of the sarcolemma of the end plate. The gap between the surfaces of the axon and muscle fiber varies in width up to 50 nm.

Sensory Nerve Endings in Striated Muscles

These are always present in considerable numbers, some in the muscular tissue, others on tendons or at muscle-tendon junctions. Some terminations are simple, others com-

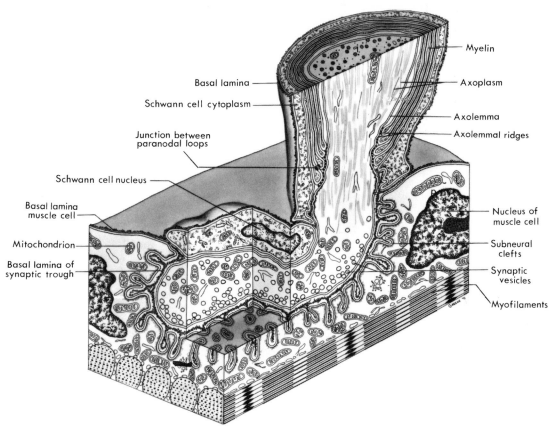

Figure 11–26. Diagrammatic representation of a myoneural junction (motor end plate), illustrating a typical chemical synapse in the peripheral nervous system. Synapses in the central nervous system have some features in common with this, but they occur between neurons and have no basal lamina or postjunctional folds. (Courtesy of D. Kent Morest.)

plex. The *interstitial terminations* are distributed in the connective tissue; the *epilemmal terminations* closely contact the muscle fibers. The interstitial terminations may be simple naked branches of the axons or encapsulated structures. The epilemmal endings likewise may be simple: one or more tortuous axons, after shedding their myelin sheath at approximately the midpoint of a muscle fiber, envelop the sarcolemma in continuous circular and spiral twists. Their varicose twigs terminate with nodular swellings. More complicated *neuromuscular spindles*, found only in higher vertebrates, are long (0.75 to 7 mm or more) narrow structures arranged parallel to the bundles of ordinary muscle fibers, and situated mainly near the junction of muscles with tendons. Each spindle, enveloped by a connective tissue capsule, consists of several long striated muscle fibers, the *intrafusal fibers,* which are shorter and thinner than the other *(extrafusal)* muscle fibers (see also Chapter 10). Midway along each fiber, the striations are replaced by a collection of nuclei,

the *nuclear bag*. Another type of intrafusal fiber displays a longitudinal array of nuclei, or *nuclear chain* in its nonstriated central portion. The intrafusal muscle fibers are attached in parallel to the extrafusal fibers and are stretched whenever the muscle is stretched. Each spindle is approached by two types of thick sensory nerve fibers. The larger axons form *annulospiral endings* around the noncontractile segment of the intrafusal fibers. This primary receptor signals both the rate and extent of muscle lengthening. Heightened activity of the primary receptors exerts an excitatory effect upon the motor neurons to the same muscle by a direct reflex connection in the CNS. The thinner axons have *flower-spray endings*, which predominantly innervate the nuclear chain fibers. This receptor signals the extent, more than the rate, of muscle lengthening.

Neuromuscular spindles are also supplied by thin motor nerves, *gamma fibers,* which emanate from small *gamma motor neurons* in the CNS. (The large motor neurons that send axons to the extrafusal muscle fibers are called *alpha motor neurons*.) The gamma fibers terminate on the intrafusal muscle fibers with typical motor end plates. These fibers effect shortening of the striated, contractile portions of the intrafusal fibers. These contractions do not contribute significantly to the tension produced by the muscle but serve instead to stretch the noncontractile region of the intrafusal fibers where the annulospiral endings are located. Such stretching causes the receptor to discharge more rapidly; hence, the function of the gamma fibers is to regulate the sensitivity of the neuromuscular spindle to stretch.

Sensory Nerve Endings in Tendons

These are of several kinds and also may be either simple or encapsulated. In simple forms, the naked nerve fibers and their branches spread over the surface of the tendon fibers in small, treelike figures of different types. Such endings in tendons and fasciae probably carry pain sensation. Composite forms, the *Golgi tendon organs*, occur at the junction of muscle fibers with intramuscular connective tissue or with tendons. They are supplied by a single sensory fiber that branches among the bundles of connective tissue fibers and terminates with small sprays of endings. In contrast to neuromuscular spindles, however, which are placed in parallel with the other muscle fibers, the Golgi tendon organs are in series with the contractile elements. These receptors respond to increase in tension; a heightened activity of the receptors exerts an inhibitory effect, through interneurons of the CNS, upon the alpha motor neurons of the same muscle.

The physiological significance of the sensory endings in muscles and tendons has been clarified greatly in recent years, as has their morphology. These receptors participate in postural and phasic adjustments of skeletal musculature. Intimate and complex connections in the CNS relate their activity to the alpha and gamma motor neurons. This activity, however, should not be described as "muscle sense" or "position sense"; awareness of the position of the body parts in space appears to be mediated by receptors located in joints.

Nerve Endings in Epithelial Tissue

Histologically, receptors and effectors can be distinguished only in rare instances. The terminations in the epithelial layers of the skin and mucous membranes are probably only sensory, and those in the epithelial glands partly secretory, partly sensory. Endings in glands (lacrimal, salivary, kidneys, and so on) are all unmyelinated sympathetic fibers forming dense nets on the outer surface of the basal lamina; branches penetrate the lamina, often forming a second network on its inner surface, and end between the gland cells.

Free sensory epithelial endings are abundant where sensitivity is highly developed: in the epithelium of the cornea, in the mucous membrane of the respiratory passages and oral cavity, and in the skin. In the epidermis, these branches do not penetrate farther than the granular layer. Free nerve endings in hair follicles are important tactile organs. There are two sets of endings—one circularly arranged in the middle layer of the dermal sheath, the other consisting of fibers running parallel to the hair shaft and terminating in the outer root sheath.

Nerve Endings in Connective Tissue

These are numerous and of many forms, particularly in the dermis, under the epithelium and mesothelium of the mucous and serous membranes, around the joints, in the endocardium, and elsewhere. They are either free or encapsulated endings, or are connected with special tactile cells of epithelial origin. More complex endings are found in skin and hypodermis, mucous and serous membranes, endocardium, cornea, sclera, and periosteum. Nonencapsulated endings are frequent in the papillary layer of the skin, connective tissue of mucous membranes (such as that of the urinary bladder), and pericardium, endocardium, and periosteum; the terminal branches form spherical or elongated structures resembling glomeruli.

Encapsulated Terminal Sensory Endings

In these, a special connective tissue capsule of varying thickness surrounds the actual nerve endings. The capsule attains its greatest thickness in the *corpuscles of Vater-Pacini* (Figs. 11–27, 11–28), found in the deeper layers of the skin, under mucous membranes, in conjunctiva, cornea, heart, mesentery, and pancreas, and in loose connective tissue. These structures are large (1 to 4 mm by 2 mm) and white in color. Each is supplied with

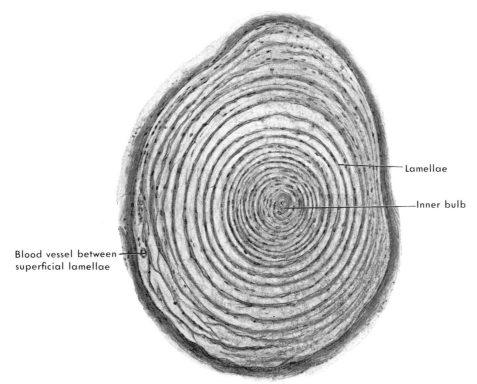

Figure 11–27. Drawing of a cross section of a corpuscle of Vater-Pacini, from the dermis of the sole of the foot. (After Schaffer.)

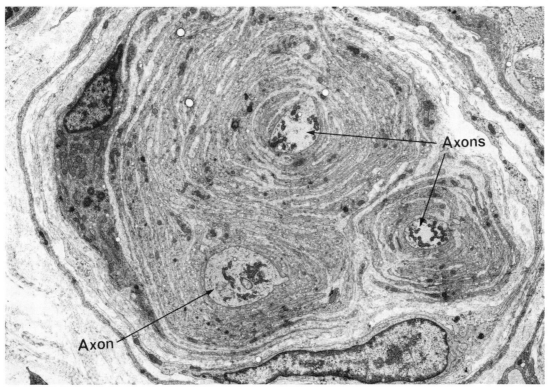

Figure 11–28. Electron micrograph of a cluster of three small encapsulated nerve endings. (Micrograph courtesy of E. Weihe.)

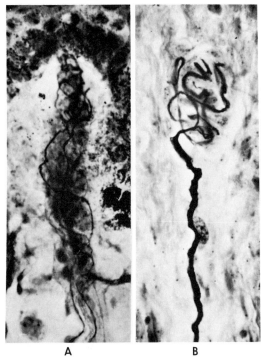

A B

Figure 11–29. *A,* Genital corpuscle from the glans penis of a 23-year-old man. Silver preparation. (Courtesy of N. Cauna.) *B,* Lingual corpuscle from a filiform papilla on the tongue of a 21-year-old woman. Silver stain. (From Cauna, N. *Anat. Rec. 124:*77, 1956.)

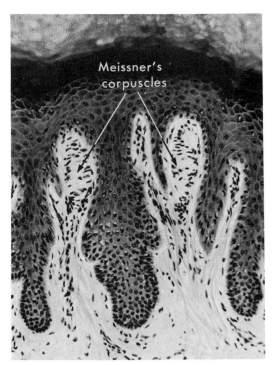

Figure 11–30. Photomicrograph of palmar digital epidermis showing Meissner's corpuscles in two neighboring dermal papillae. Hematoxylin and eosin.

one or more thick myelinated fibers, which lose myelin upon entering the corpuscle. Flattened Schwann cells surround the nerve ending, and these are in turn encircled by the lamellae of the connective tissue capsule. *Genital corpuscles,* in the skin of the external genital organs and of the nipple, are similar (Fig. 11–29A). *Meissner's corpuscles* (Figs. 11–30, 11–31, 11–32), occurring in connective tissue of the skin of the palms, soles, and tips of the fingers and toes, are elongated, pear-shaped, or elliptical formations with rounded ends, located in the cutaneous papillae, with the long axis vertical to the surface. Their size varies (40 to 100 μm by 30 to 60μm) *Corpuscles of Golgi-Mazzoni* and *terminal bulbs of Krause* resemble corpuscles of Vater-Pacini but are smaller and simpler in construction.

AUTONOMIC NERVOUS SYSTEM

Motor neurons of the central and peripheral nervous systems concerned with the regulation of visceral activities form the *auto-nomic nervous system.* This system, as defined long ago, unfortunately excludes the *visceral sensory neurons,* or interoceptive system, which form the afferent side of visceral arcs.

The autonomic nervous system includes numerous small ganglia. The *vertebral ganglia* form a chain, *the sympathetic trunk,* on either side of the spinal column; the sympathetic trunk is connected proximally with the ventral roots of the spinal nerves. Additional ganglia lie at some distance from the central nervous system in certain nerve plexuses *(collateral* or *prevertebral ganglia)* or in the walls of organs *(terminal ganglia).* The autonomic ganglia contain motor nerve cell bodies, which convey impulses originating in the brain and spinal cord to smooth muscle and glands by way of the *visceral* or *splanchnic* nerves (Fig. 11–33). Fibers of some cell bodies in the sympathetic trunk join those in the peripheral nerves and run to the sweat glands and arrector pili muscles. Whatever the destination, the autonomic nervous system mediates activity by two motor neurons placed in series; the first lies either in a nucleus of the brain stem or in a special territory of the spinal gray matter, and the second is located in a ganglion outside of the CNS. In the

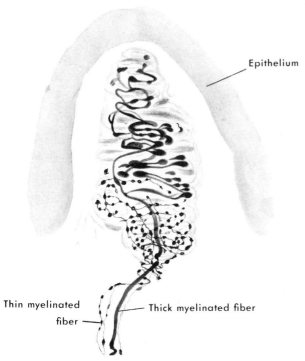

Epithelium

Thin myelinated fiber — Thick myelinated fiber

Figure 11–31

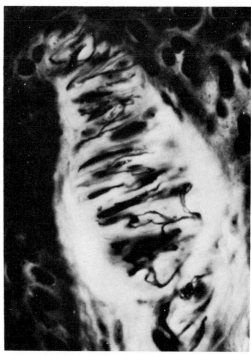

Figure 11–32

Figure 11–31. Meissner's corpuscle of a dermal papilla of a human finger. Methylene blue stain. (Redrawn after Dogiel.)

Figure 11–32. Meissner's corpuscle of an 11-year-old girl. Silver stain. (Courtesy of N. Cauna.)

peripheral nervous system, only one motor neuron transmits activity to the effector organ.

The autonomic system consists of *sympathetic (thoracolumbar)* and *parasympathetic (craniosacral)* divisions: it influences the intrinsic activity of cardiac muscle and supplies nerve fibers to smooth muscle in the viscera, salivary and sweat glands, blood vessels, and other structures. The peripheral nervous system, in contrast, innervates striated skeletal muscle. Despite these distinctions, however, the traditional concept of an autonomic nervous system is justifiable only in terms of convenience; its components and functions are inextricably bound up with the rest of the nervous system and do not possess autonomy.

The sympathetic trunks and their ganglia, as well as the collateral ganglia, are the avenues of communication for the thoracolumbar outflow between the CNS and the viscera. Each sympathetic trunk contains ganglia at the level of exit of most of the corresponding spinal nerves. The *communicating branches (rami communicantes)* pass between the trunk and the spinal nerves.

The cell bodies of the sympathetic neurons lie in the *intermediolateral gray column* of the thoracic and upper lumbar spinal cord. The axons pass into the ventral roots of spinal nerves and through the white communicating branches, to end either in a vertebral ganglion of the sympathetic trunk or in a prevertebral ganglion. Most of these axons, the *preganglionic fibers*, with thin myelin sheaths, terminate in a sympathetic ganglion. Here they synapse with secondary *visceral motor neurons*, whose axons—mostly unmyelinated postganglionic fibers—transmit activity to visceral muscles or glands. Some postganglionic fibers travel to internal viscera over sympathetic nerves, such as the cardiac or splanchnic nerves; others extend from vertebral ganglia through gray communicating branches and spinal nerves to structures of the body wall and extremities; *vasomotor fibers* chiefly to arteriolar muscles, *pilomotor fibers* to the small muscles of hair follicles, and *sudomotor fibers* to the sweat glands.

The craniosacral division of the autonomic system has preganglionic neurons in the brain and spinal cord. Axons of the cranial component emerge in the oculomotor, facial, glossopharyngeal, and vagus nerves, to synapse in terminal ganglia innervating the head and trunk. From the second, third, and fourth sacral segments of the spinal cord,

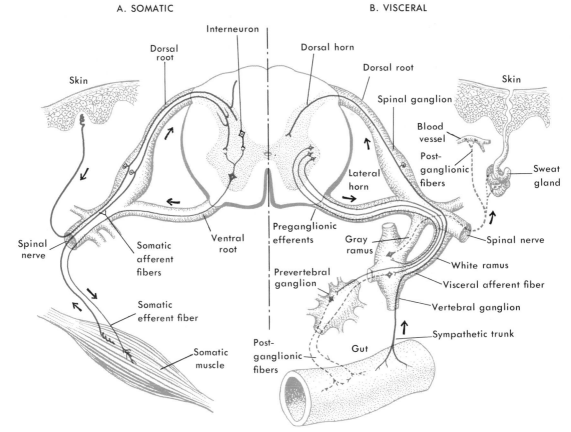

Figure 11–33. *A,* Somatic nerves. *B,* Visceral nerves. A cross section of spinal cord is shown connected via dorsal and ventral roots to the spinal nerve and to one of the ganglia of the autonomic system. The pattern of afferent (blue) and efferent (red) nerve fibers in both the somatic and visceral system may be directly compared. (From Copenhaver, W. M., and R. Bunge, eds.: Bailey's Textbook of Histology. 16th ed. Baltimore, Williams and Wilkins, 1971.)

axons leave via ventral roots and sacral nerves to reach postganglionic neurons in terminal ganglia associated with pelvic viscera.

Postganglionic neurons may exercise a local regulatory control over the viscera to which they are related, secondarily subject to control by components of the CNS.

Distributed via both divisions of the autonomic nervous system, the peripheral process of visceral sensory neurons lead from the viscera through the communicating rami, or through cranial or sacral nerves, to sensory ganglia. Their cell bodies are morphologically indistinguishable from those of the somatic sensory neurons, with which they mingle in the craniospinal ganglia.

Autonomic Nerve Cells

The cell bodies of preganglionic visceral efferent neurons are small, spindle-shaped elements in the intermediolateral gray column. Their perikarya are not studded with innumerable terminal boutons, as are the large nerve cell bodies of somatic motor neurons. Instead, a relatively small number of axodendritic endings is found.

Postganglionic neurons of the craniosacral division lie, as a rule, close to the viscera innervated. The preganglionic fibers, accordingly, are relatively long—as in the vagus nerve—and the postganglionic fibers short. On the other hand, most synapses of the thoracolumbar division are in the sympathetic trunk or collateral ganglia; therefore, the postganglionic fibers are longer.

Sympathetic ganglion cells are generally small and have diverse shapes. The cells are usually multipolar, dendrites and axon sometimes being distinguishable but in other cases showing no obvious difference. Preganglionic fibers often synapse with the dendrites of the ganglion cell in dense glomeruli. For a typical example, see the description of the postganglionic neurons of the intestine (Chap. 26).

The cell body may be encapsulated by

satellite cells, which, like those of the cranio-spinal ganglia, are ectodermal elements similar to Schwann cells in the nerve sheaths. In the outlying sympathetic ganglia these capsules may be absent, but Schwann cells accompany the peripheral sympathetic fibers everywhere.

NEUROGLIA

The number of nerve cells within the central nervous system, although enormous, is exceeded, perhaps fivefold, by the number of non-neural supportive cells, called the neuroglial cells or neuroglia. The term neuroglia is applied to the *ependyma,* which lines the ventricles of the brain and spinal cord, and to *neuroglial cells* and their processes, which mingle with neurons in the CNS and retina. The *satellite* or *capsular cells* of peripheral ganglia and the *Schwann cells* of peripheral nerves may be considered peripheral neuroglia.

Ependyma

In early embryonic stages the wall of the neural tube is a simple epithelium. Certain thin, non-nervous parts of the brain retain this structure throughout adult life, as, for example, the epithelial layer of the choroid plexus. In most other parts, the wall is greatly thickened by the accumulation of neurons and neuroglial elements. The lining of the inner surface of the ventricular cavities always retains an epithelial character. This membrane, the adult ependyma, is composed of the inner ends of epithelial cells, with their nuclei and some of their cytoplasm.

The embryonic ependyma is ciliated; in some parts of the ventricular lining, the cilia may persist into adult life. In the mature brain, the broad bases of ependymal cells taper to long, threadlike processes that branch and are lost among other elements of the brain. In a few places where the wall is thin, as in the ventral fissure of the spinal cord, some ependymal cells span the entire distance between ventricular and external surfaces, as all do in the early embryonic stages. In these cases, the ependymal cells form a dense *internal limiting membrane* at the ventricular end. At the external surface, under the *pia mater,* the ependymal threads and bars expand into pedicles that fuse into a thin, smooth, dense membrane, the *external limiting membrane* of the CNS. Similar membranes are formed around the blood vessels. The adult ependyma may represent the remaining epithelial cells of the embryonic ventricular zone (see section on development) or may be derived from a specialized subventricular zone that appears later in development and persists into adult life.

Neuroglial Cells

In any section of the central nervous system prepared by ordinary histological methods, small nuclei are seen scattered among the nerve cells and their processes. The cytoplasm and long processes of these neuroglial elements are demonstrable by special histological techniques.

Three types of neuroglia are distinguished: *astrocytes, oligodendrocytes,* and *microglia.* The first two, collectively *macroglia,* are ectodermal in origin, as are the nerve cells. The microglia are said to originate from mesodermal cells of the pia mater, which migrate into the CNS along the blood vessels.

The astrocytes are of two varieties. The *protoplasmic astrocyte* has a larger nucleus than oligodendrocytes and microglia, abundant granular cytoplasm, and numerous thick processes (Fig. 11–34A). Many processes attach to blood vessels and to the pia mater by means of expanded pedicles. In other cases, the cell body lies directly on the wall of the blood vessel or on the inner surface of the pia mater. Some of the smaller cells of this variety lie close to the bodies of the neurons and represent one type of satellite cell.

The *fibrous astrocyte* (Fig. 11–34B) is distinguished by long, relatively thin, smooth, and infrequently branched expansions. These cells also are often attached to blood vessels by means of their processes. Embedded within the cytoplasm are fibrillar structures. Electron micrographs show that the *neuroglial fibers* of light microscopy are in fact aggregation of slender filaments present in profusion in the cytoplasm. Glial filaments are distinct from neurofilaments because they are more densely packed, possess a diameter of only 8 nm, and have a different protein composition. Their main constituent is the *glial fibrillar acidic protein,* 51,000 daltons in molecular weight. Protoplasmic astrocytes are found chiefly in gray matter and fibrous astrocytes in white matter, insinuated between fascicles of nerve fibers. Mixed or *plasmatofibrous astrocytes* are occasionally encountered at the boundary between gray and

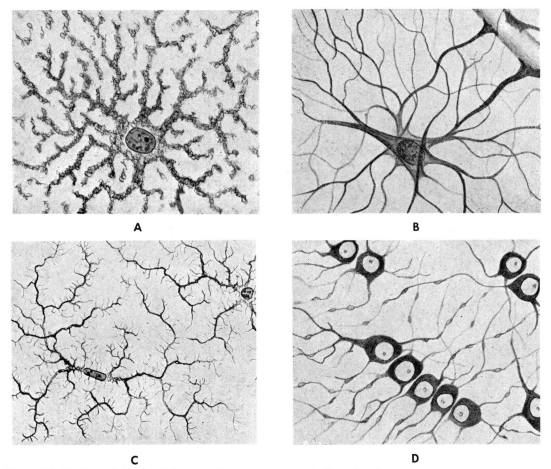

A

B

C

D

Figure 11–34. Neuroglial cells of the central nervous system. *A,* Protoplasmic astrocyte; *B,* fibrous astrocyte; *C,* microglia; *D,* oligodendroglia. (After del Rio-Hortega.)

white matter; processes that extend into the gray have a protoplasmic character whereas those that pass into the white are fibrous.

The oligodendrocytes (or oligodendroglia) (Fig. 11–34*D*) are akin to the astrocytes, which they resemble in many respects. They are usually smaller and have smaller nuclei, although there are many transitional forms. As their name implies, their few and slender processes have few branches. Oligodendrocytes relate intimately to nerve fibers, along which they form rows or columns. Although it is difficult to demonstrate the connection of the oligodendrocyte with the myelin sheath in the adult, studies on the developing nervous system show that this cell forms myelin in the CNS. Thus, it is the homologue of the neurilemmal cell of Schwann. In gray matter, oligodendrocytes adjoining nerve cells are the principal type of satellite cell. In tissue cultures, oligodendrocytes exhibit rhythmic pulsatile movements. The signifi-

cance of this behavior in relation to their normal function in the brain is not known. At the electron microscope astrocytes are pale cells with euchromatic nucleus and an inconspicuous complement of cytoplasmic organelles. Oligodendrocytes, on the other hand, have a heterochromatic nucleus, a dark cytoplasm rich in ribosomes and cisternae of granular reticulum, a large Golgi apparatus, and numerous mitochondria. Microtubules are prominent both in the perinuclear cytoplasm and in the cell processes.

In the microglia (Fig. 11–34*C*), the nucleus is small but deeply stained and surrounded by scant cytoplasm. The few processes are short and, unlike the more or less straight extensions of the astrocytes, are twisted in various ways. Also, the processes and the cell body are not smooth, but are covered with numerous tiny pointed twigs or spines. Microglia are scattered everywhere throughout the brain and spinal cord.

In the mature CNS, and also it seems now during development, neuroglia provide an extremely complex framework for the neurons, a scaffolding for migratory young neurocytes and their cell processes. Like the neurons, the supporting neuroglial cells do not form a syncytium but retain their individuality. In the chambers of a complex labyrinth of glial cells, the nerve cells and their processes are often individually encapsulated and thus insulated from one another. An interesting and probably significant fact revealed by electron microscopy is that wherever nerve cell bodies and their processes are not in synaptic contact with another neuron, they are generally enveloped by the cell bodies or processes of neuroglial cells. The distribution of these neuroglial processes thus appears neither to be random nor merely to fulfill the requirements of mechanical support and nutrition of the neurons. Early in this century, Ramón y Cajal proposed that neuroglial processes are always disposed to prevent contact between processes of nerve cells at sites other than those appropriate to their specific signaling function. On the basis of electron microscopic observations. This hypothesis has been revived. It has been shown that each neuron has a characteristic pattern of neuroglial investment complementary to the specific pattern of its synaptic connections. Only at the synapses are the neuroglial barriers interrupted, and only here is direct contact between the neurons possible. Thus, by isolating and individualizing the many diverse pathways that may converge upon a given neuron, the neuroglial cells may play an essential role in the communications function of the nervous system.

Neuroglial cells seem also to be an important mediator for the normal metabolism of neurons, although little is known in this respect. There is evidence that they remove from the extracellular space the potassium that accumulates as a result of the neuronal activity. More is known about the activity of neuroglia in states of injury or disease. Whenever neurons are affected by a local or distant pathological process, the surrounding neuroglial elements always react in some way. They are actively involved in degeneration and regeneration of the nerve fibers, in vascular disorders, and in various infectious diseases. They are the chief source of tumors of the CNS. Under certain circumstances, microglia may assume a great variety of forms, with active migration and phagocytosis.

THE SYNAPSE AND THE RELATIONSHIPS OF NEURONS

The nervous system consists of complex chains of neurons arranged to permit transmission of activity from one cell to the other. Each neuron receives excitatory and inhibitory influences from other neurons or sensory receptors, integrates them, and (depending on their balance) generates and transmits signals to other neurons or peripheral effector cells. The site of signal transmission is the *synapse.*

Two distinct modes of transmission are known: electrical and chemical. *Electrical synapses* are less common in the central nervous system of mammals; at the electron microscope they were identified as gap junctions, which permit movement of ions and thus direct spread of current from one neuron to the adjoining one.

At *chemical synapses,* the process of a neuron, called presynaptic, secretes a *neurotransmitter* substance that diffuses across the intercellular space and binds to specific receptors on the surface of a postsynaptic neuron, causing changes in ionic permeability of its membrane. Henceforth, chemical synapses will be simply referred to as synapses, because they are by far the most common site of transmission between nerve cells.

Traditionally, the synapse was described as a place of contact between two neurons; it is usually established by the terminal arborization of an axon on the dendrites *(axodendritic),* the perikaryon *(axosomatic),* or the axon *(axoaxonic)* of one or more neurons. *Dendrodendritic* synapses and synapses between the adjacent perikarya have also been found, but they are uncommon. Thus, it appears that any part of a neuron can participate in the formation of a synapse. Axons commonly end by giving rise to terminal branches that carry tiny swellings along their course *(boutons en passant)* or at their end *(boutons terminaux).* These swellings or endings are applied to the surface of the postsynaptic neuron. Sometimes, the terminal twigs may form "bouquets" or loose baskets adhering to the body or dendrites of other nerve cells. In rare instances, the axon gives rise to a single large

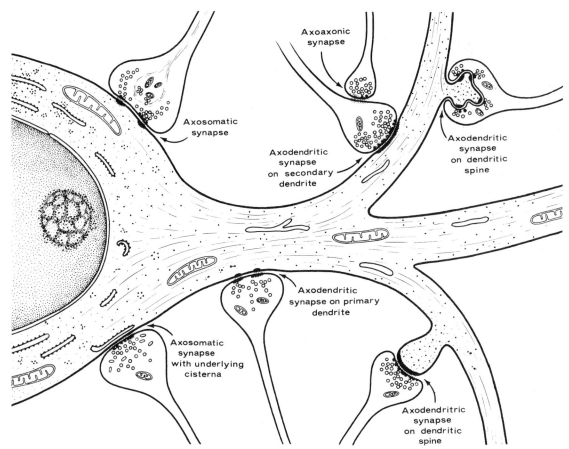

Figure 11–35. The types and terminology of the synapses occurring on various parts of the neuron. (Redrawn after Bunge, R. *In* Copenhaver, W. M., and R. Bunge, eds.: Bailey's Textbook of Histology. 16th ed. Baltimore, Williams and Wilkins, 1971.)

ending that occupies an extensive portion of the surface of the postsynaptic cell; these endings are called *end bulbs* in the ventral cochlear nucleus, and *calyces* in the nucleus of the trapezoid body. In the cerebellar and cerebral cortices, axon terminals contact the dendritic spines of the Purkinje and pyramidal cells, respectively. The number of synapses on a neuron varies enormously. Some neurons, such as the granule cell of the cerebellum, have only a few. A motor neuron may possess as many as 10,000 synapses. A Purkinje cell of the cerebellum may have 100,000 endings upon its dendrites alone.

The electron microscope demonstrates that one or more specialized junctions occur at the site of contact between presynaptic ending and postsynaptic neuron; in addition, the presynaptic ending contains a specific complement of cytoplasmic organelles (Figs. 11–36, 11–37). The synaptic junctions or complexes have the following general properties: the pre- and postsynaptic membranes

run a parallel course, often gently convex toward the presynaptic cytoplasm, and they are separated by an intercellular space or *synaptic cleft* 20 to 30 nm in width. The synaptic cleft is traversed by fine filaments and is sometimes bisected by a tenuous plaque of dense material. *Synaptic vesicles,* 40 to 60 nm in diameter, cluster near the presynaptic membrane; at this site, the membrane carries dense material on its cytoplasmic surface. Finally, the cytoplasmic aspect of the postsynaptic membrane is decorated by a layer of dense, fluffy material. The cytoplasm of the presynaptic ending contains randomly dispersed synaptic vesicles; a variable number of mitochondria, situated at some distance from the synaptic junctions; and a few cisternae and tubules of the agranular reticulum. Microtubules and neurofilaments also are occasionally present.

Certain synaptic junctions have a cleft 30 nm in width: furthermore, they are characterized by a prominent postsynaptic density

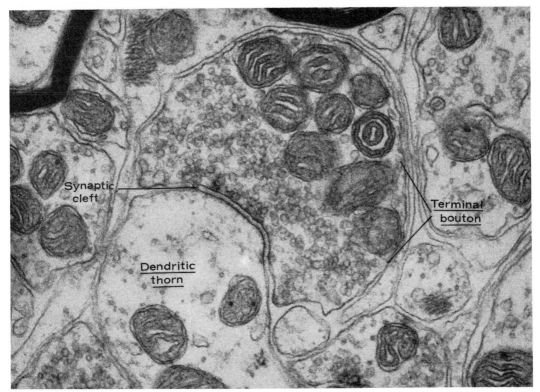

Figure 11–36. Tip of a dendritic spine, capped by a terminal bouton from the ventral horn of the spinal cord in a rat. The typical features of synapses—mitochondria, clustered vesicles, and the cleft—are well shown. The terminal is enclosed within a thin astrocytic process. (Courtesy of S. L. Palay.)

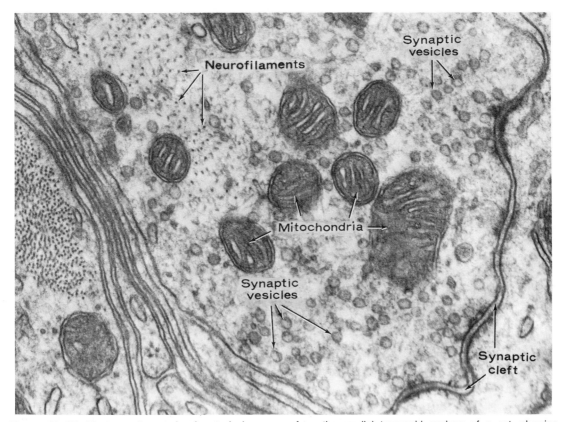

Figure 11–37. Electron micrograph of a typical synapse from the medial trapezoid nucleus of a cat, showing neurofilaments and synaptic vesicles in the nerve ending, a typical synaptic cleft between the pre- and postsynaptic membranes. (Micrograph courtesy M. Jean-Baptiste and D. Kent Morest.)

so that the contact appears asymmetrical. They are called by Gray *Type I* synapses and are consistently associated with round vesicles in the presynaptic ending. In the cerebellar cortex, they mediate excitation; thus, it is generally assumed that this type of synaptic junction has excitatory function. In other synaptic junctions, called *Type II* by Gray, the cleft is about 20 nm in width and the pre- and postsynaptic densities are nearly symmetrical. Furthermore, they may be associated with flattened synaptic vesicles in the presynaptic ending. In the cerebellar cortex, they mediate inhibition; thus, it is often assumed that Type II synapses have inhibitory function wherever they occur. It must be noted, however, that types of synaptic junctions exist whose structure is intermediate between Gray's Types I and II, so that it is impossible to infer their physiological properties solely on the basis of their morphological appearance.

Synaptic vesicles are membrane-bounded organelles that contain neurotransmitter substances. Until recently, the monoamines (norepinephrine, dopamine, and serotonin), acetylcholine, and amino acids (glycine, glutamate, and γ-aminobutyric acid or [GABA]) were thought to be the only neurotransmitters involved in synaptic transmission. More recently, a large number of peptides appear to act either as neurotransmitters or neuromodulators; i.e., substances that modify the action of classical neurotransmitters. *Substance P, hypothalamic releasing hormones, enkephalin, vasoactive intestinal polypeptide* (VIP), *cholecystokinin* (CCK), *neurotensin* are a few examples of this growing list of brain peptides involved in synaptic transmission. It is interesting to note that some of these peptides are also contained in secretory cells of the gastrointestinal tract, where they act on neighboring cells (paracrine secretion) and may be released as hormones into the bloodstream by endocrine glands or liberated from neurons into the blood of the hypophyseoportal vessels to regulate the function of the pars distalis of the pituitary (neurohormones). In all these instances the basic function of the molecule is intercellular communication, and it is not surprising that the organism exploits the same peptide for signal transmission either locally at the synapse (neurotransmitters) or at a distance (hormones). Among the large list of peptides synthesized by neurons, the best evidence

that they may act as classical neurotransmitters has been obtained for the luteinizing hormone–releasing hormone (LHRH), which, in sympathetic ganglia, acts on the postsynaptic neuron to produce a long-lasting depolarization. In addition to neurotransmitters, the synaptic vesicles may also contain enzymes involved in transmitter metabolism, such as dopamine-β-hydroxylase, which synthesizes norepinephrine.

In most synapses, the vesicles are spherical in shape and have a clear content *(agranular vesicles)*, but in some endings after aldehyde fixation and subsequent treatment with osmium tetroxide, the vesicles appear flattened. Clearly, it is a preparation artifact, for in freeze-fractured specimens all vesicles are round. As mentioned above, in the cerebellar cortex flattened vesicles are exclusively found at inhibitory synapses, whereas vesicles at excitatory synapses appear spherical. This correlation between structure and function cannot be generalized, because excitation and inhibition are the result of the action of the neurotransmitter on the postsynaptic membrane, and in different synapses the same neurotransmitter may have different postsynaptic effects.

A third variety of synaptic vesicles contain a dense core after aldehyde and especially after permanganate fixation; these *granular vesicles* are typical of nerve endings that release catecholamines as neurotransmitters. The fact that soaking the tissue in biogenic amines or their analogues causes an increase in the proportion of granular vesicles after aldehyde fixation supports the idea that the dense core indeed contain catecholamines.

The varieties of small synaptic vesicles just described are often associated with a small population of large vesicles, 80 to 120 nm in diameter, which consistently contain a core of dense material. In endings that use biogenic amines as neurotransmitters, the large dense-core vesicles probably contain catecholamines, but in endings that release different transmitters, their significance is unclear.

At the site where synaptic vesicles cluster near the presynaptic membrane, its cytoplasmic surface carries a set of dense projections arranged in a trigonal array. The vesicles of the presynaptic cluster that directly adjoin the presynaptic membrane nestle between the projections and may actually contact the plasmalemma. In rare instances, one of these vesicles is caught by the fixative fluid in the act of fusing with the presynaptic membrane; the plasmalemma becomes continuous with the vesicular membrane, and the lumen of the vesicle opens into the synaptic cleft.

Freeze-fracturing demonstrates two types of specializations in the interior of the presynaptic membrane: a population of randomly distributed large particles, and deformations of the membrane that appear as dimples or craters on the inner leaflet or P-face and protrusions on the outer leaflet or E-face. These deformations arise when the fracture plane breaks through the neck of synaptic vesicles that are fusing with the presynaptic membrane.

In addition to a cytoplasmic layer of dense material, the postsynaptic membrane may exhibit internal specializations that are revealed by the freeze-fracturing technique. In the cerebellum and olfactory bulb, excitatory synapses are characterized by a cluster of large intramembrane particles that remain consistently associated with the E-face, whereas the postsynaptic membrane of inhibitory synapses contains the usual population of randomly distributed particles, which are preferentially associated with the P-face. Synapses with a cluster of particles on the P-face of the postsynaptic membrane have also been found; examples are the neuromuscular junction, the synapses in the superior cervical ganglion, and those between photoreceptor and horizontal cells in the retina, all excitatory.

The physiological event that causes transmitter secretion is depolarization of the membrane of the presynaptic ending, produced by the arrival of a nerve impulse. As a consequence of the depolarization, calcium enters the ending and triggers release of transmitter. This is secreted in multimolecular packets or quanta of fixed size, and variations in release depend on the number of quanta secreted by the terminal. The transmitter diffuses across the synaptic cleft and combines with receptor molecules at the surface of the postsynaptic membrane. As a result of the binding of the transmitter with its receptor, ionic channels in the postsynaptic membrane open or close. In a typical excitatory synapse, the transmitter produces a simultaneous increase in the permeability to sodium and potassium, and this leads to depolarization of the postsynaptic membrane. At inhibitory synapses, the binding of the transmitter

to its receptor increases the permeability of the postsynaptic membrane to potassium or chloride, or both; this drives the membrane potential away from threshold and thus counteracts depolarization. After binding to the postsynaptic receptor, the transmitter is either degraded by enzymes or taken up again by the presynaptic ending.

The structural counterparts of these physiological events at the synapse have been actively investigated during the past decade. The specializations of the presynaptic membrane and the associated cluster of synaptic vesicles have been called the *active zone*, for it represents the site for transmitter release at the surface of the presynaptic ending. The synaptic vesicles contain the transmitter quanta, and upon calcium entry into the ending, they fuse with the plasma membrane at the synaptic junction, releasing their contents by exocytosis into the synaptic cleft. Using the technique of instantaneously freezing the presynaptic ending after the arrival of a nerve impulse, it has been shown that there is a good correlation between the number of quanta released and that of vesicles undergoing exocytosis.

The large particles within the active zone of the presynaptic membrane (Fig. 11–38) may represent the channels through which calcium enters the presynaptic ending and triggers vesicle fusion with the plasmalemma. The dense material associated with the presynaptic membrane may trap synaptic vesicles and concentrate them at the sites on the surface of the ending that face a cluster of postsynaptic receptors. It is interesting to note that there is a correlation between the configuration of this material that binds synaptic vesicles and the geometry of the synapse. In the neuromuscular junction, where acetylcholine receptors reside on the lips of the junctional folds of the muscle membrane, the dense material has the shape of a bar overlying the junctional folds. In the invaginating synapses established by the endings of the photoreceptor cells of the retina, the dense material has the shape of a thin plate or ribbon, which bisects a wedge-shaped projection of the presynaptic ending or synaptic ridge. Vesicles are thus positioned near the slopes of the ridge, opposite the postsynaptic specializations of two adjoining postsynaptic processes that belong to horizontal cells. In this fashion, two postsynaptic neurons may be activated simultaneously.

The dense material contained within the

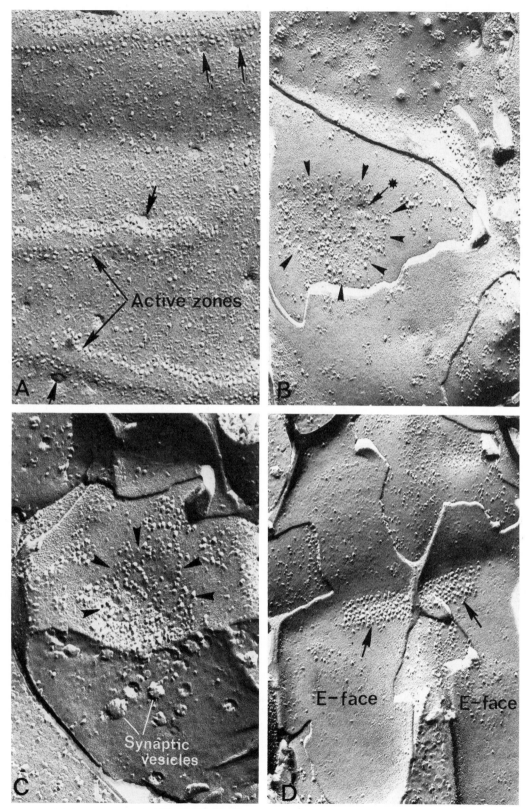

Figure 11–38. *See legend on opposite page*

synaptic cleft may provide direct mechanical coupling between the pre- and postsynaptic membranes and thus ensure cell-to-cell adhesion. In fact, a number of experiments indicate that the synaptic junction is capable of resisting stresses that elsewhere tear apart the pre- and postsynaptic surfaces. The material in the synaptic cleft may have additional important functions in synaptic transmission: in the neuromuscular junction it contains the enzyme acetylcholinesterase, which hydrolyzes the transmitter acetylcholine and thus rapidly shuts off its effect on the postsynaptic membrane.

In the Torpedo electric organ, the postsynaptic surface of the electroplax cell is covered with minute bumps that may correspond to the receptor molecules for the neurotransmitter. In the neuromuscular junction, using labeled α-bungarotoxin that irreversibly binds to acetylcholine receptors, these were localized in the regions of the postsynaptic membrane that carry a coat of dense cytoplasmic material. Thus, there is no doubt that the specialized region of the postsynaptic membrane contains the receptor-ionophore complexes responsible for the postsynaptic changes in ionic permeability. It is still unclear whether the intramembrane particles clustered within the postsynaptic membrane correspond to the ion channels that open or close after transmitter binding to its receptors.

After fusion of the synaptic vesicles with the presynaptic membrane and release of their transmitter contents into the synaptic cleft, the vesicular membrane is incorporated into the plasmalemma. According to a widely accepted hypothesis, the constituents of the vesicular membrane diffuse laterally within the plane of the plasma membrane and are finally retrieved at the periphery of the active zone through coated vesicles and smooth-surfaced cisternae (Fig. 11–39). From these endocytic organelles, new generations of synaptic vesicles are reformed and refilled with transmitter, so that the constituents of their limiting membrane are utilized many times over again by the presynaptic ending. In addition to this mechanism of local recycling of the vesicular membrane, new vesicles are certainly contributed by the neuronal soma, where they are probably formed in the Golgi apparatus and transported to the ending by the axoplasmic flow. Since agranular vesicles are rarely seen in the axoplasm, they may travel along the axon as tubules of the endoplasmic reticulum, which bud new vesicles upon their arrival to the ending.

The absence of cytoplasmic continuity between neurons forms the basic for the "neuron doctrine"—that each mature nerve cell represents a cellular unit anatomically separate from, and trophically independent of, other neurons. The processes of a neuron depend on the cell body and its nucleus. When cut off from the cell body, the processes die. New processes may, however, grow out of the perikaryon. The body and nucleus of the nerve cell are the trophic center of the entire neuron. If a nerve cell suffers irreparable injury, other nerve cells are not necessarily affected. Nevertheless, certain groups of neurons may atrophy, or degenerate, following interruption of afferent axons or death of other neurons to which they send their efferent output. This phenomenon, *transneuronal degeneration,* has been considered exceptional for many years. It was especially evident in those neuronal subsystems, notably the visual pathway, in which one group of cells along the pathway receives almost all of its input from only one other type of cell. Recently, however, it has been found that transneuronal effects are widespread, in both the central and peripheral

Figure 11–38. Freeze-fracture preparations of the synaptic membrane. *A,* Active zone in the presynaptic membrane of a myoneural junction. The pits indicated by arrows are the cross-fractured necks of synaptic vesicles discharging their transmitter. (Micrograph courtesy of Tom Reese.)

B, Synaptic junction from the inner plexiform layer of the macaque retina. The presynaptic active zone is characterized by an aggregation of large intramembrane particles *(arrowheads).* A synaptic vesicle in exocytosis is indicated by arrow with asterisk. (Micrograph courtesy of E. Raviola and G. Raviola.)

C, Specialization of the P-face of the presynaptic membrane in a synapse of the inner flexiform layer of the retina. The fracture plane has passed through the cluster of synaptic vesicles and then cleaved the presynaptic membrane, exposing its P-face at the active zone *(arrowheads).* The aggregation of large particles is in register with the underlying cluster of synaptic vesicles. (Micrograph from Raviola, E., and G. Raviola. J. Comp. Neurol. *209*:233, 1982.)

D, In one type of synapse in the central nervous system the postsynaptic membrane is characterized by an aggregation of large particles that remain associated with the E-face *(arrows).* In this synapse from the inner plexiform layer of the retina, two postsynaptic processes occur side by side, each with its aggregation of particles. (Micrograph from Raviola, E., and G. Raviola. J. Comp. Neurol. *209*:233, 1982.)

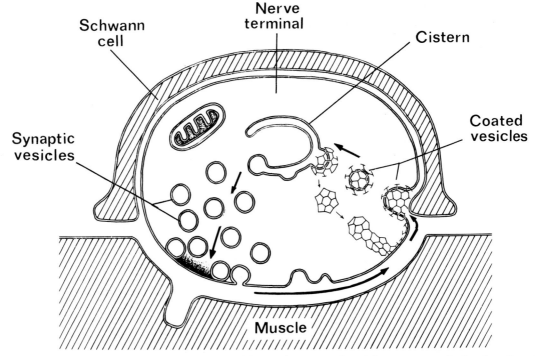

Figure 11–39. Hypothetical pathway for synaptic vesicle membrane recycling at the neuromuscular junction. Synaptic vesicles coalesce with the plasma membrane in discharging their content of transmitter. Equal amounts of membrane are retrieved by formation of clathrin-coated vesicles in regions of membrane adjacent to the Schwann sheath. The coated vesicles coalesce to form cisternae where transmitter accumulates, and new synaptic vesicles are budded off to return to the active zone of the nerve terminal. (After Heuser, J. E., and T. S. Reese. Reproduced from The Journal of Cell Biology 57:315, 1973 by copyright permission of The Rockefeller University Press.)

nervous systems. Degeneration may be *retrograde* or *anterograde,* depending on the direction, and may involve neurons more than one synapse removed; hence, it may be *primary, secondary, tertiary,* or even *quaternary.* Such findings raise important questions concerning the growth and maintenance of the nervous system, and also are crucial facts to consider in interpreting patterns of neuronal atrophy or death after natural or experimental damage to the nervous system.

Examples of Interrelationships of Neurons

Almost every neuron is connected with several or many other neurons. With the aid of the Golgi impregnation and other methods, many types of relationships between neurons have been demonstrated, ranging from complex tangles involving the processes of hundreds of cells, to a neuron synapsing upon itself. As an example of the complex type, there are attached to the body and dendrites of large motor cells in the anterior gray columns of the spinal cord hundreds of synaptic boutons of axons from neurons in

the cerebral cortex, nuclei of the medulla oblongata, and elsewhere in the spinal cord. Thus, the spinal motor cord cells serve as the *final common pathway* by which activity from many sources is transmitted to effector organs. In such arrangements, the response of the postsynaptic cell is determined by the net effect of excitation and inhibition exerted upon it by the many afferent fibers. Thus, in a spinal reflex arc the excitation of peripheral sensory elements is only one of many inputs influencing the response of the motor neurons. The intricate connections between neurons and their enormous numbers (an estimated 9×10^9 neurons in the cerebral cortex alone) indicate the complexity of neural structure and function. Details of the organization of the central nervous system are beyond the scope of this book and must be sought in textbooks of neuroanatomy. It may be instructive, however, to refer back to the photomicrographs of three different parts of the nervous system. Figure 11–13, of the spinal cord, illustrates the white matter, compromising masses of myelinated fibers that surround the relatively small amount of gray matter containing the nerve cell bodies. Figures 11–14 and 11–15 show gray matter located outside the white in the cerebral cortex and cerebellum. White matter, made up of myelinated or unmyelinated axons, serves to transmit patterns of nerve impulses from the body to the CNS or vice versa, and from one part of the brain or cord to another part. There is no evidence that any modification of the nerve impulses occurs in nerves or tracts.

In gray matter, nerve cell bodies mingle with unmyelinated and myelinated fibers. A microscopic preparation shows the bodies of the cells arranged in some order, often in layers. The space between layers, and also between individual cells, is packed with innumerable axons, dendrites, neuroglia, and blood vessels. The axons in these areas usually lack myelin sheaths, which accounts for the gray appearance in fresh condition. Innumerable reciprocal contacts between the various types of neurons permit a variety of mutual influences.

When stained with routine methods, the region between cell bodies has a punctate or stippled appearance and corresponds to the neuropil described above. In the cerebellar and cerebral cortices and in the retina, certain layers consist almost exclusively of naked neuronal and neuroglial processes. Huge numbers of synaptic contacts take place in such synaptic fields.

The pattern of the cells and fibers *(cytoarchitecture)* in gray matter varies from place to place. Every subcortical nucleus, peripheral ganglion, and locality of the cerebral cortex has architectural features of its own. Thus, the cortex in the precentral convolution of the primate brain, the so-called *motor area*, differs noticeably from that of the postcentral convolution, where *somatosensory function* is represented, and from all other parts of the cerebral cortex. One important cortical region having a characteristic cytoarchitecture is the *visual area* along the calcarine fissure of the occipital lobe. Another, in the sylvian fossa, is the *auditory area*. However, careful attempts to correlate cytoarchitectonic and functional findings have largely failed up to the present time.

Anatomical and physiological studies provide compelling evidence that the nervous system is not a random tangle of neurons and neuroglial cells and their processes. Neurons are sometimes considered redundant but in many regions display remarkable structural and functional individuality. Morphologically the individuality is expressed in the connections between particular cells and in the number, type, and location of synaptic terminals upon different parts of the same cell. Physiologically, particular neurons among the astronomical numbers making up the visual area of the cerebral cortex may respond to highly specific modes of visual stimuli to the retina. Other principles of organization of the nervous system emerge from study of neuroanatomy. Among these are the concepts that the CNS is subdivided into a series of interdependent cellular ensembles for analysis and control; that the patterns of connections often permit the reciprocal interactions necessary for modulation of both incoming and outgoing impulses; and finally, that the cells of the CNS at all levels from motor neuron to the cell of the cerebral cortex are designed for integrative action.

DEVELOPMENT OF THE NEURONS AND OF THE NERVOUS TISSUE

The neurons of the nervous system develop from embryonic ectoderm. Also of ectodermal origin are the neuroglial cells (except for the microglia), the Schwann cells of peripheral nerves and corresponding satellite cells in peripheral ganglia, and certain elements of the meninges.

In early embryonic stages, the future central nervous system separates by folding from the primitive ectoderm to form the *neural tube*. At the time the neural folds meet, some cells leave the junctional region bilaterally to form elongated cellular aggregations between the neural tube and the prospective epidermis. These bands, the *neural crests*, soon become segmented and are the precursors of the sympathetic and part of the craniospinal ganglia; cells of the meninges; the adrenal medulla; part of the cranial mesenchyme; branchial cartilages; melanocytes; and odontoblasts. Schwann cells are also generally regarded as derivatives of the neural crests. Autoradiographic studies with tritiated thymidine, however, show that some Schwann cells originate in the neural tube.

The early neural tube is a type of pseudostratified epithelium in which all cells border on the lumen. Autoradiographic and electron microscopic studies demonstrate a single type of columnar cell, now called a *ventricular cell*.

During proliferation, the nuclei of ventricular cells undergo cyclical changes of position in the ventricular zone; nuclei of premitotic cells lie deep, progressively approaching the lumen during prophase. Karyokinesis occurs only at the luminal surface, whereupon the daughter nuclei move again to deeper positions. Even before the closure of the neural tube, the nuclei of *neuroblasts* (immature neurons incapable of further division) derived from ventricular cells migrate peripherally. Later, such cells will form an *intermediate zone* (future gray matter). A *marginal zone* (future white matter) is already present; it contains the nucleus-free outer processes of the ventricular cells. Neuroglial cells in general originate also from the ventricular zone but, unlike typical neuroblasts, continue to divide after migration to the intermediate and marginal zones. In certain regions of the brain, cells are produced that retain proliferative ability after their origin in the ventricular zone; these give rise to additional neurons and glial cells. One such secondary germinal matrix forms a *subventricular zone* immediately beneath the ventricular cells; it is prominent in the lateral ventricles and persists into adult life. Its cells do not exhibit intermitotic nuclear migrations. Another, similar matrix is found in the development of the cerebellum. A transient layer is formed on the external surface of the embryonic cortex by cells that migrate from the ventricular zone of the underlying brain stem. Proliferation in this external layer produces neuroblasts that descend into the cerebellar cortex. Other cerebellar neurons and most neurons of the cerebral cortex arise directly from the ventricular zone and traverse intermediate and marginal zones to reach their destinations. Autoradiographic studies demonstrate that proliferation of neurons by the ventricular zone is a rigorously timed and highly ordered process, which is followed by active migration and frequent intermingling of neuroblasts as they proceed to their final positions.

The sensory neurons of the craniospinal nerves arise in the neural crests. The peripheral processes grow outward and become axons of the sensory nerve fibers. The dendritic region of these neurons is the receptive zone at the periphery; here, the axon develops a variable pattern of branches, which may or may not be encapsulated. The central processes enter the CNS as the axons of dorsal roots and establish connections with interneurons or motor neurons. The cell bodies of the somatic and visceral motor neurons remain within the brain or spinal cord; their axons grow out as ventral roots of the peripheral nerves and terminate in muscles or autonomic ganglia.

The protoplasm of a growing axon shows ameboid movements and insinuates itself between other tissue elements. At its advancing tip, a bulbous enlargement, or *growth cone,* thrusts slender, spinelike projections between obstructing cells and fibers. These features of neuronal development seen in fixed and stained material are confirmed in observations on living nerves in tissue culture and by studies of growing nerves in the transparent tail of the living frog tadpole. Axons of neuroblasts grow into the intercellular spaces as slender, protoplasmic strands. In peripheral nerve fibers, all newly firmed axons are at first devoid of Schwann and myelin sheaths. The earliest myelin appears near the Schwann cell nucleus, and from there it spreads proximally and distally.

The forces that direct the course of development of the complex nervous tissue of vertebrates are largely unknown. The importance of an oriented microstructure as a guide, along whose channels developing axons spread, has been confirmed. There has been no confirmation, however, of the concept of "neurobiotaxis," which assumes that differences in electric potential between dendrites and axons account for migration of nerve cell bodies in the direction of the source from which their stimuli come. No clear-cut effects of electric currents have been seen on either the rate or direction of the growth of nerves. Chemotactic influences upon growing axons have been demonstrated clearly in the optic nerve. Regenerating optic nerve fibers from different parts of the goldfish retina unerringly reach their former terminations in the optic lobes of the midbrain, even after surgical cross-union of medial and lateral optic tracts. There is evidence for refined specificities of growing axons in other regions of the CNS, but the role of chemotactic influences on the growth of peripheral nerves remains controversial. There is also evidence to show that the peripheral organs and tissues affect the development of CNS in many ways after contact has been established between the two regions. These effects are both quantitative and qualitative; they act to regulate the number and size of neurons in specific regions of the neuraxis and to influence the pattern of the connections. Another important finding has been the discovery of specific *nerve growth factors,* identified as proteins, which exert powerful effects upon the generation, growth, and maintenance of specific types of nerve cells.

Studies with the Golgi method show that many neuroblasts retain for some time the primitive distal process they possessed as ventricular cells. These studies suggest that free ameboid motion of an entire cell may not occur in neurogenesis. Instead, the nucleus may simply shift peripherally from the ventricular zone along this process until it reaches its definitive position, perhaps near the external surface of the brain wall, as in the prospective cerebral cortex. Retraction of the attachments of the internal and external processes of the neuroblast takes place from the luminal surface and basal lamina of the neural tube, respectively. Axon sprouting, growth of dendrites, and other features of neuronal differentiation appear to be independent variables. Such events occur at different times relative to the shift in position of the nucleus and in different sequences, depending on the type of nerve cell and its region of the developing CNS.

MENINGES, VENTRICLES, AND CHOROID PLEXUS

In addition to the neurons and macroglia, both of which are of ectodermal origin, the brain and spinal cord contain blood vessels derived from mesenchyme. The three layers enveloping the brain and cord are likewise composed chiefly of connective tissue. The outermost, the *dura mater* or *pachymeninx,* is dense and firm (Fig. 11–41). The inner layers, the innermost called the *pia mater* and the intermediate called the *arachnoid* (Fig. 11–40), are composed of looser connective tissue and constitute the *leptomeninges.*

Dura Mater

The dura of the spinal cord and that of the brain differ in their relationships to the surrounding bones. The inner surface of the vertebral canal is lined by its own periosteum; a separate cylindrical dural membrane loosely encloses the cord. The wide epidural space, between periosteum and dura, contains loose connective and fatty tissue and the epidural venous plexus. The dura is firmly connected to the spinal cord on each side by a series of denticulate ligaments. The inner surface of the spinal dura is lined with squamous cells. Its collagenous bundles run for the most part longitudinally. Elastic fibers are less prominent than in the cerebral dura.

The dura mater of the brain in embryonic development also has two layers, but in the adult these are closely joined. Both consist of connective tissue with elongated fibroblasts. The outer layer adheres to the skull loosely except at the sutures and the base of the skull, where it is more firmly adherent. It functions as a periosteum, is richer in cells than the inner layer, and contains many

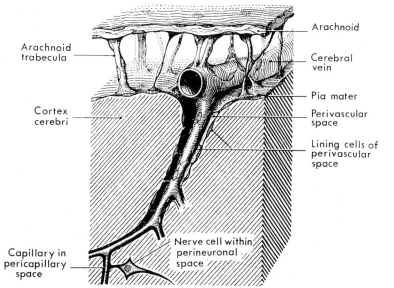

Figure 11–40. Diagram of cerebral pia-arachnoid, showing relations of the subarachnoid space, perivascular channels, and nerve cells. (From Weed, L. H. Am. J. Anat. *31.* 1922.)

Arachnoid

Arachnoid trabecula

Cerebral vein

Pia mater

Cortex cerebri

Perivascular space

Lining cells of perivascular space

Capillary in pericapillary space

Nerve cell within perineuronal space

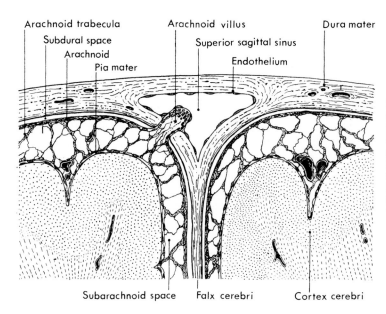

Arachnoid trabecula   Arachnoid villus   Dura mater
Subdural space   Superior sagittal sinus
Arachnoid   Endothelium
Pia mater

Subarachnoid space   Falx cerebri   Cortex cerebri

Figure 11–41. Diagram of the organization of the connective tissue sheaths of the brain. Cerebrospinal fluid formed in the choroid plexus circulates in the subarachnoid space and is absorbed by the venous sinuses through the arachnoid villi, one of which is shown here projecting into the sagittal sinus. (From Weed, L. H. Am. J. Anat. *31*, 1922.)

blood vessels; its thick collagenous fibers are arranged in bundles. The inner layer is thinner, with finer fibers forming an almost continuous sheet. Its fibers run from the frontal region backward and upward, oriented opposite to those of the outer layer. The inner surface of the dura is smooth and covered with a layer of squamous cells.

Arachnoid

The leptomeninges of the brain and spinal cord are similar in structure. The arachnoid is a thin, netlike structure devoid of blood vessels, resembling the transparent parts of the omentum. Its outer surface is smooth, but from its inner surface runs a multitude of thin, branching threads and ribbon-like strands, attached to the underlying pia. Microscopically the tissue has a cobweb-like appearance (Figs. 11–40, 11–41). The arachnoid bridges the sulci and fissures on the surface of the brain and spinal cord, forming subarachnoid spaces of various extent.

Pia Mater

This layer is a thin connective tissue net closely adherent to the surface of the brain and spinal cord. It contains a large number of blood vessels, from which most of the blood of the underlying nervous tissue is supplied. Attached to the pia are the inner fibrous strands of the arachnoid; these two membranes are so intimately related that

their histological structure can best be described together—in fact, these two membranes are often treated as a single entity, the *pia-arachnoid.*

The main elements of the arachnoid and pia are interlacing collagenous bundles surrounded by fine elastic networks. In the pia of the spinal cord an outer longitudinal and an inner circular layer can be distinguished. Among the cells are fibroblasts and macrophages; the latter are especially numerous along the pial blood vessels. They correspond to macrophages of other parts of the body, store vital dyes injected directly into the subarachnoid space, and in inflammation become large or transform into epithelioid cells. In man they often contain considerable amounts of a yellow pigment that sometimes reacts positively to tests for iron.

Along the pial vessels lie scattered single mast cells and small groups of lymphocytes. In certain pathological conditions the latter increase enormously in number and may become plasma cells. In the pia, particularly on the ventral surface of the medulla oblongata, a varying number of melanocytes can be found.

The outer and the inner surfaces of the arachnoid, its trabeculae, and the outer surface of the pia are covered with a layer of squamous epithelial cells.

During development of the meninges two zones may be distinguished: an outer zone of condensation of mesenchyme, which gives rise to the periosteum, dura, and membranous arachnoid; and an inner zone, which becomes the pia. Between these two zones the mesenchyme remains loose and later forms spongy tissue, traversing the subarachnoid spaces.

Nerves of the Meninges

The dura and pia mater are richly supplied with nerves. All vessels of the pia and of the choroid plexus are surrounded by extensive nerve plexuses in the adventitia. Axons originate in the carotid and vertebral plexuses and in certain cranial nerves and belong to the sympathetic system. Sensory, nonencapsulated nerve terminations, and even single nerve cells, are also present on the adventitia of the blood vessels.

The cerebral dura contains, besides the nerves of the vessels, numerous sensory nerve endings in its connective tissue. The cerebral pia also contains extensive nervous plexuses, especially abundant in the tela choroidea of the third ventricle. The fibers end either in large pear-shaped or bulbous swellings or in skeins and convolutions similar to those of the corpuscles of Meissner. In the spinal pia the vessels receive their nerves from the plexuses following the larger blood vessels to the cord. Afferent nerve endings are also present, but these are unevenly distributed.

Both myelinated and unmyelinated nerve fibers accompany the blood vessels into the substance of the spinal cord and the brain, ending on the muscle cells of the vessels. These come from similar nerves of the pial vessels, and the two nervous plexuses are continuous.

Meningeal Spaces

Between the dura mater and the arachnoid, the subdural space is a serous cavity containing a minimum of fluid; actually, it is scarcely more than a potential space. Between the outer sheet of arachnoid and pia is the subarachnoid space, traversed by cobwebby connective tissue trabeculae, and containing a large amount of fluid. Over the convolutions it is narrow, but in the sulci it is wide and deep. The subarachnoid space is especially wide throughout the length of the spinal cord. In the brain, it is greatly enlarged in a few places (*cisternae*) where the arachnoid is widely separated from the pia and the trabeculae are rare or absent. The largest cisterna lies above the medulla oblongata and below the posterior border of the cerebellum (*cisterna cerebellomedullaris,* or *cisterna magna*). The fourth ventricle communicates with this cisterna through three openings in the tela choroidea: a medial *foramen of Magendie,* and the two lateral *foramina of Luschka.*

Ventricles

The central nervous system begins development as a neural tube with a wide cavity throughout the length and remains a hollow organ throughout life. The *central canal* or ventricle of the spinal cord in the adult is minute, or it may be obliterated. It does not seem to perform any important function. However, in the normal adult the ventricular cavities of the brain form a continuous channel for flow of cerebrospinal fluid. If part of this channel is occluded by disease so as to prevent free circulation, intracerebral pressure increases, with resulting hydrocephalus or other serious consequences.

The ventricular cavity is dilated in four regions: the *two lateral ventricles* in the cerebral hemispheres, the *third ventricle* in the thalamic region, and the *fourth ventricle* in the medulla oblongata and pons. Choroid plexuses develop in these four regions, and most of the ventricular fluid is derived from the blood vessels of these plexuses.

Choroid Plexus

There are four places where the wall of the brain retains its embryonic character as a thin, non-nervous epithelium. This part of the brain wall is the *lamina epithelialis.* The pia mater that covers it is extremely vascular and is called the *tela choroidea.* Small arteries and capillaries of the pia form glomerular tufts of vessels, covered by the lamina epithelialis and protruding into the ventricle, constitute the *choroid plexus.*

Choroid plexuses are found in the roof of the third and fourth ventricles and in part of the wall of the two lateral ventricles. In each case, the tela choroidea is much folded and invaginated into the ventricle, so that the free surface exposed to the ventricular fluid is large, with tortuous vessels and a rich capillary net (Fig. 11–42).

The epithelium early acquires a peculiar structure, different from that of the cells lining the ventricles elsewhere. In embryonic stages it contains glycogen and carries cilia.

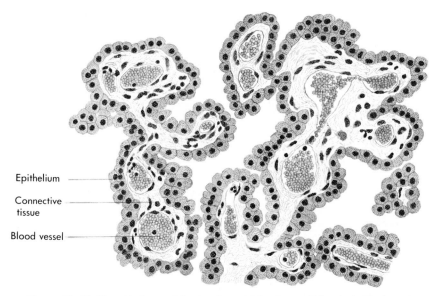

Epithelium

Connective tissue

Blood vessel

Figure 11–42. Choroid plexus of the fourth ventricle of man. (After A. A. Maximow.)

In the adult its cells are cuboidal and arranged in a single regular layer. Each contains a large round nucleus and a varying number of rod-shaped mitochondria.

On the free surface the cells have a specialized border resembling a brush border. In electron micrographs, however, this border is seen to consist of long microvilli that are irregularly oriented and often somewhat expanded at the tips (Fig. 11–43). Although possibly these terminal expansions are artifacts of fixation, microvilli of other cell types fixed similarly do not have this appearance.

In animals repeatedly injected intravenously with vital dyes, such as trypan blue, the epithelium of the choroid plexus stores large amounts of the dye. Also, in the perivascular connective tissue core of the plexus many macrophages are found, which take up and store great amounts of dye.

On the boundary between adjacent epithelial cells in electron micrographs, a juxtaluminal junctional complex appears to seal the intercellular space. The capillaries beneath the epithelium are unlike those found elsewhere in the brain; they have thin walls and fenestrations or pores closed by thin diaphragms. The junctions between endothelial cells also appear to be quite permeable. Following intravenous injection in mice, peroxidase (a protein) can be shown to cross the capillary walls and enter the stromal space. It moves between the epithelial cells but is stopped near the lumen by the junctional complex.

Cerebrospinal Fluid

The central nervous system is bathed in cerebrospinal fluid as in a water bath. This protects it from concussions and mechanical injuries and is important for its metabolism. The subarachnoid spaces freely communicate; cerebrospinal fluid may pass through them from one end to the other of the neuraxis. The amount of the fluid is variable, estimated at 80 to 100 ml, sometimes as much as 150 ml. It is limpid and slightly viscous, has a low specific gravity (1.004 to 1.008), and contains traces of proteins, small quantities of inorganic salt and dextrose, and few lymphocytes (about two or three, not more than ten, per milliliter). It resembles the aqueous humor of the eye more closely than it does any other fluid of the body.

Cerebrospinal fluid is constantly renewed. It circulates slowly through the brain ventricles and through the meshes of the subarachnoid space. If the space is opened to the outside by injury, large amounts of fluid steadily drain off—200 ml or more a day. The sources of fluid are primarily the blood vessels of the choroid plexus, the pia mater, and the brain substance. From the brain substance the flow is outward into the subarachnoid space; from the choroid plexus it is inward into the ventricles. Fluid may be added to the ventricles in a few other places, notably the area postrema at the caudal margin of the fourth ventricle. The ependymal surfaces in general do not discharge fluid

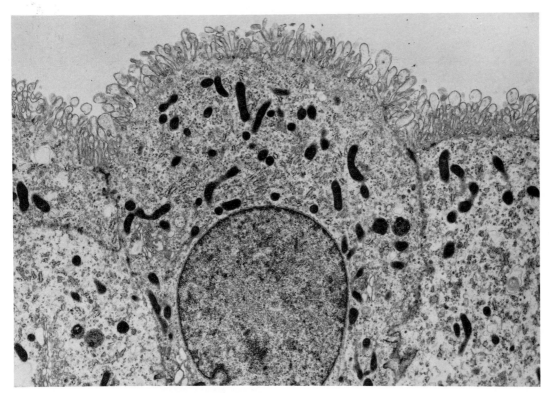

Figure 11–43. Electron micrograph of choroid plexus at higher magnification than in Figure 11–42, illustrating the unusual free border of bulbous or clavate microvilli.

into the ventricles. In contrast, absorption of fluid from the ventricles into nearby veins takes place through the ventricular wall. The plexuses are wholly secretory, not resorptive, and constitute the chief source of fluid. The major channel of ventricular fluid outward into the subarachnoid space is through specially modified places in the membranous roof of the fourth ventricle.

Ventricular fluid normally flows from the lateral ventricles of the cerebral hemispheres, where it derives chiefly from the lateral choroid plexuses, through the foramina of Monro into the third ventricle. Here fluid is added from the choroid plexus of the third ventricle and the augmented flow passes through the aqueduct of Sylvius into the fourth ventricle, where more fluid is added from the choroid plexus there. Fluid then passes into the cisterna magna and diffuses in all directions through the subarachnoid space. Some of the fluid may enter extracranial lymphatics through perineurial spaces within the cranial nerve roots, part reaching the nasal cavity along sheaths of olfactory nerve filaments. Around the spinal nerve roots, an arrangement of dural veins and

sinuses permits passage of cerebrospinal fluid directly into venous blood, rather than into lymphatics. A small amount of fluid enters lymphatics or venous vessels as just described, but most of it passes directly into the large endocranial venous sinuses through local specializations of the arachnoid called arachnoid villi.

Arachnoid Villi

The large endocranial venous sinuses are surrounded by thick walls of dura mater except in certain places, chiefly in the sagittal sinus of the falx cerebri. Here the dura is perforated by numerous protrusions of the arachnoid, through each of which a finger of arachnoid epithelium, an *arachnoid villus* (Fig. 11–41), evaginates into the lumen of the sinus. The cavity of the villus, containing a small amount of loose arachnoid tissue, communicates freely with the subarachnoid space, so that at this point fluid of the space is separated from blood in the sinus only by the thin epithelium of the arachnoid and the vascular endothelium.

Arachnoid villi have been found in dogs,

cats, monkeys, and humans. In man, with advancing age, they enlarge and become *pacchionian corpuscles* or *granulations*.

The villi provide the main pathway for outflow of cerebrospinal fluid directly into the venous circulation. This flow is rapid. Dyes and other chemicals injected into the subarachnoid space can be detected in the bloodstream in 10 to 30 seconds. After only 30 minutes they can also be found in the lymphatics.

Blood Vessels of the Central Nervous System

The arteries reach the spinal cord with the ventral and dorsal nerve roots (anterior and posterior radicular arteries) and form a dense arterial network in the spinal pia mater. Here several longitudinal arterial pathways can be distinguished (spinal arterial tracts). The most important is the anterior spinal artery; it emits many small branches (central arteries), which enter the ventral median fissure and penetrate to the right and left into the medial part of the anterior gray columns, thus supplying most of the gray matter with blood. Numerous smaller branches of the pial arterial net (peripheral arteries) penetrate the white matter along its circumference. Capillary nets in white matter are loose and have meshes drawn out longitudinally; capillaries in gray matter are much more numerous and dense. The course of the veins does not correspond to that of the arteries. Numerous venous branches emerge from the periphery of the cord and from the ventral median fissure and form a diffuse plexus in the pia, which is especially prominent on the dorsal surface of the cord. From this plexus, blood is drained by veins accompanying the ventral and dorsal roots.

The arterial supply of the brain derives almost entirely from the carotids and the large arteries at its base—the basilar artery and the circle of Willis. Most arteries from these large vessels pass superiorly in the pia mater, from which small vessels dip into the brain substance. These vessels are functionally end arteries, since few anastomoses are large enough to be effective in establishing collateral circulation.

As in the spinal cord, the capillary net in cerebral white matter is meager, with elongated meshes; in gray matter the net has a closer mesh. The density of capillaries is a crude indication of the metabolic needs of the tissue supplied. From this, it is clear that gray matter is metabolically much more active; the amount of activity, however, varies from place to place, as reflected in the density of the capillary net.

The linear extent of capillaries per unit volume of brain substance has been measured in a number of representative parts of the CNS in various animals. In the rat, parts of both white and gray matter differ in vascularity, but in all cases the gray is more vascular than the white. Motor nuclei are less vascular than sensory nuclei and groups of interneurons.

There are no lymphatics in the CNS. Fluid from the capillaries seeps through the tissue but does not collect in lymphatic channels, as in most other parts of the body. The blood vessels that penetrate from the pia are surrounded by perivascular spaces, which open freely at the brain surface into the subarachnoid space. Thus, cererospinal fluid derived from blood drains from the brain outward toward the meninges.

Blood-Brain Barrier

When certain vital dyes are introduced into the circulating blood of adult animals, the CNS remains colorless except for the choroid plexuses and certain subependymal areas, where the dyes are found within extravascular cells. Thus, a *blood-brain* or *hematoencephalic barrier* exists between the blood and the nervous system. The barrier is localized in the endothelium of the blood vessels. The zonulae occludentes between endothelial cells block movement of macromolecules along the intercellular clefts and there is little or no transport of solutes across the endothelial cells by plasmalemmal vesicles.

In young animals given intravenous dye injections, a distinct but small storage of dye does occur in cells in parts of the brain stem. The apparent impermeability of the brain to blood-borne macromolecules develops gradually.

RESPONSE OF THE NEURON TO INJURY

Two important responses of the neuron to injury are the progressive degeneration of an axon severed from its cell body and the morphological changes that occur in the perikaryon of a neuron after axonal transection. These responses, basic to neuropathology, are included here because they exemplify the neuron doctrine and illustrate the trophic influence of the nerve cell body over the axon and its other processes.

When an axon is severed, trauma occurs at both cut edges. Proximally, *primary degeneration* extends only a short distance, depending on the type of injury—one or two internodes in a clean cut, but as much as 2 or 3 cm from a gunshot wound. Damage is soon repaired and new axonal sprouts appear. Distally, however, the axon, its terminal arborizations, and the myelin sheath completely disintegrate. This *secondary,* or *wallerian, degeneration* in peripheral nerves usually proceeds simultaneously along the length of a nerve fiber distal to the point of injury, but a rapid centrifugal sweep of changes may occur, The initial changes in axonal fine structure consist in localized accumulations of mitochondria a few hours after injury; within 12 to 24 hours, neurofilaments and mitochondria vesiculate and disintegrate, and later dense granules aggregate. At about two days, the axon becomes beaded and shortly begins to fragment and dissolve. Concomitantly, myelin degeneration begins, breaking down into fatty droplets of varying size and concentric lamellar structures, often enclosing an axonal fragment. Macrophages, derived somehow from the endoneurial or Schwann cells, progressively remove the debris. In accord with the neuron doctrine, the process of degeneration does not usually spread across the synapse. Nevertheless, many exceptions are known and additional ones have been suspected. The Schwann cytoplasm remains and, after axonal and myelin degeneration, forms a tube surrounded by endoneurium and filled with fluid and scattered fragments. The wall of the tube thickens, reducing the original bore until it may be obliterated, and the tube shrinks to perhaps less than half of its original diameter; meanwhile, its constituent Schwann cell nuclei multiply. Ultimately these changes produce a solid, nucleated *band of Büngner.* As myelin disappears, a flexible, ribbon-like peripheral nerve condenses into a dull gray, hardened, and rounded cord. The bands of Büngner may remain for many months, awaiting reinnervation. If regeneration of axons does not occur, the bands gradually become reduced by encroaching endoneurial connective tissue.

Nerve fibers within the central nervous system also undergo wallerian degeneration. In young animals, degeneration is extremely rapid, but in adult man it proceeds more slowly. Loss of myelin in a heavily myelinated tract, for example, as seen in Weigert stain, may not be evident for two months. Special staining methods for normal and abnormal lipids, however, show myelin catabolism more readily. In the CNS the microglia, equivalent to macrophages elsewhere, break down and remove the myelin and axonal fragments. Whether interfascicular oligodendrocytes undertake similar functions to those of Schwann cells is not known. Wallerian degeneration is widely exploited in neuroanatomical research to trace the course of connections following experimental ablations of nuclei and tracts. Degeneration of terminal boutons, an essential part of wallerian degeneration, offers a more difficult but higher-resolution research method, since it demonstrates the termination of degenerating axons and also serves when brief survival precludes study of the slower reactions of axon or myelin.

The fleeting and restricted traumatic degeneration of the proximal stump of a peripheral nerve is usually soon followed by axonal regeneration, in the form of fine sprouts with protoplasmic *growth cones* or *filopodia* at their advancing tips. Regenerating fibers resemble embryonic ones and grow along the outer edge of a band of Büngner. There they become progressively enfolded by Schwann cells in a fashion similar to the multiple envelopment found in unmyelinated nerves. The rate of growth of the fibers is rapid—3 to 4 mm a day in mammals—but the distance that must be traversed to the terminations may be 1 m or more.

Functional recovery depends on reestablishment of appropriate sensory and motor connections at the periphery. The abundance of regenerative sprouts from the original neuron and the capacity of bands of Büngner to accommodate hundreds of fibers favor successful reinnervation. Although surgical alignment of individual axons is impossible, and regenerating sprouts can negotiate hiatuses of considerable distance, prompt approximation of the two ends of a cut peripheral nerve is nevertheless of cardinal importance. In addition to the abundance of sprouts and their accommodation by the bands of Büngner, peripheral deletion of maladaptive terminations and central remodeling of reflex arcs offer additional possibilities for functional recovery.

Following the regeneration of a peripheral nerve, the axon, myelin, and Schwann cells slowly return to their normal size and condition. During these months, large amounts of axoplasm are resynthesized—possibly 250 times that of the parent cell body.

Retrograde changes in the cell body of origin of a severed axon were first described by Nissl in 1892. Chief among these is *retrograde chromatolysis,* the apparent disappearance of the Nissl substance, obvious and well studied in motor cells, but occurring in varying extent and rate in other types of neurons. With light microscopy, breakup and dissolution of Nissl material is first seen near the axon hillock and in a rim around the nucleus, subsequently spreading to other parts of the cell. In addition, the perikaryon swells, ballooning the normally concave boundaries between dendrites, and the nucleus shifts from its usually central position to a peripheral one away from the axon hillock. Fine structural investigations have shown dispersion or disappearance of ribosomes and of the cisternal membranes of the granular endoplasmic reticulum, with appearance of numerous coarse neurofilaments. Initially the Golgi apparatus appears normal, but in later stages swarms of small dark vesicles apparently bud from its flattened profiles.

Retrograde chromatolysis begins about one day after axonal injury and is sometimes referred to as *axonal reaction;* it reaches its peak in about two weeks. Similar pathological changes in the nerve cell body may occur for other reasons. The response, like that of wallerian degeneration, offers a valuable anatomical method. In this case, the investigator can localize the origin of a tract or nerve, instead of tracing its course; to do this, however, he must be familiar with the normal pattern of Nissl substance for the neurons in the many regions under study. In practice, the neuroanatomist frequently combines anterograde and retrograde degeneration studies.

In general, the more axoplasm that is separated from the cell body, the greater is the retrograde chromatolysis. Amputation of a major process close to the perikaryon may lead to the death of the neuron, whereas section of a distal process may produce no detectable response. If the cell body survives and regeneration of the axon takes place, the retrograde changes are slowly reversed. The nucleolus becomes prominent and reconstitution of Nissl substance occurs, often in superabundance, beginning as a basophilic rim around the nucleus. Return to normal appearance takes several months. Very large amounts of axonal cytoplasm may have to be regenerated, entailing an enormous metabolic effort on the part of the cell body and synthesis of immense amounts of cytoplasm relative to the size of the perikaryon. Sensory ganglion cells react in a manner similar to motor cells, but show less obvious changes after lesions of the peripheral nerves and still slighter, perhaps undetectable, changes after section of the dorsal roots. The finely divided Nissl substance in the normal dorsal root ganglion cell and the great length of axon it possesses probably tend to minimize the visible response. In many central neurons, such as Betz cells of the cerebral cortex, retrograde chromatolysis is seldom observed. Unless destruction of the axon and all its branches takes place, intact *sustaining collaterals* are thought to remain functional and to provide enough axoplasm to offset overt retrograde cell change.

REFERENCES

Adams, R. D., and R. L. Sidman: Introduction to Neuropathology, New York, McGraw-Hill Book Co., 1968.

Angevine, J. B., Jr.: Time of neutron origin in the diencephalon of the mouse. An autoradiographic study. J. Comp. Neurol. *139*:129, 1970.

Ariëns Kappers, C. U., G. C. Huber, and E. C. Crosby: The Comparative Anatomy of the Nervous System of Vertebrates, Including Man. Vols. I and II. New York, Macmillan, 1936.

Bailey, P., and G. Von Bonin: The Isocortex of Man. Urbana, University of Illinois Press, 1951.

Boyd, I. A.: The structure and innervation of the nuclear bag muscle fiber system and the nuclear chain muscle fiber system in mammalian muscle spindles. Philos. Trans. R. Soc. B. *245*:81, 1962.

Bray, D., and D. Gilbert: Cytoskeletal elements in neurons. Annu. Rev. Neurosci. *4*:505, 1981.

Bray, G. M., M. Rasminsky, and A. J. Aguayo: Interactions between axons and their sheath cells. Annu. Rev. Neurosci. *4*:127, 1981.

Bunge, R. P.: Glial cells and the central myelin sheath. Physiol. Rev. *48*:197, 1968.

Coggeshall, R. E.: A fine structural analysis of the myelin sheath in rat spinal roots. Anat. Rec. *194*:201, 1979.

Davis H.: Some principles of sensory receptor action. Physiol. Rev. *41*:391, 1961.

Davison, A. N., and A. Peters: Myelination. Springfield, IL, Charles C Thomas, 1970.

Davison, P. F., and E. W. Taylor: Physical-chemical studies of proteins of squid nerve axoplasm, with special reference to the axon fibrous protein. J. Gen. Physiol. *43*:801, 1960.

Eccles, J. C.: The Physiology of Nerve Cells. Baltimore, Johns Hopkins Press, 1957.

Field, J., H. W. Magoun, and V. E. Hall, eds.: Handbook of Physiology. Section 1: Neurophysiology. 3 Vols. Washington DC, American Physiological Society, 1959–1961.

Fox, C. A., and J. W. Barnard: A quantitative study of the Purkinje cell dendritic branchlets and their relations to afferent fibers. J. Anat. 91:299, 1957.

Fujita, S.: Analysis of neuron differentiation in the central nervous system by tritiated thymidine autoradiography. J. Comp. Neurol. 112:311, 1964.

Furshpan, E. J.: "Electrical transmission" at an excitatory synapse in a vertebrate brain. Science 144:878, 1964.

Gerard, R. W.: Metabolism and Function in the Nervous System. In Elliott, K. A. C., I. H. Page and J. H. Quastel, eds.: Neurochemistry. Springfield, IL, Charles C Thomas, 1955.

Geren, B. B.: Structural studies of the formation of the myelin sheath in peripheral nerve fibers. In Rudnick, D., ed.: Cellular Mechanisms in Differentiation and Growth. Princeton, Princeton University Press, 1956.

Gershon, M. D.: The enteric nervous system. Annu. Rev. Neurosci. 4:227, 1981.

Glees, P.: Neuroglia: Morphology and Function. Springfield, IL, Charles C Thomas, 1955.

Glimstedt, G., and G. Wohlfort: Electron microscope studies on peripheral nerve regeneration. Lunds Universitets Arsskrift 56:1, 1960.

Grafstein, B., and D. S. Forman: Intracellular transport in neurons. Physiol. Rev. 60:1167, 1980.

Granit, R.: Receptors and Sensory Perception; A Discussion of Aims, Means, and Results of Electrophysiological Research into the Process of Reception. New Haven, Yale University Press, 1955.

Gray, E. G., and R. W. Guillery: Synaptic morphology in the normal and degenerating nervous system. Int. Rev. Cytol. 19:41, 1962.

Greenfield, J. G.: Neuropathology. Baltimore, Williams & Wilkins, 1967.

Guth, L.: Regeneration in the mammalian peripheral nervous system. Physiol. Rev. 36:441, 1956.

Harrison, R. G.: The outgrowth of the nerve fiber as a mode of protoplasmic movement. J. Exp. Zool. 9:787, 1910.

Herrick, C. J.: The Brain of the Tiger Salamander, Chicago, University of Chicago Press, 1948.

Heuser, J. E., and T. S. Reese: Structure of the synapse. Handbook of Physiology. Section 1: The Nervous System. Vol. I. Cellular Biology of Neurons, Part 1, p. 261. Bethesda, American Physiological Society, 1977.

Heuser, J. E., and T. S. Reese: Changes in structure of presynaptic membranes during transmitter secretion. In Neurobiology. New York, John Wiley & Sons, 1979.

Heuser, J. E., T. S. Reese, M. J. Dennis, Y. Yan, L. Jan, and L. Evans: Synaptic vesicle exocytosis captured by quick freezing and correlated with quantal transmitter release. J. Cell Biol. 81:275, 1979.

Hyden, H.: The Neuron. In Brachet, J., and A. E. Mirsky, eds.: The Cell; Biochemistry, Physiology, Morphology. Vol. 4. New York, Academic Press, 1960.

Katz, B.: Mechanism of Synaptic Transmission, and Nature of the Nerve Impulse. In Oncley, J. L., et al., eds.: Biophysical Science—A Study Program. New York, John Wiley & Sons, 1959.

Kuntz, A.: The Autonomic Nervous System. 4th ed. Philadelphia, Lea & Febiger, 1953.

Landis, D. M., T. S. Reese, and E. Raviola: Differences in membrane structure between excitatory and inhibitory components of the reciprocal synapse in olefactory bulb. J. Comp. Neurol. 155:67, 1974.

Lehman, H. J.: Die Nervenfaser. In von Möllendorff, W., and W. Bargmann, eds.: Handbuch der Mikroskopischen Anatomie des Menschen. Vol. 4, part 4. Berlin, Springer-Verlag, 1959.

Levi-Montalcini, R.: Events in the developing nervous system. In Purpura, D., and J. Schadé, eds.: Progress in Brain Research. Vol. 4. Amsterdam, Elsevier Publishing Co., 1964.

Ortiz-Picón, J. M.: The neuroglia of the sensory ganglia. Anat. Rec. 121:513, 1955.

Palay, S. L.: The structural basis for neural action. In Brazier, M. A. B., ed.: Brain Function. Vol. II. Berkeley, University of California Press, 1963.

Palay, S. L., and V. Chan-Palay: Cerebellar Cortex. Cytology and Organization. New York, Springer-Verlag, 1974.

Palay, S. L., and G. E. Palade: The fine structure of neurons. J. Biophys. Biochem. Cytol. 1:69, 1955

Penfield, W., ed.: Cytology and Cellular Pathology of the Nervous System. Vols. 1, 2, and 3, New York, Paul B. Hoeber, 1932.

Peters, A., S. L. Palay, and H. de F. Webster: The Fine Structure of the Nervous System. The Neurons and Supporting Cells. Philadelphia, W. B. Saunders Co., 1976.

Peterson, E. R., and M. R. Murray: Myelin sheath formation in cultures of avian spinal ganglia. Am. J. Anat. 96:319, 1955.

Polyak, S.: Vertebrate Visual System. Chicago, University of Chicago Press, 1957.

Pope, A.: Application of quantitative histochemical methods to the study of the nervous system. J. Neuropath. Exp. Neurol. 14:39, 1955.

Ramón y Cajal, S.: Histologie du Systeme Nerveux de l'Homme et des Vertébrés. Paris, A. Maloine, 1909.

Ramón y Cajal, S.: Degeneration and Regeneration of the Nervous System. London, Oxford University Press, 1929.

Raviola, E., and G. Raviola: Structure of the synaptic membranes in the inner plexiform layer of the retina. A freeze-fracture study in monkeys and rabbits. J. Comp. Neurol. 209:233, 1982.

Revel, J. P., and D. W. Hamilton: The double nature of the intermediate dense line in peripheral nerve myelin. Anat. Rec. 163:7, 1969.

Robertson, J. D.: The ultrastructure of adult vertebrate peripheral myelinated nerve fibers in relation to myelinogenesis. J. Biophys. Biochem. Cytol. 1:271, 1955.

Robertson, J. D.: The ultrastructure of Schmidt-Lantermann clefts and related shearing defects of the myelin sheath. J. Biophys. Biochem. Cytol. 4:39, 1958.

Rodriguez, L. A.: Experiments on the histologic locus of the hematoencephalic barrier. J. Comp. Neurol. 102:27, 1955.

Rich, T. C., H. D. Patton, J. W. Woodburn, and A. L. Towe: Neurophysiology, 2nd ed. Philadelphia, W. B. Saunders Co., 1965.

Schaltenbrand, G.: Plexus und Meningen. In von Möllendorff, W., and W. Bargmann, eds.: Handbuch der Mikroskopischen Anatomie des Menschen. Vol. 4, part 2. Berlin, Springer-Verlag, 1955.

Scharrer, E., and B. Scharrer: Neurosekretion. In von Möllendorff, W., and W. Bargmann, eds.: Handbuch der Mikroskopischen Anatomie des Menschen. Vol. 6, part 5. Berlin, Springer-Verlag, 1954.

Schmitt, F. O.: Molecular Organization of the Nerve Fiber. *In* Oncley, J. L., et al., eds.: Biophysical Science—A Study Program. New York, John Wiley & Sons, 1959.

Schwartz, J. H.: Axonal transport. Components, mechanisms, and specificity. Annu. Rev. Neurosci. *2*:467, 1979.

Sherrington, C. S.: The Integrative Action of the Nervous System. New Haven, Yale University Press, 1906.

Sholl, D. A.: The Organization of the Cerebral Cortex. New York, John Wiley & Sons, 1956.

Speidel, C. C.: Studies of living nerves. VII. Growth adjustments of cutaneous terminal arborizations. J. Comp. Neurol. *76*:57, 1942.

Sperry, R. W.: Chemoaffinity in the orderly growth of nerve fiber patterns and connections. Proc. Natl. Acad. Sci. U.S.A. *50*:703, 1963.

Watterson, R. L.: Structure and mitotic behavior of the early neural tube. *In* deHaan, R. L., and H. Ursprung, eds.: Organogenesis. New York, Holt, Rinehart & Winston, 1965.

Weed, L. H.: Certain anatomical and physiological aspects of the meninges and cerebrospinal fluid. Brain *58*:383, 1935.

Weiss, P., and M. W. Cavanaugh: Further evidence of perpetual growth of nerve fibers; a recovery of fiber diameter after the release of prolonged constrictions. J. Exp. Zool. *142*:461, 1959.

Weiss, P., and H. B. Hiscoe: Experiments on the mechanism of nerve growth. J. Exp. Zool. *107*:315, 1948.

Weston, J. A.: A radioautographic analysis of the migration and localization of trunk neural crest cells in the chick. Dev. Biol. *6*:279, 1963.

Willis, W. D., and R. E. Coggeshall: Sensory Mechanisms of the Spinal Cord. New York, Plenum Press, 1978.

Windle, W. F.: Regeneration of axons in the vertebrate central nervous system. Physiol. Rev. *36*:427, 1956.

Wislocki, G. B., and E. H. Leduc: Vital staining of the hematoencephalic barrier by silver nitrate and trypan blue, and cytological comparisons of neurohypophysis, pineal body, area postrema, intercolumnar tubercle and supraoptic crest. J. Comp. Neurol. *96*:371, 1952.

12

BLOOD AND LYMPH VASCULAR SYSTEMS

Multicellular animals require a mechanism for distribution of oxygen, nutritive materials, and hormones to the tissues, and to collect from them carbon dioxide and other products of metabolism for transmission to the excretory organs. In vertebrates, this function is carried out by the *blood vascular system*. This consists of a muscular pump, the *heart*, and two systems of blood vessels. One of these, the *pulmonary circulation*, carries blood to and from the lungs; the other, the *systemic circulation (peripheral circulation)*, distributes to all the other tissues and organs of the body. In both, the blood pumped from the heart passes successively through *arteries* of diminishing size to networks of minute capillaries and back to the heart via *veins* of increasing caliber.

The heart delivers about 80 ml of blood into the pulmonary artery and aorta at each beat or about 6 liters a minute. The initial velocity of flow is about 33 cm/min, but as the total cross-sectional area of the vascular system is increased by progressive dichotomous branching of the arteries, the rate of flow gradually decreases. A further expansion of the cross-sectional area of the system occurs quite abruptly at the level of the capillaries, resulting in a decrease in rate of flow to about 0.3 cm/sec. The extensive capillary networks of the body have a total surface area of 700 m² for exchange of metabolites. It is only in capillaries and small venules that the vessel walls are thin enough to permit passage of substances to and from the surrounding tissues. The other vessels are concerned with distribution of blood to the capillaries. At any given moment, only about 5 per cent of the total blood volume is in the capillaries and 95 per cent is on its way to or from them. The structure and biochemical properties of the capillary wall are subjects of great physiological importance, for it is

this portion of the circulation that carries out the primary function of the vascular system.

ARTERIES

Blood is carried from the heart to the capillary networks in the tissues and organs by arteries. These constitute an extensive system of vessels beginning with the *aorta* and *pulmonary artery*, which emerge from the left and right sides of the heart, respectively. As they course away from the heart, these vessels branch repeatedly and thus give rise to large numbers of arteries of progressively diminishing caliber.

The basic organization of the wall of all arteries is similar in that three concentric layers can be distinguished: (1) an inner layer, the *tunica intima*, consisting of an endothelial tube whose cells generally have their long axis oriented longitudinally; (2) an intermediate layer, the *tunica media*, composed predominantly of smooth muscle cells disposed circumferentially; and (3) an outer coat, the *tunica adventitia*, made up of fibroblasts and fibrous elements that are oriented, for the most part, longitudinally (Fig. 12–1). This layer gradually merges with the loose connective tissue that accompanies all blood vessels. The boundary between the tunica intima and tunica media is marked by the *internal elastic lamina (elastic interna)*, which is especially well developed in arteries of medium caliber. Between the tunica media and the tunica adventitia, a thinner *external elastic lamina (elastica externa)* is also present in many arteries.

Elastic Arteries

There is a continuous gradation in size and in character of the vessel wall from the largest

367

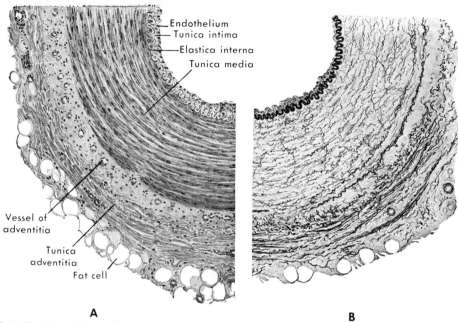

Figure 12–1. Drawings of the wall of a small artery in cross section, showing the concentric arrangement of tunica intima, media, and adventitia. *A,* Stained with hematoxylin and eosin; *B,* stained with orcein to reveal the elastic tissue component.

arteries down to the capillaries, but it is customary to designate several categories of arteries on the basis of their size, the predominant structural component of their tunica media, and their principal function in the arterial system. The large *elastic* or *conducting arteries,* such as the aorta, innominate, subclavian, common carotid, and common iliac, have walls containing many fenestrated layers of elastin in the tunica media (Fig. 12–2). Their walls may be distinctly yellow in the fresh state because of the abundance of their elastic elements. These major conducting vessels near the heart are distended during contraction of the heart (systole), and the subsequent elastic recoil of their walls during diastole serves as a subsidiary pump maintaining continuous flow in the system despite the intermittency of heartbeat.

The tunica intima of these arteries consists of the *endothelium,* a thin squamous epithelium, separated from the elastica interna by loose connective tissue containing a few fibroblasts, occasional smooth muscle cells, and sparse collagenous and elastic fibers. The endothelium provides a smooth lining layer for the vessel and a partially selective diffusion barrier between the blood and the other tunics of the vessel wall. Its cells are polygonal in outline, 10 to 15 μm wide and 25 to 50 μm long, with their long axis oriented lon-

gitudinally. Adjacent endothelial cells are attached by simple occluding junctions and occasional communicating (gap) junctions. The cells possess all of the common organelles in limited numbers, usually located in the thicker region of the cytoplasm around the flattened nucleus. The endothelium is a very slowly renewing population of cells that are rarely found in division. Their adluminal and abluminal plasmalemmae have numerous associated vesicles that are believed to be involved in transendothelial transport of water, electrolytes, and certain macromolecules. Short blunt processes occasionally extend from the base of endothelial cells through fenestrae in the elastica interna and establish communicating junctions with smooth muscle cells of the media.

Rodlike cytoplasmic inclusions are observed in electron micrographs of arterial endothelium. These were first reported 20 years ago and have since been called *Weibel-Palade bodies* after the investigators who first drew attention to them. Their chemical nature and functional significance remained obscure until recently. It was then found that their electron density diminished in response to epinephrine administration and it was postulated that they might contain a procoagulant factor. It has now been shown that a Factor VIII–related antigen (von Willebrand

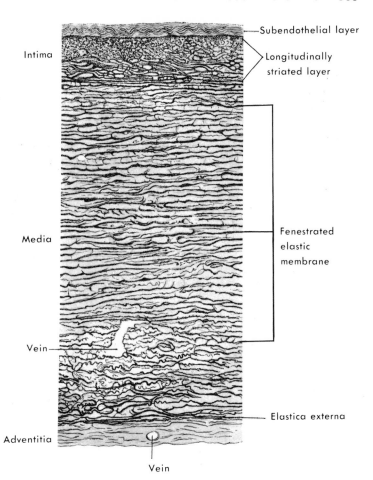

Intima

Media

Vein

Adventitia

Vein

Subendothelial layer

Longitudinally striated layer

Fenestrated elastic membrane

Elastica externa

Figure 12–2. Longitudinal section through the posterior wall of the human descending aorta. Elastic tissue is black; the other elements are not shown clearly. Elastic fiber stain. (After Kölliker and von Ebner.)

factor) can be localized immunocytochemically in the Weibel-Palade bodies. This coagulating factor is believed to be synthesized by arterial endothelial cells and secreted into the blood plasma.

The elastica interna is a less prominent feature of elastic arteries than of muscular arteries. It is merely the first of many laminae of elastin found in the media and has rather large fenestrae traversed by a network of finer elastic fibers. The media is up to 500 μm thick in the larger vessels and composed of 40 to 70 fenestrated laminae of elastin 5 to 15 μm apart and interconnected by radially oriented finer strands of elastin. The spaces between elastic laminae are occupied by long branching smooth muscle cells, occasional fibroblasts, with associated collagen fibers and other extracellular matrix components. The elastica externa is relatively thin and inconspicuous, being simply the most peripheral of the multiple elastic laminae of the media. The three-dimensional configu-

ration of the elastic component of arterial walls is difficult to visualize from study of histological sections, but it is possible to extract all other components with hot formic acid and examine the elastin with scanning electron microscopy (Fig. 12–3). In large elastic arteries, the internal elastic lamina is not as continuous a sheet as in other conducting and muscular arteries, but may have numerous large fenestrations traversed by an irregular network of elastin strands (Fig. 12–5A).

The tunica adventitia of elastic arteries is relatively thin, and consists of fibroblasts and collagen bundles of predominant longitudinal orientation and a loose network of thin elastic fibers. The walls of the larger elastic arteries are too thick to be nourished by diffusion from the vessel lumen. Such vessels have a microvasculature of their own—small vessels call *vasa vasorum* that run in the adventitia and may penetrate some distance into the media. Their penetration is deeper in large veins than in arteries.

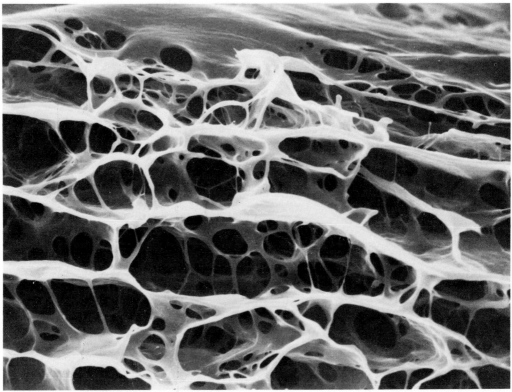

Figure 12–3. Scanning electron micrograph of the three-dimensional architecture of the elastin in a cross section of the wall of rat aorta extracted with hot formic acid to remove all other tissue components. The elastic tissue consists of multiple concentric sheets or laminae interconnected by radially oriented strands and fenestrated septa. In the intact vessel, smooth muscle cells occupy the spaces demarcated by these elastic elements. (Micrograph from Wasano, K. J. Electron Microsc. *32*:33, 1983.)

Muscular or Distributing Arteries

Elastic arteries gradually give way to *muscular* or *distributing arteries* such as the brachial, femoral, radial, popliteal, and their branches. Their tunica media consists mainly of smooth muscle that can actively change the diameter of the vessel to adjust the volume of blood delivered to meet the needs of the region supplied. This category includes the majority of the vessels in the arterial system and spans a wide range of sizes down to half a millimeter in diameter.

The intima is somewhat thinner than that of the elastic arteries and lacks smooth muscle cells but is otherwise similar in its organization. Beneath the intima is a well-developed elastica interna, which often has an undulating contour in the contracted vessels normally encountered in histological sections (Figs. 12–4, 12–6). The endothelium closely conforms to all the irregularities in the underlying elastica and sends processes through its fenestrations to establish myoendothelial junctions with the innermost smooth muscle cells of the tunica media. The fenestrations in the elastica interna are believed to be essential for nutrition of the avascular media by permitting diffusion of metabolites from the lumen. The communicating junctions of the cell processes that traverse some of the fenestrae serve to maintain metabolic coupling of the endothelium to the smooth muscle of the media.

The thickness of the media varies from 40 layers of helically or circumferentially oriented smooth muscle cells in large arteries to three or four layers in small arteries. The individual cells are surrounded and separated from one another by a moderately thick external lamina comparable with the basal lamina of epithelia (Fig. 12–7). Short processes extend from cell to cell through small discontinuities in this layer to form communicating junctions. These low-resistance junctions are probably essential for coordination of contraction throughout the media. The external lamina investing the smooth muscle

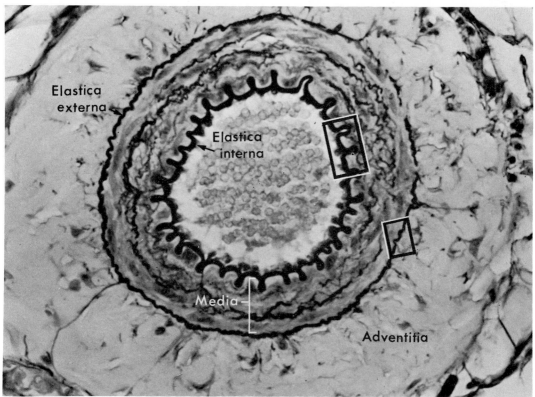

Figure 12–4. Photomicrograph of a muscular artery from the rat, showing the elastica interna, the media, the elastica externa, and a thick adventitia. Areas comparable with those enclosed in the rectangles are illustrated in electron micrographs in Figures 12–6 and 12–8. Aldehyde fuchsin stain for elastin.

cells stains deeply with the periodic acid–Schiff reaction. Embedded within this abundant interstitial material are small bundles of collagen fibrils corresponding to the network of delicate reticular fibers seen surrounding individual muscle fibers in silver-stained preparations viewed with the light microscope. Loose networks of thin elastic fibers also course circumferentially in the media and can be recognized as dark wavy lines among the smooth muscle cells in preparations stained with aldehyde-fuchsin or resorcin-fuchsin (Fig. 12–4). In electron micrographs they appear as unstained elongated profiles of irregular outline.

The elastica externa often appears in histological sections to be a continuous lamina at the boundary between the media and the adventitia (Fig. 12–4), but in electron micrographs it is an interrupted layer of irregular sheets of elastin considerably thinner than the elastica interna. Closely applied to the elastica on its outer aspect are numerous small fascicles of unmyelinated nerve axons, some containing local accumulations of mi-

tochondria and numerous synaptic vesicles. The nerves ordinarily do not penetrate into the media but appear to terminate at the elastica externa (Fig. 12–8). The neural stimulation of the muscle cells evidently results from diffusion of the neurotransmitter through fenestrations in this layer. The resulting depolarization of the peripheral muscle cells is propagated throughout the media via low-resistance cell-to-cell contacts (gap junctions or nexuses) between the muscle cells.

The tunica adventitia of muscular arteries may be thicker than the media (Figs. 12–4, 12–9) and consists of fibroblasts, elastic fibers, and bundles of collagen, oriented, for the most part, longitudinally. These continue into the surrounding connective tissue without a clearly defined boundary. The loose consistency of the tunica adventitia and predominant longitudinal orientation of its components permits the continual changes in the diameter of the vessel and limits the amount of retraction that takes place when an artery is cut.

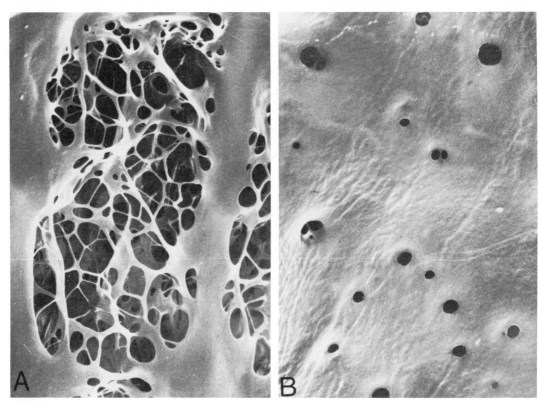

Figure 12–5. *A,* Scanning micrograph showing a surface view of the aortic internal elastic lamina of the rat. It is characterized by large fenestrations traversed by an irregular meshwork of elastin strands. *B,* In contrast, a similar view of the internal elastic lamina of the femoral artery shows small round fenestrations. (Micrographs from Wasano K. J. Electron Microsc. *32:*33, 1983.)

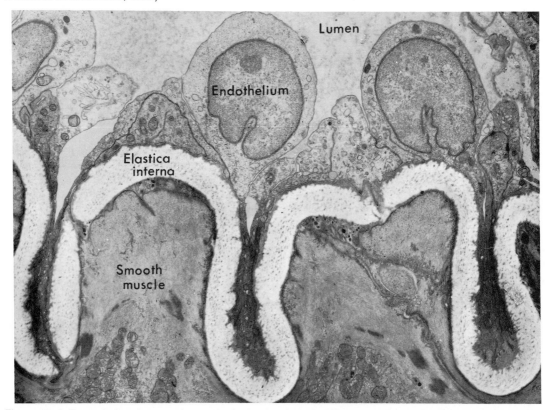

Figure 12–6. Transmission electron micrograph of a section through the wall of a small muscular artery (for orientation see upper box in Fig. 12–4). The elastica interna is scalloped owing to agonal contraction of the vessel wall. It is traversed at intervals by small fenestrations through which processes of endothelial cells extend to contact smooth muscle cells of the media.

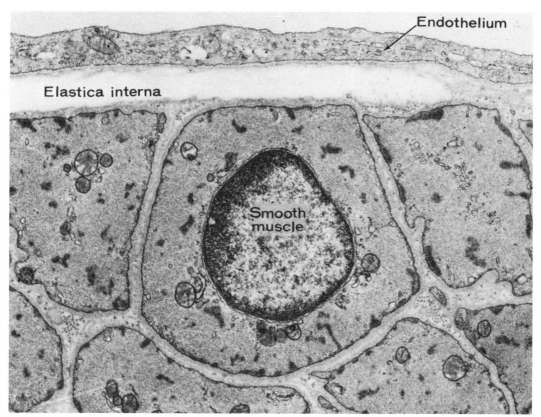

Figure 12-7. Electron micrograph of a portion of the wall of a small artery in longitudinal section. The elastica interna does not stain and therefore appears as a clear area between the endothelium and the smooth muscle of the media.

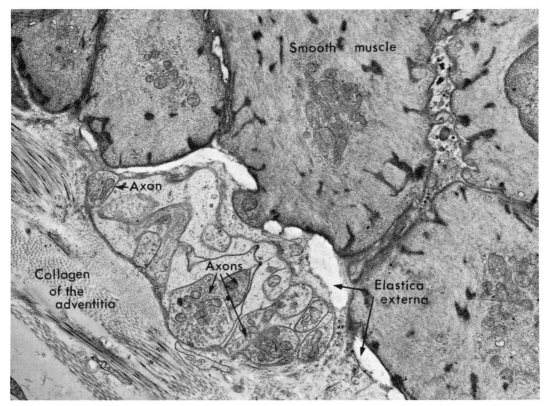

Figure 12-8. Electron micrograph of the junctional zone between the media and adventitia of a small muscular artery (see lower box in Fig. 12–4). The smooth muscle layer is limited on its outer aspect by a discontinuous elastica externa. Closely applied to this are numerous small nerves, some of whose axons contain many synaptic vesicles.

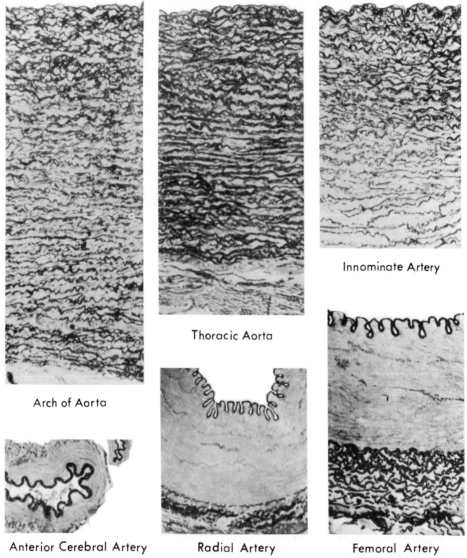

Innominate Artery

Thoracic Aorta

Arch of Aorta

Anterior Cerebral Artery   Radial Artery   Femoral Artery

Figure 12–9. Photomicrographs of the walls of elastic and muscular arteries of a macaque, illustrating variations in relative thickness and the differing amounts and distribution of elastic tissue, which has been selectively stained with resorcin fuchsin. (From Cowdry, E. V. Textbook of Histology. Philadelphia, Lea and Febiger, 1950.)

Transitional and Specialized Arteries

In the gradual transition of one type of artery to another, it is sometimes difficult to classify the intermediate region. Some arteries of intermediate caliber (e.g., popliteal, tibial) have walls that resemble larger arteries, while some large arteries (e.g., external iliac) have walls not unlike those of medium-sized arteries. The transitional regions between elastic and muscular arteries are often designated *arteries of mixed type*. Examples are the external carotid, axillary, and common iliac arteries. Their walls contain islands of smooth muscle fibers in the tunica media that

separate or interrupt the elastic laminae in many places. The visceral arteries that arise from the abdominal aorta are also of mixed type. For a varying distance, in the transitional region, the tunica media may consist of two different layers—an internal muscular layer and an external, composed of typical elastic laminae.

The thickness of the media of arteries is adapted to the internal pressure and external forces to which they are subjected. The coronary arteries of the heart are subjected to high pressure and have a wall that is thicker than other muscular arteries of comparable size. Similarly, in the arteries of the lower limbs, the tunica media is thicker than in corresponding arteries in the upper limbs.

Blood pressure in the pulmonary circulation is considerably lower than in the systemic circulation. Accordingly, the blood vessels in the lungs are relatively thin walled and distensible. A unique feature of the vessels of the lung is the presence of cardiac muscle extending from the heart a short distance into the wall of the pulmonary artery.

Within the cranial cavity, where vessels are protected from external pressures and tension, the dural and cerebral arteries have relatively thin walls. The elastica interna is well developed but the media is thin and devoid of elastic fibers (Fig. 12–9).

Where vessels are subject to bending or stretching, as in the popliteal and axillary arteries, longitudinal bundles of smooth muscle fibers may be found in the intima.

The umbilical artery, carrying blood from the fetus to the placenta, has an atypical structure. Its intima consists only of endothelium, and an internal elastic layer is lacking. The tunica media contains a few elastic fibers and two thick muscular layers that are quite distinct. The inner layer is composed of longitudinally oriented fibers; the outer layer, of circumferential fibers. In many places the longitudinal muscle raises longitudinal ridges protruding into the lumen. The extra-abdominal portion of the umbilical artery is provided with numerous rounded swellings or varicosities. In these regions the wall becomes thin and consists almost exclusively of the circularly oriented muscle.

Arterioles

The small arteries and arterioles form an important segment of the circulation, for they constitute the principal component of the peripheral resistance to flow that regulates the blood pressure. Arterioles range in diameter from 300 μm down to less than 50 μm. The tunica intima consists of a continuous endothelium, a thin basal lamina, and a very thin subendothelial layer consisting of a few reticular and elastic fibers. The elastica interna is thin and fenestrated and is absent in the terminal arterioles. The tunica media of larger arterioles may consist of two layers of smooth muscle cells, but in most arterioles there is a single layer of helically arranged smooth muscle cells (Figs. 12–10, 12–11, 12–12). In the short transitional region be-

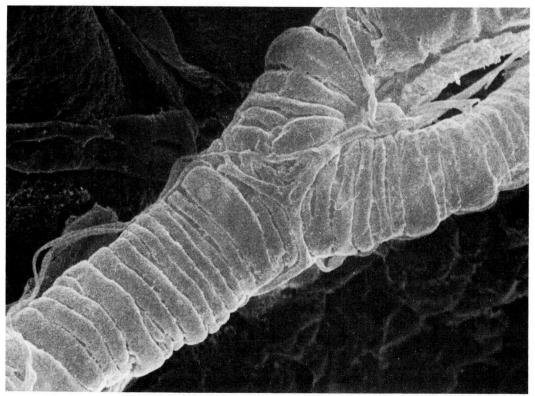

Figure 12–10. Scanning micrograph of a branching arteriole showing the circumferential arrangement of the single layer of smooth muscle cells. (Micrograph from Uehara, Y., and K. Suyama. J. Electron Microsc. 27:157, 1978.)

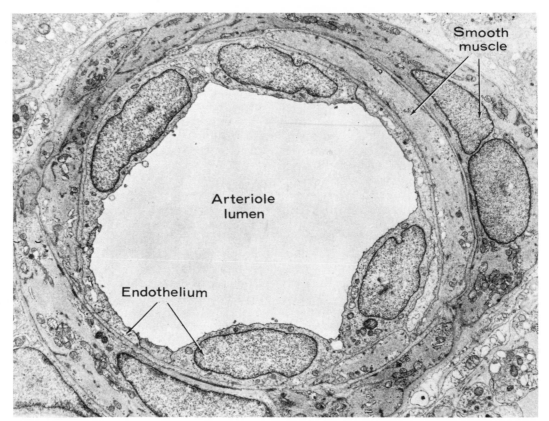

Figure 12–11. Electron micrograph of a typical small arteriole with one or two layers of smooth muscle cells around the endothelium.

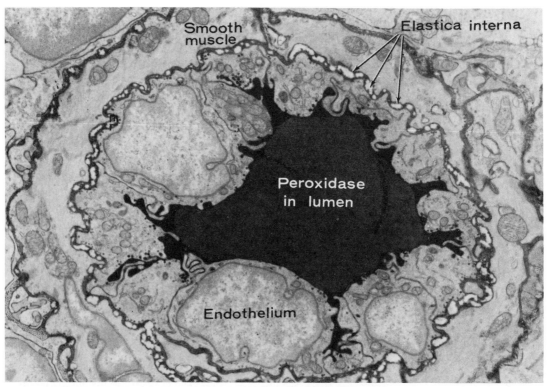

Figure 12–12. Arteriole from the corticomedullary boundary of the mouse thymus, 5 minutes after intravenous injection of peroxidase. The endothelium is freely permeable to this protein. The dense reaction product is seen in the lumen, between endothelial cells and filling the fenestrations in the elastica interna and the extracellular space around the single layer of smooth muscle cells. (Micrograph from Raviola, E., and M. J. Karnovsky. J. Exp. Med. *136*:466, 1972.)

tween arterioles and capillaries, sometimes called metarterioles, there are single muscle cells spaced at intervals. Their contraction is believed to give this region a sphincter-like function, intermittently opening and closing.

The adventitia of arterioles consists of loose connective tissue with occasional associated fibroblasts, macrophages, and small unmyelinated nerves.

Arteriovenous Anastomoses

In many parts of the body the terminal ramifications of arteries are connected with veins, not only by capillaries, but also by direct arteriovenous anastomoses of larger caliber. They usually arise as side branches from terminal arterioles and run directly to small venules. Their walls are muscular, remarkably thick for the caliber of the vessel, and richly supplied with vasomotor nerves. Observation of living vessels has shown that they contract markedly on stimulation of the sympathetic nerves. When the arteriovenous anastomosis is contracted, blood passes along the arteriole into the capillary network; when it relaxes, blood can bypass the capillaries and go directly into a thin-walled venule. The arteriovenous anastomoses are therefore considered important structures for regulating the supply of blood to many tissues.

In addition to these simple direct shunts, more highly organized connections have been described as part of a small organ called the *glomus*. These are found in the nailbed, the pads of the fingers and toes, and the ears. The afferent arteriole enters the connective tissue capsule of the glomus, loses its internal elastic lamina, and develops a heavy epithelioid muscle coat and narrow lumen. The arteriovenous anastomoses within the glomus may be branched and convoluted, and they are richly innervated by sympathetic nerves. The anastomoses empty into a short, thin-walled vein with a wide lumen, which drains into a periglomic vein and then into the ordinary veins of the skin.

Arteriovenous anastomoses are a device for shunting arterial blood directly into the venous system. By opening or closing, they can vary the amount of flow through the associated capillary bed. Their physiological significance in many organs is still poorly understood, but there is considerable evidence that those in the integument on the extremities of some species have an important role in thermoregulation. When arteriovenous anastomoses open, the rate of perfusion of the skin by blood at body temperature is increased manyfold, resulting in a greater loss of heat. Consistent with a role in temperature regulation is the finding of significant differences in distribution and numbers of arteriovenous anastomoses in various animal species related to their mode of thermal regulation. For example, in sheep in which the insulating fleece limits evaporative heat loss from much of the body surface, the ears, nose, and lower legs, which are devoid of wool, are of great importance in regulation of body temperature. The density of arteriovenous anastomoses per square centimeter of skin (72) over the lower leg is nearly five times that over the trunk (15). Similarly, in fur seals, which are provided with an internal insulating layer of subcutaneous blubber and thick fur for external insulation, the density of arteriovenous anastomoses is seven to ten times greater in the bare flippers, which can be used to dissipate heat when the seal is out of its cold aquatic environment.

Although most arterial vessels are innervated by sympathetic nerves, both adrenergic and cholinergic nerves are found in arteriovenous anastomoses, and the presence of nonadrenergic, noncholinergic nerve endings has been reported. The contractions of arteriovenous anastomoses are described as rapid, forceful, and relatively independent of the constrictions of neighboring arteries. There is evidence that they are under control of thermoregulatory centers in the central nervous system, whereas peripheral arteries are more responsive to locally generated stimuli.

The glomus type of arteriovenous anastomoses that possess modified smooth muscle cells with an epithelioid appearance, multiple convoluted channels, and an exceptionally rich innervation are considered by many investigators to be far more complex than would be required for simple shunting of blood, and are suspected of having an additional function yet to be discovered.

Sensory Organs of Arteries

Sensory nerves are associated with arteries throughout the vascular system, but at certain sites there are specialized neural organs whose function is to monitor the pressure and *composition* of the blood. These are of great importance in regulating respiration, heartbeat, and the vasomotor activity controlling blood pressure.

The *carotid bodies* are inconspicuous flattened bodies about 3 mm wide and 5 mm long, associated with the vessel walls at the bifurcation of the common carotid into internal and external carotid arteries. They are richly innervated by the carotid sinus branch of the glossopharyngeal nerve and by a plexus of sympathetic components from the vagus and glossopharyngeal nerves. The carotid bodies are highly vascular structures with a large blood flow in relation to their small volume of parenchyma. They consist of irregular clumps of pale-staining epithelioid cells in intimate relation to sinusoidal capillaries lined with fenestrated endothelium. Two types of cells can be distinguished with the light microscope on the basis of characteristic differences in their nuclei. They are more clearly distinguishable in electron micrographs.

The *Type I cell (glomus cell)* contains numerous dense-cored vesicles and occurs in clusters that are surrounded by *Type II cells,* which contain no dense-cored vesicles and are commonly regarded as sheath cells. These may yet prove to have a more significant function than is implied by that term. The Type I cells were originally considered to be a homogeneous population but subtypes have now been identified in several mammalian species. Type A cells usually have a smooth globular contour with a few processes, while Type B is irregular in outline with several long thin processes. The dense-cored vesicles of A glomus cells are twice as abundant as those of B cells and about 30 per cent larger.

Many nerves ramify throughout the carotid body and have endings rich in synaptic vesicles that terminate mainly on type A glomus cells. There is continuing controversy as to whether these nerves are afferent (conducting to the brain) or efferent (conducting to the carotid sinus). The bulk of recent evidence indicates that over 90 per cent of them are afferent and have reciprocal synapses with the glomus cells. The precise role of the glomus cell in chemoreceptor function is not clear. The traditional interpretation considered them to be chemoreceptors stimulated by hypoxia, hypercapnia, or elevated hydrogen ion concentration in the blood. They were assumed to pass information on the associated afferent nerves. An alternative interpretation postulates that the afferent nerve endings are the chemoreceptors, and that the glomus cells are dopaminergic inter-. neurons that modulate the sensitivity of chemoreceptive nerve endings. The possibility

that glomus cells also secrete a hormone cannot be ruled out. On the basis of their ultrastructure and cytochemical properties, some authors consider them paracrine cells probably secreting a polypeptide, but as yet no peptide hormone has been identified in the carotid body.

Other chemoreceptor organs, the *aortic bodies,* are situated near the arch of the aorta between the angle of the subclavian and the common carotid on the right, and medial to the origin of the subclavian artery on the left. Their structure and function appear to be identical to those of the carotid bodies.

At the bifurcation of the common carotid, the vessel exhibits a slight dilatation called the *carotid sinus.* This local specialization usually involves the proximal part of the internal carotid. The tunica media is thinner than elsewhere, while the adventitia is thicker and contains a large number of sensory nerve endings derived from the glossopharyngeal nerve. These nerve endings are stimulated by stretching. The carotid sinus therefore serves as a *baroreceptor* reacting to changes in blood pressure and initiating reflexes that bring about appropriate modifications of systemic pressure. A few baroreceptors are also found in the wall of the aorta and other large arteries in the thorax and neck, but these are not visually identifiable.

PHYSIOLOGICAL IMPLICATIONS OF THE STRUCTURE OF ARTERIES

The flow of blood in the arteries results from intermittent contraction of the heart and is therefore pulsatile. If the wall of the arteries were inflexible, the flow of blood in the capillaries would be intermittent. However, because the large arteries near the heart have distensible elastic walls, only part of the force of cardiac contraction is dissipated in advancing the column of blood in the vessels; the rest of the energy goes to expanding the walls of the large elastic arteries. The potential energy accumulated in the stretching of the walls of these vessels during contraction of the heart (systole) is dissipated in the elastic recoil of the vessel wall during the period when the heart is inactive (diastole). This release of tension in the arterial wall serves as an auxiliary pump, forcing the blood onward during diastole when no forward pressure is exerted by the heart. Thus, although the flow of blood is pulsatile throughout much of the arterial system, the elasticity of the walls of the large vessels ensures continuous flow through the capillaries.

The musculature in the media of the distributing arteries is normally in a state of partial contraction, referred to as *tone*, but the degree of contraction can be modulated in response to changes in pressure in the system and variations in activity of various tissues and organs. The *vasoconstriction* and *vasodilation* of arteries is regulated in part by the autonomic nervous system. In the majority of arteries seen in routine histological sections, the smooth muscle of the tunica media has undergone some degree of contraction, either after death or in response to the stimulus of immersion in a chemical fixative. One therefore gets a somewhat erroneous impression of the thickness of the arterial wall in relation to the size of the lumen. The remarkable capacity of the arteries to change their caliber is observed best in the living anesthetized animal. If a microdroplet of norepinephrine is placed on an artery, the underlying portion of the vessel wall will undergo marked local vasoconstriction. If the vessels are then rapidly fixed in this condition and sections are subsequently cut through the open and the adjacent constricted segments of the same vessel, one can clearly observe the great decrease in caliber of the lumen and the striking change in the character of the wall that accompanies vasomotor activity (Figs. 12–13, 12–14). Such contractions and relaxations of the muscular walls of arteries obviously influence the distribution of blood to the various organs. They also change the peripheral resistance to flow and therefore affect the blood pressure. Contraction of arteries may be the result of stimulation by sympathetic nerves, or of direct action of local products of injury. This latter effect is important in limiting hemorrhage from torn vessels in sites of tissue injury.

There are other local factors acting at the level of small arteries and arterioles that tend to regulate blood flow. If blood flow is interrupted briefly, the lack of oxygen and accumulation of carbon dioxide and lactic acid tend to cause relaxation of smooth muscle and vasodilation, so that when circulation is

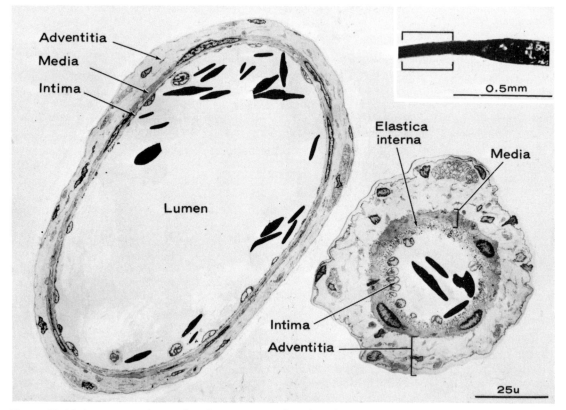

Figure 12–13. Low-power micrographs of two cross sections less than 1 mm apart in the same frog arteriole. A microdroplet applied to the living vessel caused local vasoconstriction in the area indicated by the brackets *(inset)*. The vessel was then fixed *in situ* and sectioned. The two sections offer a dramatic demonstration of the structural correlates of vasoconstriction and vasodilation. (From Phelps, P. C., and J. H. Luft. Am. J. Anat. *125*:399, 1969.)

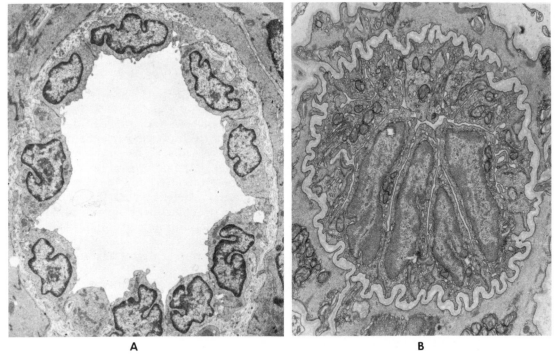

Figure 12–14. *A,* Micrograph of a typical small artery fixed with its lumen open. *B,* Micrograph of an artery of comparable size that has undergone agonal vasoconstriction. The cell bodies of the endothelial cells have increased in height, and they now almost completely occlude the lumen. Such extreme vasoconstriction probably occurs only rarely in normal physiological conditions, but it is evident that at sites of injury this could effectively reduce hemorrhage. (Micrograph courtesy of R. Bolender.)

restored the rate of flow may be two to six times greater than it was before. This important local autoregulation or reactive hyperemia correcting metabolic deficits does not depend on the nervous system.

The maintenance of normal blood pressure depends in large measure on the peripheral resistance to flow in the system, which in turn is a function of the smooth muscle tone in the walls of arterioles and small arteries. Halving the diameter of arterioles can increase the resistance as much as 16-fold, and a constriction to one fourth their original diameter may increase resistance as much as 250 times. This is the basis for the powerful effect of catecholamines and vasoactive peptides, such as angiotensin, on blood pressure.

The entire vascular system is lined by endothelium. The function of this cellular layer was long believed to be limited to providing the vessels with a smooth internal surface that would facilitate flow and prevent activation of the intrinsic coagulation mechanism of the blood. It was not thought to have significant metabolic or biosynthetic functions. This limited view of the role of the endothelium has proved to be quite erroneous. Endothelial cells have now been shown to be metabolically quite active and capable of synthesizing and releasing a variety of substances into the blood. They are believed to secrete the A and B blood-group antigens and certain of the clotting factors of the blood plasma. They also synthesize prostacyclin, a potent inhibitor of platelet aggregation. The endothelium thus contributes both to maintenance of the fluidity of the blood in the intact circulation and to the limitation of blood loss in the event of injury to the vessels. Enzymes in the plasmalemma of endothelial cells inactivate norepinephrine, serotonin, and bradykinin and transform angiotensin I to the potent vasoactive substance angiotensin II.

CHANGES IN ARTERIES WITH AGE

The structure of the wall of large arteries undergoes a gradual process of further differentiation from birth to age 25. In elastic arteries there is a progressive thickening and development of increasing numbers of elastic laminae, while in muscular arteries the thickness of the media increases with little or no addition of elastin. From middle age onward, there is a relative increase in the collagen and proteoglycans, and the walls of the larger arteries become less pliant. Perhaps the most significant age-related changes are in the intima. At birth it consists of endothelium and the internal elastic lamina, with little intervening connective tissue and only occasional smooth muscle cells. With increasing age, extracellular matrix components slowly accumulate and smooth muscle cells become more numerous.

Arteries are constantly exposed to mechanical stresses associated with oscillations of pressure and pulsatile flow in their lumen, and seem to be more subject to wear and tear than other organs. The late stages of development of their walls are not sharply differentiated from the early regressive changes associated with aging and the onset of *atherosclerosis* ("hardening of the arteries"). Some authors view these early changes as physiological; others consider them pathological. The larger arteries—particularly the aorta, iliac, femoral, coronary, and cerebral arteries—are especially prone to atherosclerosis. This disease is the principal cause of *myocardial infarction* (heart attack) and *cerebral thrombosis* (stroke) and is the leading cause of death in America and Europe. It is characterized by a patchy, irregular thickening of the intima with intracellular and extracellular deposits of lipid. The pathogenesis of the disease is still poorly understood. By the age of 10 years, small focal accumulations of intimal smooth muscle cells containing and surrounded by deposits of cholesterol-rich lipid form yellow "fatty streaks" that are visible to the naked eye on the luminal aspect of the aorta. These lesions that are asymptomatic increase to occupy 30 per cent or more of the aortic intimal surface by the age of 25. Whether these fatty streaks are invariably precursors of the more advanced lesions of atherosclerosis is still controversial. More patently pathological are lesions called *fibrous plaques* in older individuals. These are white and elevated so that they project slightly into the lumen. There is substantial agreement that these arise by proliferation of intimal smooth muscle cells and by migration of such cells from the media through fenestrations in the internal elastic lamina. Lipid accumulates in and around these cells, and their deposition of excess collagen, elastin, and

proteoglycan results in a local thickening of the intima. With progression of the disease, local extravasation of blood, necrosis, and calcification result in what are described as *complicated lesions*. These become sites of erosion of the endothelium, and aggregation of blood platelets to form a mural *thrombus* (clot). In advanced atherosclerosis, there may be necrosis and calcification of the tunica media of the muscular arteries in addition to the lesions in the intima.

The principal processes involved in arteriosclerosis thus appear to be proliferation of smooth muscle cells; their production of excess collagen, elastin, and proteoglycan; and the intracellular and extracellular accumulation of lipid. Research on the pathogenesis of the disease is now concentrating on the respective roles of the endothelial barrier; the various plasma lipoprotein fractions; and the mitogenic agents released by aggregated blood platelets.

CAPILLARIES

The branches of terminal arterioles pass through a short transitional region in which scattered smooth muscle cells persist around the endothelial tube. The vessels then continue as true *capillaries* that branch and anastomose with little or no change of diameter forming extensive capillary networks (Fig. 12–15).

The capillary wall consists of a layer of extremely attenuated endothelial cells, a basal lamina, and a sparse network of reticular fibers. Occasional undifferentiated mesenchymal cells may be associated with the capillary wall. In certain sites the pericapillary cells are more highly differentiated and have long branching processes that extend circumferentially around the capillary (Figs. 12–16, 12–17). It has been speculated that these may be contractile. It is customary to refer to all such cells as *pericytes* without attributing to them a special role in regulating the caliber of the vessel (Fig. 12–18). The endothelial cells themselves may contract after mechanical stimulation and it is therefore unnecessary to ascribe variations in size of the lumen to special cells in the capillary wall.

The caliber of the capillaries in different parts of the body varies within relatively narrow limits and averages about 8 to 12 µm, which permits unimpeded passage of the

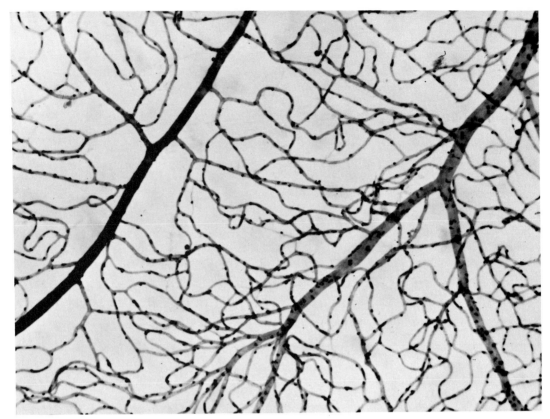

Figure 12–15. Normal human retinal blood vessels. These have been isolated by tryptic digestion of the neural and receptor elements, leaving behind only the vessels. At left is an arteriole, at right a venule, and between them is a network of capillaries of very uniform caliber. (Courtesy of T. Kuwabara.)

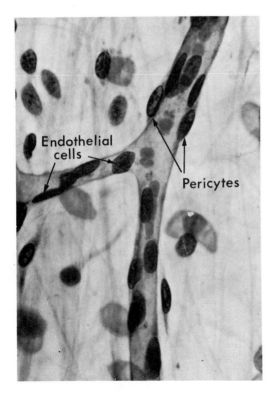

Figure 12–16. Photomicrograph of an intact capillary in a whole mount of rat mesentery. The nuclei of the flattened endothelial cells lining the capillary can be distinguished from those of the pericytes, which bulge outward. May-Grünwald-Giemsa stain.

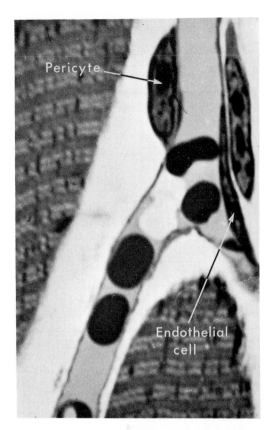

Figure 12–17. Photomicrograph of a capillary in skeletal muscle cut longitudinally. The nuclei of a pericyte, an endothelial cell, and a fibroblast can be distinguished. Several erythrocytes in the lumen give an indication of its dimensions. (Courtesy of J. Venable.)

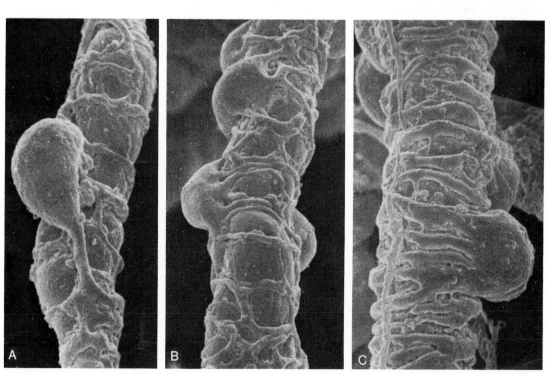

Figure 12–18. Scanning micrographs of small blood vessels showing pericytes with processes encircling the vessel wall. *A,* Pericyte of a capillary with primary processes directed longitudinally and secondary processes running circumferentially. *B,* Arterial capillary with numerous associated pericytes. *C,* Terminal arteriole with pericyte and circular smooth muscle cells. (Micrographs from Uehara, Y., and K. Suyama. J. Electron Microsc. 27:157, 1978.)

cellular elements of the blood. In organs that are in a state of minimal functional activity, many of the capillaries are narrowed so that little blood circulates through them. Normally only about 25 per cent of the total capillary bed in the body is patént, but with increased activity, these open and flow is restored to meet local needs.

In cross sections of small capillaries, a single endothelial cell may extend all around the lumen (Fig. 12–19). In larger capillaries the wall may be made up of portions of two or three cells. The nucleus of endothelial cells is greatly flattened and thus appears elliptical in section. The thicker nuclear region of the cell bulges into the lumen. The attenuated peripheral portion of the cell is extremely thin, with the adluminal and abluminal membranes separated by a layer of cytoplasm only 0.2 to 0.4 μm thick. A small Golgi complex and a few mitochondria are found in the juxtanuclear region, with meandering tubular elements of the endoplasmic reticulum extending into the thin peripheral cytoplasm. Lysosomes are rare but multivesicular bodies are not uncommon. A conspicuous feature of endothelial cells is the presence of a large population of plasmalemmal vesicles about 70 nm in diameter with narrow necks, present on both cell surfaces and opening onto the lumen and to the extravascular space (Fig. 12–20).

The luminal surface of the cells is usually smooth contoured, but edges of adjacent cells often overlap and a thin marginal ridge or flap may project a short distance into the lumen (Fig. 12–21). Desmosomes and a zonula adherens are usually absent but there is a shallow occluding junction (Fig. 12–22), which in freeze-fracture preparations exhibits one to three parallel intramembranous strands on the E-face.

At the resolution afforded by the light microscope, capillaries in different tissues and organs appear quite similar, but with the electron microscope at least two morphologically distinct types can be distinguished on the basis of differences in the endothelium (Fig. 12–23). In muscle, nervous tissue, and connective tissues of the body, the endothelium forms a thin uninterrupted layer around the entire circumference of the capillary. These are designated *continuous capillaries (muscle-type capillaries)*. In pancreas, intestinal tract, and endocrine glands the endothelium varies in thickness, and some extremely attenuated regions are interrupted

by circular fenestrations or pores 80 to 100 nm in diameter closed by a very thin pore diaphragm with a punctate central thickening (Fig. 12–24B). When seen in surface view in scanning micrographs or freeze-fracture preparations, the pores are very uniformly distributed with a center-to-center spacing of about 130 nm. In these *fenestrated capillaries (visceral capillaries)*, the areas exhibiting pores make up only a fraction of the vessel wall, the remainder resembling the endothelium of muscle-type capillaries. In this mosaic of fenestrated and unfenestrated areas, the relative proportions vary in capillaries of different organs. Among fenestrated capillaries, those of the renal glomerulus appear to be exceptional in that the pores are not closed by pore diaphragms, and their basal lamina is as much as three times thicker than that of other capillaries. Fluid traverses the wall of glomerular capillaries as much as 100 times more rapidly than in muscle capillaries.

STRUCTURAL BASIS OF TRANSENDOTHELIAL EXCHANGE

An important concern of physiologists has been the mechanism of exchange across the capillary wall. The observed rates of passage of water-soluble molecules can be accounted for by postulating two fluid-filled systems of pores traversing the endothelium: one of "small pores" about 9 nm in diameter and of relatively high frequency, and the other of "large pores" up to 70 nm in diameter and of lower frequency. Pores as such are not seen in electron micrographs of muscle capillaries and the structural equivalent of the postulated two sets of pores has been a subject of lively debate. To clarify this issue, electron-dense molecules of known dimensions greater than 10 nm are introduced into the circulation. In muscle capillaries, these molecules are rapidly taken up by open vesicles on the adluminal surface of the continuous endothelium, ferried across the cytoplasm, and discharged into the extravascular space by fusion of the vesicles with the abluminal plasmalemma (Fig. 12–26A).

The uptake of materials in small vesicles is a form of endocytosis common to many cell types and is generally referred to as *micropinocytosis*. In this process, the vesicles generally fuse with lysosomes or are incorporated in multivesicular bodies within the cytoplasm. The use of vesicles to ferry fluid and solutes

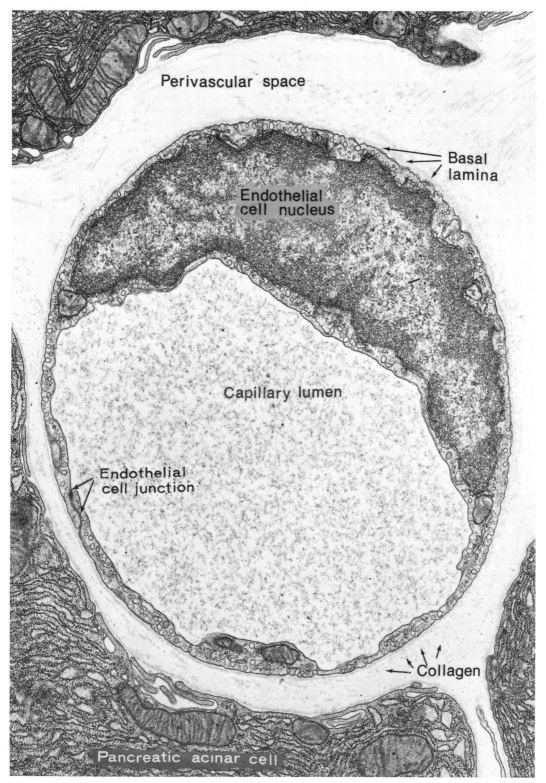

Figure 12–19. Electron micrograph of a typical capillary from guinea pig pancreas. The entire circumference is made up of a single endothelial cell. There is a thin basal lamina and a few associated collagen fibrils. No pericyte is present in this cross section. (Micrograph from Bolender, R. J. Cell Biol. 61:269, 1974.)

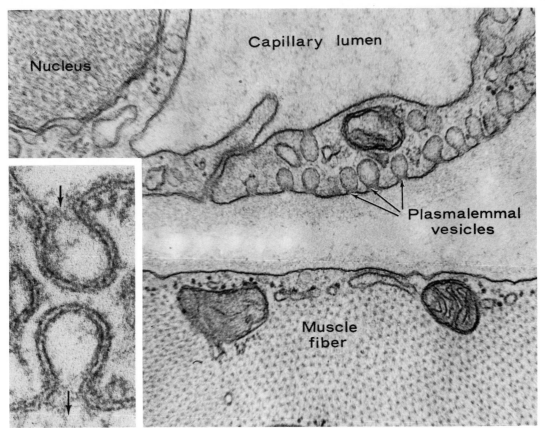

Figure 12–20. Electron micrograph of capillary endothelium, illustrating the small vesicular inpocketings of the luminal and basal surfaces that are characteristic of capillaries in muscle. (From Fawcett, D. W. J. Histochem. Cytochem. *13*:75, 1965.) Inset shows two such vesicles at high magnification. (From Bruns, R., and G. E. Palade. J. Cell. Biol. *37*:244, 1968.)

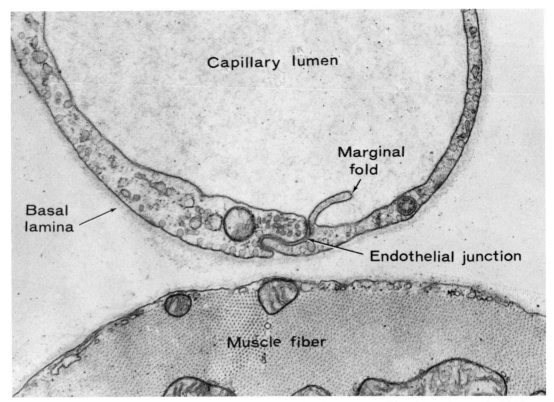

Figure 12–21. Capillary from cardiac muscle, illustrating the interdigitating cell junction and a marginal fold.

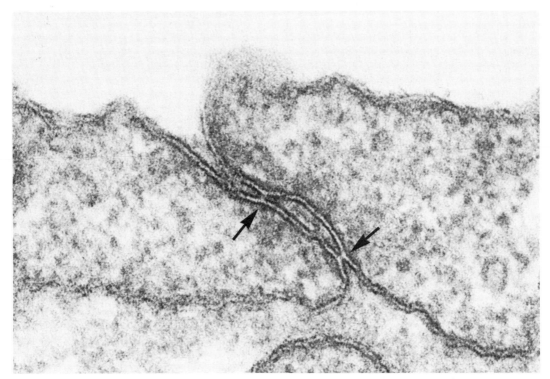

Figure 12–22. Micrograph of the junction of two endothelial cells in a muscle-type capillary. At the arrows the opposing membranes are joined to form an occluding junction. (Micrograph courtesy of E. Weihe.)

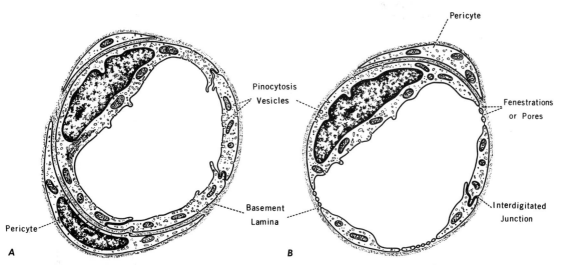

Figure 12–23. Schematic representation of the two most common types of capillaries. *A,* The continuous or muscle type with an uninterrupted endothelium. *B,* The fenestrated type, in which the endothelium varies in thickness and the thinnest areas have small pores closed by an exceedingly thin membranous diaphragm. (After Fawcett, D. W. *In* Orbison, J. L., and D. Smith, eds.: Peripheral Blood Vessels. Baltimore, Williams and Wilkins, 1962.)

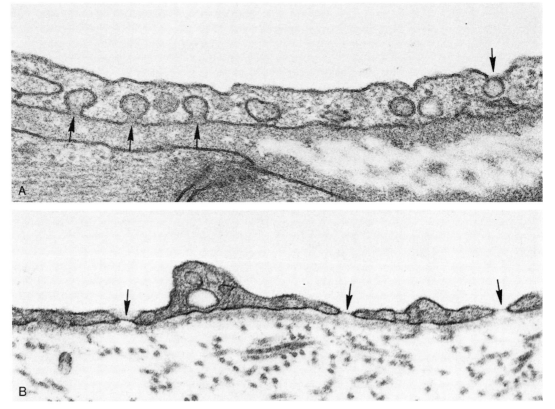

Figure 12–24. Micrographs of segments of endothelium from the two types of capillary. *A,* Endothelium of the muscle capillary endothelium has vesicular invaginations of both adluminal and abluminal plasma membranes *(at arrows). B,* Endothelium of fenestrated capillary from the lamina propria of the colon is extremely thin and has pores closed by thin diaphragms *(at arrows).* (Micrographs courtesy of E. Weihe.)

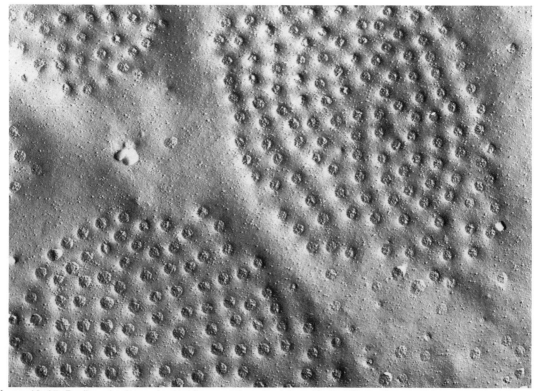

Figure 12–25. Replica of a freeze-fractured preparation of a fenestrated capillary. This extensive surface view of the cleaved membrane of an endothelial cell shows fenestrated areas separated by nonfenestrated areas. Notice the uniform size and spacing of the pores. (Micrograph courtesy of S. McNutt.)

VESICULATION OF THE PLASMALEMMA

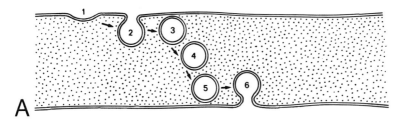

FUSION-FISSION WITHOUT MIXING OF VESICLE AND PLASMA MEMBRANES

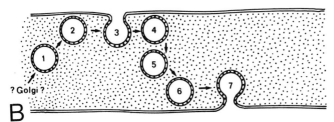

FORMATION OF CHANNELS AND FENESTRAE

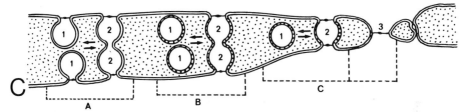

Figure 12–26. Schematic representation of alternative models for transport of water-soluble molecules across the endothelium. *A,* Continuous formation of plasmalemmal vesicles followed by detachment, transit, and fusion with the membrane on the other front of the cell. *B,* Transport mediated by a separate cytoplasmic population of vesicles, possibly of Golgi origin, which undergo transient fusion and fission first at one surface and then at the other without mixing of their membrane with the plasmalemma. This would not require massive movement of membrane from one surface to the other. *C,* Transcellular passage involving fusion of vesicles to form channels or formation of fenestrae in thin areas of endothelium. (Redrawn after Simionescu, N., and M. Simeonescu. *In* Ussing, H. H., N. B. Bindslev, and O. Sten-Knudsen, eds.: Water Transport Across Epithelia. Copenhagen, Munksgaard, 1981.)

across the cell is largely confined to endothelial cells and is an expression of their specialization for transport. The term *transcytosis* has been suggested to distinguish this process from pinocytosis. In addition to the translocation of vesicles from one surface of the endothelium to the other, serial sections reveal that transient transendothelial channels may be formed by fusion of several vesicles, or in extremely thin areas a single vesicle may open at both surfaces of the cell (Fig. 12–26C).

There is now quite general agreement that in continuous capillaries, the transcellular traffic of vesicles and the channels occasionally formed by vesicle fusion together correspond to the "large-pore" system postulated by physiologists. The process of transcytosis was originally envisioned as involving contin-

uous vesiculation of the adluminal plasmalemma, detachment, movement across the cytoplasm, and fusion with the opposite membrane. To account for the measured albumin clearance, this would involve a continuous massive translocation of membrane from the luminal to the abluminal surface of the endothelium. Some recent evidence strongly suggests that the transport vesicles are not all newly formed at the expense of the luminal plasmalemma, but may be a separate and relatively stable population, arising possibly from the Golgi complex, and simply shuttling back and forth, undergoing alternate fusion and fission without intermixing of membrane constituents at the plasmalemma (Fig. 12–26B). This model would be consistent with the images observed in electron micrographs and would not involve translocation of large amounts of membrane from the luminal to the abluminal surface of the endothelium.

There is still disagreement as to the structural equivalent of the postulated small pores in muscle capillaries, permitting passage of molecules smaller than 9 nm. Some investigators localize them in the intercellular junctions. In the case of fenestrated capillaries, there is general agreement that the fenestrae are the equivalent of the "large pores," while the "small pores" may be in the intercellular clefts or in the diaphragms of the fenestrae. The permeability properties of the pore diaphragms are still largely unexplored.

Factors other than molecular size influence transendothelial transport—the chemical nature of the molecules and their net charge, as well as the charge in the pathways involved. In general the surface of the endothelium is negatively charged. When tracers of opposite charge, such as cationized ferritin, are perfused they bind randomly on the plasmalemma, and especially tenaciously to diaphragms of fenestrae, but not to the plasmalemmal vesicles and channels involved in transcytosis, which appear to be neutral. Thus, the endothelial surface presents to the blood a mosaic of microdomains of differing charge and can probably sort macromolecules according to their differing charge. Cationic tracers are taken up mainly by adsorptive endocytosis in coated vesicles, whereas anionic or neutral tracers are shuttled across the endothelium in smooth vesicles.

There are marked differences in the permeability of capillaries of the same type in different organs. For example, intravenously injected dyes that readily escape from capillaries in most tissues are retained in the cerebral capillaries, and only a few special areas of the brain are stained. This observation, first made 70 years ago, gave rise to the concept of a *blood-brain permeability barrier*. Its structural basis was thought to reside in special relationships of the foot processes of perivascular astrocytes to each other and to the capillary walls. When this was reinvestigated by electron microscopy, the capillaries of the brain were found to have a continuous endothelium like that of muscle capillaries, but when peroxidase was administered intravascularly, the tight junctions did not permit escape of the molecules by an intercellular path. Occasional vesicles containing peroxidase were found at the luminal surface but

there was little evidence of their movement into the cytoplasm or of their discharge on the abluminal side of endothelium. Thus, the blood-brain barrier is attributable to a paucity of transport vesicles in cerebral capillaries and tighter occluding junctions than in muscle-type capillaries elsewhere in the body. A *blood-ocular barrier* and a *blood-thymus barrier* have been shown to depend on similar properties of the capillary endothelium in these organs. In the thymus, segments of the microvasculature only a few millimeters apart have different permeability properties. The endothelium prevents access of circulating macromolecules to the lymphoid cells of the cortex, while the capillaries of the medulla are freely permeable to electron-opaque probes.

SINUSOIDS

Sinusoids are endothelium-lined vascular channels of relatively large caliber and irregular cross-sectional outline. Unlike capillaries that are cylindrical, sinusoids conform in shape to the interstices among the epithelial sheets and cords of the organ they supply. Their unusual configuration is a consequence of their mode of development. Capillaries develop as dichotomously branching cellular cords that secondarily acquire a lumen, and they grow by addition of vasoformative cells at their ends. Sinusoids, on the other hand, develop during organogenesis by ingrowth of the epithelial parenchyma into large, thin-walled embryonic blood vessels. This accounts for their close conformity to the geometry of the organ. The most typical example of sinusoids is to be found in the microvasculature of the liver, but sinusoids are also found in spleen, bone marrow, adrenal cortex, adenohypophysis, and certain other endocrine glands. The sinusoidal endothelium in these organs is more active in endocytosis and has a better-developed lysosomal system than capillary endothelium elsewhere. For this reason these vessels were traditionally grouped together as elements of the so-called reticuloendothelial system.

The endothelium of sinusoids in some lymphoid organs is extremely attenuated but continuous. In endocrine glands, it is a mosaic of fenestrated and unfenestrated areas as in visceral capillaries. The endothelium of the hepatic sinusoids is unique in having large fenestrations of varying size and shape.

Here the blood plasma has direct access to the liver cells with no interposed permeability barrier.

VEINS

The blood is carried from the capillary networks toward the heart by the veins. In progressing toward the heart, they gradually increase in caliber, while their walls become thicker. The veins usually accompany their corresponding arteries (Fig. 12–27). The veins are more numerous than the arteries and their caliber is larger, so that the venous system has a much greater capacity than the arterial system. The walls of the veins are always thinner, more supple, and less elastic than those of the arteries. Thus, in sections, the veins are usually collapsed, and their lumen is irregular and slitlike unless a special effort has been made to fix them in distention.

It is customary to distinguish three types: veins of small, medium, and large caliber. This subdivision is often unsatisfactory, for the caliber and structure of the wall cannot always be correlated. Veins in the same category show much greater variations than do the arteries, and the same vein may show great differences in structure in different parts.

Most authors distinguish three layers in the walls of the veins: tunica intima, tunica media, and tunica adventitia. However, the boundaries of these layers are frequently indistinct, and in certain veins these coats, particularly the tunica media, cannot be distinguished. The muscular and elastic tissue is not nearly as well developed in the veins as in the arteries, whereas the connective tissue component is much more prominent.

Venules and Veins of Small Caliber

When several capillaries unite, they form a venule, a cylindrical vessel 15 to 20 μm in diameter, consisting of a layer of endothelium surrounded by thin, longitudinally oriented reticular fibers with occasional fibroblasts (Fig. 12–28). Although the caliber of the vessel is larger, the structure of its wall is not very different from that of a capillary (Fig. 12–29). It appears to be more permeable to intravenously injected dyes. Not all of the exchange between the blood and the tissues takes place in the capillaries. The venules appear to have a significant role in this, and they are particularly important in the changes associated with inflammation.

Early observations on the properties of venules have now been amplified by electron microscopic studies. When particulate markers are injected intravascularly, the particles are usually found not outside of the walls of the capillaries but along somewhat larger vessels interpreted as venules. This same category of vessels is also most susceptible to histamine, serotonin, and other substances

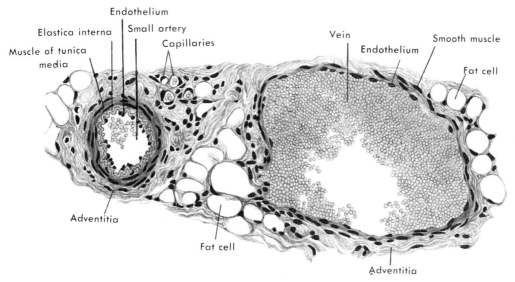

Figure 12–27. Cross section through a small artery and its accompanying vein from the submucosa of a human intestine. (After A. A. Maximow.)

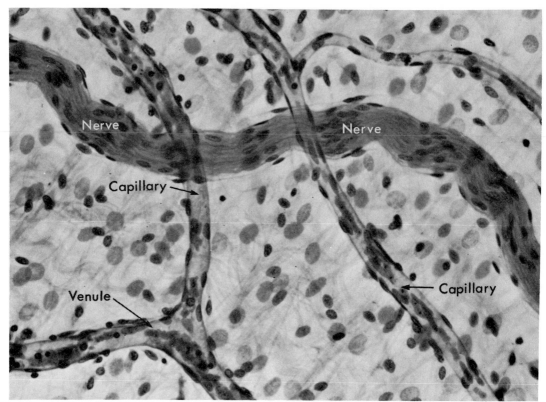

Figure 12–28. Photomicrograph of a thin-spread mesentery showing a nerve, venule, and capillaries. May-Grünwald-Giemsa stain.

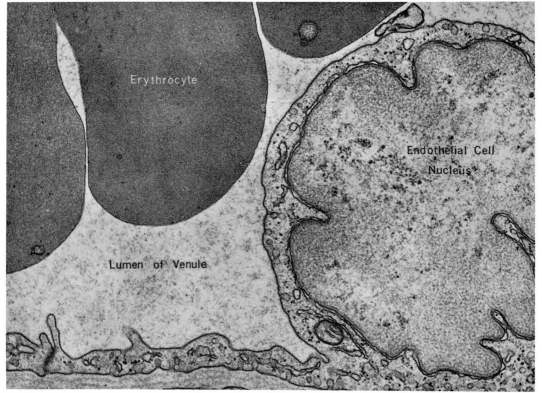

Figure 12–29. Electron micrograph of a portion of the wall of a small venule from the myocardium. The thin continuous endothelium is essentially the same as that of a capillary. The nuclear region of the endothelial cell bulges into the lumen.

known to increase vascular permeability (Fig. 12–30). If one of these substances is injected locally into an animal that has previously been injected intravenously with a particulate marker, it induces the appearance of small intercellular gaps in the endothelium. The particles, held back by the basal lamina, accumulate in the gaps, thus marking the vessels and permitting identification of the sites of increased permeability. Although leaks can occasionally be found in capillaries, the vast majority are in small venules. There seems to be a gradient of permeability from the arterial to the venous side, which reaches a maximum in the venules and then diminishes abruptly in vessels of larger size.

When the caliber of venules has increased to about 50 μm, partially differentiated smooth muscle cells appear between the endothelium and the surrounding connective tissue. These cells are at first some distance apart (Fig. 12–31). Farther along, in small veins, they become arranged closer and closer together. In small veins with a diameter of 200 μm, these elements form a more or less continuous layer and have a typical long spindle shape.

In still larger veins, thin networks of elastic fibers appear. Their tunica intima consists only of endothelium, and one or several layers of smooth muscle cells form the media. The tunica adventitia consists of fibroblasts and thin elastic and collagenous fibers. Most of these fibrous elements run longitudinally, but some penetrate among the muscle cells of the tunica media.

Veins of Medium Caliber

The veins of medium caliber (2 to 9 mm) include the cutaneous and deeper veins of the extremities distal to the brachial and the popliteal, and the veins of the viscera and head, with the exception of the main trunks. In the tunica intima of these veins, the endothelial cells in surface view are polygons with highly irregular outlines. Sometimes the tunica intima also contains an inconspicuous connective tissue layer with a few cells and thin elastic fibers. Externally, it is sometimes bounded by a network of elastic fibers. Because the tunica intima is often poorly developed, some authors consider the inner and middle coats as forming one layer.

The tunica media is much thinner than in the arteries and consists mainly of circular smooth muscle fibers separated by many longitudinal collagenous fibers and a few fibroblasts. The tunica adventitia is usually much thicker than the media and consists of loose connective tissue with thick longitudinal collagenous bundles and elastic networks. In the layers adjacent to the media, it often contains a number of longitudinal smooth muscle bundles.

Veins of Large Caliber

The tunica intima has the same structure as in the medium-sized veins. In some of the larger trunks its connective tissue layer is of considerable thickness (45 to 68 μm). The tunica media, in general, is poorly developed

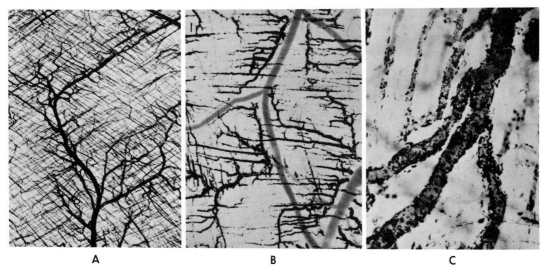

| A | B | C |

Figure 12–30. Photomicrographs illustrating the greater permeability of venules induced by serotonin. *A*, Cremaster of the normal rat injected with carbon to demonstrate the entire vascular system. *B*, Vascular labeling resulting from leakage of opaque particles from the vessels from local injection of serotonin. The black vessels are venules; the permeability of the many small capillaries visible in *A* has not been enhanced by this treatment. *C*, Higher magnification of a venule after 7 days, showing intracellular mass of particulate matter in the vascular wall. (From Majno, G., G. E. Palade, and G. I. Schoefl. J. Biophys. Biochem. Cytol. *11*:607, 1961.)

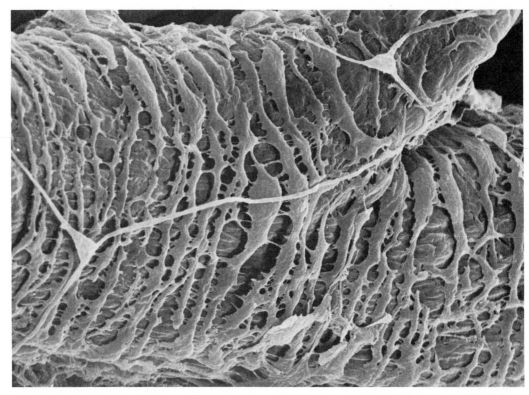

Figure 12–31. Scanning micrograph of a large venule joined by a smaller tributary at upper right. The smooth muscle cells are more irregular in shape, and are spaced farther apart than arterioles. Elements of the perivascular nerve net can be seen branching over the vessel. The fibrous and amorphous connective tissue components have been digested enzymatically in this preparation to reveal the underlying structures. (Micrograph from Uehara, Y., J. Desaki, and T. Fujiwara. Biomed. Res. 2(Suppl.):139, 1981.)

and is sometimes absent. Its structure is the same as in the veins of medium caliber. The tunica adventitia makes up the greater part of the venous wall and is usually several times as thick as the tunica media. It consists of connective tissue containing thick elastic fibers and longitudinally oriented collagenous fibers. The tunica adventitia contains prominent longitudinal bundles of smooth muscle and elastic networks. This is the structure of the inferior vena cava and of the portal, splenic, superior mesenteric, external iliac, renal, and azygos veins.

Special Types of Veins

In the iliac, femoral, popliteal, saphenous, cephalic, basilar, and umbilical veins, there are longitudinal smooth muscle fibers in the subendothelial connective tissue layer of the tunica intima. In certain veins the longitudinal orientation of cellular elements is also noticed in the innermost layers of the tunica media.

In a considerable portion of the inferior vena cava, the tunica media is absent and the well-developed longitudinal muscle bundles of the tunica adventitia are directly adjacent to the intima. In the pulmonary veins, the media is well developed, with circular smooth muscle. It is like an artery in this respect. Smooth muscle is particularly prominent in all the layers of the veins in the pregnant uterus.

Other veins are entirely devoid of smooth muscle tissue and consequently lack a tunica media. In this group belong the veins of the maternal part of the placenta, the spinal pia mater, the retina, as well as the sinuses of the dura mater, the majority of the cerebral veins, and the veins of the nailbed and the trabeculae of the spleen. The last two are simply channels lined by endothelium, with a fibrous connective tissue covering.

The adventitia of the vena cava and particularly of the pulmonary vein is provided for a considerable distance with a layer of cardiac muscle fibers arranged in a ring, with a few longitudinal fibers where these vessels enter the heart. In the rat, the pulmonary veins up to their radicles contain a considerable amount of cardiac muscle in the tunica media.

Valves of the Veins

Many veins of medium caliber, especially those of the extremities, are provided with *valves* that prevent the blood from flowing away from the heart. These are semilunar pockets on the internal surface of the wall, with their free edges pointing in the direction of the blood flow (Fig. 12–32). In man the valves are usually arranged in pairs, one opposite the other. Between the valve and the wall of the vein is the *sinus of the valve*, where the wall of the blood vessel is usually thin and somewhat distended.

The valve itself is a thin connective tissue membrane. On the side toward the lumen of the vessel, it contains a network of elastic fibers continuous with those of the tunica intima of the vein. In the thinner region of the wall, comprising the sinus of a valve, the intimal and medial tunics contain only longitudinal smooth muscle fibers. These do not enter into the substance of the valve in man.

Both surfaces of the valve are covered by endothelium. The endothelial cells lining the surface toward the lumen of the vessel are elongated in the axis of the vessel; those that line the surface of the valve facing the sinus are transversely elongated.

Portal Systems of Vessels

As a general rule, a capillary network connects the terminal ramifications of the arterial system with those of the venous system, and the transition from arterioles to capillaries to venules is gradual. In a number of regions, however, modifications of this vascular plan are adapted to the special functional requirements of the particular organ.

In one physiologically important modification of the general plan, the flow from one capillary bed passes through a larger vessel or vessels having histological characteristics of veins to a second capillary network before the blood returns to the heart via the systemic venous circulation. Such a set of vessels interposed between two capillary beds is called a *portal system*. For example, the capillary networks of the intestines and certain other abdominal viscera drain via the *portal vein* to the liver. There the portal vein ramifies into a network of sinusoids throughout the organ. Blood passes from these through a system of

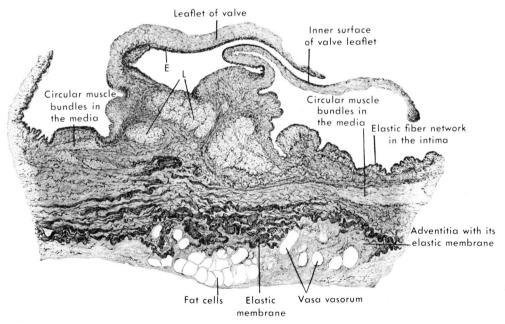

Figure 12–32. From a cross section of the femoral vein of man. The section passes through the origin of a valve. *E,* Elastic fiber network in the intima on the inner surface of the valve leaflet; *L,* longitudinal muscles of the base of the valve. Acid orecin stain. (After Schaffer.)

converging vessels of gradually increasing caliber to the hepatic vein and thence back to the heart via the inferior vena cava. This arrangement permits nutrient material absorbed in the intestines to be exposed to, and processed by, the liver cells before being distributed throughout the body by the general circulation.

The capillaries in the median eminence of the hypothalamus are continuous with a plexus of small veins, the *hypophyseoportal system*, which courses along the hypophyseal stalk and then divides into the sinusoids of the anterior lobe of the hypophysis. This arrangement permits releasing factors, which are liberated at the ends of neurosecretory axons in the hypothalamus, to be carried downstream to activate endocrine secretory cells in the hypophysis (see Chapter 19).

An artery may ramify into a set of capillaries, which are then collected into a larger arterial vessel. An example of this is found in the kidney, in which an afferent arteriole suddenly breaks up into a mass of contorted capillaries comprising the glomerulus. These capillaries do not empty into veins but coalesce to form the efferent arteriole, which goes on to ramify into another set of capillaries around the kidney tubules. In this case the efferent arteriole is a portal vessel (see Chapter 30).

THE HEART

The heart is a thick, muscular, rhythmically contracting portion of the vascular system. It lies in the pericardial cavity within the mediastinum. It is about 12 cm long, 9 cm wide, and 6 cm in its anteroposterior diameter, and consists of four chambers: a right and left *atrium* and a right and left *ventricle*. The superior and inferior venae cavae bring the venous blood from the body to the right atrium, from which it passes to the right ventricle. From here the blood is forced through the lungs, where it is aerated, and it is then brought to the left atrium. From there it passes to the left ventricle and is distributed throughout the body by the aorta and its branches. The orifices between the atria and the ventricles are closed by the *tricuspid valve* on the right and the *mitral valve* on the left side. The openings to the pulmonary artery and the aorta, from the right and left ventricles, respectively, are closed by the aortic and pulmonary *semilunar valves*.

The wall of the heart, in both the atria and the ventricles, consists of three main layers: an internal, the *endocardium;* an intermediate, the *myocardium;* and an external, the *epicardium*. The internal layer is directly exposed to the blood; the myocardium is the contractile layer, and the epicardium is the visceral layer of the *pericardium*, a serous membrane that forms the pericardial sac, the serous cavity in which the heart lies.

The endocardium is generally regarded as homologous to the tunica intima of the blood vessels, the myocardium to the tunica media, and the epicardium to the tunica adventitia.

Endocardium

The endocardium is lined with ordinary endothelium, which is continuous with that of the blood vessels entering and leaving the heart. This endothelium consists of polygonal squamous cells. Directly under the endothelium in most places is a thin *subendothelial layer* that contains fibroblasts and collagenous fibers and a few elastic fibers. External to this loose layer is a thick layer of denser connective tissue, which comprises the main mass of the endocardium and contains great numbers of elastic elements (Fig. 12–33). Bundles of smooth muscle fibers are found in varying numbers in this layer, particularly on the interventricular septum.

A *subendocardial layer*, absent from the papillary muscles and from the chordae tendineae, consists of loose connective tissue that binds the endocardium to the myocardium and is directly continuous with the interstitial tissue of the latter. It contains blood vessels, nerves, and branches of the conduction system of the heart. In the spaces between the muscular bundles of the atria, the connective tissue of the endocardium continues into that of the epicardium, and the elastic networks of the two layers intermingle.

Myocardium

The histology and fine structure of the cardiac muscle has been described in Chapter 10. In the embryos of the higher vertebrates, the myocardial fibers form a spongy network. In the adult stage, however, they are bound by connective tissue into a compact mass. This condensation of the myocardium progresses from the epicardium toward the endocardium. Many embryonic muscle fascicles remain in a more or less isolated condition on the internal surface of the walls of the

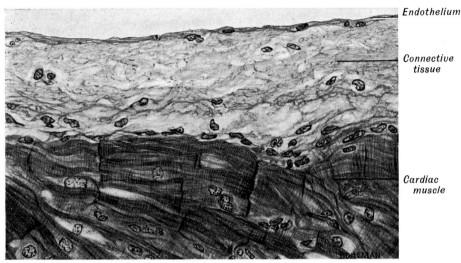

Endothelium

Connective tissue

Cardiac muscle

Figure 12–33. Section of the endocardium of the ventricle of man.

ventricular cavities. These muscle fiber bundles are covered with endocardium and are called *trabeculae carneae*.

Elastic elements are scarce in the myocardium of the ventricles of adult mammals, except in the tunica adventitia of the larger blood vessels in the walls of these chambers. In the myocardium of the atria, however, there are networks of elastic fibers, which run everywhere between the muscle fibers and are directly connected with similar networks in the endocardium and epicardium. They are also continuous with the elastic networks in the walls of the large veins. A large part of the interstitial connective tissue of the cardiac muscle consists of extensive networks of reticular fibrils.

Epicardium

The epicardium is covered on its free surface by a single layer of mesothelial cells. Beneath the mesothelium is a thin layer of connective tissue with networks of elastic fibers, blood vessels, and many nerves. In the loose connective tissue along the coronary blood vessels, considerable amounts of adipose tissue are found.

The parietal layer of the pericardium is a serous membrane of the usual type—a flat layer of connective tissue that contains elastic and collagenous fibers, fibroblasts, fixed macrophages, and a covering layer of mesothelial cells. The smooth, moist, apposed surfaces of the epicardium and the parietal pericardium permit these layers to glide freely over one another during contraction and relaxation of the heart. When they become adherent and the potential space between them is obliterated by disease (pericarditis), they may impose considerable restraint upon the action of the heart.

Cardiac Skeleton

The central supporting structure of the heart, to which most of the muscle fibers are attached and with which the valves are connected, is called rather inappropriately the *cardiac skeleton*. It has a complicated form and consists, for the most part, of dense connective tissue. Its main parts are the *septum membranaceum*, the *trigona fibrosa*, and the *annuli fibrosi* encircling the atrioventricular and arterial foramina.

In man the fibrous rings around the atrioventricular foramina contain some fat and elastic fibers but are mainly dense connective tissue. The structure of the septum membranaceum suggests that of an aponeurosis, with its more regular orientation of collagenous bundles in layers. The connective tissue of the trigona fibrosa contains islands of cartilage-like tissue (chondroid) consisting of globular cells resembling chondrocytes. The interstitial substance stains deeply with basic aniline dyes and hematoxylin, and is penetrated by collagenous fibers. In aged persons the tissue of the cardiac skeleton may become calcified in places and sometimes even ossified. In bovine species, bone is normally found in the trigona fibrosa.

Cardiac Valves

Each *atrioventricular valve* consists of a supple sheet of connective tissue, which begins at the annulus fibrosus and is reinforced internally by thin ligamentous strands. It is covered on its atrial and ventricular surfaces by a layer of endocardium. At the free edge of the value these three layers blend (Fig. 12–34).

The ground plate of connective tissue consists largely of dense chondroid tissue, with small spindle-shaped or rounded cells and a basophilic interstitial substance. The endocardial layer is thicker on the atrial side. Here the subendothelial layer has a small amount of chondroid tissue and rests upon a connective tissue layer, which contains many elastic fiber networks and some smooth muscle fi-

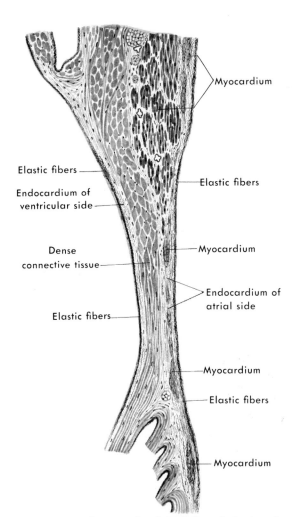

Figure 12–34. Cross section through the mitral valve of man. Atrial surface on right, ventricular on left. In upper left is the attachment of the aortic valve; on left, below, is the passage of chordae tendineae into the valve. Low magnification. (After Sato.)

bers. In the vicinity of the annulus fibrosus, the subendocardial layer is quite loose, and the musculature of the atrium penetrates far into it. On the ventricular side, the endocardial layer has a similar structure but is much thinner. In many places the chordae tendineae, which extend from the edge of the valve to the papillary muscles, enter this layer and mingle with the deeper-lying connective tissue.

The *aortic* and *pulmonic valves* have the same general structure as the atrioventricular valves. In the middle of the valves are plates of chondroid tissue with collagenous and thin elastic fibers. At the root of the valve these all continue into the annulus fibrosus. At the middle of the free edge they form a thickening called the *nodulus Arantii*.

The aortic and pulmonary valves are normally avascular structures. The mitral and tricuspid valve leaves may be penetrated by small vessels, but only to a distance of a few millimeters from their origin.

IMPULSE CONDUCTING SYSTEM

In the adult mammalian heart, the motor impulse arises in the part of the heart that develops from the embryonic sinus venosus, an area in which the superior vena cava enters the right atrium. There is a specialized mechanism by which the contraction spreads to the atria and then to the ventricles.

At the boundary between the right atrium and the superior vena cava, in the region of the sulcus terminalis, is the *sinoatrial node*, 1 cm in length and 3 to 5 mm in width. Although not sharply outlined, it can be seen with the naked eye. It consists of a dense network of interwoven Purkinje fibers. An impulse beginning at the sinoatrial node, which is the pacemaker of the heart, activates the atrial musculature and is conducted to the *atrioventricular node*. A continuous tract of atypical muscle fibers extends down the interventricular septum from this node to both ventricles, sending branches to the papillary muscles and other portions of the myocardium. This system thus serves to initiate and transmit the contractile impulse. The microscopic and submicroscopic structure of this specialized conduction tissue has been described in Chapter 10. The conduction system, even up to the terminal ramifications in the ventricles, is enclosed within a connective tissue layer that separates it from the working musculature of the myocardium.

The atrioventricular node is a flat, white structure about 6 mm long and 2 to 3 mm wide; it is located in the posterior lower part of the interatrial septum below the posterior leaf of the aortic valve. The node consists of Purkinje fibers, which form a tangled dense network whose meshes are filled with connective tissue. These fibers pass into (or between) the usual myocardial fibers, so that the boundary of the node is indistinct. Toward the ventricles the substance of the node converges abruptly into a band about 1 cm long, the *atrioventricular bundle*. It is located in the dense connective tissue of the trigonum fibrosum dextrum and continues into the septum membranaceum, where it divides into two branches.

The first branch, a cylindrical bundle 1 to 2 mm thick, runs downward along the periphery of the membranous septum and is located in part directly under the endocardium of the right ventricle. It proceeds along the interventricular septum and splits into many branches, which spread along the entire internal surface of the right ventricle and into the papillary muscles.

The left branch is a wide, flat band that comes forward under the endocardium of the left ventricle in the upper portion of the interventricular septum, under the anterior edge of the posterior cusps of the aortic valve. It divides into two main branches at the border between the upper and middle thirds of the septum; then it divides, as in the right ventricle, into numerous anastomosing thin threads, which are lost to view in the myocardium.

Blood Vessels, Lymphatics, and Nerves of the Heart

The blood supply to the heart is carried by the *coronary arteries*, usually two in number, which arise from the aorta in the sinuses behind two of the valve cusps. They are distributed to the capillaries of the myocardium. The blood from the capillaries is collected by the cardiac veins, most of which empty by way of the coronary sinus into the right atrium. A few small cardiac veins empty directly into the right atrium.

In the coronary arteries of the human heart, the tunica media, which is limited on both sides by the usual internal and external elastic membranes, is divided by a thick fenestrated membrane into an inner and an outer layer.

The conduction system and, particularly, both of its nodes are abundantly supplied with blood from special branches of the coronary arteries.

Three groups of lymphatic vessels are described in the heart: (1) large lymphatic vessels, which lie in the grooves of the heart together with the blood vessels—these drain to the lymphatic nodes beneath the arch of the aorta and at the bifurcation of the trachea; (2) lymphatic vessels of the epicardial connective tissue; and (3) lymphatic vessels of the myocardium and the endocardium.

In the subepicardial connective tissue, networks of lymphatic capillaries may easily be demonstrated and larger vessels provided with valves. Lymphatic capillaries have also been described in the atrioventricular and semilunar valves, but their presence here in the absence of blood vessels raises some doubts about the validity of these observations.

The lymphatic network in the endocardium can be confused with the finer ramifications of the sinoventricular conduction system, for both structures may be demonstrated by the same injection method. However, the conducting system forms much wider meshes, and its cross connections are thicker than those of the lymphatic network.

The myocardium is penetrated by an abundant lymphatic network, which is everywhere connected with the subendocardial plexus and also communicates with the pericardial lymphatic network.

The numerous nerves of the heart are in part ramifications of the vagus nerve and in part sympathetic nerves. Some nerve endings in the heart apparently are of effector type, while other endings are of receptor or sensory character.

HISTOGENESIS OF THE BLOOD VESSELS

In mammals the first vessels are laid down in the area vasculosa on the surface of the yolk sac, where they develop from the mesenchymal cells. In the embryo proper, the blood vessels and the heart appear later; at first they contain no blood cells. In the spaces between the germ layers, groups of mesenchymal cells flatten around spaces filled with fluid, which are thus surrounded by a thin endothelial wall. In this way, the primordia of the heart and the main blood vessels, such as the aorta and the cardinal and umbilical veins, are laid down. These originally independent primordia then rapidly unite with one another and with the vessels of the area vasculosa, after which the blood circulation is established. The endothelial cells in these first stages are merely mesenchymal cells adapted to the new function of bounding the blood vessel lumen.

After the closed blood vascular system has developed and the circulation has begun, new blood vessels always arise by "budding" from preexisting blood vessels. The new formation of blood vessels by budding may be studied in sections of young embryos or in the living condition in the margin of the tail in larval amphibians, in the mesentery of newborn mammals, or in the thin layer of inflamed tissue that grows between two coverslips introduced under the skin of an animal. A method has been devised for the continued observation of such chambers in the living rabbit for weeks and even months.

In the process of budding, a protrusion appears on the wall of the capillary and is directed into the surrounding tissues. From the beginning it often appears to be a simple, hollow expansion of the endothelial wall but in other cases it is at first a solid accumulation of endothelial cells. This *vascular bud* or sprout enlarges, elongates, and assumes many shapes. Most frequently it appears as a solid strand of cells. It later becomes hollow and thus represents a lateral extension of the blood vessel into which blood cells penetrate.

An endothelial bud may encounter another bud and fuse end on, or it may come into lateral contact with another bud or another capillary. A lumen then forms among the fused endothelial cells and unites the two capillaries. In this way a new mesh is formed in the capillary network, and blood begins to circulate through it. Later, new buds may arise from the newly formed vessels. The developing vascular buds are often accompanied by undifferentiated mesenchymal cells and fibroblasts, deployed parallel to the long axis of the buds.

Arteries and veins of all types are always formed first as capillaries. The primary endothelial tube then expands and thickens as new elements are added to the outside of the wall. These elements originate from the surrounding mesenchyme in the embryo and play an important part in the formation of new arteries and veins from capillaries, as well as in the formation of large vessels from smaller ones during the development of pathways for "collateral circulation" of the blood. The mesenchymal cells outside the endothelium become smooth muscle cells. Soon more layers of smooth muscle join the first layer; these arise in part by the addition of new mesenchymal cells and in part by division of smooth muscle cells.

The factors that cause the larger arteries and veins to develop in more or less constant patterns in particular places and in definite directions are not completely understood. It is probable that in the earliest embryonic stages the formation of the major vessels is genetically determined, while in the later stages the pattern and growth of the blood vessels are determined by local hemodynamic factors.

LYMPHATIC VESSELS

In most tissues and organs, with the exception of the central nervous system, cartilage, bone and bone marrow, thymus, teeth, and placenta, the blood capillaries are paralleled by a plexus of *lymph capillaries.* The blood vessels form a closed "circulatory system" with a central pump (the heart), an outflow tract (arteries), and a return system (veins). The lymph vascular system, on the other hand, is a "drainage system" whose smallest vessels, the lymphatic capillaries, end blindly and conduct a clear fluid, called *lymph,* from the extracellular spaces in the periphery back through successively larger *lymphatic vessels* that ultimately converge upon *lymphatic ducts* (thoracic duct and right lymphatic duct), which are confluent with the great veins at the base of the neck. Along the course of the lymphatic vessels are encapsulated accumulations of lymphoid tissue comprising small organs called *lymph nodes* (see Chapter 15). The lymph stream entering the node via *afferent lymphatic vessels* breaks up within it, percolating through a labyrinthine system of minute channels lined with endothelium and phagocytic cells. Lymph then emerges from the node through *efferent lymphatic vessels.* The lymph, exposed to an enormous number of phagocytes, is cleared of foreign matter as it filters through the lymph nodes. Many lymphocytes that enter the lymph nodes from the blood are added to the efferent lymph and are thus carried back to the bloodstream.

Lymph is essentially an ultrafiltrate of the blood plasma formed by continual seepage of fluid constituents of the blood across the capillary walls into the surrounding interstitial spaces. It contains water, electrolytes, and variable amounts of protein (2 to 5 per cent) depending upon the site and conditions of its formation. The walls of blood capillaries are normally freely permeable to water and small molecules. They are less permeable to plasma proteins, which therefore tend to maintain a significant colloid osmotic pressure in the blood. At the arterial end of blood capillaries (where the hydrostatic pressure exceeds the colloid osmotic pressure of the blood), water, solutes, and some plasma proteins move across the wall into the tissue. At the venous end, the hydrostatic pressure is lower and the colloid osmotic pressure tends to draw water, electrolytes, and products of tissue catabolism back into the blood. However, some of the fluid and much of the plasma protein that have left the blood do not return directly but are drained off in the lymph and returned to the blood via the lymph vascular system. A delicate balance is thus maintained, which keeps the volume of extracellular fluid reasonably constant and conserves the small amount of plasma protein that continually escapes through the walls of the blood capillaries.

It follows from this mechanism of lymph formation that the flow of lymph will be increased by (1) an increase in blood capillary permeability, (2) an increase in hydrostatic pressure, or (3) a decrease in colloid osmotic pressure of the blood plasma. Any of these will increase the transudation of fluid. If fluid accumulates in the tissues in excess of the capacity of lymphatic vessels to drain it away, the resulting swelling of the tissues is referred to as *edema*. Thus, increased resistance to venous return in congestive heart failure may raise pressure in the blood capillaries, resulting in edema of the ankles. Similarly, obstruction to the lymphatic vessels of an extremity owing to parasitic disease or radical surgery may result in persistent edema.

The principal function of the lymph vascular system is to return to the blood the fluid and plasma protein that escape from the circulation; to return to the blood the lymphocytes of the recirculating pool; and to add to the blood immune globulins (antibodies) that are formed in lymph nodes. We are concerned here only with the structure of the vessels; the organization of the associated lymphoid tissue will be discussed in Chapter 15.

Lymphatic Capillaries

The thin-walled, endothelium-lined lymphatic capillaries differ from blood capillaries in several respects. They branch and anastomose freely, and although they are generally cylindrical, they are far more variable in shape and caliber than are their counterparts in the blood vascular system (Figs. 12–35, 12–36). Except in the perinuclear region, the endothelium usually is extremely thin. In electron micrographs, microvilli projecting into the lumen are not uncommon. The thin edges of adjacent endothelial cells often overlap for some distance. There is a distinct intercellular cleft throughout most of this region of overlap, but one or two punctate areas of closer apposition and adherence are usually seen along the boundary. There are no pericytes associated with lymphatic capillaries, and a continuous basal lamina is usually lacking (Fig. 12–37). Extracellular bundles of filaments (5 to 10 nm) have been described, terminating on the abluminal plasma membrane of the endothelium and extending outward into the ground substance and between the collagen bundles of the surrounding connective tissue. These have been called *lymphatic anchoring filaments*, and it is suggested that they have a mechanical role in maintaining the patency of the vessels. The filaments appear to insert in the outer leaflet of the membrane or to terminate in patches of amorphous material on the outer surface of the plasmalemma. These patches bear a superficial resemblance to the material composing the continuous basal lamina of endothelium in blood capillaries. The chemical nature of the anchoring filaments has not been established, but they very closely resemble the filaments associated with elastic fibers and may possibly be identical to them.

The terminal elements of the lymphatic system are quite variable in their form from one organ to another. In the skin and mucous membranes, a plexus of tubular lymphatic capillaries generally occurs parallel to the network of blood capillaries but tends to be more deeply situated. In the lamina propria of the intestine, a single vessel or a simple network of lymphatic capillaries extends from the submucous plexus into the core of each villus and ends blindly near its tip. In the lining of the oviduct, the terminal lymphatics are not tubular but are narrow, flattened sinusoids extending for considerable

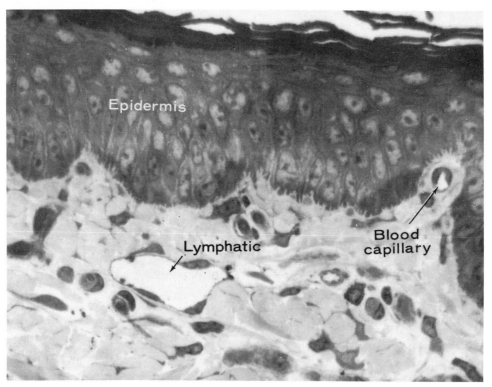

Figure 12–35. Photomicrograph of guinea pig skin, illustrating a typical lymphatic capillary in the dermis. (Photograph courtesy of L. V. Leak.)

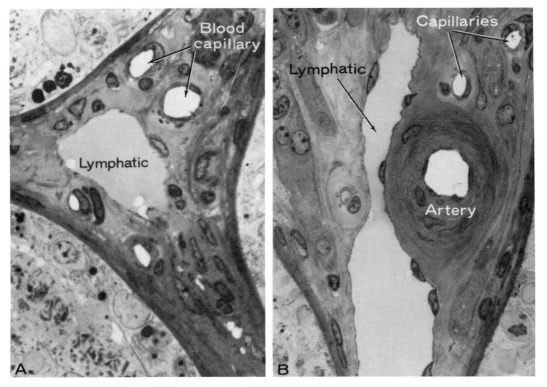

Figure 12–36. *A,* Photomicrograph of a lymphatic in the interstitial tissue of a ram testis. *B,* Lymphatic in interstitium of a bull testis. Both these preparations have been fixed by vascular perfusion. The blood capillaries are therefore empty, whereas the lymphatics have a light gray content, representing precipitated protein of the lymph. (From Fawcett, D. W., W. B. Neaves, and M. N. Flores. Biol. Reprod. *9:*500, 1973.)

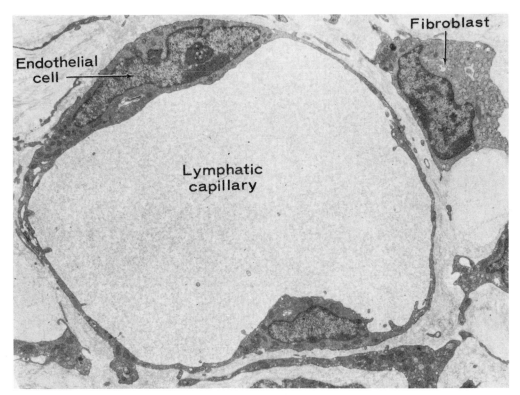

Figure 12–37. Electron micrograph of a subcutaneous lymphatic capillary from guinea pig in cross section. Notice the irregular outline, the thin wall, and the slight variations in thickness of the endothelium. The absence of a basal lamina cannot be verified at this magnification. (Micrograph courtesy of L. V. Leak.)

distances along the axis of each fold of mucous membrane. In the testis of some rodents, the lymphatics form labyrinthine peritubular sinusoids that have no consistent geometry, but conform to the shapes of the intertubular spaces that they occupy and to the contours of the blood vessels and perivascular clusters of Leydig cells that they surround. In man and other large species, the testicular lymphatics are not sinusoidal but occur as one or two tubular vessels in each interstitial space. These are usually much larger than the blood capillaries (Fig. 12–36).

Larger Lymphatic Vessels

These vessels are easily distinguished from blood vessels by the large size of their lumens in relation to the thickness of their walls. The wall is somewhat thicker than that of lymphatic capillaries and is invested by thin collagenous bundles, elastic fibers, and occasional smooth muscle cells. In lymphatics with a diameter greater than 0.2 mm, three layers of wall are recognizable corresponding to intima, media, and adventitia of blood vessels. The boundaries between the layers are often indistinct, so that the division is somewhat artificial. The intima consists of endothelium and a thin layer of interlacing longitudinal elastic fibers. The media is a layer or two of smooth muscle cells, while the adventitia is composed of elastic fibers and collagenous bundles continuous with those of the surrounding connective tissue.

Valves are a conspicuous feature of lymphatics. They occur in pairs with the two members on opposite sides of the vessel and their free edges pointing in the direction of lymph flow. As in veins, the valves are folds of the tunica intima and therefore consist of back-to-back layers of endothelium supported near their base by a thin intervening layer of connective tissue. They occur at much closer intervals along the length of the lymphatic vessel than do the valves of veins. Immediately distal to a valve, the lymphatic is often slightly expanded. The periodic fusiform expansions at the sites of valves give the lymphatic vessels a highly characteristic appearance.

The walls of lymphatic vessels are innervated and there is cinematographic evidence that, in some small mammals, rhythmic contraction of smooth muscle cells in the vessel wall helps to move the lymph along. This does not appear to be true of lymphatics in man and other larger species. Lacking a muscular pump to propel fluid through the system, the flow of lymph in these species is very dependent upon the contraction of skeletal muscles and movements of neighboring structures, which exert pressure on the thin wall of lymphatics, expressing lymph from segments of the vessel, while the presence of valves ensures its unidirectional movement. Thus, when an extremity is immobilized, as in an anesthetized animal, there is little or no lymph flow from it, but if passive movements of the extremity are initiated, a slow steady flow of lymph is reestablished comparable with that in the active unanesthetized animal.

Lymphatic Ducts

The lymphatics form progressively larger vessels by their confluence and these latter finally converge to form two main trunks: (1) the *right lymphatic duct,* which is relatively short and carries lymph drainage from the right upper portion of the body—it opens into the right brachiocephalic vein at the junction of the internal jugular and subclavian veins; and (2) the *thoracic duct,* which arises in the abdomen and courses upward along the anterior aspect of the vertebral column through the thorax and into the base of the neck, where it opens into the venous system at the junction of the left jugular and subclavian veins.

The wall of the lymphatic ducts differs from that of the great veins in the greater development of the muscles in the tunica media and by a less distinct division into three layers. The tunica intima consists of the endothelial lining and several thin layers of collagenous and elastic fibers; the latter condense into a layer similar to an internal elastic membrane near the junction with the tunica media. The smooth muscle bundles in the tunica media are penetrated by elastic fibers continuous with the elastica interna. The tunica adventitia is composed of longitudinal smooth muscle bundles, and gradually merges into the surrounding loose connective tissue. The wall of the thoracic duct is provided with small blood vessels that extend into the outer layer of the tunica media. These vessels are similar to the vasa vasorum of the larger blood vessels.

REFERENCES

BLOOD VESSELS IN GENERAL

Benninghoff, A.: *In* von Mollendorf, W., ed.: Handbuch der Mikroskopischen Anatomie des Menschen. Vol. 6, part 1. Blutgefässe und Herz. Berlin, Springer Verlag, 1939.

Brightman, M. W., and T. S. Reese: Junctions between intimately apposed cell membranes in the vertebrate brain. J. Cell. Biol., *40*:648, 1969.

Burton, A. D.: Relation of structure to function of the tissues of the wall of blood vessels. Physiol. Rev. *34*:619, 1954.

Majno, G., and I. Joris: Endothelium 1977: a review. *In* Chandler, A. B., et al., eds.: The Thrombotic Process in Atherogenesis. New York, Plenum Press, 1978.

Rhodin, J. A. G.: Fine structure of the vascular wall in mammals. Physiol. Rev. *42* (Suppl. 5):48, 1962.

Ryan, U. S., J. W. Ryan, C. Whitaker, and A. Chin: Localization of angiotensin converting enzyme (kininase II). Immunocytochemistry and immunofluorescence. Tissue Cell *8*:125, 1976.

Somlyo, A. P., and A. V. Somlyo: Vascular smooth muscle. 1. Normal structure, physiology, biochemistry and biophysics. Pharmacol. Rev. *20*:197, 1968.

Zeldis, S. M., Y. Nemerson, F. A. Pitlick, and T. L. Lenz: Tissue factor (thromboplastin). Localization to plasma membranes by peroxidase conjugated antibodies. Science *175*:755, 1972.

ARTERIES AND ARTERIOLES

Hüttner, T., M. Boutet, and R. H. Moore: Studies on protein passage through arterial endothelium. I. Structural correlates of permeability in rat arterial endothelium. Lab. Invest. *28*:272, 1973.

Movat, H. Z., and N. V. P. Fernando: The fine structure of the terminal vascular bed. 1. Small arteries with an internal elastic lamina. Exp. Mol. Pathol. *2*:549, 1963.

Phelps, P. C., and J. H. Luft: Electron microscopic study of relaxation and constriction in frog arterioles. Am. J. Anat. *125*:399, 1969.

Rhodin, J. A. G.: The ultrastructure of mammalian arterioles and precapillary sphincters. J. Ultrastruct. Res. *18*:181, 1967.

Ross, R., and J. A. Glomset: The pathogenesis of atherosclerosis. Parts I and II. N. Engl. J. Med. *295*:369, 420, 1976.

Schwartz, S. M., and E. P. Benditt: Studies on the aortic intima. 1. Structure and permeability of rat thoracic aorta intima. Am. J. Pathol. *66*:241, 1972.

Simionescu, M., N. Simionescu, and G. E. Palade: Segmental differentiations of cell junctions in the vascular endothelium. Arteries and veins. J. Cell Biol. *68*:705, 1976.

Weibel, E. R., and G. E. Palade: New cytoplasmic components in arterial endothelia. J. Cell Biol. *23*:101, 1964.

CAROTID BODY

Adams, W. E.: The Comparative Morphology of the Carotid Body and Carotid Sinus. Springfield, IL, Charles C Thomas, 1958.

Biscoe, T. J.: Carotid body. Structure and function. Physiol. Rev. *51*:437, 1971.

Boyd, J. D.: The development of the human carotid body. Carnegie Contrib. Embryol. *152*:1, 1939.

Chen, I-Li, and R. Yates: Electron microscopic radioautographic studies of the carotid body following injections of labeled biogenic amine procursors. J. Cell Biol. *42*:794, 1969.

deCastro, F.: Sur la structure et l'innervation du sinus carotidien de l'homme et des mammifères. Trav. Lab. Recherches. Biol. Univ. Madrid *25*:331, 1927.

Duncan, D., and R. Yates: Ultrastructure of the carotid body of the cat as revealed by various fixatives and the use of reserpine. Anat. Rec. *157*:667, 1967.

McDonald, C. M., and R. A. Mitchell: The innervation of glomus cells, ganglion cells and blood vessels in the rat carotid body: a quantitative structural analysis. J. Neurocytol. *4*:177, 1975.

Ross, L. L.: Electron microscopic observations of the carotid body of the cat. J. Biophys. Biochem. Cytol. *6*:253, 1959.

Yates, R. D., I-Li Chen, and D. Duncan: Effects of sinus nerve stimulation on carotid body glomus cells. J. Cell Biol. *46*:544, 1970.

ARTERIOVENOUS ANASTOMOSES

Bryden, M. M., and G. S. Molyneux: Arteriovenous anastomoses in the skin of seals. II. The California sea lion, *Zalophus californianus*, and the northern fur seal, *Callorhinus ursinus.* Anat. Rec. *191*:253, 1978.

Cauna, N.: The fine structure of the arteriovenous anastomosis and its nerve supply in the human nasal respiratory mucosa. Anat. Rec. *168*:9, 1970.

Hales, J. R., A. A. Fawcett, J. W. Bennett, and A. D. Needham: Thermal control of blood flow through capillaries and arteriovenous anastomoses in skin of sheep. Pflügers Arch. *378*:55, 1978.

Molyneux, G. S., and M. M. Bryden: Comparative aspects of arteriovenous anastomoses. *In* Harrison, R. J., ed.: Progress in Anatomy. Vol. 1. Cambridge University Press, 1981.

CAPILLARIES

Bennett, H. S., J. H. Luft, and J. C. Hampton: Morphological classification of vertebrate capillaries. Am. J. Physiol. *196*:381, 1959.

Brightman, M. W.: Morphology of the blood-brain interfaces. Eye Res. (Suppl), 1977.

Bruno, R. R., and G. E. Palade: Studies on blood capillaries. I. General organization of muscle capillaries. J. Cell Biol. *37*:244, 1968.

Florey, H.: Exchange of substances between the blood and tissues. Nature *192*:908, 1961.

Jennings, M. A., U. T. Marchesi, and H. Florey: The transport of particles across the walls of small blood vessels. Proc. R. Soc. Lond. [Biol.] *156*:14, 1962.

Karnovsky, M. G.: Morphology of capillaries with special reference to muscle capillaries. *In* Crone, C., and N. A. Lassen, eds.: Capillary Permeability. New York, Academic Press, 1970.

Maul, G. G.: Structure and formation of pores in fenestrated capillaries. J. Ultrastruct. Res. *36*:768, 1971.

Revel, J. P., and E. Raviola: Evidence for a blood-thymus barrier using electron opaque tracers. J. Exp. Med. *136*:466, 1972.

Palade, G. E.: Transport in quanta across the endothelium of blood capillaries. Anat. Rec. *136*:254, 1960.

Palade, G. E., M. Simionescu, and N. Simionescu: Structural aspects of the permeability of the microvascular endothelium. Acta Physiol. Scand. (Suppl.) *463*:11, 1979.

BLOOD-BRAIN, BLOOD-OCULAR, BLOOD-THYMUS BARRIERS

Brightman, M. W.: Morphology of blood-brain interfaces. Exp. Eye Res. 25(Suppl) 1, 1977.

Brightman, M. W., I. Klatzo, Y. Olsson, and T. Reese: The blood-brain barrier to proteins under normal and pathological conditions. J. Neurol. Sci. *10*:215, 1970.

Crerr, H. F.: Physiology of the charoid plexus. Physiol. Rev. *51*:273, 1971.

Dobbing, J.: The blood-brain barrier. Physiol. Rev. *41*:130, 1961.

Pappenheimer, J. R.: Passage of molecules through capillary walls. Physiol. Rev. *33*:387, 1953.

Rapoport, S. I.: Blood-brain barrier in physiology and medicine. New York, Raven Press, 1976.

Raviola, E., and M. J. Karnovsky: Evidence for a blood-thymus barrier using electron opaque tracers. J. Exp. Med. *136*:466, 1972.

Raviola, G.: Effects of paracentesis on the blood-aqueous barrier: an electron microscopy study on *Macaca mulatta* using horseradish peroxidase as a tracer. Invest. Ophthalmol. *13*:826, 1974.

Reese, T. G., and M. J. Karnovsky: Fine structural localization of a blood-brain barrier for exogenous peroxidase. J. Cell Biol. *34*:207, 1967.

Simionescu, N., and M. Simionescu: The hydrophilic pathway of capillary endothelium, a dynamic system. *In* Transport Across Epithelia. Copenhagen, Munksgaard, 1980.

Wissig, S. L., and M. C. Williams: Permeability of muscle capillaries to microperoxidase. J. Cell Biol. *76*:341, 1978.

VENULES AND VEINS

Majno, G., G. E. Palade, and G. Schoeffl: Studies on inflammation. II. The site of action of histamine and serotonin along the vascular tree. A topographical study. J. Biophys. Biochem. Cytol. *11*:607, 1961.

Movat, H. Z., and N. V. P. Pernando: The fine structure of the terminal vascular bed. IV. Venules and their perivascular cells. Exp. Mol. Pathol. *3*:98, 1964.

Rhodin, J. A. G.: Ultrastructure of mammalian venous capillaries, venules and small collecting venules. J. Ultrastruct. Res. *25*:452, 1968.

Simionescu, N., M. Simionescu, and G. E. Palade: Open junctions in the endothelium of post-capillary venules of the diaphragm. J. Cell Biol. *79*:27, 1978.

LYMPHATIC VESSELS

Drinker, C. K., and J. M. Yoffey: Lymphatics, Lymph and Lymphoid Tissue. Cambridge, MA, Harvard University Press, 1941.

Leak, L. V.: Normal anatomy of the lymphatic vascular system. *In* Meessen, H., ed.: Handbuch der Allgemeine Pathologie. Berlin, Springer-Verlag, 1972.

Leak, L. V.: Electron microscopic observations on lymphatic capillaries and structural components of the connective tissue-lymph interface. Microvasc. Res. *2*:361, 1970.

Rouvière, H.: Anatomie des Lymphatiques de l'Homme. Paris, Masson, 1932.

13

THE IMMUNE SYSTEM

Elio Raviola

Organisms of different species and the various individuals belonging to the same species, with the exception of genetically identical twins, possess a unique chemical identity, because the macromolecular constituents of their cells and body fluids have a different composition. The *immune system* protects the individual from exogenous macromolecules, either introduced as such into the body or deployed at the surface of invading viruses, microorganisms, or cells; furthermore, it exerts a surveillance function on the appearance in the body of endogenous, abnormal constituents. The immune system encompasses the lymphoid organs (thymus, lymph nodes, spleen, and tonsils); all the aggregates of lymphoid tissue occurring in nonlymphoid organs; the lymphocytes of the blood and lymph; and the whole population of lymphocytes and plasma cells dispersed throughout the connective and epithelial tissues of the body. The various components of the immune system are kept in communication by a continuous traffic of lymphocytes, like a mobile army continuously patrolling the body. The cells of the immune system can be thought of as having "academies," the thymus and the bursa analogue in which they are trained; their "battlefields" are the peripheral lymphoid organs and the connective tissues of the body; their "lines of communication" are the blood and lymph. They dispose of the "invaders" either by attacking them directly or through highly selective weapons, the antibodies, and they are assisted by "mercenary troops" of macrophages.

The science of immunology has developed a rather complex and specialized terminology; therefore, we must present at the outset some concepts and definitions that will be needed to understand the organization and functioning of the immune system.

Lymphocytes have the ability to recognize macromolecules on viruses, on bacteria, or on the surfaces of other cells that have chemical patterns different from the normal constituents of the individual they inhabit, and are able to set up against them a specific defensive reaction, the *immune response*. *Antigen* is the term used to define any material that bears a surface configuration *(antigenic determinant)* capable of eliciting an immune response upon entry into the internal environment of the body. The *clonal selection theory* holds that during ontogeny of the immune system, and possibly throughout life, lymphocytes arise continuously, each genetically programmed to respond to a single antigen. Thus, the versatility of the immune system in disposing of myriad endogenous or exogenous materials is innate and resides in a population of lymphocytes, all of which are identical from a morphological point of view, but each endowed with the capacity to react to a different antigen. This multiplicity of antigen specificities is generated during lymphocyte development and results from recombination of coding sequences dispersed on the lymphocyte's DNA. Upon first meeting with the appropriate antigen *(primary response)*, the lymphocyte is *stimulated* and undergoes a series of morphological and biochemical changes *(transformation)* that result in *proliferation* and *differentiation*. Proliferation leads to amplification of the population of relevant cells: this is called *clonal expansion*. Differentiation results in the appearance of both *effector cells* and *memory cells*. Effector cells *(activated lymphocytes* and *plasma cells)* are instrumental in causing antigen disposal. Memory lymphocytes revert to the inactive state, but are then capable of setting up an immune response with greater efficiency upon encountering their specific antigen again *(secondary response)*.

As lymphocytes displaying variable degrees of affinity for a given antigen may preexist in the individual, this antigen will represent

THE IMMUNE SYSTEM · 407

a better stimulus for those cells that have greater avidity for its surface determinants. Antigen, therefore, exerts a selective pressure upon lymphocyte proliferation, thus simulating on a microscopic scale "natural selection" by which the environment favors the multiplication of genetically fit individuals.

Contact with antigen, however, is not necessarily followed by lymphocyte stimulation and consequent immunization. In special circumstances, the body may become *tolerant* to the foreign material. The dose of the antigen, its degree of foreignness, and the mode of its presentation (in solution, for example, rather than at the surface of another cell) are among the factors that may result in tolerance rather than stimulation. The importance of this phenomenon is considerable, because self-tolerance rather than innate unresponsiveness is the basis for lymphocytes' inability to attack constituents of the body of which they are a part.

Antigen disposal is based on two different mechanisms: (1) in the *humoral* immunological responses, such as those evoked by most bacterial antigens, lymphocytes and plasma cells synthesize and release proteins called *antibodies,* which specifically combine with the antigen; (2) in the so-called *cellular* or *cell-mediated* immunological responses, such as those triggered by transplantation of foreign tissues, application of a chemical sensitizing agent to the skin (delayed hypersensitivity), many viral diseases, and infection with facultative intracellular bacteria (such as *Mycobacterium tuberculosis),* clones of lymphocytes arise that either release small molecules with a variety of pharmacological actions on macrophages, granulocytes, or other lymphocytes *(lymphokines)* or attack directly the foreign cells *(cytolytic lymphocytes).*

Upon binding to the antigen, antibodies may neutralize its harmful effects (if the antigen is a toxin); inhibit its entry into the cells of the body (if the antigen is a virus); enhance the uptake and destruction of bacteria by phagocytic cells such as neutrophils or macrophages (a process called *opsonization);* or induce lysis of bacteria or cells by activating *complement,* a system of proteins that are normally present in the plasma and are necessary for lysis of foreign cells in immunological defenses. Antigen-antibody reactions may also have a detrimental effect upon the host by causing either a severe inflammatory response *(Arthus reaction)* or *an-aphylaxis.* This latter is the result of release of pharmacologically active substances by tissue cells that have bound antigen-antibody complexes, the most typical example being the release of histamine by mast cells.

Antibodies are proteins found in the globulin fraction of the plasma. They are also called *immunoglobulins* and are subdivided into several classes. The immunoglobulins G (IgG) represent the bulk of the immunoglobulins of the normal human blood, and their structure is known in great detail. The IgG molecule has a weight of about 150,000 daltons. It consists of about 1400 amino acid residues and contains 2 to 3% carbohydrate. It comprises four polypeptide chains, paired in such a way that the molecule has identical halves, each consisting of one long or heavy chain (H chain) and one short or light chain (L chain). The four chains are held together by disulfide bonds and noncovalent interactions. In the free IgG molecule, the subunits are folded into a roughly cylindrical unit, about 3.5×20 nm in dimensions, but the molecule displays a considerable degree of plasticity, and upon combination with antigen it may acquire a characteristic Y or T shape. Papain splits the antibody molecule into three parts: one, the Fc fragment containing two half H chains, is crystallizable, and does not combine with the antigen. It enables the antibody molecule to bind to complement and to the surface of cells that carry appropriate membrane receptors. Each of the other two parts, the Fab fragments, contains a combining site for antigen and consists of the whole L chain and the remaining portion of the H chain; both chains contribute to the combining site for the antigen. Therefore, the IgG molecule as a whole is bivalent (i.e., it is capable of combining with two entities), and this property permits formation of polymeric aggregates of antigen and antibody, which facilitate the attachment of complement and the uptake of the complex by phagocytes. The IgG antibodies have high affinity for the antigenic determinant; thus, they are very effective in neutralizing bacterial toxins or in protecting the body against virus infections; they exchange readily between blood and extravascular space. However, they are produced late during the primary immune response and are rather ineffective in activating complement.

The immunoglobulins M (IgM) are large, complex molecules with a weight of about 900,000 daltons and a 10 per cent content of carbohydrate. They consist of 20 polypeptide chains, joined by disulfide bonds. They represent a pentamer of subunits, each resembling IgG in its general organization, but they contain an additional polypeptide chain, called J or joining chain. The IgM molecules are not as specific as IgG for the antigenic determinant and therefore are not very effective in neutralizing the harmful effects of toxic antigens. However, even a single IgM molecule is capable of activating complement; thus, IgM readily induces lysis of foreign cells. Furthermore, it is much more effective in antigen agglutination and opsonization.

The immunoglobulins A (IgA), when present in the plasma, are 170,000 daltons in molecular weight and, like IgG, consist of four polypeptide chains, but they may be linked to each other in a polymeric form. IgA is also contained in a variety of secretory products, such as colostrum, saliva, tears, and nasal and tracheobronchial mucus, and it is released into the intestinal lumen. The secretory form of IgA has a molecular weight of 390,000 daltons because two antibody molecules become united to each other by a J chain, and the resulting complex is bound to a glycoprotein with a high carbohydrate content, called the *secretory piece*, which is produced by the epithelial cells. Secretory IgA is very resistant to proteolytic enzymes; therefore, it has been speculated that the secretory piece confers stability on the immunoglobulin molecule and prevents its catabolism in the intestinal lumen. IgA probably plays a protective role at the surface of mucous membranes.

Two additional types of immunoglobulins have been described: the IgE, which induce release of histamine by mast cells and are responsible for certain allergic reactions, and the IgD, glycoproteins with a molecular weight of 170,000 to 200,000 daltons, whose concentration in the serum varies greatly in different individuals. The biological function of this serum IgD is poorly understood. However, IgD, together with monomeric IgM, is present as an integral component of the plasma membrane of one class of lymphocytes (B lymphocytes), where they function as antigen receptors. In contrast, the number of lymphocytes bearing surface IgG is very small.

Although a cellular immune response and secretion of antibody may both occur upon introduction of a single antigen, they represent the activity of two morphologically similar, but functionally distinct, classes of lymphocytes, commonly referred to as *thymus-dependent* or *T lymphocytes* and *bursa-dependent* or *B lymphocytes*. T lymphocytes have been preconditioned under the influence of the thymus to respond to antigen by differentiating into lymphokine-secreting and cytolytic lymphocytes; B lymphocytes, on the other hand, have acquired the ability to respond to antigen by differentiation into antibody-secreting lymphocytes and plasma cells. In birds, the site of production or preconditioning of B lymphocytes is the *bursa of Fabricius*, an appendix-like diverticulum of the cloaca.

Both T and B lymphocytes manifest immunological specificity; that is, both are genetically programmed to respond to a specific antigen and both carry "memory." The functions of T and B lymphocytes are not independent of each other, however, but are intimately interrelated. Only certain antigens directly stimulate B cells and lead to antibody secretion without participation of T cells. With most antigens that elicit a humoral response, T lymphocytes cooperate with B cells, helping them to become stimulated and regulating their differentiation (*"helper" T lymphocytes*). Furthermore, another class of T lymphocytes (*"suppressor" T lymphocytes*) specifically suppresses antibody responses by exerting an inhibitory feedback control on helper T lymphocytes or acting on antibody-secreting B lymphocytes. There is finally a third category of lymphocytes, which have different functional properties from both T and B lymphocytes; they have been denominated *null lymphocytes*. Their precise significance, however, is still under discussion. Although lymphocytes are the only cells that confer specificity on the immunological response, they are assisted by macrophages in the process of antigen recognition. Phagocytic cells are also involved in antigen disposal, and eosinophils seem to destroy the complexes of antibody with soluble antigens.

Lymphocytes originate from stem cell precursors which, in the embryo, arise from the mesenchyme intervening between the endoderm of the yolk sac and the splanchnopleuric mesoderm. During postnatal life, the source of the stem cells becomes the bone marrow. The differentiation of the stem cells into T lymphocytes takes place in the thymus, a *central* or *primary lymphoid organ*, made up of a special variety of *lymphoid tissue*. In birds, the differentiation of stem cells into B lymphocytes occurs in the bursa of Fabricius; in mammals, where the analogue of the bursa has not been identified, differentiation of B lymphocytes takes place in the embryonal liver and in the bone marrow. In both the thymus and the avian bursa (or its mammalian equivalent), the stem cell precursors undergo *antigen-independent* proliferation and differentiation into lymphocytes that are genetically programmed to set up a specific type of immune response upon meeting their appropriate antigen. They subsequently populate the blood and lymph, are disseminated throughout the connective tissues of the body, and infiltrate most epithelia. Together with macrophages and with plasma cells, which arise from differentiation of B lymphocytes, they become associated with reticular cells and reticular fibers, thus giving rise to a second variety of lymphoid tissue, which represents the bulk of the *peripheral* or *secondary lymphoid organs* such as the lymph nodes, spleen, and tonsils. In the secondary lymphoid organs, T and B lymphocytes undergo *antigen-dependent* proliferation and differentiation into effector and "memory" cells.

CELLS OF THE IMMUNE SYSTEM

CYTOLOGY OF THE CELLS OF THE IMMUNE SYSTEM

Lymphocytes

This cell type has already been considered as a component of the blood (Chapter 4) and connective tissue (Chapter 5), but the foregoing descriptions need review and amplification in the context of the immune system. The term "lymphocyte" actually refers to a family of cells characterized by lack of specific granules; a round, centrally located nucleus; and a cytoplasm displaying various degrees of basophilia, due to the presence of free ribosomes (Figs. 13–1 to 13–4). As previously stated, although they are morphologically similar, lymphocytes are physiologically heterogeneous; not only does this cell type include two major classes of cells, the T and B lymphocytes, but also within these two classes, individual lymphocytes have the ability to recognize different antigens and may vary in

their functional performance, life span, degree of differentiation, and sensitivity to ionizing radiations and hormones. Lymphocytes circulate with blood and lymph and infiltrate connective tissues and epithelia; they are present in the bone marrow and compose the bulk of the thymus, lymph nodes, white pulp of the spleen, and lymphoid masses associated with the digestive, respiratory, and urinary passages.

When suspended in a fluid medium, nonmotile lymphocytes are round. When crowded together in tissues, they mutually deform one another into polyhedral shapes. Motile lymphocytes display a slow, ameboid progression and conform to the shape of the interstices through which they are advancing. When moving on a solid, flat substrate, they acquire a characteristic hand-mirror shape, with the nucleus ahead, followed by a tail of cytoplasm in which most organelles are concentrated.

The size of the lymphocytes varies in different organs and in various functional situations. Lymphocytes circulating in the blood have a diameter of 4 to 8 μm but upon flattening, as when they are smeared and dried on a slide, this increases to 7 to 10 μm (Fig. 13–1A). In lymphoid organs and tissues not involved in an acute immunological response, lymphocytes range between 4 and 15 μm in diameter, the larger forms being rather uncommon. It is customary to subdivide them into small (4 to 7 μm), medium-sized (7 to 11 μm), and large lymphocytes (11 to 15 μm) on the basis of cell size, nuclear morphology, and intensity of the cytoplasmic basophilia (Fig. 13–2); such a subdivision is useful for descriptive purposes, but is rather arbitrary, because lymphocyte diameter and organization vary in a continuous fashion. According to this classification, blood lymphocytes are represented exclusively by small and medium-sized cells; lymphocytes of the lymph include a variable proportion of large cells, whereas lymphoid organs and tissues contain the whole spectrum of cell dimensions. As a consequence of stimulation by antigen, mononuclear cells arise that are up to 30 μm in diameter (Figs. 13–1C, F). These were variously termed *blast cells, immunoblasts, large pyroninophilic cells, hemocytoblasts,* and *lymphoblasts.* There is now good evidence that these large elements result from transformation of small lymphocytes and that they may in turn generate small lymphocytes. Therefore, these cells will be referred to as lymphoblasts.

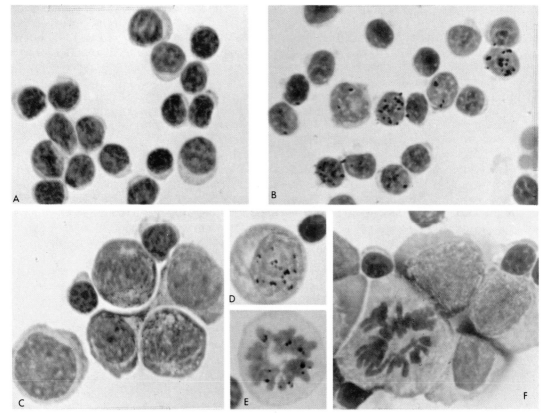

Figure 13–1. *A,* Smear preparation of small lymphocytes from the thoracic duct lymph of the rat stained with the May-Grünwald and Giemsa mixtures. *B,* Autoradiograph of rat thoracic duct lymphocytes obtained 2 weeks after ³H-thymidine administration. Only long-lived small lymphocytes are labeled. *C* and *F,* When the lymphocytes from the rat thoracic duct lymph are cultured 3 days on a monolayer of mouse embryo cells, the contact with the foreign cells stimulates a proportion of the small lymphocytes to transform into lymphoblasts and large lymphocytes. Transformation is followed by proliferation, as shown by the dividing cell in *F. D* and *E,* Autoradiograph of the transformed lymphocytes that arose from the labeled long-lived small lymphocytes of the rat after 2 days' culture on monolayer of mouse embryo cells. Note that the grain count is essentially the same as that of the labeled small lymphocytes in *B*; this shows that transformation by antigen precedes cell division. (Courtesy of N. B. Everett.)

Small lymphocytes have a dense nucleus surrounded by a thin rim of cytoplasm (Fig. 13–3). The nucleus is central, round, or slightly indented and very rich in randomly dispersed, heterochromatic masses; the nucleolus is small and scarcely identifiable in smear preparations. The cytoplasm is slightly basophilic and contains a variable number of azurophilic granules when stained with the Giemsa mixture. The electron microscope shows a diplosome located at the nuclear indentation, surrounded by a small Golgi apparatus and by a few mitochondria. Free ribosomes in moderate numbers are scattered as single units throughout the cytoplasm; cisternae of the granular endoplasmic reticulum are found only exceptionally. Small numbers of lysosomes, which represent the ultrastructural counterpart of the azurophilic granules, complete the list of cytoplasmic organelles. An occasional small lipid droplet may also be observed.

Medium-sized lymphocytes have a nucleus with a larger nucleolus and more abundant euchromatin; the cytoplasm displays more basophilia, due to a greater abundance of free ribosomes. In large lymphocytes and lymphoblasts, the nucleus is largely euchromatic and contains one or two prominent nucleoli (Fig. 13–4). The cytoplasm is abundant and intensely basophilic, owing to the presence of large numbers of free polyribosomes. Cisternae of the granular endoplasmic reticulum are, however, scarce. The Golgi apparatus is moderately enlarged and mitochondria and lysosomes are slightly increased in number.

Plasma Cells (Plasmacytes)

The term "plasma cell" includes a range of immature and mature elements, characterized by the presence of considerable but varying numbers of cisternae of the granular

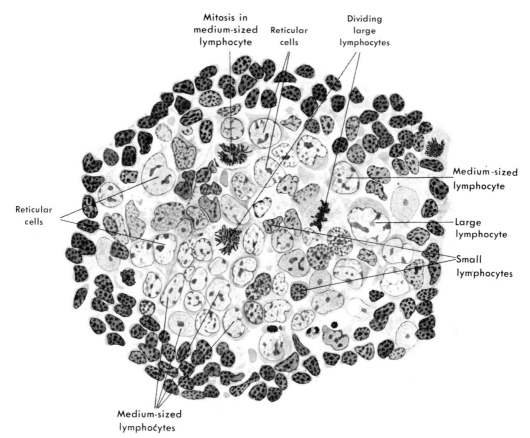

Figure 13–2. Various types of lymphocytes in a section of a human lymph node. Hematoxylin-eosin-azure II. (After A. A. Maximow.)

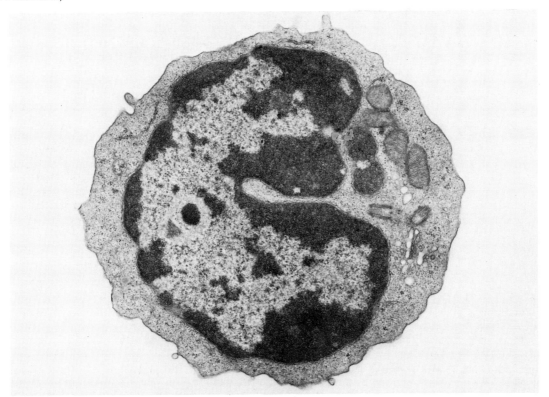

Figure 13–3. A typical lymphocyte from blood. The nucleus has a coarse pattern of heterochromatin and has an indentation that is not obvious with the light microscope. A pair of centrioles and a small Golgi complex are located in or near the concavity of the nucleus.

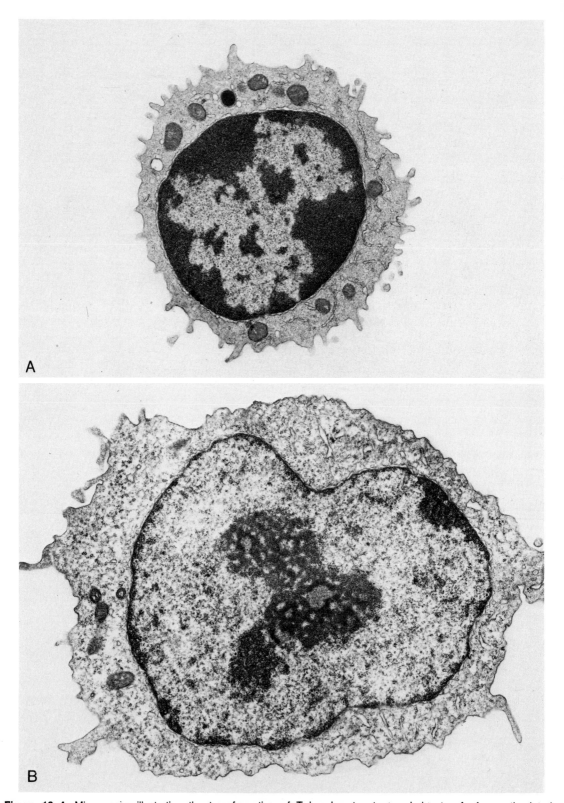

Figure 13–4. Micrographs illustrating the transformation of T lymphocytes to lymphoblasts. *A,* An unstimulated lymphocyte. *B,* From the same culture, a lymphoblast 36 hours after transformation induced by treatment with the lectin concanavalin A. These micrographs at the same magnification show the great increase in cell volume and development of a euchromatic nucleus with a prominent nucleolus. Transformation induced by phytohemagglutinin or concanavalin A is similar to that which occurs in response to antigenic stimulation.

endoplasmic reticulum. Their function is the synthesis and release (secretion) of antibody. They represent the late stages of differentiation of the B lymphocytes. Plasma cells are found in the medullary cords of resting lymph nodes, in the marginal zone and cords of the resting spleen, and scattered throughout the connective tissues of the body. They are especially numerous in the lamina propria of the intestinal mucosa, where most of them have been shown by immunofluorescent methods to produce immunoglobulins A. During the acute phase of a humoral immune response, large numbers of immature plasma cells appear in the deep portion of the cortex of lymph nodes and at the boundary between white and red pulp of the spleen. Mature plasma cells are sessile elements and apparently never enter blood and lymph. After an antigenic challenge, however, immature forms appear in the lymph; furthermore, a limited number of elements appear in the blood that at the light microscope level resemble lymphocytes in size and

have a centrally located nucleus, but which in electron micrographs display the abundant granular endoplasmic reticulum typical of the plasma cell line (Fig. 13–5).

Plasma cells are 6 to 20 μm in diameter and have a rounded, elongate, or polyhedral form, depending on their location. Seen with the light microscope, mature elements are small; they possess an eccentric, rounded nucleus with a small nucleolus and radially arranged coarse heterochromatic masses adjacent to the nuclear envelope, resulting in a cartwheel configuration. The cytoplasm is strongly basophilic, except for a conspicuous juxtanuclear, pale area, which contains the diplosome and surrounding Golgi apparatus.

It is evident in electron micrographs that the cytoplasmic basophilia of plasma cells is due to their highly developed granular endoplasmic reticulum, often distended with flocculent material (Fig. 13–6). Experiments involving immunolabeling with ferritin or horseradish peroxidase have shown that the content of the cisternae of the granular retic-

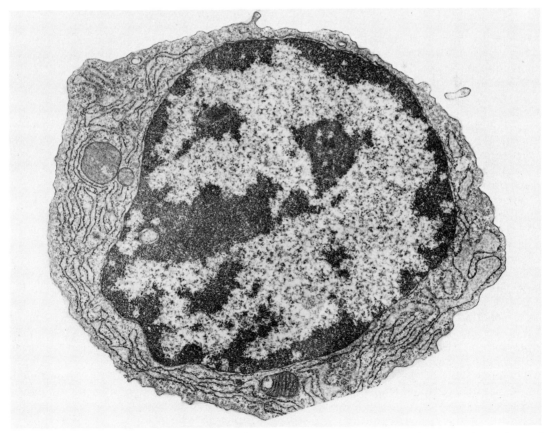

Figure 13–5. An immature plasma cell from peripheral blood. The cell has developed an extensive endoplasmic reticulum. In its further maturation the pattern of nuclear chromatin would become coarser, the cytoplasm would increase in volume, and the reticulum would become ordered into closely spaced, parallel arrays of cisternae. For an illustration of a mature plasma cell, see Figure 5–20.

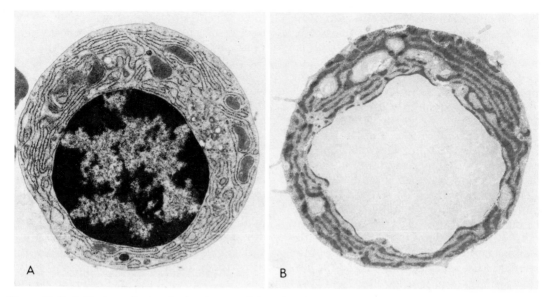

Figure 13–6. *A,* Electron micrograph of a plasma cell from the rabbit spleen. The eccentric, rounded nucleus contains masses of heterochromatin adjacent to the nuclear envelope. The cytoplasm displays a highly developed granular endoplasmic reticulum. *B,* Plasma cell from the spleen of a rabbit, which was injected with the enzyme horseradish peroxidase as an antigen. The antibody-containing spleen cells were subsequently treated with the antigen and stained with the histochemical method for demonstration of peroxidase activity. Dense reaction product is seen in the lumen of the cisternae of the granular endoplasmic reticulum, indicating the presence of anti–horseradish peroxidase antibody. (Courtesy of E. H. Leduc and S. Avrameas.)

ulum consists largely of antibody. The Golgi apparatus of mature plasma cells is large; the mitochondria are few and unremarkable in their internal structure. In a small percentage of plasma cells, one or more cisternae of the granular reticulum are greatly distended with a mass of dense material. These inclusions (Russell bodies) are readily seen with the light microscope and consist of incomplete immunoglobulin molecules. It has been suggested that Russell bodies are indicative of an aberrant synthesis or faulty intracellular transport of antibody, but this speculation lacks conclusive evidence.

Very immature precursors of the plasma cell line *(plasmablasts)* are difficult to distinguish from lymphoblasts or large lymphocytes. The nucleus is rich in euchromatin and provided with a large nucleolus; the cytoplasm contains many free polyribosomes as well as narrow cisternae of the granular endoplasmic reticulum. The transition from plasmablasts to plasmacyte involves progressive condensation of the chromatin, reduction in size and complexity of the nucleolus, disappearance of the free polyribosomes, enlargement of the Golgi apparatus, and appearance of a highly organized granular endoplasmic reticulum. The cisternae of the reticulum may form parallel, concentric arrays or become distended with accumulated antibody. The intermediate stages in the course of this differentiation are often referred to as *proplasmacytes.*

Macrophages

The structure of macrophages was discussed in Chapter 5 and will not be repeated here.

HISTOPHYSIOLOGY

Surface Properties of T and B Lymphocytes

The terms "T" and "B lymphocyte" describe two functionally distinct types of lymphocytes that circulate with blood and lymph and inhabit the peripheral lymphoid tissues. The lymphocytes of the thymus have different properties from those of T lymphocytes, but they represent the precursors of the T cells. Although B lymphocytes cannot be distinguished from T lymphocytes by light or transmission electron microscopy, they have distinct surface properties demonstrable by indirect methods. If antibody is produced against immunoglobulins by injecting the antibody of one species into an animal of a different species, the anti-immunoglobulin

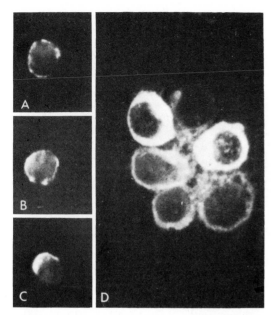

Figure 13–7. *A, B,* and *C,* B lymphocytes from the mouse spleen stained with anti-immunoglubulin antibody conjugated to fluorescein isothyocyanate and photographed with the fluorescence microscope. In *A,* the lymphocyte was reacted with the labeled antibody at 4° C. The anti-immunoglobulin is dispersed over the entire cell surface, although some patching of the marker is already in progress. *B,* and *C,* Upon warming at 37° C, the fluorescent antibody becomes concentrated over one pole of the cell (capping). For comparison, *D* illustrates the intense staining of the antibody in the cytoplasm of splenic plasma cells treated with fluorescent anti-immunoglobulin. (Courtesy of E. R. Unanue.)

antibody produced by the recipient can be isolated, purified, and conjugated to a visible marker. For example, the anti-immunoglobulin antibody can be conjugated with a fluorescent dye and then, after interaction with the lymphocyte surface, it can be localized with the fluorescence microscope (Fig. 13–7*A, B, C*). Alternatively, the antibody can be labeled with radioiodine and its localization studied with light or electron microscopic autoradiography (Fig. 13–8); finally, in a third method, the antibody can be conjugated to the electron-opaque particulate ferritin or hemocyanin (Figs. 13–9, 13–10) or to the enzyme horseradish peroxidase, and visualized with the electron microscope either directly or after appropriate histochemical reaction. With these techniques, it has been shown that B lymphocytes incubated at 0° C with labeled anti-immunoglobulin bind the antibody over their entire surface (Figs. 13–7*A*, 13–8). This property is attributable to the presence of immunoglobulins, predominantly monomeric IgM and IgD, bound to

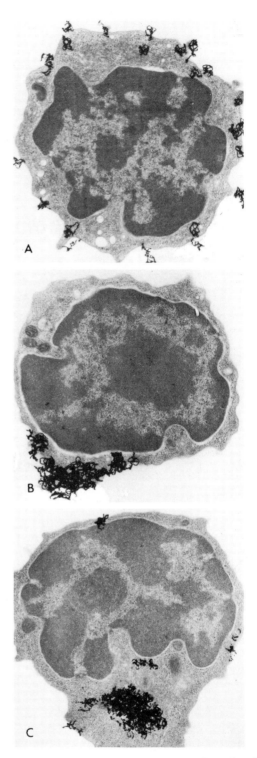

Figure 13–8. Electron microscope autoradiography of mouse spleen B lymphocytes treated with ^{125}I-labeled rabbit anti-immunoglobulin antibody. *A,* At 4° C the marker is randomly distributed over the entire cell membrane. *B,* When the lymphocytes are incubated at 37° C, the label becomes concentrated at one pole of the cell, forming a cap. *C,* Finally, the label is interiorized by endocytosis. (From Unanue, E. R., et al. *J. Exp. Med. 136*:885, 1972.)

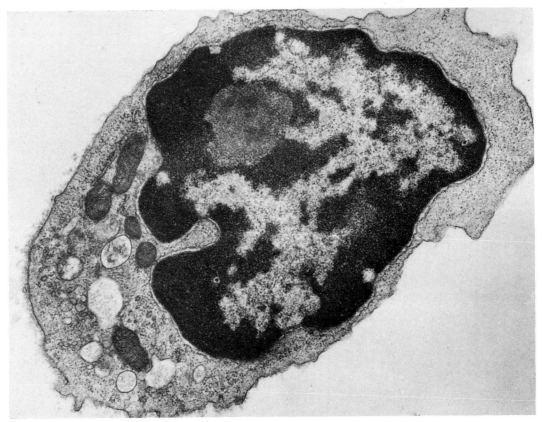

Figure 13–9. B lymphocyte of the mouse spleen treated with rabbit anti-immunoglobulin antibody conjugated with hemocyanin, a respiratory pigment present in the hemolymph of many invertebrates. The hemocyanin molecule has the shape of a short cylinder and is readily recognized with the electron microscope. This lymphocyte was reacted with the labeled anti-immunoglobulin at 4° C and then warmed to 37° C for 10 min. The label is concentrated in a cap over the cell pole in which the Golgi apparatus is contained. (From Karnovsky, M. J., et al. J. Exp. Med. *136*:907, 1972.)

the cell membrane. Compared with the secreted, pentameric IgM, the heavy chain of the surface IgM has an added hydrophobic sequence, which anchors the molecule to the plasmalemma. There is evidence that this antibody at the cell surface represents the receptor that combines with antigen. The plasma membrane of B cells is also able to bind antibody by means of the Fc fragment of their molecule and the C3b component of the complement system.

B cells have lower electrophoretic mobility and lower density than T cells, and they adhere preferentially to nylon wool at 37°C in the presence of serum. These properties have been exploited in attempts to separate the B- from the T-cell components of a mixed lymphocyte population.

T lymphocytes do not possess immunoglobulins as integral membrane proteins. Their antigen receptor is a polypeptide chain consisting of a constant and a variable region, similar or identical to the antigen-combining

moiety of the antibody heavy chain. Some T lymphocytes have surface receptors for the Fc region of IgM and others for the Fc region of IgG; a few have receptors for the C3b component of complement. In the human, a large proportion of T lymphocytes, and possibly all of them, bind sheep erythrocytes, and to a lesser extent pig erythrocytes, forming characteristic clusters or rosettes. The significance of this phenomenon, which lacks immunological specificity, is poorly understood. Nevertheless, spontaneous rosette formation provides a reliable clinical test for evaluation of the size of the T cell population in human patients.

When T lymphocytes are transferred from a donor mouse into a recipient of the same species but with a slightly different genetic constitution, they elicit production of antibodies that combine with T but not with B lymphocytes. Thus, murine T cells possess a surface antigenic determinant called Thy-1 or *theta,* which is lacking on B cells. Anti-

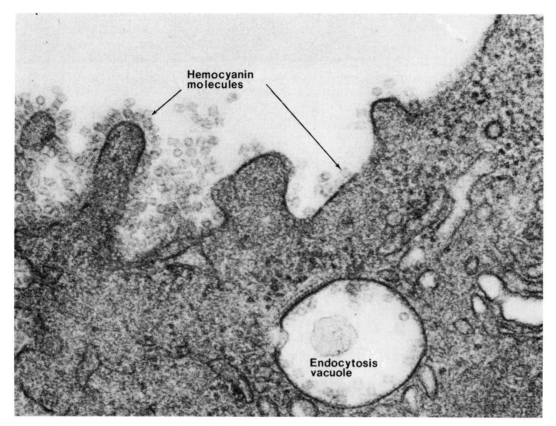

Figure 13–10. Same specimen as in Figure 13–9. Hemocyanin-labeled anti-immunoglobulin antibody is attached to the membrane immunoglobulins of the B lymphocyte. The cell has begun to interiorize the label in endocytotic vacuoles. (From Karnovsky, M. J., et al. J. Exp. Med. *136*:907, 1972.)

Thy-1 antibodies, when injected into mice belonging to the strain whose T lymphocytes carry the Thy-1 antigen, lead to specific complement-mediated destruction of T cells. It is thus possible to study the distribution of T lymphocytes in the immune system and the functional impairment caused by their selective elimination. Furthermore, anti-Thy-1 antibody conjugated to a visible marker, such as fluorochrome or ferritin, or labeled with radioiodine, binds to the surface of T lymphocytes and permits their morphological identification. Other antigens expressed on the surface of T lymphocytes belong to the Ly (lymphocyte) system. Of the peripheral murine T lymphocytes, about 50 per cent bear Ly 1,2 antigens, 30 to 40 per cent the Ly 1 antigen, and 10 per cent the Ly 2 antigen. Helper and lymphokine-secreting T lymphocytes express the Ly $+1,-2$ phenotype, suppressor and cytolytic T lymphocytes express the Ly $-1,+2$ phenotype, and both differentiate from Ly $+1,+2$ lymphocytes.

The different reactivity of T and B lymphocytes to various mitogens, to x-ray irra-

diation, and to cortisone; their distinctive distribution in the organs of the immune system; and their different pattern of recirculation are discussed on later pages.

Response of T Lymphocytes to Antigen

Both T and B lymphocytes manifest immunological specificity; i.e., both are genetically programmed to respond to an antigen that is specific for each individual cell. This commitment is expressed by the presence of receptors on the lymphocyte plasma membrane, which combine with the antigenic determinants. This process of specific binding is called *antigen recognition.* Antigen binding by T lymphocytes can be studied in laboratory rodents by mixing lymphocyte suspensions with foreign erythrocytes, usually those of sheep. This technique cannot be applied to human T cells because most of them bind sheep erythrocytes nonspecifically. Antigen-binding T cells of laboratory rodents can also be studied by combined autoradiography and immunofluorescence, using radioiodine-labeled antigen and fluorochrome-conjugated anti-Thy-1 antibody. It has been shown by these experimental strategies that antigen-binding T lymphocytes in animals not previously exposed to the antigen are very few in number and belong to the category of the small or medium-sized lymphocytes. They increase in number following immunization, probably because the challenge with the antigen induces amplification of the small fraction of the lymphocyte population that carries surface receptors specific for that particular antigen. The number of receptor sites for antigen on the membrane of T lymphocytes is very small, probably a few hundred, in contrast to the several thousands on B lymphocytes.

To become stimulated, T lymphocytes must interact with histocompatibility molecules, a class of membrane glycoproteins, which are present on the surface of eukaryotic cells and are coded by a set of genes known as *major histocompatibility complex*. Histocompatibility molecules belong to two types, one expressed on the surface of all cells and the other exclusively represented on the cells of the immune system. Those expressed on the surface of all cells differ from individual to individual and their genetic diversity provides biological uniqueness for every subject in a normal population. They represent the specific antigen recognized by T lymphocytes in graft rejection and activate T cells directly, without participation of macrophages as a third partner cell. The other type of histocompatibility molecules, named Ia in the mouse, are expressed on the surface of macrophages, B lymphocytes, and some activated T lymphocytes. When the antigen is a foreign substance, different from the histocompatibility molecules recognized in graft rejection, it can stimulate T lymphocytes only when deployed at the surface of a cell in association with an autologous Ia molecule. This requirement is met by macrophages, which present the T lymphocyte with the antigen bound to their plasma membrane and their own surface histocompatibility molecules. These observations explain why eukaryotic cells can stimulate T cells directly, whereas soluble, particulate, or bacterial antigen requires the participation of macrophages for effective immunization.

The sequence of events following antigen binding by T lymphocytes is not fully understood. However, circumstantial evidence favors the view that antigen, upon combining with its receptor at the cell surface, somehow triggers the transformation of the small lymphocyte into a proliferating lymphoblast (Figs. 13–1, 13–4). The size of the cell increases, its nucleus becomes euchromatic, the nucleolus enlarges, a great number of polyribosomes appear in the cytoplasm, and the Golgi apparatus becomes more prominent. Probably related to antigen recognition are the behavioral phenomena called *peripolesis* and *emperipolesis*—i.e., the tendency of lymphocytes in cell culture to move about, indenting and even penetrating other cells.

Antigens that elicit a humoral response stimulate a class of T lymphocytes characterized by the Ly $+1, -2$ phenotype and these, called *helper T lymphocytes,* at some stage of their transformation into lymphoblasts, interact with B lymphocytes and trigger their differentiation into antibody-secreting cells. The mechanism underlying this cooperation is not fully understood; it involves intimate surface association and complex interactions among antigen, macrophages, T cells, and B cells. At the onset, the helper T cell is activated by the antigen presented by a macrophage in association with an autologous histocompatibility molecule. The activated helper T cell releases factors that stimulate the resting B cell, in turn bearing antigen bound to the plasma membrane through its IgM and IgD receptors. The B cell transforms into a lymphoblast that has receptors for soluble growth factors. During a subsequent phase, which is antigen independent, the interacting T lymphocyte and macrophage produce growth factors that stimulate the B lymphoblast to proliferate and mature into antibody-secreting effector cells. Proliferation of the helper T lymphocytes leads to amplification of the response and to the differentiation of memory T cells, which revert to the state of small lymphocytes.

Antigens that elicit a delayed type of hypersensitivity reaction, such as chemical skin-sensitizing agents or products of facultative intracellular bacteria, are presented by macrophages to another class of T lymphocytes, which also express the Ly $+1, -2$ phenotype, and stimulate them to transform into lymphoblasts. As a result of this transformation, T cells begin to produce lymphocyte mediators or lymphokines. Lymphokines are molecules of 8000 to 80,000 daltons in molecular weight, which display a great variety of pharmacological activities; they are not immunoglobulins and their biochemical characterization is still incomplete. The best known lymphokine identified to date is the *macrophage inhibitory factor* (MIF), a glycoprotein 20,000 to 40,000 daltons in molecular weight, which immobilizes macrophages and may possibly lead to accumulation of these cells at the site of the antigen. A *macrophage-activating factor* enhances the bactericidal capacity of macrophages. A *chemotactic factor* recruits phagocytes to the site of the antigen, and *lymphotoxin* causes cell lysis.

Antigens such as tissue grafts and cells bearing tumor antigens or infected with viruses stimulate directly (i.e., without participation of macrophages) a third class of T lymphocytes, which express the Ly $-1, +2$ phenotype. In this instance, lymphoblast proliferation and differentiation lead to the appearance of cytolytic lymphocytes, which have the ability to cause the lysis of the foreign or altered cells after making contact with their surface. The mechanism of this direct cytotoxicity is poorly understood; it is specific for the cells that caused immunization, for nearby cellular elements are not affected and it requires close cell-to-cell contact. Three phases have been identified in the interaction between cytolytic T lymphocytes and target cells; the first is *adhesion:* it is temperature dependent and requires the presence of Mg^{++}, but not Ca^{++}. Adhesion is prevented by drugs that affect the cytoskeleton, inhibitors of ATP production, and local anesthetics. The second phase has been termed the *lethal hit:* during this stage the cytolytic T lymphocyte causes irreversible damage to the membrane of the target cell. It is temperature dependent and requires Ca^{++} but not protein synthesis. The third phase, called *killer cell independent lysis,* is characterized by the osmotic swelling of the target cell as a result of the membrane lesions caused by the lethal hit. The activity of helper T cells has been extended in the recent past to other immune responses in addition to antibody production. Thus, the development of Ly $-1, +2$ cytolytic T cells is enhanced by the influence of specific Ly $+1, -2$ T cells, which therefore regulate most immune responses positively.

Antigen also stimulates a separate T cell population with a suppressor function that belongs to the Ly $-1, +2$ phenotype. Two types of suppressor T cells have been identified: those that specifically suppress the immune response to the antigen that stimulated their development and those that suppress all antibody responses. The mechanism of action of suppressor T cells has not yet been fully elucidated: they elaborate mediators, 10,000 to 50,000 daltons in molecular weight, which have the ability to bind to the antigen that stimulated their production. In humoral immunity, they exert an inhibitory feedback on helper T cells or act on antibody-secreting B cells and plasma cells, decreasing their immunoglobulin secretion. Suppressor T cells also participate in cellular immune responses, such as delayed hypersensitivity, and responses to tumor antigens.

Response of B Lymphocytes to Antigen

Antigen receptors on the surface of B lymphocytes are clearly immunoglobulins, for it can be shown that specific binding of radioactive antigen to the cell membrane is blocked by anti-immunoglobulin antibody. The number of immunoglobulin receptors varies between 50,000 and 150,000 per cell; thus, the number of sites is much higher than on T lymphocytes. Despite the abundance of binding sites at the cell surface, direct stimulation of B lymphocytes is possible only by polymeric antigens—i.e., by molecules that display identical groupings in a linear, repetitive sequence such as the pneumococcal polysaccharide. Furthermore, the response only occurs within a narrow range of antigen dose and results predominantly, if not solely, in production of IgM antibodies. With most antigens that elicit a humoral response, B-cell stimulation also requires the participation of helper T lymphocytes and macrophages. The influence of helper T lymphocytes is also necessary for efficient production of IgG antibodies and for differentiation of memory cells within the B-cell population.

As a result of the cooperation between stimulated T and B lymphocytes, antibody is secreted and plasma cells appear. That plasma cells synthesize and release antibody has been firmly established by comparative immunological and histological studies, by immunofluorescent (Fig. 13–7) and autoradiographic techniques, and by antibody assay in microdroplets containing individual plasma cells. However, B lymphocytes are also capable of synthesizing and releasing antibody. Evidence for this was obtained from antibody assay in microdroplets containing single cells and from electron microscopic identification of single cells that had demonstrated their capacity to produce hemolytic antibody by forming a plaque of lysis in a layer of erythrocytes dispersed in agar (Figs. 13–11, 13–12). Antibody-producing lymphocytes are typical lymphoblasts or large cells that in addition to polyribosomes contain a small amount of cisternae of the granular endoplasmic reticulum. These cells have been regarded as transitional forms between lymphocytes and immature plasma cells.

Two schools of thought have developed on the interrelationships between lymphocytes and plasma cells, one regarding the lymphocyte as the ancestor of the plasma cell, the other considering plasma cells as a separate cell line arising from independent, still unidentified, stem cell precursors. A great deal of circumstantial evidence, however, favors the view that lymphocytes represent the precursors of the plasma cells. Especially persuasive are the fact that lymphocytes can also secrete antibody and the observation that during the immune response transitional

forms having cytological characteristics intermediate between lymphoblasts and immature plasma cells are found consistently. Furthermore, all experiments in which lymphocyte populations have been transferred from immunized animals into syngeneic* unprimed recipients, or from unprimed donors into allogeneic recipients, have led to the appearance of plasma cells in the recipient.

It is thus widely accepted that the small lymphocytes of the B type, stimulated by antigen under the influence of T lymphocytes, undergo transformation into lymphoblasts. During this process, antibody having identical specificity to that deployed on the cell surface is synthesized in increasing amounts and is released as a secretory product instead of being inserted into the plasma

---

Syngeneic in the field of transplantation immunity refers to individuals of the same species that are genetically identical, such as monozygotic twins or inbred laboratory animals. *Allogeneic* refers to individuals of the same species that are not genetically identical.

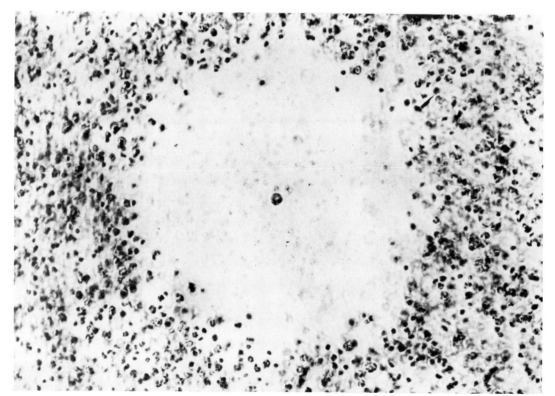

Figure 13–11. Hemolytic plaque-forming cell. A diluted suspension of lymphoid cells from an animal immunized with foreign erythrocytes was plated in agar along with the erythrocytes that served as antigen. The lymphoid cell at the center has synthetized and released hemolytic antibody into the surrounding agar, and the antibody has combined with the erythrocytes embedded in it. Complement has subsequently been added and the erythrocytes carrying the antibody have lysed, leaving a clear halo or plaque around the antibody-secreting cell. (Courtesy of A. A. Nordin and N. K. Jerne.)

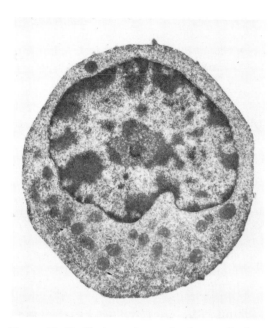

Figure 13–12. Electron micrograph of an antibody-secreting cell from the rabbit popliteal lymph node identified by the hemolytic-antibody plaque technique illustrated in Figure 13–11. The cell has the morphology of a large lymphocyte with euchromatic nucleus, prominent nucleolus, and abundant cytoplasm lacking an organized granular endoplasmic reticulum. (From Harris, T. N., et al. J. Exp. Med. *123*:161, 1966.)

membrane. Antibody-secreting lymphoblasts are actively proliferating cells; their progeny include (1) memory B cells, which revert to the state of small lymphocytes; and (2) transitional elements, which display an enlarged Golgi apparatus and increasing amounts of granular endoplasmic reticulum. These transitional cells, in turn, undergo further differentiation into plasma cells, passing through the stages in which they are identified as plasmablasts and proplasmacytes. Differentiation into plasma cells is accompanied by decrease in amount of surface membrane-bounded immunoglobulins, loss of proliferative capacity, and loss of motility. Experiments involving labeling with ^{3}H-thymidine indicate that the process of differentiation of lymphocytes into plasma cells takes about one day. The life span of plasma cells is a few weeks. Lymphoblasts and immature plasma cells also have the capacity to enter the efferent lymph of the lymph nodes draining the site of antigen injection and to colonize additional lymph nodes along the same path of lymphatic drainage. There are also indications that they may transform into smaller cells with central nucleus, scanty cytoplasm, but abundant granular endoplasmic reticulum, and that these cells enter the blood and propagate the response throughout the body (Fig. 13–5).

During the primary response to antigen, the first antibody to appear in the blood belongs to the IgM type; later, much larger amounts of the more efficient IgG are produced. The switch from IgM to IgG production is dependent on the regulatory influence of T lymphocytes. Both types of immunoglobulins can be produced by either lymphocytes or plasma cells.

Antibody synthesis and release involve an intracellular pathway that has been found to be typical of all other protein-secreting cells studied to date. The heavy and light chains are transcribed from separate messengers on polyribosomes bound to the membranes of the granular endoplasmic reticulum. They are subsequently transferred into the lumen of the cisternae, either free or combined with each other. In lymphocytes, the first detectable antibody appears in the perinuclear cisterna and later, as differentiation to plasma cells proceeds, antibody is produced and stored throughout the granular endoplasmic reticulum. In mature plasma cells, antibody is no longer detected in the space within the nuclear envelope and it disappears from some of the cisternae of the granular endoplasmic reticulum. Some carbohydrate components of the antibody molecules (e.g., *N*-acetylglucosamine) are incorporated into the nascent H chain. The polypeptide backbone, carrying part of the carbohydrate moiety, is subsequently transported to the Golgi apparatus, where additional saccharides (e.g., galactose) are added. From the Golgi, antibody is carried to the cell surface by some unknown mechanism and is released from the cell.

The amount of antibody produced by lymphocytes may be smaller than that produced by plasma cells, but it is released at an early stage of the response and at the very site of antigen stimulation, where it can be much more effective than the circulating antibody, which is confined largely to the intravascular space. Plasma cells may synthesize much larger amounts of antibody, but they store a large proportion of this immunoglobulin in the distended cisternae of their granular reticulum and may release it only upon cell death and disintegration.

The Role of Macrophages in Immune Responses

The only immune responses in which lymphocytes are directly stimulated by antigen are those triggered by eukaryotic cells carrying histocompatibility molecules on their surface, and the special case of certain polymeric antigens that stimulate B cells directly, without participation of helper T cells. In all other instances, effective immunization requires an additional cell that carries the antigen on its surface and presents it to the T lymphocyte in association with autologous histocompatibility molecules. However, the specificity of the immune response is determined by the lymphocyte, since other cells are unable to distinguish foreign determinants from the normal body constituents. A subject of controversy over the past few years concerns the question whether macrophages belonging to the mononuclear phagocyte lineage represent the partner cell that collaborates with the lymphocyte during the inductive phase of the immune response. Since this view is widely accepted by immunologists, it will be discussed first.

The need for macrophage participation in the initiation of immune responses has emerged from a wide variety of experiments, all showing that antigens which are avidly taken up by macrophages are good immunogens, whereas those which are not phagocytized are poor immunogens. Blockade of the macrophages of the body by administration of inert particulate suspensions significantly depresses the immune response. If a donor animal is injected with an antigen that is feebly immunogenic, and its macrophages are then transferred to a syngeneic recipient, this latter responds with a vigorous immune response, possibly because the small amount of antigen bound to the surface of the macrophages is a much stronger immunogen than the antigen in its original dispersed form. The strongest evidence for macrophage participation in lymphocyte stimulation comes from experiments in which the response to antigen has been reproduced in vitro; in these systems it has been clearly shown that in addition to T and B lymphocytes, a third partner cell is required. This cell has many properties of macrophages; it is radioresistant, adheres to glass surfaces, and does not synthesize antibodies.

The precise mechanism of macrophage function in the induction of an immune response by lymphocytes is poorly understood.

Macrophages certainly act in general by removing and digesting excess of antigen. If antigen interacts indiscriminately with lymphocytes in a location unfavorable for cell cooperation, tolerance is induced instead of immunity. Thus, only a small fraction of the antigen escapes destruction by macrophages and triggers immunization. Macrophages, however, seem to play a more intimate and important role in lymphocyte stimulation by antigen. According to a widely accepted hypothesis, in addition to ingesting and destroying antigen, macrophages retain a small amount of antigen bound to their surface and present it in a concentrated form to lymphocytes (a phenomenon referred to as *antigen presentation*). In addition, to be immunogenic antigen must be presented by macrophages in association with their surface histocompatibility molecules (Ia molecules in the mouse); only macrophages that possess Ia molecules are capable of cooperating with T lymphocytes. The function of the histocompatibility molecules is to mediate in some way the recognition of antigen by T cells, either by ensuring cell-to-cell contact or by binding the antigen at the macrophage surface. This function implies close topographical relationships between macrophages and lymphoid cells, and this intimate association has been demonstrated with the electron microscope in the cell clusters that produce antibody against foreign red blood cells in vitro.

As a result of the interaction among antigen, macrophage, and T lymphocyte, it has been suggested the macrophages secrete growth and differentiation factors that affect the adjacent lymphocytes.

These views on the identification of macrophages as partner cells for the lymphocytes in immune induction are vigorously challenged by some cell biologists, who regard the evidence presented by immunologists as inconclusive. According to these investigators, radioresistance and adherence to glass surfaces are not sufficient criteria for identification of the partner cell as a macrophage. They also argue that macrophages completely degrade the ingested material, that the membrane of their lysosomes is impermeable to macromolecules, and that they are unable to release undigested material by exocytosis. Thus, they deem it unlikely that in macrophages a small fraction of the antigen escapes destruction and is transferred to the cell surface for presentation to the lymphocyte.

THE IMMUNE SYSTEM ·

Candidates for the antigen-presenting cells in immune induction are the *lymphoid dendritic cells,* identified in cell suspensions of lymphoid organs. These cells are provided with numerous irregular processes, which may appear as spiny branches, blunt pseudopods, or thin veils. The cytoplasm has many mitochondria, but few ribosomes, lysosomes, or secretory inclusions. The nucleus is irregular in shape, lined with a rim of heterochromatin, and provided with distinct nucleoli. Dendritic cells adhere to plastic or glass during the first few hours in culture, but show little or no phagocytic activity. They derive from the bone marrow, possess histocompatibility (Ia) molecules at their surface, and seem capable of cooperating with lymphocytes in the induction phase of certain immune responses. Possibly related to lymphoid dendritic cells are other cell types, all characterized by irregular shape, inconspicuous cell organelles, and lack of phagocytic activity. These include the *follicular dendritic cells,* identified in germinal centers, which retain antigen-antibody complexes on their surface; the *interdigitating cells,* identified in the thymus-dependent areas of lymph nodes and spleen; the *"veiled" cells,* identified in the afferent lymph of lymph nodes in rodents and man; and the *Langerhans cells* of the epidermis. At present, it is unclear whether all these dendritic cells represent a homogeneous population with novel biological properties and important functions in immune induction, or a subpopulation of macrophages in a special state of differentiation.

Macrophages are certainly involved in the terminal events of antigen disposal. Their role includes removal of foreign cells or bacteria whose viability has been impaired by lymphocytes or lytic antibody in presence of complement. Furthermore, phagocytosis of foreign material, cells, and bacteria is powerfully enhanced when the antigenic determinants are opsonized, i.e., complexed with antibody or with antibody and complement. Opsonization depends on the presence of receptors on the macrophage membrane that bind the Fc part of the antibody molecule or the C3b component of the complement system. Only certain classes of immunoglobulins bind directly to the macrophage surface (IgG in humans, IgG and IgM in mice), and the interaction is especially strong when they are combined with antigen. IgM, which does not bind to the membrane of human macrophages directly, becomes cytophilic in the presence of complement.

The enhancement of phagocytosis by antibody and complement is not an exclusive property of macrophages; granulocytes also have an enhanced capacity for engulfing bacteria when the bacteria are complexed with antibody and complement.

The effect on macrophages of the lymphokines released by T cells in the course of delayed hypersensitivity reactions has been discussed previously (p. 418).

Nonspecific Stimulation of Lymphocytes

A number of agents besides antigen, commonly referred to as *mitogens,* stimulate lymphocytes, inducing their transformation into actively proliferating lymphoblasts. The major difference between antigen and mitogens resides in the fact that the former reacts with individual lymphocytes that on a genetic basis have developed membrane receptors specific for its surface determinants, whereas mitogens are effective on much larger lymphocyte populations. Mitogens include a variety of substances extracted from plants or seeds, constituents of bacteria or products of their metabolism, and antilymphocyte sera, produced by immunizing animals with exogenous lymphocytes. All mitogens whose mechanism of action has been studied in detail have the capacity to bind chemical groupings on the plasma membrane of lymphocytes; many of them also combine with the surface of other cells, but only lymphocytes respond with transformation and mitosis. As agents also exist that bind to the surface of lymphocytes without stimulating them, mitogens can be regarded as belonging to a larger class of substances whose common property is an affinity for chemical groupings on the surfaces of cells, and which are therefore generically named *ligands.* The effects of mitogenic ligands on lymphocytes has great theoretical importance because their mechanism of action, although nonspecific, appears to be identical to that of antigens. Therefore, they have become a useful laboratory tool in studies aimed at an understanding of lymphocyte stimulation. Especially well studied are the chemical and biological properties of extracts of certain plants or seeds, which have long been known to cause agglutination of erythrocytes and leukocytes. These substances are called *lectins.* Agglutination depends on the fact that lectins are multivalent ligands and thus form bridges between neighboring cells, causing formation of clumps. Plant lectins are proteins or glycoproteins that have strong chemical affinity for the oligosaccharide residues on the plasma membrane of mammalian cells. They can be conjugated to an ultrastructural marker such as ferritin or hemocyanin, and in this way the distribution of the lectin-binding oligosaccharides at the cell surface can be visualized with the electron microscope.

Ligands do not stimulate all lymphocytes indiscriminately. Phytohemagglutinin (PHA), a lectin extracted from the red kidney bean *(Phaseolus vulgaris)*, and concanavalin A (Con A), extracted from the jackbean *(Canavalia ensiformis)*, stimulate T lymphocytes. Pokeweed mitogen (PWM), extracted from the root of *Phytolacca americana*, activates both T and B cells, whereas a lipopolysaccharide extracted from the bacterium *Escherichia coli* (LPS) is specific for B cells.

T lymphocyte stimulation by PHA has been studied in great detail and provides a satisfactory means of imitating the morphological and biochemical phenomena that follow combination of antigen with T cells. The earliest event after addition of PHA to a culture of small lymphocytes (15 min) is enhanced endocytotic activity, as evidenced by increased uptake of neutral red, and increased synthesis of RNA (15 to 30 min). Soon afterward, the nucleolus begins to enlarge (four hours). At 24 to 36 hours, the nucleus becomes more euchromatic, the nucleolonema is clearly visible in the nucleolus, and the cell volume increases. The cell begins DNA synthesis, thus entering the S phase of the cell cycle, which lasts six to ten hours. Then, it enters the G2 phase, characterized by active RNA and protein synthesis. There is a striking concomitant increase in cytoplasmic polyribosomes, whereas the granular endoplasmic reticulum remains relatively sparse. The Golgi apparatus enlarges and the lysosomes are moderately increased in number. At the end of G2, which lasts two to four hours, the lymphocyte has undergone a fourfold increase in volume and enters mitosis. DNA synthesis in cultures of PHA-stimulated lymphocytes reaches a peak at 72 to 120 hours, then slowly declines over a period of five to seven days. Beginning at about 24 hours after PHA exposure, the T lymphocyte develops the capacity to impair nonspecifically the viability of other cells, such as fibroblasts. This property is mediated by production and release into the culture medium of various lymphokines. The effects of lectins on B lymphocytes are poorly understood, but there is evidence that in seven- to ten-day-old cultures of PWM-stimulated lymphocytes, plasma cells develop.

It is evident that binding of molecules to the plasma membrane is not effective *per se* in causing lymphocyte stimulation, but saturation of specific chemical groupings at the cell surface is probably required. Once a mitogenic ligand has bound to the plasma membrane, it somehow triggers lymphocyte transformation. Lymphocytes are unique among mammalian cells in that they respond with cell division and differentiation to a variety of exogenous substances, including the antigen for which they carry specific receptors.

Studies using ligands conjugated to a visible marker have cast some light upon the cellular events that immediately follow the ligand's combination with the lymphocyte membrane (Figs. 13–7 to 13–10). When anti-immunoglobulin antibody conjugated to a fluorescent dye (or to ferritin or hemocyanin) is reacted at 4° C with a B lymphocyte bearing the immunoglobulin, the label appears uniformly dispersed over the entire cell surface. This demonstrates that antibody molecules on B cells are uniformly distributed throughout the plasma membrane. With the passage of time, the marker becomes aggregated, resulting in formation of interconnected patches. This phenomenon, called *patching*, depends on the fact that surface immunoglobulins move randomly in the fluid domain of the plasma membrane and that when they approach sufficiently close to one another, they are cross-linked by the multivalent anti-immunoglobulin antibody. However, if the cell suspension is warmed to 37° C, the marker molecules become aggregated to form a continuous cap localized in the region of the cell surface overlying the Golgi apparatus, a behavior called *capping*. That portion of the plasma membrane bearing the marker subsequently becomes interiorized by endocytosis, or the label is shed from the cell surface. This process leaves the B lymphocyte denuded of its surface immunoglobulins and antigen receptors for several hours.

Capping is an energy-dependent process by which the cell eliminates the ligand bound to its surface; its relationship to lymphocyte stimulation is still poorly understood. Probably, capping occurs upon binding of antigen to the surface of the B lymphocyte, but stimulation also requires the cooperative interaction with helper T cells.

Other Functional Properties of Lymphocytes

Lymphocyte heterogeneity is not limited to the three classes of T, B, and null cells. Within each class, lymphocytes may differ considerably in other functional properties, such as immunocompetence, life span, and sensitivity to ionizing radiation or to adrenal steroids. In T lymphocytes, which have been more thoroughly studied, these functional differences are related to the degree of cell differentiation. Most lymphocytes of the thymus, which represent the precursors of the T lymphocyte, are not immunocompetent— i.e., they lack the capacity to respond to antigen or to lectins such as PHA by transformation and proliferation. They are also readily destroyed by x-ray irradiation or administration of cortisone; furthermore, some of the thymic lymphocytes have a very short life span (see Chapter 14). Upon leaving the thymus, T lymphocytes become immunocompetent and more resistant to irradiation and cortisone. Their life span is unknown, but upon interaction with antigen they can give rise to memory cells, which have the morphology of small lymphocytes and a life span in man of up to several years.

The changes in functional properties of B lymphocytes during their development are still poorly understood. There is evidence, however, that their bone marrow precursors are resistant to corticosteroids, whereas peripheral B lymphocytes are sensitive to both x-ray irradiation and adrenal steroids. Memory cells of the B type also have a long life span.

An important property of lymphocytes is their motility, which enables them to cross the walls of the postcapillary venules in order to enter or leave the bloodstream. They also move about in the parenchyma of lymph nodes and can leave the nodes by migrating into the lymph. They penetrate epithelia and freely wander through the connective tissues of the body. Differentiation into plasma cells is accompanied by a loss of motility.

LYMPHOID TISSUE

Lymphocytes occur as individual cells in blood, in lymph, and throughout the connective and epithelial tissues of the body. However, in most organs, but especially in the lamina propria of the digestive and respiratory tracts, they occur together with plasma cells and macrophages as densely packed masses in loose connective tissue. Furthermore, the thymus, lymph nodes, white pulp of the spleen, and tonsils consist mainly of lymphocytes. The terms "lymphoid" and "lymphatic tissue" have been widely employed to define the common features of all aggregates of lymphocytes and lymphocyte-rich organs. Although in the past these terms were often used with quite different connotations, modern advances in immunology have rendered the traditional distinctions obsolete. On the other hand, our knowledge of the cell-to-cell interactions at a tissue or organ level is still largely incomplete, and a solid basis for a rational classification of the lymphocyte collections of the body is lacking. The term "lymphoid tissue" or "lymphoid organ" will be used here to define regions of the body in which lymphocytes, with or without associated plasma cells, represent the chief cellular constituent. It must be emphasized, however, that this definition is purely descriptive and includes cell aggregates that may have very different functions.

One morphologically and functionally distinct type of lymphoid tissue is that found in the thymus and in the medulla of the nodules of the avian bursa of Fabricius. It consists of lymphocytes and a few macrophages, contained in the meshes of a tridimensional network of stellate cells joined by desmosomes. These stellate stromal elements are called *reticular cells* simply because they form a network. Unlike the mesenchymal stroma of most other organs, these cells arise from an epithelial outgrowth of the endoderm, which becomes secondarily invaded by lymphopoietic stem cells. Reticular fibers are scarce in this variety of lymphoid tissue.

A much more common type of lymphoid tissue makes up the bulk of the lymph nodes, the white pulp of the spleen, and the tonsils and forms more or less discrete masses scattered in the connective tissues of the body. From a descriptive point of view, "diffuse" and "nodular" subvarieties of this second type of lymphoid tissue can be distinguished (Fig. 13–13).

Diffuse Lymphoid Tissue

Lymphoid tissue of this description is typically found in the internodular, deep cortical, and medullary regions of lymph nodes, in the periarterial lymphoid sheaths of the

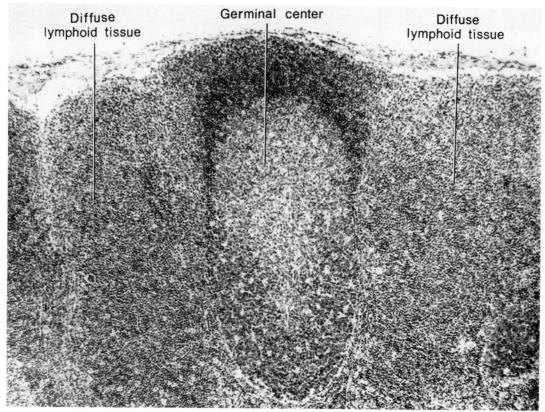

Figure 13–13. Diffuse lymphoid tissue and a germinal center in the outer cortex of a mesenteric lymph node of a dog. Hematoxylin-eosin.

spleen, and in the internodular regions of the tonsils and Peyer's patches. It consists of a spongelike stroma with lymphocytes in the meshes. The stroma, in turn, is made up of reticular fibers and reticular cells of mesenchymal origin (Fig. 13–14). Reticular fibers, best shown by the silver impregnation methods, are intimately associated with the reticular cells and often occupy deep recesses or grooves in their surface. In ordinary histological preparations the reticular cells appear as stellate or elongate elements with oval, euchromatic nucleus and scanty acidophilic cytoplasm. In vitally stained animals, some of the reticular cells take up colloidal dyes avidly while others do not. By this functional criterion, some of them can actually be regarded as macrophages. With the electron microscope, reticular cells display cisternae of granular endoplasmic reticulum in varying amounts and a moderately well-developed Golgi apparatus, whereas the other cell organelles are inconspicuous. The cell periphery is often devoid of organelles and inclusions and contains bundles of filaments. Thus, some of the reticular cells of the dif-

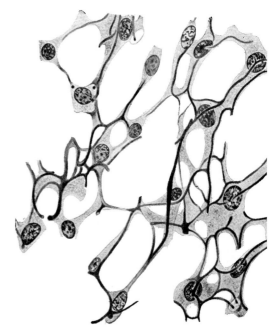

Figure 13–14. Section of a lymph node after the lymphocytes have been removed, showing the network of reticular cells and their intimate relations with the reticular fibers. Mallory-azan stain. (Redrawn after Heidenhain.)

fuse lymphoid tissue are tissue macrophages, while others are not very different from the fibroblasts of the connective tissues elsewhere in the body. Experiments involving labeling with ^{3}H-thymidine have shown that in lymph nodes, reticular cells have a very slow turnover rate. Moreover, during the regeneration of the lymph node following irradiation, no transformation of labeled reticular cells to the free elements of the lymphoid parenchyma is seen. Thus, contrary to the traditional teaching, it seems unlikely that reticular cells can give rise to other cell types. There seems to be no evidence supporting the time-honored view that reticular cells are primitive or undifferentiated elements, capable of giving rise to lymphocytes or other connective tissue elements. It now appears that reticular cells, as seen with the light microscope, represent either fibroblasts, concerned with the synthesis and maintenance of the reticular fibers, or occasional tissue phagocytes, belonging to the mononuclear phagocyte system. The free cells of the diffuse lymphoid tissue are lymphocytes of various sizes, macrophages, and a variable number of plasma cells.

Lymphoid Nodules

Lymphoid nodules or follicles are compact, circumscribed collections of cells within the diffuse lymphoid tissue. They are typically found in the cortex of lymph nodes, at the periphery of the white pulp of the spleen, and in the lamina propria of the digestive and respiratory passages. They are very numerous in the tonsils, Peyer's patches, and appendix. There is much disagreement in the literature as to the nomenclature for lymphoid nodules, since the terms "primary" and "secondary nodule" and "germinal center" have been used to define different entities. *Primary nodule* is most commonly employed to designate a rounded collection of tightly packed small lymphocytes, whereas *secondary nodule* (also called *germinal center)* describes ovoid structures consisting of a spherical cluster of larger, pale-staining cells invested by a cap of small lymphocytes. The precise significance of primary nodules is unknown; moreover, there is no evidence that secondary nodules, with their cap of small lymphocytes, arise by transformation of preexisting primary nodules, as the terms would imply. Thus, the term "secondary nodule" does not seem to be justified experimen-

tally and should be discarded in favor of "germinal center."

Germinal centers are a highly organized, widely distributed component of the lymphoid tissue absent only in the normal thymus (Figs. 13–15, 13–16). In their fully developed form, the germinal centers appear as a spherical mass with a dark, or densely populated, pole and a pale, or less densely populated, pole. The germinal center is surrounded by a capsule of elongated cells, which is in turn partially invested by a crescentic cap of small lymphocytes. Germinal centers display a clear-cut morphological polarity, inasmuch as the lymphocyte cap is especially thick over the light region and becomes gradually thinner toward the darker pole. Furthermore, they show a consistent orientation with respect to the neighboring structures. In the lymph nodes, the light region and lymphocyte cap of the germinal centers are directed toward the marginal sinus; in the spleen they are directed toward the red pulp. In the digestive and respiratory passages they are oriented toward the nearest epithelial surface. When the plane of a histological section passes through a germinal center in a direction perpendicular to its axis of symmetry, the polarity just described is not seen, for the cap of small lymphocytes appears as a circular rim of uniform width surrounding the germinal center. For this reason, the cap has often been described as a mantle or corona.

In the dark region of the germinal center (Fig. 13–15), the intense staining results from the nuclei and basophilic cytoplasm of numerous closely packed elements of the lymphoid cell line—namely, lymphoblasts, large and medium-sized lymphocytes, and cells in transition to the plasma cell line. All these cells are actively proliferating and they contain antibody within the perinuclear space and occasional cisternae of the granular endoplasmic reticulum. In the dark zone, macrophages are also found consistently, loaded with debris of phagocytized lymphocytes. The free cells are contained in the meshes of a cellular framework composed of stellate elements joined by desmosomes. These cells display little cytoplasmic specialization; they are stained by silver methods and were called dendritic cells because of their numerous radiating processes. The transition between the light and the dark region at the equator of the germinal center is a gradual one; the large basophilic cells of the lymphoid line progressively give way to small lymphocytes,

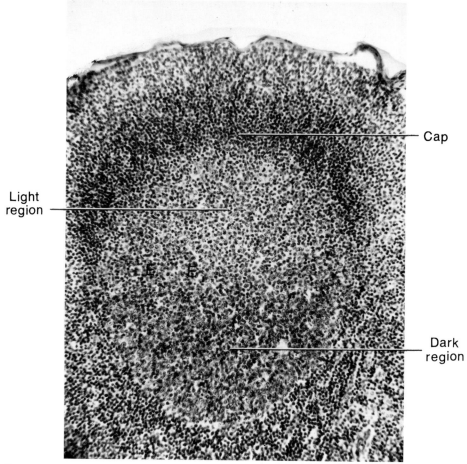

Figure 13–15. Germinal center in the outer cortex of an inguinal node of a dog. Hematoxylin-eosin.

mitotic figures disappear, and macrophages decrease in number. The dendritic cells acquire abundant eosinophilic cytoplasm and myriad peripheral interdigitating processes.

The capsule of the germinal center consists of a few layers of flattened reticular cells joined by desmosomes. This investment is disorganized over the light pole because of the presence of many highly deformed small lymphocytes, allegedly fixed in the course of their migration toward or from the overlying small lymphocyte cap. Mature plasma cells are scarce in germinal centers except in those of the tonsils. Reticular fibers are sparse within the center, but they form a concentric envelope around its periphery.

Germinal centers are thought to pass through a sequence of developmental changes and ultimately to involute and disappear. They seem to arise from small nests of large lymphocytes or lymphoblasts, which progressively gain in size and complexity to form aggregations, up to 1 mm in diameter.

In very large germinal centers, lymphocyte phagocytosis is intense; thus, they acquire a characteristic appearance with the light microscope, because the macrophages loaded with residual bodies are seen as light areas on a background of tightly packed nuclei (starry sky). The life span of germinal centers and the precise sequence of events leading to their disappearance are unknown.

Very little is understood about the function of germinal centers. They are the site of active production of lymphocytes, but a proportion of the newly formed cells die locally and are disposed of by macrophages; the fate of the survivors is unknown. On the one hand, autoradiographic studies on the tonsil after ^{3}H-thymidine injection seem to indicate that lymphocytes arise in the germinal center, move outward entering the small lymphocyte cap, and finally migrate into the overlying epithelium. On the other hand, in the germinal centers of lymph nodes and spleen, no such centrifugal cell movement is observed

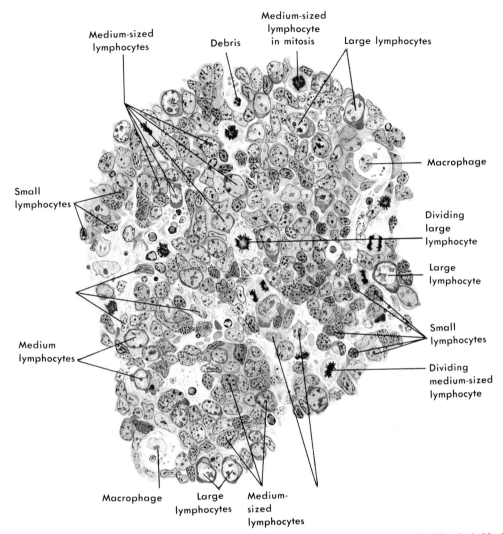

Figure 13–16. Portion of a germinal center of a human lymph node. Hematoxylin-eosin-azure II. (After A. A. Maximow.)

and the small lymphocytes of the cap seem to belong to the long-lived variety.

The functional significance of the dendritic cells is not clear. They do not seem to be capable of phagocytosis, for which reason the term "dendritic macrophages" originally applied to these cells is no longer tenable. However, they have been shown to trap antigen in the presence of antibody and to retain the antigen-antibody complex for long periods of time. It has been suggested that the numerous peripheral processes of these cells bind the complex to their surface membrane, but inert particles such as carbon, titanium oxide, and saccharated iron oxide are also retained. The possibility that dendritic cells may participate in immune induction has been discussed previously.

Germinal centers also develop in rodents

thymectomized at birth and in patients with congenital thymic aplasia. In birds, their appearance is prevented by bursectomy, and they are absent in humans with congenital agammaglobulinemia. Intravenously injected B lymphocytes localize both in germinal centers and in their small lymphocyte cap. Thus, they are probably involved in some stage of the development or functional differentiation of B lymphocytes.

The appearance of germinal centers is closely correlated with the evolution of humoral immunological responses. They are formed *de novo* during the primary response to antigen and increase explosively in number during the secondary response, whereas they are very few in animals reared in a germ-free environment. Furthermore, their lymphoid cells synthesize antibody of the IgG variety, although they do not differentiate into plasma cells or do so only to a very limited extent. Each germinal center seems to produce monospecific antibody; thus, the suggestion has been advanced that the whole lymphoid population of an individual germinal center may represent a clone of cells, all committed in the response to a single antigen. Despite the good correlation between the appearance of germinal centers and the humoral response to antigen, germinal centers are not essential for antibody production nor for plasma cell formation. In the human fetus, there is antibody secretion before germinal centers develop; in the course of the primary response to antigen, antibody appears in the blood and plasma cells develop before antibody-producing germinal centers can be demonstrated. It has been claimed, however, that during the secondary response, germinal center formation precedes the rise of circulating antibody. On the basis of this observation and experiments on antibody secretion in vitro, transfer of immune responses, and effects of drugs or x-ray irradiation, it has been speculated that germinal centers develop following repeated contact with antigens eliciting antibody secretion and that they may therefore be involved in the long-term memory of the IgG response. At the present state of our knowledge, however, it must be admitted that the precise function of the germinal center, a conspicuous and ubiquitous component of the lymphoid tissue, is still unknown.

HISTOPHYSIOLOGICAL OVERVIEW OF THE IMMUNE SYSTEM

LYMPHOCYTE CIRCULATION

The immune system consists of (1) specific lymphoid organs, (2) masses of lymphoid tissue embedded in other organs, (3) isolated lymphoid cells infiltrating the epithelial and connective tissues of the body, and (4) lymphocytes circulating with blood and lymph. Among the organs of the immune system, the thymus and lymph nodes are composed exclusively of lymphoid tissue, whereas the spleen possesses an additional component, the red pulp, which is primarily concerned with nonimmune functions. Aggregates of lymphoid tissue and lymphoid cells can be found anywhere in the body, with the single exception of the central nervous system. A special situation is found in the bone marrow, which *in sensu stricto* does not belong to the immune system, but which represents the only source for the stem cell precursors of lymphocytes in late fetal and postnatal life. The various regions of the immune system have precise functional interrelationships and are interconnected by an orderly traffic of lymphocytes, which exploit blood and lymph as circulatory pathways. To understand these relationships, one must first recapitulate the developmental history of the lymphocyte; stem cell precursors arising from the yolk sac in the embryo and from the bone marrow in the adult migrate through the bloodstream into the thymus and the unknown mammalian analogue of the avian bursa of Fabricius. Under the influence of thymus and bursa equivalent, these stem cell precursors undergo antigen-independent proliferation and differentiate into immunocompetent T and B lymphocytes, respectively. These reenter the bloodstream and populate the lymph nodes, the spleen, and the connective tissues of the body. Upon meeting their appropriate antigen, T and B lymphocytes are stimulated to transform, proliferate, and differentiate, thus giving rise to activated T lymphocytes and antibody-secreting B lymphocytes and plasma cells. As a result of antigen stimulation, lymphocytes also arise that propagate the response throughout the immune system or carry memory of the primary response, and these are capable of mounting an enhanced reaction upon successive exposures to the same antigen.

An efficient immunological surveillance of the body is only possible if lymphocytes, each endowed with the property to respond to a single antigen, are able to move freely throughout the body, thus increasing the chance for them to encounter their appropriate antigen. That this is the case has been proved by a series of elegant studies that have disclosed the existence of a continuous traffic of lymphocytes between the various lymphoid organs via the blood and lymph. There are two main patterns of migration of lymphocytes through the body—slow and fast (Fig. 13–17). The movement of stem cells from bone marrow to thymus and bursa and the subsequent seeding of lymphocytes to the peripheral lymphoid organs are measured in weeks, during which cells undergo sequential steps of differentiation. Superimposed upon

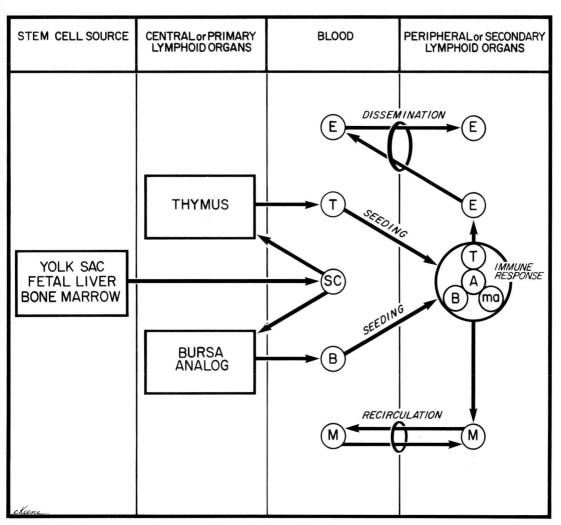

Figure 13–17. Diagram of lymphocyte circulation and differentiation. Stem cell precursors arising from the yolk sac in the embryo or the bone marrow in the adult enter the blood and migrate into the thymus and the unknown mammalian analogue of the avian bursa. Here they proliferate and differentiate into T and B lymphocytes. These enter the blood and seed the peripheral lymphoid organs (lymph nodes, spleen, gut-associated lymphoid tissue), where they undergo antigen-dependent proliferation and differentiation. SC, stem cell; T, thymus-dependent lymphocyte; B, bursa-dependent lymphocyte; A, antigen; M, memory lymphocyte; E, effector lymphocyte, which propagates the immune response throughout the body; ma, macrophage.

this slow traffic is a second type of migratory phenomenon, by which long-lived small lymphocytes rapidly move from blood to peripheral lymphoid organs and tissues and back into the blood. This latter process, called *recirculation*, does not involve lymphocyte proliferation and is measured in hours. Finally, there are hints of a third pattern of cell migration, which may be especially prominent in the course of an acute immune response; effector lymphocytes and plasma cell precursors are seeded by lymph and blood throughout the immune system and connective tissues of the body, thus bringing about a propagation of the immune response.

The plasma cell precursors localize in great numbers in the lamina propria of the mucosa of the gut, where they undergo differentiation into mature plasma cells; a proportion of them may be involved in synthesis and release of immunoglobulins A.

Recirculation was demonstrated by experimental drainage of lymphocytes from a chronic fistula of the thoracic duct. This lymphatic channel collects most of the lymph of the body and returns it to the bloodstream; the thoracic duct lymph contains variable numbers of cells in different mammals (2 to $30 \times 10^3/mm^3$ in man) predominantly represented by small lymphocytes (90 to 95 per cent) (Fig. 13–1A). The remaining cells are large lymphocytes that do not recirculate and possibly represent plasma cell precursors that are released into the blood and later selectively localize in the mucosa of the gut. The output of small lymphocytes from the thoracic duct is sufficient to replace all blood lymphocytes several times daily; thus, since the number of blood lymphocytes remains constant, they must continuously leave the blood at the same rate as they enter it through the thoracic duct.

Prolonged drainage of the thoracic duct lymph causes pronounced lymphopenia and extreme depletion of the lymphocyte population of the spleen, lymph nodes, and gut-associated lymphoid tissue. The bone marrow is not affected; the thymus responds with a decrease in weight, but this effect seems to be nonspecific.

If thoracic duct lymphocytes are recovered, labeled radioactively in vitro, and injected intravenously into a syngeneic recipient, it can be shown that they rapidly leave the bloodstream and localize in the peripheral lymphoid organs. They do not enter either the thymus or the bone marrow. The idea therefore emerged that a pool of small lymphocytes continuously migrate from the blood into the peripheral lymphoid organs and tissues, but leave them again to reenter the blood, either directly or through the lymphatic system. This being true, it should be possible to deplete the recirculating pool by destroying lymphocytes at any point along their migratory pathway. This has been shown to be the case through local irradiation of the hilus of the spleen.

Recirculation is very rapid, as the average transit time of the small lymphocytes through the blood is 0.6 hours; transit time through the spleen is five to six hours, and through the lymph nodes 15 to 20 hours. Recirculating lymphocytes represent a substantial fraction of the body's small lymphocyte population (about half of it in rats); most, if not all, of these cells are long-lived (Fig. 13–1B). Since the blood contains a much higher proportion of short-lived small lymphocytes (30 to 50 per cent in rats) than the thoracic duct lymph, only part of the blood lymphocytes must belong to the recirculating pool. The origin and fate of these short-lived blood lymphocytes are poorly understood. The vast majority of the recirculating lymphocytes belongs to T variety (85 per cent in mice), the remaining being B lymphocytes. These latter

seem to recirculate at a slower rate than T cells and are mobilized with difficulty by prolonged drainage of the thoracic duct lymph, possibly because they are inherently sluggish or because they are somewhat segregated from the main recirculatory pathway.

Drainage of the thoracic duct lymph causes a selective lymphocyte depletion in specific territories of the lymphoid organs and tissues: at the beginning of the experiment, lymphocytes disappear from the deep cortex of the lymph nodes, the central region of the periarterial lymphoid sheaths of the spleen, and the internodular regions of Peyer's patches. These territories are the same that appear devoid of lymphocytes in neonatally thymectomized rodents and which were therefore designated *thymus dependent*. This observation can be explained by the fact that T lymphocytes represent the main component of the recirculating pool and that they are rapidly mobilized from the peripheral lymphoid organs. More prolonged drainage of the thoracic duct lymph leads to lymphocyte depletion of the *thymus-independent* territories of the peripheral lymphoid organs: namely, the superficial cortex and medullary cords of lymph nodes and the peripheral regions of the white pulp of the spleen. This finding may reflect the late mobilization of the recirculating B lymphocytes. The recirculating T and B lymphocytes, labelled in vitro and injected into a syngeneic recipient, localize respectively in the thymus-dependent and thymus-independent (or bursa-dependent) territories of the peripheral lymphoid organs. The mechanism by which recirculating small lymphocytes leave and subsequently reenter the bloodstream in the spleen or leave the blood and enter the lymph in lymph nodes will be discussed in the chapters devoted to these organs (Chapters 15 and 16).

In normal subjects, despite the continuous exchange of lymphocytes between the various districts of the immune system, a steady state is reached that ensures a consistent proportion of T and B lymphocytes in blood, lymph, and major lymphoid organs. Thus, in the mouse, 65 to 85 per cent of the small lymphocytes of the lymph nodes and thoracic duct lymph and 30 to 50 per cent of those in the spleen belong to the T variety. In the human blood, 69 to 82 per cent of the lymphocyte population are T and the remaining 20 to 30 per cent are B lymphocytes. The significance of the recirculation of the small lymphocytes is still open to investigation, but it has been speculated that they represent, at least in part, memory cells "patrolling" the immune system, ready quickly and efficiently to set up a secondary response upon meeting their appropriate antigen.

REFERENCES

SYMPOSIA, JOURNALS, AND BOOKS

In seeking detailed information on lymphocyte physiology, the student should consult a modern textbook of immunology. Topics of current interest on the cells of the immune system are reviewed in specific journals such as *Advances in Immunology* and *Transplantation Reviews*. Additional books and symposia are listed below:

Benacerraf, B., and E. R. Unanue: Textbook of Immunology. Baltimore, Williams and Wilkins, 1984.

Burnet, Sir F. McF.: Cellular Immunology. Melbourne, Australia, Melbourne University Press, 1969.

Cottier, H., N. Odartchenko, R. Schindler, and C. C. Congdon, eds.: Germinal Centers in Immune Responses. New York, Springer, 1967.

Good, R. A., and D. W. Fisher, eds.: Immunobiology. Stamford, CT, Sinauer Associates, 1971.

Lawrence, H. S., and M. Landy: Mediators of Cellular Immunity. New York, Academic Press, 1969.

Roitt, I. M.: Essential Immunology. Oxford, Blackwell, 1980.

Weiss, L.: The Cells and Tissues of the Immune System: Structure, Functions, Interactions. Englewood Cliffs, NJ, Prentice-Hall, 1972.

REVIEWS AND ORIGINAL ARTICLES

Ada, G. L.: Antigen binding cells in tolerance and immunity. Transplant. Rev. 5:105, 1970.

Andersson, J., O. Sjöberg, and G. Möller: Mitogens as probes for immunocyte activation and cellular cooperation. Transplant. Rev. 11:131, 1972.

Aoki, T., U. Hämmerling, E. de Harven, E. A. Boyse, and L. J. Old: Antigenic structure of cell surfaces: an immunoferritin study of the occurrence and topology of H-2, θ, and TL alloantigens on mouse cells. J. Exp. Med. 130:979, 1969.

Attardi, G., M. Cohn, K. Horibata, and E. S. Lennox: Antibody formation by rabbit lymph node cells. II. Further observations on the behavior of single antibody-producing cells with respect to their synthetic capacity and morphology. J. Immunol. 92:346, 1964.

Avrameas, S., and E. H. Leduc: Detection of simultaneous antibody synthesis in plasma cells and specialized lymphocytes in rabbit lymph nodes. J. Exp. Med. 131:1137, 1970.

Balfour, B. M., E. H. Cooper, and E. L. Alpen: Morphological and kinetic studies on antibody-producing cells in rat lymph nodes. Immunology 8:230, 1965.

Baney, R. N., J. J. Vazquez, and F. J. Dixon: Cellular proliferation in relation to antibody synthesis. Proc. Soc. Exp. Biol. Med. 109:1, 1962.

Benacerraf, B., and M. I. Greene: The thymus, transplantation, and immunity. *In* Benacerraf, B., ed.: Immunogenetics and Immune Regulation. Milano, Masson, 1982.

Berenbaum, M. C.: The autoradiographic localization of intracellular antibody. Immunology 2:71, 1959.

Björneboe, M., and H. Gormsen: Experimental studies on the role of plasma cells as antibody producers. Acta Pathol. Microbiol. Scand. 20:649, 1943.

Bussard, A. E., and J. L. Binet: Electron micrography of antibody-producing cells. Nature 205:675, 1965.

Cantor, H., and E. Boyse: Lymphocytes as models for the study of mammalian cellular differentiation. Immunol. Rev. 33:105, 1977.

Carr, I.: The fine structure of the mammalian lymphoreticular system. Int. Rev. Cytol. 27:283, 1970.

Cerottini, J. C., and K. T. Brunner: Cell-mediated cytotoxicity, allograft rejection, and tumor immunity. Adv. Immunol. 18:67, 1974.

Chang, T. S., B. Glick, and A. R. Winter: The significance of the bursa of Fabricius of chickens in antibody production. Poultry Sci. 34:1187, 1955.

Chen, L. T., A. Eden, V. Nussenzweig, and L. Weiss: Electron microscopic study of the lymphocytes capable of binding antigen-antibody-complement complexes. Cell. Immunol. 4:279, 1972.

Clark, S. L., Jr.: The synthesis and storage of protein by isolated lymphoid cells, examined by autoradiography with the electron microscope. Am. J. Anat. 119:375, 1966.

Cohn, Z. A.: The structure and function of monocytes and macrophages. Adv. Immunol. 9:163, 1968.

Coons, A. H.: Some reactions of lymphoid tissues to stimulation by antigens. Harvey Lect. Ser. 53:113, 1957–58.

Coons, A. H., E. H. Leduc, and J. M. Connolly: Studies on antibody production. I. A method for the histochemical demonstration of specific antibody and its application to a study of the hyperimmune rabbit. J. Exp. Med. 102:49, 1955.

Cooper, M. D., R. D. A. Peterson, M. A. South, and R. A. Good: The function of the thymus system and bursa system in the chicken. J. Exp. Med. 123:75, 1966.

Craddock, C. G., R. Longmire, and R. McMillan: Lymphocytes and the immune response. N. Engl. J. Med. 285:324, 378, 1971.

de Petris, S., G. Karlsbad, and B. Pernis: Localization of antibodies in plasma cells by electron microscopy. J. Exp. Med. 117:849, 1963.

Dougherty, T. F., J. H. Chase, and A. White: The demonstration of antibodies in lymphocytes. Proc. Soc. Exp. Biol. Med. 57:295, 1944.

Douglas, S. D.: Human lymphocyte growth *in vitro*: morphologic, biochemical, and immunologic significance. Int. Rev. Exp. Pathol. 10:41, 1971.

Dutton, R. W.: *In vitro* studies of immunological responses of lymphoid cells. Adv. Immunol. 6:253, 1967.

Everett, N. B., and R. W. Tyler: Lymphopoiesis in the thymus and other tissues: functional implications. Int. Rev. Cytol. 22:205, 1967.

Fagraeus, A.: Antibody production in relation to the development of plasma cells; *in vivo* and *in vitro* experiments. Acta Med. Scand. 130(Suppl 204):3, 1948.

Feldman, J. D.: Ultrastructure of immunologic processes. Adv. Immunol. 4:175, 1964.

Fitch, F. W., D. A. Rowley, and S. Coulthard: Ultrastructure of antibody-forming cells. Nature 207:994, 1965.

Ford, W. L., and J. L. Gowans: The traffic of lymphocytes. Sem. Hematol. 6:67, 1969.

Gengozian, N.: Heterotransplantation of human antibody-forming cells in diffusion chambers. Ann. N.Y. Acad. Sci. *120*:91, 1964.

Gowans, J. L.: The effect of the continuous reinfusion of lymph and lymphocytes on the output of lymphocytes from the thoracic duct of unanaesthetized rats. Br. J. Exp. Pathol. *38*:67, 1957.

Gowans, J. L.: The recirculation of lymphocytes from blood to lymph in the rat. J. Physiol. *146*:54, 1959.

Gowans, J. L., and E. J. Knight: The route of recirculation of lymphocytes in the rat. Proc. R. Soc. B *159*:257, 1964.

Green, N. M.: Electron microscopy of the immunoglobulins. Adv. Immunol. *11*:1, 1969.

Gudat, F. G., T. N. Harris, S. Harris, and K. Hummeler: Studies on antibody-producing cells. I. Ultrastructure of 19S and 7S antibody-producing cells. J. Exp. Med. *132*:448, 1970.

Gudat, F. G., T. N. Harris, S. Harris, and K. Hummeler: Studies on antibody-producing cells. II. Appearance of ³H-thymidine-labeled rosette-forming cells. J. Exp. Med. *133*:305, 1971.

Gudat, F. G., T. N. Harris, S. Harris, and K. Hummeler: Studies on antibody-producing cells. III. Identification of young plaque-forming cells by thymidine-³H labeling. J. Exp. Med. *134*:1155, 1971.

Hall, J. G., B. Morris, G. D. Moreno, and M. C. Bessis: The ultrastructure and function of the cells in lymph following antigenic stimulation. J. Exp. Med. *125*:91, 1967.

Harris, S., and T. N. Harris: Influenzal antibodies in lymphocytes of rabbits following the local injection of virus. J. Immunol. *61*:193, 1949.

Harris, T. N., E. Grimm, E. Mertens, and W. E. Ehrich: The role of the lymphocyte in antibody formation. J. Exp. Med. *81*:73, 1945.

Harris, T. N., and S. Harris: The genesis of antibodies. Am. J. Med. *20*:114, 1956.

Harris, T. N., K. Hummeler, and S. Harris: Electron microscopic observations on antibody-producing lymph node cells. J. Exp. Med. *123*:161, 1966.

Holub, M.: Potentialities of the small lymphocyte as revealed by homotransplantation and autotransplantation experiments in diffusion chambers. Ann. N.Y. Acad. Sci. *99*:477, 1962.

Hummeler, K., T. N. Harris, N. Tomassini, M. Hechtel, and M. B. Farber: Electron microscopic observations on antibody-producing cells in lymph and blood. J. Exp. Med. *124*:255, 1966.

Ingraham, J., and A. Bussard: Application of localized hemolysin reaction for specific detection of individual antibody-forming cells. J. Exp. Med. *119*:667, 1964.

Jerne, N. K., and A. A. Nordin: Plaque formation in agar by single antibody-producing cells. Science *140*:405, 1963.

Karnovsky, M. J., E. R. Unanue, and M. Leventhal: Ligand-induced movement of lymphocyte membrane macromolecules. II. Mapping of surface moieties. J. Exp. Med. *136*:907, 1972.

Katz, D. H., and B. Benacerraf: The regulatory influence of activated T cells on B cell responses to antigen. Adv. Immunol. *15*:1, 1972.

Leduc, E. H., S. Avrameas, and M. Bouteille: Ultrastructural localization of antibody in differentiating plasma cells. J. Exp. Med. *127*:109, 1968.

Leduc, E. H., A. H. Coons, and J. M. Connolly: Studies on antibody production. II. The primary and secondary responses in the popliteal lymph node of the rabbit. J. Exp. Med. *102*:61, 1955.

Lin, P. S., A. G. Cooper, and H. H. Wortis: Scanning electron microscopy of human T-cell and B-cell rosettes. N. Engl. J. Med. *289*:548, 1973.

Mäkelä, O., and G. J. V. Nossal: Bacterial adherence: a method for detecting antibody production by single cells. J. Immunol. *87*:447, 1961.

McGregor, D. D., and J. L. Gowans: The antibody response of rats depleted of lymphocytes by chronic drainage from the thoracic duct. J. Exp. Med. *117*:303, 1963.

McIntyre, J. A., and C. W. Pierce: Immune responses *in vitro*. IX. Role of cell clusters. J. Immunol. *111*:1526, 1973.

McMaster, P. D., and S. S. Hudack: The formation of agglutinins within lymph nodes. J. Exp. Med. *61*:783, 1935.

Miller, J. F. A. P., and G. F. Mitchell: Thymus and antigen-reactive cells. Transplant. Rev. *1*:3, 1969.

Millikin, P.: Anatomy of germinal centers in human lymphoid tissue. Arch. Pathol. *82*:499, 1966.

Mills, J. A., and S. R. Cooperband: Lymphocyte physiology. Annu. Rev. Med. *22*:185, 1971.

Mishell, R. I., and R. W. Dutton: Immunization of dissociated spleen cell cultures from normal mice. J. Exp. Med. *126*:423, 1967.

Moore, M. A. S., and J. J. T. Owen: Experimental studies on the development of the bursa of Fabricius. Dev. Biol. *14*:40, 1966.

Moore, M. A. S., and J. J. T. Owen: Experimental studies on the development of the thymus. J. Exp. Med. *126*:715, 1967.

Mosier, D. E., and L. W. Coppleson: A three-cell interaction required for the induction of the primary immune response *in vitro*. Proc. Natl. Acad. Sci. U.S.A. *61*:542, 1968.

Movat, H. Z., and N. V. P. Fernando: The fine structure of lymphoid tissue. Exp. Mol. Pathol. *3*:546, 1964.

Movat, H. Z., and N. V. P. Fernando: The fine structure of the lymphoid tissue during antibody formation. Exp. Mol. Pathol. *4*:155, 1965.

Murphy, M. J., J. B. Hay, B. Morris, and M. C. Bessis: Ultrastructural analysis of antibody synthesis in cells from lymph and lymph nodes. Am. J. Pathol. *66*:25, 1972.

Neil, A. L., and F. J. Dixon: Immunohistochemical detection of antibody in cell-transfer studies. Arch. Pathol. *67*:643, 1959.

Nieuwenhuis, P., and W. L. Ford: Comparative migration of B- and T-lymphocytes in the rat spleen and lymph nodes. Cell. Immunol. *23*:254, 1976.

Nossal, G. J. V.: Antibody production by single cells. III. The histology of antibody production. Br. J. Exp. Pathol. *40*:25, 1959.

Nossal, G. J. V.: Cellular genetics of immune responses. Adv. Immunol. *2*:163, 1962.

Ortega, L. G., and R. C. Mellors: Cellular sites of formation of gamma globulin. J. Exp. Med. *106*:627, 1957.

Perkins, W. D., M. J. Karnovsky, and E. R. Unanue: An ultrastructural study of lymphocytes with surface-bound immunoglobulin. J. Exp. Med. *135*:267, 1972.

Pernis, B., L. Forni, and L. Amante: Immunoglobulin spots on the surface of rabbit lymphocytes. J. Exp. Med. *132*:1001, 1970.

Polliack, A., N. Lampen, B. D. Clarkson, and E. de Harven: Identification of human B and T lymphocytes by scanning electron microscopy. J. Exp. Med. *138*:607, 1973.

Rabellino, E., S. Colon, H. M. Grey, and E. R. Unanue:

Immunoglobulins on the surface of lymphocytes. I. Distribution and quantitation. J. Exp. Med. *133*:156, 1971.

Raff, M. C.: Theta isoantigen as a marker of thymus-derived lymphocytes in mice. Nature *224*:378, 1969.

Raff, M. C.: Two distinct populations of peripheral lymphocytes in mice distinguishable by immuno-fluorescence. Immunology *19*:637, 1970.

Raff, M. C., M. Sternberg, and R. B. Taylor: Immuno-globulin determinants on the surface of mouse lymphoid cells. Nature *255*:553, 1970.

Reiss, E., E. Mertens, and W. E. Ehrich: Agglutination of bacteria by lymphoid cells *in vitro*. Proc. Soc. Exp. Biol. Med. *74*:732, 1950.

Roelants, G.: Antigen recognition by B and T lympho-cytes. Curr. Top. Microbiol. Immunol. *59*:135, 1972.

Saunders, G. C., and W. S. Hammond: Ultrastructural analysis of hemolysin-forming cell clusters. I. Pre-liminary observations. J. Immunol. *105*:1299, 1970.

Sordat, B., M. Sordat, M. W. Hess, R. D. Stoner, and H. Cottier: Specific antibody within lymphoid germinal center cells of mice after primary immunization with horseradish peroxidase: a light and electron micro-scopic study. J. Exp. Med. *131*:77, 1970.

Sprent, J.: Circulating T and B lymphocytes of the mouse. I. Migratory properties. Cell. Immunol. 7:10, 1973.

Sprent, J., and A. Basten: Circulating T and B lympho-cytes of the mouse. II. Lifespan. Cell. Immunol. 7:40, 1973.

Stackpole, C. W., T. Aoki, E. A. Boyse, L. J. Old, J. Lumley-Frank, and E. de Harven: Cell surface an-tigens: serial sectioning of single cells as an approach to topographical analysis. Science *172*:472, 1971.

Steinman, R. M.: Dendritic cells. Transplantation *31*:151, 1981.

Steinman, R. M., and M. C. Nussenzweig: Dendritic cells: features and functions. Immunol. Rev. *53*:127, 1980.

Taylor, R. B., P. H. Duffus, M. C. Raff, and S. de Petris: Redistribution and pinocytosis of lymphocyte sur-face immunoglobulin molecules induced by anti-immunoglobulin antibody. Nature New Biol. *233*:225, 1971.

Tew, J. G., G. J. Thorbecke, and R. M. Steinman: Dendritic cells in the immune response: character-istics and recommended nomenclature (a report from the Reticuloendothelial Society Committee on Nomenclature). J. Reticuloendothel. Soc. *31*:371, 1982.

Uhr, J. W.: Intracellular events underlying synthesis and secretion of immunoglobulin. Cell. Immunol. *1*:228, 1970.

Unanue, E. R.: The regulatory role of macrophages in antigenic stimulation. Adv. Immunol. *15*:95, 1972.

Unanue, E. R.: Cooperation between mononuclear phagocytes and lymphocytes in immunity. N. Engl. J. Med. *303*:977, 1980.

Unanue, E. R., W. D. Perkins, and M. J. Karnovsky: Ligand-induced movement of lymphocyte mem-brane macromolecules. J. Exp. Med. *136*:885, 1972.

Unanue, E. R., W. D. Perkins, and M. J. Karnovsky: Endocytosis by lymphocytes of complexes of anti-Ig with membrane-bound Ig. J. Immunol. *108*:569, 1972.

Urso, P., and T. Makinodan: The roles of cellular division and maturation in the formation of precip-itating antibody. J. Immunol. *90*:897, 1963.

van Furth, R., Z. A. Cohn, J. G. Hirsch, J. H. Humphrey, W. G. Spector, and H. L. Langevoort: The mono-nuclear phagocyte system: a new classification of macrophages, monocytes, and their precursor cells. Bull. WHO *46*:845, 1972.

White, R. G., A. H. Coons, and J. M. Connolly: Studies on antibody production. III. The alum granuloma. J. Exp. Med. *102*:73, 1955.

Wybran, J., and H. H. Fudenberg: Thymus-derived rosette-forming cells. N. Engl. J. Med. *288*:1072, 1973.

Zagury, D., J. W. Uhr, J. D. Jamieson, and G. E. Palade: Immunoglobulin synthesis and secretion. II. Ra-dioautographic studies of sites of addition of car-bohydrate moieties and intracellular transport. J. Cell Biol. *46*:52, 1970.

Zlotnik, A., J. J. Vazquez, and F. J. Dixon: Mitotic activity of immunologically competent lymphoid cells trans-ferred into X-irradiated recipients. Lab. Invest. *11*:493, 1962.

14

THYMUS

Elio Raviola

The thymus is a median organ situated in the superior mediastinum anterior to the great vessels as they emerge from the heart. It extends from the pericardial sac, caudally, to the root of the neck, cranially. It consists of two lobes, arising in the embryo as separate primordia on each side of the midline, but later becoming closely joined by connective tissue. The thymus attains its greatest relative weight at the end of fetal life, but its absolute weight continues to increase, reaching 30 to 40 g at about the time of puberty. It then begins to undergo an involution that progresses rapidly until in the adult the organ becomes largely replaced by adipose cells.

The thymus is the only primary lymphoid organ thus far identified in mammals. It is the first organ to become lymphoid during embryonic life, being seeded by blood-borne stem cells from the yolk sac, which then differentiate into lymphocytes within the special environment of the thymus. Thymic lymphocytes undergo intensive, antigen-independent proliferation. For reasons that are not understood, a portion of them degenerate within the organ, while the remainder enter the bloodstream, populate the peripheral lymphoid organs, and ultimately differentiate into thymus-dependent or T lymphocytes. These are capable of performing a variety of immunological functions that collectively constitute the cellular immune responses, and they also cooperate with B lymphocytes in humoral responses. Germinal centers are lacking in the thymus and there is no antibody production. Although the majority of the thymic lymphocytes have not yet acquired immunological competence, the removal of the organ before the immune system has completed development causes a specific irretrievable impairment of the body's immunological defenses.

HISTOLOGICAL ORGANIZATION

Each thymic lobe is invested by a thin capsule of loose connective tissue and is subdivided by primary connective tissue septa that carry blood vessels into a number of parenchymal lobules that appear polyhedral in shape and are 0.5 to 2 mm in diameter (Fig. 14–1). The thymic lobules are not, however, completely independent of one another. By serial sectioning, one can demonstrate continuity from lobule to lobule via narrow parenchymal bridges. Thus, each lobe of the thymus actually consists of a convoluted parenchymal strand with irregular expansions corresponding to the lobules.

The principal cellular constituents of the thymus are lymphocytes (thymocytes), reticular cells, and a smaller number of macrophages. At the periphery of the lobule, lymphocytes are numerous and densely packed, whereas at the center of the lobule, lymphocytes are fewer in number and reticular cells have more abundant acidophilic cytoplasm. Thus, each lobule comprises a darkly stained, peripheral region, the *cortex*, and a lighter staining central portion, the *medulla* (Figs. 14–1,14–2). Secondary connective tissue septa, carrying blood vessels, extend inward from the surface of the cortex and reach as far as the corticomedullary boundary.

The thymic parenchyma consists of a tridimensional network of stellate reticular cells bounding irregular compartments filled with lymphocytes that are closely aggregated and in direct contact with each other, without intervening connective tissue. This compact cellular mass is comparable to an epithelium or to the brain in its paucity of intercellular substance, but small blood vessels do thread

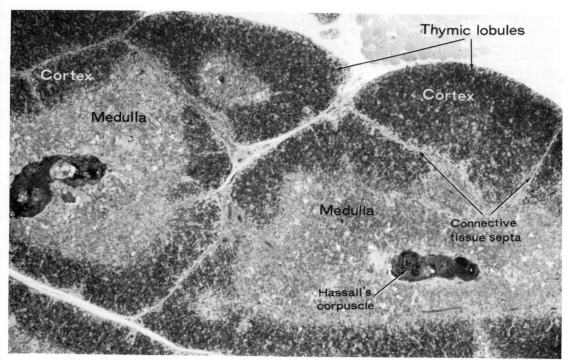

Figure 14–1. Section through the thymus of a guinea pig. The thymic lobes consist of polyhedral lobules separated from each other by connective tissue septa. Each lobule comprises a densely staining peripheral region or cortex and a lighter staining central portion, the medulla. The dark areas in the medulla are Hassall's bodies or corpuscles. Toluidine blue. (Courtesy of G. B. Schneider and S. Clark, Jr.)

their way through it bringing a minimal amount of connective tissue in their adventitia.

The reticular cells of the thymus, like those of the lymph nodes and spleen, are stellate in shape, but their embryonal origin is endodermal instead of mesenchymal. They are in places associated with connective tissue fibers of the reticular type. They occasionally display more obvious epithelial features in the medulla of the lobule, where they may bound cysts or be organized into concentric arrays of squamous epithelial cells, comprising the *Hassall's bodies* or *thymic corpuscles*. The thymic reticulum is often referred to as cytoreticulum, to emphasize the cellular nature of the parenchymal framework of the thymic lobules. Thymic lymphocytes are morphologically indistinguishable from the lymphocytes of the blood, lymph, and peripheral lymphoid organs.

The thymic lobule is a highly dynamic structure. Lymphocytes are continuously produced in the cortex; some of them die and are destroyed by macrophages, others migrate toward the medulla and enter the bloodstream through the walls of the postcapillary venules.

The Cortex

The stellate reticular cells in the cortex have a scanty acidophilic cytoplasm and a large, oval nucleus, 7 to 11 μm in diameter, which is smooth-contoured, is lightly staining, and contains one or two small nucleoli. In electron micrographs (Figs. 14–3,14–4), the processes of the reticular cells are seen to be joined by small desmosomes. Their cytoplasm contains bundles of intermediate filaments, some of which seem to insert on the desmosomes. Their cytoplasmic organelles are unremarkable: sparse mitochondria, a few ribosomes, either free or attached to rare cisternae of the granular endoplasmic reticulum, and a small Golgi apparatus. Membrane-bounded vacuoles that contain a transparent matrix and a variable amount of debris are also found. Although these are scarce in the fetal thymus and in the superficial cortex, they increase in number with age, especially in the deep cortical regions of the lobule. They are probably lysosomes, but their significance is obscure, inasmuch as reticular cells are incapable of phagocytosis.

At the periphery of the cortex (Fig. 14–3) and around the blood vessels, attenuated

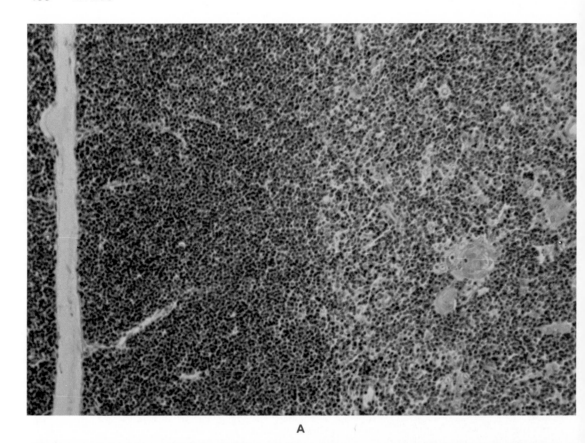

A

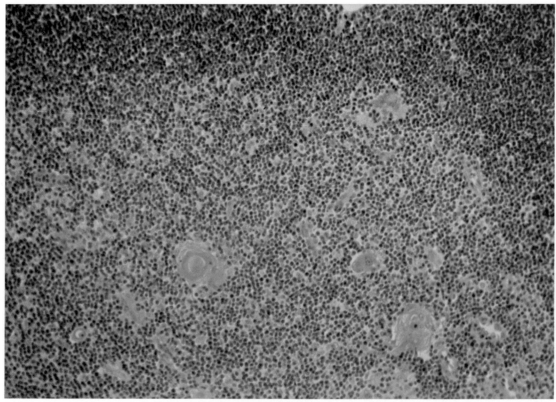

B

Figure 14–2. *See legend on opposite page*

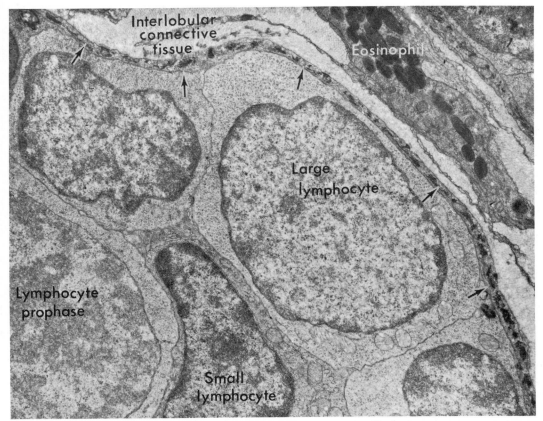

Figure 14–3. Electron micrograph of the periphery of a rat thymic lobule. Large and small lymphocytes are seen in the superficial portion of the cortex. These are separated from the connective tissue of the interlobular septum by a continuous layer of attenuated processes of the reticular cells *(arrows)*. (Courtesy of E. Raviola.)

reticular cell processes form a continuous limiting sheath that separates the thymic parenchyma from the interlobular and adventitial connective tissue. A boundary layer of amorphous material analogous to the basal lamina of epithelia intervenes between this limiting cellular sheath and the connective tissue.

The vast majority of the cell population of the cortex is made up of lymphocytes. These include large, medium-sized, and small forms. The largest lymphocytes have a round or oval nucleus, 9 μm in diameter, rich in euchromatin, and containing one or two prominent nucleoli. The cytoplasm is relatively abundant and strongly basophilic. In electron micrographs (Fig. 14–3), the most prominent feature of the cytoplasm of large lymphocytes is the abundance of free poly-

ribosomes, whereas cisternae of the granular endoplasmic reticulum are exceedingly rare. A diplosome surrounded by a small Golgi apparatus is located near a slight indentation of the nuclear envelope. Mitochondria are few and tend to be grouped near the Golgi apparatus. Multivesicular bodies, small dense granules, and lipid droplets are seen only exceptionally. The small lymphocytes (Fig. 14–4) have a round, darkly staining nucleus, 4 to 5 μm in diameter, with a small nucleolus. The rim of cytoplasm is very thin and contains a few free ribosomes, mostly dispersed as single units. The cytocentrum and associated minute Golgi apparatus slightly indent the nucleus. Mitochondria and granular endoplasmic reticulum are encountered even less often than in large lymphocytes. Occasional multivesicular bodies, a rare lipid

Figure 14–2. Sections through the thymus of monkey. *A,* On left is the cortex of a lobule with densely packed lymphocytes. On right, and in *B,* is the medulla; the lymphocytes are fewer in number and the reticular cells have more abundant acidophilic cytoplasm. The pink, homogenous areas are Hassall's bodies. Hematoxylin-eosin.

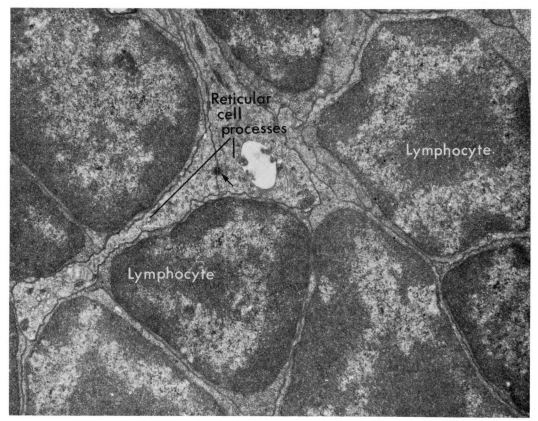

Figure 14–4. Electron micrograph from the deep cortex of a rat thymic lobule, showing among the crowded small lymphocytes two reticular cell processes joined by a desmosome *(at arrow)*. (Courtesy of E. Raviola.)

droplet, and small dense granules complete the list of cytoplasmic organelles. Large and small lymphocytes are at the extremes of a continuous spectrum of cells displaying intermediate gradations of nuclear and cytoplasmic organization. Consistent features of cortical lymphocytes are their smooth surface contour and their polyhedral shape, due to mutual deformation.

Large lymphocytes make up only a small proportion of the lymphoid population of the lobule and tend to be concentrated at the periphery of the cortex; progressively smaller forms are found in increasing number toward the center of the lobule, and the deep cortex consists chiefly of tightly packed small lymphocytes. Both dividing and degenerating lymphocytes are commonly found in the cortex. Mitoses are more frequent at the periphery of the lobule, whereas degenerating cells with pyknotic nuclei are most abundant in the deep cortical areas.

The macrophages represent a minor but consistent component of the cell population of the cortex. They are scattered throughout the cortex, and in most mammals except the mouse, they increase in number at the boundary region between the cortex and the medulla. With the light microscope, they are distinguished from reticular cells with some difficulty, but with the electron microscope, they can be easily recognized by their lack of desmosomes and the presence within the cytoplasm of phagocytized lymphocytes or the remnants of their digestion. The cells that have been described by light microscopists as containing PAS-positive inclusions are actually macrophages loaded with residual bodies.

A few plasma cells are present within the parenchyma and the interstitial connective tissue of the involuting thymus. They occur at the extreme periphery of the cortex and along the blood vessels; their significance is not known. Mast cells may also be found, but they are mainly extralobular.

The Medulla

In the medulla, the reticular cells are extremely pleomorphic. In some areas they maintain a stellate shape and contain numerous bundles of intermediate filaments (Fig. 14–5); in other areas, they are much larger and have a pale cytoplasm and myriad cytoplasmic processes. Some of them contain granules of unknown nature; others are filled with vacuoles. Some are rounded; others are flattened and wrapped around one another, giving rise to the structures known as thymic corpuscles or Hassall's bodies (Fig. 14–6). These may reach 100 μm or more in diameter, and consist of a concentric array of squamous cells joined by many desmosomes and containing keratohyalin granules and conspicuous bundles of cytoplasmic filaments. The cells in the central part of a Hassall's corpuscle may degenerate or become calcified.

Lymphocytes are much less abundant than in the cortex and are predominantly of the small variety. They also differ from cortical small lymphocytes in their irregular shape and have a somewhat greater amount of cytoplasm containing relatively few ribosomes.

Macrophages are only rarely found in the medulla of the thymus. Granulocytes, especially eosinophils, may be found in small numbers. Plasma cells are absent from the medulla.

The significance of the pleomorphism of reticular cells in the medulla is not understood. It may well represent an abnormal, local response of the thymic reticulum to the loss of surface relationships with the lymphocytes.

In the thymus of nonmammalian vertebrates, especially reptiles and birds (and also rarely in mammals), the medulla of the thymic lobules displays an extraordinary congeries of seemingly extraneous components, such as striated muscle cells (Hammar's myoid cells); cysts lined by epithelial cells provided with a brush border or with cilia;

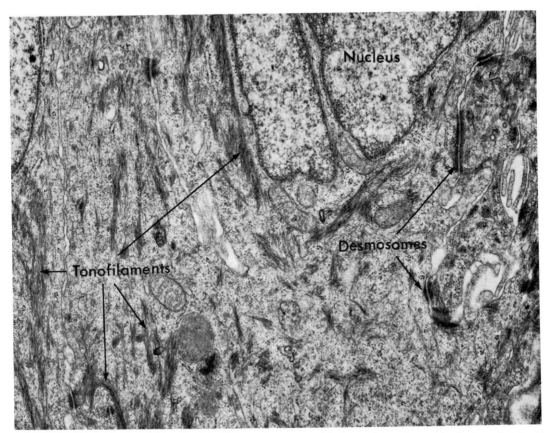

Figure 14–5. Electron micrograph from the medulla of rat thymus, showing portions of several reticular cells joined by desmosomes and containing conspicuous bundles of tonofilaments. (Courtesy of E. Raviola.)

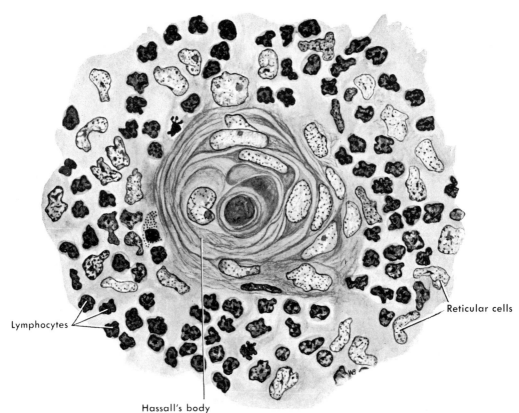

Figure 14–6. Hassall's body in the medulla of the thymus of an 8-year-old boy. It consists of a concentric array of squamous reticular cells. Eosin-azure.

mucus-secreting cells; and reticular cells with large vacuoles lined by microvilli. It is not clear whether these unusual constituents have functional significance or are simply embryonic rests or errors of differentiation.

Germinal centers may appear in the medullary region of the lobules as a consequence of certain diseases for which an autoimmune pathogenesis has been postulated.

Vessels and Nerves

The arteries supplying the thymus arise from the internal thoracic arteries and their mediastinal and pericardiacophrenic branches. They ramify in the interlobular connective tissue, and their ultimate subdivisions follow the secondary connective tissue septa, which extend inward from the surface of the lobules; thus, they penetrate the lobule at the corticomedullary boundary, without coursing through the cortex. The arterioles, following the boundary between cortex and medulla, give off capillaries that ascend into the cortex, joined to each other by collateral anastomoses. At the periphery of the cortex, but still within the cortical parenchyma, the capillaries form a network of branching and anastomosing arcades and turn back toward the interior of the lobule. In their recurrent course through the cortex, the capillaries join to form larger vessels, which can still be classified as capillaries on the basis of their fine structure. These vessels are confluent with postcapillary venules at the corticomedullary boundary and in the medulla. As an exception to this basic pattern, capillaries may leave the periphery of the cortex and join superficial veins coursing within the interlobular connective tissue. The postcapillary venules of the corticomedullary boundary and medulla leave the thymic parenchyma via the secondary connective tissue septa and join to form interlobular veins. The majority of these are ultimately drained by a single thymic vein, a tributary of the left brachiocephalic vein.

Because of the peculiar arrangement of the parenchymal blood vessels, the various segments of the vascular tree appear to be spatially segregated within the lobules, the cortex being exclusively supplied by capillaries, and the corticomedullary boundary and the medulla also containing arterioles and venules. There is very little movement of macromolecules from blood to thymic parenchyma across the capillary walls in the cortex (Fig. 14–7), whereas the large medullary vessels are highly permeable to substances in the plasma. Thus, only the lymphoid population of the cortex is protected from the influence of circulating macromolecules. This is the structural basis for the so-called *blood-thymus barrier* to antigens.

Great numbers of lymphocytes enter the bloodstream by traversing the walls of the postcapillary venules of the corticomedullary junction and those of the medulla. The endothelium of these venules is low, in contrast to the cuboidal endothelium of the postcapillary venules of lymph nodes. It must be noted, however, that in lymph nodes lymphocytes migrate in the opposite direction, namely from blood to parenchyma.

Lymphatics are found in the connective tissue septa, but they seem to be lacking within the lobular parenchyma; their lymph is drained by the sternal, tracheobronchial, and anterior mediastinal nodes.

The thymus receives branches from the vagus and sympathetic nerves. Sympathetic fibers are distributed to the blood vessels, but the manner of termination of the vagal fibers is unknown.

Histogenesis

In man, the thymus arises from an outgrowth of the endodermal lining of the third branchial pouch on each side of the midline; the fourth branchial pouch often gives rise to some thymic tissue. The primordium has a cleftlike lumen continuous with that of the embryonic pharynx and a wall composed of several layers of columnar epithelium. The lumen disappears as the endodermal bud proliferates, giving rise to solid epithelial outgrowths that invade the surrounding mesenchyme. Round, basophilic cells have been described in the mesenchyme surrounding the thymic rudiment at very early stages of development.

The two separate primordia, after considerable elongation caudally and medially, meet in the midline in embryos of about eight weeks and acquire a common mesenchymal investment. At about the same time, lymphocytes appear within the epithelium. Studies using both the chromosomal marker technique and antisera to surface antigens on thymic lymphocytes have clearly shown that the blood-borne stem cells originating from the yolk sac in the embryo migrate into the thymic primordium and there differentiate into lymphocytes. These subsequently increase in number, blood vessels penetrate the rudiment, and the parenchyma is gradually converted into a meshwork of stellate cells of endodermal origin attached by desmosomes and bounding a labyrinthine system of spaces occupied by proliferating lymphocytes. The medulla arises relatively late in the deep region of the lobules, by disappearance of many lymphocytes and an enlargement of the reticular cells.

In man, the thymus is the first organ of the immune system in which lymphocytes appear, and it continues to be the most active lymphocytopoietic tissue of the body throughout embryonal life. The rate of growth of the thymus, when expressed in relation to the body weight, levels off at the beginning of the third fetal trimester; a gradual decline follows, which is already perceptible at birth, and continues thereafter. In laboratory rodents, on the other hand, the thymus continues to grow until the second week of postnatal life.

NORMAL, ACCIDENTAL, AND EXPERIMENTAL INVOLUTION

The thymus undergoes a slow physiological process of involution with age; lymphocyte production declines, the cortex becomes thinner, and the parenchyma shrinks and becomes replaced by adipose tissue, which is thought to arise from precursors in the interlobular connective tissue. It is generally assumed that the onset of this normal process of *age involution* is coincidental with puberty, but if relative reduction of the cortical parenchyma is taken as an index of declining functional activity, age involution in humans actually begins in early childhood. In adults, the thymus is transformed into a mass of adipose tissue, containing scattered islands of parenchyma consisting mainly of enlarged reticular cells. The parenchyma, however, does not disappear completely, even in old age. Moreover, experiments involving thymectomy in adult rodents that have been deprived of their lymphoid population show that the thymus maintains its functional com-

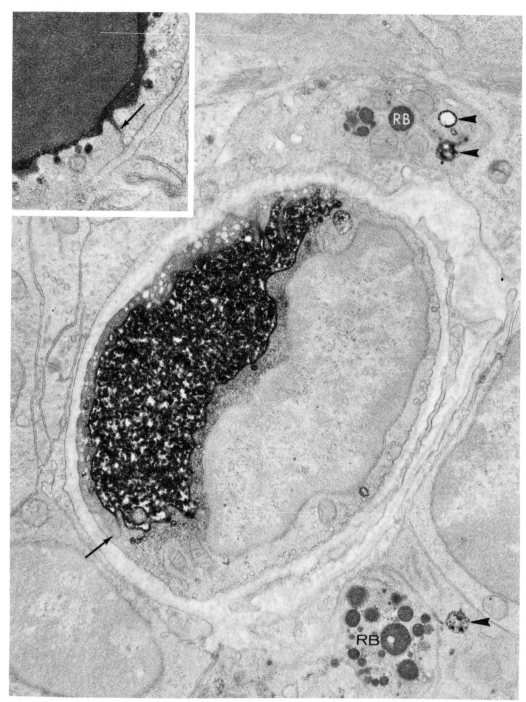

Figure 14–7. Cortical capillary in the mouse thymus. When horseradish peroxidase (molecular weight, 40,000 daltons) is injected as a tracer into the bloodstream, its progression along the intercellular clefts of the capillary endothelium is blocked by an impermeable tight junction *(arrow)*. Very little tracer is transported across the endothelium by micropinocytotic vesicles, and this is readily sequestrated by perivascular macrophages *(arrowheads)*. *RB,* residual bodies. *Inset.* In addition, a much smaller molecule, such as cytochrome *c* (molecular weight, 12,000 daltons), is arrested by the interendothelial junctions *(arrow)*. (From Raviola, E., and M. J. Karnovsky. J. Exp. Med. *136*:466, 1972.)

petence throughout life and can reacquire full lymphocytopoietic capacity. The same may be true in man, although it has not been demonstrated.

The process of gradual age involution can be complicated or accelerated by acute involutional changes constituting the so-called *accidental involution,* which occurs in response to a wide variety of stimuli, such as disease, severe stress, dietary deficiencies, ionizing radiation, injection of colloidal substances, bacterial endotoxin, adrenocorticotrophic hormone, and adrenal and gonadal steroids. Under these conditions, the thymus rapidly diminishes in size, primarily because of massive death of cortical small lymphocytes and their destruction by macrophages. Medullary lymphocytes are less sensitive, so that the usual pattern of the lobule, with a densely staining cortex and a lighter medulla, may be reversed. Acute involution in experimental animals is followed by intensive regeneration, so that the thymus rapidly returns to its former size.

HISTOPHYSIOLOGY

The thymus is essential to the development of the class of lymphocytes that is responsible for cellular or cell-mediated immunological responses, i.e., homograft rejection, delayed cutaneous reactions to protein antigens (delayed hypersensitivity), immune attack of a nonresponsive host (graft-versus-host reaction), and immune response to fungi, facultative intracellular bacteria, and certain viruses. Thymus-dependent lymphocytes do not release conventional antibody, but act as helper cells in humoral responses. All these functions are carried out by lymphocytes that are circulating in the blood and lymph or residing in the spleen, lymph nodes, and connective tissues of the body. The vast majority of the lymphocytes located in the thymus are functionally inert. There is evidence that thymic lymphocytes become immunocompetent when they move into the blood or peripheral lymphoid organs, but the mechanism triggering this further differentiation is unknown. Thus, the thymic lymphocyte or thymocyte must be regarded as a type of cell functionally distinct from the peripheral thymus-dependent (T) lymphocyte, but it represents the immature precursor of the latter.

Much of the current knowledge on the functions of the thymus began with experiments in rodents involving thymectomy at a critical stage of the development of the immune system. The removal of the thymus in adult animals has but little effect on peripheral lymphocyte populations or immune responsiveness, but in newborn rodents, thymectomy causes lymphocytopenia, marked decrease in the population of long-lived recirculating lymphocytes, impairment of cellular immune reactions, and severe depression of those antibody responses requiring the cooperative participation of the thymus-dependent lymphocyte. The inner cortex of the lymph nodes and the periarterial lymphoid sheaths in the spleen fail to develop, but plasmacytopoiesis and germinal center formation are not affected.

In neonatal rodents, the thymus has completed development, but the peripheral population of thymus-dependent lymphocytes has not yet been established. The appearance of this population is therefore prevented by removal of the thymus. Once the periphery has become populated with T lymphocytes, thymectomy is no longer followed by a dramatic deficiency of cellular immune responses, unless the peripheral stock of thymus-dependent lymphocytes is destroyed by sublethal, total body irradiation. A notable exception to this rule is represented by *suppressor T cells,* which are short-lived and continuously generated in the adult thymus. Adult thymectomy therefore abolishes T-cell suppressor functions, whereas helper, lymphokine-producing, and cytolytic T lymphocytes can only be depleted by neonatal thymectomy. In other mammals, including man, the immune system is fully mature at birth and less dependent on the integrity of the thymus.

In neonatally thymectomized rodents, the immunological defect can be corrected by grafting a thymus or injecting lymph node or spleen cells. Injection of thymic cell suspensions, on the other hand, is relatively ineffective, probably because very few mature lymphocytes are present in the thymus. Experiments in animals that were thymectomized, irradiated, "reconstituted" with bone marrow cells bearing a chromosomal marker, and grafted with an unmarked thymus have shown that the original lymphocyte population of the grafted thymus is replaced by a new population of cells bearing the bone marrow karyotype; this provides further evidence that the lymphocyte population of the thymus arises from immigration and differentiation of blood-borne stem cell precursors, arising in this instance from the bone marrow.

Two possible explanations exist for the results of the reconstitution experiments. (1) The thymus may provide stem cell precursors immigrating from the embryonic yolk sac or postnatal marrow with a uniquely favorable environment for differentiation into peripheral, thymus-dependent lymphocytes. The thymus would therefore seed the immune system with lymphocytes capable of expressing the thymus-dependent immune functions. (2) Alternatively, the thymus may produce one or more factors that act at the periphery on stem cell precursors, triggering their differentiation into thymus-dependent lymphocytes. Whereas little doubt exists that the thymus seeds the peripheral lymphoid organs with lymphocytes, no definitive evidence is available so far that thymic factors are released into the circulation and act on a peripheral target.

Once stem cells have migrated into the thymus, they differentiate into thymic lymphocytes, possibly under local inductive influences, and begin a sustained proliferation. At the peak of its activity, which corresponds to the perinatal period in laboratory rodents, the thymus has the highest rate of lymphocyte production in the whole immune system. Larger lymphocytes proliferate in the superficial cortex and give rise to generations of smaller cells that accumulate in the deep cortical areas of the lobule. This lymphocyte proliferation does not depend on antigen stimulation, in contrast with the situation in peripheral lymphoid organs. However, the mechanism controlling the rate of lymphocyte production is unknown.

The intrathymic life span of the newly formed small lymphocytes has been shown to be very short (two to three days). It follows that lymphocytes either die within the organ or migrate out of the thymus. Lymphocyte death does occur in the cortex, and these cells are disposed of by macrophages. The extent of this cell death and its physiological significance are not understood. However, evidence coming from autoradiographic and chromosome marker labeling, from experiments involving thymectomy, and from lymphocyte counts in arterial and thymic venous blood shows that a proportion of the thymic lymphocytes do migrate from the cortex to the medulla of the lobule and there enter the bloodstream through the walls of the postcapillary venules.

The lymphocytes that leave the thymus "home in" to the so-called thymus-dependent regions of the peripheral lymphoid organs, namely, the inner cortex of lymph nodes, the periarterial lymphoid sheaths of the spleen, and the internodular areas of the tonsils, appendix, and Peyer's patches. All these regions represent the portal of entry of blood-borne lymphocytes into the peripheral stations of the immune system and the sites in which the thymus-dependent lymphocytes are preferentially concentrated.

Although the vast majority of thymocytes are not immunocompetent, a small proportion of them seem to be capable of transformation upon interaction with phytohemagglutinin or allogeneic cells. These lymphocytes are less sensitive to x-ray irradiation and to the cytolytic effect of adrenal steroids, and they have therefore been identified with the lymphocytes located in the medulla of the lobule. These observations seem to suggest that the small lymphocytes of the cortex of the lobule are functionally inert and acquire immunological competence as they migrate to the medulla.

Indirect evidence supporting this hypothesis comes from a growing body of animal experiments with antisera to surface antigens on the thymic or thymus-derived lymphocytes. In the mouse, thymus lymphocytes possess membrane constituents, such as the *Thy-1, TL, GIX, and Ly antigens*, which can be detected by immunological methods; their significance is poorly understood, but they can be usefully employed as cell markers for investigating cell interactions, differentiation, and migration. Stem cells lack these surface antigens; as they move into the thymus and differentiate into thymic lymphocytes or thymocytes, they acquire the Thy-1, TL, GIX, and Ly 1,2 surface antigens. Upon migration out of the thymus and differentiation into peripheral T cells, the Thy-1 antigen decreases in amount on the lymphocyte surface, TL and GIX disappear altogether, and Ly 1,2 persists on about 50 per cent of the peripheral T lymphocytes. Ly $+1,+2$ lymphocytes undergo further differentiation at the periphery into Ly $+1,-2$ cells, which can either express helper function or produce lymphokines, and into Ly $-1,+2$ cells, which can express either cytolytic or suppressor functions. From these studies the hypothesis has emerged that the differentiation of thymic lymphocytes into peripheral, thymus-dependent lymphocytes consists of an orderly succession of maturational steps: first, undifferentiated stem cell precursors of yolk sac or bone marrow origin enter the thymus and differentiate into thymic lymphocytes. These proliferate in the cortex, then move to the medulla and acquire immunocompetence either at the very moment of leaving the organ or after they have entered the bloodstream through the wall of the postcapillary venules.

It was reported that immunological responsiveness can be partially restored in thymectomized animals by grafts of thymus enclosed in chambers that are permeable to molecules but not to cells. In addition, active factors were isolated, which simulate the function of the thymus both in vivo and in vitro, and were variously called *thymosin, thymopoietin, thymic humoral factor,* and *thymic serum factor* (FTS). Of these, FTS was characterized biochemically as a nonapeptide 847 daltons in molecular weight and localized in the thymic reticular cells by immunocytochemistry. It has been claimed that these factors are actually hormones and that the thymus exerts its functions on the immune system by releasing them into the bloodstream as an endocrine gland. The evidence supporting this view is controversial, however, and it seems more likely that the various thymic factors act within the organ as mediators of short-range cellular interactions.

REFERENCES

Abe, K., and T. Ito: Fine structure of small lymphocytes in the thymus of the mouse: qualitative and quantitative analysis by electron microscopy. Z. Zellforsch. *110*:321, 1970.

Bach, J. F., and M. Dardenne: Studies on thymus products. II. Demonstration and characterization of a circulating thymic hormone. Immunology *25*:353, 1973.

Bargmann, W.: Der Thymus. *In* von Mollendorff, W., and Bargmann, W. (eds.): Handbuch der Mikroskopischen Anatomie des Menschen. Vol. 6, Part 4. Berlin, Julius Springer, 1943.

Benacerraf, B., and M. I. Greene: The thymus, transplantation, and immunity. *In* Benacerraf, B., ed.: Immunogenetics and Immune Regulation. Milano, Masson, 1982.

Blomgren, H., and B. Andersson: Evidence for a small pool of immunocompetent cells in the mouse thymus. Exp. Cell Res. *57*:185, 1969.

Cantor, H., and E. Boyse: Lymphocytes as models for the study of mammalian cellular differentiation. Immunol. Rev. *33*:105, 1977.

Cantor, H., M. A. Mandel, and R. Asofsky: Studies of thoracic duct lymphocytes of mice. II. A quantitative comparison of the capacity of thoracic duct lymphocytes and other lymphoid cells to induce graft-versus-host reactions. J. Immunol. *104*:409, 1970.

Claman, H. N., and F. H. Brunstetter: The response of cultured human thymus cells to phytohemagglutinin. J. Immunol. *100*:1127, 1968.

Claman, H. N., and F. H. Brunstetter: Effects of antilymphocyte serum and phytohemagglutinin upon cultures of human thymus and peripheral blood lymphoid cells. I. Morphologic and biochemical studies of thymus and blood lymphoid cells. Lab. Invest. *18*:757, 1968.

Clark, S. L., Jr.: The thymus in mice of strain 129/J studied with the electron microscope. Am. J. Anat. *112*:1, 1963.

Clark, S. L., Jr.: Incorporation of sulfate by the mouse thymus: its relation to secretion by medullary epithelial cells and to thymic lymphopoiesis. J. Exp. Med. *128*:927, 1968.

Cohen, M. W., G. J. Thorbecke, G. M. Hochwald, and E. B. Jacobson: Induction of graft-versus-host reaction in newborn mice by injection of newborn or adult homologous thymus cells. Proc. Soc. Exp. Biol. Med. *114*:242, 1963.

Colley, D. G., A. Malakian, and B. H. Waksman: Cellular differentiation in the thymus. II. Thymus-specific antigens in rat thymus and peripheral lymphoid cells. J. Immunol. *104*:585, 1970.

Colley, D. G., A. Y. Shih Wu, and B. H. Waksman: Cellular differentiation in the thymus. III. Surface properties of rat thymus and lymph node cells separated on density gradients. J. Exp. Med. *132*:1107, 1970.

Dardenne, M., and J. F. Bach: Studies on thymus products. I. Modification of rosette-forming cells by thymic extracts. Determination of the target RFC subpopulation. Immunology *25*:343, 1973.

Davies, A. J. S., E. Leuchars, V. Wallis, R. Marchant, and E. V. Elliott: The failure of thymus-derived cells to produce antibody. Transplantation *5*:222, 1967.

Defendi, V., and D. Metcalf, eds.: The Thymus. The Wistar Institute Symposium, Monograph No. 2. Philadelphia, Wistar Institute Press, 1964.

Doenhoff, M. J., A. J. S. Davies, E. Leuchars, and V. Wallis: The thymus and circulating lymphocytes of mice. Proc. R. Soc. B *176*:69, 1970.

Ernström, U., and B. Larsson: Thymic export of lymphocytes 3 days after labelling with tritiated thymidine. Nature *222*:279, 1969.

Ford, W. L., and J. L. Gowans: The traffic of lymphocytes. Semin. Hematol. *6*:67, 1969.

Goldschneider, I., and D. D. McGregor: Migration of lymphocytes and thymocytes in the rat. I. The route of migration from blood to spleen and lymph nodes. J. Exp. Med. *127*:155, 1968.

Goldstein, A. L., F. D. Slater, and A. White: Preparation, assay, and partial purification of a thymic lymphocytopoietic factor (thymosin). Proc. Natl. Acad. Sci. U.S.A. *56*:1010, 1966.

Good, R. A., and A. E. Gabrielsen, eds.: The Thymus in Immunobiology. New York, Hoeber Medical Division, Harper & Row, 1964.

Haelst, U. van: Light and electron microscopic study of the normal and pathological thymus of the rat. I. The normal thymus. Z. Zellforsch. 77:534, 1967.

Hoshino, T., M. Takeda, K. Abe, and T. Ito: Early development of thymic lymphocytes in mice, studied by light and electron microscopy. Anat. Rec. 164:47, 1969.

Ishidate, M., and D. Metcalf: The pattern of lymphopoiesis in the mouse thymus after cortisone administration or adrenalectomy. Aust. J. Exp. Biol. Med. Sci. 41:637, 1963.

Izard, J.: Ultrastructure of the thymic reticulum in guinea pig. Cytological aspects of the problem of the thymic secretion. Anat. Rec. 155:117, 1966.

Kennedy, J. C., L. Siminovitch, J. E. Till, and E. A. McCulloch: A transplantation assay for mouse cells responsive to antigenic stimulation by sheep erythrocytes. Proc. Soc. Exp. Biol. Med. 120:868, 1965.

Leckband, E., and E. A. Boyse: Immunocompetent cells among mouse thymocytes: a minor population. Science 172:1258, 1971.

Lundin, P. M., and U. Schelin: Ultrastructure of the rat thymus. Acta Pathol. Microbiol. Scand. 65:379, 1965.

Mandel, T.: The development and structure of Hassall's corpuscles in the guinea pig. Z. Zellforsch. 89:180, 1968.

Mandel, T.: Ultrastructure of epithelial cells in the cortex of guinea pig thymus. Z. Zellforsch. 92:159, 1968.

Miller, H. C., S. K. Schmiege, and A. Rule: Production of functional T cells after treatment of bone marrow with thymic factor. J. Immunol. 111:1005, 1973.

Miller, J. F. A. P., and P. Dukor: Die Biologie des Thymus nach dem Heutigen Stande der Forschung. Basel, Karger, 1964.

Miller, J. F. A. P., and D. Osoba: Current concepts of the immunological function of the thymus. Physiol. Rev. 47:437, 1967.

Mitchell, G. F., and J. F. A. P. Miller: Immunological activity of thymus and thoracic-duct lymphocytes. Proc. Natl. Acad. Sci. U.S.A. 59:296, 1968.

Moore, M. A. S., and J. J. T. Owen: Experimental studies on the development of the thymus. J. Exp. Med. 126:715, 1967.

Murray, R. G., A. Murray, and A. Pizzo: The fine structure of the thymocytes of young rats. Anat. Rec. 151:17, 1965.

Order, S. E., and B. H. Waksman: Cellular differentiation in the thymus. Changes in size, antigenic character, and stem cell function of thymocytes during thymus repopulation following irradiation. Transplantation 8:783, 1969.

Owen, J. J. T., and M. C. Raff: Studies on the differentiation of thymus-derived lymphocytes. J. Exp. Med. 132:1216, 1970.

Owen, J. J. T., and M. A. Ritter: Tissue interaction in the development of thymus lymphocytes. J. Exp. Med. 129:431, 1969.

Parrott, D. M. V., M. A. B. de Sousa, and J. East: Thymus-dependent areas in the lymphoid organs of neonatally thymectomized mice. J. Exp. Med. 123:191, 1966.

Raff, M. C.: Evidence for subpopulation of mature lymphocytes within mouse thymus. Nature New Biol. 229:182, 1971.

Raviola, E., and M. J. Karnovsky: Evidence for a bloodthymus barrier using electron-opaque tracers. J. Exp. Med. 136:466, 1972.

Raviola, E., and G. Raviola: Striated muscle cells in the thymus of reptiles and birds: an electron microscopic study. Am. J. Anat. 121:623, 1967.

Sainte-Marie, G., and F. S. Peng: Emigration of thymocytes from the thymus: a review and study of the problem. Rev. Can. Biol. 30:51, 1971.

Sanel, F. T.: Ultrastructure of differentiating cells during thymus histogenesis. Z. Zellforsch. 83:8, 1967.

Schwarz, M. R.: Transformation of rat small lymphocytes with allogeneic lymphoid cells. Am. J. Anat. 121:559, 1967.

Small, M., and N. Trainin: Contribution of a thymic humoral factor to the development of an immunologically competent population from cells of mouse bone marrow. J. Exp. Med. 134:786, 1971.

Warner, N. L.: The immunological role of different lymphoid organs in the chicken. II. The immunological competence of thymic cell suspensions. Aust. J. Exp. Biol. Med. Sci. 42:401, 1964.

Weber, W. T.: Difference between medullary and cortical thymic lymphocytes of the pig in their response to phytohemagglutinin. J. Cell Physiol. 68:117, 1966.

Weiss, L.: The Cells and Tissues of the Immune System. Structure, Functions, Interactions. Englewood Cliffs, NJ, Prentice-Hall, 1972.

Weissman, I. L.: Thymus cell migration. J. Exp. Med. 126:291, 1967.

Williams, R. M., A. D. Chanana, E. P. Cronkite, and B. H. Waksmann: Antigenic markers on cells leaving calf thymus by way of the efferent lymph and venous blood. J. Immunol. 106:1143, 1971.

Winkelstein, A., and C. G. Craddock: Comparative response of normal human thymus and lymph node cells to phytohemagglutinin in culture. Blood 29:594, 1967.

Wolstenholme, G. E. W., and R. Porter, eds.: The Thymus: Experimental and Clinical Studies. Ciba Foundation Symposium. Boston, Little, Brown & Co., 1966.

15

LYMPH NODES

Elio Raviola

Lymph nodes are small organs occurring in series along the course of lymphatic vessels. Their parenchyma consists of a highly organized accumulation of lymphoid tissue, which recognizes antigenic materials in the lymph that percolates through the node, and builds up against them a specific immune reaction. Lymph nodes are also very rich in macrophages, which clear the lymph of undesirable cells, invading microorganisms, and other particulate matter.

Large numbers of lymph nodes occur, usually in groups, scattered throughout the prevertebral region, along the large blood vessels of the thoracic and abdominal cavities, between the leaves of the mesentery, and in the loose connective tissue of the neck, axilla, and groin. They are commonly flattened and ovoid or reniform in shape, varying from 1 to 25 mm in diameter, with a slight indentation, the *hilus,* where blood vessels enter or leave the organ. In most mammals, as *afferent lymphatic vessels* approach the node they give rise to a number of branches that enter the node at multiple sites over its convex surface (Fig. 15–1). A smaller number of *efferent lymphatic vessels* leave the node at the hilus. The afferent vessels are provided with valves that open toward the node, whereas the valves of the efferent lymphatics point away from the hilus. This arrangement of valves ensures unidirectional lymph flow through the node.

Lymph nodes vary somewhat in their structure from species to species, but their variation in appearance within species depends primarily upon their state of activity. In a healthy subject, each lymph node reflects in its organization both the background activity of the immune system as a whole and the local response of the node to small amounts of antigens reaching it from the body territory drained by its afferent lymphatics. Resting lymph nodes therefore show pronounced structural differences according to their location in the body. Extreme examples are, on the one hand, the small, poorly developed popliteal node of unstimulated laboratory rodents and, on the other hand, the highly organized human mesenteric nodes, which are continuously bombarded by a variety of antigens of intestinal origin. If, however, microorganisms or a high dose of any foreign macromolecule is injected subcutaneously, or if a foreign tissue is transplanted into the body, the lymph nodes draining the site of injection or grafting undergo profound structural changes typical of an acute primary or secondary immune response.

HISTOLOGICAL ORGANIZATION

The lymph node consists basically of a parenchymal mass of lymphoid tissue, traversed by specialized lymph vessels or *sinuses* (Figs. 15–1, 15–2). Its collagenous framework consists of a *capsule,* which invests the whole organ, but which is greatly thickened at the hilus. From the capsule a variable number of branching connective tissue *trabeculae* extend into the substance of the node. The lymphoid parenchyma between the trabeculae is supported by a tridimensional network of reticular fibers with associated reticular cells. The meshes of this network are filled with lymphocytes, plasma cells, and macrophages. The lymph sinuses are irregular channels transformed into a labyrinth of intercommunicating chambers by a loose network of tissue strands that traverse their lumen.

Under low magnification, the sectioned lymph node is seen to have an outer, densely staining *cortex* and an inner, paler *medulla.* The difference in appearance of these two regions is due mainly to differences in num-

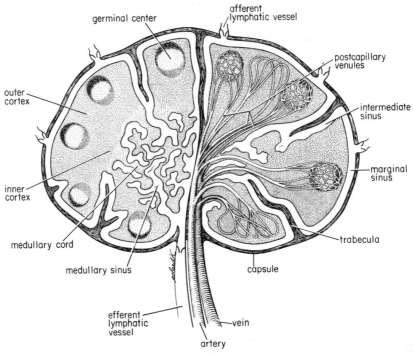

Figure 15–1. Diagram of lymph node. Blood supply is depicted on right side.

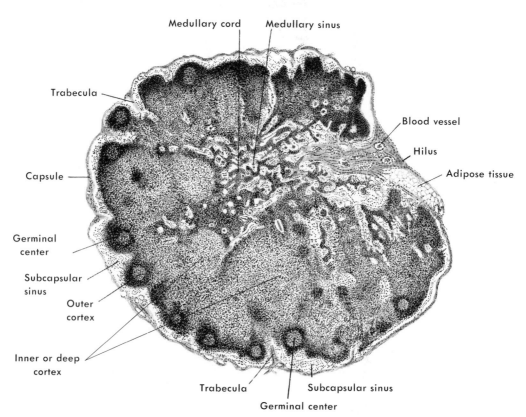

Figure 15–2. Section through small jugular lymph node of man. (Redrawn and slightly modified from Sobotta.)

ber, diameter, and arrangement of the lymph sinuses. The relative amounts of cortical and medullary substance and their distribution vary within wide limits. The nodes of the abdominal cavity are especially rich in medullary substance. The cortical substance in some nodes may surround the medulla completely, but in others the medullary substance may border directly on the capsule for long distances. In some cases the medulla and cortex may accumulate at opposite poles of the node. In the pig, the "cortical" substance is collected in the central portion of the node, while "medullary" tissue is located at the periphery. In the ox, the cortex is extensively compartmentalized by numerous trabeculae, whereas in man trabeculae are poorly developed and the cortex appears as a diffuse, continuous mass. The trabeculae are prominent in large lymph nodes, but in small nodes they are thin and frequently interrupted.

Nodes deep in the body, as in the abdominal cavity, are distinguished by the relatively poor development of their trabeculae compared with that of the more peripheral nodes. In some cases, a hilus may be absent; in others, it is highly developed, with its connective tissue penetrating far into the node and partitioning it extensively.

Lymph Sinuses

The afferent lymphatic vessels approach the convex surface of the node, pierce its capsule obliquely, and open into the *marginal* or *subcapsular sinus* (Figs. 15–3, 15–4). This is not a cylindrical channel, but a bowl-shaped cavity, which separates the capsule from the cortical parenchyma. It is traversed by the collagenous trabeculae and communicates at the hilus with the lumen of the efferent lymph vessels. Arising from the marginal

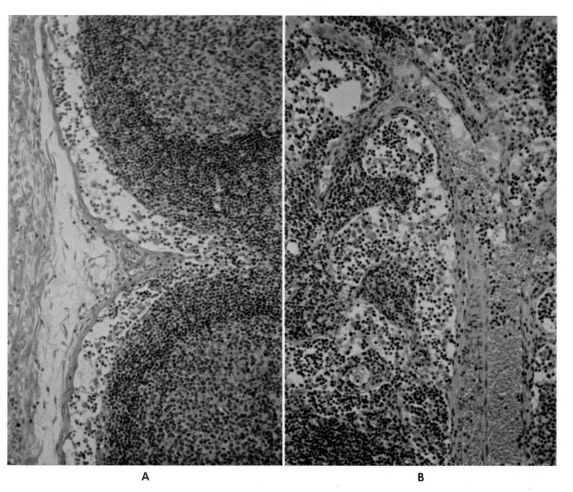

A	B

Figure 15–3. *A,* Capsule, marginal sinus, and part of two germinal centers in a mesenteric lymph node of a dog. *B,* Medullary sinuses and cords from a mesenteric lymph node of a dog. A trabecula is seen on the right carrying an artery and a vein; the vein receives tributaries from neighboring medullary cords. Hematoxylin-eosin.

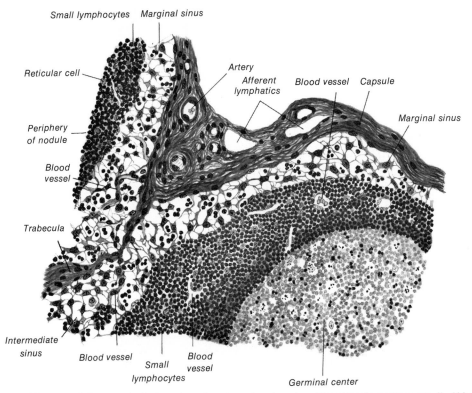

Figure 15–4. Diagram of the marginal sinus in a lymph node of a dog. Hematoxylin-eosin-azure II. (After A. A. Maximow.)

sinus are radially directed lymph channels called the *intermediate* or *cortical sinuses,* which penetrate the cortical parenchyma, usually following along the collagenous trabeculae. The compact appearance of the cortex is primarily due to the relatively small number and narrow lumen of the intermediate sinuses. These continue into the medulla as *medullary sinuses*—large, tortuous, irregular channels, that branch and anastomose repeatedly, thus fragmenting the lymphoid parenchyma into a number of *medullary cords* (Figs. 15–3, 15–5). The sinuses of the medullary substance are confluent with the marginal sinus at the hilus and form there a plexus of tortuous vessels, which penetrate the thickened capsule of this region and continue into the efferent lymphatics.

Seen with the scanning electron microscope (Fig. 15–6), the sinuses appear as tunnels lined by a layer of attenuated cells, but their lumen is bridged by a meshwork of stellate cells, which are connected to each other and to the opposite walls of the sinus via slender cell processes. Projecting from the sinus walls and luminal network of stellate elements are rounded macrophages, hirsute with myriad surface protrusions. Also present are smaller cells, probably lymphocytes. The framework of the sinus walls is a layer of reticular fibers, continuous with the parenchymal reticulum. These fibers directly underlie the sinus lining cells without any intervening basal lamina. The intraluminal network of cell processes is supported by a skeleton of reticular and elastic fibers anchored to the reticulum of the sinus walls and suspended from the collagenous framework of the capsule and the trabeculae. The fibers traversing the sinuses are not directly exposed to the lymph, but are completely invested by the luminal stellate cells, often lying embedded in deep invaginations of the cell surface.

There is no doubt that the wall of the sinuses is freely permeable to the constituents of the lymph and is continually crossed by wandering cells, which move freely between lymph and lymphoid parenchyma. However, the nature and physiological properties of the cells lining the walls of the sinuses and those traversing their lumens have long been subjects of controversy and are far from being settled satisfactorily. Traditionally,

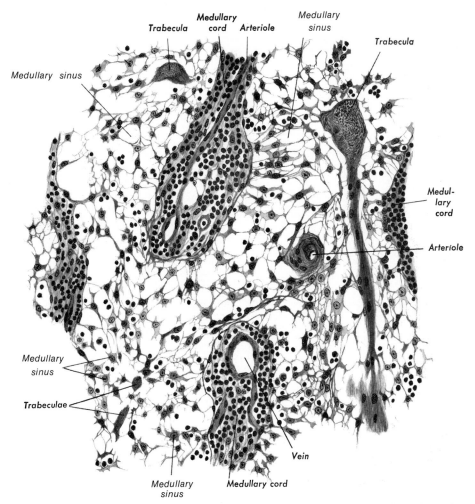

Figure 15–5. Diagram of medulla in a lymph node of a dog. Hematoxylin-eosin-azure II. (After A. A. Maximow.)

these cells were identified with the "reticular cells" of the lymphoid parenchyma and were thought to be capable of phagocytosis. At present, however, there are indications that there are two distinct categories of lining cells: macrophages and flattened or stellate endothelial cells. These latter have an inconspicuous complement of cell organelles. They are connected to each other by specialized junctions and they take up only small amounts of particulate matter by endocytosis, like the endothelium of blood vessels generally. Macrophages are inserted into the sinus wall or trapped in the meshes of the luminal network of tissue strands, apparently stuck to the surface of the endothelial cells. They lack specialized intercellular junctions, do not invest the reticular fibers, and contain the pleomorphic complement of cell organelles and residual bodies typical of phagocytic

cells. The source of the macrophages is still unknown. Nor is it clear whether they are permanently associated with the endothelium (tissue macrophages), having migrated from the parenchyma into the sinuses, or are lymph-borne elements that secondarily took up residence in the sinus walls and acquired phagocytic properties.

The relative proportions of macrophages and endothelial cells vary in different regions of the node. The capsular wall of the marginal sinus and the wall of the intermediate sinuses adjacent to the collagenous trabeculae are composed exclusively of flattened endothelial cells, whose outlines are easily stained by treatment with silver nitrate. On the other hand, macrophages are especially numerous in medullary sinuses, and there the outlines of endothelial cells usually cannot be demonstrated by silver nitrate.

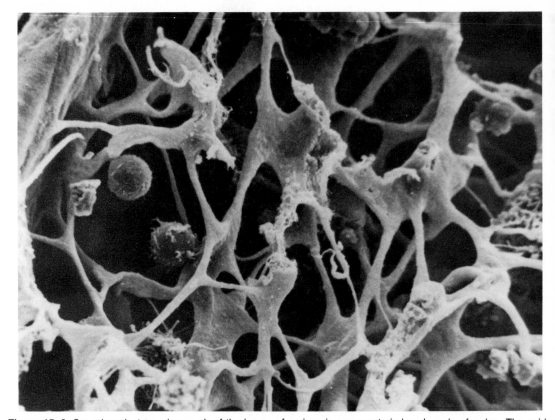

Figure 15–6. Scanning electron micrograph of the lumen of a sinus in a mesenteric lymph node of a dog. The spider web of luminal stellate cells acts as a multitude of microscopic baffles that generate turbulence in the lymph and facilitate the monitoring function of the macrophages deployed along the sinus walls. On left, two rounded cells, probably lymphocytes, were trapped in the lumen of the sinus. (From Fujita, T., et al. Z. Zellforsch. *133*:147, 1972.)

The organization of the lymph sinuses is well suited to the filtering function of the lymph node. The lymph entering the organ through the afferent vessels floods the marginal sinus and slowly percolates through the intermediate and medullary sinuses, freely exchanging with the lymphoid parenchyma substances in solution, particulate matter, and cells. The system of sinuses functions as a "trap" or "settling chamber," with the intraluminal tissue strands acting as a multitude of microscopic baffles that increase the surface exposed to the lymph, generate turbulence, and facilitate the monitoring function of the macrophages deployed along the sinus walls.

Cortex

The cortical parenchyma appears with the light microscope as a dense mass of lymphoid cells, traversed in places by the collagenous trabeculae and intermediate sinuses. It has been customary to classify certain regional differentiations in the cortical parenchyma as *primary lymphoid nodules, secondary nodules,* and *diffuse lymphoid tissue.* Secondary nodule is a term that has been used to describe either the *germinal centers* proper or the germinal centers together with their cap of small lymphocytes. Primary nodules and germinal centers are usually located at the periphery of the node and together comprise the *outer cortex,* whereas the *inner* or *deep cortex* (also called the paracortical area) consists of diffuse lymphoid tissue (Fig. 15–7). No clearcut boundary exists between outer and deep cortex, and the latter continues without demarcation into the medullary cords. Furthermore, the relative proportions of the two zones are quite variable in different lymph nodes and in various functional states. This subdivision does, however, have considerable physiological importance, because only the deep cortex is populated by lymphocytes of the recirculating pool and it contains postcap-

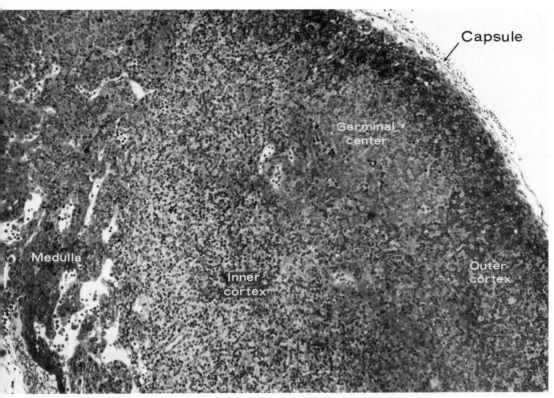

Figure 15–7. Portion of the auricular lymph node of a mouse. Notice the considerable thickness of the inner cortex. Toluidine blue. (Courtesy of G. B. Schneider.)

llary venules with cuboidal endothelium, which represent the portal of entry of blood-borne lymphocytes into the node.

Primary nodules are not clearly defined morphological entities. In man and laboratory rodents, they consist merely of the lymphoid tissue intervening between the germinal centers of the outer cortex. Only in species such as the ox, whose lymph nodes possess a well-developed system of trabeculae and intermediate sinuses, does the parenchyma of the outer cortex appear subdivided into discrete, rounded aggregates, projecting slightly at the surface of the organ. The stroma of the primary nodules consists of a rather loose network of reticular fibers and associated reticular cells. The labyrinthine interstices of this reticulum are occupied by small lymphocytes. Both large lymphocytes and macrophages are rare; mature plasma cells are usually lacking.

Germinal centers occur in variable numbers in the outer cortex, are less commonly found deeper in the cortex, and are only exceptionally present in the medullary cords. Those located at the lymph node periphery are polarized in such a way that their light regions, invested by the small lymphocyte cap, point toward the marginal sinus that receives the incoming lymph (Fig. 15–8). In the lymph nodes of the pig, these relationships are reversed, with the germinal centers pointing toward the central sinus, which in this species receives the incoming lymph. In germinal centers situated deep in the cortex, the orientation of the light pole and lymphocytic cap is either random or toward a neighboring intermediate sinus. The structure of germinal centers conforms to the general description provided in Chapter 13.

In the deep cortex, cells are more loosely packed than in the outer cortex. Small lymphocytes predominate, while large lymphocytes, macrophages, and plasma cells are found only occasionally. Reticular fibers are more abundant than in the outer cortex and increase additionally in number at the junction of the cortex with the medulla. Considerable attention has been paid in the recent past to a type of cells normally found in the resting lymph node, which are characterized by euchromatic nucleus, pale cytoplasm, few

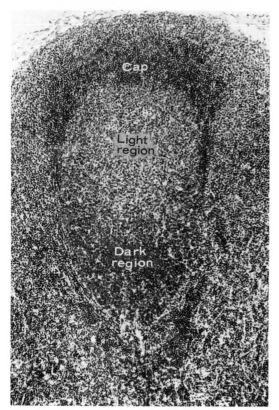

Figure 15–8. Germinal center in the outer cortex of a mesenteric lymph node of a dog. Hematoxylin-eosin.

cell organelles, and numerous surface processes that interdigitate with those of the adjoining lymphocytes. They are called *interdigitating cells* and are localized in the deep cortex. In places, they contain granules that have the same structure as those present in the cytoplasm of the Langerhans cells in the epidermis. Furthermore, cells with numerous surface ruffles have been isolated from the afferent lymph *(veiled cells)*; they are contained in the lumen of the sinuses or appear to be migrating across the endothelium of the marginal sinus. Veiled cells may contain Langerhans-type granules in their cytoplasm. Their relationships with interdigitating cells and the dendritic cells of the germinal centers are unclear.

Medulla

The medullary cords consist of aggregations of lymphoid tissue organized around small blood vessels. The cords branch and anastomose freely with one another, and near the hilus they terminate blindly or, more frequently, they form loops that continue into other cords. The medullary cords are not very prominent in resting lymph nodes. They consist of a rich network of reticular fibers and reticular cells, enclosing small lymphocytes, mature plasma cells, and macrophages.

The lymph node parenchyma contains variable, but usually small numbers of granulocytes and erythrocytes. The number of these cellular elements may, however, be greatly increased upon stimulation or in pathological states.

Capsule and Trabeculae

The capsule of the lymph node consists of dense collagenous fibers with a few fibroblasts and, especially on its inner surface, networks of thin elastic fibers. A few smooth muscle cells are also found in the capsule around the points of entry and exit of the afferent and efferent lymph vessels. The outer aspect of the capsule blends into the fat or loose connective tissue surrounding the lymph node, whereas its inner aspect is more sharply defined and is lined by the endothelium of the marginal sinus, except where it gives rise to the cortical trabeculae. The trabeculae do not represent complete septa, but cylindrical or flattened beams of dense connective tissue; they traverse the node completely ensheathed by the intermediate and medullary lymph sinuses, and, near the hilus, they carry the major blood vessels.

Blood Vessels and Nerves

Almost all the blood vessels destined for the lymph node enter the organ through the hilus, with only occasional small ones entering through the rest of the capsule (Fig. 15–1). The larger arterial branches initially run within the trabeculae, but they soon enter the medullary cords and supply their capillary networks. Passing along the cords, the arteries reach the cortex, where they distribute to capillary plexuses of the diffuse cortical parenchyma and around the germinal centers. Special *postcapillary venules* with cuboidal endothelium arise from these peripheral capillary plexuses and course radially through the deep cortex to enter the medullary cords. Here they give rise to small veins lined with normal endothelium. These in turn are tributaries of the larger venous channels that

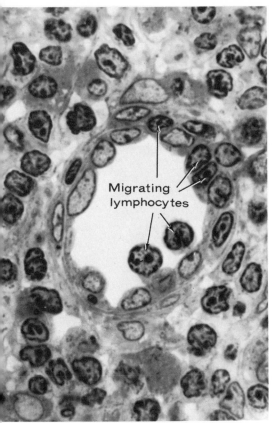

Figure 15–9. Small lymphocytes migrating through the endothelium of a postcapillary venule in the popliteal lymph node of a rabbit. Toluidine blue. (Courtesy of C. Compton.)

They have tall endothelial cells and no muscular coat, and their wall is traversed by great numbers of blood-borne small lymphocytes, which migrate into the lymph node parenchyma either by perforating the endothelial cells or by insinuating themselves into the interendothelial clefts. Similar vessels occur in certain segments of the vascular tree of the tonsils, Peyer's patches, and appendix. The exact significance of the cuboidal endothelium is obscure, but it has been suggested that the compliant endothelial cells adapt their surface contours to the shape of the wandering lymphocytes, thus limiting the plasma loss that might otherwise be associated with cell migration. Circulating lymphocytes seem to be capable of specifically recognizing this segment of the vascular tree as the portal of entry into the lymph node parenchyma. The mechanism of this remarkable phenomenon is unknown, but it may imply some sort of specific surface interaction between lymphocytes and cuboidal endothelial cells. Experiments involving enzymatic digestion suggest that carbohydrate moieties of membrane glycoproteins are the essential component of the recognition sites on the surface of the lymphocytes. On the other hand, immunoglobulins have been demonstrated at the surface of the endothelial cells, and these might also be the basis for selective capture of circulating lymphocytes.

Nerves enter the hilus of the node with the blood vessels, forming perivascular plexuses. In the trabeculae and medullary cords, nerve fibers are observed that are independent of the vessels, but in the cortex all nerves are probably of vasomotor type.

accompany the major arterial trunks in the interior of the collagenous trabeculae.

The postcapillary venules of the deep cortex are of special interest (Figs. 15–9, 15–10).

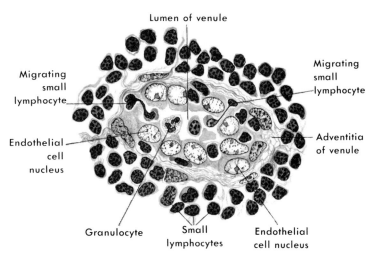

Figure 15–10. Diagram of lymphocyte migration through the walls of the postcapillary venules. (After A. A. Maximow.)

Lumen of venule

Migrating small lymphocyte

Migrating small lymphocyte

Endothelial cell nucleus

Adventitia of venule

Granulocyte

Small lymphocytes

Endothelial cell nucleus

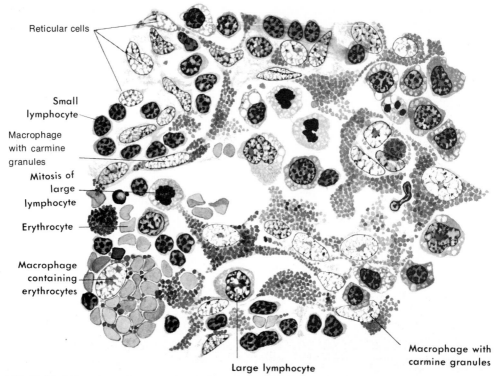

Reticular cells

Small
lymphocyte

Macrophage
with carmine
granules

Mitosis of
large
lymphocyte

Erythrocyte

Macrophage
containing
erythrocytes

Large lymphocyte

Macrophage with
carmine granules

Figure 15–11. Medullary sinus of mesenteric lymph node of a rabbit that had repeated intravenous injections of lithium carmine. Hematoxylin-eosin-azure II. (After A. A. Maximow.)

HISTOPHYSIOLOGY OF LYMPH NODES

The delicate walls of the lymphatic capillaries are easily penetrated by macromolecules, particulate matter, and wandering cells of the connective tissue. Furthermore, bacterial cells may cross the epidermis or the epithelium of the mucous membranes lining the body cavities. Escaping destruction by local or blood-borne phagocytes, they may proliferate and release toxins. Both microorganisms and their toxins easily gain access to the lymph. Lymph nodes intercalated along the path of lymph drainage prevent entry into the bloodstream of potentially harmful macromolecules, particulate matter, and bacteria carried by the lymph, and exert immunological surveillance on their antigenic determinants.

The filtering capacity of the lymph nodes, recognized long ago by Virchow and substantiated by experiments involving perfusion with particulate matter and bacterial cells, is based on both mechanical and biological mechanisms. The labyrinthine configuration of the sinuses favors arrest of the particles suspended in the lymph, and the macrophages of the sinus walls remove them by phagocytosis (Fig. 15–11). Lymph nodes, however, represent a much less efficient barrier for lymph-borne cells and may even facilitate dissemination of certain viruses. Erythrocytes injected into the afferent lymphatic vessels are effectively retained by the node, although the filtering efficiency decreases when very large numbers of red blood cells are infused. On the other hand, lymph nodes retain only a small proportion of lymph-borne cancer cells. Viruses that are capable of proliferating in the lymph node cells are quickly disseminated throughout the body, possibly carried by the recirculating lymphocytes.

The function of the lymph nodes in the immunological defenses of the body is a property of their lymphocyte and plasma cell populations, assisted by the macrophages in both the preliminary phase of antigen recognition and the terminal phase of antigen disposal. To initiate a primary immune response, uncommitted T and B lymphocytes must be present in the resting lymph node, whereas memory cells are required for a secondary response. Upon interaction with antigens that elicit a humoral response, lymphocytes are activated and undergo antigen-dependent proliferation and differentiation. As a consequence, plasma cells appear in the node and antibody is synthesized and released into the efferent lymph, together with lymphoid cells that propagate the response throughout the body. In cellular immune responses, lymphocyte activation and differentiation lead to the development and systemic dissemination of lymphokine-producing and cytolytic lymphocytes. Although these events are known to occur in the lymph node, the precise location of the relevant cell populations within the organ and the ultrastructural details of their antigen-dependent differentiation are poorly understood.

In resting peripheral lymph nodes, such as the popliteal node of the sheep, which has been studied in some detail, the afferent lymph contains very few cells. Among these are lymphocytes, macrophages, and occasional granulocytes. The efferent lymph contains 20 to 75 times more cells than the afferent lymph, and these are predominantly small lymphocytes (98 per cent). Only a very small fraction of the small lymphocytes emerging with the efferent lymph actually arise from division of precursors in the node, the vast majority (95 per cent) being derived from the bloodstream. These lymphocytes belong to the recirculating pool and enter the node through the cuboidal endothelium of the postcapillary venules in the deep cortex. Blood-borne small lymphocytes are selectively trapped by these vessels, whereas granulocytes and monocytes are specifically excluded. Most of the recirculating lymphocytes are thymus dependent and, upon entering the node, they localize in the deep cortex. Shortly thereafter, they migrate into the sinus lymph and leave the organ through the efferent lymphatic vessels. The fate of the small component of the recirculating pool that consists of B lymphocytes is poorly understood. B cells recirculate at a slower rate than T cells, either because they are inherently sluggish or because they are somehow separated from the main recirculatory pathway. Thoracic duct cells of animals congenitally or experimentally deprived of T lymphocytes cross the endothelium of the postcapillary venules and are initially localized in the deep cortex. Subsequently, however, they "home in" to the outer cortex and medullary cords. In the outer cortex, they take residence in the primary nodules and lymphocyte cap of the germinal centers.

Lymph nodes are also likely to be seeded with cells that have just emerged from the thymus or the bone marrow. Neonatal thymectomy is followed by a deficit of small lymphocytes in the deep cortex of lymph nodes, whereas outer cortex and medullary cords are unaffected; furthermore, experiments involving careful infusion of radioactive label into the thymus show that thymic lymphocytes specifically "home in" to the deep cortex. Lymphocytes of bone marrow origin also appear to migrate continuously into the resting lymph node; they do not seem to localize in specific regions of the organ, but instead become distributed throughout cortex and medulla. It is still a matter of conjecture whether or not this direct inflow of lymphocytes from thymus and bone marrow endows the lymph node with a complement of newly formed, uncommitted elements, capable of reacting to antigens never experienced previously by the immune system. Also unknown is the life span of these cells and their contribution to the recirculating pool.

Observations on the effects of thymectomy and the selective "homing" of both thymic and thoracic duct lymphocytes have given rise to the concept that the parenchyma of the lymph nodes consists of a thymus-dependent area, the deep cortex, and a bursa-dependent area, which includes the medullary cords and the outer cortex with its germinal centers. This postulated compartmentalization of the lymph node is easily understood in view of the facts that the deep cortex is the major traffic area of the lymph node and that the vast majority of the recirculating lymphocytes are thymus dependent. Less clear is the functional significance of the outer cortex and medullary cords, regions that seem to be inhabited by a population of lymphocytes that are either sessile or sluggishly migratory, and whose functional properties are still poorly understood.

The lymphocytopoietic activity of a quiescent lymph node seems to be slight, for 75 per cent of the lymphocytes of the mesenteric nodes of the rat belong to the long-lived variety. The only sites of sustained lymphocyte proliferation in the lymph nodes are the germinal centers, but the fate of the lymphocytes produced by these enigmatic structures is still not known. Of the remaining cellular elements of the resting node, the plasma cells located in the medulla are sessile, effete elements, which either arose locally as a consequence of a previous antigenic stimulation or differentiated from ancestors seeded throughout the body from a distant focus of immune activity. The macrophages of the lymph node parenchyma are probably of monocytic origin, although definitive evidence on this point has not yet been obtained. In contrast to the ideas prevailing in the past, autoradiographic studies show that the turnover of the reticular cells is extremely slow and not influenced by experimental procedures that deplete the lymphocyte population of the node. Thus, the claim that they represent primitive precursors of lymphocytes, plasma cells, or macrophages is devoid of experimental foundation. Detailed and systematic studies on the ultrastructure and functional properties of the reticular cells are still lacking. They probably are not a homogeneous class of cells but may include fibroblasts responsible for the synthesis of the reticular fibers, tissue macrophages, and dendritic cells. The term dendritic cell encompasses a seemingly heterogeneous population of lymph node constituents, which includes the "follicular dendritic cells" of germinal centers, the interdigitating cells of the deep cortex, and the veiled cells of the afferent lymph and lymphatic sinuses. All these cells have irregular shape, with numerous branching processes radiating in all directions. They are not phagocytic and have an inconspicuous complement of cell organelles, except for the occasional presence of granules identical to those typical of the Langerhans cells of the epidermis. The dendritic cells of the germinal centers have the property of retaining for long periods of time antigen-antibody complexes in the labyrinth of clefts bounded by their surface processes. Interdigitating cells do not carry receptors for antibody molecules, but share with Langerhans cells the presence of histocompatibility (Ia) molecules on their surface. It is presently debated whether dendritic cells, including the Langerhans cells of the epidermis, are a novel cell type whose function is to present antigen to T lymphocytes during the inductive phase of the immune response.

After administration of an antigen that elicits antibody production, the primary response of the lymph node draining the site of injection is characterized, during the first day, by an increase in number of granulocytes in both the parenchyma and lymph sinuses. Simultaneously, large and medium-sized basophilic mononuclear cells appear in the deep cortex. The antigen can be demonstrated in phagocytic vacuoles of the macrophages lining the sinuses of the medulla and is retained in the intercellular clefts of the outer cortex. On days 2 and 3, granulocytes usually disappear and the large basophilic or pyroninophilic cells proliferate and greatly increase in number. The lymph node enlarges, and the deep cortex seems to spread, invading the whole organ. Preexisting germinal centers usually disappear and the medullary cords are greatly reduced in length or are no longer evident. With the electron microscope, the newly formed population of basophilic cells appears to include lymphoblasts and transitional forms between the lymphocytic and plasmocytic lines. The lymphoblasts have a pale nucleus, a prominent nucleolus, and a profusion of cytoplasmic polyribosomes. Cisternae of the granular endoplasmic reticulum are only exceptionally found in these cells, and mitochondria are few, whereas the Golgi apparatus is well developed but lacking the dense granules typical of this organelle in cells of the plasmocytic series. The transitional cells display increasing amounts of granular endoplasmic reticulum, suggestive of a differentiation into immature plasma cells. Both the lymphoblasts and the transitional elements have been shown to produce antibody.

Later on, immature members of the plasma cell family become more and more numerous, with their eccentric nucleus, condensed chromatin, and large amounts of granular endoplasmic reticulum. Antibody is actively synthesized at this stage and appears in both efferent lymph and blood. Furthermore, well-circumscribed nests of small to large lymphocytes appear near the surface of the node. These probably represent early developmental stages of new germinal centers.

Toward the end of the first week after the injection, the lymph node begins to reacquire its normal architecture. Numerous newly formed germinal centers have appeared in the cortex; medullary cords are prominent again near the hilus and contain abundant immature and mature plasma cells.

During the second week after antigenic challenge, plasma cells begin to decrease in number and become exclusively confined to the medullary cords. Antigen is still present in the node, confined both to the residual bodies of medullary macrophages and to the intercellular clefts between the dendritic cells of the germinal centers.

These events in the lymph node are accompanied by characteristic changes in the efferent lymph. During the first 24 hours that follow antigen administration, the output of cells from the node decreases. Blood lymphocytes keep entering the node, but are retained in it by some unknown mechanism. From two to five days after antigen administration, cell release by the node doubles, because more lymphocytes are crossing from the blood, but are no longer retained in the node. The lymphocytes, however, which have been stimulated by the antigen, do not appear yet in the efferent lymph. After five days, the output of cells declines, but the newly emerging population contains a large proportion of activated lymphocytes. These appear as large lymphocytes, with euchromatic nucleus, prominent nucleoli, and abundant cytoplasm very rich in polyribosomes. They have only a few elements of the granular endoplasmic reticulum even though they are actively producing antibody; they are motile and capable of incorporating DNA precursors into their chromatin. The remaining cells leaving the stimulated node include antibody-producing small lymphocytes and immature elements of the plasma cell line. The antibody-producing cells of the efferent lymph are thought to colonize successive lymph nodes along the chain and, by entering the bloodstream through the thoracic duct, may propagate the immune response throughout the body. In fact, if the efferent lymphatic vessel of a locally stimulated node is cannulated and its lymph drained off, antibody fails to appear in the blood and the dissemination of the immune response is prevented. If the cells leaving a stimulated node are recovered from the efferent lymph, labeled radioactively in vitro, and reinfused into an afferent lymphatic of a quiescent node, they localize in the medullary cords, proliferate, and finally differentiate into mature plasma cells. Antibody-producing cells have also been demonstrated in the thoracic duct lymph. The fate of these cells has been studied after in vitro labeling and intravenous injection into a syngeneic animal. They are retained transiently in the lung, liver, and spleen, but later they localize in the spleen, lymph nodes, and gut-associated lymphoid structures and especially in the lamina propria of the small intestine.

The antibody-producing cells appearing in the thoracic duct lymph after local stimulation of a lymph node seem to undergo further modulation as they enter the bloodstream. Here, they appear as elements with a central nucleus, an inconspicuous nucleolus, and a narrow rim of cytoplasm, filled by parallel arrays of cisternae of the granular endoplasmic reticulum.

During the secondary response, the lymph node undergoes changes that resemble those following the first exposure to antigen, but they occur earlier and are much more pronounced.

When a lymph node is involved in a cellular immune response, it undergoes morphological changes that are not strikingly different from those typical of a humoral response. If skin is grafted from a donor onto an allogeneic recipient (allograft or homograft) or if delayed hypersensitivity is induced by application of a chemical sensitizing agent to the skin, the draining node enlarges markedly and the deep cortex becomes very thick. Lymphoblasts with pale nucleus, prominent nucleoli, and abundant basophilic cytoplasm (large pyroninophilic cells) appear in the deep cortex. With the electron microscope, they display abundant cytoplasmic polyribosomes, minimal amounts of granular endoplasmic reticulum, a small Golgi apparatus, and a few mitochondria. These are actively dividing cells, and their number in the deep cortex increases rapidly, reaching a maximum toward the end of the first week. At the beginning of the second week, the number of lymphoblasts declines rapidly and a second phase in the response becomes apparent: newly formed germinal centers appear in the outer cortex, and immature and mature plasma cells become localized in the medullary cords. At the same time, humoral antibody is detected in the blood.

After a slight time lag with respect to the appearance of the lymphoblasts in the deep cortex of the draining node, lymphocytes and macrophages begin to infiltrate the graft or the sensitized skin region. The peripheral response reaches its peak and the graft is rejected when the number of lymphoblasts has already begun to decline in the draining node, but before antibody is produced in significant amounts.

The mechanism of the cellular response is poorly understood. Antigens from the homograft or the site of application of the sensitizing agent may reach the regional lymph node through the afferent lymph. Small lymphocytes in the deep cortex may react with the antigens and differentiate into proliferating lymphoblasts; these in turn produce lymphocytes of decreasing size, which emigrate from the regional node, circulate in the blood, and are disseminated throughout the immune system. They invade the graft and destroy it or mediate the skin lesion typical of a delayed hypersensitivity reaction (contact dermatitis or erythematous papule). The antibody response that accompanies the cellular immune reaction seems to contribute but little to the rejection process, at least in laboratory rodents.

Neonatal thymectomy prevents the appearance of the lymphoblasts in the deep cortex in response to homologous transplantation and prolongs the survival of the graft. Thus, the lymphoblasts appearing in the deep cortex are likely to be thymus dependent.

Hemal Nodes

Even in normal lymph nodes, varying numbers of erythrocytes are found. These have either entered the lymph from the afferent vessels or come from the blood vessels of the node. Some of them pass with the lymph into the efferent vessels, but most of them are engulfed by macrophages. Some nodes, however, called *hemal nodes,* are characterized by the exceptionally high content of erythrocytes. They are most numerous and best defined in the ruminants (sheep); they probably do not occur in man. They vary from minute bodies scarcely noticeable to the size of a pea or larger, and are scattered along large blood vessels from the neck to the pelvic inlet. They are also found near the kidneys and spleen, where they are believed by some to be accessory spleens. Each hemal node is covered by a dense capsule loosely connected to the surrounding tissue. At the hilus a small artery and a large vein enter and leave. The nodes are devoid of afferent lymphatics and have postcapillary venules with walls infiltrated by migrating lymphocytes. In the pig, a special type of hemal node has characteristics intermediate between the ordinary lymph node and the typical hemal node. It has blood vessels as well as lymphatic vessels, and the contents of both types of vessels mix in the sinuses. The functions of the hemal nodes are probably comparable with those of the spleen.

REFERENCES

Ada, G. L., G. J. V. Nossal, and J. Pye: Antigens in immunity. III. Distribution of iodinated antigens following injection into rats via the hind footpads. Aust. J. Exp. Biol. Med. Sci. *42*:295, 1964.

Borum, K., and M. H. Claesson: Histology of the induction phase of the primary immune response in lymph nodes of germfree mice. Acta Pathol. Microbiol. Scand. [A] *79*:561, 1971.

Brahim, F., and D. G. Osmond: The migration of lymphocytes from bone marrow to popliteal lymph nodes demonstrated by selective bone marrow labeling with ³H-thymidine *in vivo.* Anat. Rec. *175*:737, 1973.

Caffery, R. W., N. B. Everett, and W. O. Rieke: Radioautographic studies of reticular and blast cells in the hemopoietic tissues of the rat. Anat. Rec. *155*:41, 1966.

Cahill, R. N. P., H. Frost, and Z. Trnka: The effects of antigen on the migration of recirculating lymphocytes through single lymph nodes. J. Exp. Med. *143*:870, 1976.

Carr, I.: The fine structure of the mammalian lymphoreticular system. Int. Rev. Cytol. *27*:283, 1970.

Claésson, M. H., O. Jørgensen, and C. Röpke: Light and electron microscopic studies of the paracortical postcapillary high-endothelial venules. Z. Zellforsch. *119*:195, 1971.

Clark, S. L., Jr.: The reticulum of lymph nodes in mice studied with the electron microscope. Am. J. Anat. *110*:217, 1962.

Cohen, S., P. Vassalli, B. Benacerraf, and R. T. McCluskey: The distribution of antigenic and nonantigenic compounds within draining lymph nodes. Lab. Invest. *15*:1143, 1966.

Conway, E. A.: Cyclic changes in lymphatic nodules. Anat. Rec. *69*:487, 1937.

Dougherty, T. F., M. L. Berliner, G. L. Schneebell, and D. L. Berliner: Hormonal control of lymphatic structure and function. *In* Bierman, H. R., ed.: Leukopoiesis in Health and Disease. Ann. N. Y. Acad. Sci. *113*:511, 1964.

Downey, H.: The structure and origin of the lymph sinuses of mammalian lymph nodes and their relations to endothelium and reticulum. Haematologica *3*:431, 1922.

Downey, H., ed.: Handbook of Hematology. New York, Paul B. Hoeber, 1938.

Drinker, C. K., M. E. Field, and H. K. Ward: The filtering capacity of lymph nodes. J. Exp. Med. *59*:393, 1934.

Farr, A. G., Y. Cho, and P. P. H. DeBruyn: The structure of the sinus wall of the lymph node relative to its endocytic properties and transmural cell passage. Am. J. Anat. *157*:265, 1980.

Fisher, B., and E. R. Fisher: Barrier function of lymph node to tumor cells and erythrocytes. I. Normal nodes. Cancer *20*:1907, 1967.

Ford, W. L., and J. L. Gowans: The traffic of lymphocytes. Semin. Hematol. *6*:67, 1969.

Forkert, P.-G., J. A. Thliveris, and F. D. Bertalanffy: Structure of sinuses in the human lymph node. Cell Tissue Res. *183*:115, 1977.

Fossum, S.: The architecture of rat lymph nodes. II. Lymph node compartments. Scand. J. Immunol. *12*:411, 1980.

Fossum, S.: The architecture of rat lymph nodes. IV. Distribution of ferritin and colloidal carbon in the draining lymph nodes after foot-pad injection. Scand. J. Immunol. *12*:433, 1980.

Fujita, T., M. Miyoshi, and T. Murakami: Scanning electron microscope observation of the dog mesenteric lymph node. Z. Zellforsch. *133*:147, 1972.

Goldschneider, I., and D. D. McGregor: Migration of lymphocytes and thymocytes in the rat. I. The route of migration from blood to spleen and lymph nodes. J. Exp. Med. *127*:155, 1968.

Gowans, J. L., and E. J. Knight: The route of recirculation of lymphocytes in the rat. Proc. R. Soc. B *159*:257, 1964.

Hall, J. G., and B. Morris: The output of cells in lymph from the popliteal node of sheep. Q. J. Exp. Physiol. *47*:360, 1962.

Hall, J. G., and B. Morris: The lymph-borne cells of the immune response. Q. J. Exp. Physiol. *48*:235, 1963.

Hall, J. G., B. Morris, G. D. Moreno, and M. C. Bessis: The ultrastructure and function of the cells in lymph following antigenic stimulation. J. Exp. Med. *125*:91, 1967.

Han, S. S.: The ultrastructure of the mesenteric lymph node of the rat. Am. J. Anat. *109*:183, 1961.

Harris, T. N., K. Hummeler, and S. Harris: Electron microscopic observations on antibody-producing lymph node cells. J. Exp. Med. *123*:161, 1966.

Hay, J. B., M. J. Murphy, B. Morris, and M. C. Bessis: Quantitative studies on the proliferation and differentiation of antibody-forming cells in lymph. Am. J. Pathol. *66*:1, 1972.

Hostetler, J. R., and G. A. Ackerman: Lymphopoiesis and lymph node histogenesis in the embryonic and neonatal rabbit. Am. J. Anat. *124*:57, 1969.

Hummeler, K., T. N. Harris, N. Tomassini, M. Hechtel, and M. B. Farber: Electron microscopic observations on antibody-producing cells in lymph and blood. J. Exp. Med. *124*:255, 1966.

Leduc, E. H., A. H. Coons, and J. M. Connolly: Studies on antibody production. II. The primary and secondary responses in the popliteal lymph node of the rabbit. J. Exp. Med. *102*:61, 1955.

Marchesi, V. T., and J. L. Gowans: The migration of lymphocytes through the endothelium of venules in lymph nodes: an electron microscope study. Proc. R. Soc. B *159*:283, 1964.

Mikata, A., and R. Niki: Permeability of postcapillary venules of the lymph node. An electron microscopic study. Exp. Mol. Pathol. *14*:289, 1971.

Miller, J. J., and G. J. V. Nossal: Antigens in immunity. VI. The phagocytic reticulum of lymph node follicles. J. Exp. Med. *120*:1075, 1964.

Millikin, P. D.: Anatomy of germinal centers in human lymphoid tissue. Arch. Pathol. *82*:499, 1966.

Moe, R. E.: Fine structure of the reticulum and sinuses of lymph nodes. Am. J. Anat. *112*:311, 1963.

Moe, R. E.: Electron microscopic appearance of the parenchyma of lymph nodes. Am. J. Anat. *114*:341, 1964.

Mori, Y., and K. Lennert: Electron Microscopic Atlas of Lymph Node Cytology and Pathology. Berlin, Springer Verlag, 1969.

Movat, H. Z., and N. V. P. Fernando: The fine structure of lymphoid tissue. Exp. Mol. Pathol. *3*:546, 1964.

Movat, H. Z., and N. V. P. Fernando: The fine structure of the lymphoid tissue during antibody formation. Exp. Mol. Pathol. *4*:155, 1965.

Murphy, M. J., J. B. Hay, B. Morris, and M. C. Bessis: Ultrastructural analysis of antibody synthesis in cells from lymph and lymph nodes. Am. J. Pathol. *66*:25, 1972.

Nieuwenhuis, P., and W. L. Ford: Comparative migration of B- and T-lymphocytes in the rat spleen and lymph nodes. Cell. Immunol. *23*:254, 1976.

Nopajaroonsri, C., S. C. Luk, and G. T. Simon: Ultrastructure of the normal lymph node. Am. J. Pathol. *65*:1, 1971.

Nopajaroonsri, C., and G. T. Simon: Phagocytosis of colloidal carbon in a lymph node. Am. J. Pathol. *65*:25, 1971.

Nossal, G. J. V., A. Abbot, and J. Mitchell: Antigens in immunity. XIV. Electron microscopic radioautographic studies of antigen capture in the lymph node medulla. J. Exp. Med. *127*:263, 1968.

Nossal, G. J. V., A. Abbot, J. Mitchell, and Z. Lummus: Antigens in immunity. XV. Ultrastructural features of antigen capture in primary and secondary lymphoid follicles. J. Exp. Med. *127*:277, 1968.

Nossal, G. J. V., G. L. Ada, and C. M. Austin: Antigens in immunity. IV. Cellular localization of [125]I- and ^{131}I-labelled flagella in lymph nodes. Aust. J. Exp. Biol. Med. Sci. *42*:311, 1964.

Nossal, G. J. V., G. L. Ada, C. M. Austin, and J. Pye: Antigens in immunity. VIII. Localization of ^{125}I-labelled antigens in the secondary response. Immunology *9*:349, 1965.

Parrott, D. M. V., M. A. B. de Sousa, and J. East: Thymus-dependent areas in the lymphoid organs of neonatally thymectomized mice. J. Exp. Med. *123*:191, 1966.

Röpke, C., O. Jørgensen, and M. H. Claësson: Histochemical studies of high-endothelial venules of lymph nodes and Peyer's patches in the mouse. Z. Zellforsch. *131*:287, 1972.

Sainte-Marie, G., and Y. M. Sin: Structures of the lymph node and their possible function during the immune response. Rev. Can. Biol. 27:191, 1968.

Schoefl, G. I.: The migration of lymphocytes across the vascular endothelium in lymphoid tissues. A reexamination. J. Exp. Med. *136*:568, 1972.

Sordat, B., M. W. Hess, and H. Cottier: IgG immunoglobulin in the wall of post-capillary venules: possible relationship to lymphocyte recirculation. Immunology *20*:115, 1971.

Sorenson, G. D.: An electron microscopic study of popliteal lymph nodes from rabbits. Am. J. Anat. *107*:73, 1960.

Sprent, J.: Circulating T and B lymphocytes of the mouse. I. Migratory properties. Cell. Immunol 7:10, 1973.

Steinman, R. M.: Dendritic cells. Transplantation *31*:151, 1981.

Steinman, R. M., and M. C. Nussenzweig: Dendritic cells: features and functions. Immunol. Rev. *53*:127, 1980.

Straus, W.: Localization of the antigen in popliteal lymph nodes of rabbits during the formation of antibodies to horseradish peroxidase. J. Histochem. Cytochem. *18*:131, 1970.

Tew, J. G., G. J. Thorbecke, and R. M. Steinman: Dendritic cells in the immune response: Characteristics and recommended nomenclature (a report from the Reticuloendothelial Society Committee on Nomenclature). J. Reticuloendothel. Soc. *31*:371, 1982.

van Deurs, B., C. Ropke, and E. Westergaard: Ultrastructure and permeability of lymph node microvasculature in the mouse. Cell Tissue Res. *168*:507, 1976.

Weiss, L.: The Cells and Tissues of the Immune System. Structure, Functions, Interactions. Englewood Cliffs, NJ, Prentice-Hall, 1972.

Yoffey, J. M., and F. C. Courtice: Lymphatics, Lymph and Lymphoid Tissue. Cambridge, Harvard University Press, 1956.

Zimmermann, A. A.: Origin and development of the lymphatic system in the opossum. Illinois Medical and Dental Monographs, Vol. 3, Nos. 1 and 2, 1940.

16

SPLEEN

Elio Raviola

The spleen is an abdominal organ situated in the left hypochondrium beneath the diaphragm; largely invested by visceral peritoneum, it is connected to the stomach, diaphragm, and left kidney by peritoneal folds, called gastrolienal, phrenicolienal, and lienorenal ligaments. The lienorenal ligament carries the splenic blood vessels, lymphatics, and nerves. The spleen is a complex filter interposed in the bloodstream. It is concerned with clearing the blood of particulate matter and effete cells, and with immune defense against blood-borne antigens. In many vertebrates, but not in man, the spleen is also involved in formation of erythrocytes, granulocytes, and platelets, and in certain mammals it acts as a reservoir for mature erythrocytes that can be added to the circulation in response to unusual demands. The spleen contains a large amount of lymphoid tissue and possesses a peculiar type of blood vessel that allows the circulating blood to come into contact with great numbers of macrophages.

HISTOLOGICAL ORGANIZATION

On the freshly sectioned surface of the spleen, elongate or rounded gray areas, 0.2 to 0.7 mm in diameter, are visible with the naked eye (Fig. 16–1). Together these compose the *white pulp;* they are scattered throughout a soft, dark red mass, the *red pulp,* which can easily be scraped from the cut surface of the organ. The white areas, often called *malpighian bodies,* consist of diffuse and nodular lymphoid tissue. The red pulp consists of irregularly shaped blood vessels of large caliber (the *venous sinuses*) and the tissue occupying the spaces between them (the *splenic cords of Billroth*). The color of the

red pulp is due to the abundance of the erythrocytes that fill the lumen of the sinuses and infiltrate the splenic cords.

The spleen, much like the lymph nodes, has a collagenous *capsule* with inward extensions called *trabeculae* (Fig. 16–1). This capsule is continuous with a delicate reticular framework that occupies the rest of the interior of the organ and holds in its meshes the free cells of the splenic tissue. The *capsule* is thickened at the hilus of the organ, where it is attached to the peritoneal ligaments and where arteries and nerves enter and veins and lymphatic vessels leave the viscus.

The structure of the spleen and the relationships between the red and white pulp depend on the distribution of the blood vessels. They differ markedly in different animal species and change in the course of immune responses or disturbances of blood cell formation and destruction. Animal species with a large blood volume (horse, ruminants, carnivores) have scanty white pulp and a robust connective tissue and muscular framework. Species with a relatively small blood volume (man, rabbit, laboratory rodents) have abundant white pulp, a less prominent connective tissue framework, and poorly developed smooth musculature. In the splenic parenchyma, the white pulp is organized around the arteries and the red pulp fills the interstices among the venous sinuses.

White Pulp

The white pulp forms periarterial lymphoid *sheaths* (PALS) about the arteries where these leave the trabeculae to penetrate the parenchyma (Figs. 16–1, 16–6). The periarterial lymphoid sheaths follow peripherally along the vessels almost to the point where they break up into capillaries. In many places along their course the sheaths contain ger-

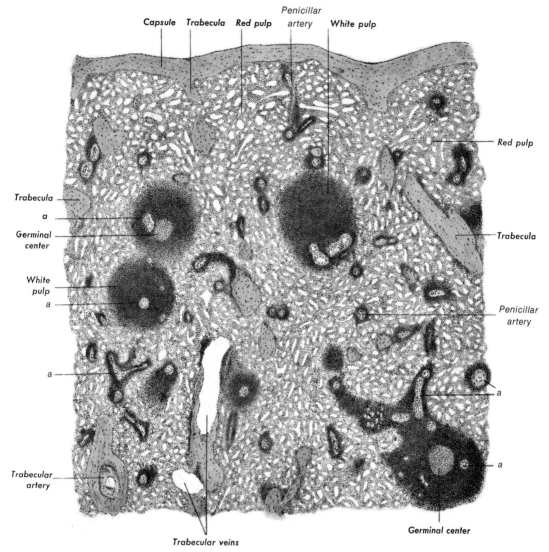

Capsule   Trabecula   Red pulp   *Penicillar artery*   White pulp

Red pulp

Trabecula

Penicillar artery

Trabecula

a

Germinal center

White pulp

a

a

a

a

Trabecular artery

Germinal center

Trabecular veins

Figure 16–1. Section of human spleen. *A,* Central arteries of the white pulp. (After A. A. Maximow.)

minal centers. Although both the periarterial lymphoid sheaths and the germinal centers consist of lymphoid tissue, they differ in their physiological significance; the former, in fact, consist predominantly of lymphocytes belonging to the recirculating pool, whereas the germinal centers are bursa-dependent structures, whose function is still poorly understood.

The periarterial lymphoid sheaths display an organization similar to the deep cortex of the lymph nodes. They have a loose, irregular framework of reticular fibers with associated reticular cells. At the periphery of the sheath, the reticular fibers become circumferentially arranged, and flattened reticular cells form concentric layers that delimit the lymphoid tissue from the surrounding red pulp. Near the central artery, a few elastic fibers are interspersed among the reticular fibers. The meshes of the reticular framework are occupied by lymphocytes, predominantly belonging to the small and medium-sized variety, in places associated with interdigitating cells (see Chap. 13). Plasma cells and macrophages are only occasionally found but increase in number toward the periphery of the sheath. Erythrocytes are rare, but they may occur at the boundary between white and red pulp. In the course of immune responses to blood-borne antigens, great numbers of large lymphocytes, lymphoblasts,

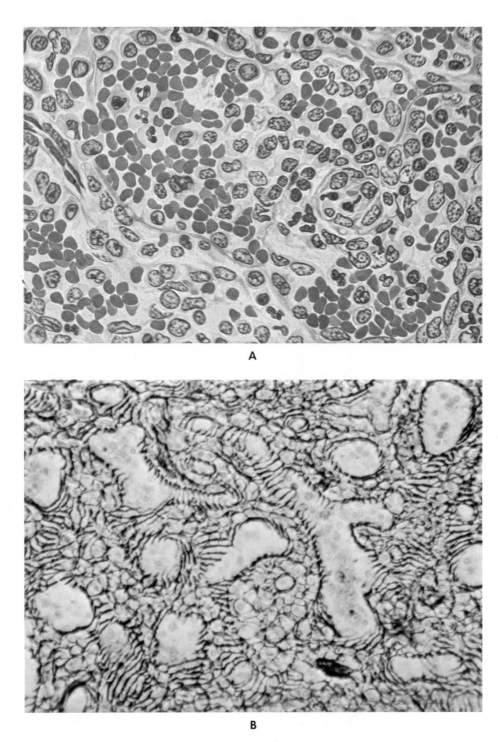

A

B

Figure 16–2. *A,* Drawing of red pulp of the human spleen. Venous sinuses filled with erythrocytes are separated from each other by the pulp cords. Hematoxylin-eosin. (After W. Bloom.) *B,* Photomicrograph of a silver impregnation of the reticular fibers of the spleen. The regularly spaced, circumferential ribs encircling the sinus endothelium are readily distinguished from the randomly distributed reticular fibers of the surrounding splenic cords. (Preparation by K. Richardson.)

and immature plasma cells appear in the periarterial lymphoid sheaths and soon become concentrated at their periphery.

The germinal centers display the usual architecture (see Chap. 13); they are eccentrically situated within the sheath and, when fully developed, their light region and cap of small lymphocytes are directed toward the red pulp. Their number varies in different animal species and tends to decrease progressively with age.

Red Pulp

The red pulp consists of a network of branching and anastomosing, tortuous sinuses, separated from each other by highly cellular partitions, the splenic or pulp cords (Figs. 16–2,16–3). The venous sinuses are discussed with the blood vessels of the spleen. The splenic cords vary in thickness but typically form a spongy cellular mass supported by a framework of reticular fibers (Fig. 16–2). The collagenous fibers of the trabeculae continue directly into the reticular fibers of the red pulp. As elsewhere in the body, the reticular fibers as seen with the electron microscope consist of collagen fibrils embedded in a finely filamentous matrix. They are completely invested by stellate reticular cells (Fig. 16–4), which resemble fibroblasts in their complement of organelles except for an uncommon abundance of filaments in their cytoplasm. Some of the reticular cells, as seen with the light microscope, may actually represent tissue macrophages of monocytic origin. The reticular fibers of the red pulp merge with ribs of basal lamina–like material that support the sinus endothelium. Their investing reticular cells are in turn anchored to the sinus walls through footlike processes, which are directed perpendicularly to the long axis of the sinuses.

The meshes of reticulum in the pulp cords are filled with great numbers of free cells, which include macrophages; all the cellular elements circulating in the blood, including great numbers of erythrocytes and platelets; and a few plasma cells (Figs. 16–3,16–8). With the light microscope the macrophages are readily recognized as large, rounded, or irregularly shaped cells, with a vesicular nucleus and abundant cytoplasm. They often contain engulfed erythrocytes, neutrophils, and platelets, or are loaded with masses of a yellowish-brown pigment that stains for iron

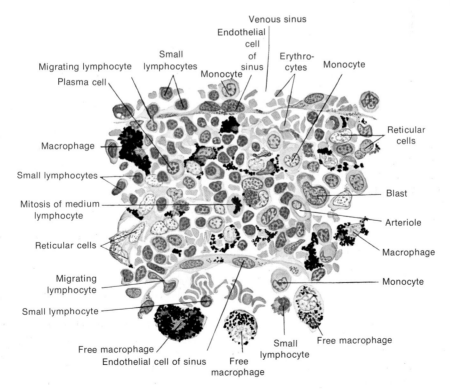

Figure 16–3. Cross section of splenic cord lying between two venous sinuses, from spleen of a rabbit injected with lithium carmine and India ink. Hematoxylin-eosin-azure II stain. (After A. A. Maximow.)

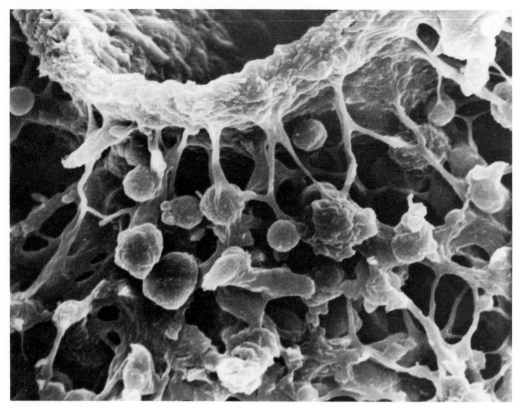

Figure 16–4. Scanning electron micrograph of a splenic cord adjacent to a pulp vein in the dog. Spleen perfusion with physiological salt solution has removed most of the free cells, thus exposing the three-dimensional network formed by the reticular cells. (From Miyoshi, M., and T. Fujita. Arch. Histol. Jpn. *33*:225, 1971.)

with the Prussian blue reaction and gives a positive reaction for the lysosomal enzyme acid phosphatase. This pigment represents the undigestible residues of phagocytized materials, especially red blood cells. Its iron, in the form of ferritin or hemosiderin, comes from the degradation of hemoglobin. In many mammalian species (laboratory rodents, hedgehog) and in the embryonic spleen, the red pulp contains groups of erythroblasts of various sizes, myeloblasts, myelocytes, and megakaryocytes. In adult man, these islands of hemopoietic tissue are lacking, but in certain infections, in some of the anemias, in leukemias, and in poisoning with certain blood-destroying agents, they may reappear, a condition described as *myeloid metaplasia.*

Immediately peripheral to the white pulp is an 80- to 100-μm transitional region between lymphoid tissue and red pulp, called the *marginal zone;* it contains smaller venous sinuses, circumferentially oriented around the white pulp. In the marginal zone, the reticular fibers of the cords form a closely knit concentric network, and the meshes of the cords have a greater content of small lymphocytes and plasma cells than the rest of the red pulp. The marginal zone is the region of the red pulp that receives the incoming arterial blood; thus, it is the site where blood-borne cells and particulate matter first contact the splenic parenchyma. Here, the lymphocytes of the recirculating pool leave the blood of the sinuses to enter the periarterial lymphoid sheaths.

Capsule and Trabeculae

The capsule and the trabeculae of the spleen consist of dense connective tissue, smooth muscle cells, and elastic networks. The external surface of the capsule is covered by a layer of flattened mesothelium, which is part of the general peritoneum. In man, rabbits, and laboratory rodents, the capsule is rich in elastic fibers, especially in its deep layers, and in addition to typical fibroblasts it contains a small number of stellate elements that display cytological characteristics intermediate between smooth muscle cells and fibroblasts, having filamentous cytoplasm and abundant glycogen. Smooth muscle cells are especially abundant in the splenic capsule of the horse, ruminants, and carnivores.

The trabeculae are flattened or cylindrical strands that carry arteries, veins, and lymphatics. They contain a larger number of elastic fibers than the capsule and varying amounts of smooth muscle cells (Fig. 16–5). Smooth muscle cells are sparse in the human spleen. In those species in which muscle is prominent, changes in the volume of the organ, either spontaneous or induced by injection of epinephrine, are due to contraction of the smooth muscle in the capsule and trabeculae, as well as to vasomotor changes in the amount of blood in the organ.

Arteries

The branches of the splenic artery enter the hilus and pass along the trabeculae, within which they branch repeatedly, becoming smaller in diameter (Fig. 16–6). They are muscular arteries of medium caliber and have a loose tunica adventitia surrounded by the dense connective tissue of the trabeculae. When the arterial branches have been reduced by progressive dichotomous branching to a diameter of approximately 0.2 mm, they leave the trabeculae. At this point, the tunica adventitia is replaced by a cylindrical sheath of lymphoid tissue, and the artery is designated the *central artery*. Where germinal cen-

ters are embedded in the periarterial lymphoid sheath, the artery is displaced to one side, thus losing its central position. It almost never passes through the center of the nodules. The central artery is a muscular artery with tall endothelial cells and one or two layers of smooth muscle cells. Throughout its course within the white pulp, the artery gives off numerous collateral capillaries, which supply the lymphoid tissue of the sheath. Initially, the capillary wall consists of tall endothelial cells, basal lamina, and an investment of pericytes; farther on, the endothelium becomes low and the pericytes disappear. Around the capillaries, the reticular meshwork of the white pulp is condensed and contains a few elastic fibers. These collateral capillaries, after coursing through the white pulp, pass into the surrounding marginal zone; how they end is uncertain.

The central artery continues to branch and becomes thinner. On reaching a diameter of 40 to 50 μm, its lymphoid sheath appears greatly reduced in thickness and the artery suddenly branches into two to six vessels, called *penicillar arteries* (Latin, penicillus = a painter's brush) or *arteries of the red pulp*. These pursue a radiating course still invested by one or two layers of lymphocytes that represent a greatly attenuated terminal extension of the periarterial lymphoid sheaths. The penicillar arteries are 0.6 to 0.7 mm in

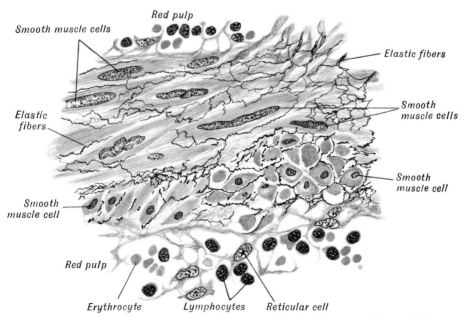

Figure 16–5. Portion of a trabecula from the spleen of a cat. Elastic fiber stain. (After A. A. Maximow.)

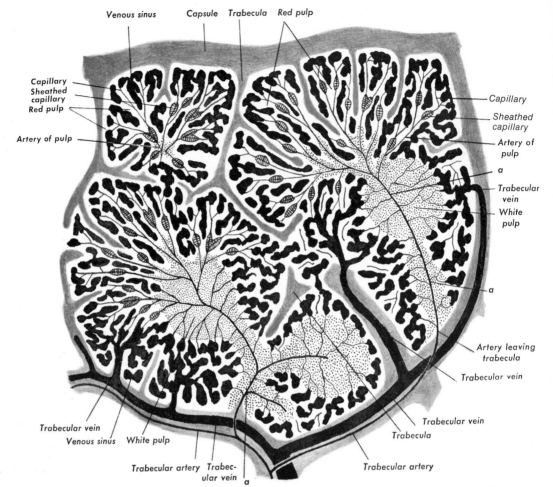

Figure 16–6. Diagram of the vascular tree of the spleen. Capillaries are depicted as communicating with the venous sinuses, according to the "closed circulation" theory. *A,* Central arteries. (After A. A. Maximow.)

length and have a tall endothelium resting on a continuous basal lamina, but they lack an elastica interna. Their media consists of one layer of smooth muscle cells; they lack an elastica externa and have a thin adventitia of collagenous and elastic fibers.

Upon entering the red pulp, each penicillar artery as a rule branches into two to three capillaries, which may exhibit a characteristic thickening of their walls, called the ellipsoidal or Schweigger-Seidel sheath (Fig. 16–7). The capillaries are therefore named *sheathed capillaries.* The endothelium of these vessels consists of tall, fusiform cells arranged parallel to the long axis of the vessel. They are in places connected by intercellular junctions and in other places separated by gaps through which blood cells can pass from the lumen. They contain abundant intermediate

filaments and rest on a discontinuous basal lamina. In man, the sheath is tubular and fairly thin (50 to 100 μm in length and 20 to 30 μm in diameter), but in certain species it is very prominent and ellipsoidal or spherical in shape (pig, dog, and cat). Sheathed capillaries are lacking in the spleen of laboratory rodents. Not all capillaries arising from a penicillar artery are sheathed, and most commonly only one sheath is associated with the terminal branches of a penicillar artery. Occasionally, multiple vessels (two to five) are invested by a single sheath, and sometimes two to three sheaths are arranged in series along a single branch of a penicillar artery. The sheath consists of a closely knit network of reticular fibers and cells. Most cells belong to two varieties, reticular cells and macrophages, but elements of the circulating blood

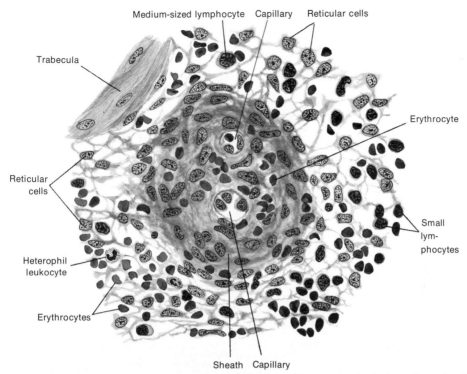

Medium-sized lymphocyte   Capillary   Reticular cells

Trabecula

Reticular cells

Heterophil leukocyte

Erythrocytes

Erythrocyte

Small lymphocytes

Sheath   Capillary

Figure 16–7. Cross section of a Schweigger-Seidel sheath surrounding two capillaries in the spleen of a dog. Eosin-azure stain. (After A. A. Maximow.)

are also present. Reticular cells are stellate in shape, are associated with the reticular fibers, and, in addition to the usual organelles, contain abundant cytoplasmic filaments: intermediate filaments coursing throughout the cytoplasm and a feltwork of thin filaments on the inner surface of the plasmalemma. Macrophages contain residual bodies and occasional phagocytized red blood cells. Upon intravenous injection of particulate matter they become avidly phagocytic; thus, there is no doubt that they belong to the mononuclear phagocyte system. Red blood cells are always present, in large or small numbers, among the cells of the sheath. There is general consensus that ellipsoidal sheaths function as filters that clear the blood of particulate materials, yet the reasons for their location around arterial capillaries remain unclear.

The sheathed capillaries continue as simple capillaries that either do not divide or bifurcate only once. Their mode of termination is unknown and will be discussed below after the venous sinuses have been described.

Venous Sinuses and Veins

The venous sinuses permeate the entire red pulp and are especially numerous around the white pulp (Fig. 16–8). These vessels are called sinuses because they have a wide (12 to 40 μm), irregular lumen, which varies in size depending on the amount of blood in the organ. The sinuses, even when only moderately distended, occupy more space than the splenic cords between them. Venous sinuses are missing in the mouse and cat spleen and substituted for by conventional venules.

Unlike true veins, the walls of the sinuses lack a muscular coat and display a unique arrangement of endothelium and basal lamina. The endothelial cells are fusiform elements, about 100 μm long, oriented parallel to the longitudinal axis of the sinus (Fig. 16–9). The central nuclear region of the cell body is thick and tapers toward the ends; they are in contact with each other laterally but lack typical intercellular junctions. Micropinocytotic vesicles are plentiful on both the luminal and lateral surfaces, and the cyto-

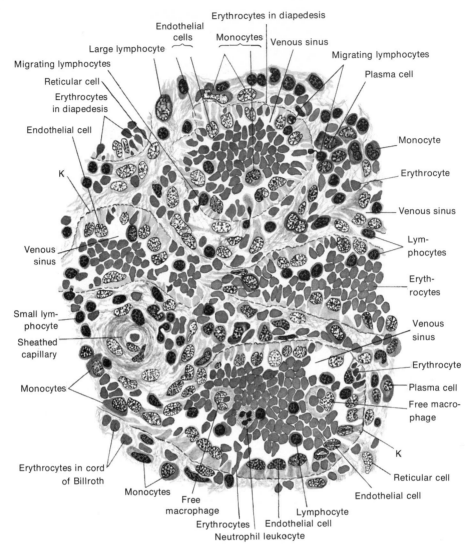

Figure 16–8. Venous sinuses in the red pulp of the human spleen. Note the cuboidal shape of the cross-sectioned endothelial cells. The cytoplasmic densities at the base of the cells (K) probably correspond to the condensations of finely filamentous material revealed by the electron microscope. Eosin-azure stain. (After A. A. Maximow.)

plasm contains, in addition to the usual complement of organelles, two types of filaments, both oriented parallel to the long axis of the cells. There are loosely packed intermediate filaments, free in the cytoplasmic matrix, and denser bands of finely filamentous material in the basal region of the cell. These latter seem to run from one rib of the basal lamina to the next, where they insert on the inner aspect of the plasma membrane; they are probably responsible for the longitudinal basal striations of the endothelium seen in specimens stained with iron hematoxylin. Except for their unusual shape, lack of intercellular junctions, and abundance of filaments, the sinus-lining cells resemble endothelial cells elsewhere in the body. Like other endothelial cells, they display only a limited capacity to take up particulate matter injected into the bloodstream. Thus, the traditional interpretation of the sinus-lining cells of the spleen as tissue macrophages is no longer tenable.

Outside the endothelium, the wall of the sinuses is supported by a system of circumferential ribs, about 1 μm in thickness, encircling the endothelial cells as the hoops embrace the staves of a barrel (Fig. 16–2). The ribs are spaced 2 to 5 μm apart and are interconnected by relatively few thin, longitudinal strands. At the light microscope level, they are observed to stain with silver impreg-

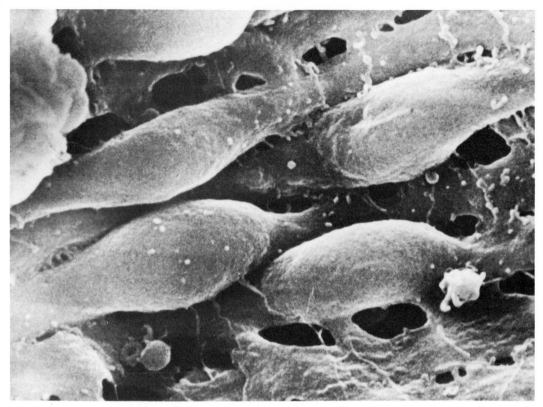

Figure 16–9. Surface view of the endothelial cells of a venous sinus in the rabbit spleen as seen with the scanning electron microscope. As the specimen was air-dried, cells have pulled apart, exposing the fenestrations of the basal lamina. (From Miyoshi, M., et al. Arch. Histol. Jpn. 32:289, 1970.)

nation methods and with histochemical methods for carbohydrates. In electron micrographs, they appear to consist of finely filamentous material with a few embedded collagen fibrils. Thus, in their fine structure, they correspond to an unusually thick, fenestrated basal lamina. The ribs are continuous with the reticular fibers of the splenic cords and are interposed between the endothelium on one side and the foot processes of the reticular cells of the cords on the other. Cellular elements of the circulating blood can easily migrate through the sinus wall, traversing the interendothelial clefts and the fenestrations of the basal lamina. Furthermore, cordal macrophages are frequently seen extending processes through the sinus walls into the lumen and they may also migrate into the blood within the sinus.

The venous sinuses empty into the *veins of the pulp*, whose walls consist of elongated, slender endothelial cells, a continuous basal lamina, and a thin layer of smooth muscle. They are supported externally by a condensation of the stroma of the red pulp and by a few elastic fibers. The pulp veins coalesce

to form the veins of the trabeculae; in turn, these are drained by the veins at the hilus of the spleen, which are tributaries of the splenic vein.

Union of the Arteries with the Veins

In almost all other organs of the body, the arterial is joined to the venous system by a continuous capillary network, in which the vascular lumen is completely enclosed. In the spleen, however, the connection of arterial and venous systems may be different, and its details are still subject to dispute. There are three main theories as to how blood gets from the arteries to the venous sinuses (Fig. 16–10). (1) The "open circulation" theory holds that the capillaries open directly into the spaces among the reticular cells of the splenic cords, and that the blood gradually filters into the venous sinuses. (2) The "closed circulation" theory holds that the capillaries communicate directly with the lumen of the venous sinuses. (3) A compromise interpretation holds that both types of circulation are present at the same time. One of the variants

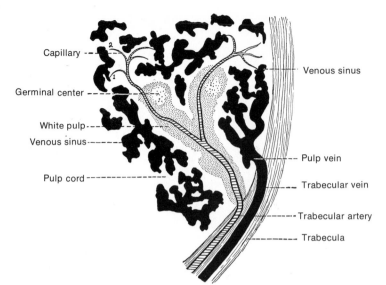

Capillary

Germinal center

White pulp

Venous sinus

Pulp cord

Venous sinus

Pulp vein

Trabecular vein

Trabecular artery

Trabecula

Figure 16–10. Diagram to show closed (1) and open (2) circulation through the spleen.

of this theory contends that a "closed" circulation in a contracted spleen may become an "open" circulation when the organ is distended.

The opposing theories are based on the following observations. (1) There are always many erythrocytes scattered throughout the tissue spaces of the splenic cords. Since in most species there is little or no erythropoiesis in the cords, it is concluded that the red blood cells have come from the circulating blood through gaps in the vascular segment between arterioles and venous sinuses. Those who maintain that the circulation is "closed" hold that the number of erythrocytes in the splenic cords is much smaller than it would be if the capillaries opened directly into the pulp. They argue that if the capillaries were open, the red pulp would be completely filled with blood, as in hemorrhages of the spleen. (2) When the splenic arteries are injected even at low pressures with dye solutions, India ink, or avian erythrocytes, the foreign materials readily gain access to the tissue spaces of the splenic cords, particularly in the marginal zone. Only later do they reach the venous sinuses. When the splenic vein is injected, the venous sinuses and the meshes of the stroma can be filled easily, but the arteries cannot. Those who favor a closed circulation believe that this injection of the red pulp by foreign materials is an artificial situation resulting from the rupture of the delicate vascular walls. (3) In every freshly fixed spleen, granulocytes, lymphocytes, and erythrocytes can be found passing through

the walls of the venous sinuses. According to the "open circulation" theory, these cells are returning to the bloodstream from the extravascular spaces of the splenic cords. According to the "closed circulation" theory, both plasma and cells of the blood are believed to pass into the cordal spaces at the arterial end of the sinuses and to return to the circulation at their venous end, driven by a pressure gradient that may exist between the two ends of these blood vessels. (4) Studies with the electron microscope seem to favor the view that the circulation is open, for it has been reported that arterial capillaries directly open into the red pulp, whereas endothelial continuity between arterial and venous vessels has never been shown. (5) The problem of the circulation in the spleen would seem to be an ideal one for solution by direct observation of the living organ. Unfortunately, the techniques available for this are difficult, and the reports made on such studies are contradictory. According to one group, the circulation in the spleen appears to be closed, there is a marked intermittency of circulation, there is extensive filtering of the liquid portion of the blood from the sinuses into the splenic cords, and erythrocytes normally leave the sinuses by diapedesis.

These conclusions are contradicted by another group of observers who report the circulation to be open—i.e., without preformed connections between the arterial and venous systems, so that the blood from the terminations of the arterial tree percolates between the reticular cells and macrophages of the splenic cords and finds its way through openings in the wall of the sinuses.

Lymphatic Vessels and Nerves

In man, lymphatic vessels are poorly developed and are found only in the capsule of the spleen and in the thickest trabeculae, particularly those in the vicinity of the hilus. In some mammals, true lymphatic vessels follow the arteries of the white pulp. Networks of nerves that originate from the celiac plexus and consist almost entirely of unmyelinated fibers accompany the splenic artery and penetrate into the hilus of the spleen. In the sheep and ox, these nerves form trunks of considerable thickness. The nerve bundles mainly follow the ramifications of the arteries and form networks that can be followed as far as the central arteries of the white pulp and even along the branches of the penicillar arteries. The terminal branches usually end with button-like thickenings on the smooth muscles of the arteries and of the trabeculae. Apparently many branches penetrate into the red as well as the white pulp, but their endings here are not definitely established.

HISTOPHYSIOLOGY

The filtering function of the spleen depends upon the abundant population of macrophages of the splenic cords, which arise from blood monocytes. Upon intravenous injection, particulate matter or macromolecular antigen first localize in the macrophages of the marginal zone and subsequently spread to the phagocytes of the rest of the red pulp. Neither the endothelial cells of the sinuses nor the fibroblast-like reticular cells of the splenic cords contribute significantly to clearing the blood of foreign material. Very little particulate matter enters the white pulp, but in the presence of antibody, antigen may be trapped for long periods of time in the germinal centers. When lipid in the blood is increased in amount, the macrophages of the spleen, like the other phagocytes of the body, have the capacity to remove it from the circulation. In this process, the macrophages enlarge and become filled with lipid droplets, thus acquiring a foamy appearance. This phenomenon is observed in diabetic hyperlipemia in man and in experimental hypercholesterolemia of rabbits.

The destruction of aged, abnormal, or damaged blood cells and platelets takes place in the meshes of the cords of the red pulp. How blood-borne elements and especially erythrocytes, which lack motility, reach the tissue spaces of the cords is still a matter of controversy. According to the "open circulation" theory, the capillaries deliver the blood directly to the pulp cords; this being true, the constituents of the plasma and the cells of the blood can freely percolate through the interstitial spaces between cord macrophages and reticular cells and finally reenter the blood through the walls of the venous sinuses. In a "closed" vascular system, one must postulate either that the pressure gradient between the arterial and venous ends of the sinuses drives plasma and erythrocytes into the cord spaces and then back into the blood, or that rhythmic contractions of the sinus endothelium squeeze the blood out of the vascular bed; this latter hypothesis implies the existence of a sphincteric mechanism at the venous end of the sinuses. With either theory, both plasma and blood cells establish extensive contact with the macrophages of the cords, which can then remove any undesirable component. Unphagocytosed cells can freely return to the intravascular compartment through the fenestrations of the basal lamina and the interendothelial clefts of the sinuses. The precise role of the spleen in removing aged erythrocytes, as well as the extent to which this function is shared with bone marrow and liver, is poorly understood. Splenectomy does not seem to affect the average life span of red blood cells significantly. There is no doubt, however, that the spleen plays a major role in destroying pathological or defective blood elements. When abnormal or experimentally damaged erythrocytes are perfused through the spleen, they are retained by this organ, whereas normal erythrocytes are not. Granulocytes damaged by endotoxin have also been shown to be destroyed in the spleen. Moreover, splenectomy is followed by the appearance in the bloodstream of defective erythrocytes containing remnants of the nucleus or cytoplasmic organelles. The mechanism by which macrophages recognize old or abnormal blood cells is unknown. It has been postulated that the immune system may react to changes in the erythrocyte surface and tag pathological cells with opsonizing antibody. In normal subjects, no lysis or fragmentation of red blood cells is observed either in the lumen of the sinuses or in the cord spaces, and erythrocytes seem to be phagocytized intact by macrophages. In pathological conditions, however, extracellular disintegration of red blood cells has been described.

Closely connected with erythrocyte destruction by the macrophages is the function of the spleen in hemoglobin degradation and iron metabolism. In the lysosomes of the macrophages, the iron of hemoglobin is freed and stored by the cell as ferritin or hemosiderin, readily available to the body for synthesis of new hemoglobin by bone marrow erythroblasts. The heme moiety of hemoglobin is degraded by macrophages to bilirubin, which enters the plasma, where it binds to albumin. It is then captured by the liver, conjugated to glucuronic acid, and secreted in the bile.

In animal species in which the capsule and trabeculae are rich in smooth muscle cells, the spleen can act as a store for red blood cells; large numbers of them in fact can be retained in the red pulp and then given up to the bloodstream when they are needed in the circulation. This may also occur experimentally following injection of drugs, such as epinephrine, that induce contraction of the splenic smooth muscle. The human spleen has little storage capacity (about 30 to 40 ml of erythrocytes), but it temporarily sequesters reticulocytes so that they can complete their maturation; in addition, it traps a large fraction of blood platelets in a reserve pool available to meet physiological demands or emergency conditions.

Although in the embryo the spleen contains immature precursors of the circulating blood elements, the erythrocytes found in the red pulp in the normal, adult human are never formed there. In some pathological conditions, especially myeloid leukemia, the red pulp of the spleen undergoes myeloid metaplasia, after which a large number of erythroblasts, megakaryocytes, and myelocytes appear in the tissue, so that the red pulp acquires a structure resembling that of the red bone marrow. In many other adult mammals, some myelocytes and erythroblasts may be found normally in the red pulp, and megakaryocytes are consistently present in the spleen of rats and mice.

The spleen has great physiological importance in the immune response to bacteria, viruses, and foreign macromolecules that have invaded the circulation. In an animal not involved in an acute response to antigen, it is evident from the small arteriovenous difference in lymphocyte counts on splenic blood that only a small fraction of the lymphocytes that leave the spleen via the veins arise from division of precursors in that organ. A large fraction of splenic lymphocytes belong to the recirculating pool and they are specifically localized in the periarterial lymphoid sheaths. This has been shown by experiments involving drainage of the thoracic duct lymph and reinjection of thoracic duct lymphocytes after labeling in vitro. Drainage of the thoracic duct lymph initially affects the central region of the periarterial lymphoid sheaths; only after prolonged drainage do the peripheral regions of the white pulp also become depleted of lymphocytes. This finding has been interpreted as evidence favoring the idea that the rapidly recirculating T lymphocytes localize close to the central artery, whereas the sluggishly migrating B cells assume a more peripheral position in the periarterial lymphoid sheaths. After intravenous injection, labeled thoracic duct cells, which are predominantly T lymphocytes, first localize in the marginal zone of the red pulp, but a few hours later they have migrated throughout the periarterial lymphoid sheaths. Labeled B lymphocytes first appear in the marginal zone, then reside for a few hours at the periphery of the sheaths, and finally migrate to the cap of the germinal centers. Thus, the suggestion has been advanced that the periarterial lymphoid sheaths consist of a central, thymus-dependent region and a peripheral, bursa-dependent region. In neonatally thymectomized rodents, the periarterial lymphoid sheaths are poorly populated with lymphocytes; thus, the vast majority of their lymphocytes are represented by T cells.

The transit time of the recirculating lymphocytes through the spleen is very short and may be as brief as two hours. The pathway followed by the lymphocytes in entering and leaving the periarterial lymphoid sheaths is poorly understood. They probably enter the cords of the marginal zone by crossing the walls of the venous sinuses and subsequently migrate into the white pulp. The route by which the lymphocytes reenter the blood is unknown; it has been suggested that they follow the lymphatic vessels that accompany the central artery, but these vessels do not seem to be found consistently in the splenic white pulp of all mammals.

Upon introduction into the bloodstream of an antigen that elicits a humoral response, morphological changes are first seen in the periarterial lymphoid sheaths. One day after the injection, proliferating lymphoblasts appear, scattered throughout the sheaths. They increase in number during the following one or two days and become more concentrated toward the periphery of the sheaths. At the same time, antibody first appears in the bloodstream. Lymphoblasts also occur around the small arteries of the red pulp. These may have developed from the terminal extensions of the periarterial lymphoid sheaths that surround the penicillar arteries. On days 4 to 6, an increasing number of immature plasma cells appear at the periphery of the periarterial lymphoid sheaths and along the penicillar arteries; mature plasma cells are also found, but in very small numbers. At this stage, morphological changes in germinal centers are first seen; they contain many proliferating lymphoblasts and macrophages loaded with debris of phagocytized lymphocytes. At the end of the first week, lymphoblasts and immature plasma cells begin to decrease in number in the periarterial lymphoid sheaths, and mature plasma cells are more numerous at the boundary between white and red pulp and along the penicillar arteries. They also occur in the cords of the red pulp and not infrequently free in the sinus lumen. During the second week after the introduction of the antigen, the structure of the spleen reverts to normal, except for the germinal centers, which continue to remain prominent for about one month.

During the secondary response, the spleen undergoes changes that resemble those following the first exposure to antigen, but they occur earlier and are much more dramatic. At the beginning of the response the spleen is, per unit weight, the most active organ of the body in antibody secretion, but it rapidly falls off in production as the response becomes propagated throughout the other peripheral lymphoid tissues and organs of the body.

Inasmuch as macrophages and lymphocytes are not restricted to the spleen, it is not surprising that the effects of splenectomy are transient and largely disappear as splenic functions are assumed by other organs.

REFERENCES

Blue, J., and L. Weiss: Periarterial macrophage sheaths (ellipsoids) in cat spleen—an electron microscope study. Am. J. Anat. *161*:115, 1981.

Blue, J., and L. Weiss: Vascular pathways in nonsinusal red pulp—an electron microscope study of the cat spleen. Am. J. Anat. *161*:135, 1981.

Blue, J., and L. Weiss: Species variation in the structure and function of the marginal zone—an electron microscope study of cat spleen. Am. J. Anat. *161*:169, 1981.

Blue, J., and L. Weiss: Electron microscopy of the red pulp of the dog spleen including vascular arrangements, periarterial macrophage sheaths (ellipsoids), and the contractile, innervated reticular meshwork. Am. J. Anat. *161*:189, 1981.

Burke, J. S., and G. T. Simon: Electron microscopy of the spleen. I. Anatomy and microcirculation. Am. J. Pathol. *58*:127, 1970.

Burke, J. S., and G. T. Simon: Electron microscopy of the spleen. II. Phagocytosis of colloidal carbon. Am. J. Pathol. *58*:157, 1970.

Carr, I.: The fine structure of the mammalian lymphoreticular system. Int. Rev. Cytol. 27:283, 1970.

Chen, L-T., and L. Weiss: Electron microscopy of the red pulp of human spleen. Am. J. Anat. *134*:425, 1972.

Coons, A. H.: Some reactions of lymphoid tissues to stimulation by antigen. Harvey Lect. *53*:113, 1959.

Edwards, V. D., and G. T. Simon: Ultrastructural aspects of red cell destruction in the normal rat spleen. J. Ultrastruct. Res. *33*:187, 1970.

Ernstrom, U., and G. Sandberg: Migration of splenic lymphocytes. Acta Pathol. Microbiol. Scand. *72*:379, 1968.

Ford, W. L., and J. L. Gowans: The traffic of lymphocytes. Semin. Hematol. *6*:67, 1969.

Galindo, B., and T. Imaeda: Electron microscope study of the white pulp of the mouse spleen. Anat. Rec. *143*:399, 1962.

Goldschneider, I., and D. D. McGregor: Migration of lymphocytes and thymocytes in the rat. I. The route of migration from blood to spleen and lymph nodes. J. Exp. Med. *127*:155, 1968.

Hanna, M. G., Jr., and A. K. Szakal: Localization of ^{125}I-labeled antigen in germinal centers of mouse spleen: histologic and ultrastructural autoradiographic studies of the secondary immune reaction. J. Immunol. *101*:949, 1968.

Jacobsen, G.: Morphological-histochemical comparison of dog and cat splenic ellipsoid sheaths. Anat. Rec. *169*:105, 1971.

Jacobson, L. O., E. K. Marks, M. J. Robson, E. Gaston, and R. E. Zirkle: The effect of spleen protection on mortality following x-irradiation. J. Lab. Clin. Med. *34*:1538, 1949.

Klemperer, P.: The Spleen. *In* Downey, H., ed.: Handbook of Hematology. New York, Paul B. Hoeber, 1938.

Knisely, M. H.: Spleen studies. I. Microscopic observations of the circulatory system of living unstimulated mammalian spleens. Anat. Rec. *65*:23, 1936.

Langevoort, H. L.: The histophysiology of the antibody response. I. Histogenesis of the plasma cell reaction in rabbit spleen. Lab. Invest. *12*:106, 1963.

Lewis, O. J.: The blood vessels of the adult mammalian spleen. J. Anat. *91*:245, 1957.

MacKenzie, D. W., Jr., A. O. Whipple, and M. P. Wintersteiner: Studies on the microscopic anatomy and physiology of living transilluminated mammalian spleens. Am. J. Anat. *68*:397, 1941.

McCuskey, R. S., and P. A. McCuskey: In vivo microscopy of the spleen. Bibl. Anat. *16*:121, 1977.

Miyoshi, M., and T. Fujita: Stereo-fine structure of the splenic red pulp. A combined scanning and transmission electron microscope study on dog and rat spleen. Arch. Histol. Jpn. *33*:225, 1971.

Miyoshi, M., T. Fujita, and J. Tokunaga: The red pulp

of the rabbit spleen studied under the scanning electron microscope. Arch. Histol. Jpn. *32*:289, 1970.

Mollier, S.: Uber den Bau der Capillaren Milzvenen (Milzsinus). Arch. f. Mikros. Anat. *76*:608, 1911.

Movat, H. Z., and N. V. P. Fernando: The fine structure of lymphoid tissue. Exp. Mol. Pathol. *3*:546, 1964.

Movat, H. Z., and N. V. P. Fernando: The fine structure of the lymphoid tissue during antibody formation. Exp. Mol. Pathol. *4*:155, 1965.

Nieuwenhuis, P., and W. L. Ford: Comparative migration of B- and T-lymphocytes in the rat spleen and lymph nodes. Cell. Immunol. *23*:254, 1976.

Peck, H. M., and N. L. Hoerr: The intermediary circulation in the red pulp of the mouse spleen. Anat. Rec. *109*:447, 1951.

Pictet, R., L. Orci, W. G. Forssmann, and L. Girardier: An electron microscope study of the perfusion-fixed spleen. I. The splenic circulation and the RES concept. Z. Zellforsch. *96*:372, 1969.

Robinson, W.: The vascular mechanism of the spleen. Am. J. Pathol. *2*:341, 1926.

Simon, G. T., and J. S. Burke: Electron microscopy of the spleen. III. Erythroleukophagocytosis. Am. J. Pathol. *58*:451, 1970.

Snodgrass, M. J.: A study of some histochemical and phagocytic reactions of the sinus lining cells of the rabbit's spleen. Anat. Rec. *161*:353, 1968.

Snook, T.: A comparative study of the vascular arrangements in mammalian spleens. Am. J. Anat. *87*:31, 1950.

Solnitzky, O.: The Schweigger-Seidel sheath (ellipsoid) of the spleen. Anat. Rec. *69*:55, 1937.

Sprent, J.: Circulating T and B lymphocytes of the mouse. I. Migratory properties. Cell. Immunol. *7*:10, 1973.

Stutte, H. J.: Nature of human spleen red pulp cells with special reference to sinus lining cells. Z. Zellforsch. *91*:300, 1968.

Sussdorf, D. H., and L. R. Draper: The primary hemolysin response in rabbits following shielding from x-rays or x-irradiation of the spleen, appendix, liver or hind legs. J. Infect. Dis. *99*:129, 1956.

Szakal, A. K., and M. G. Hanna, Jr.: The ultrastructure of antigen localization and virus-like particles in mouse spleen germinal centers. Exp. Mol. Pathol. *8*:75, 1968.

Thiel, G. A., and H. Downey: The development of the mammalian spleen, with special reference to its hematopoietic activity. Am. J. Anat. *28*:279, 1921.

Weidenreich, F.: Das Gefässsystem der menschlichen Milz. Arch. Mikros. Anat. *58*:247, 1901.

Weiss, L.: An experimental study of the organization of the reticuloendothelial system in the red pulp of the spleen. J. Anat. *93*:465, 1959.

Weiss, L.: The structure of fine splenic arterial vessels in relation to hemoconcentration and red cell destruction. Am. J. Anat. *111*:131, 1962.

Weiss, L.: The structure of intermediate vascular pathways in the spleen of rabbits. Am. J. Anat. *113*:51, 1963.

Weiss, L.: The Cells and Tissues of the Immune System. Structure, Functions, Interactions. Englewood Cliffs, NJ, Prentice-Hall, 1972.

Weiss, L.: The development of the primary vascular reticulum in the spleen of human fetuses (38 to 57 mm. crown-rump length). Am. J. Anat. *136*:315, 1973.

Weiss, L., and M. Tavassoli: Anatomical hazards to the passage of erythrocytes through the spleen. Semin. Hematol. *7*:372, 1970.

Wennberg, E., and L. Weiss: The structure of the spleen and hemolysis. Annu. Rev. Med. *20*:29, 1969.

17

HYPOPHYSIS

The hypophysis or pituitary is an endocrine gland located at the base of the brain. It is about 1 cm in length, 1 to 1.5 cm in width, and about 0.5 cm deep. It weighs about 0.5 g in men and slightly more in women. Despite its small size it is one of the most important organs in the body, producing at least nine hormones and having many reciprocal relations with other endocrine glands. It also has neural and vascular connections with the brain, to which it is attached by a slender stalk. By virtue of these connections, the hypophysis occupies a key position in the interplay of the nervous system and the endocrine system—the two great integrating systems of the body.

The hypophysis has two major subdivisions: the *neurohypophysis,* which develops as a process growing downward from the floor of the diencephalon, and the *adenohypophysis,* which originates in the embryo as a dorsal outpocketing of the roof of the embryonic pharynx. There are three subdivisions of the adenohypophysis: the *pars distalis* or anterior lobe, the *pars infundibularis (pars tuberalis),* and the *pars intermedia.* The neurohypophysis generally is divided into three regions: the *median eminence,* a funnel-shaped extension of the tuber cinereum; the *infundibular stalk;*

and the *infundibular process.* The relations of these components are depicted in Figure 17–3. In many species, the pars intermedia is closely adherent to the infundibular process to form the so-called *posterior lobe,* separated by a cleft from the pars distalis or anterior lobe. In man the cleft is largely obliterated in late fetal and postnatal life, so that the anterior and posterior lobes are in continuity. The subdivisions of the hypophysis and the accepted descriptive terminology are presented in tabular form in Figure 17–1.

The hypophysis is lodged in a deep depression in the sphenoid bone, the *sella turcica,* and is covered by a tough diaphragm, the *diaphragma sellae.* This barrier between the sella turcica and the intracranial cavity is often incomplete, being penetrated by an opening 5 mm or more in diameter around the hypophyseal stalk. Some of the pia-arachnoid may extend through this opening and occupy the narrow space between the diaphragm and the connective tissue capsule of the gland. Elsewhere the dense collagenous capsule is separated from the periosteum of the sphenoid bone by a looser layer of connective tissue containing numerous veins. This layer appears to be separate from the pia-arachnoid. In mammals other than man,

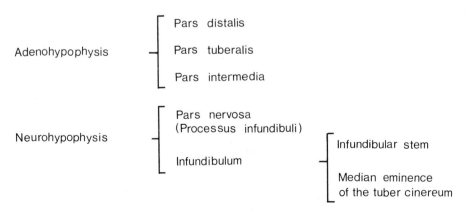

Figure 17–1. Terminology of the divisions and subdivisions of the hypophysis. In addition, the pars intermedia and pars nervosa together are sometimes called the posterior lobe, and the pars distalis and pars tuberalis are collectively called the anterior lobe.

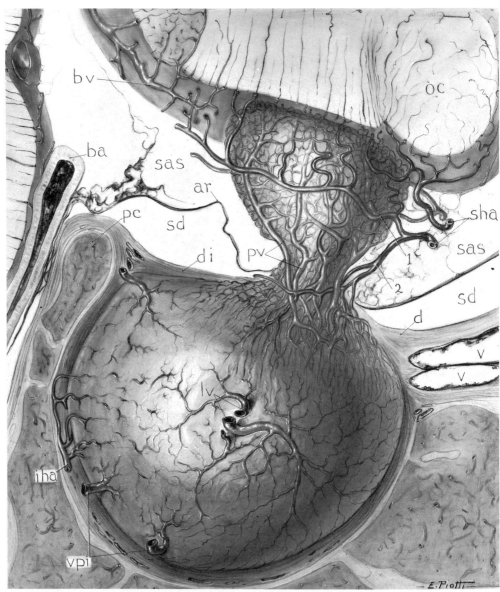

Figure 17–2. Schematic drawing of the hypophysis of an adult rhesus monkey, showing its relation to the sella turcica of the sphenoid bone. Also depicted are the superior and inferior hypophyseal arteries (*sha* and *iha*) and the important portal venules *(pv)* coursing down the infundibular stalk. The superior hypophyseal artery usually sends an ascending branch *(1)* to the proximal part of the infundibular stalk and median eminence and a descending branch *(2)* coursing distally. *ar*, Arachnoid membrane; *ba*, basilar artery; *bv*, basilar veins; *d*, dura; *di*, sellar diaphragm; *lv*, lateral hypophyseal veins; *oc*, optic chiasm; *pc*, posterior clinoid process; *sas*, subarachnoid space; *sd*, subdural space; *v*, dural vein; *vpi*, veins of the infundibular process. (After Wislocki, G. B. Proc. Assoc. Res. Nerv. Ment. Dis. *17*:48, 1936.)

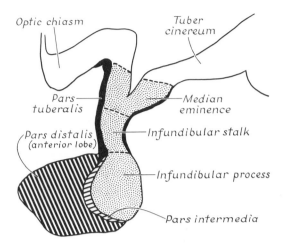

Figure 17–3. Diagram of midsagittal section of hypothalamus and hypophysis of man to show relations of major divisions and subdivisions of the gland to the hypothalamus. (Modified from Tilney.)

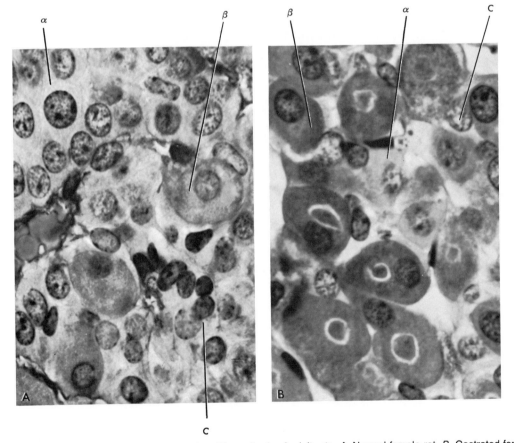

Figure 17–4. Photomicrographs of anterior lobe of hypophysis of adult rats. *A,* Normal female rat. *B,* Castrated female rat of same age. Hypertrophy of basophil cells *(β),* with enlargement of the Golgi complexes (here shown next to each nucleus as a negative image and appearing as a clear halo), and reduction in acidophil *(α)* and chromophobe (C) cells follow castration. Zenker-formol, Mallory-azan. × 1300. (Courtesy of I. Gersh.)

the diaphragma sellae is commonly incomplete.

PARS DISTALIS

The pars distalis or anterior lobe is the largest subdivision of the hypophysis. It is composed of glandular cells arranged in irregular cords and clumps. These are intimately related to an extensive system of thin-walled sinusoids of the blood vascular system. The anterior lobe is largely enclosed by a dense collagenous capsule. The stroma of the gland is not abundant, but some collagenous fibers, which accompany the superior hypophyseal arteries and the portal venules, penetrate the anterior lobe at the pole adjacent to the pars tuberalis and fan out bilaterally, extending about a third of the way into the gland. There they become continuous with reticular fibers that surround the cords of parenchymal cells and support the small branches of the hypophyseal artery and the sinusoids. The sinusoids at the periphery of the gland continue into collecting venules that join an extensive venous plexus in the capsule. The endothelium lining the sinusoids was formerly considered to be phagocytic and was classified as a component of the reticuloendothelial system. This interpretation is not borne out by electron microscopy. Uptake of particulate tracers in the gland is confined to extravascular tissue macrophages.

The glandular cells are classified as *chromophilic* or *chromophobic* on the basis of their avidity or lack of affinity for the dyes used in routine staining of histological sections. The chromophilic cells were originally subdivided into *acidophilic cells* or *basophilic cells,* according to the tinctorial reactions of their specific granules in sections stained with eosin and alum-hematoxylin or with other combinations of an acidic and a basic dye.

It is important to realize that the terms acidophilic and basophilic as used by the pituitary cytologist do not have the same connotation with respect to the chemistry of the cytoplasm that they generally have in other fields of cytology. The basophilia of the granules in the pituitary basophilic cell is not to be confused with that attributable to cytoplasmic ribonucleoprotein in other glandular cells. In the naming of the pituitary cells, *acidophilic* and *basophilic* refer only to

the staining affinities of the specific granules. Historically these terms were reasonable and served to distinguish two major classes of chromophilic cells at a time when there were only a few empirically developed staining combinations in routine use, and when the great diversity of pituitary functions was not yet appreciated. As time has passed, the number of hormones known to be secreted by the adenohypophysis has increased to six. The effort to identify cell types to which synthesis of each of these hormones could be attributed led to the development of numerous staining methods. The terminological problem has been greatly aggravated by the fact that most of the staining procedures now considered useful for the study of the adenohypophysis do not make use of an acid and a basic dye but involve mixtures of acid dyes. With many of these methods, staining does not depend on the binding of a dye by a tissue component of opposite charge, and no conclusion as to the chemical nature of the granules can be drawn from their color in sections stained in this way. The color of specific granules of the same cell type may be red, orange, purple, or blue, depending on the combination of acid dyes used. With the trichrome staining methods, it has been necessary to establish the relation of the cell types to the traditional acidophilic, basophilic, and chromophobic categories by comparison of the same cells in consecutive sections stained with trichrome mixtures and with hematoxylin and eosin.

The most meaningful histochemical method for identification of cell categories is the periodic acid–Schiff (PAS) reaction, which selectively stains the granules of basophils because of their content of glycoprotein. Another approach of proven value for identification of the cell of origin of various hormones involves the use of immunohistochemical procedures. In these methods, antibodies to a specific hormone are induced in another species and are conjugated with fluorescent dyes or with horseradish peroxidase. These labeled antibodies are then reacted with sections of hypophysis and the sites of the antigen in the tissue are localized by fluorescence microscopy or by the histochemical method for peroxidase.

Electron microscopic studies have shown that the specific granules of the cells in the adenohypophysis differ significantly in their size. Granule size and shape are therefore valuable criteria for distinguishing cell types in electron micrographs.

Various systems of nomenclature based on Greek letter designations have been proposed to avoid the inconsistency involved in continued use of acidophil and basophil, but none of these has gained widespread acceptance. The terminology now in general use is therefore a confusing mixture of terms in which acidophil, basophil, and chromophobe are used to designate three major classes of cells in the adenohypophysis, while various Greek letters or adjectives referring to distinctive tinctorial reactions are used to identify specific cell types within these classes. In recent years it has become common practice to substitute terms that identify the target organ stimulated (e.g., *thyrotroph, gonadotroph, corticotroph*) or the hormone secreted (e.g., *TSH cell, FSH/LH cell, ACTH cell*).

The description of the ultrastructure of the cells that follows relies heavily upon studies of the rat, because comparable investigations of the human gland are few as yet. Although there are interspecific differences, the general principles are the same.

ACIDOPHILS (ALPHA CELLS)

Acidophils in the human hypophysis are most numerous in the posterolateral portions of the pars distalis. They are small rounded cells 14 to 19 μm in diameter, with a well-developed juxtanuclear Golgi complex and small rod-shaped mitochondria. They stain with eosin in routine histological sections, and their granules are large enough to be resolved with the light microscope. Two categories of acidophils can be distinguished by selective staining methods, and with greater precision by immunocytochemical procedures using antibodies to specific hormones.

Somatotrophs

These acidophils, occurring in groups along the sinusoids, secrete growth hormone (*somatotropin*) and are therefore called *somatotrophs* (*STH cells*). They contain very numerous spherical granules 300 to 350 nm in diameter (Figs. 17–5, 17–6), which are selectively stained by antibody against growth hormone. The cisternae of their well-developed endoplasmic reticulum tend to be arranged parallel to the cell surface.

Human *pituitary gigantism* resulting from excess production of growth hormone is associated with a tumor of the pars distalis composed of acidophils having these ultra-structural features and immunohistochemical staining properties.

Mammotrophs (Prolactin Cells)

Acidophils of this type tend to be distributed individually in the interior of the cell cords. They secrete the hormone *prolactin*, which stimulates the mammary gland. They contain numerous small granules about 200 nm in diameter.

In the nonlactating, sexually mature female they are relatively small cells with a few short cisternae of reticulum near the cell periphery. In pregnancy they are stimulated by the elevated level of circulating estrogens, and undergo considerable hypertrophy. In this condition they stain with azocarmine or erythrosin in trichrome stains, and they were formerly called "pregnancy cells." Their Golgi complex enlarges and the endoplasmic reticulum becomes more extensive, forming multiple layers parallel to the plasmalemma, and the granules become larger, 550 to 600 nm in diameter and often irregular in outline (Fig. 17–7).

The period of greatest activity of the mammotrophs is during the postpartum prolactin secretion necessary to initiate and maintain lactation. When suckling is terminated, lysosomes have an important role in the elimination of excess secretory granules and the hypertrophied cellular organelles involved in the earlier period of active protein synthesis. Lysosomes fuse with the secretory granules to form autophagic vacuoles in which the granules are degraded by hydrolytic enzymes (Fig. 17–8). This method of disposal of secretory product no longer needed is called *crinophagy*. Excess cytomembranes and ribosomes are also enclosed in vacuoles and degraded by autophagy until the mammotrophs have reverted to the relatively inactive state characteristic of the normal cycling female.

BASOPHILS (BETA CELLS)

This category of cells in the anterior pituitary stains poorly with hematoxylin and is less easily identified in routine preparations than are the eosinophils. Basophils do stain well with the aniline blue of Mallory's trichrome stain and with resorcin-fuchsin. They are most easily distinguished from eosinophils by their pink staining with the PAS

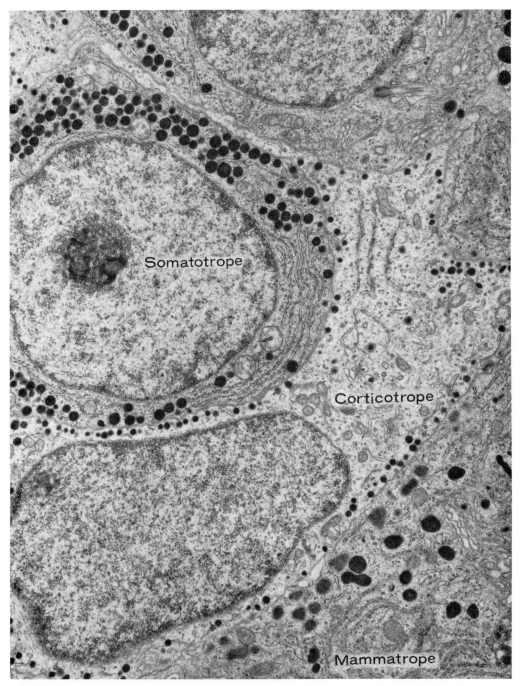

Figure 17–5. Electron micrograph of an area of the pars distalis of rat hypophysis illustrating the fine structure and relative size of the specific granules of a somatotrope, mammatrope, and corticotrope. (Micrograph from Nakayama, I., F. A. Nickerson, and F. R. Shelton. Lab. Invest. *21*:169, 1969.)

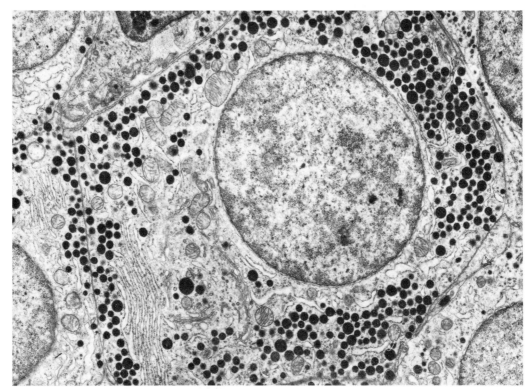

Figure 17–6. A typical somatotrope, showing numerous cisternae of endoplasmic reticulum, a well-developed Golgi complex, and many specific granules about 350 nm in diameter. (Micrograph courtesy of M. Farquhar.)

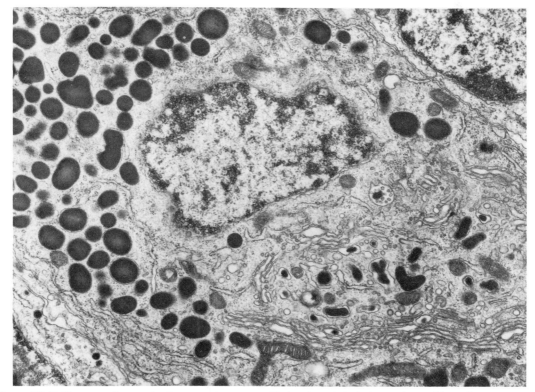

Figure 17–7. Electron micrograph of a rat mammatrope. Notice the relatively large size and irregular shape of the granules. A number of developing granules are associated with a large Golgi complex at lower right of figure. (Micrograph courtesy of M. Farquhar and T. Kanaseki.)

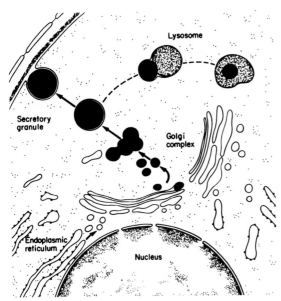

Figure 17–8. Diagram illustrating the secretory pathway of a mammatrope. Small granules are formed in the Golgi complex and subsequently fuse to form larger granules, often of irregular outline. During lactation, they are discharged by exocytosis, but after the young are weaned, excess granules fuse with lysosomes and are destroyed by autophagy. (After Smith, R. E., and M. G. Farquhar. J. Cell Biol. 31:319, 1966.)

reaction for carbohydrates. There are three distinct types of basophils.

Thyrotrophs (Beta Basophils, TSH Cells)

The cells that secrete *thyroid stimulating hormone* (TSH) are elongated or polygonal in shape and arranged in clusters in the anteromedial portion of the anterior lobe. They tend to be deeply situated in the cell cords, not in contact with the sinusoids. They can be distinguished from other basophils by the selective staining of their granules with aldehyde thionin. In electron micrographs they have the smallest granules of any cell in the pituitary, 140 to 160 nm in diameter. They are less dense than the granules of other basophils and tend to congregate at the periphery of the cell. They stain immunocytochemically with anti-TSH antibody.

Thyrotrophs hypertrophy following thyroidectomy and atrophy after thyroxin administration.

Corticotrophs (Corticotropes, ACTH Cells)

These cells secrete *adrenocorticotropic hormone* (ACTH) and *lipotropic hormone* (LPH).

In the human they are round or oval, are distributed throughout the anteromedial portion of the pars distalis, and commonly invade a short distance into the neural lobe.

They contain granules that are intensely stained with the PAS reaction. The granule size 200 to 250 nm does not differ significantly from that of gonadotrophs and is not a reliable criterion for identification. In rodents these cells are irregularly stellate in shape, with cell processes that extend between neighboring cells to end adjacent to sinusoids. Their cytoplasm is of low density with a rather sparse endoplasmic reticulum (Fig. 17–5). The granules tend to be located adjacent to the cell membrane. The small granules are not easily resolved with the light microscope and these cells were often misidentified as chromophobes. The most dependable criterion for their identification is immunocytochemical staining with anti-ACTH or anti-LPH.

It was long believed that there was one cell type for each pituitary hormone. It is now known that the corticotrophs synthesize a 31,000-M.W. glycoprotein prohormone that includes the amino acid sequences of ACTH and LPH. This molecule undergoes posttranslational cleavage to yield these two hormones. In pig and rat, and possibly in other species, the LPH is further processed to yield *beta endorphin,* an opiate-like peptide with potent analgesic activity.

Following adrenalectomy, corticotrophs become more numerous and larger, and contain greater numbers of granules. After prolonged administration of cortisol, they decrease in size and stain only faintly.

Gonadotrophs (Delta Basophils, Gonadotropes, FSH/LH Cells)

These rounded cells are usually situated adjacent to sinusoids. They secrete two hormones, *follicle stimulating hormone* (FSH) and *luteinizing hormone* (LH). They are PAS positive but do not stain with aldehyde fuchsin. In electron micrographs there is a prominent juxtanuclear Golgi complex and a well-developed endoplasmic reticulum with meandering cisternae that are often distended with a homogeneous content of low density (Fig. 17–9). The granules are spherical and vary over a wide range, 200 to 400 nm in diameter. Whether there are two gonadotrophs, one secreting FSH and the other LH, has long been a subject of controversy. Certainly they exhibit considerable cytological varia-

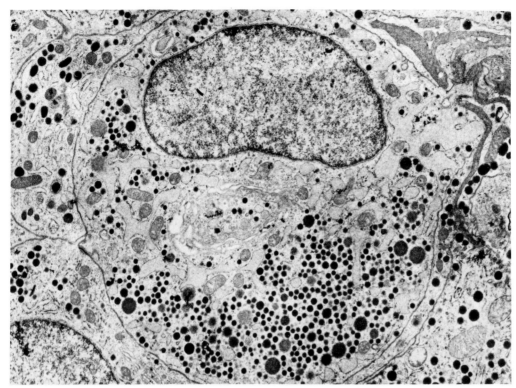

Figure 17–9. Gonadotrope with granules of relatively smaller size than the somatotrope (see Fig. 17–6) but displaying considerable variability. The endoplasmic reticulum is typically distended with an amorphous material of low density. (Micrograph courtesy of M. Farquhar.)

tion. Some are ovoid with a population of small granules; others are angular or stellate and contain only small granules, 200 to 220 nm. Some stain immunocytochemically only with anti-FSH, others with anti-LH, and still others react to both antibodies. It remains unsettled whether both hormones are found in the same granule or in different populations of granules. It seems likely that the varying cytological features observed represent different physiological states of the same cell type.

CHROMOPHOBES (RESERVE CELLS)

Chromophobes are usually small cells located in groups in the interior of the cell cords. They generally have less cytoplasm than the chromophilic cells but may rarely reach the dimensions of acidophils or basophils. Traditionally, chromophobes have been considered to be devoid of specific granules, but electron micrographs reveal relatively few cells with no specific granules. The cells of the pars distalis are believed to have cyclic secretory activity, first accumulating and then releasing their specific granules. It

seems likely that many of the cells identified as chromophobes with the light microscope are, in fact, partially degranulated chromophil cells.

Mitoses are relatively few in the anterior lobe. For this reason, it was formerly thought that the shifts in proportions of the three major cell categories were the result of transformations of one cell type to another. Investigations of these population shifts led to proposals of several cell lineages based upon observation of what were presumed to be morphological transition stages. The most widely accepted of these schemes considered the chromophobes to be a reserve population of relatively undifferentiated cells capable of differentiating into either acidophils or basophils. It has become increasingly apparent that the cells classified as chromophobes by light microscopy are not a homogeneous population. Some are evidently chromophils degranulated to the point at which their specific nature is not detectable. There seems to be a considerable degree of cytological specialization among the cells normally classified as chromophobes. Some are said to have a Golgi apparatus characteristic of acidophils, while in others the Golgi apparatus resembles that

Hormones	Cell Type		Staining reactions*		Electron microscopic description
	General	Specific	AF	PAS	
Growth or somato-tropic hormone (STH)	Acidophil	Somatotrope	−	−	350 nm. granules, cells columnar and arranged in groups on sinusoids
Lactogenic or luteo-tropic hormone (LTH)	Acidophil	Mammotrope or luteotrope	−	−	600 nm. elliptical gran-ules, cells located indi-vidually in interior of cell cords
Thyrotropic hormone (TSH)	Basophil	Thyrotrope	+	+	140 nm. granules, cells angular and not usually located on sinusoids
Follicle stimulating hormone (FSH)	Basophil	FSH Gonadotrope	−	+	200 nm. granules, cells located on sinusoids and are usually rounded
Luteinizing hormone (LH)	Basophil	LH Gonadotrope	−	+	200 nm. granules, cells usually located on sinusoids, rounded and contain bizarre cyto-plasmic formations
Adrenocorticotropic hormone (ACTH)	Chromophobe	Corticotrope	−	−	200–250 nm. granules, cells pale, stellate. Few granules at cell periphery
No specific hormone	Chromophobe	Acidophilic chromophobe Basophilic chromophobe	−	−	Few characteristic granules

*AF, Aldehyde fuchsin; PAS, periodic acid–Schiff.

Figure 17–10. Summary of current views of rat anterior pituitary cell types and their secretions. (Modified from McShan W. H., and M. W. Hartley. Ergebn. Physiol. *56*:264, 1965.)

of basophils. It is probable that many of the apparent chromophobes are already deter-mined and capable of differentiating into only one of the chromophil types.

With the light microscope, chromophobes were formerly estimated to make up 65 per cent of the cells in the pars distalis. It is now evident that the great majority of these were degranulated secretory cells with so few re-maining granules that their affinity for stains was below a detectable level. If chromo-phobes that are nonspecific stem cells exist at all, they are evidently much less numerous than they were formerly thought to be.

FOLLICULAR CELLS (STELLATE CELLS)

The principal nonsecretory cells of the anterior pituitary are *follicular cells,* so named because they often adopt an epithelial mode of association, lining small cystlike follicles containing colloidal material of low electron density. In this form the cells have microvilli and occasional tufts of cilia on their luminal surface. The apical plasma membrane has a prominent surface coat and the cells are joined by juxtaluminal junctional complexes. Unlike other epithelia, these cells have long basal processes that extend outward between the neighboring glandular cells. Their cyto-plasm contains the usual complement of or-ganelles, occasional lipid droplets, numerous polyribosomes, and beta particles of glyco-gen. They may also occur as *stellate cells* that do not line follicles but extend branching processes among the secretory cells. Similar interstitial stellate cells form a loose mesh-work throughout the pars intermedia. Their function is poorly understood. They are re-ported to be phagocytic in in vitro studies, surrounding and ingesting dead cells and cellular debris. There is evidence that they have a similar scavenger function in vivo. The filaments in their processes react with antibody to gliofibrillar acid protein, and it has been suggested that they may have a nurse cell function comparable with that of the glial cells of the central nervous system.

NERVES

The secretory activity of the pars distalis is controlled primarily by releasing hormones generated in the hypothalamus and carried to it in the blood. Therefore, one would not expect to find nerves in the gland. There are, however, isolated reports of the occurrence, in some species, of rare bundles of unmyelinated axons found in the perisinusoidal connective tissue and in the delicate septa between clusters of secretory cells. The axons are described as having varicosities containing small clear vesicles and large dense-cored vesicles. Some appear to terminate in close association with somatotrophs. It remains unclear whether these are functionally significant or represent aberrant invasion of the pars distalis by nerves from the pars intermedia and pars tuberalis. There is as yet no supporting physiological evidence of neural control of secretion in the pars distalis.

BLOOD SUPPLY

The blood supply of the hypophysis is unusual and is intimately involved in the control of the secretory activity of the gland. Two *inferior hypophyseal* arteries from the internal carotid arborize within the capsule of the gland, sending branches to the posterior lobe and to a lesser extent to the sinusoids of the anterior lobe. Several *superior hypophyseal* arteries arise from the internal carotid artery and posterior communicating artery of the circle of Willis and anastomose freely in the region of the median eminence of the hypothalamus and base of the pituitary stalk (Figs. 17–2, 17–11). From these vessels, capillaries comprising the so-called *primary plexus* extend into the median eminence and are then returned to the surface, where they are col-

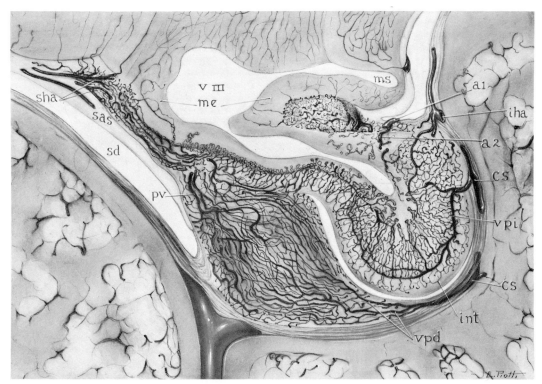

Figure 17–11. Drawing of a thick median sagittal section of a cat's hypophysis after injection of the blood vascular system with India ink. The main blood supply is via the superior hypophyseal artery *(sha)* and inferior hypophyseal arteries *(iha)*. The venous drainage is via systemic veins from the pars distalis *(vpd)* and the pars nervosa *(vpi)*. Portal veins arising in capillaries in the median eminence and pars tuberalis *(pv)* carry the neurohumoral releasing hormones from the median eminence of the hypothalamus *(me)* to the pars distalis. *sas*, Subarachnoid space; *sd*, subdural space; *V iii*, third ventricle; *a1* and *a2*, branches of inferior hypophyseal artery; *cs*, capsular venous sinuses; *int*, pars intermedia. (From Wislocki, G. B. Anat. Rec. *69*:361, 1937.)

lected into veins that run downward around the hypophyseal stalk to supply the sinusoids of the adenohypophysis below. The venules connecting capillaries in the median eminence with the sinusoidal capillaries of the anterior lobe constitute the *hypophyseoportal* system. The venous drainage of the hypophysis is chiefly through vessels that run in the vascular layer of the capsule to the diaphragm of the sella turcica and thence into adjacent dural sinuses. Some venous blood may also enter sinuses in the sphenoid bone. It is firmly established that neurohumoral substances (*releasing factors* or *hypophyseotropic hormones*) released by nerves in the median eminence of the hypothalamus are carried in the blood via the hypophyseoportal system to the adenohypophysis, where they stimulate the cells to release their specific hormones.

HISTOPHYSIOLOGY OF THE PARS DISTALIS

The pars distalis or anterior lobe of the hypophysis secretes at least six hormones that stimulate several target organs—thyroid, adrenal cortex, ovaries, testicles, and mammary glands. It is an indispensable organ control-

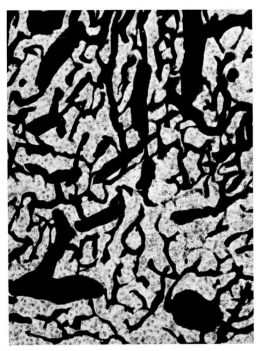

Figure 17–12. Photomicrograph of anterior lobe of hypophysis of monkey injected intravenously with India ink to show the irregular, richly anastomotic sinusoids. × 165. (Courtesy of I. Gersh.)

ling many different physiological processes. Its surgical removal results in cessation of growth in young animals; atrophy of the gonads, thyroid gland, and adrenal cortex; and disturbances of carbohydrate, protein, and lipid metabolism. These profound and potentially fatal effects of hypophysectomy are the collective consequences of eliminating the source of the hormones whose individual functions are described below.

Growth Hormone (Somatotropin, GH, STH)

Growth hormone is a small protein consisting of about 190 amino acids and no carbohydrate component. Unlike the other hormones of the anterior lobe, it does not have a specific target organ but has a generalized effect upon cells throughout the body, increasing their rate of protein synthesis. Other metabolic effects include increased mobilization of fatty acids from adipose tissue and a decreased rate of utilization of glucose. Its most conspicuous effect is upon the rate of growth of young animals. Absence of growth hormone results in *pituitary dwarfism*. Excess secretion leads to *pituitary gigantism*. Growth hormone produced in excess by a pituitary tumor in adult life results in *acromegaly*, a condition characterized by disproportionate thickening of the bones. Its effect upon growth in stature in childhood is mediated by smaller proteins, *somatomedins*, which are synthesized in the liver and elsewhere in response to growth hormone. The somatomedins in turn stimulate the proliferation of cartilage that is necessary for growth in length of the long bones.

Prolactin

The lactogenic hormone *prolactin* is a protein with a molecular weight of about 25,000 consisting of a single chain of 205 amino acids. Its principal function is the promotion of mammary gland development and lactation. In pregnancy its concentration in the blood rises progressively from the fifth week until full term when it reaches levels ten times that of the nonpregnant woman. This stimulates development of the mammary gland, but the lactogenic effect of the hormone is suppressed by high levels of estrogen and progesterone until birth of the baby. Thereafter the precipitous fall of these ovarian hormones allows the lactogenic effect of prolactin to be expressed.

In rodents prolactin also participates in maintenance of the corpus luteum of pregnancy. Because of this function it has also been called *luteotropin* (LTH).

Thyrotropin (Thyroid Stimulating Hormones, TSH)

Thyroid stimulating hormone is a glycoprotein with a molecular weight of about 28,000. It appears to exert its effect exclusively upon the thyroid gland where it promotes proteolysis of thyroglobulin and release of thyroid hormone into the blood. It also causes hypertrophy of the thyroid cells and increases their rate of synthesis of thyroid hormone.

Gonadotropins: Follicle Stimulating Hormone (FSH) and Luteinizing Hormone (LH)

These two hormones are produced by the cells of the anterior lobe called gonadotrophs. As indicated earlier in this chapter, the question is moot whether they are produced in the same cell concurrently, or in a different phase of a secretory cycle, or by two subpopulations of the same cell type.

Follicle stimulating hormone (FSH) is a glycoprotein with a molecular weight of about 30,000. In the female there is a cyclic increase and decrease in the secretion of FSH each month. A rising level stimulates the development of several follicles in the ovary in preparation for ovulation of one, or occasionally two, at midcycle. In the male, FSH plays an important role in the initiation of spermatogenesis at puberty. Its function in the adult is less clear, but it has been shown to act upon the Sertoli cells of the seminiferous epithelium to promote the synthesis of an androgen-binding protein.

Luteinizing hormone (LH) is also a glycoprotein, having a molecular weight of about 26,000. In the female it acts upon the ovary, promoting secretion of estrogen by the developing follicles. It is necessary for maturation of the follicle, and a midcycle surge of LH release triggers ovulation. The common oral contraceptives act by inhibiting this peak of LH. After ovulation the hormone causes differentiation of lutein cells that form the corpus luteum.

In the male, LH stimulates the interstitial cells of the testis to secrete testosterone, which is essential for maintenance of spermatogenesis.

Adrenocorticotropin (Adrenocorticotropic Hormone, ACTH)

Adrenocorticotropin is a straight chained polypeptide with 39 amino acids and a molecular weight of about 4500. It stimulates the adrenal cortex to secrete cortisol. It is produced in the corticotrophs by proteolytic cleavage of a larger precursor molecule, *pro-opiocortin* or *pro-opiomelanocortin*. Another cleavage product, *beta-lipotropic hormone* (LPH), is secreted with ACTH, but no peripheral physiological effects of LPH have yet been identified. LPH may be further cleaved to yield *melanocyte stimulating hormone* (MSH), and beta endorphin. The physiological role of these peptides is still unclear.

Occurrence of Pituitary Hormones in Other Organs

It has long been assumed that the hormones of the adenohypophysis were produced only by specific cells in that gland. As sensitive radioimmunoassays for their detection and immunocytochemical methods for their localization have developed, all the hormones of the anterior and intermediate lobe, except the gonadotropins, have been found within the central nervous system of several species including humans. Although some investigators insist that all such hormones are of pituitary origin, evidence is accumulating to indicate that they are of neural origin. This interpretation is supported by the finding that the concentration of ACTH, α-MSH, β endorphin, and growth hormone in certain areas of the brain remain unchanged or increase after hypophysectomy. Moreover, brain slices or dispersed central nervous system cells maintained in culture secrete into the medium a greater amount of hormone than was present in the tissue when explanted.

There is now great interest in the possible functions of these molecules in the nervous system. Effects of some of these peptides on learning and behavior of experimental animals have been reported, and it is speculated that they may function as neurotransmitters or may modulate the effects of classical neurotransmitters on the receptors of specific sets of target neurons.

ACTH immunoreactivity has also been detected in certain cells in the gastrointestinal tract and in neoplasms of the lung that are thought to arise from neuroepithelial bodies in the bronchial epithelium. One explanation advanced for the synthesis of similar peptides in neurons and endocrine cells postulates that both are specialized ectodermal cells arising from the epiblast of the embryo and have similar potential because of their common origin.

Histophysiological Correlations

The cell types believed to be responsible for secretion of the hypophyseal hormones have already been identified. Elaboration of somatotropin and prolactin is attributed to two morphologically distinct types of acidophil. The glycoprotein gonadotropic hormones FSH and LH are assigned to the PAS-positive basophils. There is reason to believe that basophils that also stain with aldehyde-fuchsin are responsible for secretion of thyrotropin. In addition to the histochemical and biochemical evidence relating these hormones to the basophils, there is experimental evidence based upon the negative feedback mechanisms that operate in the regulation of hormone release. Endocrine glands that are under the direct control of the anterior lobe hormones usually exert a reciprocal inhibiting effect upon hypophyseal function via the hypothalamus. Removal of the target organ therefore results in hypertrophy of those cells in the adenohypophysis responsible for elaboration of the corresponding tropic hormone. After castration, the rat hypophysis contains increased amounts of gonadotropic hormones, and at the same time the basophils become markedly enlarged and vacuolated in a characteristic way (castration cells, Fig. 17–4). Thyroidectomy also results in an increase in the percentage of another type of basophil, thyroidectomy cells.

Control of Anterior Lobe Function

If the pituitary is severed from the hypothalamus and transplanted elsewhere in the body, its cells remain viable but the rates of secretion of all the hormones except prolactin fall nearly to zero. However, if the anterior lobe is placed in tissue culture together with fragments of the ventral hypothalamus, secretory function of the pituitary cells is better maintained. These and other experiments clearly indicated that the control of pituitary function depended on the existence of secretory products of hypothalamic neurons that are carried to the pars distalis in the hypothalamohypophyseal portal system of blood vessels.

Prodigious efforts to identify these substances culminated in 1968 in the isolation from 300,000 sheep hypothalami of 1 mg of a hypophyseotropic peptide designated thyrotropin releasing factor (TRF), now more commonly called thyrotropin releasing hormone (TRH)—a peptide of only three amino acids. This was the first of a series of similar efforts that led to isolation, sequencing, and synthesis of other releasing hormones: gonadotropin releasing hormone (GnRH), a decapeptide that causes release of both FSH and LH; and corticotropin releasing hormone (CRH), a 41 amino acid polypeptide releasing ACTH. Hypothalamic inhibiting hormones have also been isolated and characterized: prolactin inhibiting hormone (PIH), which suppresses prolactin secretion; and growth hormone inhibiting hormone (GHIH), also known as somatostatin. The latter is less specific in its action than the others, inhibiting secretion of glucagon, insulin, and other hormones of the gastrointestinal tract in addition to growth hormone.

Thus, nearly all the functions of the adenohypophysis depend on peptide signals received from the hypothalamus in the portal blood. Secretion of TSH, FSH, LH, and ACTH occurs in response to releasing hormones. Prolactin, on the other hand, seems to be under tonic inhibition by the hypothalamus. Therefore, its secretion by mammatrophs is enhanced by pituitary transplantation or explantation to tissue culture, while other cell types atrophy.

PARS INTERMEDIA

In many mammals, the pars distalis is separated from the neurohypophysis by a cleft, lined on the juxtaneural side by a multilayered epithelium of basophilic cells making up the pars intermedia. There is considerable variation among species in the degree of development of the pars intermedia. In rats and mice, dogs, cats, and oxen it forms a multilayered epithelium of basophilic cells. In marsupials it is reduced to a layer only one or two cells deep, and in cetacea, sirenia, and some birds it is absent. In the human fetus it is represented by a typical stratified epithelium adjacent to the infundibular process and may constitute 3 per cent of the glandular portion of the hypophysis, but in he adult it is no longer identifiable as a distinct layer. In the great majority of humans the hypophyseal cleft becomes discontinuous in postnatal life and is represented in the adult by a zone of cysts (Rathke's cysts). These are often lined by ciliated epithelium and contain a colorless or pale yellow colloid that varies in consistency but is often a highly viscous fluid. With the disappearance of the cleft, the epithelium of the pars intermedia becomes discontinuous and the isolated cells or groups of cells that remain may extend some distance into the neural tissue of the infundibular process, where they are often overlooked in routine histological preparations but can be detected immunohistochemically. Thus, the pars intermedia of humans differs from that of most mammals in several respects: the cleft is rarely complete; cysts are of common occurrence; and the remaining basophilic cells are few and may extend into the neural lobe to a surprising degree. In rodents such as the mouse, on the other hand, the pars intermedia constitutes 19 per cent of the hypophysis. The following description of its ultrastructure is based mainly on studies of the rodent hypophysis.

The principal cells of the pars intermedia secrete *melanocyte stimulating hormone* (MSH). They are large polygonal epithelial cells, rich in mitochondria and possessing a well-developed rough endoplasmic reticulum and Golgi complex. Numerous small secretory granules 200 to 300 nm in diameter are distributed throughout the cytoplasm. Some of these are electron dense and others are quite pale. Their variation in density is attributed to partial extraction of their contents, which are not adequately preserved by osmium fixation. Although the granules are inconspicuous at the light microscope level, the cells stain with the PAS reaction. The hormone secreted is a simple polypeptide, but the carbohydrate staining of the granules is consistent with biochemical evidence that the precursor is a high-molecular-weight glycoprotein.

In addition to the MSH-secreting cells there is a limited number of cells in the pars intermedia that have all the ultrastructural characteristics of the ACTH-secreting cells of the pars distalis. They are smaller than the MSH cells, are irregular in outline, and have dense, 200-nm secretory granules located mainly at the periphery adjacent to the plasma membrane. These cells react with anti-ACTH antibody as intensely as the corticotrophs of the pars distalis. Cells with sim-ilar ultrastructure and immunohistochemical properties may also be found scattered in neighboring regions of the neural lobe.

Nonsecretory *stellate cells* extend long branching processes around and between the glandular cells, forming a loose meshwork throughout the pars intermedia. These cells react strongly with antibody to glial fibrillar acid protein, and their membranes exhibit Na^+,K^+-ATPase activity. They are therefore similar to the astrocytes of the median eminence and hypophyseal stalk and may conceivably play some role in regulation of the secretory activity of the MSH cells.

The pars intermedia is poorly vascularized but richly innervated. Numerous axons contain dense-cored vesicles 80 to 120 nm in diameter and are believed to be dopaminergic fibers originating in the rostral arcuate nucleus.

HISTOPHYSIOLOGY OF THE PARS INTERMEDIA

The role of the hypophysis in the control of pigmentation in fish and amphibia was discovered over 50 years ago. Removal of the gland in frogs resulted in lightening of skin color, and when the anterior and intermediate lobes were then transplanted separately into tadpoles, only the transplants of the pars intermedia resulted in skin darkening. The rapid color change induced by the hormone in lower vertebrates is caused by centrifugal dispersion of the pigment granules into the radiating processes of their melanophores.

It was long assumed that pigmentation in mammals was not under pituitary control, but the hormone of the intermediate lobe has been shown to induce synthesis of melanin in melanoma cells grown in vitro. The increased pigmentation that occurs in humans suffering from degeneration of the adrenal cortex (Addison's disease) is now attributed to release of excess MSH and ACTH from the hypophysis. The darkening of the skin observed in human pregnancy may also result from enhanced release of one or both of these hormones.

A highly basic melanocyte stimulating polypeptide was isolated in 1954 from pig pituitary glands and called α-MSH. A slightly acidic polypeptide was subsequently isolated from the same source and designated β-MSH. Analysis of the amino acid sequences and synthesis of α- and β-MSH was soon achieved; α-MSH contains 13 amino acids in a sequence identical to that of one portion of the molecule of ACTH. β-MSH contains 18 amino acids, of which seven are in a sequence similar to a part of the ACTH molecule. The cells of the pars intermedia have also been found to release significant amounts of a *corticotropin-like intermediate lobe peptide* (CLIP) and of β *endorphin,* an opiate-like peptide.

It has now been found that melanotrophs of the pars intermedia, corticotrophs of the pars distalis, certain neurons of the hypothalamus, and cells in the placenta synthesize a high-molecular-weight parent molecule variously called *protropin, pro-opiocortin,* or *pro-opiomelanocortin.* Proteolytic cleavage of this glycosylated common precursor molecule gives rise to ACTH, lipotropic peptide hormone (β-LPH), melanotropin (α-MSH), and endorphins.

Different modes of post-translational processing of the precursor molecule in the several cell types yield different ratios of the cleavage products. Some of these function as active hormones and others may serve as potentiators or inhibitors of other hormones. As yet, little is known about the interactions and target cells of these peptides.

Melanotropin, the principal product of the pars intermedia, acts primarily upon melanocytes, but a variety of nonpigmentary effects have been described. Systemic administration of MSH to rats has been shown to affect avoidance responses and induce other behavioral changes. It is also reported to improve attention and vigilance in humans. The neurons in certain regions of the brain are immunoreactive to β-LPH, α-MSH, endorphins, and a number of other peptides. Optimal brain function may ultimately prove to depend on a delicate balance between the amounts of various endogenous neuropeptides.

PARS INFUNDIBULARIS OR TUBERALIS

Like the pars intermedia, the pars tuberalis constitutes only a small part of the hypophysis. Both are adjacent to and continuous with the anterior lobe. The pars tuberalis is 25 to 60 μm thick and forms a sleeve around the stalk, the thickest portion being on its anterior surface (Fig. 17–3). It is frequently incomplete on the posterior surface of the stalk. The distinctive morphological characteristic of the pars tuberalis is the longitudinal arrangement of its cords of epithelial cells which occupy the interstices between the longitudinally oriented blood vessels.

The pars tuberalis is the most highly vascularized subdivision of the hypophysis, because it is traversed by the major arterial supply for the anterior lobe and the hypothalamohypophyseal venous portal system. The pars tuberalis is separated from the infundibular stalk by a thin layer of connective tissue continuous with the pia. On the outside, the connective tissue is typical arachnoidal membrane. Between these, the blood vessels and groups of epithelial cells are supported by reticular fibers.

The epithelial cells of the pars tuberalis include undifferentiated cells and some small acidophilic and basophilic cells. The main component is a cuboidal or columnar cell which may reach 12 to 18 μm in size and contains numerous small granules or sometimes fine colloid droplets. The mitochondria are short rods, and numerous small lipid droplets may be present. These are the only cells in the adult hypophysis containing large amounts of glycogen. The cells may be arranged to form follicle-like structures. Islands of squamous epithelial cells may also be present. Despite the occurrence of a pars tuberalis in all vertebrates studied, the epithelial cells are not known to have any distinctive hormonal function.

NEUROHYPOPHYSIS

The neurohypophysis consists of the median eminence of the tuber cinereum, the infundibular stalk, and the infundibular process (Fig. 17–3). Much of its substance consists of axons of neurons whose cell bodies are located at a higher level in the hypothalamus. Therefore, the organization and function of the neural lobe cannot be adequately described without inclusion of the cell bodies that are situated beyond its anatomical boundaries.

The hypothalamus is the major neuroendocrine regulatory center of the brain. Within it, two principal neurosecretory systems are recognized. In one, designated the *parvicellular system,* axons extend from the cell bodies to the median eminence, where they secrete the releasing and inhibiting hormones

...at control the levels of all the hormones of ...e adenohypophysis. The other, the *magno-cellular neurosecretory system*, consists of neu-onal cell bodies located in the *supraoptic nucleus* and *paraventricular nucleus*, and their unmyelinated axons form the *hypothalamohy-pophyseal tract*, which descends into, and makes up the bulk of, the substance of the neural lobe of the hypophysis. This system secretes the hormones *oxytocin* and *vasopressin*. In addition to the axons of hypothalamic neurosecretory cells, the neural lobe contains an intrinsic population of cells called *pitui-cytes*, which do not appear to be secretory.

The cells of the hypothalamic nuclei are large neurons with few processes, an eccen-tric nucleus, and abundant cytoplasm. The endoplasmic reticulum tends to occur in par-allel cisternae at the periphery of the peri-karyon. There is a well-developed juxtanu-clear Golgi complex, which forms small (120–200 nm) neurosecretory granules. Neurotu-bules and neurofilaments converge upon the axon and form an axial bundle in its center along which the neurosecretory granules are transported to the neural lobe at a rate of 1 to 4 mm an hour. Labeled precursors of the hormones injected intracisternally can be de-tected in the neural lobe in one to two hours.

In histological preparations stained with chrome-alum hematoxylin, deeply stained material is seen in aggregations of varying size throughout the infundibular process and neural lobe. These were traditionally called *Herring bodies* (Fig. 17–13). In electron micro-graphs they are found to be large aggrega-tions of the small secretory granules. The axons of the neurosecretory neurons are un-usual in that they vary greatly in caliber and have numerous dilatations along their length. It is in these that the bulk of the neurosecre-tory material is stored. It is estimated that each axon has up to 4.4×10^2 of these expansions along its course holding an aver-age of 2.2×10^3 neurosecretory granules. About 60 per cent of all neurosecretory ma-terial resides in these dilatations, and about 40 per cent in axon endings associated with the walls of fenestrated capillaries. Endings are distinguishable from other axon dilata-tions by the presence of numerous small spherical vesicles in addition to the secretory granules. These are similar in appearance to the synaptic vesicles of cholinergic nerve end-ings but there is no evidence that they contain neurotransmitter. Instead they are usually interpreted as agents of membrane retrieval after exocytosis of neurosecretory granules.

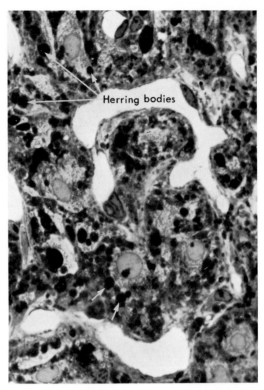

Figure 17–13. Photomicrograph of rat neurohypophysis fixed by perfusion. The large clear areas are capillaries. The dark rounded masses indicated by arrows are Herring bodies. In electron micrographs these are resolved as accumulations of neurosecretory material in dilatation of nerve axons. × 950. (Courtesy of P. Orkand and S. L. Palay.)

Pituicytes

Pituicytes have slender processes that are joined to processes of neighboring cells of the same type to form a three-dimensional network ensheathing the neuronal elements. In the human they are highly variable in size and shape and commonly contain lipochrome pigment granules and lipid droplets. Their cytoplasmic processes meander among groups of preterminal secretory axons and often intimately envelop their granule-filled terminal expansions. The structural relation-ship of pituicytes to the nerve fibers is thus similar to that of the neuroglial cells of the brain. They occupy 25 to 30 per cent of the volume of the neural lobe. Their function is poorly understood. The processes of pitui-cytes are connected by gap junctions, which may provide for their metabolic coupling. Cholinesterase has been localized in or on them, but no physiological interactions be-tween pituicytes and axons have yet been demonstrated. They are assigned no role in the secretory process, but are generally be-

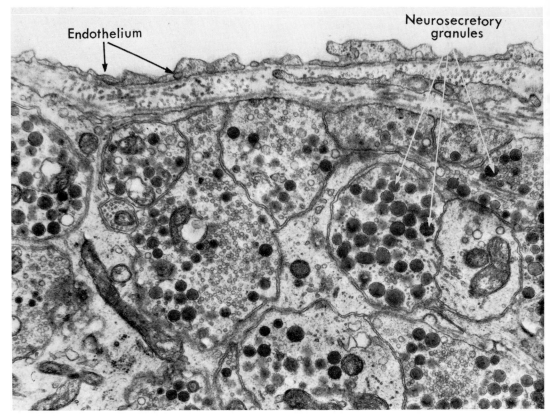

Figure 17–14. Electron micrograph of rat neurohypophysis, showing neurosecretory granules and small vesicles in the axoplasm of fibers of the hypothalamo-hypophyseal tract ending in close relation to a capillary. × 22,000. (Courtesy of P. Orkand and S. L. Palay.)

lieved to have a trophic and supportive function and to maintain the appropriate ionic composition of the extracellular fluid compartment.

HISTOPHYSIOLOGY OF THE NEURAL LOBE

The two hormones of the neural lobe, *oxytocin* and *vasopressin (antidiuretic hormone, ADH)*, are similar polypeptides both consisting of nine amino acids and differing from each other in only two amino acids. They were formerly thought to be produced in separate hypothalamic nuclei—oxytocin in the paraventricular nuclei and vasopressin in the supraoptic nucleus. Although they are synthesized in separate neurons, both types are now known to be present in the supraoptic and paraventricular nuclei. They are first synthesized in the form of a larger precursor molecule, which is subsequently cleaved enzymatically to yield active hormone. Oxytocin

and vasopressin are associated with proteins called *neurophysins,* which are immunologically and biochemically distinct. During exocytosis of the neurosecretory granules, hormone and neurophysins are both released, but the latter have no known physiological effect.

Vasopressin

Vasopressin acts upon vascular smooth muscle, causing constriction of the arterioles, thereby increasing peripheral resistance and raising blood pressure. Loss of blood is a potent stimulus for increased secretion of vasopressin. Severe hemorrhage may result in secretion of the hormone at 50 times the normal rate. Diminished blood volume is sensed by pressure receptors in the carotid artery and aorta that exert reflex control over vasopressin secretion.

Vasopressin is also called antidiuretic hormone (ADH) because of its important role in

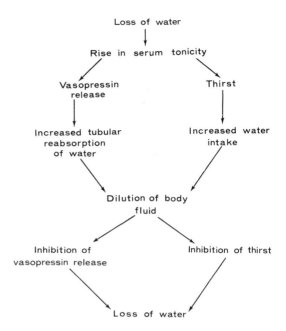

Figure 17–15. Diagram of the role of vasopressin or antidiuretic hormone of the neurohypophysis in regulation of the concentration of body fluids. Interaction of the neurohypophysis, the thirst center of the hypothalamus, and renal tubules results in maintenance of a constant osmolarity of the body fluids. (After Leaf, A., and C. H. Coggins. *In* Williams, R. H. Textbook of Endocrinology. 4th ed. Philadelphia, W. B. Saunders Co., 1968.)

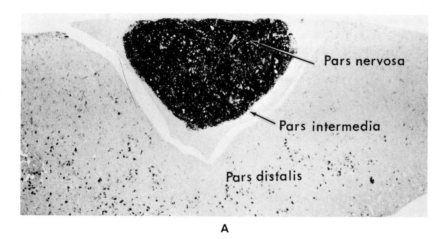

A

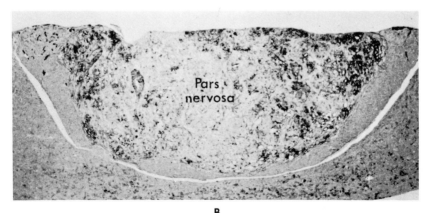

B

Figure 17–16. Photomicrograph of cross sections of rat hypophysis stained with paraldehyde-fuchsin. *A,* Hypophysis of a normal control rat showing abundant, densely stained neurosecretory material in the neurohypophysis. *B,* Hypophysis of a rat of the Brattleboro strain with hypothalamic diabetes insipidus. The neurohypophysis is unusually large but contains very little neurosecretion *(black).* × 40. (After Sokol, H. W., and H. Valtin. Endocrinology 77:692, 1965.)

water conservation (Fig. 17–15). Its administration in minute amounts greatly decreases excretion of water by the kidneys. The hormone increases the permeability of the collecting ducts to water and permits reabsorption of most of the water in tubule fluid, by an osmotic gradient existing between the lumen and the interstitial fluid of the renal papilla. The urine is concentrated and water conserved. In the absence of ADH, the distal tubules and collecting ducts are relatively impermeable to water and concentration of the urine does not occur. In dehydration or osmotic stress induced by high intake of salt, the neurons in the supraoptic and paraventricular nuclei send impulses along their axons to the posterior lobe, releasing large amounts of stored ADH. If the osmotic stress is of longer duration, the hypothalamic neurons enlarge and develop a more extensive endoplasmic reticulum for enhanced synthesis of hormone.

In humans who have a tumor in the hypothalamus, the supraoptic and paraventricular nuclei may be invaded and destroyed. Such patients are unable to secrete ADH and develop *diabetes insipidus*, a condition characterized by constant thirst and drinking of large amounts of water (polydipsia) and by excessive urination (polyuria). Much of our understanding of the physiology of the hypothalamoneurohypophyseal system has been gained by study of a convenient animal model of this disease—the Brattleboro rat. This strain of rats inherit diabetes insipidus as a recessive trait. They excrete every day a volume of urine equivalent to 80 per cent of their body weight and drink correspondingly large amounts of water. Their posterior pituitary is unusually large but contains very little stainable neurosecretory material (Fig. 17–16) and no immunocytochemically demonstrable ADH. The failure of their hypothalamic neurons to synthesize the hormone was long attributed to a simple deletion of the vasopressin gene. It has been found, however, that Brattleboro rats do synthesize vasopressin in their ovaries and adrenals. Thus, it appears that their hypothalamic disorder is an inherited, tissue-specific, post-translational defect instead of a gene deletion. The occurrence of vasopressin in the ovaries and adrenals of normal animals of several species is a relatively recent finding and its physiological significance is not understood. Immunoreactive vasopressin is also found in occasional tumors of the lungs and gastrointestinal tract.

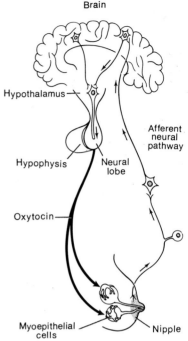

Figure 17–17. Diagram illustrating the role of oxytocin the suckling reflex. Stimulation of the nipples generat sensory impulses that pass to the brain via dorsal r ganglia. In the brain, these impulses are relayed to t hypothalamus, where they activate neurosecretory ce whose processes extend into the pars nervosa of t hypophysis. Stimulation of these cells results in relea of the hormone oxytocin, which is carried in the blood the mammary gland, where it causes contraction of my epithelial cells, causing milk to be expressed.

Oxytocin

A principal target of this hormone is tl myometrium of the pregnant uterus. It stin ulates contraction of uterine smooth musc! Its concentration in the blood increases du ing the late stages of labor and it is believe to have a significant role in parturition.

Oxytocin is also responsible for milk eje tion in the lactating mammary gland (Fi 17–17). Stimulation of the nipple by the suc! ling infant sends afferent impulses to tl brain stem and onward to neurons in tl supraoptic and paraventricular nuclei, whic respond by releasing oxytocin into the capi laries of the neurohypophysis. Blood-born oxytocin then stimulates contraction of my epithelial cells in the alveoli of the mamma gland, ejecting milk into the ducts. Milk b gins to flow from the nipples about or minute after the onset of suckling.

REFERENCES

PARS DISTALIS

Baker, B. L. Functional cytology of the hypophyseal pa distalis and pars intermedia. *In* Greep, R. O., ar

E. B. Astwood, eds.: Handbook of Physiology. Sect. 7, Vol. 4, part 1. Washington, DC, American Physiological Society, 1974.

Duello, T. M., and N. S. Halmi: Ultrastructural immunocytolochemical localization of growth hormone and prolactin in human pituitaries. J. Clin. Endocrinol. 49:189, 1979.

Farquhar, M. G.: Processing of secretory products by cells of the anterior pituitary gland. Mem. Soc. Endocrinol. 19:79, 1971.

Farquhar, M. G., E. H. Skutelsky, and C. R. Hopkins: Structure and function of the anterior pituitary and dispersed pituitary cells in in vitro studies. In Anterior Pituitary. San Francisco, Academic Press, 1975.

Guillemin, R.: Control of adenohypophysial functions by peptides of the central nervous system. Harvey Lect. Series 71, 1975–1976.

Herlant, M.: The cells of the adenohypophysis and their functional significance. Int. Rev. Cytol. 17:299, 1964.

Kurosumi, K., and T. Kobayaski: Corticotrophs in the anterior pituitary glands of normal and adrenalectomized rats as revealed by electron microscopy. Endocrinology 78:745, 1966.

Moriarty, G. C.: Adenohypophysis: ultrastructural cytochemistry. A review. J. Histochem. Cytochem. 21:855, 1973.

Moriarty, G. C.: Immunocytochemistry of the pituitary glycoprotein hormones. J. Histochem. Cytochem. 24:846, 1976.

Nakane, P.: Classification of anterior pituitary cell types with immunoenzyme histochemistry. J. Histochem. Cytochem. 18:9, 1970.

Pelletier, G., F. Robert, and J. Hardy: Identification of human pituitary cell types by immunoelectron microscopy. J. Clin. Endocrinol. Metab. 46:534, 1978.

Phifer, R. F., A. R. Midgley, and S. S. Spicer. Immunohistologic and histologic evidence that follicle-stimulating and luteinizing hormones are present in the same cell types in the human pars distalis. J. Clin. Endocrinol. Metab. 36:125, 1973.

Phifer, R. F., and S. S. Spicer. Immunohistochemical and histologic demonstration of thyrotropic cells of the human adenohypophysis. J. Clin. Endocrinol. Metab. 36:1210, 1973.

Shiino, M., A. Arimura, A. V. Schally, and E. G. Rennels: Ultrastructural observations of granule extrusion from rat anterior pituitary cells after injection of LH-releasing hormone. Z. Zellforsch. Mikrosk. Anat. 128:152, 1972.

Shiino, M., M. G. Williams, and E. G. Rennels: Ultrastructural observation of pituitary release of prolactin in the rat by suckling stimulus. Endocrinology 90:176, 1972.

PARS INTERMEDIA

Hadley, M. E., C. B. Heward, V. J. Hruby, T. K. Sawyer, and Y. C. S. Yong: Biological actions of melanocyte-stimulating hormone. In Peptides of the Pars Intermedia. Ciba Foundation Symposium 81. London, Pitman Medical, 1981.

Jackson, S., J. Hope, F. Estivarex, and P. J. Lowry: Nature and control of peptide release from the pars intermedia. In Peptides and the Pars Intermedia. Ciba Foundation Symposium 81. London, Pitman Medical, 1981.

Lerner, A. B., and J. S. McGuire: Effects of alpha- and beta-melanocyte stimulating hormones on skin colour in man. Nature 189:176, 1961.

Lerner, A. B., and Y. Takahashi: Hormonal control of melanin pigmentation. Recent Prog. Horm. Res. 12:203, 1956.

Stoeckel, M. E., G. Schmitt, and A. Porte: Fine structure and cytochemistry of the mammalian pars intermedia. In Peptides of the Pars Intermedia. Ciba Foundation Symposium 81. London, Pitman Medical, 1981.

NEUROHYPOPHYSIS

Baker, B. J., W. C. Dermody, and J. R. Reed: Distribution of gonadotropin releasing hormone in the rat brain as observed by immunocytochemistry. Endocrinology 97:125, 1975.

Barer, R., and K. Lederis: Ultrastructure of the rabbit neurohypophysis with special reference to the release of hormones. Zeitschr. Zellforsch. 75:201, 1966.

Bargmann, W.: Neurosecretion. Int. Rev. Cytol. 19:183, 1966.

Bodian, D.: Cytological aspects of neurosecretion in opossum neurohypophysis. Bull. Johns Hopkins Hosp. 113:57, 1963.

Bonner, T. I., and M. J. Brownstein: Vasopressin, tissue-specific defects and the Brattleboro rat. Nature 310:17, 1984.

Dierickx, K., and F. Vandesande: Immunocytochemical localization of the vasopressinergic and oxytocinergic neurons in the human hypothalamus. Cell Tissue Res. 184:15, 1977.

Dierickx, K., and F. Vandesande: Immunocytochemical demonstration of separate vasopressin-neurophysin and oxytocin-neurophysin neurones in the human hypothalamus. Cell Tissue Res. 196:203, 1979.

du Vigneaud, V.: Trail of sulfur research from insulin to oxytocin. Science 123:967, 1956.

Gainer, H., Y. Sarne, and M. J. Brownstein: Biosynthesis and axon transport of rat neurohypophyseal protein and peptides. J. Cell Biol. 73:366, 1977.

Morris, J. F., J. J. Nordmann, and R. E. Dyball: Structure-function correlation in mammalian neurosecretion. Int. Rev. Exp. Pathol. 18:1, 1973.

Sawyer, W. H.: Vertebrate neurohypophyseal principles. Endocrinology 75:981, 1964.

Sokol, H. W., and H. Valtin: Morphology of the neurosecretory system in rats homozygous and heterozygous for hypothalamic diabetes insipidus (Brattleboro strain). Endocrinology 77:692, 1965.

BLOOD VESSELS

Bergland, R. M., and R. B. Page: Pituitary-brain vascular relations: a new paradigm. Science 204:18, 1979.

Farquhar, M. G.: Fine structure and function in capillaries of the anterior pituitary gland. Angiology 12:270, 1961.

Green, J. D.: The comparative anatomy of the portal vascular system and of the innervation of the hypophysis. In Harris, G. W., and B. T. Donovan, eds.: The Pituitary Gland. Berkeley, CA, University of California Press, 1966.

Green, J. D., and G. W. Harris: The neurovascular link between the neurohypophysis and adenohypophysis. J. Endocrinol. 5:136, 1949.

Wislocki, G. B.: The vascular supply of the hypophysis cerebri of the rhesus monkey and man. Proc. Assoc. Res. Nerv. Ment. Dis. 17:48, 1938.

18

THE THYROID GLAND

The thyroid gland situated in the anterior part of the neck weighs 25 to 40 g. It consists of two *lateral lobes* connected by a narrow *isthmus,* which crosses the trachea just below the cricoid cartilage. In about one third of the persons examined, a *pyramidal lobe* extends upward from the isthmus near the left lobe.

The gland is enclosed in a connective tissue capsule that is continuous with the surrounding cervical fascia. This outer capsule is loosely connected on its deep surface to another layer of moderately dense connective tissue that is intimately adherent to the gland. This separation of the capsule into two layers creates a plane of cleavage between the two, which facilitates surgical access in subtotal thyroidectomy.

The function of the thyroid is to elaborate, store, and release into the bloodstream *thyroid hormones,* which are concerned with the regulation of metabolic rate. The thyroid differs from other endocrine glands in that a mechanism for extracellular storage of its hormones is highly developed, whereas in other endocrine glands there are only rather limited provisions for intracellular storage.

HISTOLOGICAL ORGANIZATION

The gland is composed of spherical, cyst-like follicles 0.02 to 0.9 mm in diameter, lined with a simple epithelium and containing a gelatinous *colloid* (Figs. 18–1, 18–2). This represents the stored product of secretory activity by the epithelium lining the follicle. In the human there is great variability in the size of the follicles, but the small predominate over the large. In other species the follicles are of more uniform size. In the rat and guinea pig, those at the periphery of the gland are larger than those more centrally situated.

The follicles are surrounded by an extremely thin basal lamina, which usually is not resolved with the light microscope. With silver stains the follicles are seen to be enclosed by a delicate network of reticular fibers. A close-meshed plexus of capillaries surrounds each follicle (Fig. 18–3). Between the capillary nets of adjacent follicles are the blind terminations of lymphatic vessels, and in some rodent species lymphatics form extensive perifollicular sinusoids. Numerous nerve fibers accompany the blood vessels as they ramify among the follicles. These seem to terminate mainly along the vessels, but in some instances they appear to end in direct contact with the base of the thyroid epithelial cells. The nerves entering the thyroid are postganglionic sympathetic fibers originating in the middle and superior cervical ganglia. There are also preganglionic parasympathetic fibers, and ganglion cells may occasionally be encountered within the thyroid. The nerves to the thyroid are presumed to be mainly vasomotor, inasmuch as transplanted thyroid tissue functions adequately, suggesting that an intact nerve supply is not necessary for secretion.

The epithelial cells vary in height but are commonly low cuboidal to squamous. In general, the epithelium tends to be squamous when the gland is underactive and columnar when it is overactive, but there are many exceptions, and an accurate assessment of the functional activity of the gland cannot be based on histological examination alone.

The nucleus of the cells is spheroidal, centrally situated, and poor in chromatin and contains one or more nucleoli. The cytoplasm is basophilic; the mitochondria are thin rods and the Golgi apparatus is usually supranuclear. Lipid droplets are common, and "clear droplets" have been described by various workers using the light microscope, and interpreted as intracellular globules of colloid. They stain with aniline blue and with the periodic acid–Schiff (PAS) reaction in much

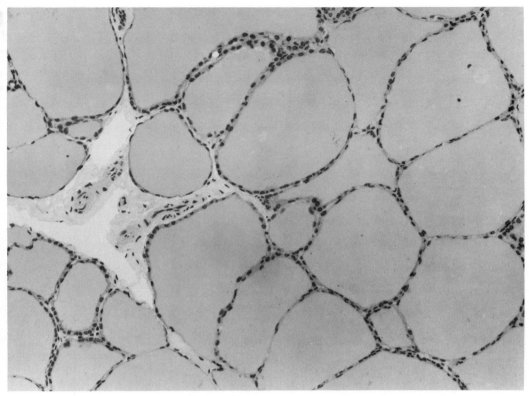

Figure 18–1. Photomicrograph of monkey thyroid showing variations in size of the follicles.

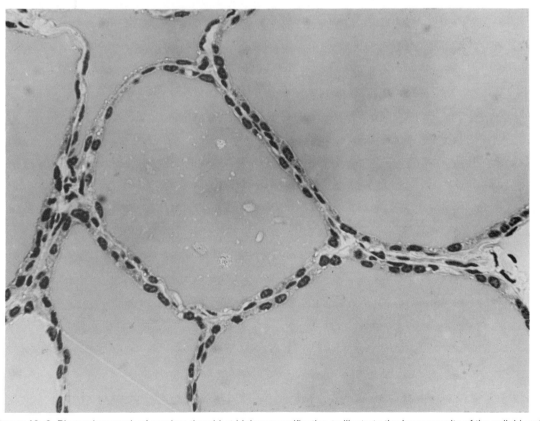

Figure 18–2. Photomicrograph of monkey thyroid at higher magnification to illustrate the homogeneity of the colloid and the character of the epithelium.

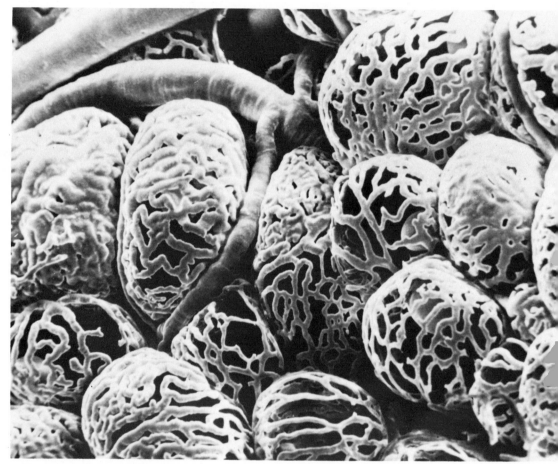

Figure 18–3. Scanning electron micrograph of a monkey thyroid in which the blood vessels have been injected with plastic and the tissue digested away. Each spherical follicle is surrounded by a dense network of capillaries. (Micrograph from Fujita, H., and T. Murakami. Arch. Histol. Jpn. *36*:181, 1974.)

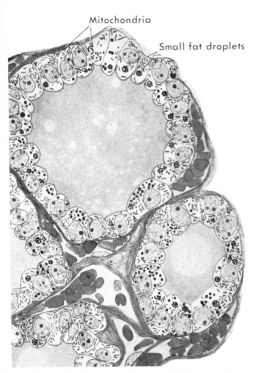

Mitochondria

Small fat droplets

igure 18–4. Section through several follicles of human ʰyroid. Aniline-acid fuchsin. (Courtesy of R. R. Bensley.)

he same way as the colloid in the lumen of ʰe follicle. Granules of varying size, located ʰainly in the apical cytoplasm, give positive ʰaining reactions for acid phosphatase and ʰsterase and are therefore considered to be ʰsosomes.

The unfixed colloid is optically homoge-ʰeous, except for occasional desquamated ʰells and rare macrophages. After fixation, ʰe colloid stains with either acid or basic ʰyes, and with the trichrome stains it is not ʰncommon for different follicles or even ʰifferent areas of the colloid in the same ʰollicle to be colored differently. Although ʰhysiological significance has been erro-ʰeously ascribed to this multiple staining, the ʰaried patterns observed appear to be due to ʰcal differences in concentration of protein ʰat depend on the direction and rate of ʰenetration of fixative into the tissue block. ʰhe colloid stains intensely with the PAS ʰeaction, because the *thyroglobulin* secreted by ʰe thyroid is a glycoprotein containing about ʰ per cent carbohydrate. The thyroglobulin ʰf the colloid also contains various iodinated ʰmino acids. Among these are *thyroxin* (tetra-ʰodothyronine) and *triiodothyronine,* which are ʰe *thyroid hormones.* The presence of these ʰompounds in the colloid has been demon-ʰtrated by microchemical analysis, by ultra-

violet absorption spectrophotometry, and by the use of radioactive ^{131}I (Fig. 18–5). The follicle cells were formerly believed to secrete into the colloid a protease that split thyro-globulin into smaller molecules and liberated the biologically active thyroxin and triiodo-thyronine. It is now widely accepted that the proteases act within the thyroid cells upon stored thyroglobulin taken up from the lu-men of the follicle.

In electron micrographs the follicles of the human thyroid are found to be composed of a single layer of low cuboidal cells surround-ing a homogeneous, moderately dense col-loid. A thin, continuous basal lamina about 50 nm thick surrounds the entire follicle. In the interfollicular spaces are numerous cap-illaries of the fenestrated type, occasional fibroblasts, and small bundles of collagen fibrils. The follicle cells are joined laterally by typical junctional complexes, and the free surfaces bear a small number of short, irreg-ularly oriented microvilli. In follicles with cuboidal epithelium, the microvilli are some-what more numerous. The basal plasma membrane is smoothly contoured and not infolded. The relatively large nucleus is cen-trally placed and has an eccentric nucleolus. The mitochondria are relatively few and uni-formly distributed. Their cristae are not es-pecially numerous. The endoplasmic reticu-

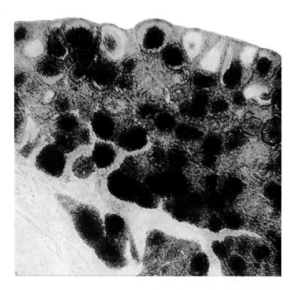

Figure 18–5. Low-power photomicrograph of autoradio-graph of thyroid gland of rat previously injected with ^{131}I. Blackened areas represent sites of deposition of the radioactive material. There is great variability in the con-tent of the isotope in the several follicles. In a few places the epithelium is blackened. (Courtesy of C. P. Leblond, D. Findlay, and S. Gross.)

lum varies in its degree of development. In the squamous cells there are only a few elongated cisternal profiles, but in the cuboidal cells the reticulum is well developed (Fig. 18–6). The Golgi apparatus is in a supranuclear or paranuclear position and is composed of flattened or dilated saccules, vacuoles, and small vesicles. Small vesicles similar to those of the Golgi apparatus are present in abundance throughout the cytoplasm. Multivesicular bodies are also common. Membrane-limited dense bodies 0.5 to 0.7 μm in diameter are plentiful in the apical cytoplasm. These are lysosomes.

In addition to the principal cells of the thyroid follicles, there is another, smaller population of cells, present both in the follicular epithelium and in the interfollicular spaces. These cells were first described by Baker (1877) and Hürthle (1894) and studied in greater detail by Nonidez (1931) (Figs. 18–7, 18–8), but evidence permitting assignment of a function to them was not forthcoming until 30 years later. They are variously designated as *parafollicular cells, light cells, mito-*

chondria-rich cells, C cells, and *ultimobranchial cells.* The term "parafollicular cell" was introduced to distinguish these cells from other interfollicular cells, some of which may be undifferentiated embryonal elements or connective tissue cells. They arise during embryonic life from the last pair of pharyngeal pouches. In fishes, amphibians, reptiles, and birds, they form discrete epithelial cell masses called *ultimobranchial bodies,* located in the neck or mediastinum. In mammals, they are incorporated into the thyroid. They are often larger than the principal cells, and in routine histological preparations they stain less deeply. They can be selectively stained by the silver nitrate method of Cajal, which reveals the presence of brown or black cytoplasmic granules (Figs. 18–7, 18–8). The granules exhibit an affinity for aniline blue in trichrome stains. Cytochemically they are distinguished from follicular cells by their high level of activity of the mitochondrial enzyme α-glycerophosphate dehydrogenase.

Where the parafollicular cells are intercalated among the principal cells of the follicle

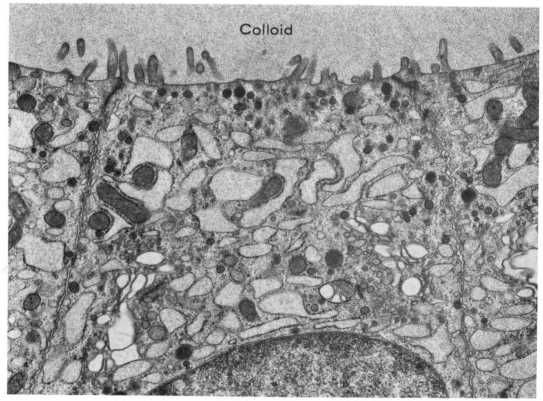

Figure 18–6. Electron micrograph of the apical half of an epithelial cell from rat thyroid gland. The free surface of the cell is provided with numerous short microvilli that project into the colloid of the follicle. The endoplasmic reticulum is well developed and its cisternae are distended with an amorphous content of low density. The small dense granules are lysosomes. (Micrograph courtesy of S. Wissig.)

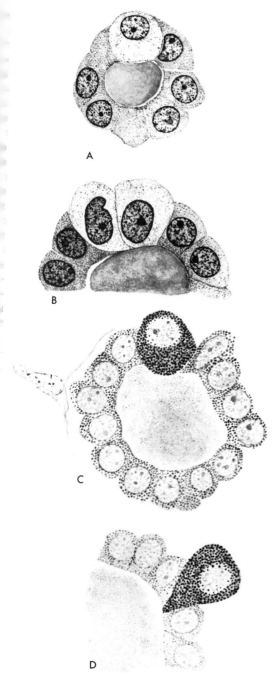

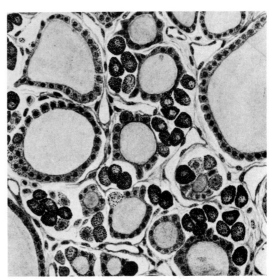

Figure 18–8. Drawing of an area occupied by small and medium-sized follicles in the thyroid of an adult dog. Numerous parafollicular cells are seen in clusters in the interfollicular spaces. Cajal stain. (After Nonidez, J. F. Anat. Rec. *53*:339, 1932.)

ture. They are now adequately preserved by aldehyde fixatives and appear as membrane-limited, dense, spherical granules 0.1 to 0.4 μm in diameter (Fig. 18–9). The parafollicular cells elaborate and secrete *calcitonin*, a hormone that lowers blood calcium concentration.

HISTOPHYSIOLOGY

The function of the thyroid gland is to synthesize, store, and release hormones concerned with the regulation of metabolic rate (thyroxin and triiodothyronine) and with maintenance of blood calcium levels within tolerable limits (calcitonin). The function related to metabolic rate resides in the follicular epithelial cells, whereas the calcium-regulating action resides in the parafollicular cells.

THE PRINCIPAL CELLS

The thyroid is the only endocrine gland that stores its product extracellularly. The secretory process is therefore somewhat more complex than that in other glands. It involves (1) synthesis of the large glycoprotein thyroglobulin (2) iodination of tyrosine molecules that are important constituents of thyroglobulin (3) release of thyroglobulin into the lumen of the follicle for storage (4) reabsorp-

Figure 18–7. Parafollicular cells in thyroid follicles. *A, B,* Cat thyroid, Ehrlich's hematoxylin; *C, D,* dog thyroid (35-day-old puppy), Cajal silver nitrate method. (After Nonidez, J. F. Am. J. Anat. *49*:479, 1932.)

they are close to the base of the epithelium. They never border directly on the lumen but are separated from it by overarching processes of neighboring principal cells (Fig. 18–9). The secretory granules are not easily preserved and were overlooked in the early descriptions of parafollicular cell ultrastruc-

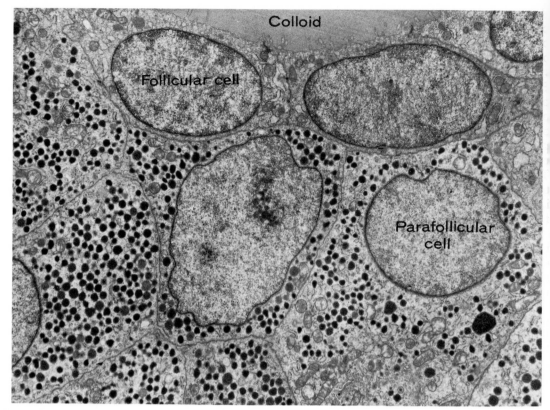

Figure 18–9. Electron micrograph of follicular and parafollicular cells of normal cat thyroid. The granular parafollicular cells do not border on the lumen but are usually separated from the colloid by follicular cells. When adequately fixed, the parafollicular cells contain many dense spherical secretory granules. (Micrograph courtesy of S. Wissig.)

tion of thyroglobulin into the follicular epithelial cells (5) hydrolysis of thyroglobulin to liberate thyroxin and triiodothyronine and (6) release of these hormones into the perifollicular capillaries and lymphatics.

Synthesis of thyroglobulin involves the same intracellular pathway described for other protein-secreting cells. Amino acids are assembled into polypeptides on ribosomes of the endoplasmic reticulum, then transported to the Golgi complex. Since thyroglobulin is a glycoprotein, the glycosyltransferases of the Golgi apparatus no doubt play a role in synthesis and conjugation of its carbohydrate components. From the Golgi complex, the product is transported in small vesicles to the apical surface of the cell, where it is discharged by exocytosis.

The thyroid has the capacity to concentrate iodine to several hundred thousand times the concentration of this element in the blood plasma. After an injection of inorganic iodide, 40 per cent of the circulating ion is concentrated in the thyroid gland within ten minutes. The iodine is used to iodinate tyrosine molecules that are ultimately incor-

porated into the thyroglobulin. The synthesis of thyroglobulin and its iodination are apparently independent, and while the sites of synthesis of the glycoprotein are well known, the site of its iodination has been a subject of controversy—some believe that it takes place in the cells, whereas others contend that it occurs in the lumen of the follicle. After iodine is actively transported from the blood into the cells, it is oxidized in the presence of hydrogen peroxide to a different ionic species. The oxidized iodide ion subsequently iodinates the tyrosine residues of thyroglobulin to form mono- and diiodotyrosine. Triiodothyronine is formed when one molecule each of monoiodotyrosine and diiodotyrosine are coupled. Thyroxin is formed when two molecules of diiodotyrosine are joined. Since both the initial oxidation of iodide and the subsequent iodination of tyrosine may be catalyzed by the enzyme peroxidase, histochemical localization of this enzyme seemed a reasonable approach for determining the site of iodination. Peroxidase is found in the perinuclear cisternae, endoplasmic reticulum, inner lamellae of the Golgi, apical vesiles, and external surfaces of the microvilli projecting into the colloid. The reaction product observed in the membranous cell organelles is believed to represent continuous synthesis of peroxidase by the thyroid cells. Peroxidase transported along this pathway is probably incorporated into the cell surface membrane. It is now believed that the principal site of iodination of thyroglobulin is probably the microvillous border of the thyroid cells, and possibly the apical vesicles. This interpretation is in agreement with autoradiographic studies localizing radioactive iodine at early time intervals over the interface between the epithelium and the colloid.

The uptake of colloid from the lumen of the follicle has been studied mainly in animals strongly stimulated to release hormone by administration of thyroid stimulating hormone (TSH) of the hypophysis (Fig. 18–10). Under these conditions, large droplets containing colloid appear in the apical cytoplasm. By microinjection of ferritin into follicles before administration of TSH, it was shown that the large colloid droplets which appear in the cells after stimulation contain ferritin

and hence represent colloid taken up from the lumen, not newly synthesized thyroglobulin.

The hydrolysis of thyroglobulin, formerly attributed to proteases in the lumen of the follicles, is now known to be a function of lysosomes in the epithelial cells. Lysosomes coalesce with the endocytosis vacuoles containing reabsorbed colloid, and add to their contents cathepsins that hydrolyze thyroglobulin. The tetraiodothyronine and triiodothyronine liberated apparently diffuse into the cytoplasmic matrix and through the cell base to enter the blood. This phase of the process cannot be visualized with the electron microscope. As in other endocrine glands, the capillaries of the thyroid are of the fenestrated type and offer little or no barrier to passage of hormones to the blood. Whereas the blood vascular system is undoubtedly the most important avenue of egress of thyroid hormones because of the high rate of blood flow, it has been shown that concentration of hormone in the lymph draining the gland is as much as 100 times greater than the concentration in venous blood. Thus, the lym-

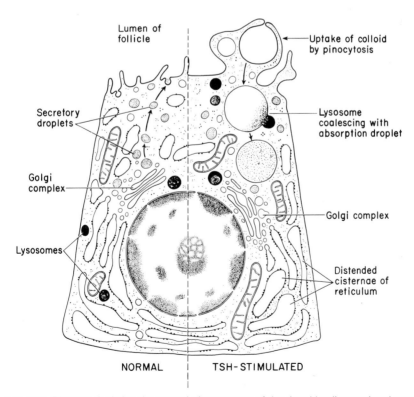

Lumen of follicle

Uptake of colloid by pinocytosis

Secretory droplets

Lysosome coalescing with absorption droplet

Golgi complex

Golgi complex

Lysosomes

Distended cisternae of reticulum

NORMAL | TSH-STIMULATED

Figure 18–10. *Left side,* Diagram depicting the normal ultrastructure of the thyroid cell secreting thyroglobulin into the lumen of the follicle. *Right side,* The uptake of colloid by pinocytosis after stimulation with thyroid-stimulating hormone, and the lysosomal degradation of thyroglobulin to release thyroxin. (From Fawcett, D. W., J. A. Long, and A. L. Jones. Recent Prog. Horm. Res. 25:315, 1969.)

phatics must be considered a significant pathway for transport of hormone to the circulating blood.

The activity of the thyroid is regulated by the thyrotropic hormone (TSH) of the anterior lobe of the hypophysis, and this in turn is controlled by thyrotropin releasing factor (TRF) of the hypothalamus. Lowered levels of thyroid hormone in the blood stimulates the hypothalamus to secrete TRF, which results in increased thyrotropin secretion. Excess circulating thyroid hormone depresses thyrotropin secretion. Chronic hypersecretion of thyrotropin results in a highly vascular gland with columnar follicular epithelial cells and relatively little colloid. After hypophysectomy, the thyroid is no longer capable of accumulating significant amounts of ^{131}I, and only traces of thyroid hormone appear in the blood.

The most striking effect of thyroid secretion is its control of the *metabolic rate* of the body. When a deficiency of thyroid hormone occurs, the metabolic rate falls below normal; when there is an excess, the metabolic rate rises above normal. When *hypothyroidism* begins in infancy and persists, it leads to *cretinism*, a condition attended by stunting of physical and mental development. When hypofunction begins in adulthood and persists, it leads to *myxedema*, a disorder characterized by a sallow, puffy appearance; dry, sparse hair; lethargy; and slow cerebration. In both conditions the basal metabolic rate is reduced, and in both the symptoms may be relieved through timely oral administration of dried thyroid gland.

Enlargement of the thyroid gland is called *goiter,* and any substance that causes enlargement of the thyroid is called a *goitrogen.* When iodine is deficient in the diet, as it tends to be in a number of geographical regions, there is an excess production and accumulation of colloid, but in the absence of sufficient iodine, relatively little active hormone is produced. This compensatory enlargement of the gland is called *colloid goiter.* Antithyroid substances occur naturally in some plants used for food. Excess consumption of these goitrogens may interfere with iodination in the thyroid and result in enlargement.

A common form of *hyperthyroidism* in the human is *Graves' disease* or *exophthalmic goiter.* The follicles become enlarged, with tall cells and papillary projections into the lumen. The mitochondria increase in number, the Golgi apparatus hypertrophies, and colloid is diminished or absent. Such hyperplastic thyroids may secrete thyroxin at five to ten times the normal rate. The patient suffers weight loss, nervousness, weakness, rapid heart rate, intolerance of heat, and tremor. The increased metabolic rate and associated symptoms return temporarily to normal after administration of iodine and of antithyroid agents, such as thiouracil. The exact cause of Graves' disease is poorly understood, but the blood of patients suffering from it often contains an immunoglobulin of the IgG type, which is a long-acting thyroid stimulator (LATS). This substance may play a role in the pathogenesis of the disease.

THE PARAFOLLICULAR CELLS

When it was first detected in the outflow from a preparation of dog thyroid and parathyroid glands perfused with hypercalcemic blood, calcitonin was believed to come from the parathyroids. It was later shown to be present only in the thyroid, and several lines of evidence associated it with the parafollicular cells: (1) sustained elevation of calcium results in degranulation of these cells; (2) extractable calcitonin correlates well with the presence and number of such cells; (3) human medullary carcinomas of the thyroid, which are thought to arise from the parafollicular cells, contain 100 to 10,000 times as much calcitonin as normal thyroid tissue; (4) fluorescent antibodies to calcitonin bind selectively to the parafollicular cells.

The hormone was extracted in pure form from pig thyroid glands by 1968, and it was found to be a polypeptide consisting of a single chain of 32 amino acids. The sequence of the amino acids has been worked out, and the hormone has now been synthesized. Calcitonin of human thyroid origin differs slightly from the porcine hormone.

Calcitonin appears to exert its effect by suppressing release of calcium into the blood from resorption of bone. Bone is constantly undergoing internal remodeling (see Chapter 9). Parathyroid hormone tends to alter the balance between bone deposition and bone absorption so as to cause increased resorption. The calcium released from bone enters the blood, raising the blood calcium level. Parathyroid hormone acts upon osteocytes and osteoclasts, accelerating osteolysis. Calcitonin appears to have an opposite effect upon these cells, decreasing bone resorption and thus lowering the blood calcium level.

The role of calcitonin in normal human blood calcium regulation is less well established than in experimental animals. However, hypercalcitonism is thought to occur in medullary carcinoma and in certain adenomas of the human thyroid.

REFERENCES

Anast, C. S.: Thyrocalcitonin—a review. Clin. Orthop. *47*:179, 1966.

Andros, G., and S. H. Wollman: Autoradiographic localization of iodine[125] in the thyroid epithelial cell. Proc. Soc. Exp. Biol. Med. *115*:775, 1964.

Baghdiantz, A., G. V. Foster, A. Edwards, M. A. Kumar, E. Slack, H. A. Soliman, and I. MacIntyre: Extraction and purification of calcitonin. Nature *203*:1927, 1964.

Bargmann, W.: Schildrüse. *In* von Möllendorff, W., and W. Bargmann, eds.: Handbuch der Mikroskopischen Anatomie des Menschen. Vol. 6, part 2. Berlin, Julius Springer, 1939.

Bogdanove, E. M.: Regulation of TSH secretion. Fed. Proc. *21*:633, 1962.

Bussolati, G., and A. G. E. Pearse: Immunofluorescence localization of calcitonin in the C-cells of pig and dog's thyroid. J. Endocrinol. *37*:205, 1967.

Copp, D. H., E. C. Cameron, B. A. Cheney, A. G. F. Davidson, and K. G. Henze: Evidence for calcitonin—a new hormone from the parathyroid that lowers blood calcium. Endocrinology *70*:637, 1962.

Daniel, P. M., Plaskett, L. G., and Pratt, O. E.: The lymphatic and venous pathways for the outflow of thyroxine, iodoprotein and inorganic iodide from the thyroid gland. J. Physiol. (Lond.) *188*:25, 1967.

Degroot, L. J., and H. Niepomniszeze: Biosynthesis of thyroid hormone: basic and clinical aspects. Metabolism *26*:665, 1977.

Dempsey, E. W., and R. R. Peterson: Electron microscopic observations on the thyroid glands of normal, hypophysectomized, cold-exposed and thiouracil-treated rats. Endocrinology *56*:46, 1955.

Ekholm, R., and L. E. Ericson: Ultrastructure of the parafollicular cells of the rat J. Ultrastruct. Res. *23*:378, 1968.

Falck, B., B. Larsen, C. v. Mecklenburg, C. Rosengren, and K. Svenaeus: On the presence of a second specific cell system in mammalian thyroid gland. Acta Physiol. Scand. *62*:491, 1964.

Foster, G. V., A. Baghdiantz, M. A. Kumar, E. Slack, H. A. Soliman, and I. MacIntyre: Thyroid origin of calcitonin. Nature *202*:1303, 1964.

Foster, G. V., I. MacIntyre, and A. G. E. Pearse: Calcitonin production and the mitochondrion-rich cells of the dog thyroid. Nature *203*:1029, 1964.

Fujita, H.: Outline of the fine structural aspects of synthesis and release of thyroid hormone. Gunma Symposium on Endocrinology *7*:49, 1970.

Fujita, H., and T. Murakami: Scanning electron microscopy on the distribution of the minute blood vessels of the dog, rat and Rhesus monkey. Arch. Histol. Jpn. *36*:181, 1974.

Gittes, R. F., and G. L. Irvin: Thyroid and parathyroid roles in hypercalcemia: evidence for a thyrocalcitonin releasing factor. Science *148*:1737, 1965.

Gross, J., and R. Pitt-Rivers: 3:5:3'-Triiodothyronine. 1.

Isolation from thyroid gland and synthesis. 2. Physiological activity. Biochem. J. *53*:645, 652, 1953.

Heimann, P.: Ultrastructure of the human thyroid. A study of normal thyroid, untreated and treated toxic goiter. Acta Endocrinol. *53*(Suppl. 110):5, 1966.

Hilfer, R. S.: Follicle formation in embryonic chick thyroid. I. Early morphogenesis. J. Morphol. *115*:135, 1964.

Hirsch, P. F., F. F. Gauthier, and P. L. Munson: Thyroid hypocalcemic principle and recurrent laryngeal nerve injury as factors affecting the response to parathyroidectomy in rats. Endocrinology *73*:244, 1963.

Hirsch, P. F., and Munson, P. L.: Thyrocalcitonin. Physiol. Rev. 49:548, 1969.

Kumar, M. A., E. Slack, A. Edwards, H. A. Soliman, A. Baghdiantz, G. V. Foster, and I. MacIntyre: A biological assay for calcitonin. J. Endocrinol. *33*:469, 1965.

Leblond, C. P., and J. Gross: Thyroglobulin formation in the thyroid follicle visualized by the "coated autograph" technique. Endocrinology *43*:306, 1948.

MacIntyre, I., G. V. Foster, and M. A. Kumar: The thyroid origin of calcitonin. *In* Gaillard, P. J., R. V. Talmage, and A. M. Budy, eds.: The Parathyroid Glands: Ultrastructure, Secretion and Function. Chicago, University of Chicago Press, 1965.

Nadler, N. J., S. K. Sarkar, and C. P. Leblond: Origin of intracellular colloid droplets in the rat thyroid. Endocrinology *71*:120, 1962.

Nadler, N. J., B. A. Young, C. P. Leblond, and B. Mitmaker: Elaboration of thyroglobulin in the thyroid follicle. Endocrinology *74*:333, 1964.

Nonidez, J. F.: The origin of the parafollicular cell, a second epithelial component of the thyroid gland of the dog. Am. J. Anat. *49*:479, 1932.

Nonidez, J. F.: Further observations on the parafollicular cells of the mammalian thyroid. Anat. Rec. *53*:339, 1932.

Pearse, A. G. E.: The cytochemistry of the thyroid C cells and their relationship to calcitonin. Proc. R. Soc. B *164*:478, 1966.

Pitt-Rivers, R.: Mode of action of antithyroid compounds. Physiol. Rev. *30*:194, 1950.

Pitt-Rivers, R., and W. R. Trotter, eds.: The Thyroid. London, Butterworths, 1964.

Seljelid, R.: Electron microscopic localization of acid phosphatase in rat thyroid follicle cells after stimulation with thyrotropic hormone. J. Histochem. Cytochem. *13*:687, 1965.

Seljelid, R.: Endocytosis in thyroid follicle cells. II. A microinjection study of the origin of colloid droplets. J. Ultrastruct. Res. *17*:401, 1967.

Seljelid, R., A. Reith, and N. F. Nakken: The early phase of endocytosis in the rat thyroid follicle cell. Lab. Invest. *23*:595, 1970.

Strum, J. M., and M. J. Karnovsky: Cytochemical localization of endogenous peroxidase in thyroid follicular cells. J. Cell Biol. *44*:655, 1970.

Taurog, A.: Thyroid hormone synthesis and release. *In* Werner, S. C., and Ingbar, S. H. eds.: The Thyroid. A Fundamental and Clinical Test. New York, Harper & Row, 1978.

Turner, C. D., and J. T. Bagnara: General Endocrinology. 5th ed. Philadelphia, W. B. Saunders Co., 1971.

Welzel, B. K., S. S. Spicer, and S. H. Wollman: Changes in fine structure and acid phosphatase localization in rat thyroid cells following thyrotrophin administration. J. Cell Biol. *25*:593, 1965.

Whur, P., A. Herscovics, and C. P. Leblond: Radioautographic visualization of the incorporation of galactose-^{3}H and mannose-^{3}H by rat thyroids in vitro in relation to the stages of thyroglobulin synthesis. J. Cell Biol. *43*:289, 1969.

Wissig, S. L.: The anatomy of secretion in the follicular cells of the thyroid gland; the fine structure of the gland in the normal rat. J. Biophys. Biochem. Cytol. 7:419, 1960.

Wissig, S. L.: The anatomy of secretion in the follicular cells of the thyroid gland. II. The effect of acute thyrotrophic hormone stimulation on the secretory apparatus. J. Cell Biol. *16*:93, 1963.

Wolman, S. H., S. S. Spicer, and M. S. Burstone: Localization of esterase and acid phosphatase in granules and colloid droplets in rat thyroid epithelium. J. Cell Biol. *21*:191, 1964.

19

PARATHYROID GLANDS

The *parathyroid glands* are endocrine glands producing a hormone that is essential for maintaining the normal concentration of calcium in the blood and extracellular fluid of the body. In most mammalian species their removal results in a precipitous fall in blood calcium, leading to violent spasm of skeletal muscle (tetany) and ultimately to death. In the human there are usually four parathyroid glands but accessory glands are common. They are small, yellow-brown, oval bodies adhering to the posterior surface of the thyroid gland. Their total weight varies from 0.05 to 0.3 g. They may range from 3 to 8 mm in length, 2 to 5 mm in width, and 0.5 to 2 mm in thickness. Most of the glands are associated with the middle third of the thyroid, a smaller number with the inferior third. In 5 to 10 per cent of cases one or more parathyroids are associated with the thymus and may therefore be deep in the anterior mediastinum. This association of the parathyroid glands with the thymus stems from their common origin from the same pharyngeal pouch in the embryo.

Most parathyroid glands lie in the capsule of the thyroid, but they may be embedded within the gland (Fig. 19–1). In either case, they are separated from the substance of thyroid by a thin connective tissue capsule. The capsular connective tissue extends into the parathyroid gland, and it is via these trabeculae that the larger branches of blood vessels, nerves, and lymphatics enter. Between the gland cells is a framework of reticular fibers. These support the rich capillary network and the nerve fibers. The connective tissue stroma may contain numerous fat cells and these may occupy half the volume of the gland in elderly individuals.

The parenchyma of the parathyroid glands consists of densely packed groups of cells, which may form a compact mass or may be arranged as anastomosing cords, or less commonly as follicles with a small amount of colloidal material in the lumen. Two main types of epithelial cells have been described in man: *principal cells* and *oxyphilic cells* (Fig. 19–2).

The Principal Cells (Chief Cells)

The principal cells are polygonal and 7 to 10 μm in diameter, with a centrally placed vesicular nucleus and a pale, slightly acidophilic cytoplasm that tends to shrink during fixation. There is a small juxtanuclear Golgi apparatus and a number of elongated mitochondria. Coarse granular deposits of fluorescent lipofuscin pigment are often present, and when the cells are appropriately stained, a considerable amount of glycogen is found. In addition to these components, small granules have been described that stain with iron-hematoxylin and exhibit argyrophilia with the Bodian stain. These have been interpreted by some investigators as secretory granules.

Electron microscopic studies reaffirm the presence of all the components enumerated above and reveal, in addition, cisternal profiles of the granular endoplasmic reticulum, sometimes aggregated in conspicuous parallel arrays. The argyrophilic granules at this level of resolution have irregular outlines, are limited by a membrane, and have a dense granular content. They appear to arise in the Golgi apparatus and tend to accumulate at the periphery of the cell. A single abortive cilium is often found projecting from the principal cell into the narrow intercellular space.

A second category of principal cells is distinguished at the electron microscope level. These have a smaller Golgi apparatus, few dense "secretory" granules, and large lakes of glycogen. These cells appear to be physiologically less active than those described above and may outnumber them.

The Oxyphilic Cells

The oxyphilic cells are greatly in the minority and occur singly or in small groups.

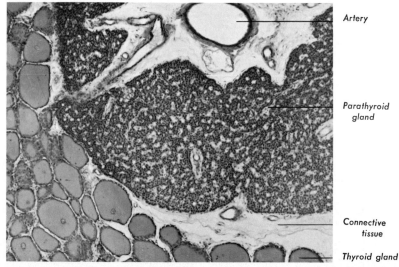

Artery

Parathyroid gland

Connective tissue

Thyroid gland

Figure 19–1. Photomicrograph of section of thyroid and parathyroid glands of *Macacus rhesus.* × 80.

They are distinctly larger than the principal cells. They have a small, darkly staining nucleus and a strongly acidophilic cytoplasm. When stained by the aniline-acid fuchsin method, they are found to have many more mitochondria than the principal cells. This is borne out in electron micrographs, which show a remarkable concentration of elon-gated mitochondria with numerous closely spaced cristae. In the interstices among the mitochondria are numerous glycogen particles, but these do not form large masses as they do in the less active principal cells. The Golgi apparatus is inconspicuous and the endoplasmic reticulum sparse. The eosino-philic granulation formerly described by light

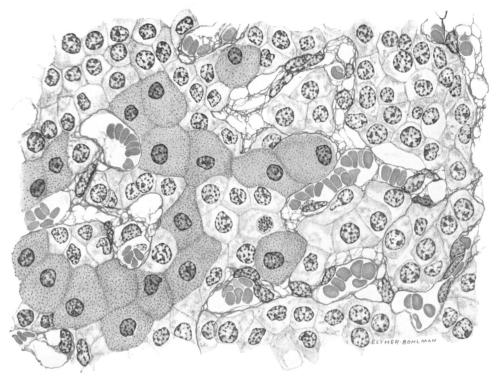

Figure 19–2. Section through human parathyroid gland showing the small principal cells, often vacuolated, and the large oxyphilic cells with fine purplish granules. Zenker-formol fixation. Mallory-azan stain. × 960.

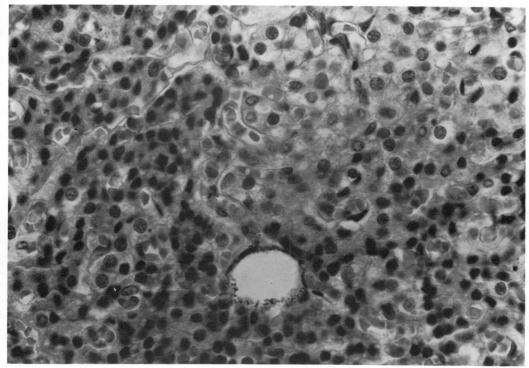

jure 19–3. Photomicrograph of human parathyroid. Only one adipose cell is shown in this field, but such cells may very numerous. (Courtesy of S. I. Roth.)

icroscopists must be attributed to the abun-
ant mitochondria, for granules resembling
cretory granules are rarely encountered in
ectron micrographs.

Another type of cell, intermediate between
e oxyphilic and principal cells, has been
scribed. It has a fine granular cytoplasm,
nich stains faintly with acid dyes, and a
ucleus that is smaller and stains darker than
at of the principal cells. Also, "water-clear"
lls and "dark oxyphilic" cells have been
scribed, but it is not clear to what extent
ese latter types are to be attributed to
garies of fixation.

The parathyroid glands show certain
anges with increasing age: (1) an increase
the amount of connective tissue, including
creased numbers of fat cells; (2) the oxy-
ilic cells are said to appear at the age of
½ to 7 years and to increase in number,
pecially after puberty; (3) in the closely
cked masses of gland cells, some cords and
llicles appear in the 1-year-old infant, and
ey increase thereafter; colloid accumula-
n in the lumen of the follicles shows the
me tendency.

When rats are given injections of a large
se of parathyroid extract, the cells of the
rathyroid glands become smaller; the Golgi

apparatus also becomes smaller and more
compact. Both changes are suggestive of decreased functional activity. After two weeks
the cells return to normal, both in size and
in morphology of the Golgi apparatus, suggesting a resumption of normal secretory
activity. During the hypertrophy of the parathyroid glands in rickets, the Golgi apparatus
is described as undergoing changes that indicate great secretory activity in comparison
with normal cells. It is not possible to extend
these conclusions to the human gland, for it
has yet to be clearly shown which cells in man
are equivalent to those in laboratory animals.

HISTOPHYSIOLOGY

The function of *parathyroid hormone* is to
maintain the normal concentration of calcium in the extracellular fluid. It does this by
acting directly upon the osteocytes and osteoclasts in bone, which is the principal store of
calcium in the body. Its initial rapid effect is
to increase the rate of release of calcium
from bone mineral. This appears to be a
result of stimulation of osteocytic osteolysis
(Fig. 19–4). If the increase in circulating

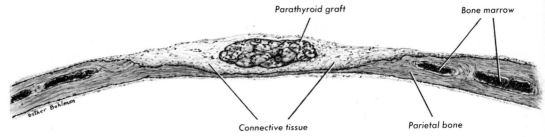

Figure 19–4. Section of parietal bone of rat 14 days after autogenous transplantation of parathyroid gland. The bon[e] beneath the graft has been nearly completely resorbed. × 50. (From a preparation by H. Chang.)

parathyroid hormone continues for some time, there is an acceleration of the rate of internal remodeling of bone, which is a function of the osteoclasts.

Parathyroid hormone also acts directly upon the kidney to minimize calcium loss in the urine. Within a few minutes after administration of the hormone to a parathyroidectomized animal, there is an increase in excretion of phosphate, sodium, and potassium in the urine and a decrease in clearance of calcium. The hormone also influences the synthesis, in the intestine, of a form of vitamin D_3 that increases the efficiency of calcium absorption from dietary sources.

The secretion of parathyroid hormone is under feedback control by the concentration of calcium in the blood and extracellular fluid. In response to a marked fall in the blood calcium, the rate of hormone secretion may reach 50 to 100 times the normal level.

The first biologically active extracts of the parathyroid were prepared 70 years ago by Collip. A highly purified fraction of the hormone was produced by Rasmussen in 1960 and its complete primary structure was determined by Brewer and Ronan in 1970. It is a polypeptide of 84 amino acids. More recent investigations have concentrated upon elucidating its intracellular biosynthetic pathway and upon identifying its precursors. Many proteins produced by cells are first synthesized in the form of large precursor molecules that are subsequently cleaved intra- or extracellularly to yield the biologically active product. Discovery of the precursors of parathyroid hormone was somewhat delayed because the very small size of the gland made it difficult to obtain sufficient material for analysis. One or two milligrams of a precursor fraction were ultimately isolated from several kilograms of bovine parathyroids and sequenced in 1972. This *propara-thyroid hormone* consisted of the 84 amino acid chain of parathyroid hormone with an addi-

tional hexapeptide at one end. This prove[d] to be only an intermediate in the biosyntheti[c] process, and a still larger precursor of 11[5] amino acids, called *pre-proparathyroid hormon[e]* was soon identified. This appears to be th[e] initial product resulting from transcriptio[n] of the specific messenger RNA. A sho[rt] amino acid "signal" sequence serves to attac[h] the polyribosomes to the membrane of th[e] endoplasmic reticulum. As the nascent poly[-] peptide chain extends through the mem[-] brane into the lumen, a specific peptidas[e] cleaves off the signal peptide, yielding pr[o] parathyroid hormone. This is channele[d] through the reticulum to the Golgi comple[x] where the aminoterminal hexapeptide is re[-] moved to form the final product *parathyro[id] hormone.*

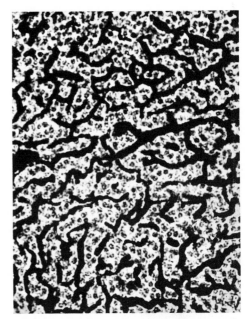

Figure 19–5. Photomicrograph of parathyroid gland [of] monkey injected intravenously with India ink to show th[e] extensively anastomotic capillary network in intimate co[n-] tact with the gland cells. × 165. (Courtesy of I. Gersh.)

There is relatively little storage of hormone in the parathyroid. The amount accumulated intracellularly in bovine glands is estimated to be sufficient for only five to six hours of basal demand or 1½ hours under maximal stimulation. Increased demand for hormone must be met by active synthesis, and the intracellular mechanisms that couple secretory activity to synthesis are poorly understood.

The precise mechanism by which parathyroid hormone exerts its effect upon bone and kidney cells has yet to be completely worked out. There are strong indications, however, that activation of adenyl cyclase and elevated intracellular concentrations of cyclic AMP are involved. The concentration of cyclic AMP in the urine rises within minutes after administration of the hormone to intact animals. In vitro, an increased activity of adenyl cyclase in kidney and bone can be demonstrated within 15 seconds after adding parathyroid hormone to the system.

The parathyroids may give rise to tumors in which the cells produce excessive amounts of hormone, resulting in *primary hyperparathyroidism.* Such patients have high blood calcium levels, rarefaction of their bones (osteitis fibrosa), low blood phosphate level, kidney stones, and deposits of calcium in other soft tissues. In *rickets,* calcium and phosphate are not adequately absorbed from the diet, owing to a deficiency of vitamin D. The resulting low blood calcium results in a compensatory activation of the parathyroids called *secondary hyperparathyroidism.* Similarly, in severe kidney disease, there may be phosphate retention, resulting in low blood calcium, and consequent hypertrophy of the parathyroids.

REFERENCES

Abe, M., and L. M. Sherwood: Regulation of parathyroid secretion by adenyl cyclase. Biochem. Biophys. Res. Commun. *48*:396, 1972.

Aurbach, G. D., R. Marcus, J. Heersche, S. Marx, H. Niall, G. W. Tregear, H. T. Keutmann, and J. T. Potts, Jr.: Hormones and other factors regulating calcium metabolism. *In* Robison, G. A., et al., eds.: Cyclic AMP and Cell Function. Ann. N. Y. Acad. Sci. *185*:386, 1971.

Barnicot, N. A.: The local action of the parathyroid and other tissues on bone in intracerebral grafts. J. Anat. *82*:233, 1948.

Chang, H. Y.: Grafts of parathyroid and other tissues to bone. Anat. Rec. *111*:23, 1951.

Collip, J. B.: The extraction of a parathyroid hormone which will prevent or control tetany and which regulates the level of blood calcium. J. Biol. Chem. *63*:395, 1925.

Davis, R., and A. C. Enders: Light and electron microscope studies on the parathyroid gland. *In* Greep, R. O., and R. V. Talmage, eds.: The Parathyroids. Springfield, IL, Charles C Thomas, 1961, p. 76.

DeRobertis, E.: The cytology of the parathyroid gland of rats injected with parathyroid extract. Anat. Rec. *78*:473, 1940.

Gaillard, P. J.: Parathyroid gland tissue and bone *in vitro.* Exp. Cell Res. *3*(Suppl.):154, 1955.

Gaillard, P. J.: Parathyroid and bone in tissue culture. *In* Greep, R. O., and R. V. Talmage, eds.: The Parathyroids. Springfield, IL, Charles C Thomas, 1961, p. 20.

Grafflin, A. L.: Cytological evidence of secretory activity in the mammalian parathyroid. Endocrinology *26*:857, 1940.

Greep, R. O.: Parathyroid glands. *In* von Euler, U.S., and H. Heller, eds.: The Parathyroids. Comparative Endocrinology. Vol. I. New York, Academic Press, 1963, p. 235.

Greep, R. O., and R. V. Talmage, eds.: The Parathyroids. Springfield, IL, Charles C Thomas, 1961.

Habener, J. F. and J. T. Potts, Jr.: Biosynthesis of parathyroid hormone. Parts 1 and 2. N. Engl. J. Med. *299*:580, 635, 1978.

Habener, J. F., D. Powell, T. M. Murray, G. P. Mayer, and J. T. Potts, Jr.: Parathyroid hormone: secretion and metabolism in vivo. Proc. Natl. Acad. Sci. U.S.A. *68*:2896, 1971.

Kemper, B., J. F. Habener, R. C. Mulligan, J. T. Potts, and A. Rich: Pre-proparathyroid hormone: a direct translation product of parathyroid messenger RNA. Proc. Natl. Acad. Sci. U.S.A. *71*:3731, 1974.

Munger, B. L., and S. I. Roth: The cytology of the normal parathyroid glands of man and Virginia deer: a light and electron microscopic study with morphologic evidence of secretory activity. J. Cell Biol. *16*:379, 1963.

Potts, J. T., Jr., and L. J. Deftos: Parathyroid hormone, thyrocalcitonin, vitamin D and diseases of bone and bone mineral metabolism. *In* Bondy, P. K., ed.: Duncan's Diseases of Metabolism. 6th ed. Philadelphia, W. B. Saunders Co., 1969.

Potts, J. T., Jr., T. Murray, M. Peacock, H. D. Niall, G. W. Tregear, H. T. Keutmann, D. Powell, and L. J. Deftos: Parathyroid hormone: sequence, synthesis, immunoassay studies. Am. J. Med. *50*:639, 1971.

Rasmussen, H.: Chemistry of parathyroid hormone. *In* Greep, R. O., and R. V. Talmage, eds.: The Parathyroids. Springfield, IL, Charles C Thomas, 1961, p. 60.

Rasmussen, H., and L. C. Craig: Isolation and characterization of bovine parathyroid hormone. J. Biol. Chem. *236*:759, 1961.

Roth, S. I.: Pathology of the parathyroids in hyperparathyroidism with a discussion of recent advances in the anatomy and pathology of the parathyroid glands. Arch. Pathol. *73*:492, 1962.

Trier, J. S.: The fine structure of the parathyroid gland. J. Biophys. Biochem. Cytol. *4*:13, 1958.

Weymouth, R. J., and B. L. Baker: The presence of argyrophilic granules in the parenchymal cells of the parathyroid glands. Anat. Rec. *119*:519, 1954.

20

ADRENAL GLANDS AND PARAGANGLIA

The paired *adrenal* or *suprarenal* glands are roughly triangular, flattened organs embedded in the retroperitoneal adipose tissue at the cranial pole of each kidney. They measure approximately 5 by 3 by less than 1 cm and together weigh about 15 g. Both weight and size may vary considerably, depending on the age and physiological condition of the individual. The cut surface of the transected gland presents a bright yellow *cortex* in its outer part, with a reddish brown inner zone adjacent to the thin, gray *medulla*.

The adrenal glands comprise two distinct endocrine organs that differ in their embryological origin, type of secretion, and function—the *interrenal tissue* and the *chromaffin tissue.* In mammals these are arranged as cortex and medulla respectively, but in other vertebrate classes they may be intermingled in a variety of patterns or may be entirely dissociated.

THE ADRENAL CORTEX

The cortex, which forms the bulk of the gland, has three distinguishable concentric zones—a thin, outer *zona glomerulosa* adjacent to the capsule; a thick middle layer, the *zona fasciculata;* and a moderately thick, inner *zona reticularis* contiguous with the medulla (Figs. 20–1, 20–2). In man these make up respectively 15, 78, and 7 per cent of the total cortical volume. The transition from one zone to another in histological sections is gradual but may appear sharper in preparations injected to show the vascular pattern.

The zona glomerulosa consists of closely packed clusters and arcades of columnar cells that are continuous with the cell columns of the zona fasciculata (Fig. 20–3). The spherical nuclei stain deeply and contain one or two nucleoli. The cytoplasm is less abundant than in the cells of the other zones and is generally acidophilic, but it contains some basophilic material, which is usually disposed in clumps. Lipid droplets are small and relatively scarce in this zone in most species but may be numerous in others. Mitochondria are filamentous. The compact Golgi apparatus is juxtanuclear and in some animals may be polarized toward the nearest vascular channel.

At the electron microscopic level, the most characteristic feature of the cytoplasm is its smooth-surfaced endoplasmic reticulum, which forms an anastomosing network of tubules throughout the cell body. Profiles of granular endoplasmic reticulum are also present in limited numbers, and there are many polyribosomes free in the cytoplasmic matrix. There is nothing unusual in the organization of the Golgi complex or in the centrioles that are associated with it. The mitochondria as a rule have lamellar cristae like those of most other organs. The plasma membrane is smoothly contoured over most of the cell body but may have a few folds or microvilli on the surface bordering on a perivascular space and at the junctions where several cells meet.

The zona fasciculata consists of polyhedral cells considerably larger than those of the glomerulosa and arranged in long cords disposed radially with respect to the medulla (Fig. 20–4). The cords are usually one cell thick and separated by sinusoidal blood vessels. The nucleus is central, and binucleate cells are common. The cytoplasm is generally acidophilic but may contain basophilic masses, particularly in the peripheral portion of the zone. The cells are crowded with lipid droplets in the fresh condition, but after treatment with the organic solvents used in preparation of routine histological sections,

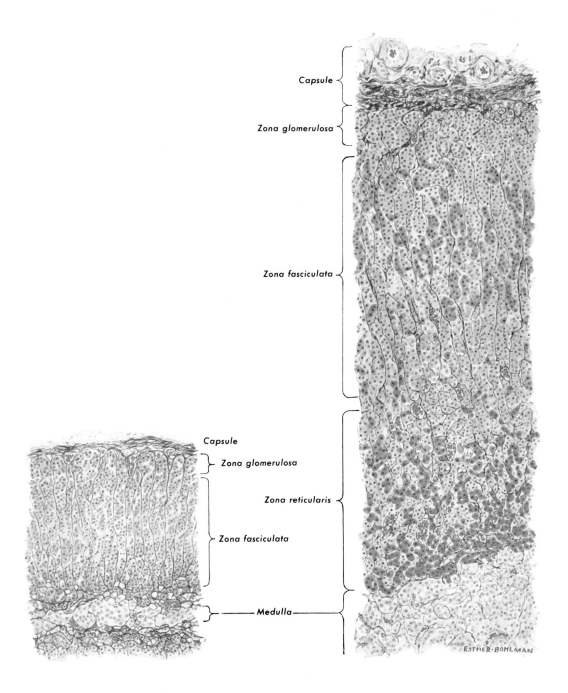

Capsule

Zona glomerulosa

Zona fasciculata

Capsule

Zona glomerulosa

Zona reticularis

Zona fasciculata

Medulla

ESTHER·BOHLMAN

Figure 20–1. Sections through the adrenal glands of a 6-month-old infant *(left)* and of a man *(right)*. Mallory-azan stain. × 110.

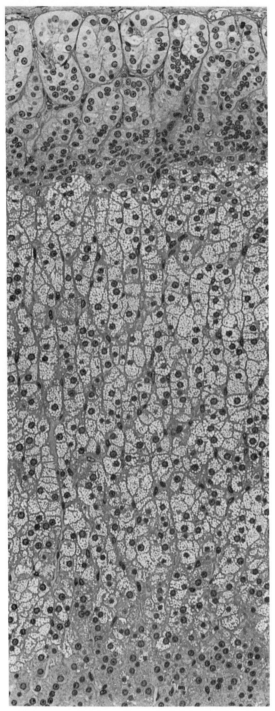

Figure 20–2. Photomicrograph of the full thickness of the adrenal cortex of a rhesus monkey, showing from the top downward the zona glomerulosa, zona fasciculata, and zona reticularis.

of the cortex, and in such places the zona fasciculata is found immediately beneath the cortex, but this is not common. There may also be a thin transitional region between the zona glomerulosa and zona fasciculata that is relatively free of lipid droplets. Such a sudanophobic *zona intermedia* is particularly obvious in the rat adrenal.

In electron micrographs, cells of the zona fasciculata have a round nucleus, a prominent nucleolus, and clumps of heterochromatin distributed at the periphery. In the human the nuclear envelope has a distinct internal fibrous lamina. The most conspicuous ultrastructural feature of the cells is a very extensive smooth endoplasmic reticulum in the form of branching and anastomosing tubules (Figs. 20–5, 20–6, 20–7). This organelle occupies 40 to 45 per cent of the cell volume. Occasional parallel arrays of cisternae of rough endoplasmic reticulum are found in the zona fasciculata of the human adrenal but rarely in other species. The Golgi complex is well developed and has multiple stacks of cisternae and associated vesicles.

The mitochondria are numerous, occupying 26 to 36 per cent of the cell volume. They are elongate in humans but generally spherical in common laboratory rodents. The matrix is of low density and the cristae are atypical in form. In the rat they appear to be spherical vesicles 60 to 70 nm in diameter, while in the human they are described as tubulovesicular—short tubules with vesicular dilatations along their length. In the hamster they are slender tubules of uniform caliber. Cristae of tubular form are also found in other steroid-secreting cells.

Small dense bodies of irregular shape, assumed to be lysosomes, are present in small numbers throughout the cytoplasm, and microperoxisomes have been identified with the diaminobenzidene reaction. Deposits of lipochrome pigment are common in the human adrenal.

Lipid droplets are usually present but there is considerable interspecific variation in their abundance. They occupy 10 to 15 per cent of the cell volume in the rat, and are numerous in the human and other primates but usually absent in the ox and hamster.

The relationships between cell ultrastructure and function in adrenocortical cells is better understood than in many other cell types. The enzymes involved in biosynthesis of steroid hormones are located in the extensive smooth endoplasmic reticulum and in the numerous mitochondria. The varying

the cytoplasm has a foamy appearance due to the numerous clear vacuoles left by extraction of lipid (Fig. 20–4). In man, the zona glomerulosa may be absent in restricted areas

Text continued on page 524

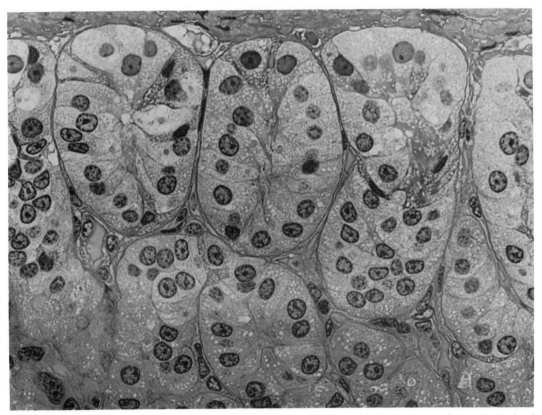

Figure 20–3. Photomicrograph of the monkey zona glomerulosa at higher magnification than in Figure 20–2, showing the alveolar or glomerular arrangement of cells. These cells have relatively few vacuoles, representing extracted lipid.

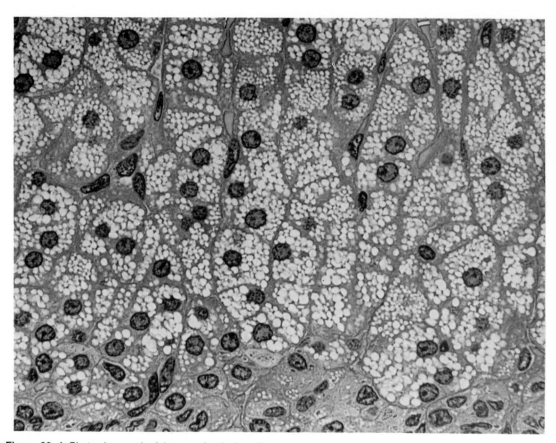

Figure 20–4. Photomicrograph of the zona fasciculata. This zone consists of cords of cells filled with spherical vacuoles resulting from extraction of the abundant lipid droplets characteristic of this zone.

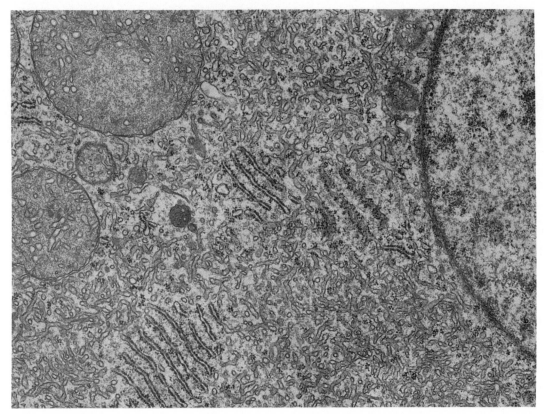

Figure 20–5. Electron micrograph of a portion of a cell from the human fetal adrenal cortex, showing large spherical mitochondria with tubular cristae, a few parallel arrays of cisternae of granular reticulum, and an extraordinary abundance of smooth endoplasmic reticulum. (Micrograph courtesy of A. L. Jones and S. McNutt.)

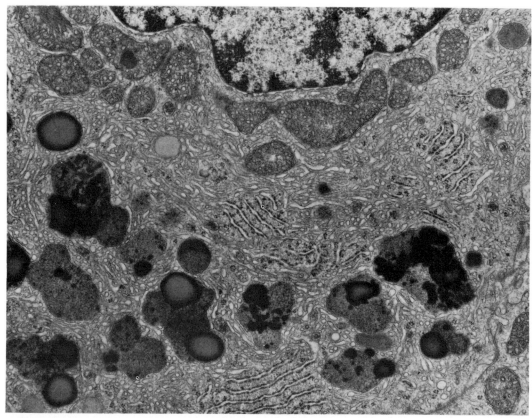

Figure 20–6. Electron micrograph of a juxtanuclear area of a cortical cell from an adult human adrenal. The smooth reticulum remains abundant, the mitochondria are variable in size and shape, and they generally have tubular cristae. There is a marked tendency for accumulation of irregular dense masses of lipochrome pigment. (Micrograph courtesy of J. Long.)

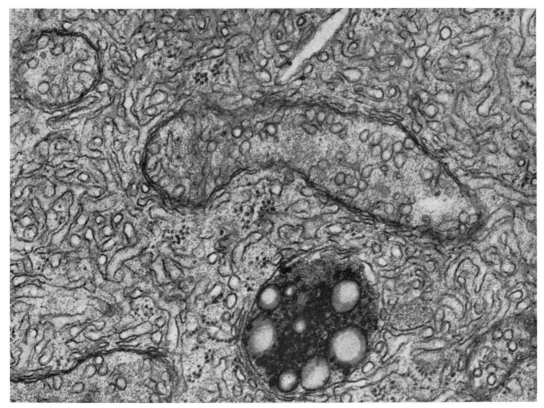

Figure 20–7. Electron micrograph of an area of cytoplasm of an adult adrenocortical cell at high magnification, illustrating the tubular nature of the smooth reticulum and the fine structure of the mitochondria. (Micrograph courtesy of J. Long.)

abundance of lipid in different species is correlated with the degree to which cholesterol, the precursor of steroid synthesis, is taken up from the blood or is synthesized from acetate in the smooth reticulum of the adrenocortical cells. Cholesterol stored in the lipid droplets is released by cholesterol esterase and enters mitochondria, where it undergoes side-chain cleavage to yield pregnenolone. Transferred from mitochondria to endoplasmic reticulum, pregnenolone is converted to progesterone and then to 11-deoxycorticosterone or 17-deoxycorticosterone. These intermediate products are converted to the steroid hormones *deoxycorticosterone* and *cortisol*, respectively, by enzymes located in the mitochondria. The biosynthetic pathway thus involves transfer of precursor molecules and intermediate products to and fro between mitochondria and smooth endoplasmic reticulum. Little is known as to how these translocations occur.

The stimulatory effect of adrenocorticotropic hormone (ACTH) is mediated by cyclic AMP. Upon binding of the hormone to receptors in the membrane of the cells in the zona fasciculata, adenyl cyclase is activated to catalyze the formation of cyclic AMP from ATP. This in turn activates cholesterol esterase, which hydrolyzes cholesterol ester stored in lipid droplets, making free cholesterol available for steroid hormone biosynthesis. There is some evidence of ACTH enhancement of transcription and translation, possibly related to synthesis of carrier proteins involved in transfer of intermediate products between organelles.

The morphological correlates of prolonged ACTH stimulation are depletion of lipid droplets; increase in smooth endoplasmic reticulum; proliferation of mitochondria; and enlargement of the Golgi complex. Unlike many other glandular cells, steroid-secreting cells do not store their product in secretory granules formed in the Golgi complex. The role of the Golgi in steroid-secreting cells remains unclear, but it is speculated that it may be involved in sulfation of intermediate steroid molecules or their conjugation to carrier proteins.

In the absence of unambiguous evidence of vesicular transport and exocytosis, the mechanism of hormone release by adrenocortical cells is controversial. A majority of investigators favor simple diffusion through the aqueous phase of the cytoplasm and across the lipid bilayer of the cell membrane.

Others believe this requires modification of the steroid molecule by sulfation or binding to a carrier molecule. Evidence has recently accumulated suggesting that some of the small dense bodies that have usually been interpreted as lysosomes or microperoxisomes are in fact secretory granules formed in the Golgi and released by exocytosis as rapidly as they are formed. In support of this interpretation is the observation that in ACTH-stimulated cells that have been exposed to vinblastin to block the microtubule transport mechanism commonly associated with exocytosis, there is an increase in small dense bodies in the cytoplasm and a tenfold increase in intracellular corticosterone.

In the zona reticularis, the regular parallel arrangement of cell cords gives way to an anastomosing network of cell cords. The transition from the fasciculata is gradual, the cells differing but little. The cytoplasm contains fewer lipid droplets. Toward the medulla there is a variable number of "light" and "dark" cells. The nuclei of the light cells are pale-staining; those of the dark cells are hyperchromatic and shrunken. The physiological significance of these differences in staining affinity is not known. In other organs, this appearance is often a fixation artifact. It is so common in the zona reticularis, however, that some interpret these cells as degenerative. The cells of this zone, particularly the dark cells, contain large accumulations of lipofuscin pigment. Apart from the presence of light and dark cells and the greater amount of pigment, the cells of the zona reticularis resemble those of the fasciculata and, like them, have an abundance of agranular reticulum.

THE ADRENAL MEDULLA

The boundary between the zona reticularis and medulla is usually irregular in the human adult, with columns of cortical cells projecting some distance into the medulla. In other animals, the boundary may be quite sharp. The medulla is composed of large epithelioid cells arranged in rounded groups or short cords in intimate relation to blood capillaries and venules (Fig. 20–8). When the tissue is fixed in a solution containing potassium bichromate, these cells are seen to be filled with fine brown granules. This browning of the cytoplasmic granules with chromium salts is

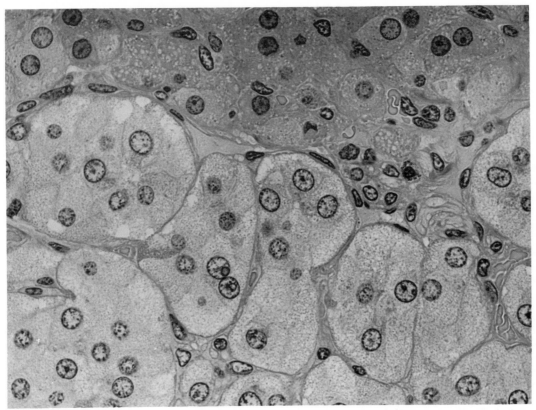

Figure 20–8. Photomicrograph of the junction of the zona reticularis *(above)* with the clusters of large pale cells of the adrenal medulla *(below)*. Catecholamine granules ordinarily are not visible with the light microscope in the cells of the medulla.

called the *chromaffin reaction* and is thought to result from the oxidation and polymerization of the catecholamines *epinephrine* and *norepinephrine* contained within the granules of the cells. The medulla is colored green after treatment with ferric chloride—apparently for the same reason. There are other cells in the body that give a similar reaction, notably some of the argentaffin cells of the gastrointestinal tract and the mast cells, which are reactive because of their content of 5-hydroxytryptamine. The chromaffin cells of the adrenal medulla, however, are derived from neuroectoderm, secrete catecholamines, and are innervated by preganglionic sympathetic fibers.

In most species the application of a group of histochemical methods to the chromaffin cells permits the identification of two types of cells, one containing norepinephrine and the other epinephrine. The norepinephrine storing cells are autofluorescent, give argentaffin and potassium iodate reactions, exhibit a low affinity for azocarmine, and give a negative acid phosphatase reaction. The epinephrine-storing cells have a high staining affinity for azocarmine and a positive acid phosphatase reaction, and are not fluorescent or reactive with iodate or silver.

In electron micrographs, the most prominent feature of the cells of the adrenal medulla is the presence of large numbers of membrane-bounded dense granules 100 to 300 nm in diameter (Fig. 20–9). The granules are bounded by a membrane separated from the dense content by an electron-lucent gap. When tissue is fixed in glutaraldehyde, two populations of cells are distinguishable on the basis of the character of their granules. Cells that store norepinephrine have granules that contain a very electron-dense core, often eccentric in its location within the membrane-limited vesicle. Cells that store epinephrine have granules that are relatively homogeneous and less electron dense. The mitochondria are not remarkable. The cisternae of the granular endoplasmic reticulum form small parallel arrays. The juxtanuclear Golgi apparatus frequently contains in its cisternae dense material interpreted as a precursor of the granules.

It has been established by cell fractionation

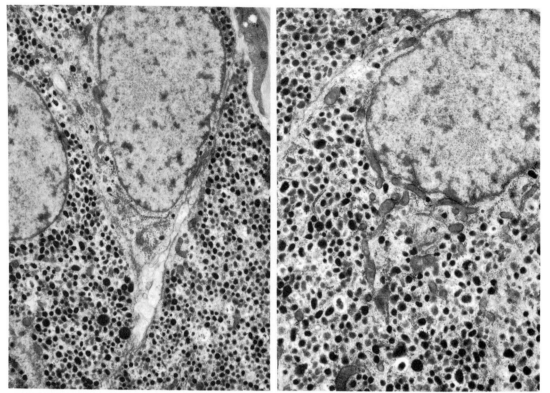

Figure 20–9. Electron micrographs of cells from the adrenal medulla of the cat, showing the abundant, membrane-bounded, dense granules that are the sites of storage of catecholamines. × 9600 and × 13,600. (Courtesy or R. Yates.)

and density gradient centrifugation that the hormones are contained within the secretory granules. The granules may contain as much as 20 per cent by weight of the hormone. Although they also contain a significant amount of protein, much of this is the soluble protein *chromogranin.* The catecholamines do not seem to be bound to a specific protein, as are the hormones of the neurohypophysis and other neurosecretory cells. Therefore, it is not entirely clear how such low-molecular-weight substances are retained in the granules. According to one hypothesis, the hormone forms high-molecular-weight aggregates with adenosine triphosphate (ATP) and divalent cations, both of which are present in the granules. The active uptake of catecholamine by the granules appears to be the result of an active transport mechanism dependent on magnesium-activated ATPase in the limiting membrane. Thus, the ability of secretory granules in the adrenal medulla to retain hormones in vivo probably depends on (1) micelle formation between ATP and hormone and (2) an active transport mechanism in the membrane limiting the granules. The depletion of catecholamines by the phar-

macologically active substance *reserpine* may be the result of inhibition of the active transport mechanism.

For some time there was a divergence of opinion as to whether the granules of the adrenal medulla are released by exocytosis, as are protein hormones, or whether the smaller molecules of catecholamines are released from the granules within the cytoplasm and diffuse out of the cell. It now seems to have been well established experimentally that all or nearly all of the hormones of the adrenal medulla are discharged by exocytosis. Evidence for this resides not only in morphological observations but in the physiological finding that a perfusate of a stimulated gland contains not only catecholamines but also soluble protein constituents of the granules (chromogranin) and ATP, in the same proportions that occur in a lysate of isolated granules, whereas the insoluble constituents associated with the membranes of the granules are retained within the gland.

In addition to the chromaffin cells, sympathetic ganglion cells occur singly or in small groups in the adrenal medulla.

The adrenal is enclosed by a thick capsule

of collagenous connective tissue that extends into the cortex to varying depths as trabeculae. Most of the rest of the supporting framework of the cortex consists of reticular fibers that lie between the sinusoids and the cell cords and penetrate to some extent between the gland cells. Reticular fibers also enclose the cell clusters in the medulla and support the capillaries, veins, and nerves. Collagenous fibers appear around the larger tributaries of the veins and merge with the capsular connective tissue.

BLOOD SUPPLY AND LYMPHATIC DRAINAGE OF THE ADRENAL

The gland is richly supplied by a number of arteries that enter at various points around the periphery. Three principal groups are recognized. The *superior suprarenal arteries* arising from the inferior phrenic artery appear to be the major source, but in addition there are the *middle suprarenals* arising from the aorta and the *inferior suprarenals,* which are branches of the renal artery. Arteries from these several sources form a plexus in the capsule. The *cortical arteries* arise from this capsular plexus and distribute to the anastomosing network of sinusoids surrounding the cords of parenchymal cells in the cortex (Fig. 20–10). The sinusoids of a given region converge in the zona reticularis upon a collecting vein at the corticomedullary junction. There is no venous system in the cortex.

Some major arterial branches from the capsule penetrate the connective tissue trabeculae and pass directly through the cortex, giving off few or no branches until they reach the medulla. In the medulla, they branch repeatedly to form the rich capillary net around the clumps and cords of chromaffin cells. The medulla thus has a dual blood supply—via the cortical sinusoids that anastomose with its capillary bed across the corticomedullary junction, and via the medullary arteries that course from the capsule directly to the medulla. The capillaries of the medulla empty into the same venous system that drains the cortex. The multiple venules ultimately join to form the large central veins of the medulla, which emerge from the gland as the *suprarenal vein.*

This pattern of vascularization has impor-

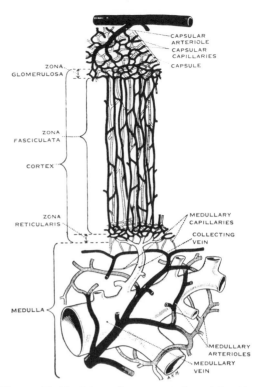

Figure 20–10. Schematic representation of the blood supply of the adrenal, showing how blood from capsular arterioles traverses the cortex and continues into capillaries and venules in the medulla. This arrangement carries blood rich in cortical steroids to the catecholamine-synthesizing cells in the medulla. (From Hamilton, W. J., ed.: Textbook of Human Anatomy. London, St. Martin's Press, Macmillan and Co., 1957.)

tant physiological consequences. The blood reaching the medulla via the sinusoids has traversed the cortex and is rich in cortical steroid hormones. There is evidence that high concentration of glucocorticoids may be required for induction and maintenance of the enzyme phenylethanolamine-*N*-methyl transferase, which is necessary for the synthesis of epinephrine. Thus, the adrenocortical steroids have a local downstream effect on the medulla, as well as a general systemic effect. Indeed, whether a medullary cell secretes norepinephrine or epinephrine may be determined by where it is situated with respect to steroid-rich blood from the cortex that regulates the synthesis of the enzyme necessary for conversion of norepinephrine to epinephrine.

The cells lining the capillaries of the medulla are typical endothelium. The nature of the lining of the sinusoids in the cortex is still a subject of debate. These cells have been reported to take up colloidal vital dyes, such as lithium carmine and trypan blue, and on this basis they have been regarded as belonging to the reticuloendothelial system. Subsequent studies suggest that these substances simply adhere to the cell surface or that they are taken up by macrophages lying between the endothelium and the parenchymal cells. Electron microscopic observations have failed to reveal any evidence of phagocytosis by the endothelial cells of the sinusoids. Except in the regions occupied by the nucleus and cell center, the endothelium is extremely attenuated and interrupted at intervals by small circular pores or fenestrae closed only by a very thin diaphragm. There is a continuous basal lamina supported at intervals by small bundles of collagen fibrils corresponding to the reticulum of light microscopy.

Lymphatics are limited to the capsule and its cortical trabeculae, and to the connective tissue around the large veins.

NERVES OF THE ADRENAL

The cells of the adrenal cortex apparently are not innervated. Those of the zona fasciculata are stimulated by circulating adrenocorticotropic hormone (ACTH) of the pituitary; those of the glomerulosa are responsive to changes in extracellular fluid volume or changes in concentration of sodium and potassium in the blood, possibly acting indirectly via a hypothetical hormone of the diencephalon, *aldosterone-stimulating factor*.

Preganglionic sympathetic nerve fibers arising from cell bodies in the intermediolateral column of the spinal cord in the lower thoracic and lumbar regions of the spinal cord pass through the sympathetic chain and via splanchnic nerves to the capsule of the adrenal, where they form a rich nerve plexus, including a few sympathetic ganglion cells. From this plexus preganglionic nerves turn inward, traverse the cortex, and end in the medulla around the cells that secrete epinephrine and norepinephrine. These cells are derived embryologically from the nervous system in early development and are analogous to postganglionic neurons. The nerve terminals form typical synapses with the cells, in which the pre- and postsynaptic membranes are separated by a cleft of 15 to 20 nm. The nerve terminals are cholinergic and contain multiple clear synaptic vesicles.

HISTOPHYSIOLOGY OF THE ADRENAL CORTEX

The adrenal cortex is involved in a wide variety of body functions, including maintenance of fluid and electrolyte balance, maintenance of carbohydrate balance, and maintenance of the normal function of certain cellular elements of the connective tissues. It is essential for life. Its removal or destruction leads ultimately to death unless the patient is given exogenous adrenocortical hormones.

The widely accepted zonal hypothesis of adrenal function affirms that different functions can be ascribed to the morphologically recognizable zones of the adrenal cortex. The zona glomerulosa secretes hormones collectively called *mineralocorticoids* (aldosterone and deoxycorticosterone), which are concerned with fluid and electrolyte balance. The zona fasciculata and zona reticularis secrete hormones collectively referred to as *glucocorticoids* (cortisol, cortisone, and corticosterone), which are concerned with metabolism of carbohydrates, proteins, and fat. The concept of a separate function of the zona glomerulosa and the inner zones of the cortex is supported by abundant experimental evidence. There is as yet no clear-cut evidence of qualitative functional differences between the zona fasciculata and zona reticularis.

The most important hormone of the zona glomerulosa is *aldosterone*. When released in the body or administered exogenously, it has three basic effects: it increases reabsorption of sodium by the tubules of the kidney; it increases the excretion of potassium by the kidney; and it appears to increase both the movement of sodium into the cells of the body and the associated transfer of potassium out of the cells. If the secretion of this hormone is eliminated by disease or surgical removal of the adrenal, the sodium and chloride concentrations of the extracellular fluid decrease markedly, the volume of extracellular fluid is greatly diminished, and the patient goes into a shocklike state that is followed by death within a few days, unless treated by salt replacement or administration of exogenous mineralocorticoids.

As in other parts of the endocrine system, the secretion of aldosterone is carefully regulated to maintain constancy of the internal environment of the cells of the body. If for some reason the extracellular sodium concentration falls, or if potassium rises, or extra-cellular fluid volume is dangerously diminished, this is reflected in the concentration in the blood and detected by centers in the midbrain. These, in turn, release a hormone that stimulates the zona glomerulosa to release aldosterone, which acts upon the kidney tubules to increase sodium absorption and decrease potassium resorption, thus correcting the imbalance. If increased demands are placed upon the homeostatic mechanisms for maintaining electrolyte balance by giving an animal either an excess of potassium or a sodium-deficient diet, there is a selective hypertrophy of the zona glomerulosa and an increase in the abundance of smooth endoplasmic reticulum in its cells. Conversely, injection of large doses of aldosterone or deoxycorticosterone results in atrophy of this zone.

The glucocorticoids secreted by the two inner zones of the cortex are almost as important in sustaining life as are the mineralocorticoids. Secretion or administration of cortisol results in a great increase in the formation of glucose in the liver and its intracellular storage as glycogen. Excess glucose is also released into the blood, producing a condition comparable with diabetes. The hormone also causes a decrease in the rate of protein synthesis and an increase in the rate of protein breakdown in the cells of the body. Therefore, the level of amino acids in the blood increases. Finally, cortisol acts upon adipose tissue, increasing both the rate at which lipid is accumulated in the fat cells and the rate at which the lipids are mobilized from those cells.

The control of the secretion of glucocorticoids is quite independent of that of the mineralocorticoids. The maintenance of the inner zones of the cortex depends on secretion of ACTH by the anterior lobe of the hypophysis. Hypophysectomy results in a marked atrophy of the zona fasciculata and zona reticularis but has little effect on the zona glomerulosa. This atrophy of the inner zones can be prevented or reversed by injection of ACTH. Conversely, administration of large doses of cortisol to an intact animal suppresses hypophyseal secretion of ACTH and results in atrophy of the inner zones of the adrenal cortex.

The mechanisms of control of glucocorticoid secretion have already been presented in Chapter 3 but, briefly restated, many different kinds of alarming or stressful situations, such as pain, fear, and rage result in passage of nerve impulses to the hypothalamus that initiate secretion of corticotropin releasing factor (CRF) into the hypophyseoportal vessels. Carried to the anterior lobe of the hypophysis, this promotes adrenocorticotropin release, which in turn causes discharge of glucocorticoids from the adrenal. The resulting increase in blood amino acid and glucose levels makes available to the cells the energy-rich substrates that may be needed for combat, flight, or other responses to stress.

The glucocorticoids also have effects upon inflammatory responses of the connective tissues and upon the immune system. The mechanisms of these actions are poorly understood but they are widely utilized in the treatment of allergies, arthritis, rheumatic fever, and many other inflammatory diseases. Cortisol somehow reduces the severity of allergic reactions and suppresses the inflammation. Among other effects it causes destruction of lymphocytes, atrophy of lymphoid tissue, and a decrease in level of circulating eosinophils. Therefore, in surgical grafting of organs, cortisol is often given to suppress the rejection reaction.

There is also a relationship between the adrenal cortex and the reproductive system. Adrenalectomy is followed by loss of libido in the male and abnormal cycles in the female. Removal of the adrenal interrupts lactation. Whether or not these effects are mediated via the adenohypophysis is not clear. It is known that under normal conditions, small amounts of estrogens and androgens are produced in the two inner zones of the cortex. In the pathological condition known as *adrenogenital syndrome*, the inner zones of the cortex are hypertrophic, and high levels of circulating androgens may result in precocious puberty, increased hirsutism, and other manifestations of virilism.

Hyperadrenocorticism or *Cushing's disease* is a condition in which the adrenal cortex is hyperplastic, as a result of stimulation by pituitary or other tumors producing excessive amounts of ACTH. It is characterized by obesity, particularly over the nape of the neck; hirsutism; impotence or amenorrhea; abdominal striae; and a characteristic round "moon face." *Hypoadrenocorticism* or *Addison's disease* is due to destruction of the adrenal cortex by tuberculosis or other infection of the gland, resulting in chronic insufficiency of hormone production. It is characterized by generalized weakness, weight loss, low blood pressure, and abnormal pigmentation, and leads ultimately to death if hormone replacement therapy is not undertaken.

HISTOPHYSIOLOGY OF THE ADRENAL MEDULLA

The adrenal medulla is not essential for life. Animals that have had their adrenal medullas removed can survive under ordinary circumstances but are unable to respond normally to emergency situations. The hormones of the medulla, *epinephrine* and *norepinephrine,* are catecholamines, and unlike the steroid hormones of the cortex, they accumulate in high concentration in the cells. The granules of the cells are the site of storage of catecholamines. The two hormones are produced in different proportions depending upon the species. Aggressive and predatory animals tend to secrete large amounts of norepinephrine, whereas the more timid and placid species produce relatively less.

Although the two hormones are very closely related chemically, there are important qualitative and quantitative differences in their physiological effects.

Epinephrine increases the heart rate and cardiac output without significantly increasing the blood pressure, and may increase the blood flow through some organs by as much as 100 per cent. It has effect on the cardiovascular system in very low concentrations. The denervated mammalian heart, for example, is accelerated by as little as one part epinephrine in 1.4 billion parts of fluid medium. Epinephrine also has a marked effect upon metabolism. It increases oxygen consumption and basal metabolic rate. It elevates the blood sugar level by mobilizing the carbohydrate stores of the liver; by promoting the conversion of muscle glycogen into lactic acid, from which new carbohydrate can be made in the liver; and by causing the release of ACTH from the hypophysis, which in turn affects gluconeogenesis by stimulating secretion of glucocorticoids from the adrenal cortex. The mobilization of glucose from the liver by epinephrine appears to result from its activation of the enzyme phosphorylase, which accelerates the first step in the breakdown of glycogen to glucose.

Norepinephrine has relatively little effect upon metabolism but causes a marked elevation of the blood pressure with very little effect upon heart rate or cardiac output. The effect of norepinephrine on the blood pressure is not due to an action upon the heartbeat but is primarily a consequence of the vasoconstriction it brings about in the peripheral portion of the arterial system. Both epinephrine and norepinephrine cause lipolysis and release of unesterified fatty acid from adipose tissue isolated in vitro.

Norepinephrine is not confined to the adrenal medulla but is present in the brain and in most of the innervated peripheral tissues, where it is localized mainly in the sympathetic nerve endings. It has been established as the principal transmitter substance of adrenergic neurons. Thus it is a *neurohumor.* Neurohumors such as norepinephrine, acetylcholine, and serotinin are released by nerve cells, usually at their endings, and affect other neurons or muscles or glands. In general they act transiently and at very short range, being destroyed enzymatically before they reach effective concentrations in the circulation. The norepinephrine released into the bloodstream by the adrenal medulla is somewhat exceptional among neurohumors in that it does reach effective levels in the blood and acts at a distance. On the other hand, the *neurosecretory substances,* such as the oxytocin and vasopressin of the posterior lobe of the hypophysis, are long-acting products of nerve cells that act at long range.

Although the adrenomedullary hormones are not essential for life, it appears that in times of stress they do help to maintain homeostasis and to prepare the organism to meet emergency situations. Epinephrine accomplishes this by elevating blood glucose levels, increasing cardiac output, and redistributing blood within the circulation to ensure continuing rapid flow to those organs vital for survival. Norepinephrine is less important in these emergency adjustments, but, as the mediator of adrenergic nerve impulses throughout the body, it acts continuously on the blood vessels of the normal animal to maintain blood pressure.

Hyperfunction of the adrenal medulla in man occurs with certain rare tumors of the medulla or of extramedullary chromaffin tissues. In such cases there may be attacks of sweating, mydriasis, hypertension, and hyperglycemia, terminating suddenly in death. The paroxysmal hypertension (acute high blood pressure) of adrenomedullary tumors is decreased or abolished by intravenous administration of a series of compounds that have an epinephrine-inhibiting action.

The cells of the adrenal medulla are regarded as modified postganglionic neurons, and their secretory activity seems to be largely, if not entirely, under nervous control. Hormones of the medulla are increased in the blood of the adrenal veins after stimulation of the splanchnic nerves, and secretion is prevented by sectioning these nerves. After splanchnic nerve stimulation, about 75 per cent of the secretion is norepinephrine and 25 per cent epinephrine. Certain centers in the posterior hypothalamus are known to relay impulses to the adrenal medulla by way of the splanchnic nerves. In the intact animal, certain kinds of emotional stimuli are especially effective in releasing norepinephrine, and other kinds of stimuli, such as pain or hypoglycemia, promote the release of epinephrine. For this reason, it is believed that the cells producing epinephrine and those producing norepinephrine receive different innervation and secrete their hormones independently.

HISTOGENESIS OF THE ADRENAL GLANDS

The cortex develops from the coelomic mesoderm on the medial side of the urogenital ridge of the embryo. Mesothelial cells near the cranial pole of the mesonephros in 8- to 10-mm human fetuses proliferate and penetrate the subjacent, highly vascular mesenchyme. These cells ultimately form the *fetal cortex*. A second proliferation of the coelomic mesothelium taking place in 14-mm embryos later forms the definitive or *permanent cortex*. The adrenal gland in the fetus is relatively large, with the fetal zone composing about 80 per cent of the cortex. The cells of this zone are large and stain intensely with eosin. After birth the fetal cortex undergoes a rapid degeneration and the permanent cortex enlarges. Associated with these changes is a 50 per cent decline in the absolute weight of the adrenal during the first few postnatal weeks.

The adrenal in the fetus is functional and under the control of ACTH secreted by the hypophysis. Monstrous anencephalic fetuses, which lack a normal hypophysis, have very small adrenal glands with no *fetal zone*. The physiological role of this zone during intrauterine life is not well understood. Progress in this area is hampered by the fact that none

of the common laboratory animals has a comparable fetal zone. In the mouse, the so-called *X zone* differentiates postnatally and regresses at puberty in the male or at the time of the first pregnancy in the female. The hormonal factors controlling it appear to be different from those affecting the human fetal zone.

The medulla arises from the ectodermal neural crest tissue, which also gives rise to sympathetic ganglion cells. Strands of these sympathochromaffin cells migrate ventrally and penetrate the anlagen of the adrenal cortex on its medial side to take up a central position in the organ rudiment.

Cell Renewal and Regeneration in the Adrenal Cortex

There have long been divergent views as to the mode of growth and repair of the adrenal cortex. It was formerly believed that the cells arose either from fibroblast-like cells in the capsule or by division of the cells in the zona glomerulosa, and that they gradually moved through the zona fasciculata and degenerated in the zona reticularis. The dark cells of this zone were interpreted as cells undergoing regressive changes. During their migration, the cells were believed to go through one cycle of secretion.

The bulk of the evidence now seems to favor the view that, once formed, the cells of the glomerulosa and fasciculata do not move appreciably and that replacement and repair take place as a result of local mitotic activity. After injection of colchicine to arrest cell division at metaphase, mitotic figures are not confined to any one region but are found throughout the cortex, the majority being in the zona fasciculata. Autoradiographic studies after administration of tritiated thymidine have produced equivocal results but, on the whole, they provide little evidence of extensive cell migration.

In experimental animals the adrenal cortex has a considerable capacity for regeneration. If the gland is incised and all of the tissue in its interior removed, leaving behind only the capsule and a few adherent granulosal cells, the whole cortex will be regenerated. The medulla is not restored. Studies of the steroids elaborated during regeneration of the cortex show that an adequate level of secretion of mineralocorticoids is established early, although the secretion of glucocorticoids does not occur until one to two weeks later. Thus, in the regenerating gland, cells func-

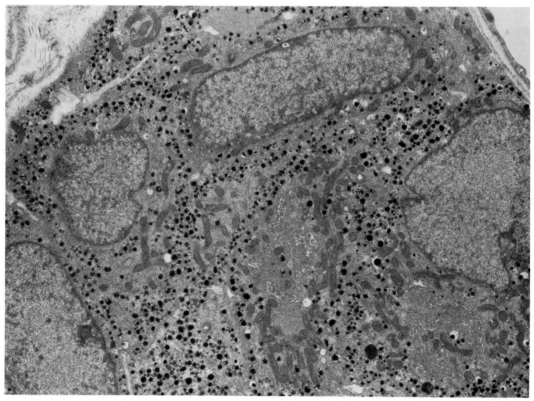

Figure 20–11. Cells of a paraganglion from the rabbit, showing chief cells, which contain numerous catecholamine-storing granules resembling those of the adrenal medulla. (Micrograph courtesy of R. Yates.)

tionally similar to those of the normal zonae fasciculata and reticularis differentiate from cells of the zona glomerulosa.

Phylogeny of the Adrenal Gland

Chromaffin tissue that yields epinephrine-like activity is present in the central nervous system of leeches and also in the mantles of certain molluscs. In cyclostomes and teleosts, the *interrenal bodies* (which are homologous with the cortex) are separate from the discrete chromaffin bodies. In amphibians the two components are in juxtaposition, or they may be intermingled; in reptiles and birds they are commonly intermingled. The well-known cortex and medulla relationship first appears in mammals, where this is the predominant form of organization.

THE PARAGANGLIA

The term *paraganglia* is used to describe small clusters of epithelioid cells that give a chromaffin reaction. They are found rather widely scattered in the retroperitoneal tissue. Some of them are associated with sympathetic ganglia, others with branches of the parasympathetic nerves. The cells of the paraganglia and those of the adrenal medulla are morphologically similar and of similar embryonic origin. Together they make up the *chromaffin system*. In ordinary histological preparations the cells of paraganglia appear pale or clear, but they are stained by the chromaffin reaction.

These cells found in the ganglia and along the nerves of the sympathetic nervous system have now been studied electron microscopically and by histochemical procedures for the identification of catecholamines. The paraganglia are surrounded by a rather thick investment of collagenous connective tissue that extends inward between clumps of parenchymal cells. Two types of parenchymal cells are distinguishable, the chief cells and supporting cells. The chief cells are irregular in shape, with a single nucleus and well-developed juxtanuclear Golgi complex. The endoplasmic reticulum is sparse, but occasional parallel associations of cisternae are observed. Glycogen particles are present in small numbers scattered through the cytoplasmic matrix. In addition, there are numerous membrane-limited, electron-opaque granules 50 to 200 nm, closely resembling those of the adrenal medulla (Fig. 20–11). Histochemical methods indicate that these granules contain catecholamines, principally if not exclusively norepinephrine. The supporting cells partially or completely surround each of the chief cells. The nucleus of these cells is elongated in section and frequently deeply infolded. The cytoplasm is devoid of secretory granules and is otherwise unremarkable.

The paraganglia are richly vascularized by capillaries lined by very attenuated endothelial cells, occasionally exhibiting fenestrated regions. The chief cells are usually separated from the blood by a barrier consisting of a thin intervening supporting cell, two basal laminae, and the endothelium, but there are areas in which the supporting cell is absent and the chief cells are in close relation to the capillary wall. These vascular relationships are of some significance, for it is not yet clear whether the paraganglion cells have an endocrine function, releasing catecholamine into the blood, or whether the chief cells are essentially interneurons synapsing on sympathetic neurons and exerting an inhibitory effect on transmission in sympathetic ganglia.

The parasympathetic paraganglia often do not give a conspicuous chromaffin reaction and they were formerly classified by light microscopists as "achromaffin paraganglia" to distinguish them from those associated with the sympathetic ganglia. It was even suggested by some that they probably elaborated acetylcholine. This distinction between chromaffin and achromaffin paraganglia receives no support from electron microscopic studies and should probably be abandoned. The chief cells of vagal paraganglia contain 50- to 200-nm electron-opaque granules that tend to be at the cell periphery or in its processes. The supporting cells are somewhat less numerous than in sympathetic paraganglia, and chief cells may adjoin one another and be attached by desmosomes. Nerve terminals apposed to the surface of the chief cells contain numerous clear synaptic vesicles.

REFERENCES

ADRENAL CORTEX

Baxter, J. D., and G. G. Rousseau: Glucocorticoid hormone action: an overview. *In* Baxter, J. D., and G. G. Rousseau, eds.: Glucocorticoid Hormone Action. Monogr. Endocrinol. *12*:1, 1979.

Black, V. H., E. Robbins, E. McNamara, and T. Huima: A correlated thin-section and freeze fracture analysis of guinea pig adrenocortical cells. Am. J. Anat. *156*:453, 1979.

Brown, M. S., P. T. Kovanen, and J. L. Goldstein: Receptor mediated uptake of lipoprotein-cholesterol and its utilization for steroid synthesis in the adrenal cortex. Recent Prog. Horm. Res. *35*:215, 1979.

Gill, G. N.: ACTH regulation of the adrenal cortex. Pharmacol. Ther. [B] *2*:313, 1976.

Griffiths, K., and E. H. D. Cameron: Steroid biosynthetic pathways in the human adrenal. Adv. Steroid Biochem. Pharmacol. *2*:223, 1970.

Lanman, J. T.: The fetal zone of the adrenal gland. Medicine *32*:389, 1953.

Long, J. A.: Zonation of the mammalian adrenal cortex. *In* Blaschko, H., G. Sayers, and A. D. Smith, eds.: Handbook of Physiology. Sect. 7, Endocrinology, Vol. 6. Washington, DC, American Physiological Society, 1975, p. 13.

Long, J. A., and A. L. Jones: Observations on the fine structure of the adrenal cortex of man. Lab. Invest. *17*:355, 1967.

Nussdorfer, G. G., G. Mazzocchi, and V. Meneghelli: Cytophysiology of the adrenal zone fasciculata. Int. Rev. Cytol. *55*:291, 1978.

Pohorecky, L. A., and R. J. Wurtman: Adrenocortical control of epinephrine synthesis. Pharmacol. Rev. *27*:1, 1971.

ADRENAL MEDULLA

Benedeczky, I., and A. D. Smith: Ultrastructural studies on the adrenal medulla of the hamster. Origin and fats of secretory granules. Zeitschr. Zellforsch. *124*:367, 1972.

Bennett, H. S.: Cytological manifestations of secretion in the adrenal medulla of the cat. Am. J. Anat. *69*:333, 1941.

Blaschko, H., G. Sayers, and A. D. Smith: Adrenal gland. *In* Handbook of Physiology. Sect. 7, Endocrinology, Vol. 6. Washington, DC, American Physiological Society, 1975.

Coupland, R. E.: Electron microscopic observations on the structure of the rat adrenal medulla. I. Ultrastructure and organization of chromaffin cells in the normal adrenal medulla. J. Anat. *99*:231, 1965.

Landsberg, L., and J. B. Young: Catecholamines and the adrenal medulla. *In* Bondy, P. K., and L. E. Rosenberg, eds.: Metabolic Control and Disease. 8th ed. Philadelphia, W. B. Saunders Co., 1980, p. 1621.

Smith, A. D., and H. Winkler: Catecholamines. *In* Blaschko, H., and E. Muschelli, eds.: Handbook of Experimental Pharmacology. Vol. 33. Berlin, Springer Verlag, 1972, p. 538.

Wurtman, R. J., and L. A. Pohorecky: Adrenal cortical control of epinephrine in health and disease. Adv. Metab. Disord. *5*:53, 1971.

Yates, R. D.: A light and electron microscopic study correlating the chromaffin reaction and granule ultrastructure in the adrenal medulla of the Syrian hamster. Anat. Rec. *149*:237, 1964.

PARAGANGLIA AND PARA-AORTIC BODIES

Brudin, T.: Catecholamines in the pre-aortic paraganglia of fetal rabbits. Acta Physiol. Scand. *64*:287, 1965.

Chen, I., and R. D. Yates: Ultrastructural studies of vagal paraganglia in Syrian hamsters. Zeitschr. Zellforsch. *108*:309, 1970.

Coupland, R. E., and B. S. Weakley: Electron microscopic observations on the adrenal medulla and extra-adrenal chromaffin tissue in the post-natal rabbit. J. Anat. *106*:213, 1970.

Mascorro, J. A., and R. D. Yates: Microscopic observations on abdominal sympathetic paraganglia. Tex. Rep. Biol. Med. *28*:59, 1970.

21

PINEAL GLAND

The *pineal gland (epiphysis cerebri)* is an endocrine gland that modulates the function of the reproductive system. In seasonal breeding species it responds to changes in day length and regulates gonadal activity. It is of less importance in species that breed continuously. In the human brain it is a conical gray body measuring 5 to 8 mm in length and 3 to 5 mm in its greatest width. It lies above the roof of the diencephalon at the posterior extremity of the third ventricle. A small ependyma-lined recess of the third ventricle extends into a short stalk, which joins the pineal body to the diencephalic roof (Fig. 21–1).

HISTOLOGICAL ORGANIZATION

The organ is invested by pia mater, from which connective tissue septa containing many blood vessels penetrate into the pineal tissue and surround its clusters of epithelioid cells. In sections stained with hematoxylin and eosin, the pineal body is seen to consist of cords of pale-staining epithelioid cells. Their large nuclei are often irregularly infolded or lobulated and have prominent nucleoli. These cells, making up the bulk of the organ, are called *pinealocytes*. When appropriately stained, the cytoplasm is moderately basophilic and often contains lipid droplets. As described by del Rio-Hortega, who used silver impregnation methods for their demonstration, human pinealocytes are cells with long tortuous processes, which radiate from the cords toward the connective tissue septa where they end in bulbous swellings on or near blood vessels (see Fig. 21–5). Such processes are visualized with some difficulty in routine preparations.

In electron micrographs the pinealocytes have nuclei of irregular outline with peripherally distributed heterochromatin. The cytoplasm contains occasional short profiles of rough endoplasmic reticulum and numerous free polyribosomes. More abundant than the granular endoplasmic reticulum are tubular and vesicular elements of an atypical smooth endoplasmic reticulum (Fig. 21–6). Mitochondria are numerous in the perikaryon and quite variable in form. The Golgi complex is moderately well developed and many coated and smooth vesicles are associated with it. Some of these contain dense cores.

In addition to the usual organelles, the pinealocytes contain peculiar *synaptic ribbons,* which consist of a dense rod or lamella surrounded by small vesicles that resemble the synaptic vesicles of nerve endings. Similar organelles are found in the photoreceptor cells of the retina; in the organ of Corti in the inner ear; and in certain other sensory organs where they are involved in synaptic transmission. It has been proposed that the pinealocytes of mammals originate from a sensory cell line that evolved from the pineal photoreceptors of lower vertebrates. This interpretation fostered the belief that the synaptic ribbons were phylogenetic relics with no functional significance. This view is no longer espoused for it has been shown that there is a good correlation between the number of synaptic ribbons and the state of physiological activity of the gland. Their function in the pineal is unknown. Where they occur in sensory organs, synaptic ribbons are part of the presynaptic complex and are thought to play a role in the transport of vesicles to the active sites of neurotransmitter release at the cell membrane. In the pinealocyte, they show no consistent relationship to other cellular elements and may be found adjacent to other pinealocytes or glial cells, or in areas of the cell surface exposed to extracellular spaces. They may be involved in transport and release of chemical mediators but they do not appear to have a synaptic relationship to other cells.

Where synaptic ribbons are found in sensory organs they occur singly or in pairs, but in pinealocytes they may be numerous. The

535

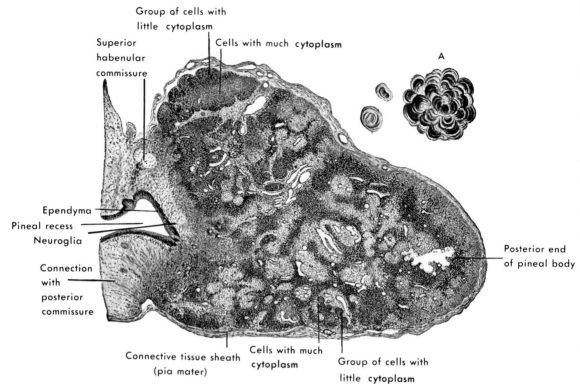

Group of cells with
little cytoplasm

Cells with much cytoplasm

Superior
habenular
commissure

A

Ependyma

Pineal recess

Neuroglia

Connection
with
posterior
commissure

Posterior end
of pineal body

Connective tissue sheath
(pia mater)

Cells with much
cytoplasm

Group of cells with
little cytoplasm

Figure 21–1. Median section through pineal body of a newborn child. Blood vessels empty. × 32. *A,* Corpora arenacea (sand granules) from the pineal body of a 69-year-old woman. × 160. (After Schaffer.)

pineal exhibits a circadian cycle of activity related to the periods of light and darkness. In the dark phase of the cycle, when it is most active, there may be a marked increase in the length of the synaptic rods or ribbons and a two- to threefold increase in their number. They may assemble in sizable aggregations, called *synaptic ribbon fields,* containing 20 or more of these organelles.

The pinealocytes arise from a neuroepithelium and have numerous gap junctions that provide for electrical and metabolic coupling of groups of cells. The cytoplasm often contains lipid droplets and deposits of lipochrome pigment, and is usually rich in microtubules and intermediate filaments. The microtubules are randomly oriented in the cell body but become associated in parallel arrays in the cell processes. The shorter processes end blindly among the surrounding cells, while the longer ones have bulbous terminal expansions in close proximity to fenestrated blood capillaries or near ependymal cells lining the pineal recess. The endings may contain small dense-cored vesicles that are believed to contain monoamines or peptide hormones conjugated to specific car-

rier proteins called *neuroepiphysins* to distinguish them from neurophysins, which are the carrier proteins of the neural lobe of the pituitary. When the vesicles are discharged by exocytosis, the hormones become dissociated from the carrier protein and diffuse into the capillaries or the cerebrospinal fluid.

The pineal body in humans and in cattle contains extracellular concretions called *corpora arenacea* or "brain sand" (Fig. 21–2). These are composed of calcium phosphates and carbonates in an organic matrix deposited in concentric layers. Their significance and mode of formation are poorly understood. They are not regarded as pathological but rather as biproducts of secretory activity. It is suggested that the carrier proteins released during exocytosis bind calcium and become deposited in concentric layers around portions of cellular debris that serve as nucleation sites. The calcified corpora arenacea increase with age and are visible in x-ray films or CAT scans of the head in 80 per cent of individuals over 30 years of age. They are useful to the roentgenologist in the diagnosis and localization of tumors or other expanding lesions in either hemisphere of the brain, which may displace the pineal from its normal midline position toward the opposite side.

The second cell type of the pineal is the *interstitial cell.* These cells occur in the perivascular areas and between the clusters of pinealocytes. Their nuclei are elongated and stain more deeply than those of the parenchymal cells. The cytoplasm is somewhat more basophilic and drawn out into long processes. In electron micrographs the granular endoplasmic reticulum is well represented, and free ribosomes are numerous. In addition, occasional deposits of glycogen are found. Rare microtubules are present, but these are overshadowed by a profusion of cytoplasmic filaments 5 to 6 nm in diameter and of indeterminate length. They may occur in large bundles or as single, randomly oriented filaments.

Some workers consider the interstitial cells, which represent about 5 per cent of the cells in the pineal, to be glial elements. The abundance of filaments in their cytoplasm is indeed reminiscent of the fine structure of astrocytes. The presence in rat pineal of stellate cells that stain strongly with the acid hematin method has been reported, but whether these represent a cell type distinct from interstitial cells is not yet clear.

Histogenesis

The pineal body first appears at about 36 days of gestation as a prominent thickening of the ependyma in the posterior part of the roof of the diencephalon. Cells migrate from this ependymal thickening to form a segregated mantle layer, whose cells tend to assume a follicular arrangement that is gradually transformed into the cordlike arrangement seen in later stages of development. By the end of the sixth month, interstitial and pineal parenchymal cells have differentiated.

It is generally believed that the pineal body increases in size until about 7 years of age.

Innervation

Nerves are found throughout the organ in silver-impregnated specimens. As the nerve fibers penetrate into the organ, their myelin sheaths terminate and the bare axons continue among the pinealocytes. Some of these contain many small vesicles in the size range

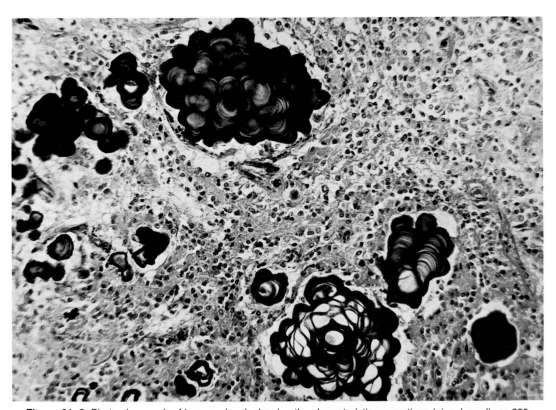

Figure 21–2. Photomicrograph of human pineal, showing the characteristic concretions (pineal sand). × 200.

of synaptic vesicles, suggesting that the nerves have functional endings in close relation to the parenchymal cells. The innervation appears to be exclusively via autonomic fibers originating in the superior cervical sympathetic ganglion.

Pineal System of Lower Vertebrates

In contrast to the single, relatively solid mass of tissue making up the pineal body in adult mammals, the organs in most lower vertebrates remain saccular throughout life and are somewhat more complex. The pineal system may consist of a single pineal sac (the intracranial epiphysis), as in most fishes and tailed amphibians, or it may be double. In the latter case (primitive fishes, tailless amphibians, and lizards) a second, *parapineal* organ results either from elaboration of an anterior end vesicle of the epiphysis, or from a separate evagination from the diencephalic roof situated more anteriorly. In frogs, the parapineal component (the frontal organ) comes to lie subepidermally and is discernible externally on the median dorsal aspect of the head. It is connected with the intracranial epiphysis by a long pineal nerve. While many nerve fibers and their endings are readily demonstrable in pineal systems of lower vertebrates, there is no evidence that any are sympathetic.

Electron microscopic examination of adult saccular pineal systems reveals that, in most lower vertebrates, the principal cell type is an apparent photoreceptor. This cell closely resembles a retinal rod or cone, both in the form of the membranous lamellated modified flagellum that protrudes from the cell apex into the pineal lumen and in the presence of characteristic receptor synapses at the cell base. Physiological data indicate that, in these species, impulses course along pineal tracts to surrounding brain regions in response to darkness or to light of various wavelengths. The most elaborate pineal photoreceptor systems are found in certain lizards, such as the Tuatara (*Sphenodon*), in which, in addition to a photoreceptor-type intracranial epiphysis, the parapineal component (or parietal "eye") is specialized to the extent of possessing a distinct lens and a retina composed of photoreceptor cells backed by supportive cells containing pigment. Photoreceptor cells have not been distinguished in mammalian pineal systems.

HISTOPHYSIOLOGY

The pineal in mammals was long considered to be a vestigial organ of little functional significance, but experimental investigations of the past 20 years have firmly established it as an endocrine gland whose primary function is the modulation of reproduction.

The pineal secretes an indolamine hormone, *melatonin*. The gland contains a higher concentration of serotonin than any other organ. Serotonin is converted by the enzyme serotonin N-acetyltransferase to N-acetylserotonin, which in turn is converted to melatonin by hydroxyindole-O-methyltransferase. A unique feature of the pineal is that its

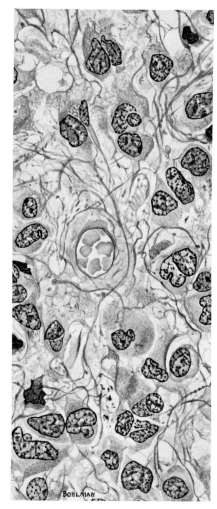

Figure 21–3. Section of pineal body of man stained with hematoxylin and eosin, showing irregularly shaped cells and their processes. Note the blood vessel in the center. Compare with Figure 21–5.

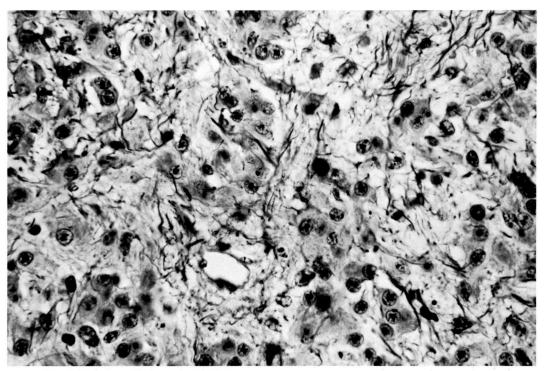

Figure 21–4. Photomicrograph of bovine pineal. The pinealocytes have large nuclei with prominent nucleoli. The outlines of the stellate cells are not easily distinguished. Many densely stained processes are visible in this preparation, but it is not possible to determine which belong to pinealocytes and which to interstitial cells. Iron hematoxylin stain. × 500. (Courtesy of E. Anderson.)

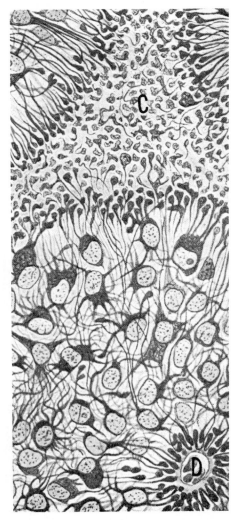

Figure 21–5. Specifically impregnated section of the pineal body of a young boy, showing interlobular tissue (C) and vessel (D) with club-shaped processes of specific cells in its adventitia. Note parenchymatous cells and their claviform processes bordering on C. (After del Rio-Hortega.)

the evidence is not compelling. Various peptides normally found in the hypothalamo-hypophyseal system have also been reported in the pineal, but their localization and pineal origin are disputed.

The pineal is involved in the reproductive process to varying degree in different mammalian species. The reproductive system of the laboratory rat responds little and inconsistently to experimental manipulation of the pineal. This may be a consequence of being inbred for many generations under unnatural conditions that may have led to loss of mechanisms essential for survival of a species in the wild. The scientific community's heavy reliance upon the laboratory rat no doubt contributed to slow progress in defining the role of the pineal in reproduction. Many species that inhabit temperate or arctic zones are seasonal breeders, and it is important for the young to be born in the spring to ensure an appropriate ambient temperature and the availability of food for their survival. At other seasons of the year the gonads may regress and only regain reproductive competence with the approach of spring. In such animals the critical environmental factor regulating their seasonal pattern of reproduction is day length (photoperiod). Information about the photoperiod is transmitted to the reproductive system via the pineal.

The photoreceptors for light detection are in the retina. Information is carried from the eyes over a neural pathway involving retinohypothalamic fibers, the suprachiasmatic nuclei, the hypothalamospinal fibers, and thence to the sympathetic nervous system and via the cervical sympathetic ganglion to the pineal. Interruption of this pathway severs the link between photoperiod and pineal function.

The influence of the pineal on reproduction has been most thoroughly studied in the Syrian hamster, a species adopted as a laboratory animal more recently than the rat. Either cutting the optic nerves or exposure of intact hamsters to a short photoperiod (less than 12.5 hours daily) for four weeks or longer enhances melatonin secretion by the pineal and results in atrophy of the testes. Either pinealectomy or superior cervical ganglionectomy prevents the gonadal atrophy normally induced by shortening the photoperiod.

In the annual cycle of seasonal breeders, the shortening of the day as autumn approaches leads to enhanced melatonin secretion by the pineal and atrophy of the gonads, which remain inactive through the winter

biosynthetic activity exhibits a diurnal rhythmicity correlated with the periods of daylight and darkness. Melatonin concentrations in the gland and in the blood increase during the dark phase of the diurnal cycle and there is evidence of seasonal variations. When applied to the skin of amphibians, the hormone causes aggregation of pigment granules in melanophores and results in blanching. Its effect is therefore opposite to that of melanocyte stimulating hormone of the pituitary. In mammals it has an antigonadotropic action.

The gland may also produce physiologically active peptides. The most studied of these is *arginine vasotocin*, which is reported to have anti-FSH and anti-LH activity, but

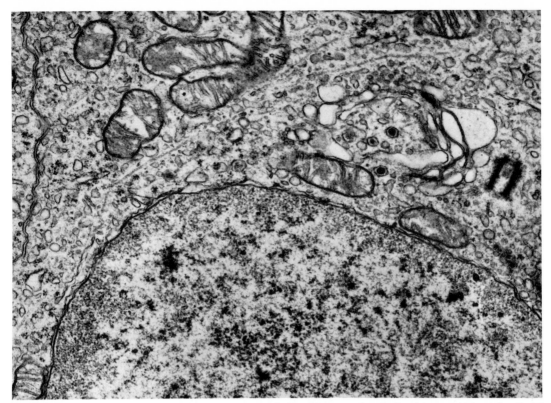

Figure 21–6. Electron micrograph of a juxtanuclear area of pinealocyte cytoplasm, showing a centriole and part of the Golgi complex, with associated vesicles with dense osmiophilic content. The cytoplasm generally contains abundant small vesicles and numerous microtubules. × 30,000. (Courtesy of E. Anderson.)

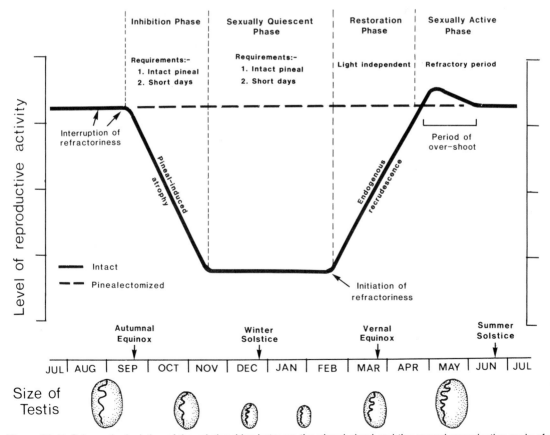

Figure 21–7. Schematic depiction of the relationships between the pineal gland and the annual reproductive cycle of a seasonal breeding species such as the hamster. (From Reiter, R. J. Endocr. Rev. *1*:109, 1980.)

(Fig. 21–7). Although the pineal continues to secrete melatonin in this period, the neuroendocrine reproductive complex appears to become refractory to its suppressive effect, and recrudescence of the reproductive organs begins in the latter part of winter. This ensures that the animals will be sexually competent when they emerge from hibernation in the spring. The refractory state subsides during the long days of the summer months and the system again becomes responsive to the antigonadotropic action of the pineal. All the effects of the naturally occurring changes in photoperiod can be duplicated in the laboratory by administration of melatonin at the appropriate time and dosage. It is not yet clear whether the pineal hormone brings about reproductive incompetence by acting upon the hypothalamus or directly upon the gonads, and the mechanisms for development of, and recovery from, the refractory state have yet to be elucidated. It is likely that, with minor variations, the relationship of the pineal to the control of the annual reproductive cycle in the hamster will be found to apply to other species living in climatic zones where survival of the young requires restriction of breeding to a favorable time of year.

The degree of pineal participation in the reproduction of humans and other continuous breeders is less clear. There is no doubt, however, that the pineal exerts some degree of antigonadotropic influence in these species also. Pinealectomy or superior cervical ganglionectomy in young rats leads to enlargement of the reproductive organs and precocious puberty. Conversely, sustained injection of melatonin delays puberty. Young boys with brain tumors that destroy the pineal also exhibit precocious puberty.

REFERENCES

Ariens-Kappers, J., and J. P. Schade, eds.: Structure and function of the epiphysis cerebri. *In* Progress in Brain Research. Vol. 10. Amsterdam, Elsevier Publishing Co., 1965.

Arstila, A. U.: Electron microscopic studies on the structure and histochemistry of the pineal gland of the rat. Neuroendocrinology (Suppl.) 2:1, 1967.

Axelrod, J., and H. Weissbach: Purification and properties of hydroxyindole-*O*-methyl transferase. J. Biol. Chem. 236:216, 1961.

Benson, B.: Current status of pineal peptides. Neuroendocrinology 24:241, 1977.

Fiske, V. M., J. Pound, and K. Putnam: Effect of light on the weight of the pineal organ in hypophysectomized, gonadectomized, adrenalectomized or thiouracil-fed rats. Endocrinology 71:130, 1962.

Kelly, D. E.: Pineal organs: photoreception, secretion and development. Am. Sci. 50:597, 1962.

Kitay, J. I., and M. D. Altschule: The Pineal Gland; A Review of the Physiologic Literature. Cambridge, Harvard University Press, 1954.

Knight, B. K., M. M. Hayes, and R. B. Symington: The pineal gland—a synopsis of present knowledge with particular emphasis on its possible role in control of gonadotrophin functions. S. Afr. J. Anim. Sci. 3:143, 1973.

Kumado, K., and W. Mori: A morphological study of the circadian cycle of the pineal gland of the rat. Cell Tissue Res. 182:565, 1977.

Lerner, A. B., and J. D. Case: Pigment cell regulatory factors. J. Invest. Dermatol. 32:221, 1959.

Lukaszyk, A., and R. J. Reiter: Histophysiologic evidence for the secretion of polypeptides by the pineal gland. Am. J. Anat. 143:451, 1975.

Matsushima, S., Y. Morisawa, I. Aida, and K. Abe: Circadian variations in pinealocytes of the Chinese hamster *Cricetus griseus*. Cell Tissue Res. 228:231, 1983.

Oksche, A.: Survey of the development and comparative morphology of the pineal organ. Prog. Brain Res. 10:3, 1965.

Quay, W. B.: Reduction of mammalian pineal weight and lipid during continuous light. Gen. Comp. Endocrinol. 1:211, 1961.

Quay, W. B.: Experimental and cytological studies of pineal cells staining with acid hematin in the rat. Acta Morphol. Neerl. Scand. 5:87, 1962.

Quay, W. B.: Circadian rhythm in rat serotonin and its modification by estrous cycles and photoperiod. Gen. Comp. Endocrinol. 3:473, 1963.

Quay, W. B.: Retinal and pineal hydroxyindole-*O*-methyl transferase activity in vertebrates. Life Sci. 4:983, 1965.

Reiter, R. J.: Comparative physiology: pineal gland. Annu. Rev. Physiol. 35:305, 1973.

Reiter, R. J.: Pineal control of seasonal reproductive rhythm in male golden hamsters exposed to natural daylight and temperature. Endocrinology 92:423, 1973.

Reiter, R. J.: The pineal and its hormones in the control of reproduction in mammals. Endocr. Rev. 1:109, 1980.

Roth, W. D., R. J. Wurtman, and M. D. Altschule: Morphologic changes in the pineal parenchymal cells of rats exposed to continuous light or darkness. Endocrinology 71:888, 1962.

Soriano, F. M., H. A. Wether, and L. Volbrath: Correlation of the number of pineal "synaptic" ribbons and spherules with the level of serum melatonin over a 24-hour period in male rabbits. Cell Tissue Res. 236:555, 1984.

Theron, J. J., R. Biagio, and A. C. Meyer: Circadian changes in microtubules, synaptic ribbons and synaptic ribbon fields in the pinealocytes of the baboon *Papio ursinus*. Cell Tissue Res. 217:405, 1981.

Wartenberg, H.: The mammalian pineal organ: electron microscopic studies on the fine structure of pinealocytes, glial cells, and on the perivascular component. Z. Zellforsch. 86:74, 1968.

Wetterberg, L.: Melatonin in humans. Physiological and clinical studies. J. Neural Transm. (Suppl.) 13:289, 1978.

Wolstenholme, G. E., and J. Knight, eds.: The Pineal Gland. Ciba Foundation Symposium. London, Churchill, 1971.

Wurtman, R. J.: Effects of light and visual stimuli on endocrine function. *In* Ganong, W. F., and L. Martini, eds.: Neuroendocrinology. New York, Academic Press, 1966.

22

SKIN

The skin covers the surface of the body and consists of two main layers, the surface epithelium, or *epidermis*, and the subjacent connective tissue layer, the *corium* or *dermis* (Figs. 22–1, 22–2). Beneath the dermis is a looser connective tissue layer, the superficial fascia, or *hypodermis*, which in many places is largely transformed into subcutaneous adipose tissue. The hypodermis is loosely connected to underlying deep fascia, aponeurosis, or periosteum. The skin is continuous with several mucous membranes at *mucocutaneous junctions*. Such junctions are found at the lips, nares, eyelids, vulva, prepuce, and anus.

The skin is one of the largest of the organs, making up some 16 per cent of the body weight. Its functions are several. It protects the organism from injury and desiccation; it receives stimuli from the environment; it excretes various substances; and, in warm-blooded animals, it takes part in thermoregulation and maintenance of water balance. The subcutaneous adipose tissue has an important role in fat metabolism.

The specific functions of the skin depend largely upon the properties of the epidermis. This epithelium forms an uninterrupted cellular investment covering the entire outer surface of the body, but it is also locally specialized to form the various skin appendages: *hair, nails,* and *glands.* Its cells produce the fibrous protein *keratin*, which is essential to the protective function of the skin, and *melanin*, the pigment that protects against ultraviolet irradiation. The epidermis gives rise to two main types of glands, one of which produces the watery secretion *sweat* and the other the oily secretion *sebum*.

The free surface of the skin is not smooth but is marked by delicate grooves or flexure lines, which create patterns that vary from region to region. They are deeper on non-hairy areas, such as knees and elbows, palms and soles. The most familiar of the surface patterns are those responsible for the finger-prints. It is well known that the complicated patterns of ridges found on the fingers are subject to such marked variations that their impressions are a dependable means for identification of individuals. The same degree of variation holds for skin patterns in other regions, but these are less commonly used.

The interface of the epidermis and the dermis is also uneven. A pattern of ridges and grooves on the deep surface of the epidermis fits a complementary pattern of corrugations on the underlying dermis. The projections of the dermis have traditionally been described as *dermal papillae* and those of the epidermis as *epidermal ridges*, owing to their respective appearances in vertical sections of skin. As will be seen later, these terms are not always accurately descriptive of their three-dimensional configuration as seen in whole mounts.

Although the boundary between the epithelial and the connective tissue portions of the skin is sharp, the fibrous elements of the dermis merge with those of the hypodermis, so that there is no clear-cut boundary between these layers.

THE EPIDERMIS

The epidermis is a stratified squamous epithelium composed of cells of two distinct lineages. Those comprising the bulk of the epithelium undergo keratinization and form the dead superficial layers of the skin. They are derivatives of the ectoderm covering the embryo, and they constitute the *keratinizing system*. There are also cells in the deeper layers of the epidermis that do not keratinize but are capable of producing the pigment melanin. These are the *melanocytes*, which arise from the embryonic neural crest and invade the skin in the third to sixth months of intrauterine life. Collectively these cells

543

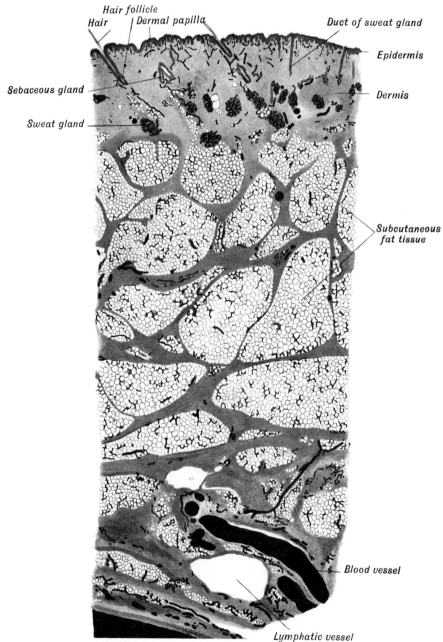

Figure 22–1. Section through human thigh perpendicular to the surface of the skin. Blood vessels are injected and appear black. Low magnification. (After A. A. Maximow.)

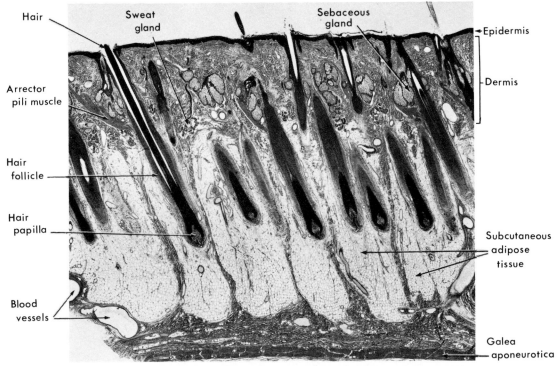

Hair

Sweat gland

Sebaceous gland

Epidermis

Arrector pili muscle

Dermis

Hair follicle

Hair papilla

Subcutaneous adipose tissue

Blood vessels

Galea aponeurotica

Figure 22–2. Section of the skin of the scalp. × 15. (Courtesy of H. Mizoguchi.)

comprise the *pigmentary system* of the skin. In addition, there are two other cell types, not part of the keratinizing system. These are the *Langerhans cells* and the *Merkel cells*.

The epidermis varies from 0.07 to 0.12 mm in thickness over most of the body, but it may reach a thickness of 0.8 mm on the palms and 1.4 mm on the soles. In the fetus, these sites are already appreciably thicker than other areas of skin, but continuous friction or pressure in postnatal life may cause considerable additional thickening of the outer layer of the epidermis on exposed areas of the body surface.

The superficial keratinized cells of the skin are continually exfoliated from the surface and are replaced by cells that arise from mitotic activity in the basal layer of the epidermis. The cells produced there are displaced to successively higher levels by the generation of new cells below them. As they move upward, they elaborate keratin, which accumulates in their interior until it largely replaces all metabolically active cytoplasm. The cell dies and its nucleus and other organelles disappear. It is finally shed as a flakelike, lifeless residue of a cell. This sequence of changes, referred to as the *cytomorphosis* of the keratinocyte, takes from 15 to 30 days, depending on the region of the body and a number of other factors.

Epidermis of the Palms and Soles

The structural organization of the epidermis can be studied to advantage in those areas of the skin where it attains its greatest thickness—namely, the palm of the hand and the sole of the foot. In sections perpendicular to the surface (Figs. 22–3, 22–4), four principal layers can be distinguished—*stratum basale, stratum spinosum, stratum granulosum,* and *stratum corneum.*

The *stratum basale* consists of a single layer of cells resting upon the basal lamina and underlying dermis. Its cells are cuboidal or low columnar. The nucleus is relatively large, the cytoplasm basophilic. In electron micrographs, there are a few profiles of rough endoplasmic reticulum, and a small Golgi complex. The cytoplasmic matrix is rich in ribosomes and contains abundant 10-nm filaments occurring singly or in conspicuous bundles. Desmosomes attach neighboring cells, and hemidesmosomes are found along the membrane adhering to the basal lamina.

Mitotic figures are common in this layer, formerly called the *stratum germinativum* be-

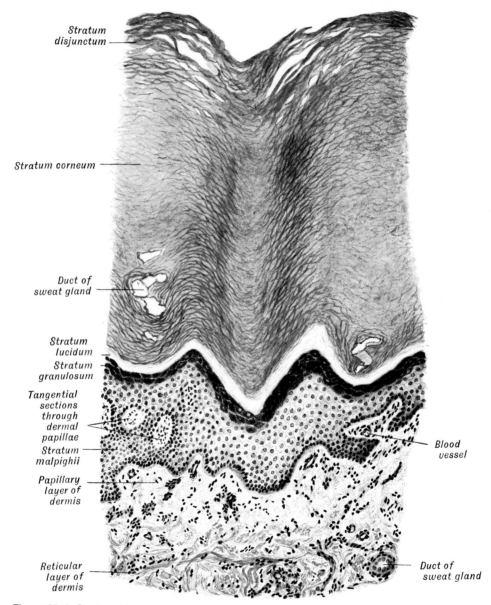

Stratum
disjunctum

Stratum corneum

Duct of
sweat gland

Stratum
lucidum
Stratum
granulosum

Tangential
sections
through
dermal
papillae
Stratum
malpighii

Papillary
layer of
dermis

Reticular
layer of
dermis

Blood
vessel

Duct of
sweat gland

Figure 22–3. Section of human sole perpendicular to the free surface. × 100. (After A. A. Maximow.)

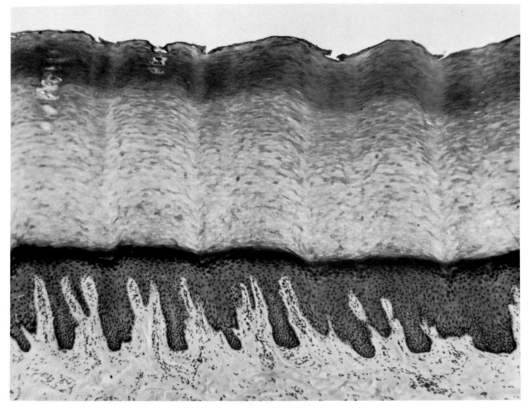

Figure 22–4. Skin of the human finger tip, illustrating a very thick stratum corneum. Hematoxylin and eosin. × 65.

cause the proliferation of its cells is mainly responsible for the continual renewal of the epidermis. As the cells generated here move up into the stratum spinosum, they assume a flattened, polyhedral form with their long axis parallel to the surface and their nucleus somewhat elongated in this direction.

The cells of the *stratum spinosum* are somewhat basophilic and have the same complement of organelles as their precursors. In addition, electron micrographs show numerous small granules with a distinctive substructure, called *lamellated granules* or *membrane-coating granules*. These ovoid, membrane-bounded granules are 0.1 to 0.5 μm in diameter, containing parallel lamellae about 2 nm thick, usually oriented transverse to the long axis. The lamellar structure consists of alternating electron-lucent and -dense layers. Bundles of 10-nm filaments, corresponding to the *tonofibrils* seen with the light microscope, are a prominent feature of these cells. They extend into the spinous processes and terminate in the dense plaques of the desmosomes (Fig. 22–6).

The *stratum granulosum* consists of three to five layers of flattened cells whose distinguishing feature is the presence of irregularly shaped coarse granules that stain intensely with basic dyes and·hematoxylin. These *keratohyalin granules* have no limiting membrane and consist of closely packed, dense, 2-nm subunits (Fig. 22–8). Tonofilaments may pass through them or be partially incorporated in their periphery. The origin and chemical nature of keratohyalin granules have not been clearly established. They were formerly believed to be associated with the process of keratinization, but this is questioned because they are not found in all keratinizing epithelia. They are absent in finger- and toenails, for example, but abundant in the epidermis forming the hooves of cattle.

The lamellar bodies that first appear in the stratum spinosum increase in number in the stratum granulosum, where they collect at the cell periphery, and their contents are secreted into the intercellular spaces. In the granular layer, they occupy as much as 15 per cent of the cytoplasmic volume. The lamellar bodies contain little phospholipid but appear to be rich in glycolipids and sterols. When released into the intercellular spaces, they form multiple membrane bilayers arranged in broad sheets between the cells. Correlated with release of the contents

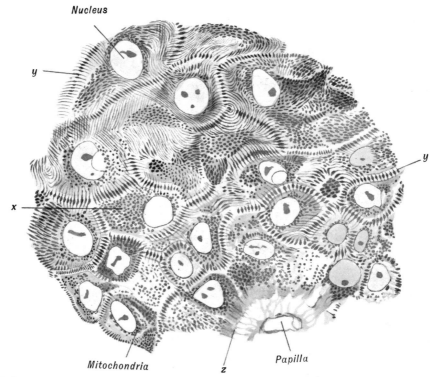

Nucleus

y

x

Mitochondria

z

Papilla

y

Figure 22–5. Section tangential to the surface, of the malpighian layer of epidermis of human palm, showing fibrils and so-called "intercellular bridges" in cross section at *x* and in longitudinal section at *y*. The junction of the scalloped lower surface of the epithelial cells with the dermis is at *z*.

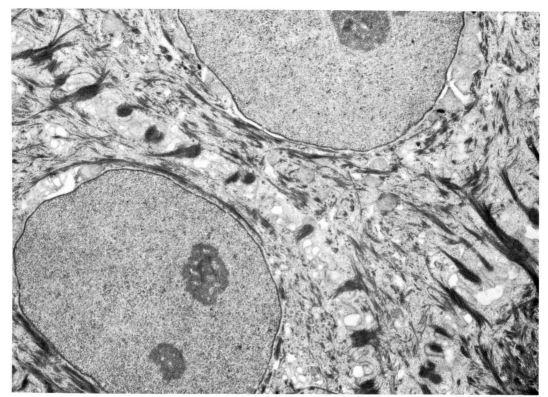

Figure 22–6. Electron micrograph of parts of three cells from the stratum germinativum of human epidermis. × 12,000. (Courtesy of G. Odland.)

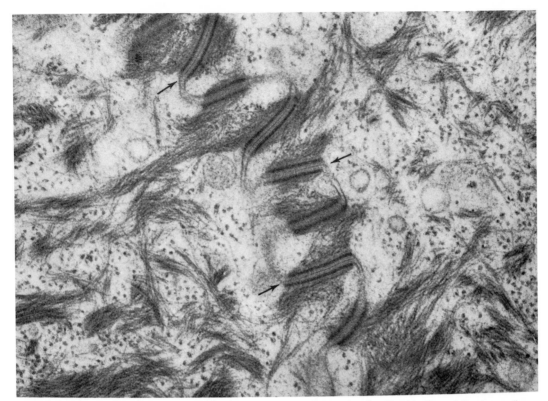

Figure 22–7. Electron micrograph of portions of two adjoining epidermal cells. The junction of the two cells runs diagonally across the figure. Desmosomes attaching the apposed cell surfaces are indicated by the arrows. Bundles of epidermal filaments run in various directions in the cytoplasm and terminate in desmosomes. × 50,000. (Courtesy of G. Odland.)

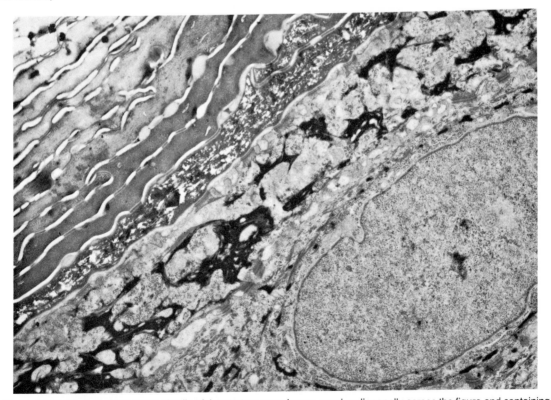

Figure 22–8. Electron micrograph of cells of the stratum granulosum, running diagonally across the figure and containing irregularly shaped keratohyalin granules. At upper left are several cell layers of the stratum corneum. × 12,000. (Courtesy of G. Odland.)

of the lamellar bodies is an increase in the volume of the intercellular space from less than 1 per cent to 5 to 30 per cent of the total tissue volume. The release of the content of the lamellar bodies appears to provide waterproofing intercellular lipids that are essential to the barrier function of the epidermis.

The *stratum corneum* consists of many layers of flat, cornified cells (Figs. 22–4, 22–10). The processes by which the cells were joined in the spiny layer are no longer present. The cells lack a nucleus, and few remnants of organelles remain, nearly all of the cytoplasm having been replaced by 8- to 10-nm filaments of keratin embedded in an amorphous matrix. The plasma membrane appears thickened because of deposition of a layer of dense nonkeratinous material on its inner aspect, and is highly corrugated, its ridges interdigitating with the grooves of adjacent cells. The abundant desmosomes present in the granular layer are still detectable but greatly modified, with their two halves often widely separated. The intercellular spaces are occupied by lipid-containing material derived from the lamellar granules of the strata spinosum and granulosum.

Two additional layers are recognized by some histologists in the stratum corneum. The *stratum lucidum* consists of a few layers of closely compacted, highly refractile eosinophilic cells on its deep surface. It appears in histological sections as a wavy clear stripe immediately above the stratum granulosum. The nucleus of the cells has already disappeared and keratinization of the cells is well advanced. The outermost layers of the stratum corneum, where the fully keratinized, lifeless cells are loosening and desquamating, is sometimes referred to as the *stratum disjunctum*. Electron micrographs reveal no distinctive cytological features of the cells in these regions, and their designation as separate layers of the stratum corneum probably serves no useful purpose.

Epidermis of the Body in General

On the rest of the body the epidermis is much thinner and simpler in its structure (Figs. 22–11, 22–12). The stratum spinosum

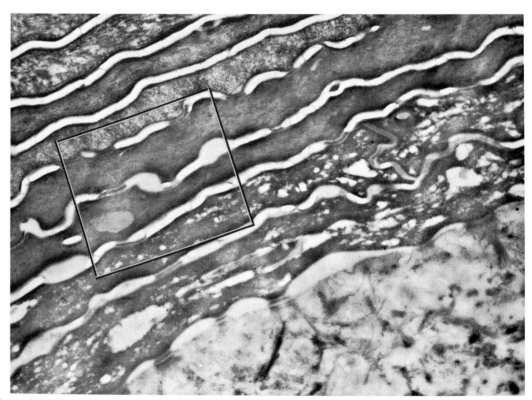

Figure 22–9. Electron micrograph showing a portion of a cell of the granular layer *(lower right)* and several layers of flattened cells of the stratum corneum *(upper left)*. Area enclosed in rectangle is shown at higher magnification in Figure 22–10. Osmium fixation. × 22,500. (Courtesy of G. Odland.)

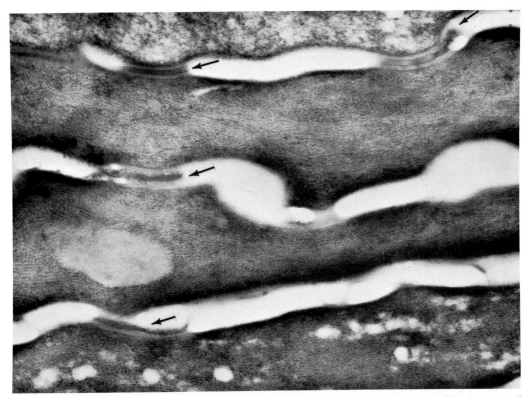

Figure 22–10. Electron micrograph of the area of stratum corneum of human epidermis enclosed in the rectangle in Figure 22–9. The cytoplasm of the flat keratinized cells appears devoid of organelles and seems to consist mainly of closely packed, fine filaments embedded in a rather dense matrix. The desmosomes, indicated by arrows, have an unusually thick, dense intermediate layer. The clear spaces between the cells are, in part, artifacts of specimen preparation. Osmium fixation. × 62,000. (Courtesy of G. Odland.)

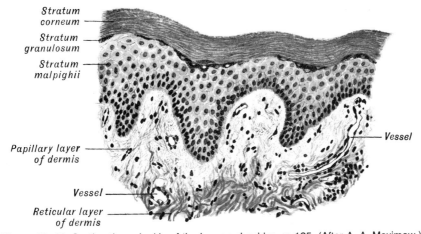

Figure 22–11. Section through skin of the human shoulder. × 125. (After A. A. Maximow.)

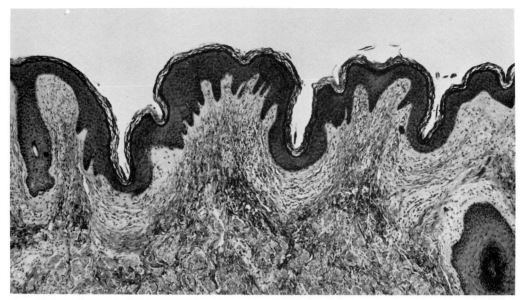

Figure 22–12. Photomicrograph of skin of the abdomen. Compare the thickness of the stratum corneum with that of the finger tip in Figure 22–4. × 60.

and stratum corneum are always present, although the latter may be relatively thin. A granular layer consisting of two or three layers of cells is usually identifiable, but a definite stratum lucidum is seldom seen in the thinner epidermis of the general body surface.

The epidermis is entirely devoid of blood vessels; it is nourished from capillaries in the underlying connective tissue by diffusion through tissue fluid, which occupies an extensive system of intercellular spaces. Human skin, unlike that of practically all other vertebrates, blisters after exposure to thermal and certain chemical stimuli.

CELL TYPES OF THE EPIDERMIS

Keratinocytes

The principal cell type of the epidermis and of other stratified squamous epithelia is now called the *keratinocyte*, because of its capacity to synthesize keratin. While keratin filaments are a component of the cytoskeleton of most epithelia, it is most abundant in the keratinocytes of the epidermis. As these cells differentiate and move upward in the epithelium, their content of keratins steadily increases, ultimately constituting 85 per cent of the total protein of the stratum corneum. Keratin is not a single protein but a family of polypeptides ranging from 40,000 to 70,000 M.W., which are products of different

genes and mRNAs. At different stages of their cytomorphosis, the keratinocytes produce different keratins. The cells in the basal layer contain only keratins of low molecular weight, but as they move upward they produce increasing amounts of the larger keratins that make up the bulk of the cornified layer. In this layer, the keratins are also extensively cross-linked by disulfide bonds.

Another characteristic feature of keratinocytes late in their differentiation is the pres-

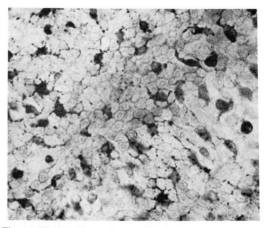

Figure 22–13. Photomicrograph of a whole mount of a sheet of epidermis from the thigh spread upon a slide and viewed from the underside to illustrate the melanocytes. The epidermis was separated from the dermis by treatment of the excised skin with trypsin. The epidermal sheet was then incubated in 1,3,4-dihydroxyphenylalanine (DOPA), which selectively stains the melanocytes. Notice their branching process. × 300. (Courtesy of G. Szabo.)

SPECIES	AREA AND NUMBER OF INDIVIDUALS	NUMBER OF MELANOCYTES (PER mm.^{2} ± s.e.)
Man[1]		
Caucasoid	Thigh (35)	1000 ± 70
Mongoloid	Thigh (3)	1290 ± 45
Negroid	Thigh (7)	1415 ± 255
Guinea Pig[2]		
Black	Ear (8)	920 ± 145
Red	Ear (8)	865 ± 100
Mouse[3]		
C57 Black	Tail (4)	590 ± 65
DBL Dilute	Tail (4)	590 ± 165

Figure 22–14. Comparison of melanocyte numbers among color variants of mammals.

[1] Szabo (1969) and Szabo; Gerald et al. (1971).
[2] Billingham and Medawar (1953).
[3] Gerson and Szabo (1969).

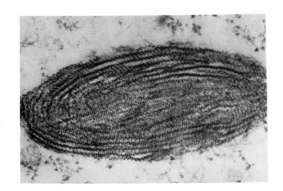

Figure 22–15. Electron micrograph of a developing human melanosome from the retina, showing the periodicity in its structural framework. When the melanosome is fully developed, its interior structure is obscured by the accumulated melanin. (Courtesy of A. Breathnach.)

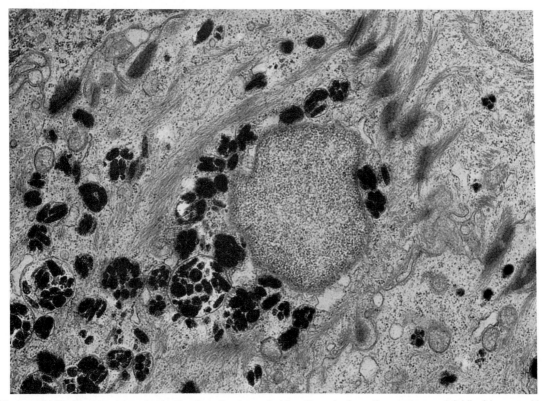

Figure 22–16. Electron micrograph of a heavily pigmented keratinocyte from the stratum malpighii of human skin. Whereas the melanosomes of melanocytes occur singly, those of keratinocytes are found in clusters of varying size enclosed by a membrane. (Courtesy of G. Szabo.)

553

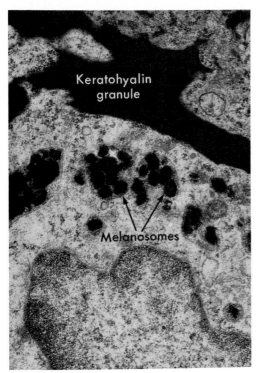

Figure 22–17. Micrograph of a portion of a cell from the stratum granulosum, showing dense keratohyalin granules and several clusters of melanosomes. (Courtesy of G. Szabo.)

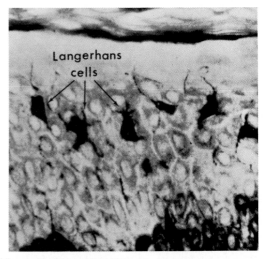

Figure 22–18. Section of human epidermis, showing gold impregnated Langerhans cells at a high level in the stratum malpighii. Gairn's gold chloride technique. (After Breathnach, A. S. Int. Rev. Cytol. *18*:1, 1965.)

ence of a dense layer (12 nm) of an insoluble protein deposited on the inner aspect of the plasma membrane. In the deposition of this layer, a soluble protein precursor called *involucrin* is cross-linked by isopeptide bonds to form an insoluble envelope. As in the case of the large keratins, involucrin is absent in the basal layers but appears as the cells move toward the free surface of the epithelium.

Langerhans Cells

Throughout the epidermis, but particularly in the upper layers of the stratum spinosum, there are peculiar dendritic cells first described by Langerhans in 1868 (Fig. 22–18). In routine hematoxylin and eosin preparations, they have a dark-staining nucleus surrounded by a pale clear cytoplasm. When stained by the gold chloride method, they are blackened and their stellate or dendritic form is revealed. Their slender processes extend into the intercellular spaces among the cells of the stratum spinosum and appear to form an almost continuous network in the epidermis. In electron micrographs, the nucleus is highly irregular in outline, and the cytoplasm is of low density and contains rel-

atively few organelles (Fig. 22–19). The absence of desmosomes, melanosomes, and bundles of tonofilaments serves to distinguish them from the other cells of the epidermis. They contain numerous small vesicles, multivesicular bodies, and a few dense granules, possibly lysosomes. Their most distinguishing characteristic is the presence of peculiar, membrane-bounded, rod-shaped granules variously called *Birbeck granules, Langerhans cell granules,* or *vermiform granules.* These are 15 to 50 nm long, 4 nm wide, with a centrally placed linear density and faint striations radiating from it to the enclosing membrane (Fig. 22–20).

Dendritic cells containing similar granules have been identified in lymph nodes, spleen, and thymus. The Langerhans cells of the skin have been shown to migrate from the skin to regional lymph nodes. The origin and function of these cells has long been controversial. Evidence has recently accumulated indicating that they may participate in the body's immune responses. They have been shown to possess surface Ia, Fc, and C_3 receptors in common with macrophages. At sites of allergic contact, cutaneous hypersensitivity lymphocytes are observed to gather around Langerhans cells in close apposition to their surface soon after antigenic challenge. It is believed that Langerhans cells may be involved in presentation of antigen to lymphocytes and may participate in immunoproliferative processes in the regional lymph nodes. The Langerhans cells are now believed to be important agents in contact

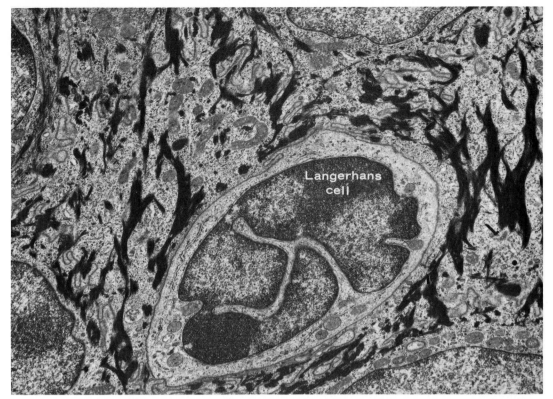

Figure 22–19. Electron micrograph of a Langerhans cell surrounded by keratinocytes containing dense bundles of filaments. The polymorphous appearance of the nucleus is typical. The stellate form of the cell is not evident here because none of the processes is included in the plane of section. (Courtesy of G. Szabo.)

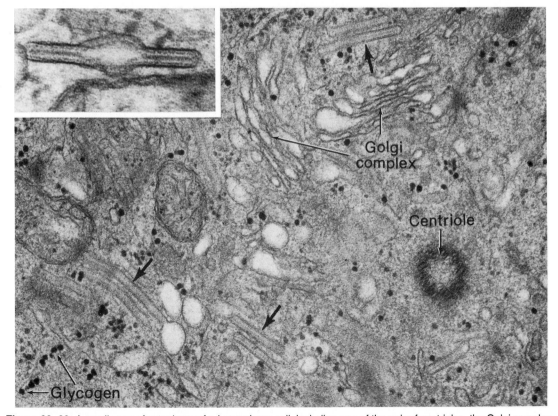

Figure 22–20. A small area of cytoplasm of a Langerhans cell, including one of the pair of centrioles, the Golgi complex, and several vermiform granules *(at heavy arrows)*. One of these is shown at higher magnification in the inset. The dense granules in the cytoplasmic matrix are glycogen. (Courtesy of G. Szabo.)

allergic responses and other cell-mediated reactions of the skin.

Merkel Cell

The Merkel cell occurs in small numbers in the basal portion of the epidermis. It bears a superficial resemblance to the keratinocytes to which it may be attached by desmosomes. The nucleus is deeply invaginated (Figs. 22–21, 22–22) and occasionally contains a peculiar inclusion consisting of a fascicle of straight parallel filaments. The cytoplasm contains bundles of filaments in the perinuclear zone and at the periphery but these are less abundant than in the keratinocytes. A few transferred melanosomes may be present. The most distinctive feature of the Merkel cell is the presence in the cytoplasm of 80-nm dense-cored vesicles resembling those found in cells of the adrenal medulla or carotid body. However, it has not been established that these contain catecholamines.

The Merkel cells tend to be associated with areas where the dermis is especially well vascularized and richly innervated. Unmyelinated axons are found in close relationship to these cells and appear to form expanded endings applied to their surface. The nerve endings contain no synaptic vesicles and are presumed to be sensory. Because of their content of dense-cored vesicles and their intimate relationship to nerve terminals, the Merkel cells are now considered to be paraneurones involved in sensory reception.

Melanocyte

The color of the skin is the resultant of three components. The tissue has an inherent yellowish color, attributable in part to *carotene*. The *oxyhemoglobin* in the underlying vascular bed imparts a reddish hue, and shades of brown to black are contributed by varying amounts of *melanin*. Of these three colored substances, only the melanin is produced in the skin. It is the product of specialized cells with elaborately branching processes called *melanocytes*, which are located in the basal layer of the epidermis or in the underlying connective tissue of the dermis. Although melanin granules are also found in the keratinocytes, they are formed only by the epidermal melanocytes, for these cells alone pos-

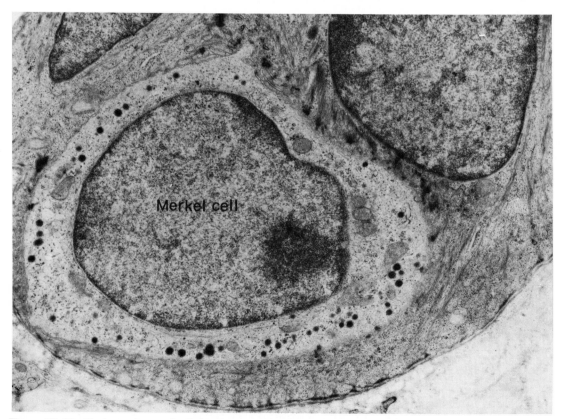

Figure 22–21. Electron micrograph of the base of the human epidermis, showing a Merkel cell surrounded by keratinocytes. Notice its pale cytoplasm and characteristic dense granules. (Courtesy of G. Szabo.)

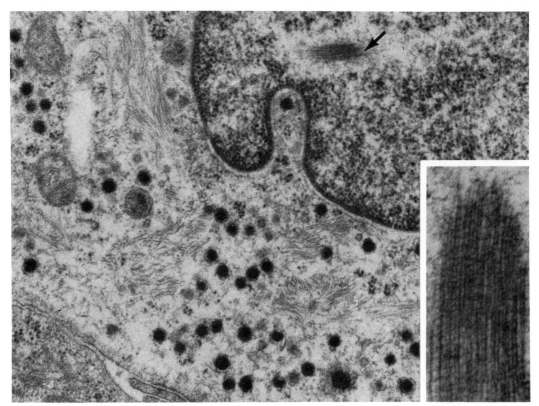

Figure 22–22. Portion of a Merkel cell from human gingival epithelium. The cytoplasm contains numerous dense granules and filaments. The nucleoplasm may contain an unusual inclusion consisting of paracrystalline aggregations of slender filamentous subunits *(inset)*. (Micrograph courtesy of R. Winkelmann.)

sess the enzyme tyrosinase that is necessary for synthesis of the pigment. The fully formed melanin granules are transferred from the melanocytes to the keratinocytes by an unusual form of activity sometimes referred to as *cytocrine* secretion. The melanocytes are commonly located at the dermo-epidermal junction with their pigment-containing processes extending for long distances upward into the interstices among the keratinocytes. They are not attached to the other cells by desmosomes, and in specimen preparation they may shrink away so that they are surrounded by a clear space. Because of their tendency to pass pigment to the keratinocytes, the melanocytes may actually contain less melanin than the neighboring epidermal cells, and their processes (or dendrites) are very difficult to identify in sections stained with hematoxylin and eosin. They are best studied in whole mounts of separated epidermis that have been treated with 1,3,4-dihydroxyphenylalanine (DOPA) (Fig. 22–13). In such preparations, the melanocytes are blackened and appear as highly branched cells. The ratio of melanocytes to

basal epidermal cells varies between 1 to 4 and 1 to 10, depending on the region of the body. The melanocytes in the cheek and forehead and in the genital, nasal, and oral epithelium are about twice as numerous as in other parts of the body surface. It is also of interest that the number of melanocytes is approximately the same in all human races. Racial differences in color are attributable to differences in the amount of pigment that these cells produce and transfer to the keratinocytes (Fig. 22–14).

Melanin is formed in a specific cell particle, the *melanosome*. In the human it is an elongated body with rounded ends, measuring about 0.2 by 0.6 μm, with a fibrillar or lamellar internal structure exhibiting characteristic periodic density variations along its length in early stages of development. This internal structure tends to be obscured by accumulation of dense melanin in the mature melanosome. The size, shape, and internal structure of the melanosomes vary with the animal species and are characteristic of particular genotypes within the same species. In the human, however, melanosomes are uniformly elongated (Figs. 22–16, 22–17) except in red-haired individuals, in whom they tend to be spherical. Melanosomes are somewhat larger in the skin of Australoids, Negroids, and Mongoloids than they are in Caucasoids. Within the same individual they tend to be larger in the hair follicles than in the skin.

Lack of melanin in the epidermis of some areas of the skin of animals may be due either to absence of melanocytes or, as in *albinism*, to the inability of the melanocytes to form pigmented melanosomes. In humans the entire integument normally possesses functioning melanocytes. Their activity is influenced by hormones and by factors in the physical environment. During pregnancy, the pigmentation of the areola of the nipples increases. Freckles are intensified and some individuals develop *cloasma*, the so-called "mask of pregnancy," consisting of a pigmented area over the malar eminences and a brownish discoloration of the forehead. This gradually disappears after delivery. The phenomenon of *tanning* on exposure to sunlight results from an immediate darkening of the existing melanin and, after a few days, an enhanced tyrosinase activity in the melanocytes that leads to the formation of new melanin. The pigmentation of the skin is believed to protect the underlying tissues against the potentially harmful effects of solar radiation. In the human, small melanosomes often aggregate to form melanosome complexes within the keratinocytes (Fig. 22–16), whereas large melanosomes usually are individually distributed. A more effective protective layer against ultraviolet radiation results.

Melanin is also found in the retinal pigment epithelium of the eye (Fig. 22–15) and in dermal melanocytes and melanophores of cold-blooded vertebrates. In the latter they constitute the pigmentary effector system responsible for rapid changes of color for purposes of camouflage and concealment. The "ink" of squid and other cephalopods consists of small spherical melanosomes that are produced in a special ink gland, stored in the ink sac, and squirted out to blacken the water and conceal the animal threatened by a predator.

MUCOCUTANEOUS JUNCTIONS

These are transitions between the mucous membranes and skin. Their epithelium is thicker than that of the adjacent skin and is more like that of a mucosa. They may have a thin, rudimentary, cornified layer. Normally they do not contain sweat glands, hair follicles, hairs, or sebaceous glands, but are moistened by mucous glands situated within the body orifices. Since the keratinized layer is thin or may even be absent, the redness of the blood in the underlying capillaries shows through and gives the junction region a red color as exemplified in the lips.

THE DERMIS

The thickness of the dermis cannot be measured exactly, because it passes over into the subcutaneous layer without a sharp boundary. The average thickness is approximately 1 to 2 mm; it is less on the eyelids and the prepuce (0.6 mm or less) but reaches a thickness of 3 mm or more on the soles and palms. On the ventral surface of the body and the appendages it is generally thinner than on the dorsal surface. It is thinner in women than in men.

The outer surface of the dermis in contact with the epidermis is usually uneven and is elevated into papillae that project into concavities between the ridges on the deep surface of the epidermis. This sculptured surface of the dermis is called the *papillary layer*, and the deeper main portion of the dermis is called the *reticular layer*. There is no distinct boundary between them.

The reticular layer consists of rather dense connective tissue. Its collagenous fibers form a feltwork with bundles running in various directions but, for the most part, more or less parallel to the surface. Occasional bundles are oriented almost perpendicular to the majority. The papillary layer and its papillae consist of looser connective tissue with much thinner collagenous bundles.

The elastic fibers of the dermis form abundant, thick networks between the collagenous bundles and are condensed about the hair follicles and the sebaceous and sweat glands. In the papillary layer they are much thinner and form a continuous fine network in the papillae beneath the epithelium. The cells of the dermis are more abundant in the papillary than in the reticular layer and are similar to those of the subcutaneous layer except for the relative paucity of fat cells.

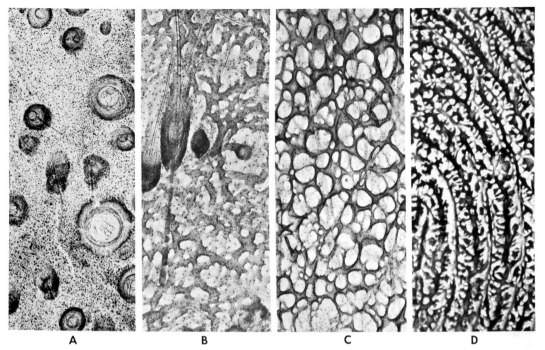

Figure 22–23. The pattern formed at a dermoepidermal junction shows marked regional variations. The figures shown here are views of the undersurface of separated sheets of epidermis stained with carmine. The light areas are the depressions occupied in life by the dermal papillae. *A,* From the cheek; the undersurface of the epidermis is smooth, except for the hair follicles. *B,* From the back. *C,* The breast. *D,* The elaborate pattern of concavities occupied by the dermal papillae of a finger pad. (Courtesy of G. Szabo.)

Within the deep parts of the reticular layer in the areolae, penis, perineum, and scrotum, numerous smooth muscle cells form a loose plexus. Such portions of the skin become wrinkled during contraction of these muscles. Smooth muscle cells forming the so-called *arrector pili* muscles are also connected with the hairs (Figs. 22–24, 22–25). In many places in the skin of the face, cross-striated muscle fibers terminate in the dermis. These are the *muscles of facial expression.* They are responsible for smiling, frowning, and the voluntary movement of the ears and scalp. These represent vestiges of a more extensive subcutaneous layer of muscle that is present in many mammals, called the *panniculus carnosus.* This layer is responsible for the voluntary movement of large segments of the integument, which can be observed when animals attempt to dislodge insects from their skin or to shake dry when they emerge from the water. The absence of this layer over most of the body in the human is disadvantageous in that, after wounds, the skin is likely to become immobile and bound down to the underlying structures because of shrinkage of scar tissue. Greater disfigurement results than in other mammals with more mobile skin.

At various levels of the dermis are the hair follicles and the sweat and sebaceous glands, which are epidermal derivatives extending down into the dermis. Blood vessels, nerves, and nerve endings are also abundant in this layer of the skin.

Hypodermis

The subcutaneous layer consists of loose connective tissue and is a deeper continuation of the dermis. Its collagenous and elastic fibers are directly continuous with those of the dermis and run in all directions but mainly parallel to the surface of the skin. Where the skin is flexible or freely movable, these fibers are few, but where it is closely attached to the underlying parts, as on the soles and palms, they are thick and numerous.

Depending on the portion of the body and the nutrition of the organism, varying numbers of fat cells develop in the subcutaneous layer. These are also found in clusters in the deep layers of the dermis. The fatty tissue of the subcutaneous layer on the abdomen may reach a thickness of 3 cm or more, but in the

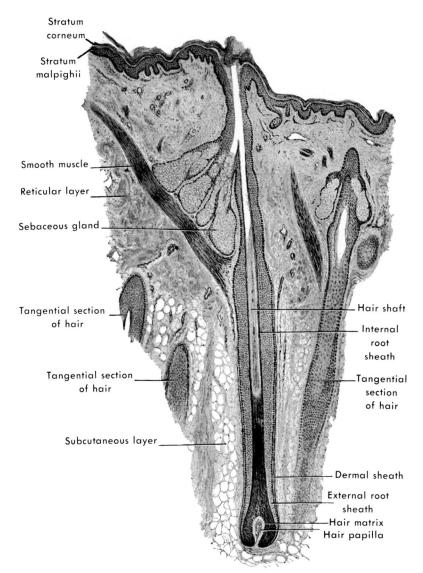

Figure 22–24. Section of the scalp of a man, showing the root of a hair in longitudinal section. × 32. (After Schaffer.)

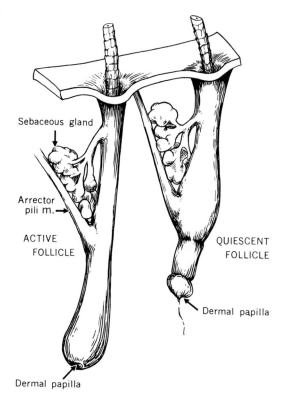

Sebaceous gland

Arrector
pili m.

ACTIVE
FOLLICLE

QUIESCENT
FOLLICLE

Dermal papilla

Dermal papilla

Figure 22–25. Diagrammatic representation of an actively growing and a quiescent hair follicle and the accessory structures. (Redrawn after Montagna, W. *In* Structure and Function of Skin. New York, Academic Press, 1956.)

eyelids and on the penis the subcutaneous layer does not contain fat cells.

The subcutaneous layer is penetrated everywhere by large blood vessels and nerve trunks and contains many nerve endings.

HAIRS

The hairs are slender keratinous filaments that develop from the matrix cells of follicular invaginations of the epidermal epithelium. They vary from several millimeters to over a meter in length and from 0.005 to 0.6 mm in thickness. They are distributed in varying numbers (Fig. 22–40) and in variable thickness and length on the whole surface of the skin, except on the palms, the soles, the sides of fingers and toes, the lateral surface of the feet below the ankles, the lip, the glans penis, the prepuce, the clitoris, the labia minora, and the internal surface of the labia majora.

Each hair arises in a tubular invagination of the epidermis, the *hair follicle*, which ex-

tends down into the dermis, where it is surrounded by connective tissue (Figs. 22–2, 22–24, 22–25). The active follicle has a bulbous terminal expansion with a concavity in its underside occupied by a connective tissue *papilla* (Figs. 22–24, 22–29). The papilla is covered by epithelial *matrix cells* of hair and root sheath. The cells on the dome of the convexity form the hair *root*, which develops into the hair *shaft*. The free end of the shaft protrudes beyond the surface of the skin.

The hair is not a continuously growing organ but has phases of growth that alternate with periods of rest. The structure of the hair follicle varies markedly according to the stage of hair growth (Fig. 22–25). In the resting hair (club hair), the follicle is relatively short, its epithelium is more or less similar to the surface epidermis, and the hair shaft is firmly anchored into the follicle by fine filaments of keratin that penetrate between the follicular cells. A cluster of dermal cells attached to the end of the follicular epithelium is the remnant of the dermal papilla of the growing hair and will again develop into a typical dermal papilla at the next period of hair generation (Figs. 22–25, 22–30).

In a phase of growth the follicle elongates and the epithelium again surrounds the dermal papilla. The epithelial cells around the papilla (the matrix) differentiate into several types. (1) In certain types of coarse hairs, the central matrix cells on top of the convexity of the papilla develop into the *medulla* of the hair shaft. The cells are large and vacuolated and eventually keratinize. This central part of the hair shaft is not demonstrable in thinner hairs. (2) The next concentric layer of matrix cells keratinize and develop into the *cortex* of the hair, the main constituent of the shaft. Its cells are heavily keratinized and tightly compacted, and they carry most of the pigment of the hair (Fig. 22–27). (3) Peripheral to the matrix cells of the cortex lie those of the *cuticle* of the hair (Figs. 22–27, 22–28). These cells of the outermost layer are the most heavily keratinized and their imbrication (Fig. 22–26) prevents matting of the erupted hairs. These three layers of cellular components all undergo keratinization in the so-called *keratogenous zone* of the follicle, immediately above the dome of the dermal papilla, and form the solid hair shaft (Figs. 22–29, 22–31).

The more peripheral concentric rows of matrix cells produce the *internal root sheath*, a transient structure surrounding the hair

Text continued on page 566

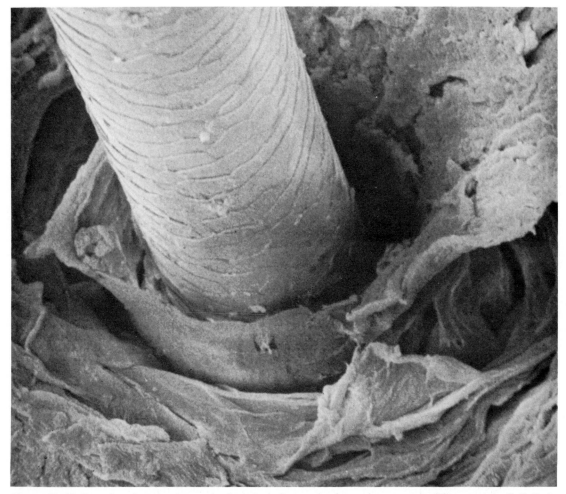

Figure 22–26. Scanning electron micrograph of a hair shaft emerging from a human scalp. (Micrograph by T. Fujita.)

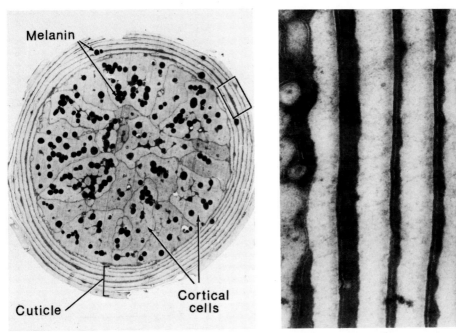

Figure 22–27   **Figure 22–28**

Figure 22–27. Electron micrograph of a mature black hair of a guinea pig in transverse section, showing a few melanin granules in the concentrically arranged flattened cuticle cells, and a large number in the cortical cells in the interior of the hair. No medullary cells are present at this level in the hair. For higher magnification of the area in the rectangle, see Figure 22–28. (From Snell, R. J. Invest. Dermatol. *58*:47, 1972.)

Figure 22–28. Higher magnification of the cuticle of a hair in an area similar to that in the rectangle in Figure 22–27. The markedly flattened cuticle cells are separated with intercellular spaces filled with electron-dense amorphous material. (From Snell, R. J. Invest. Dermatol. *58*:47, 1972.)

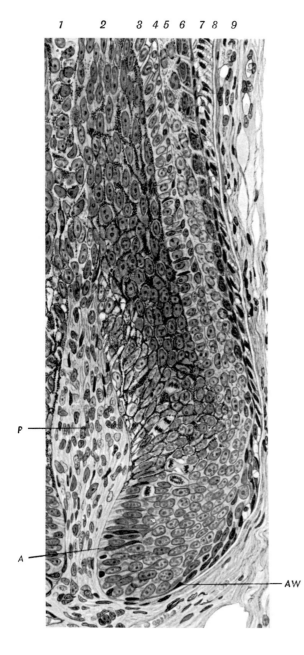

Figure 22–29. Longitudinal section through a hair from the head of a 22-year-old man. *1,* Medulla; *2,* cortex; *3,* hair cuticle; *4,* inner sheath cuticle; *5,* Huxley's layer; *6,* Henle's layer; *7,* external root sheath; *8,* glassy membrane; *9,* connective tissue of the hair follicle; *A,* matrix; *AW,* external root sheath at the bulb; *P,* papilla. × 350. (After Hoepke.)

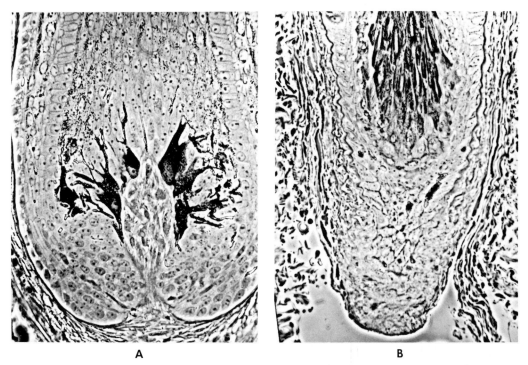

Figure 22–30. Unstained plastic sections of hair follicles. *A,* Active hair, showing large melanocytes and their processes contributing pigment to the hair. *B,* Inactive or club hair. × 200. (Courtesy of R. Mitchell and G. Szabo.)

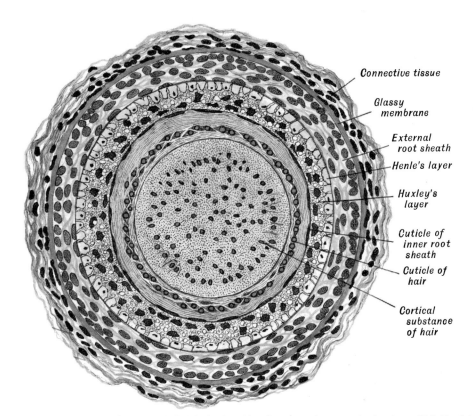

Figure 22–31. Cross section through a hair follicle in the skin of a pig embryo, at the level at which Henle's layer is completely cornified. × 375.

shaft below the level of the sebaceous glands, which is presumed to facilitate the movement of the growing hair shaft. It consists of three layers. The *cuticle of the internal root sheath*, like the cuticle of the hair, consists of overlapping thin scales with their free margins directed toward the bottom of the follicle. *Huxley's layer* consists of one to three layers of cornified cells, and *Henle's layer* is a single layer of elongated cells closely adherent to the external sheath (Fig. 22–31). These three layers form "trichohyalin" granules and keratinize, but they do not form a compact enduring structure, and they finally desquamate at the level of the opening of the sebaceous glands.

The outermost layer of the follicle, the *outer root sheath*, is basically similar to the unspecialized epidermal epithelium and is continuous with it above. At the neck of the papilla it is one layer of flat cells. It becomes two-layered at the level of the middle third of the papilla, and higher up it becomes stratified.

The *glassy membrane*, which is a part of the dermis, separates the epithelial from the connective tissue portion of the follicle. The latter portion is made up of two layers, a thin internal layer formed by circular fibers and an external, poorly outlined layer consisting of longitudinal collagenous and elastic fibers.

The hair matrix cells are analogous to the germinal cells of the epidermis insofar as the life cycle of each ends with formation of cornified cells. However, the epidermis produces a relatively soft keratinous material that is steadily shed, whereas in the hair, the product of the matrix cells, is a hard, cohesive, nonshedding, keratinous structure consisting of cells that accumulate in numerous concentric layers.

Since the hair is not perpendicular to the skin surface but inclined, it is very difficult to find a perfect longitudinal section of a follicle that displays these concentric layers well. The student will therefore have difficulty in identifying all of the structures described here. For this purpose the follicle needs to be reconstructed from serial sections.

It is well to bear in mind certain differences between the keratinizing epidermis and the keratinizing hair follicle. In the epidermis this process is general and continuous. In the case of the hair follicle it is intermittent and localized to a particular portion of the dermis—the dermal papilla, which has an inductive influence on the formation of the hair. If for any reason the dermal papilla is destroyed in postnatal life, no hair is formed. It is noteworthy, too, that there is a greater diversity of specialization and division of labor among the epidermal cells of the hair matrix with respect to their fate in the process of keratinization. In electron micrographs, the cells of the medulla, the cortex, and the internal and external root sheaths can all be distinguished by characteristic differences in their granules and their mode of keratinization.

The pigmentation of the hair is attributable to epidermal melanocytes located over the tip of the dermal papilla, a site corresponding to their location in the base of the epidermis generally (Fig. 22–30*A*). These melanocytes donate their pigment to the cells of the hair matrix and cortex. The melanosomes of the hair are usually larger than those found in the skin of the same individual. The melanocytes of the hair follicle function only at the beginning of the growing phase of the hair cycle, the onset of hair growth usually being heralded by increased melanogenic activity. In later stages of the growing phase or in the resting hair, melanocytes cannot be distinguished in the follicle.

In young rodents, hair growth is synchronized and spreads over the body in a *wave pattern*. Later in life, however, this process gives way to a *mosaic pattern*, hair growth beginning in isolated islands here and there. In man the mosaic growth pattern prevails, and the duration of the growing and resting phases varies from one region to another. In the case of scalp hair the growing phase is very long (several years), whereas the resting phase is of the order of three months.

Among mammals, humans are exceptional in that their skin is not furry. It is by no means hairless, however (see Fig. 22–40 for numbers of hair follicles per square centimeter). In accordance with its relative paucity of hairs, the human epidermis is generally thicker than that of other mammals. The architectural pattern of the dermoepidermal junction varies greatly from region to region. It is almost flat on the cheek, whereas deep dermal ridges occur on the soles and palms (Fig. 22–23).

The human hairy coat also exhibits regional differences in the competence of the hair follicles to respond to male sex hormones. At the onset of puberty in males, the areas of the mustache and the beard produce strongly pigmented thick hairs. The same areas in the female, although they contain the same number of hair follicles, continue to produce fine hair. In other places, however, such as the axillae and the pubic regions, hair appears in both sexes at the onset of puberty. In males, there is often a characteristic regression of the scalp hair with age, which varies in degree according to genotype. In its extreme form, this male pattern of changing hair distribution progresses so far that all the hair follicles are lost (baldness) or only a few are left and produce very fine hair.

One or more *sebaceous glands* are associated with each hair follicle. They discharge their holocrine secretory product through a short duct into the upper portion of the follicular canal.

A band of smooth muscle cells, the hair muscle or *arrector pili muscle*, is attached at one end to the papillary layer of the dermis and at the other to the connective tissue sheath of the hair follicle (Figs. 22–24, 22–25). When this muscle contracts in response to cold, fear, or anger, it moves the hair into a more vertical position while depressing the skin in the region of its attachment and elevating the region immediately around the hair. This is responsible for the erection of hairs in animals and for the so-called "goose flesh" in man.

NAILS

The nails are horny plates on the dorsal surfaces of the terminal phalanges of the fingers and toes. The surface of the skin covered by them is the *nail bed*. It is surrounded laterally and proximally by a fold of skin, the *nail wall*. The slit between the wall and the bed is the *nail groove*. The proximal edge of the *nail plate* is the *root* of the nail. The visible part of the nail plate, called the *body of the nail*, is surrounded by the nail wall. The distal portion, becoming free of the nail bed, extends forward and is gradually worn off or is cut off. The nail is semitransparent and permits the color of the underlying tissue, rich in blood vessels, to show through. Near the root, the nail has a whitish color. This crescentic portion, the *lunula*, is usually covered by the proximal portion of the nail fold.

The nail plate consists of closely compacted scales, the dead residues of cornified epithelial cells so arranged that in section the nail appears longitudinally striated. The nail wall has the structure of skin, with all its layers. Turning inward into the nail groove, it loses its papillae, and the epidermis loses its cornified, clear, and granular layers. Under the proximal fold, the stratum corneum spreads onto the free surface of the nail body as the *eponychium* (Fig. 22–32). The stratum lucidum and the stratum granulosum also reach far inside the groove but do not continue along the lower surface of the nail plate. On the surface of the nail bed, only the stratum basale and stratum spinosum of the epidermis are present.

In the nail bed the dermis is directly fused with the periosteum of the phalanx. The surface of the dermis under the proximal edge of the nail is provided with rather low papillae, but under the distal half of the lunula this surface is quite smooth. At the distal margin of the lunula, longitudinal, parallel ridges project instead of papillae. The

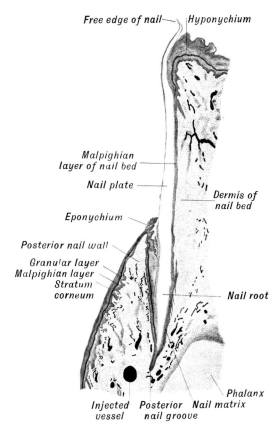

Figure 22–32. Longitudinal section of the nail of a newborn infant. (After A. A. Maximow.)

boundary between the epithelium and the dermis of the nail bed is, therefore, scalloped in a perpendicular section (Fig. 22–33), whereas it is smooth in longitudinal sections. Beyond the free edge of the nail the dermal ridges are replaced by cylindrical papillae.

The epithelium of the nail bed distal to the lunula retains the typical structure of the basal layers of the epidermis. The epithelium is thicker between the ridges of the dermis than over them. The upper layer of cells, which touches the substance of the nail, is separated from it in places by an even line, while in others it is jagged. Under the free edge of the nail the usual cornified layer again begins; it is thickened at this place and is called *hyponychium* (Fig. 22–32).

The epithelium that lines the proximal portion of the nail bed and corresponds roughly in distribution with the lunula on the upper surface is particularly thick distally and its upper portion gradually passes over into the substance of the nail plate. Here the new formation of the nail substance proceeds; accordingly, this region of the epithelium is called the *nail matrix* (Fig. 22–33). The cells of the deepest layer are low columnar and mitoses can be observed frequently in them. Above these are six to ten layers of polyhedral cells joined by three to 12 layers of more flattened cells. This entire mass is penetrated by parallel fibrils of a special "onychogenic" substance. On passing into the proximal edge of the nail plate, these cells cornify and become homogeneous.

As new formation of the nail takes place in the matrix, the nail moves forward. Most authors deny the participation of the epithelium of the other portions of the nail bed in the formation of the nail substance, believing that the nail simply glides forward over this region.

GLANDS

The glands of the skin include the sebaceous, sweat, and mammary glands. The last will be described in Chapter 33.

Sebaceous Glands

The *sebaceous glands* are scattered over the entire integument except in the palms, the soles, and the sides of the feet, where there are no hairs. They vary from 0.2 to 2 mm in diameter. They lie in the dermis, and their excretory ducts open into the necks of hair follicles. When several glands are connected with one hair, they lie at the same level. On the lips, around the corners of the mouth, on the glans penis and the internal fold of the prepuce, on the labia minora, and on the mammary papilla, the sebaceous glands are independent of hairs and open directly onto the surface of the skin. To this category also belong the *meibomian glands* of the eyelids. The sebaceous glands in mucocutaneous

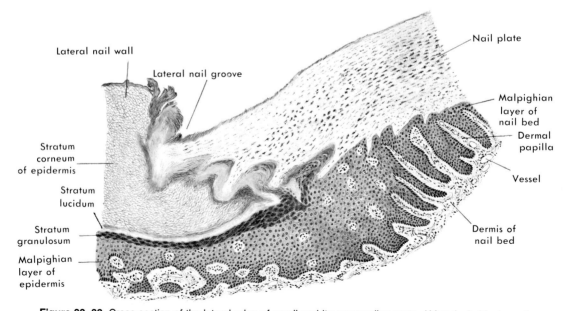

Figure 22–33. Cross section of the lateral edge of a nail and its surrounding parts. (After A. A. Maximow.)

junctions are more superficial than those that are associated with hairs.

The secretory portions of the sebaceous glands are rounded sacs (alveoli). As a rule, several adjacent alveoli form a mass like a bunch of grapes, and all of them open into a short duct (Figs. 22–24, 22–25). A simple branched gland results. Much less frequently, only one alveolus is present. In the meibomian glands of the eyelids there is one long, straight duct, from which a row of alveoli project.

The walls of the alveoli are formed by a basal lamina supported by a thin layer of fibrillar connective tissue. Along the internal surface is a single layer of thin cells with round nuclei. Toward the center of the alveoli a few cells keratinize, but most of them become larger and polyhedral, gradually fill with fat droplets, and resemble multilocular fat cells. The nuclei gradually shrink and then disappear, and the cells break down into fatty detritus. This is the oily secretion of the gland, and it is secreted onto the hair and upon the surface of the epidermis. The ducts of sebaceous glands are lined by stratified squamous epithelium continuous with the external root sheath of the hair and with the malpighian layer of the epidermis.

In sebaceous glands, the secretion results from the destruction of the epithelial cells and is therefore of the holocrine type. It is accompanied by a regenerative multiplication of epithelial elements. In the body of the gland, mitoses are rare in the cells lying on the basal lamina. They are numerous, however, in the cells close to the walls of the ducts, whence the new cells move into the secretory regions.

The so-called *uropygial* or *preen glands* of birds, especially aquatic birds, are specialized sebaceous glands. They produce oily material that is spread with the beak over the surface of the feathers to make them impervious to water.

Eccrine Sweat Glands

The *eccrine sweat glands* have not received investigative attention commensurate with their physiological importance. The human skin contains 3 to 4 $\times$ 10^6 eccrine sweat glands distributed over nearly the entire surface of the body. Each weighs 30 to 40 μg and their aggregate weight is roughly that of a kidney. A human can perspire as much as 10 liters a day, a rate of secretion exceeding that of many exocrine glands that have been studied in great detail.

The eccrine sweat glands are simple, coiled, tubular glands. Their secretory portion is a tube convoluted into a ball, and the duct is a slender unbranched tube (Fig. 22–35, 22–36). The bulk of the secretory portion is in the dermis, and the duct ascends through the epidermis to open at the skin surface. In response to stimulation by cholinergic nerves, the secretory portion forms a precursor fluid with a composition similar to an ultrafiltrate of blood plasma. Sodium and excess water are reabsorbed in the duct, producing a hypotonic sweat released at the skin surface.

The secretory coil is composed of three cell types: *clear cells, dark cells,* and *myoepithelial cells.* The dark cells border nearly all of the luminal surface of the tubule and are either cuboidal in shape or pyramidal, with a broad adluminal end and a narrower portion extending downward between the apices of the clear cells, which rest upon a thick basal

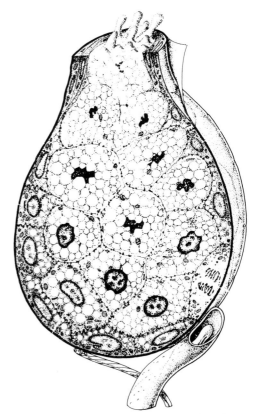

Figure 22–34. Drawing of a portion of a human sweat gland. (From Krstić, R. V. Die Gewebe des Menschen und der Saugetiere. Berlin, Springer Verlag, 1978.)

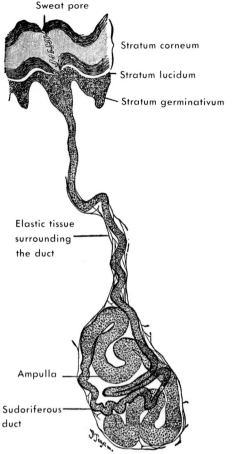

Figure 22–35. Sweat gland from the palmar surface of an index finger. The drawing was based on study of sections and a teased preparation. × 45. (Slightly modified from von Brunn.)

lamina. The dark cells do not reach the basal lamina. In electron micrographs they contain abundant ribosomes and secretory granules with glycoprotein staining characteristics.

These cells are believed to secrete a mucoid substance but its biochemical properties have not been analyzed. Glycogen, fat droplets, and pigment deposits may also occur in the cytoplasm. The clear cells rest directly on the basal lamina or on the myoepithelial cells. Intercellular canaliculi lined with microvilli occur between adjacent clear cells and provide the only egress from these cells to the lumen of the gland. The commissures of canaliculi are closed by occluding junctions between the apposed membranes of neighboring clear cells. These cells are rich in mitochondria, but poor in endoplasmic reticulum. Their cytoplasm contains varying amounts of glycogen. The basal plasma membrane is elaborately infolded as in other cell types involved in secretion of water and electrolytes. Myoepithelial cells occur at intervals between the clear cells and the basal lamina. Their function is not clear, for the lumen of the gland is collapsed in the resting gland and contains no accumulated fluid that could be expressed by their contraction. There is no evidence of their pulsatile contraction in the stimulated gland.

At the transition from the secretory portion of the gland, the tube narrows and its lumen takes on a slitlike or star-shaped configuration in cross section. The glandular and myoepithelial cells are replaced by a double layer of cuboidal cells. The peripheral row of cells have comparatively large nuclei and abundant mitochondria (Fig. 22–39). The adluminal cells have large, irregularly shaped nuclei and relatively little cytoplasm. The membranous organelles of the cytoplasm are poorly developed. Immediately beneath their luminal surface is a remarkable condensation of filaments constituting a conspicuous ter-

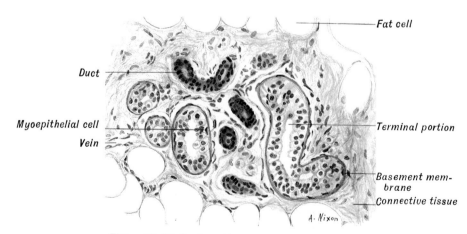

Figure 22–36. Section of human sweat gland. × 120.

minal web. This was formerly referred to as a "cuticular border," but this is erroneous, since the cuticle of such borders is outside of the plasmalemma whereas this specialization is in the apical cytoplasm.

As the ducts pass through the dermis and epidermis, they take a curved, loosely helical course, so that in sections they tend to appear discontinuous at sites where they curve out of the plane of section. In the epidermis they are surrounded by concentrically arranged keratinocytes. On the palms and soles and volar surface of the fingers, the rows of ducts open on the epidermal ridges with funnel-shaped openings that are easily seen with a magnifying glass.

Histophysiology of Eccrine Glands. The sweat glands play an important role in the control of body temperature. Heat is produced continuously as a by-product of metabolism and is continually being lost to the environment by radiation, conduction, and evaporation. Of these, evaporation is perhaps the most important and the only one subject to physiological control. When the environment is warmer than body temperature, evaporation is the only way in which the body can dissipate heat. Under normal conditions there is a continuous evaporative heat loss of about 600 ml per day from the lungs and skin over which there is no control. At high environmental temperatures, loss of heat by evaporation can be regulated by varying the rate of sweating. The eccrine glands do not function simultaneously or under the same conditions on all parts of the body. When the human body is exposed to excessive heat, sweating begins on the forehead and spreads to the face, and then to the rest of the body. Finally, the palms and the soles will show increased sweat production. Under nervous strain, however, palms and soles may start to sweat first.

It has been shown that the glandular portion of the eccrine sweat gland excretes more electrolytes than are finally found at the surface of the skin. It is assumed that an absorption of electrolytes takes place in the duct portion of the gland.

Sweating is controlled by centers in the preoptic area of the hypothalamus that function like a thermostat to regulate body temperature. An increase in body temperature may increase the rate of discharge of heat-sensitive neurons in these centers by as much as tenfold. This is accompanied by vasodilation and profuse sweating. Impulses from the hypothalamic nucleus are conducted over autonomic pathways through the brain stem and spinal cord and to the periphery over postganglionic sympathetic fibers that terminate in unmyelinated axons around the eccrine sweat glands. These are generally believed to be cholinergic. However, a loose network of catecholamine-containing nerves has been demonstrated in the sweat glands of the palm in monkeys, and it is quite possible that the sweat glands of the palms and soles of humans may also have adrenergic as well as cholinergic innervation. This may explain the localized "emotional sweating" that is generally confined to the palms, soles, axillae, and forehead under emotionally charged circumstances that activate the adrenergic portions of the sympathetic nervous system.

Apocrine Sweat Glands

A second type of sweat gland occurs in the axilla (Fig. 22-37), the mons pubis, the areola of the mammary gland, and the circumanal area. These are called *apocrine sweat glands* and are larger than the eccrine; their coiled secretory portion may reach 3 to 5 mm in diameter compared with 0.3 to 0.4 mm for eccrine glands. They are located deep in the subcutaneous connective tissue and each opens into a hair follicle. They arise during fetal life as an epithelial bud from the side of the hair follicle, whereas the eccrine glands develop from cords of epithelial cells that grow downward from the epidermal ridges. Eccrine sweat glands become functional in the neonatal period, but secretory function does not begin in apocrine sweat glands until puberty. The designation apocrine implies that a portion of the apical cytoplasm of the cells is shed in the secretory process. However, the mechanism of secretion of apocrine glands has not been established to everyone's satisfaction. The protein and electrolyte composition of apocrine sweat in humans has not been determined.

In certain parts of the skin the sweat glands have a peculiar arrangement and function. Such are the glands that produce *cerumen* "wax" in the external auditory meatus. They reach a considerable size and extend to the perichondrium. The secretory portions of the *ceruminous glands* branch, and the ducts, which sometimes also branch, may open together with the ducts of the adjacent sebaceous glands into the hair sacs of the fine

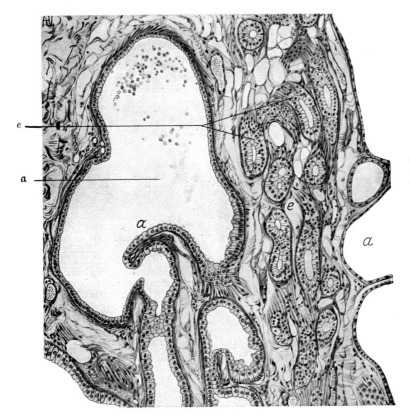

e

a

α

e

α

α

Figure 22–37. Axillary glands from a 37-year-old woman during the premenstruum. *a*, Greatly enlarged glands that change with the menstrual cycle. *e*, Glands that do not change. Resorcin-fuchsin stain for elastic fibers. Preparation of Loescke. × 110. (After Hoepke.)

hairs. In the terminal portions are highly developed smooth muscle cells; the glandular cells located upon them are particularly rich in pigment granules containing lipid.

Moll's glands of the margin of the eyelid are also a special kind of sweat gland, with terminal portions that do not form a ball but are irregularly twisted and provided with a wide lumen. The excretory ducts open onto the free surface or into the hair sacs of the eyelashes.

The secretion of the sweat glands is not the same everywhere. True sweat, a transparent, watery liquid, is excreted mainly by the small sweat glands, while a thicker secretion of complex composition is produced by the apocrine glands of the axilla and about the anus. In women, the apocrine sweat glands of the axilla show periodic changes with the menstrual cycle. These changes consist mainly of enlargement of the epithelial cells and of the lumens of the glands in the premenstrual period, followed by regressive changes during the period of menstruation.

The differences between the eccrine and apocrine sweat glands are as follows. The eccrine glands have no connections with hair follicles; they function throughout life, producing a watery secretion; and they are in-nervated mainly by cholinergic nerves. The apocrine glands are connected with hair follicles; they begin to function at puberty, producing a more viscous secretion; and they are supplied by adrenergic nerves.

BLOOD AND LYMPHATIC VESSELS

The arteries that supply the skin are located in the subcutaneous layer. Their branches, reaching upward, form a network (rete cutaneum) parallel to the surface on the boundary line between the dermis and the hypodermis. From one side of this network, branches are given off that nourish the subcutaneous stratum with its fat cells, the sweat glands, and the deeper portions of the hair follicles. From the other side of this network, vessels enter the dermis. At the boundary between the papillary and reticular layers they form the denser, subpapillary network or the rete subpapillare (Fig. 22–41). This gives off thin branches to the papillae. Each papilla has a single loop of capillary vessels with an ascending arterial and descending venous limb.

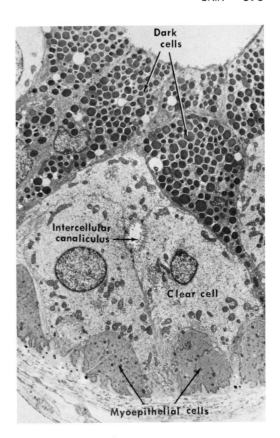

Figure 22–38. Electron micrograph of a sector of the secretory coil of a normal eccrine sweat gland. Mucigenous, "dark" cells border the lumen, while "clear" serous cells are more deeply situated and surround intercellular canaliculi. The myoepithelial cells form an incomplete layer at the periphery of the tubule. × 3400. (Courtesy of R. E. Ellis.)

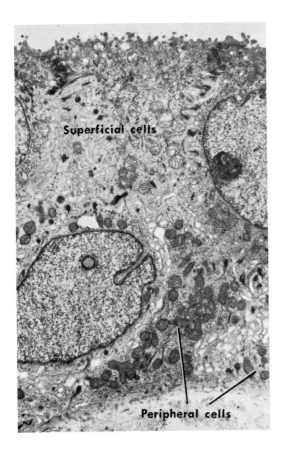

Figure 22–39. Electron micrograph of a portion of the wall of the coiled duct of an eccrine sweat gland. The luminal margin of the superficial cells contains a concentration of filaments formerly described as a "cuticular border." The peripheral cells have elaborately convoluted surfaces and contain many mitochondria. × 4000. (Courtesy of R. A. Ellis.)

	AVERAGE NUMBERS, ± S.E. OF MEAN.		
	HAIR FOLLICLES PER SQUARE CENTIMETER	SWEAT GLANDS PER SQUARE CENTIMETER	MELANOCYTES PER SQUARE MILLIMETER
Face	700 ± 40	270 ± 25	2120 ± 90
Trunk	70 ± 10	175 ± 20	890 ± 70
Arm	65 ± 5	175 ± 15	1160 ± 40
Leg	·55 ± 5	130 ± 10	1130 ± 60
Average	330 ± 20	212 ± 15	1560 ± 110

Figure 22–40. Regional anatomy of the human integument. (After G. Szabo.)

The veins that collect the blood from the capillaries in the papillae form the first network of thin veins immediately beneath the papillae. Then follow three flat networks of gradually enlarging veins on the boundary line between the papillary and reticular layers. In the middle section of the dermis and also at the boundary between the dermis and the subcutaneous tissue, the venous network is on the same level as the arterial rete cutaneum. Into this network the veins of the sebaceous and the sweat glands enter. From the deeper network the large, independent, subcutaneous veins pass, as well as the deep veins accompanying the arteries.

There are direct connections between the arterial and venous circulation in the skin without intervening capillary networks. These so-called arteriovenous anastomoses play a vital role in thermoregulation in the body.

Each hair follicle has its own blood vessels. It is supplied with blood from three sources: a special small artery that gives off a capillary network into the papilla; the rete subpapillare toward the sides of the hair sac; and several other small arteries that form a dense capillary network in the connective tissue layer of the follicle.

There is a dense network of capillaries outside the basal lamina of the sebaceous and, particularly, of the sweat glands.

The skin is rich in lymphatic vessels. In the papillary layer they form a dense meshwork of lymphatic capillaries. They begin in the papillae as networks or blind outgrowths, which are always deeper than the blood vessels. From this peripheral network, branches pass to the deeper network, which lies on the boundary between the dermis and the hypodermis; under the rete cutaneum it has much wider meshes, and its vessels are provided with valves. From the deeper network, large subcutaneous lymphatic vessels originate and follow the blood vessels. Lymphatic

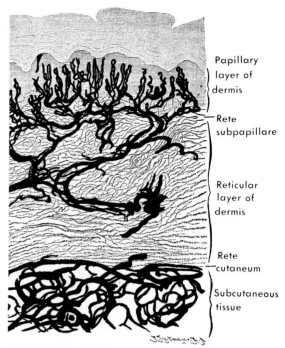

Papillary layer of dermis

Rete subpapillare

Reticular layer of dermis

Rete cutaneum

Subcutaneous tissue

Figure 22–41. Distribution of blood vessels in the skin. (Modified slightly from von Brunn.)

vessels are not associated with the hairs or glands of the skin.

NERVES

The skin is the most extensive sense organ in the body, receiving stimuli from the external environment, and it is therefore abundantly supplied with sensory nerves. In addition, it contains nerves that supply blood vessels, sweat glands, and the arrector pili muscles.

Firmly entrenched in the literature of physiology is the concept that the skin possesses four distinct types of sensory nerve endings, each responding to a specific kind of stimulus: touch, heat, cold, or pain. However, histologists to date have been unable to identify four kinds of receptor organs to match the four sensory modalities.

Two broad categories can be recognized: (1) the corpuscular receptors and (2) free nerve endings. The specialized corpuscular endings include the Meissner, Merkel, pacinian, and genital corpuscles, which are described in the chapter on the nervous system (Chapter 11). It will suffice here to state that all of these possess non-neural cellular and extracellular components arranged in such a way as to convey mechanical stimuli to the associated nerve axons. The free nerve endings are simpler in structure and require special silver staining techniques or electron microscopy for their demonstration. The skin on the palmar surface of the fingers is especially sensitive and has a high concentration of both corpuscular and free sensory receptors. The skin there has about 80 dermal papillae per square micrometer, and some 60 per cent of all papillae contain one or more free nerve endings, resulting in up to 100 endings per μm^2. These approach the epidermis vertically, providing a punctate distribution ensuring sensitive point-to-point discrimination. It is important to understand that the term "free" nerve ending signifies only the absence of a corpuscular receptor specialization; it does not imply a naked axon. The terminal cell of the Schwann sheath sends multiple cytoplasmic processes that provide a thin covering for the axon and its branches to their blind ends in the dermal papillae.

In addition to the vertically oriented papillary endings, there is an extensive horizontal nerve plexus underlying the dermal-epidermal junction. This network consists of ramifying subunits arising from nonmyelinated preterminal fibers. Because of their tuftlike pattern of arborization, these units have been termed *penicillate endings*. In each, the terminal cell of the Schwann sheath, located 2 to 6 μm beneath the epidermis, is highly branched and supplies cytoplasmic sheaths for single or multiple axons that fan out from the parent nerve fiber. Communicating branches from adjacent penicillate units permit exchange of axons and establish horizontal continuity of the subepidermal plexus. It is not clear which sensory modality is served by these endings, but their overlapping and ramification over relatively large areas could not provide highly localized sensation.

Where the skin bears even fine hairs, these are important adjuncts to tactile sensation. The myelin sheath of nerve fibers in dermis terminates as they approach hair follicles, and the branching axons that continue are individually ensheathed in processes of the terminal Schwann cell. They terminate in multiple fusiform endings applied to the root sheath of the sloping hair shaft on its underside just below the sebaceous glands. In this position, the spindle endings are strategically placed to sense deformation resulting from the lever-like action of the stiff, keratinized hair shaft whenever the free portion of the hair is touched. The hair and its associated nerve endings thus form a sensitive mechanoreceptor. Other nerve fibers bypass the deeper region of the hair and form papillary endings around the orifice through which it emerges from the epidermis.

HISTOGENESIS OF THE SKIN AND ITS ACCESSORIES

The epidermis develops from the ectoderm, and the dermis arises from the mesenchyme. The *epidermis* in the human embryo, during the first two months, is a double-layered epithelium. The basal layer, which lies on the mesenchyme, consists of cuboidal or cylindrical cells that multiply rapidly. The peripheral layer consists of flat cells that are constantly formed anew from the elements of the deeper layer. Beginning with the third month, the epidermis becomes triple layered. The new intermediate layer above the basal cells consists of polygonal cells, which increase in number and develop the surface projections formerly interpreted as intercellular bridges. At the end of the third month, in the peripheral portions of the intermediate layer, cornification begins and leads to the formation of the layers found in the adult. The cornified scales are desquamated and form part of the vernix caseosa.

The irregularities on the lower surface of the epidermis arise at the end of the third month on the inner surfaces of the fingers, palms, and soles as parallel ridges protruding into the dermis. From the beginning they show a characteristic pattern, and from them sweat glands develop.

The regional specificity of the epidermis has been the subject of detailed embryological study. It has been shown that maintenance of the adult specificity of the epidermis depends on the dermis. When the dermis and epidermis are separated and epidermis from the ear is implanted on dermis from the sole, thick epidermis will develop. If a composite graft from sole epidermis is maintained with ear dermis, the originally thick epidermis becomes thinner and hair follicles develop.

The *dermis* and *hypodermis* consist during the first six weeks of mesenchyme with wandering cells. From the second month on, the collagenous fibers appear and elastic fibers follow. In still later stages, the mesenchyme divides into a peripheral dense layer with a compact arrangement of its elements—the dermis—and a deep loose layer, the future subcutaneous layer. In the dermis, in turn, the peripheral papillary layer differentiates.

Hair first appears in the eyebrows and on the chin and upper lip, at the end of the second month. At first, in the deep layer of the epidermis, a group of dividing cells appear. These grow into the underlying connective tissue and produce a gradually elongating epithelial cylinder. This is the primordium of a hair follicle, the so-called "hair germ"; it is rounded on its end. Under the latter an accumulation of condensed connective tissue appears early. From it the hair papilla forms and protrudes into the epithelial mass of the bulb. The epithelial cells at the surface of the connective tissue papilla represent the matrix of the future hair. The connective tissue that surrounds the bulb later forms the connective tissue portions of the hair follicle. On the surface of the epithelial hair bulb, two projections arise. The upper represents the primordium of the sebaceous gland; its central cells early undergo a fatty transformation. The lower protuberance becomes the insertion of the arrector pili muscle on the hair sac. In the mass of epithelium that forms the hair primordium, a layer of rapidly cornifying cells differentiates into the layers of matrix, cortex, and inner and outer root sheaths. The shaft of the new hair elongates, owing to the multiplication of the cells of the matrix on the summit of the papilla, and perforates the top of the hollow cone of Henle's sheath. The tip of the hair moves upward, pierces the epidermis, and protrudes above the surface of the skin.

The development of the *nails* begins in the third month by the formation, on the back of the terminal phalanx of each finger, of a flat area, the *primary nail field,* which is surrounded by a fold of the skin. In the region of the nail the epithelium has three or four layers. The true nail substance is laid down during the fifth month in the portion of the nail bed near the proximal nail groove. Here the deep layer of the epidermis is transformed into the nail matrix, and its cells become flat, adjoin one another closely, and give rise to the true nail plate. In the beginning it is still thin and is entirely buried in the epidermis of the nail field or bed. It gradually moves in the distal direction. The

layers of epidermis that cover the plate eventually desquamate.

The development of the eccrine *sweat glands* proceeds independently of that of the hairs. The first primordia appear during the fifth month on the palms and soles and the lower surface of the fingers. At first they are similar to the primordia of the hairs. An epithelial shaft with a terminal thickening grows into the underlying connective tissue. But, unlike that around the hairs, the connective tissue here does not condense about the epithelium. The shaft gradually elongates and becomes cylindrical, and its lower portion curls in the form of a ball. Beginning in the seventh month, an irregular lumen forms in this lower portion, which constitutes the secretory part; along the course of the future excretory duct another lumen develops and later unites with the first one. In the secretory portion, the epithelium around the lumen forms two layers, which differentiate into an external layer of myoepithelial elements and an internal layer of glandular cells.

Quantitative investigations have shown that in the embryo the density of the skin appendages, regardless of whether they are hair or eccrine glands, is originally the same. A large proportion of these appendages on the head, however, will become hairs and a large proportion of them on the rest of the body will become eccrine sweat glands. No hairs will be found on the palms and the soles. Due to the differential rate of growth of the body surface, the original uniform density changes because no new hair follicles or eccrine sweat glands form after the original population is established. These appendages subsequently become widely spaced in the trunk and in the extremities, which grow to a surface area about three times as great as that of the head. In wound healing, usually no new hair follicles are formed.

REFERENCES

GENERAL

Montagna, W. W., and P. F. Parakkal: The Structure and Function of Skin. 3rd ed. New York, Academic Press, 1974.

Rothman, S.: Physiology and Biochemistry of the Skin. Chicago, University of Chicago Press, 1954.

EPIDERMIS AND KERATINIZATION

Allen, T. D., and C. S. Pottan: Desmosomal form, fate and function in mammalian epidermis. J. Ultrastruct Res. *51*:94,1975.

De Bersaques, J.: Keratin and its formation. Curr. Probl. Dermatol. *6*:34, 1976.

Elias, P. M.: Epidermal lipids, membranes, and keratinization. Int. J. Dermatol. *20*:1, 1981.

Elias, P. J., J. Goerke, and D. S. Friend: Permeability barrier lipids: composition and influence on epidermal structure. J. Invest. Dermatol. *69*:535, 1977.

Franke, W. W., E. Schmid, C. Grund, H. Muller, I. Engelbrecht, R. Moll, J. Stadler, and E. D. Jarash: Antibodies to high molecular weight polypeptides of desmosomes: specific localization of a class of junctional proteins in cells and tissues. Differentiation *20*:217, 1981.

Green, H.: The keratinocyte as differentiated cell type. Harvey Lect. *74*:101, 1980.

Green, H., E. Fuchs, and F. Watt: Differentiated structural components of the keratinocyte. Cold Spring Harbor Symp. Quant. Biol. *46*:293, 1982.

MacKenzie, I. C.: The ordered structure of mammalian epidermis. *In* Maiback, H. I., and Rovee, D. T., eds.: Epidermal Wound Healing. Chicago, Year Book Medical Publishers, 1972, p. 5.

Matoltsy, A. G.: Desmosomes, filaments, and keratohyalin granules: their role in the stabilization and keratinization of the epidermis. J. Invest. Dermatol. *65*:127, 1975.

Matoltsy, A. G., and M. Matoltsy: The chemical nature of keratohyalin granules of the epidermis. J. Cell Biol. *47*:593, 1970.

Matoltsy, A. G., and P. E. Parakkal: Membrane-coating granules of keratinizing epithelia. J. Cell Biol. *24*:297, 1965.

Menton, D. N.: A minimum surface mechanism to account for the organization of cells into columns in the mammalian epidermis. Am. J. Anat. *145*:1, 1976.

Montagna, W., and W. C. Lobitz, eds.: The Epidermis. New York, Academic Press, 1964.

Rice, R. H., and H. Green: Presence in human epidermal cells of a soluble protein precursor of the cross-linked envelope. Activation of the cross linking by calcium ions. Cell *18*:681, 1979.

Sun, T. T., and H. Green: Keratin filaments of cultured human epidermal cells. Formation of intermolecular disulfide bonds during terminal differentiation. J. Biol. Chem. *253*:2053, 1978.

LANGERHANS CELLS

Breathnach, A. S.: The cell of Langerhans. Int. Rev. Cytol. *18*:1, 1965.

Katz, S., K. Tamaki, and D. H. Sacks. Epidermal Langerhans cells are derived from cells originating in the bone marrow. Nature (Lond.) *282*:324, 1979.

Rowden, G.: Immunoelectron microscopic studies of surface receptors and antigens of human Langerhans cells. Br. J. Dermatol. *97*:593, 1977.

Shelley, W. B., and J. Lennart: The Langerhans cell: its origin, nature, and function. Acta Dermatol. (Stockh.) Suppl. *79*:7, 1978.

Silberberg, I., R. L. Baer, and S. A. Rosenthal: The role of Langerhans cells in allergic contact hypersensitivity. A review of findings in man and guinea pigs. J. Invest. Dermatol. *66*:210, 1976.

Stingl, G., S. I. Katz, L. Clement, I. Green, and E. M. Shevack: Immunologic functions of Ia-bearing epidermal Langerhans cells. J. Immunol. *121*:2005, 1978.

Tew, J. G., J. Thorbecke, and R. M. Steinman: Dendritic cells in immune response. J. Reticuloendothel. Soc. *31*:371, 1982.

Wolff, K., and E. Scheimer: Uptake, intracellular transport and degradation of exogenous protein by Langerhans cells. J. Invest. Dermatol *54*:37, 1970.

Wolff, K., and R. K. Winkelmann: Quantitative studies on the Langerhans cell population of guinea pig epidermis. J. Invest. Dermatol *48*:504, 1967.

MERKEL CELL

Hashimoto, K.: Fine structure of the Merkel cell in human oral mucosa. J. Invest. Dermatol *58*:381, 1972.

Kurosumi, K., V. Kurosumi, and K. Inoue. Morphological and morphometric studies on the Merkel cells and associated nerve terminals of normal and denervated skin. Arch. Histol. Jpn. *42*:243, 1979.

Mihara, M., K. Hashimoto, K. Ueda, and M. Kumakiri: The specialized junctions between Merkel cell and neurite: an electron microscopic study. J. Invest. Dermatol *73*:325, 1979.

Winkelmann, R. K.: The Merkel cell system and a comparison between it and the neurosecretory or APUD cell system. J. Invest. Dermatol *69*:41, 1977.

MELANOCYTES

Billingham, R. E., and W. K. Silvers: The melanocytes of mammals. Qt. Rev. Biol. *35*:1, 1960.

Drochmans, P.: On melanin granules. Int. Rev. Exp. Pathol. *2*:357, 1963.

Fitzpatrick, T. B., G. Szabo, M. Seiji, and W. C. Quevedo: Biology of the melanin pigmentary system. *In* Fitzpatrick, T. B., et al., eds: Dermatology in General Medicine 2nd ed. New York, McGraw-Hill Book Co., 1979, p. 131.

Snell, R. S.: An electron microscopic study of melanin in the hair and hair follicles. J. Invest. Dermatol *58*:218, 1972.

Szabo, G.: The regional anatomy of the human integument with special reference to the distribution of hair follicles, sweat glands and melanocytes. Philos. Trans. R. Soc. Lond. [B]. *252*:447, 1967.

DERMIS AND EPIDERMAL-DERMAL JUNCTION

Briggaman, R. A.: Biochemical composition of the epidermal-dermal junction and other basement membranes. J. Invest. Dermatol. *78*:1, 1982.

Briggaman, R. A., and C. E. Wheeler: The epidermal-dermal junction. J. Invest. Dermatol. *65*:71, 1975.

Montagna, W., J. P. Bentley, and R. L. Robson. The dermis. Adv. Biol. Skin 10, 1970.

HAIR AND NAILS

Ebling, F. J.: Hair. J. Invest. Dermatol *67*:98, 1976.

Montagna, W., and R. L. Robson, eds.: Hair growth. Adv. Biol. Skin 9, 1969.

Orwin, D. F.: The cytology and cytochemistry of the wool follicles. Int. Rev. Cytol. *60*:331, 1979.

Wyatt, E. H., and J. M. Riggot: Scanning electron microscopy of hair. Observations on surface morphology with respect to site, sex, and age in man. Br. J. Dermatol. *96*:627, 1977.

Zaias, N. J., and Alvarez, J.: The formation of the primate nail plate. An autoradiographic study in the squirrel monkey. J. Invest. Dermatol. *51*:120, 1968.

SEBACEOUS GLANDS

Bell, M. A.: A comparative study of sebaceous gland ultrastructure in sub-human primates. Anat. Rec. *170*:331, 1971.

Rupec, M.: Zur Ultrastruktur der Talgdrüsenzelle. Arch. Klin. Exp. Derm. *234*:273, 1969.

SWEAT GLANDS

Cage, G. W., and R. L. Dobson: Sodium secretion and reabsorption in the human eccrine sweat gland. J. Clin. Invest. *44*:1270, 1965.

Dobson, R. I.: The correlation of structure and function in the human eccrine sweat gland. *In* Montagna, W., R. A. Ellis, and A. F. Silver, eds.: Advances in Biology of Skin. Vol. III. New York, Appleton-Century-Crofts, 1962, pp. 54–75.

Dole, V. P., and J. H. Thaysen: Variation in the functional power of human sweat glands. J. Exp. Med. *98*:129, 1953.

Ellis, R. A.: Eccrine sweat glands. *In* Jadassohn, J., ed.: Handbuch der Haut und Geschlechtskrankheiten I. Band. Normale und Pathologische Anatomie der Haut. Berlin–Heidelberg–New York, Springer, 1967.

Forstrom, L., M. E. Goldyne, and R. K. Winkelmann: Ig E in human eccrine sweat. J. Invest. Dermatol. *64*:156, 1975.

Haimovici, H.: Evidence for adrenergic sweating in man. J. Appl. Physiol. *2*:512, 1950.

Kuno, Y.: Human Perspiration. Springfield, Il, Charles C Thomas, 1956.

Lloyd, D. P. C.: Secretion and reabsorption in eccrine sweat gland. *In* Montagna, W., ed.: Advances in Biology of Skin. Oxford–London–New York, Pergamon Press, 1962, pp. 127–151.

Montgomery, I., D. M. Jenkinson, and H. Y. Elder: The effects of thermal stimulation on the ultrastructure of the fundus and duct of the equine sweat gland. J. Anat. *134*:741, 1982.

Munger, B. L.: The ultrastructure and histophysiology of human eccrine sweat glands. J. Biophys. Biochem. Cytol. *11*:385, 1961.

Robertshaw, D., C. R. Taylor, and L. M. Mazia: Sweating in primates: secretion by adrenal medulla during exercise. Am. J. Physiol. *224*:678, 1973.

Sato, K.: The physiology, pharmacology, and biochemistry of the eccrine sweat gland. Rev. Physiol. Biochem. Pharmacol. *79*:51, 1977.

Sato, K., and R. L. Dobson: Regional and individual variations in the function of the human eccrine sweat gland. J. Invest. Dermatol. *54*:443, 1970.

Schaumberg-Lever, G., and W. F. Lever: Secretion from human apocrine glands: an electron microscopic study. J. Invest. Dermatol. *64*:38, 1975.

Szabo, G.: The number of eccrine sweat glands in human skin. *In* Montagna, W., R. Ellis, and A. Silver, eds.: Advances in Biology of Skin. Vol. III. New York, Pergamon Press, 1962, pp. 1–5.

Terzakis, J. A.: The ultrastructure of monkey eccrine sweat glands. Z. Zellforsch. *64*:493, 1964.

Uno, H., and W. Montagna: Catecholamine containing nerve terminals in the eccrine sweat glands of macaques. Cell Tissue Res. *158*:1, 1975.

BLOOD VESSELS AND INNERVATION

Braverman, I. M., and A. Yen: Ultrastructure of the human dermal microcirculation. II The capillary loops of the dermal papillae. J. Invest. Dermatol. *68*:44, 1977.

Montagna, W. W., and J. M. Brookhart: Cutaneous innervation and modalities of cutaneous sensibility. J. Invest. Dermatol. *60*:3, 1977.

Odland, G. F.: The fine structure of cutaneous capillaries. *In* Montagna, W., and R. A. Ellis, eds.: Advances in Biology of the Skin. Vol. 2, New York, Pergamon Press, 1961, p. 57.

Winkelmann, R. K.: Nerve Endings in Normal and Pathological Skin. Springfield, IL, Charles C Thomas, 1960.

23

ORAL CAVITY AND ASSOCIATED GLANDS

The oral cavity is the entrance to the long tubular *digestive system*, which consists of the lips, mouth, pharynx, esophagus, stomach, small and large intestine, rectum, and anus. On its way through this tract, the food undergoes mechanical fragmentation and chemical digestion. Products of degradation of the food are absorbed through the wall of the intestine into the blood, which carries them to the tissues for utilization or storage. The undigested residue of the food is eliminated as feces.

The inner surface of the digestive tube is lined with a mucous membrane or *mucosa*, which consists of a superficial layer of epithelium regionally specialized for different digestive functions; and a supporting layer of loose connective tissue, the *lamina propria*. The peripheral layers of the wall of the digestive tube are smooth muscle making up the *muscularis externa* (Fig. 23–1). In most parts of the tract, the outer limit of the mucosa is demarcated by a thin layer of smooth muscle, the *muscularis mucosae*. Between it and the muscularis externa is a layer of loose connective tissue, the *submucosa*. Numerous blood vessels, nerves, lymphatics, and lymphoid nodules are to be found in this layer. Where a muscularis mucosae is absent, there is a gradual transition from the lamina propria to the submucosa.

The mucosa of the developing gastrointestinal tract evaginates to form *folds* and *villi* that project into the lumen and increase the surface area of the absorptive epithelium. It also invaginates to form tubular *crypts* or *glands* whose lining cells produce mucus, digestive enzymes, and hormones. The majority of these outgrowths remain confined to the thickness of the mucosa. Other evaginations proliferate to such an extent during embryonic development that they give rise to separate organs, the accessory glands of the gastrointestinal tract, such as the salivary glands, liver, and pancreas. However, these remain connected by long ducts to the epithelial surface from which they originated in embryonic life.

In the oral cavity, esophagus, and rectum, the wall of the digestive tube is surrounded by a layer of connective tissue that attaches it to the adjacent structures. The stomach and intestines, on the other hand, are suspended in the abdominal cavity by mesenteries, and their surface is covered by a moist serous membrane, the *serosa* or *peritoneum*, which permits these organs to slide freely over one another within the cavity during the peristaltic movements of the digestive tract.

The wall of the digestive tube is richly provided with blood vessels that bring to it oxygen and the metabolites necessary to sustain its secretory activities. The veins and lymphatics also carry away the absorbed products of digestion. In addition, the wall of the digestive tract contains an intricate system of sympathetic ganglia and nerve plexuses concerned with coordination of the movements of the digestive tube.

THE ORAL CAVITY

The epithelium of the mucous membrane in the mouth is of stratified squamous type, like that of the skin. However, in the human, it normally does not undergo complete keratinization. The nuclei of the cells of the superficial layers condense and become metabolically inert, but do not disappear, and the cell bodies do not reach the same degree of flatness as in the epidermis. The superficial cells are continually exfoliating in great numbers and are found in the saliva. In some

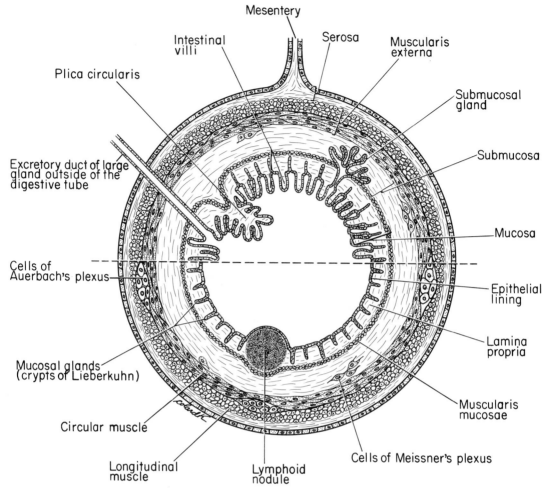

Figure 23–1. Schematic representation of the general features of organization in the gastrointestinal tract. The concentric layers of serosa, muscularis, and mucosa are common to virtually all regions of the tract. In the upper half of the drawing, the mucosa is depicted with glands and villi, as in the small intestine; in the lower half, it is shown with glands only, as in the colon.

places they contain granules of keratohyalin, and glycogen is present in the superficial and middle layers of the epithelium. In many animal species, particularly ruminants, the epithelium of the oral cavity undergoes extensive keratinization.

The lamina propria, in most places, extends into concavities in the deep surface of the epithelium forming connective tissue papillae similar to those associated with the epidermis of the skin. Their structure is, however, more delicate, and the collagenous and elastic fibers are thinner than in the dermis. In the posterior region of the oral cavity the lamina propria contains many lymphocytes, which are often found migrating into and through the epithelium.

The arrangement of the blood vessels is similar to that in the skin. There is a deep submucous plexus of large vessels, from which arise branches that form a second plexus in the lamina propria. This in turn sends capillaries into the papillae. The lymphatics also show an arrangement similar to that in the skin, and begin with blind capillary outgrowths in the papillae.

The oral mucous membrane is very sensitive and is provided with many nerve endings derived from the sensory branches of the trigeminal nerve. On that portion covering the tongue it also contains the specific end organs of the sense of taste. Under the lamina propria, especially in the cheeks and on the soft palate, there is a loose submucosa, which gradually merges with the denser connective tissue of the mucosa. In regions with a well-developed submucosa the mucous membrane can be easily lifted into folds, whereas in those places against which the food is crushed and rubbed, as on the hard palate, there is no submucosa, and the mucous membrane is firmly bound to the periosteum of the underlying bone.

The inner zone of the lip margin in the newborn is considerably thickened and provided with many high papillae and numerous sebaceous glands that are not associated with hairs (Fig. 23–2). These structural features seem to facilitate the process of suckling.

The soft palate consists of layers of striated muscle and fibrous connective tissue covered with mucous membrane. On the oral surface the latter has the structure typical of the oral cavity–a stratified squamous epithelium, with high papillae, and associated mucous glands. The glands are surrounded by adipose tissue and are scattered in a loose submucous layer separated from the lamina propria by dense elastic networks. This oral type of mucous membrane also covers the posterior margin of the soft palate and continues for some

distance onto its nasal surface. On this surface, at varying distances from its posterior margin, the stratified epithelium is replaced by pseudostratified, ciliated, columnar epithelium, which rests on a thickened basal lamina. The lamina propria contains small glands of the mixed type, but no adipose tissue, and it is heavily infiltrated with lymphocytes. A dense layer of elastic fibers is found between the glands and the underlying muscle. A submucosa is not present.

Most of the structures in the oral cavity—the salivary glands, the lining of the palate, the anterior two thirds of the tongue, and the vestibule of the nose—are derived from the embryonic ectoderm. The tooth enamel is said to be a neural crest derivative, whereas the dentin and pulp originate from mesenchyme. Endodermal derivatives include the tonsils, the epithelium of the posterior third of the tongue, the pharyngeal tonsils, and the remainder of the gastrointestinal tract and its associated glands.

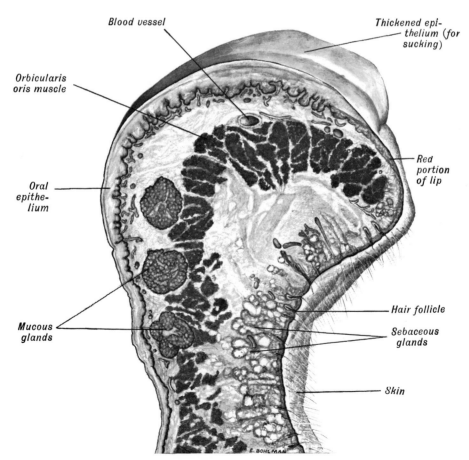

Figure 23–2. Camera lucida drawing of sagittal section through lip of a newborn infant. Stained with hematoxylin. × 10.

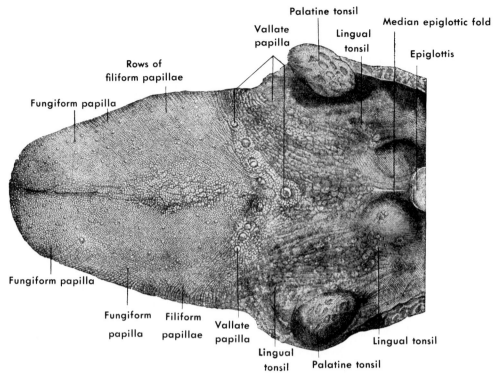

Figure 23–3. Surface of dorsum and root of human tongue. (After Sappey, from Schumacher.)

THE TONGUE

The tongue consists of interlacing bundles of striated muscle that run in three planes and cross one another at right angles. The muscular mass is covered by a tightly adherent mucous membrane. The dense lamina propria is continuous with the interstitial connective tissue of the muscle. A submucous layer is present only on the smooth ventral surface of the tongue. The dorsal surface is covered in its anterior two thirds by a multitude of small excrescences—the *lingual papillae*—whereas in its posterior one third it presents only irregular bulges of larger size. The boundary line between the two regions is V-shaped, with the opening of the angle directed forward (Fig. 23–3). At the apex of the angle is a small invagination, the *foramen caecum*. It is the rudiment of the thyroglossal duct, which in early embryonic stages connects the thyroid gland primordium with the epithelium of the oral cavity.

Papillae

Four types of papillae are present on the tongue: filiform, fungiform, circumvallate, and foliate. The *filiform papillae* are arranged in more or less distinct rows diverging to the right and left from the middle line and parallel to the V-shaped boundary between anterior and posterior regions of the tongue. The *fungiform papillae* are scattered singly among the filiform papillae and are especially numerous near the tip of the tongue. The *circumvallate papillae*, numbering only 10 to 12 in man, are distributed along the diverging arms of the V-shaped boundary (Fig. 23–3). The paired *foliate papillae* are found on the dorsolateral aspect of the posterior part of the tongue.

The filiform papillae are 2 to 3 mm long. Their connective tissue core forms secondary papillae with pointed ends (Fig. 23–4). The epithelium covering these connective tissue outgrowths also forms short processes, which taper to a point (Fig. 23–6). The superficial squamous cells are transformed into hard scales containing shrunken nuclei. The axial parts of the scales at the point of the papilla are connected with its solid axial core and their lower edges project from the surface of the papilla like the branches of a fir tree. When digestion is disturbed in illness, the normal shedding of these scales is delayed.

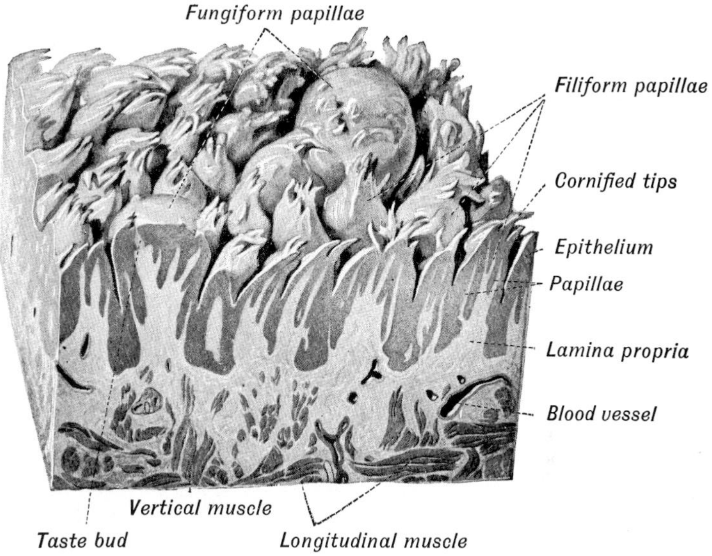

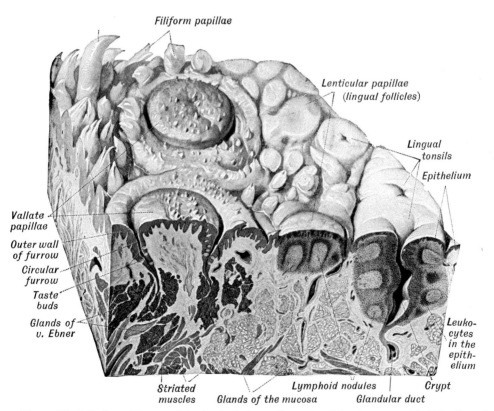

Fungiform papillae

Filiform papillae

Cornified tips

Epithelium

Papillae

Lamina propria

Blood vessel

Figure 23–4. Surface of dorsum of tongue, drawn from a combined study using the binocular microscope and from sections. The anterior cut surface corresponds with the long axis of the tongue—the tip of the tongue being to the reader's left. × 16. (After Braus.)

Vertical muscle

Taste bud

Longitudinal muscle

Filiform papillae

Lenticular papillae (lingual follicles)

Lingual tonsils

Epithelium

Vallate papillae

Outer wall of furrow

Circular furrow

Taste buds

Glands of v. Ebner

Leuko-cytes in the epith-elium

Striated muscles

Glands of the mucosa

Lymphoid nodules

Glandular duct

Crypt

Figure 23–5. Surface of tongue at the border between the root and the dorsum. × 16. (After Braus.)

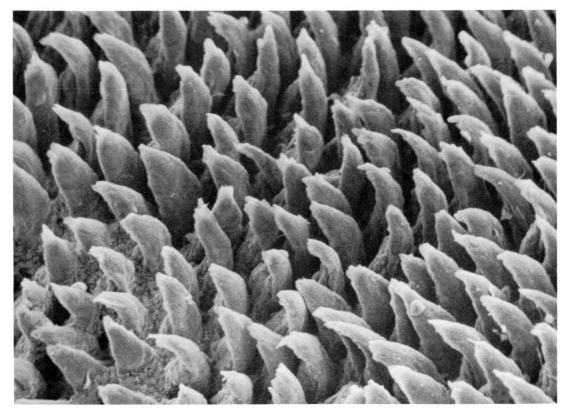

Figure 23–6. Scanning electron micrograph of the filiform papillae of rabbit tongue. (Micrograph courtesy of F. Fujita.)

They then accumulate, in layers mixed with bacteria, on the surface of the tongue, which becomes covered with a gray film—the "coated" tongue.

The fungiform papillae have a short, slightly constricted stalk and a slightly flattened hemispherical upper part. The connective tissue core forms secondary papillae that project into recesses in the underside of the epithelium, which has a smooth free surface (Figs. 23–4, 23–7). On many of the fungiform papillae the epithelium associated with the secondary papillae contains *taste buds*. Because the core is rich in blood vessels and the epithelium is relatively thin, the fungiform papillae have a distinct red color.

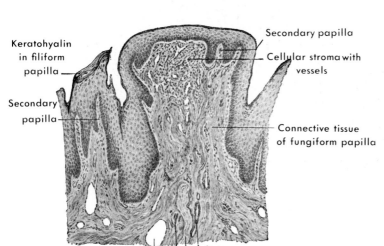

Figure 23–7. Perpendicular section through a fungiform papilla. × 46. (After Schaffer, from Schumacher.)

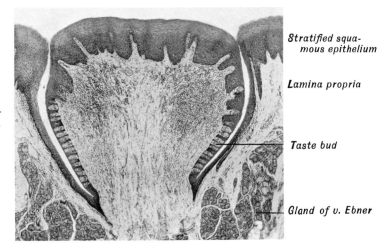

Stratified squamous epithelium

Lamina propria

Taste bud

Gland of v. Ebner

Figure 23–8. Section through circumvallate papilla of *Macacus rhesus.* Photomicrograph, × 42.

The circumvallate papillae are recessed into the surface of the mucous membrane, and each is surrounded by a deep, circular furrow. The connective tissue core forms secondary papillae only on the upper surface. The covering epithelium is smooth contoured, whereas that of the lateral surfaces of the papillae contains many taste buds (Fig. 23–8). In vertical sections, 10 to 12 of them can often be seen aligned on the lateral surface of the papilla. A few may be present in the outer wall of the groove surrounding the papilla. The number of taste buds in a single papilla is subject to great variations, but it has been estimated to average 250. Connected with the circumvallate papillae are glands of the serous type (*glands of von Ebner*), which are embedded deep in the underlying

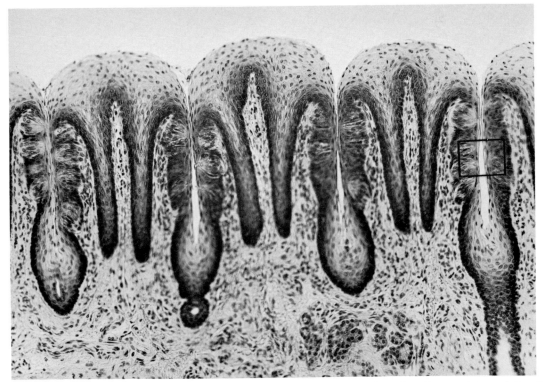

Figure 23–9. Photomicrograph of the foliate papillae of a rabbit, showing the alternating ridges and deep clefts with numerous taste buds on either side of the cleft. × 150. An area such as that enclosed in the rectangle is shown at higher magnification in Figure 23–10.

muscular tissue and whose excretory ducts open into the bottom of the circumferential furrow.

In the human, foliate papillae are rudimentary, but in many animals they are the site of the main aggregations of taste receptors (Fig. 23–9). The fully developed foliate papillae in the rabbit, for example, are oval bulgings on the mucous membrane, consisting of alternating parallel ridges and grooves. The epithelium of the sides of the ridges contains great numbers of taste buds. Small serous glands open into the bottom of the grooves between the folia.

Taste buds are also found on the glossopalatine arch, on the soft palate, on the posterior surface of the epiglottis, and on the posterior wall of the pharynx as far down as the inferior edge of the cricoid cartilage.

The nodular bulges on the root of the tongue are caused by lymphatic nodules, forming the *lingual tonsils* (Fig. 23–3). On the free surface of each lingual tonsil a small opening leads into a deep invagination, the *crypt*, lined with stratified squamous epithelium. The crypt is surrounded by lymphoid tissue. Innumerable lymphocytes infiltrate the epithelium and congregate in the lumen of the crypt, where they degenerate and form masses of detritus with the desquamated epithelial cells and bacteria. The lingual tonsils are often associated with mucous glands embedded in the underlying muscle tissue. The ducts of the latter open either into the crypt or onto the free surface.

Taste Buds

The taste buds are seen in sections under low power as pale, oval bodies in the darker-stained epithelium (Fig. 23–9). Their long axis averages 72 μm. They extend from the basal lamina almost to the surface. The epithelium over each taste bud is pierced by a small opening—the *taste pore* (Figs. 23–10, 23–11, 23–12).

Light microscopists distinguished two types of cells among the constituents of taste buds, the dark *supporting cells* (Type I) and the light *neuroepithelial cells* (Type II). Electron microscopists have confirmed the existence of two cell types but are not able to assign a functional role to them with any certainty and have therefore adopted the designation Type I and Type II to avoid functional implications. A Type III cell structurally comparable with the Type I cell has been identified in

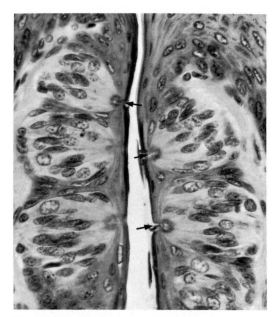

Figure 23–10. Photomicrograph of taste buds from the foliate papillae of a rabbit. × 450. See Figure 23–9 for location. Arrows indicate the taste pores.

the taste buds of the rabbit. Typical synapses of nerves with the epithelial cells of taste buds have been observed only on Type III cells. *Basal cells* and *peripheral cells* have also been described, and these are believed to be undifferentiated progenitor cells of the taste buds.

Both Type I and Type II cells have large microvilli that projects into the taste pore, where they are embedded in a rather amorphous extracellular substance. Material of similar density and texture is found in membrane-bounded vesicles in the apical cytoplasm of Type I cells. It is presumed to be a secretory product of these cells. The *taste hairs* described by light microscopists were no doubt the clusters of coarse microvilli found in the pore region in electron micrographs. Zonulae occludentes are present on the boundaries between cells near the free surface. The lateral surfaces of the cells below the junctional complexes may be folded and interdigitated. The cytoplasm of the lighter Type II cells has a rather extensive smooth endoplasmic reticulum, which is not observed in Type I cells.

There are only four fundamental taste sensations: sweet, bitter, acid, and salty. It has been shown by the application of substances to individual fungiform papillae that they differ widely in their receptive properties. Some do not give any taste sensations,

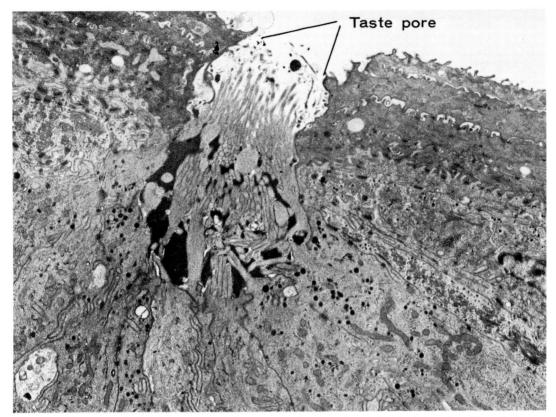

Figure 23–11. Electron micrograph of the pore region of a rabbit taste bud. Notice the large microvilli on the sensory cells, surrounded by a dense amorphous secretory product. For a surface view of the pore, see Figure 23–12. (Micrograph courtesy of M. Coppe.)

whereas others give sensations of one or more of the four taste qualities. No structural differences in the various taste buds have been found, in spite of the differences in sensation mediated. There is, moreover, a general chemical sensitivity in regions of the mouth where there are no taste buds.

Nerves

The anterior two thirds of the tongue is innervated by the lingual nerve, which contains fibers of general sensibility from the fifth cranial nerve (trigeminal) and fibers of gustatory sensibility from the seventh cranial nerve (facialis). The latter enter the lingual nerve from the chorda tympani. The posterior third of the tongue is innervated by the glossopharyngeal nerve for both general and gustatory sensibility. Taste buds of the epiglottis and lower pharynx are innervated by the vagus. These nerve fibers are lightly myelinated. They branch profusely under the basal lamina, lose their myelin, and form a subepithelial plexus, from which fibers penetrate the epithelium. Some terminate as *intergemmal fibers* by free arborization between the taste buds. Others, the *perigemmal fibers*, closely envelop the taste buds; and still others, the *intragemmal fibers*, penetrate the taste buds and end with small terminal enlargements in intimate contact with certain of the taste bud cells. The functional significance of these different nerve endings is unknown.

GLANDS OF THE ORAL CAVITY

General Description

Numerous *salivary glands* open into the oral cavity. Many of them are small glands in the mucosa or submucosa and are named according to their location. They seem to secrete continuously and furnish a liquid, the *saliva*, which moistens the oral mucous membrane.

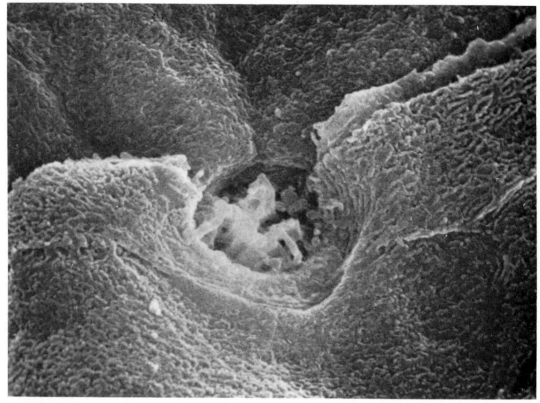

Figure 23–12. Scanning micrograph of the pore of a taste bud opening onto the surface of the epithelium. (Micrograph courtesy of M. Coppe.)

In addition, there are three pairs of large glands, which constitute the salivary glands proper. They are the *parotid*, the *submandibular (submaxillary)*, and the *sublingual* glands. They secrete only when mechanical, thermal, or chemical stimuli act upon the nerve endings in the oral mucous membrane, or as the result of certain psychic or olfactory stimuli.

The saliva collected from the oral cavity is a mixture of the secretions of the various salivary glands. It is a viscous, colorless, opalescent liquid that contains water, mucoprotein, immunoglobulins, carbohydrates, and a number of inorganic components, including calcium, phosphorus, sodium, potassium, magnesium, chloride, and traces of iron and iodine. Enzymes are also present, especially amylase (ptyalin), which splits starch into smaller, water-soluble carbohydrates. Saliva always contains desquamated squamous epithelial cells and the so-called *salivary corpuscles*. The latter originate in the lymphoid nodules of the tongue and in the tonsils, and are degenerating lymphocytes or granulocytes.

The composition of the saliva collected from the oral cavity varies, depending on the degree of participation of the various salivary glands in its formation. But even the secretions of the same gland may change considerably with variations in the stimuli acting upon the oral mucous membrane, as, for instance, with different kinds of food.

The salivary glands may be classified in three categories, according to the type of their secretory cells. The glands containing only *mucous* cells elaborate a viscid secretion that consists almost exclusively of mucin. In glands with only *serous* cells, the secretion is a watery liquid that lacks mucus but contains salts, proteins, and the enzymes amylase, lysozyme, peroxidase, DNase, and RNase. In the *mixed glands*, containing serous and mucous cells, the secretion is a viscid liquid containing mucin, salts, and enzymes.

All glands of the oral cavity have a system of branching ducts. The secretory portions or acini of the pure mucous glands are usually long, branching tubules. In the pure serous and mixed glands, the secretory portions vary from simple oval acini to tubulo-acinar forms.

The initial intralobular ducts are thin, branched tubules called the *necks*, or *intercalated ducts*. Branches of the next larger order, also intralobular, have a vertically striated epithelium. These segments are called *striated ducts*. Then follow the larger branches. Among them, lobular, interlobular, and primary ducts may be distinguished in the large glands.

Mucous Cells

In the pure mucous glands, the cells are arranged in a layer against the basal lamina and have an irregularly cuboidal form. In fresh state their cytoplasm contains many pale droplets of *mucigen*, the antecedent of mucin. In fixed and stained sections, the droplets of mucigen are usually extracted so that the cell body appears clear and contains only a loose network of cytoplasm and traces of precipitated mucigen. This material stains red with mucicarmine, or metachromatically with thionine. The nucleus is near the base of the cell and usually appears angular and compressed when there is a large accumula-

tion of mucigen. The Golgi apparatus, mitochondria, and rough endoplasmic reticulum are located toward the cell base, below the mucigen granules. The amount of endoplasmic reticulum varies with the phase of the cell's secretory cycle. The juxtaluminal region of the epithelium is provided with a network of occluding junctions. Secretory canaliculi are absent. The lumen of the terminal portions of the glands is large and usually filled with masses of mucin.

When the secretion has been discharged, the cell collapses, and only a few granules of mucigen may remain near its free surface. In this depleted condition the mucous cells may be mistaken for serous cells, but the absence of intercellular secretory canaliculi always distinguishes mucous from serous glands. The demonstration of these canaliculi, however, requires special staining methods or electron microscopy. With the initiation of the secretory cycle, the cell organelles undergo morphological changes correlated with the cell's activity. Rarely under physiological conditions do the mucous cells discharge all of their granules. The cells, as a

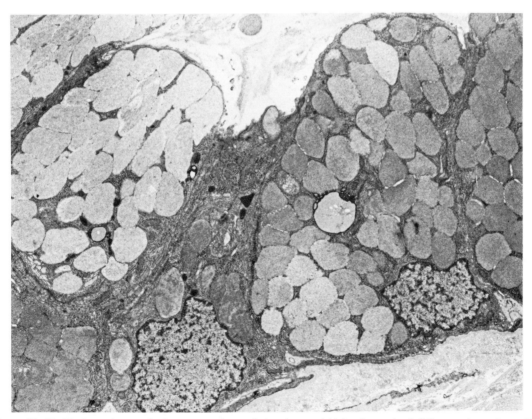

Figure 23–13. Electron micrograph of mucous acinar cells in a human labial salivary gland. (Micrograph courtesy of B. Tandler.)

rule, do not show any signs of degeneration and apparently recover completely from discharge of their secretion. Mitoses have occasionally been observed in them.

Serous Cells

These cells are roughly cuboidal and surround a small tubular lumen. In an unfixed resting gland they contain numerous highly refractile secretion granules that accumulate between the nucleus and the free surface. After the gland has secreted for a certain period, the serous cells diminish in size and their few remaining granules are confined to the juxtaluminal cytoplasm. The Golgi complex is usually found in an apical or paranuclear position, and cisternae of endoplasmic reticulum are abundant toward the cell base. Mitochondria are scattered among the cisternae at the base and in the apical cytoplasm as well. The luminal surface of the serous cells has sparse microvilli, and intercellular canaliculi lined with microvilli are found between the cells. In human submandibular glands, the serous acinar cells have numerous basal processes that interdigitate to form a complex basal labyrinth typical of cells transporting fluid and electrolytes.

The serous cells in the various oral glands have a similar microscopic structure even though they are not functionally identical (Figs. 23–17, 23–18). They are grouped together under a general heading because histological methods are not able to demonstrate differences corresponding to the variations in the nature of their secretions.

Salivary glands exhibit considerable interspecific variation in their cytology. In some, including the human parotid gland, cells with the appearance of serous cells have secretory granules that stain with the periodic acid–Schiff (PAS) reaction for carbohydrates and contain sialomucin and sulfomucin in addition to enzyme proteins. Such cells are termed *seromucous* cells.

Cells in the Mixed Glands

The relative numbers of the two kinds of glandular cells in the mixed glands vary within wide limits. In some cases the serous cells are far more numerous than the mucous cells, whereas in other glands the reverse is true. In still other instances, both cell types are present in about equal numbers. The mucous and serous cells line different parts of the terminal secretory portion of the

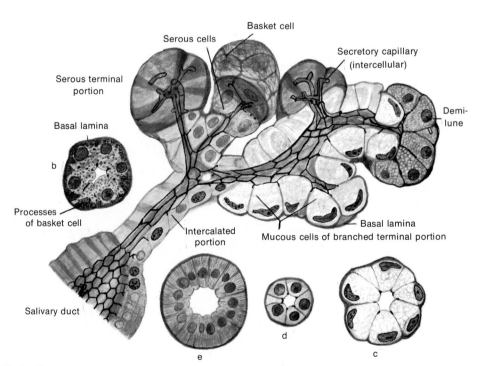

Figure 23–14. Reconstruction of a terminal portion of a submandibular gland with its duct. *b,* Cross section of a purely serous terminal portion, showing basal lamina; *c,* cross section through a purely mucous terminal portion; *d,* cross section through an intercalated portion; *e,* cross section through a salivary duct. (Redrawn and modified after a reconstruction by Vierling, from Braus.)

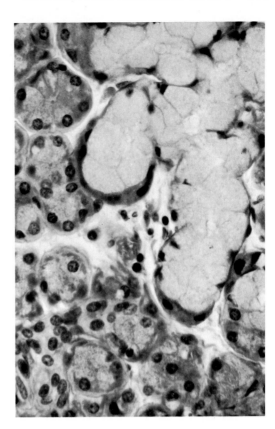

Figure 23–15. Photomicrograph of the human submandibular gland, a mixed gland, showing serous acini at lower left and mucous acini with serous demilunes at upper right. × 475.

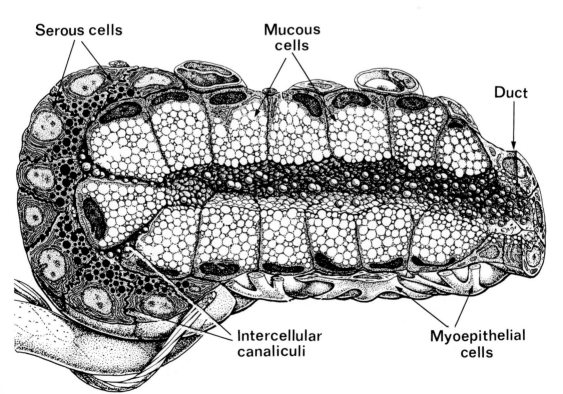

Figure 23–16. Drawing of a tubuloalveolar end piece in a mixed salivary gland showing mucous cells capped by a serous demilune. Human submandibular gland. (From Krstić, R.V. Die Gewebe des Menschen und der Säugetiere. Berlin, Springer Verlag, 1978.)

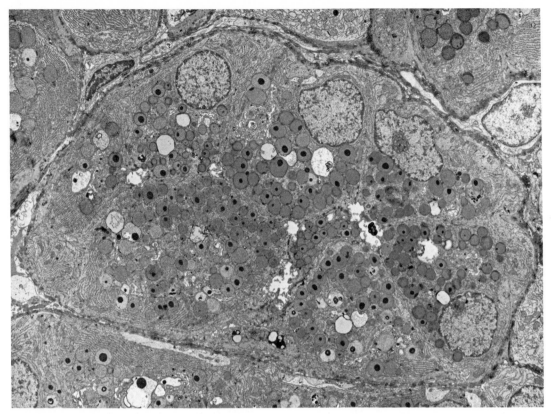

Figure 23–17. Electron micrograph of a serous acinus from human submandibular gland. (From Tandler, B., and R. A. Erlandson. Am. J. Anat. *135*:419, 1972.)

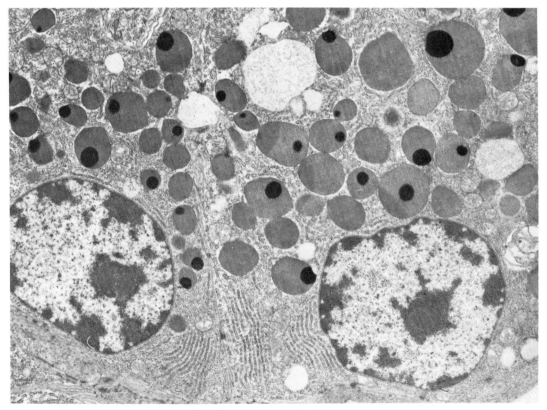

Figure 23–18. Electron micrograph of serous cells from submandibular gland of rhesus monkey. Notice the nonhomogeneity of the secretory granules, with dense and less dense regions. (Micrograph courtesy of A. Ichikawa.)

gland. In those mixed glands in which the serous cells predominate, some of the terminal portions may be exclusively serous (Fig. 23–15). In others a part of the secretory portion is lined with mucous cells and a part is lined with serous cells. In sections the mucous portions can usually be recognized by the clear, empty appearance of their cytoplasm, but they are identified more certainly by their color after staining of the mucus with the PAS reaction.

As a rule, the mucous cells are located nearer the ducts, whereas the serous cells are located at the end of the terminal secretory portion. It is quite probable that the mucous cells in mixed glands arise by differentiation of the cells in the smallest ducts. Sometimes single mucous cells are scattered among the unspecialized cells of the neck of the gland. In other cases where the mucous transformation affects all the cells, the neck of the duct ceases to exist as such. If the mucous cells are not numerous, the secretory portion of the gland will show an irregular mixture of the pale mucous and dark serous cells.

If the mucous cells predominate, the serous cells are displaced to the terminal portion or into saccular outpocketings of the acinus. Here they form small groups, which in sections appear as darkly staining crescents (*demilunes of Giannuzzi*) surrounding the ends of the tubules of mucous cells (Figs. 23–14, 23–15, 23–16). In the demilunes the serous cells are small and flattened and often seem to be entirely separated from the lumen by the large mucous cells. However, there are always secretory canaliculi that conduct the secretion through clefts between the mucous cells into the lumen (Fig. 23–16).

Basal Myoepithelial Cells

In all the glands of the oral cavity, the epithelium in the terminal portion, as well as in the ducts, is provided with basal cells. They lie between the glandular cells and the basal lamina and appear as slender, spindle-shaped or stellate elements (Fig. 23–16). Usually, only their nuclei can be discerned in sections. When seen from the surface, they exhibit a stellate cell body with processes containing many cytoplasmic filaments. In their ultrastructure, they resemble smooth muscle cells, and are presumed to be contractile and to facilitate the movement of the secretion into the ducts. They are considered to be myoepithelial cells and resemble those of the sweat glands and mammary gland.

Ducts of the Glands

The ducts of the glands of the oral cavity are of variable length and have a low cuboidal epithelium. Between the lining cells and the basal lamina are scattered myoepithelial cells. The epithelium of the necks may show varying degrees of transformation to mucous cells.

In the columnar epithelium of the striated segments of the ducts, the lower parts of the cell bodies exhibit a parallel striation, attributable to vertical orientation of mitochondria in slender compartments formed by infolding of the basal cell membrane (Fig. 23–19, 23–20, 23–21). The numerous infoldings of the basal surface of the cells in the striated ducts are not resolved with the light microscope but are visible with the electron microscope, as they are in other epithelia in which there is rapid transport of water and ions.

In the larger ducts the epithelium is columnar and pseudostratified, and occasionally contains goblet cells. Nearing the opening on the mucous membrane, it becomes stratified for a short distance and is then succeeded by stratified squamous epithelium.

Glands Opening into the Vestibule

Scattered in the mucous membrane of the upper and lower lips are small *labial glands* (Fig. 23–13). Similar glands associated with the mucous membrane of the cheeks are called *buccal glands*. Both of these are glands of mixed type. The secretory portion sometimes contains only seromucinous cells, but in most cases these are confined to the blind ends of the glands, with the remainder lined with mucous cells. Since the necks of the glands are short and branch very little, the mucous secretory portions often pass directly into striated ducts.

By far the largest salivary glands opening into the vestibule are the two *parotid glands*. Situated subcutaneously on either side of the face just in front of the ear, they extend from the zygomatic arch above to below the angle of the jaw. Each is connected to the vestibule by a long parotid duct (*Stenson's duct*), which emerges from the anterior border of the gland and courses forward and then through the cheek to open into the mouth opposite the second upper molar tooth. In the adult human, the gland is largely serous in its histological appearance. However, in large areas of the gland the cells have a positive staining reaction for carbohydrate and therefore must be interpreted as seromucous.

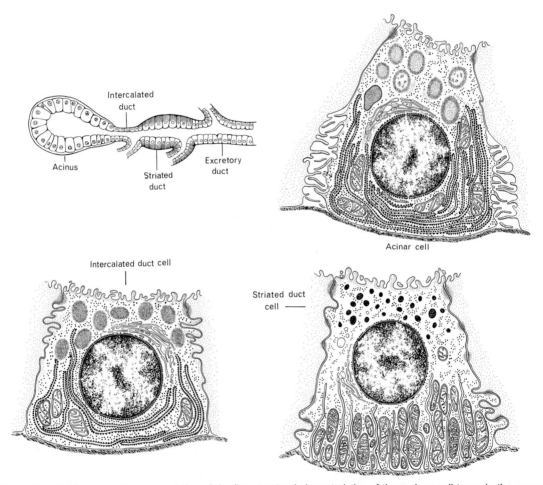

Figure 23–19. Diagrammatic representation of the fine structural characteristics of the various cell types in the mouse submandibular gland. (Redrawn after U. Rutberg.)

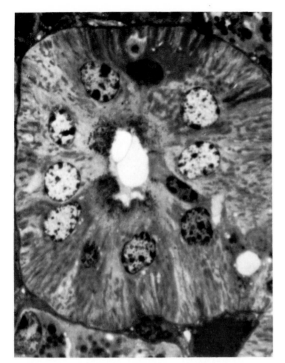

Figure 23–20. Photomicrograph of a striated duct from the parotid gland of a marmoset. Notice the orientation of mitochondria parallel to the cell axis, giving the basal cytoplasm a vertically striated appearance. (Micrograph courtesy of B. Tandler.)

Glands Opening on the Floor of the Mouth

In the space between the mandible and the muscles forming the floor of the mouth, on either side, is a large *submandibular gland*. Its duct (*Wharton's duct*), about 5 cm. long, leaves the deep surface of the gland and runs forward to open at the tip of the sublingual papilla on the floor of the mouth adjacent to the frenulum of the tongue. The secretory portion of the gland is mainly seromucous, but some parts are mucous, with serous cells at the blind ends. Typical serous demilunes (crescents of Giannuzzi) are less common in the submandibular gland of the human than in other species. Striated ducts are numerous and long and have many branches.

Deep to the mucous membrane on the underside of the tongue, there is a large *sublingual gland*, 3 to 4 cm long, on either side of the frenulum, and a number of smaller sublingual glands (Fig. 23–22). The ducts of the large glands open into the ducts of the submandibular gland. The small glands open separately along a fold of mucous membrane called the plica sublingualis.

At the posterior end of these is another group of small glands called the *glossopalatine glands*.

In the sublingual glands, mucous cells are far more numerous than in the submandibular glands. There are no acini formed exclusively of serous cells. For the most part these are arranged in thick demilunes. The gland consists of about 60 per cent mucous cells and 30 per cent serous cells. The striated ducts are few and short and are sometimes represented only by small groups of basally striated cells in the epithelium of the interlobular ducts. The glossopalatine glands are pure mucous glands.

Glands of the Tongue

On either side of the midline near the tip of the tongue is an *anterior lingual gland* (gland of Blandin or Nuhn). The anterior portion of this gland contains secretory tubules with seromucous cells only. Its posterior part consists of mixed branching tubules that contain mucous cells and, on their blind ends, thin demilunes of seromucous cells.

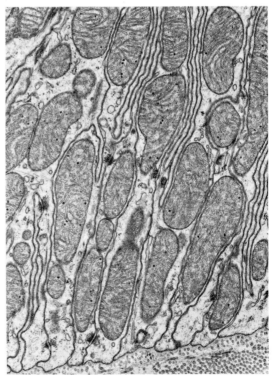

Figure 23–21. Electron micrograph of basal region of striated duct cells from cat submandibular gland. Notice the desmosomes joining the interdigitating processes of neighboring cells. (Micrograph courtesy of B. Tandler.)

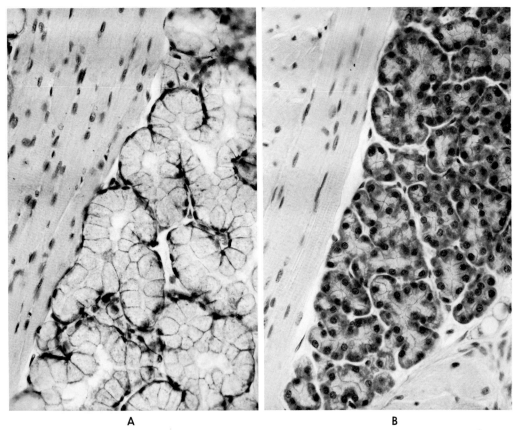

A   B

Figure 23–22. Lingual glands, situated among the bundles of striated muscle in rabbit tongue. *A,* Mucous glands. *B,* Serous glands. × 300.

The posterior lingual glands comprise the *glands of von Ebner* that open into the groove around the circumvallate papillae and the *mucous glands of the root of the tongue.* The long secretory portions of von Ebner's glands are branching tubules that contain only serous cells. Rarely these show a slight reaction for mucus. The system of ducts is poorly developed; isthmuses are absent. These glands form a thin serous secretion that evidently serves to wash out the circumvallate groove and the associated taste buds.

The *glands of the root of the tongue* and the *palatine glands* are of the pure mucous variety. Short isthmuses have been found in the latter group.

Blood and Lymphatic Vessels

In the interstitial reticular connective tissue of the salivary glands are fibroblasts and macrophages, with fat cells scattered singly or in small groups. Plasma cells are of common occurrence and, occasionally, small lymphocytes are also found. The larger blood vessels follow the larger ducts. Loose capillary

networks surround the ducts and the terminal portions. The lymph vessels are relatively scarce.

Nerves

Each salivary gland is provided with sensory nerve endings and two kinds of efferent secretory nerves, parasympathetic and sympathetic. The parasympathetic preganglionic fibers for the submandibular and sublingual glands run in the chorda tympani nerve to the submaxillary ganglion. The sympathetic preganglionic fibers go to the superior cervical ganglion. From here the postganglionic fibers follow along the carotid artery. The vasodilators are believed to be included in the chorda tympani, the vasoconstrictors in the sympathetic nerves.

The parotid gland receives its secretory fibers from the glossopharyngeal nerve. In the interstitial tissue, along the course of its blood vessels, are found plexuses of myelinated (preganglionic and sensory) and nonmyelinated fibers, and groups of sympathetic multipolar nerve cells close to the larger ducts. On the outer surface of the terminal portions, nonmyelinated fibers form a network that sends small branches through the basal lamina. These branches form a second network, from which branches penetrate between the glandular cells, ramify, and end on the surfaces of the glandular cells with small, terminal thickenings.

Stimulation of the parasympathetic nerves of the submandibular gland causes the secretion of an abundant thin saliva, rich in water and salts but poor in organic substances. Stimulation of the sympathetic nerve, on the contrary, yields a small quantity of thick saliva, with a high content of organic substances. The mechanism of action of the nerves upon the glandular cells and the role of the vasodilators in secretion are not known. The presence of different kinds of nerve endings has not been proved. It is even doubtful whether the secretory fibers in the chorda tympani and in the sympathetic nerve are of different nature.

After sectioning of the chorda tympani nerve in the dog, the so-called "paralytic" secretion in the corresponding submandibular and retrolingual glands occurs. This secretion is accompanied by intense degeneration and atrophy of the gland cells, especially of the mucous elements in the retrolingual gland.

HISTOPHYSIOLOGY OF THE SALIVARY GLANDS

The human salivary glands continually secrete at a basal rate of 0.5 to 1 ml per minute, and this is increased manyfold during meals. The total daily flow is about 1200 ml. The saliva serves to moisten and lubricate ingested food, and its enzyme α-amylase initiates the digestive process by hydrolyzing starch to soluble sugars.

The saliva also plays an important role in controlling the bacterial flora of the oral cavity. The mouth is always inhabited by a very large number and variety of pathogenic bacteria. Some of these contribute to the degradative processes of dental caries; others are capable of initiating ulcers and severe periodontal inflammation. They are held in check by the continual secretion and swallowing of saliva, which dislodges residual food particles and bacteria and sweeps them on down the alimentary tract. In addition to these mechanical effects, the saliva has bac-

tericidal properties. The principal function of the enzyme *lysozyme*, secreted by serous cells of salivary glands, is hydrolysis of bacterial cell walls. Deprived of their walls, the bacteria are more easily penetrated and killed by thiocyanate ions present in saliva.

The connective tissue of the stroma and interlobular septa of the glands contain lymphocytes and plasma cells. The latter produce immunoglobulins, mainly IgA. This forms a complex with a *secretory piece* synthesized in the serous cells of the acini, and the IgA–secretory piece complex is released into the saliva where it is believed to participate in immunological defense against bacteria in the oral cavity.

The salivary acini elaborate a *primary secretion* consisting of mucus, enzymes, and ions. The ionic concentration of this fluid is not significantly different from that of the extracellular fluid, but as it flows through the ducts it is greatly modified by active transport of certain ions by the epithelium lining the ducts. Bicarbonate ion is actively secreted by duct cells near the acini that contain carbonic anhydrase catalyzing the combination of water and carbon dioxide to form carbonic acid. The resulting bicarbonate ions are secreted and chloride ions absorbed in this region. Potassium ions are actively secreted, and sodium ions reabsorbed throughout the duct system. As a result of these active transport processes and ion exchanges, the sodium and chloride concentration of the saliva is only about one eighth that of blood plasma while the potassium concentration is seven times, and bicarbonate three times, greater than in plasma. Aldosterone, the adrenal hormone that controls absorption of sodium and excretion of potassium in the kidney, also influences the electrolyte concentration of the saliva. Acting upon the salivary duct system, it greatly increases reabsorption of sodium and the excretion of potassium.

TONSILS

The aperture through which the oral cavity communicates with the pharynx is called the *fauces*. In this region the mucous membrane of the digestive tract contains accumulations of lymphoid tissue. In addition to small infiltrations of lymphocytes, which may occur anywhere in this part of the mucous membrane, there are well-outlined organs of lymphoid tissue. The surface epithelium invaginates into them, and they are called *tonsils*. The lingual tonsils have been described above.

Between the glossopalatine and the pharyngopalatine arches are the *palatine tonsils*, two large oval accumulations of lymphoid tissue in the connective tissue beneath the mucous membrane. The overlying epithelium invaginates to form 10 to 20 deep *tonsillar crypts*. The stratified squamous epithelium of the free surface overlies a thin layer of connective tissue. The crypts reach almost to the connective tissue *capsule* and are of simple or branching form (Fig. 23–23).

The nodules with their prominent germinal centers are embedded in a diffuse mass of lymphoid tissue 1 to 2 mm thick, and are usually arranged in a single layer under the epithelium. The epithelial crypts with their surrounding sheaths of lymphoid tissue are partially separated from one another by thin partitions of loose connective tissue that extend inward from the capsule. In this connective tissue there are always numerous lymphocytes of various sizes, mast cells, and plasma cells. The presence of large numbers of polymorphonuclear leukocytes is indica-

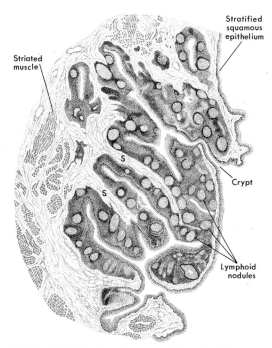

Figure 23–23. Section through palatine tonsil of man, showing crypts penetrating the tonsil from the free surface, and connective tissue septa *(S)* penetrating the lymphoid tissue from beneath. × 6. (Redrawn and modified from Sobotta.)

tive of inflammation, which is very common in tonsils. Occasionally islands of cartilage or bone are found, which are probably late sequelae of earlier pathological processes in the tonsils. In the deeper portions of the crypts, the limit between the epithelium and the lymphoid tissue is obscured by an intense infiltration of the epithelium with lymphocytes. The epithelial cells are pushed aside and distorted, so that only a few recognizable epithelial cells remain on the surface (Fig. 23–24). Plasma cells are common here.

The lymphocytes and neutrophils that pass through the epithelium are found in the saliva as the *salivary corpuscles*. They appear there as degenerating vesicular elements with a pyknotic nucleus surrounded by a clear vesicle containing granules that show brownian movement. The salivary corpuscles that originate from polymorphonuclear leukocytes are recognized by the remnants of their specific granules and their polymorphous nucleus.

The lumen of the crypts may contain large accumulations of living and degenerated lymphocytes mixed with desquamated squamous epithelial cells, granular detritus, and microorganisms. These masses may increase in size and form cheesy plugs, which are ultimately eliminated. If they remain for a long time, they may calcify. The microorganisms are sometimes the cause of inflammation and suppuration, and, carried to other parts of the body, they may be responsible for some general infections.

Many small glands are connected with the palatine tonsils. Their bodies are outside the capsule, and their ducts open for the most part on the free surface. Openings into the crypts seem rare.

In the roof and posterior wall of the nasopharynx is the unpaired *pharyngeal tonsil*. The epithelium on the surface of this tonsil is the same as in the rest of the respiratory passages—pseudostratified ciliated columnar epithelium with many goblet cells. Small patches of stratified squamous epithelium are common, however. The epithelium is not invaginated to form crypts like those of the palatine tonsil but is plicated to form numerous surface folds. It is abundantly infiltrated with lymphocytes, especially on the crests of the folds. A 2-mm thick layer of diffuse and nodular lymphoid tissue is found under the epithelium and participates in the formation of the folds. The lymphoid tissue of the tonsil is separated from the surrounding parts by

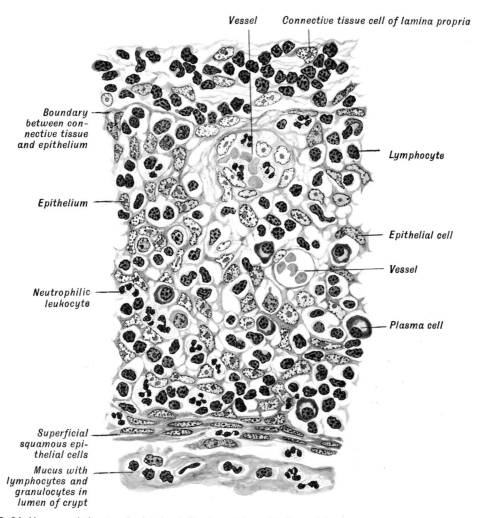

Vessel   Connective tissue cell of lamina propria

Boundary
between con-
nective tissue
and epithelium

Epithelium

Neutrophilic
leukocyte

Superficial
squamous epi-
thelial cells

Mucus with
lymphocytes and
granulocytes in
lumen of crypt

Lymphocyte

Epithelial cell

Vessel

Plasma cell

Figure 23–24. Human palatine tonsil, showing infiltration of the epithelium of the crypt with lymphocytes, neutrophilic (heterophilic) granular leukocytes, and plasma cells. Hematoxylin-eosin-azure stain. × 520. (After A. A. Maximow.)

a thin connective tissue capsule, which sends thin partitions into the core of each fold. Outside the capsule are small glands of mixed character. Their ducts—often markedly dilated—traverse the lymphoid tissue and empty into the furrows or on the folds.

Other small accumulations of lymphoid tissue occur in the mucous membrane of the pharynx, especially around the orifices of the eustachian tubes, behind the pharyngopalatine arches, and in the posterior wall.

Unlike the lymph nodes, the tonsils do not have lymphatic sinuses, and lymph is not filtered through them. However, plexuses of blindly ending lymph capillaries surround their outer surface.

The tonsils generally reach their maximal development in childhood. The involution of the palatine tonsils begins about the age of

15 or earlier, though the nodules on the root of the tongue persist longer. The pharyngeal tonsil is usually found in an atrophic condition in the adult, with its ciliated epithelium largely replaced by stratified squamous epithelium.

THE PHARYNX

The posterior continuation of the oral cavity is the pharynx. In this region of the digestive tract, the respiratory passage and the pathway for food merge and cross. The upper part of the pharynx is the *nasal*, the middle the *oral*, and the lower the *laryngeal* portion. In the upper part its structure resembles that of the respiratory system,

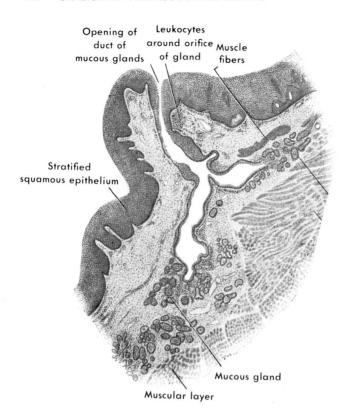

Opening of duct of mucous glands

Leukocytes around orifice of gland

Muscle fibers

Stratified squamous epithelium

Mucous gland

Muscular layer

Figure 23–25. Longitudinal section of the wall of the pharynx of an 11-year-old girl. × 27. (After Schaffer.)

whereas in the lower part it corresponds more closely to the general plan of the digestive tube.

Instead of a muscularis mucosae, the mucous membrane is provided with a thick, dense, elastic layer. A loose submucous layer is well developed only in the lateral wall of the nasopharynx and where the pharynx continues into the esophagus; here the elastic layer becomes thinner. In all other places, the mucous membrane is directly adjacent to the muscular wall, which consists of an inner longitudinal and an outer oblique or circular layer of striated muscle. The elastic layer fuses with the interstitial tissue of the muscle and sends strands of elastic fibers between the muscular bundles. In the fornix it is fused with the periosteum of the base of the skull.

The lamina propria mucosae consists of dense connective tissue containing fine elastic networks. Those areas covered with stratified squamous epithelium are provided with small papillae. In the area covered with pseudo-stratified ciliated columnar epithelium there are no papillae.

The two lower sections of the pharynx and a part of the nasal region have stratified squamous epithelium. Toward the roof of the pharynx its epithelium becomes stratified columnar ciliated, with many goblet cells. On the lateral sides of the nasopharynx this ciliated epithelium continues downward beyond the aperture of the eustachian tube. With age, the ciliated epithelium may be replaced by stratified squamous epithelium over large areas.

Glands of a pure mucous type are found in those places lined with stratified squamous epithelium (Fig. 23–25). They are always located under the elastic layer, sometimes penetrating deep into the muscle. Glands of mixed type, similar to those of the dorsal surface of the soft palate, are confined to the regions covered with ciliated epithelium.

REFERENCES

TONGUE AND TASTE BUDS

Beidler, L. M., and R. L. Smallman: Renewal of cells with the taste buds. J. Cell Biol. *27*:263, 1965.

Farbman, A. I.: Fine structure of the taste bud. J. Ultrastruct. Res. *12*:328, 1965.

Hodgson, E. S.: Taste receptors. Sci. Am. *204*:135, 1961.

Murray, R. G., and S. Fujimoto: Fine structure of gustatory cells in the rabbit taste buds. J. Ultrastruct Res. *27*:444, 1969.

Oakley, B., and R. P. Benjamin: Neural mechanisms of taste. Physiol. Rev. *46*:173, 1966.

Tucker, D., and J. Smith: The chemical senses. Annu. Rev. Psychol. *20*:129, 1969.

Zotterman, Y.: Olefaction and Taste. New York, Macmillan Co., 1963.

SALIVARY GLANDS

Amsterdam, A., I. Ohad, and M. Schramm: Dynamic changes in the ultrastructure of the acinar cell of the rat parotid gland during the secretory cycle. J. Cell Biol. *41*:753, 1969.

Amsterdam, A., M. Schramm, I. Ohad, et al.: Concomitant syntheses of membrane protein and exportable protein of the secretory granules in rat parotid gland. J. Cell Biol. *40*:187, 1971.

Castle, J. D., J. D. Jamieson, and G. E. Palade: Radioautographic analysis of the secretory process in the parotid acinar cell of the rabbit. J. Cell Biol. *53*:290, 1972.

Junquiera, L. C., and F. F. de Moraes: Comparative aspects of the vertebrate major salivary glands biology. *In* Wohlfarth-Botterman, K. E., ed.: Functionelle und Morphologische Organization der Zelle: Sekretion und Excretion. Heidelberg–Berlin–New York, Springer Verlag, 1965.

Leeson, C. R.: Structure of the salivary glands. *In* Handbook of Physiology. Vol. 2, Sect. 6. Washington, DC, American Physiological Society, 1967.

Mason, D. K., and D. M. Chisholm: Salivary Glands in Health and Disease. London, W. B. Saunders Co., 1975.

Shackleford, J., and C. E. Klapper: Structure and carbohydrate histochemistry of mammalian salivary glands. Am. J. Anat. *111*:25, 1962.

Spicer, S. G., and L. Warren: The histochemistry of sialic acid containing mucoproteins. J. Histochem. Cytochem. *8*:135, 1960.

Strum, J. M., and M. J. Karmovsky: Ultrastructural localization of peroxidase in submaxillary acinar cells. J. Ultrastruct. Res. *16*:320, 1970.

Tamarin, A., and L. Screenby: The rat submaxillary gland. A comparative study by light and electron microscopy. J. Morphol. *117*:295, 1965.

Tandler, B.: Ultrastructure of human submaxillary gland. I. Architecture and histological relationships of the secretory cells. Am. J. Anat. *111*:287, 1962.

Tandler, B.: Ultrastructure of human submaxillary gland. II. The base of the striated duct cells. J. Ultrastruct Res. *9*:165, 1963.

Tandler, B., C. R. Denning, I. D. Mandel, and A. H. Kutscher: Ultrastructure of human labial salivary glands. III. Myoepithelium and ducts. J. Morphol. *130*:227, 1970.

Young, J. A.: Salivary secretion of inorganic electrolytes. Int. Rev. Physiol. *19*:1, 1979.

Young, J. A., and E. W. van Lennep: Morphology and physiology of salivary myoepithelial cells. Int. Rev. Physiol. *12*:105, 1977.

24

THE TEETH

The adult human has 32 teeth of which 16 are in the alveolar process of the maxilla and 16 in the mandible. These permanent teeth are preceded by a set of 20 *deciduous teeth* that begin to erupt about seven months after birth and reach their full complement at 6 to 8 years of age. These are shed between the sixth and 13th year and are gradually replaced by the permanent or *succedaneous teeth.* This process of replacement extends over a period of about 12 years, and full dentition is usually attained by the age of 18 with the eruption of the third molars. Each of the several types of teeth in each set has a distinctive form adapted to its specific function. Thus, the *incisors* are specialized for cutting or shearing; the pointed *canines* for puncturing and holding; and the *molars* for crushing and grinding.

All teeth consist of a *crown* projecting above the gum or gingiva and one or more tapering *roots* that occupy conforming sockets or *alveoli* in the bone of the maxilla or of the mandible. The junctional region between the crown and the root is called the *neck* or *cervix.* Incisors have a single root, lower molars two, and upper molars three. The tooth contains a small central *pulp chamber* or *cavity* that corresponds roughly in its shape to the outer form of the tooth. This continues downward into each root as a narrow canal that communicates with the *periodontal membrane* through an *apical foramen* at the tip of the root.

The hard portions of a tooth consist of three different tissues: *dentin, enamel,* and *cementum* (Fig. 24–1). The bulk of the tooth is formed of the *dentin,* which surrounds the pulp chamber. It is thickest in the crown and gradually tapers as it reaches the apex of the root. Its outer surface is covered, in the region of the crown, by a layer of *enamel,* which is thinnest in the cervical region. On the root the tooth is covered by a thin layer of *cementum,* which extends from the neck to the apical foramina.

The soft parts associated with the tooth are the *pulp,* which fills the pulp chamber; the *periodontal membrane,* which connects the cementum-covered surface of the root with the alveolar bone; and the *gingiva,* that portion of the oral mucous membrane surrounding the tooth. In young persons the gingiva is attached to the enamel; with increasing age it gradually recedes from the enamel, and in old people it is attached to the cementum.

Dentin

Dentin makes up the bulk of the tooth. It is formed by a layer of *odontoblasts* that lines the pulp cavity. Dentin is yellowish in color and semitranslucent in the fresh condition. Although it resembles bone in structure and chemical composition, it is harder than compact bone. It consists of 20 per cent organic and 80 per cent inorganic matter. The organic part is 92 per cent collagen, and most of the inorganic components are in the form of hydroxyapatite crystals. Upon decalcification in acids, only the organic part remains and the substance of the tooth becomes soft. Upon incineration, only the inorganic mate-

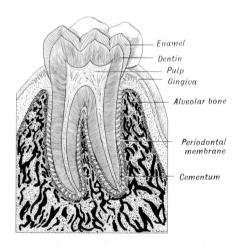

Figure 24–1. Diagram of sagittal section of adult human lower first permanent molar. (Courtesy of I. Schour.)

rial remains. The inorganic material is much the same as in bone, except that it is denser and more insoluble. The organic part, like other collagen-rich tissues, also contains glycosaminoglycan–protein complexes.

In a ground section passing through the axis of an extracted tooth, the dentin has a radially striated appearance (Fig. 24–2). This is attributable to the presence of innumerable minute canals, the *dentinal tubules,* which radiate from the pulp cavity toward the periphery. Apical cytoplasmic processes from the formative cells, called odontoblasts, extend into these minute tubules. Near the pulp, their diameter is 3 to 4 μm, but in the outer

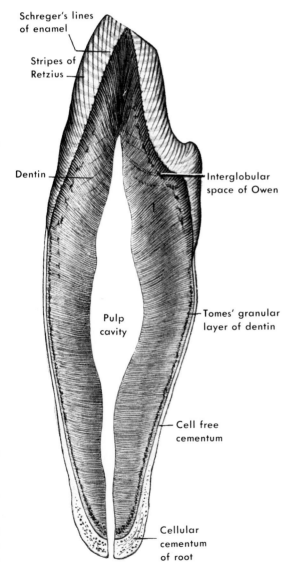

Figure 24–2. Longitudinal ground section of human cuspid. The top of the crown has been abraded. × 7. (After von Ebner, from Schaffer.)

Labels on figure:
Schreger's lines of enamel
Stripes of Retzius
Dentin
Pulp cavity
Interglobular space of Owen
Tomes' granular layer of dentin
Cell free cementum
Cellular cementum of root

portions they become narrower. In their outward course from the pulp cavity, most of the dentinal tubules describe an S-shaped curve. The layer of dentin immediately surrounding each tubule, the *sheath of Neumann,* differs from the rest of the dentin in its high refringence and denser staining in decalcified specimens.

Between the dentinal tubules are bundles of collagenous fibrils corresponding to the collagenous fibrils within bone. They are embedded in a ground substance consisting of glycosaminoglycans and protein. The course of the fibrillar bundles is, in general, parallel to the long axis of the tooth and perpendicular to the dentinal tubules. Some investigators distinguish a peripheral layer, the *cover* or *mantle dentin,* characterized by a branching pattern of dentinal tubules, and a thicker inner layer, the *circumpulpar dentin,* with thinner, straighter tubules.

The calcification of the developing dentin is not always complete and uniform. The mineral deposits that appear during development in the organic ground substance have the form of spherical aggregations of apatite crystals, which gradually gain in size and finally fuse. These nuclei of mineralization are found initially in rows or chains on and within collagen fibrils. In incompletely calcified regions, between the calcified spheres, there remain angular "interglobular" spaces that contain only the organic matrix of the dentin (Fig. 24–3). The dentinal tubules continue uninterrupted through the spheres and interglobular spaces. In a macerated tooth from which all organic parts have been extracted, the tubules, as well as the interglobular spaces, are filled with air and appear dark in transmitted light. In many normal human teeth there are layers of large interglobular spaces in the deeper parts of the dentin of the crown. Mineralization in dentin is not uniform, and as a result, curvilinear lines of appositional growth are apparent. These are called the *contour lines of Owen.* Immediately under the dentinocemental junction in the root there is always a layer of small interglobular spaces, the *granular layer of Tomes* (Fig. 24–2).

In sections through a decalcified tooth, each dentinal tubule contains a slender cytoplasmic process, *Tomes' fiber,* which in life probably completely fills the lumen of the tubule, but which in fixed preparations appears shrunken away from the wall. When the tubules are seen in cross section, each

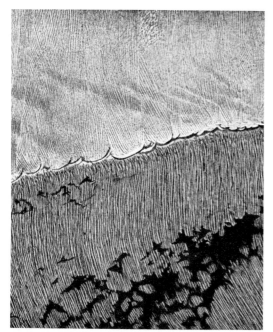

Figure 24-3. Dentinoenamel junction of a tooth of a man; ground section. The enamel prisms appear as a fine, wavy striation. The interglobular spaces in the dentin are black (air filled). Between these lacunae are the dentinal tubules. × 80. (After Braus.)

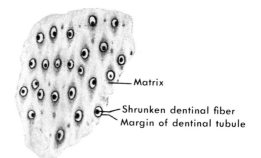

Figure 24-4. Tangential section through the root of a molar of an ape. The margin of the dentinal tubule is also called the sheath of Neumann. The dot in the center of each dentinal tubule is a somewhat shrunken Tomes' fiber. × 740. (After Schaffer.)

small oval contains a dark dot (Fig. 24-4). These Tomes' fibers are the processes of the *odontoblasts.* Dentin continues to be formed very slowly throughout life, and the pulp cavity is therefore progressively narrowed with advancing age.

The dentin is sensitive to touch, to cold, to acid-containing foods, and the like. Only occasional nerve fibers penetrate for short distances into the dentin. It has been suggested that the odontoblastic processes may transmit sensory stimulation to the pulp, which is richly innervated.

In old age the dentinal tubules are often obliterated through calcification. The dentin then becomes more transparent. When the dentin is exposed by extensive abrasion of the enamel of the crown, or when the outside of the tooth is irritated, a production of new or "secondary" dentin of irregular structure may often be observed on the wall of the pulp chamber. This may be so extensive as to fill the chamber completely.

Enamel

Enamel is the hardest substance found in the body. It is bluish white and transparent in thin-ground sections. When fully devel-

oped, enamel consists almost entirely of calcium salts in the form of large apatite crystals; only 0.5 per cent is organic substance. The protein matrix of enamel, secreted by cells called *ameloblasts,* has been isolated, and oriented samples have been subjected to x-ray diffraction analysis. The protein was found to be in the cross-β configuration. Complete amino acid analysis revealed that one fourth of the amino acid residues are proline. The protein therefore cannot be either keratin or collagen. Relatively high concentrations of

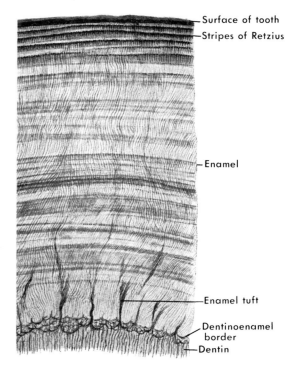

Figure 24-5. Portion of a ground cross section of crown of a human cuspid. × 80. (After Schaffer.)

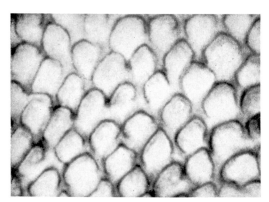

Figure 24–6. Enamel rods of human tooth in cross section. The dark lines are the interprismatic substance between the pale rods. Photomicrograph at high magnification. (Courtesy of B. Orban.)

organic-bound phosphorus have been found in bovine enamel organ matrix. This may play a role in the initiation of enamel calcification. After decalcification of a fully developed tooth, the enamel, as a rule, is completely dissolved.

As seen with the light microscope, the enamel consists of thin rods or prisms that stand upright on the surface of the dentin, usually with a pronounced inclination toward the incisal or occlusal edge (Fig. 24–5). Between the rods is "interprismatic substance," which has a substructure identical to that of the rods but is oriented in a different direction. Surrounding each rod is a clear area of organic matrix called the *enamel sheath* or *prismatic rod sheath* (Fig. 24–6). Every rod runs through the whole thickness of the enamel layer. This, however, cannot be seen in sections of the enamel, because the rods are twisted and soon pass out of the plane of section. In a ground preparation, the substance of a rod in its longitudinal section seems homogeneous. However, after acid acts upon such a section, a distinct cross striation appears in the rods; this indicates that the calcification probably proceeds layer by layer.

Studies with the electron microscope show that the *enamel rods* or *prisms* and the interprismatic substance are both composed of apatite crystals and organic material. The relations of the crystals in the prisms and in

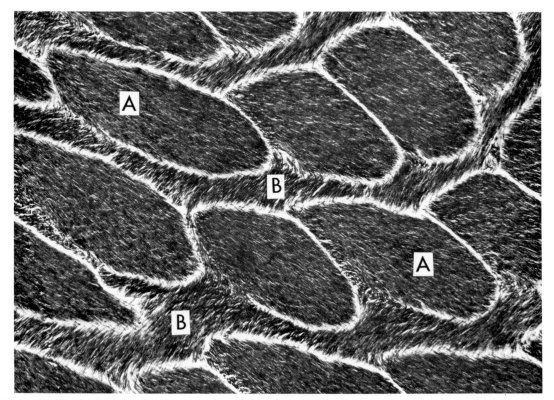

Figure 24–7. Slightly oblique section of undecalcified calf enamel, showing the roughly ovoid enamel prisms *(A)* and the interprismatic substance *(B)*. Note the remarkable orientation of the apatite crystals within the individual prisms, and the different orientation of the crystals in the interprismatic substance. Note also the clear areas that define the prisms. Embedded in methacrylate and sectioned with the diamond knife. Osmium fixation. × 18,000. (Courtesy of E. J. Daniel and M. J. Glimcher.)

the interprismatic substance are clearly shown in Figures 24–7 and 24–8.

In the human tooth, most of the rods in cross section have the form of fluted semicircles. The convex surfaces of all rods face the dentin, and their cross sections have a scale-like appearance (Fig. 24–6). The three-dimensional configuration and arrangement of the enamel rods in human teeth is still controversial. Some investigators report that in electron micrographs the enamel rods in cross section have a keyhole shape, and that the asymmetrical projection is what others call interprismatic substance. This form and arrangement are explained by calcification beginning earlier on the side of the rods that lies nearest the dentin. This inner, harder side is supposed to press into the softer side of the adjacent rod, compressing it and leaving one or two groovelike impressions.

The exact course of the enamel rods is extremely complicated but seems to be perfectly adapted to the mechanical requirements of the grinding and crushing of food. Starting from the dentin, the rods run perpendicular to its surface; in the middle zone of the enamel they bend helically, and in the outer zone they again assume a direction perpendicular to the surface. In addition, the rods show numerous small, wavy curves. On the lateral surfaces of the crown the rods are arranged in zones that encircle the tooth in horizontal planes. The bends of the rods in two neighboring zones cross one another. In axial, longitudinal ground sections, the crossing of groups of rods appears in reflected light as light and dark lines, more or less perpendicular to the surface—the *lines of Schreger* (Fig. 24–2).

In a cross section of the crown, the enamel shows concentric lines, which are brown in transmitted light and colorless in reflected light. In longitudinal, undecalcified axial sections they are seen to run obliquely inward from the surface and toward the root. They are called the *lines of Retzius* or *incremental lines of Retzius* and are connected with the circular striation on the surface of the crown (Fig. 24–2). They are believed to result from rhythmic deposition and mineralization of enamel matrix.

The free surface of the enamel is covered

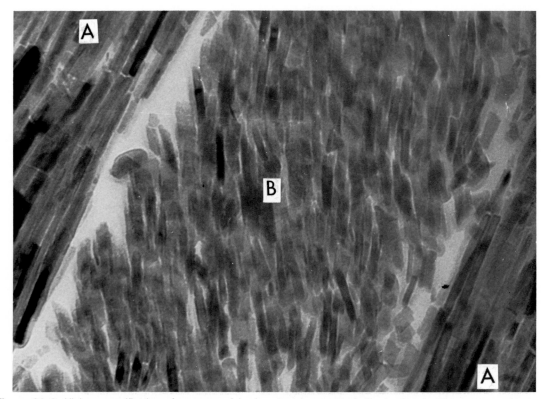

Figure 24–8. Higher magnification of an area of bovine dental enamel similar to that in Figure 24–7, showing longitudinally oriented prismatic crystals *(A)* with the interprismatic crystals *(B)* oriented approximately 30 degrees to the direction of the crystals within the prism. Osmium fixation. × 100,000. (Courtesy of E. J. Daniel and M. J. Glimcher.)

by two thin layers. The inner *enamel cuticle* (formerly called Nasmyth's membrane) is about one micron thick, and appears to be the final product of the activity of the enamel-forming ameloblasts before they disappear. The outer is an acellular layer, probably derived from the keratinized remnants of the dental sac of the developing tooth. It is continuous with the cementum covering the root and is similar in composition and histological structure. This layer is tenaciously adherent to the tooth and is distinct from the connective tissue of the gingiva. It may persist for some time after eruption of the tooth.

In an axial section of the tooth, the line of junction between the dentin and the enamel *(dentinoenamel junction)* is uneven and scalloped. Pointed or spindle-shaped processes of dentin penetrate the enamel. The spindle-shaped processes of the dentinal matrix penetrating a short distance into the enamel are called *enamel spindles.*

Local disturbances of the enamel during development cause the so-called *enamel lamellae* and *tufts.* These lamellae, usually found in cervical enamel, are organic material extending from the surface of the enamel toward and sometimes into the dentin. The tufts extend from the dentinoenamel junction into the enamel for one third of its thickness. The tuftlike shape, however, is an optical illusion, due to the projection, into one plane, of fibers lying in different planes. They are groups of poorly calcified, twisted enamel rods with abundant cementing substance between them.

Cementum

The *cementum* covering most of the root is coarsely fibrillar bone substance. The periodontal ligament attaches to it and to the alveolar bone. Of all the dental hard tissues, cementum is the closest to bone in physical and chemical characteristics. In the adult the organic matrix is elaborated by the *cementocytes* embedded in the apical cementum. The cervical portion of the cementum is acellular, whereas at the apex there is only a thin layer of *acellular cementum* adjacent to the dentin. The remainder of the cementum in this region is *cellular cementum.* Canaliculi, haversian systems, and blood vessels are normally absent. The layer of cementum increases in thickness with age, especially near the end of the root, and then haversian systems with blood vessels may appear.

Coarse collagenous bundles from the periodontal membrane penetrate the cementum. These fibers, corresponding to Sharpey's fibers of bone, remain uncalcified and in ground sections of a tooth appear as empty canals.

Not infrequently, epithelial cells are found in cementum. These are thought to be remnants of *Hertwig's epithelial root sheath.*

Unlike the dentin, which may remain unchanged even after the destruction of the pulp and the odontoblasts and after the "filling" of the pulp cavity, the cementum readily undergoes necrosis when the periodontal membrane is destroyed. On the other hand, new layers of cementum may be deposited on the surface of the root. This deposition is called *cementum hyperplasia* when it becomes excessive and is considered to be a reaction to chronic irritation.

Pulp

The *pulp* occupies the pulp cavity of the tooth and is the connective tissue that formed the dental papilla during embryonic development. In the adult it has an abundant, gelatinous, metachromatic ground substance similar to that of mucoid connective tissue. It contains a multitude of thin collagenous fibrils running in all directions and not aggregated into bundles. Elastic fibers are found only in the walls of the afferent vasculature.

The odontoblasts are the cells of the pulp adjacent to the dentin. Beneath the layer of odontoblasts is a relatively cell-free area, *the zone of Weil.* With silver impregnation techniques, bundles of reticular fibers *(Korff's fibers)* are found in this zone (Fig. 24–9). These fibers, described by light microscopists, pass from the pulp into interstices between the odontoblasts and their distal ends are incorporated in the dentinal matrix. Occasional cells are found in the zone of Weil, and capillaries and nerves are plentiful. Adjacent to this cell-poor zone, at the periphery of the pulp proper, is a cell-rich zone. Spindle-shaped or stellate fibroblasts are the predominant cell type of the pulp. Other cells present in limited numbers include mesenchymal cells, macrophages, lymphocytes, plasma cells, and eosinophils.

The pulp continues into the narrow root canal, where it surrounds the blood vessels and nerves, and continues through the openings in the root apex into the periodontal

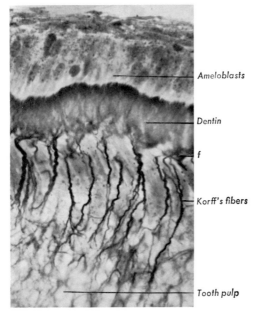

Ameloblasts

Dentin

f

Korff's fibers

Tooth pulp

Figure 24–9. Continuation of Korff's fibers of the pulp into the matrix of the dentin at *(f)*. Photomicrograph. × 700. (Courtesy of B. Orban.)

membrane. The pulp contains blood vessels and lymphatics, which enter and leave the pulp through the apical foramen. The circulation of the pulp consists of a system of arterioles and capillaries close to the bases of the odontoblasts. These drain into small veins more centrally situated in the pulp. Arteriovenous anastomoses are readily demonstrable in the pulp. Numerous bundles of myelinated nerve fibers, which arise from small cells in the gasserian ganglion, enter the pulp cavity through the canal of the root. They form a plexus in the pulp, from which arises a finer plexus of nonmyelinated fibers in the peripheral layers. Nerve endings have been described between the odontoblasts.

Periodontal Membrane

The *periodontal membrane,* which also serves as periosteum to the alveolar bone, furnishes a firm fibrous attachment of the root to the bone. It differs from the usual periosteum by the absence of elastic fibers. It consists, in part, of thick collagenous bundles, that run from the alveolar wall into the cementum of the roots. The orientation of the fibers varies at different levels in the alveolus. From root tip to neck, there are the *cementoalveolar fibers,* which are variously designated as *apical,* *oblique,* or *horizontal,* and *alveolar crest fibers.* The terms describe their direction or their

attachments. The fiber bundles of the periodontal membrane have a slightly wavy course. When the tooth is not functioning, they are slack and permit it to move slightly on the application of stress. The ligament adjacent to the cementum contains only *cementoblasts* and the usual complement of connective tissue cells. On the alveolar bone side of the periodontal ligament, osteoblasts and osteoclasts may be found.

Scattered in many places in the periodontal membrane, especially near the surface of the cementum, are blood and lymph vessels and nerves embedded in a thin layer of loose connective tissue, and small islands of epithelium. These islands are vestiges of the epithelial sheath of Hertwig, which will be described below in the section on the histogenesis of teeth. The epithelial rests frequently degenerate and undergo calcification, giving rise to the *cementicles.*

The Gingiva

The gum or *gingiva* is that part of the mucous membrane that is firmly connected with the periosteum at the crest of the alveolar bone. It is a keratinized stratified squamous epithelium with numerous connective tissue papillae projecting into its base. It is also linked to the surface of the tooth by the *epithelial attachment of Gottlieb,* which gradually recedes with advancing age, moving toward the root.

Although the gingiva generally has high papillae, the epithelial attachment to a tooth is devoid of papillae except when chronically inflamed. Between the epithelium and the enamel there is a small furrow surrounding the crown, the *gingival crevice,* which is lined by a nonkeratinizing stratified squamous epithelium. The *crevicular margin* of the epithelial attachment is the junction between the attached gingiva and the *marginal gingiva,* which surrounds the tooth like a collar about 1 mm wide.

The thinner portions of the gingival epithelium covering the papillae protrude slightly, giving a nubbled appearance to the otherwise smooth free surface. The crevicular epithelium is devoid of papillae except when chronically inflamed. Three groups of collagenous fibers are associated with the gingiva: the gingivodental group, the cuticular group, and the transseptal group, the latter usually being associated with the fibers of the periodontal ligament. Small aggregates of lymphocytes and plasma cells are usually found in the lamina propria at the base of the gingival crevice.

Alveolar Bone

As the teeth are formed, so is the bone that supports them, and it is to this bone that the principal fibers of the periodontal ligament attach. This *alveolar bone* consists of cancellous bone between two layers of cortical bone. The outer cortical plate is a continuation of the cortical layer of the maxilla or mandible. The inner cortical plate adjacent to the periodontal membrane is referred to by radiologists as the *lamina dura*. It surrounds the roots of the teeth to form the socket. The vessels and nerves to the teeth course through the alveolar bone to the apical foramina of the roots where they enter into the pulp chamber. Considerable resorption of alveolar bone can occur after loss of permanent teeth or as a result of periodontitis (inflammation of the supporting tissues of the teeth). Alveolar bone is very labile and serves as a readily available source of calcium to maintain blood levels. The cancellous trabeculae buttressed by the labial and lingual cortical plates aid in support of the teeth during mastication.

HISTOGENESIS OF THE TEETH

The teeth are derivatives of the oral mucous membrane. They may be considered to be modified papillae of the epithelium that have been covered by a thick layer of calcified material originating in part from the epithelium and in part from the underlying connective tissue. The most primitive toothlike structures are the placoid scales found in the integument of elasmobranch fish, where their derivation from papillae of the epidermis is quite evident.

In human embryos of the fifth week, the ectodermal epithelium lining the oral cavity presents a thickening along the edge of the future upper and lower jaws. The thickening consists of two parallel epithelial ridges that extend into the subjacent mesenchyme. Of these, the labial ridge later splits and forms the space between lip and alveolar process of the jaw. The lingual ridge, nearer the tongue, produces teeth and is called the *dental lamina*.

The edge of the dental lamina extends into the mesenchyme of the jaw and shows at several points budlike thickenings, the *tooth germs,* that are the primordia of the teeth (Fig. 24–10*A,B*). There are ten tooth germs in each jaw, one for each deciduous tooth. In each germ a group of epithelial cells becomes conspicuous as the *enamel knot* or *cord*, a temporary structure that later disappears (Fig. 24–11). The cells of the mesenchyme under the enamel knot aggregate in a dense group to form the primordium of the papilla (Figs. 24–10*C*, 24–11, 24–12). The dental lamina then extends posteriorly beyond the last deciduous tooth germ and slowly forms germs of the permanent molars, which are not preceded by corresponding deciduous teeth.

Beginning with the 10th to 12th weeks, the remainder of the dental lamina again produces solid epithelial buds—the *germs for the permanent teeth*—one on the lingual side of each deciduous germ (Fig. 24–13). After the formation of the permanent tooth germs, the dental lamina disappears. The germs of the permanent teeth undergo the same transformations as do those of the deciduous teeth.

The papilla enlarges and invaginates into the base of the epithelial tooth germ (Figs. 24–10*C,D*, 24–11, 24–12). The latter, while still connected by an epithelial strand with the dental lamina, becomes bell shaped and caps the convex upper surface of the papilla. Thenceforth it is called the *enamel organ,* because in its further development it produces the enamel. Both the papilla and the enamel organ gradually gain in height, and the latter soon acquires approximately the shape of the future tooth.

A concentric layer of connective tissue, the *dental sac*, develops around the tooth primordium and interrupts its epithelial connection with the oral cavity. Around the sac, and at a certain distance from it, the maxillary or mandibular bone develops (Fig. 24–12).

The peripheral cells of the enamel organ are arranged in a regular, radial fashion. On the convex outer surface of the enamel organ, the cells remain small and cuboidal. On its invaginated base, the cells of the inner enamel epithelium become tall and columnar and differentiate into *ameloblasts* that elaborate the enamel. In the interior of the enamel organ a clear liquid accumulates between the cell bodies, which remain connected by long processes. This tissue of epithelial origin thus acquires a reticular appearance like that of connective tissue and forms the *stellate reticulum* of the enamel pulp (Fig. 24–12).

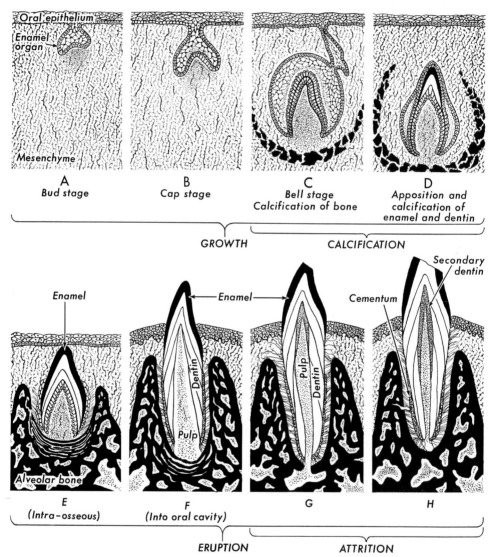

Figure 24–10. Diagram of life cycle of a human deciduous incisor. The normal resorption of the root is not indicated. Enamel and bone are drawn in black. (Redrawn and modified from Schour and Massler.)

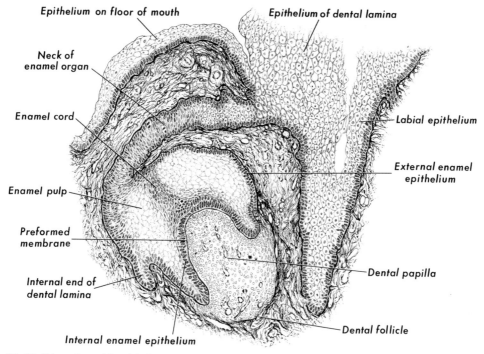

Figure 24–11. Primordium of the right lower central incisor of a human fetus of 91 days, in sagittal section. Collagenous fibers are black. Mallory's connective tissue stain. × 80. (Redrawn and modified from Schaffer.)

Epithelium on floor of mouth

Epithelium of dental lamina

Neck of enamel organ

Enamel cord

Labial epithelium

External enamel epithelium

Enamel pulp

Preformed membrane

Internal end of dental lamina

Dental papilla

Internal enamel epithelium

Dental follicle

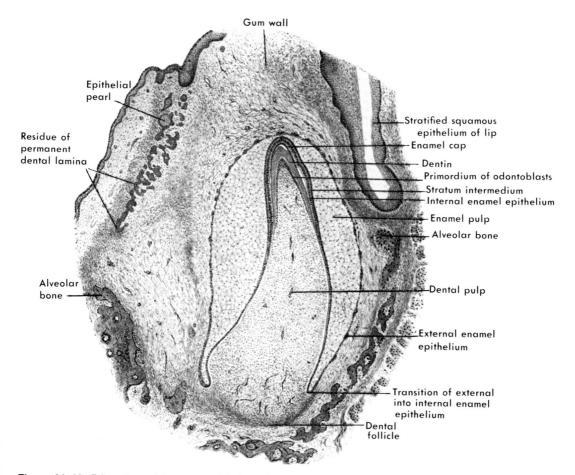

Gum wall

Epithelial pearl

Residue of permanent dental lamina

Stratified squamous epithelium of lip

Enamel cap

Dentin

Primordium of odontoblasts

Stratum intermedium

Internal enamel epithelium

Enamel pulp

Alveolar bone

Alveolar bone

Dental pulp

External enamel epithelium

Transition of external into internal enamel epithelium

Dental follicle

Figure 24–12. Primordium of lower central incisor of a 5-month fetus, in sagittal section. × 30. (After Schaffer.) Compare with photomicrographs in Figure 24–14.

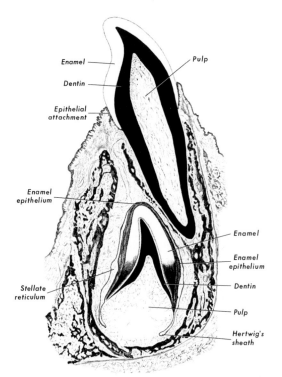

Enamel

Pulp

Dentin

Epithelial attachment

Enamel epithelium

Enamel

Enamel epithelium

Dentin

Stellate reticulum

Pulp

Hertwig's sheath

Figure 24–13. Diagram of deciduous tooth and the tooth germ *(below)* of its corresponding permanent tooth. Note the surrounding alveolar bone. × 5. (Redrawn from a photograph by B. Orban.)

When the formation of the hard substances of the tooth begins in fetuses of about 20 weeks, the mesenchyme of the dental papilla contains numerous blood vessels and a few reticular fibrils between its cells. The pulp cells adjacent to the layer of ameloblasts become transformed into *odontoblasts* (Figs. 24–12, 24–14).

The odontoblasts that form the dentin are tall columnar cells with their base toward the interior of the pulp and their tapering apical processes embedded in a layer of *predentin* (Figs. 24–15, 24–16). The long, slender extensions of their apical processes continue into the dentinal tubules. The layer of odontoblasts is epithelioid in appearance but the cells are not in as close apposition laterally as in typical epithelium, and capillaries may penetrate between them nearly to the predentin. These cells have an extensive rough endoplasmic reticulum and a large supranuclear Golgi complex. Condensing vacuoles associated with the transface of the Golgi contain filamentous material that has been identified immunocytochemically as procollagen. After their condensation the secretory granules are distributed along the odonto-

blast process where they discharge their content by exocytosis. The tropocollagen then polymerizes extracellularly to form the striated collagen fibers of the dentin matrix.

The odontoblasts are unusual among collagen-secreting cells in their polarization. In fibroblasts, procollagen is released anywhere on the cell surface. Exocytosis in odontoblasts is confined to the apical process. The secretory pathway is clearly demonstrated in radioautographs. When radioactively labeled precursors of collagen are administered, the grains first appear in autoradiographs over the endoplasmic reticulum of the odontoblasts. At later time intervals they are concentrated over the Golgi complex and then over the cell apex. In a few hours they are located predominantly over the predentin.

Newly formed predentin around the tapering apical processes of the odontoblasts is unmineralized. It stains poorly in routine histological sections and is apparently devoid of glycoprotein, for it is not stained by the PAS reaction. The transition from predentin to dentin is abrupt. Beyond this line the matrix is PAS positive, and the collagen fibers are larger and heavily encrusted with hydroxyapatite crystals.

The dentin first appears as a thick limiting layer between ameloblasts and odontoblasts, sometimes called the *membrana perforata*. The layer of dentin extends down the slopes of the dental papillae (Fig. 24–14). It gradually grows thicker and is transformed into a solid cap of dentin by the apposition of new layers on its concave surface. As the odontoblasts recede with the deposition of new dentin, thin processes of their apical cytoplasm remain in the deposited dentin as the odontoblastic processes.

When the dentin first appears, it is a soft fibrillar substance. The fibrils are continuations of the fibrils of the papilla. They are argyrophilic and are generally called *Korff's fibers*. They enter the dentin, spread out fanlike, and are incorporated into the fibrillar collagenous matrix of the dentin (Fig. 24–9). Mantle dentin is formed first, followed by formation of circumpulpar dentin.

In dentin formation, calcification follows closely the deposition of the fibrillar organic matrix. During the whole process, however, there is always a thin layer of uncalcified predentin adjacent to the odontoblasts (Fig. 24–15).

Almost immediately after the appearance of the first calcified dentin on the papilla, the ameloblasts begin the elaboration of enamel

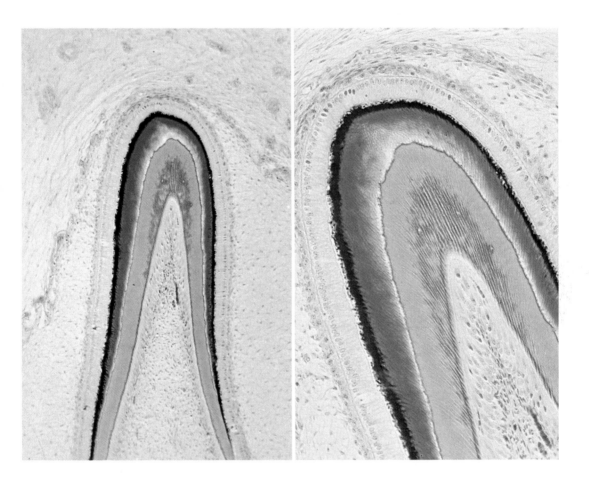

Figure 24–14. Photomicrographs of a portion of a developing tooth, showing the enamel stained red and dentin stained blue near the dental pulp and pink near the dentinoenamel junction. The columnar epithelium of ameloblasts is closely applied to the enamel. Peripheral to this epithelium are the stellate cells of the enamel pulp. The dental pulp is limited by an epithelial layer of odontoblasts depositing dentin. For further orientation, see Figure 24–12.

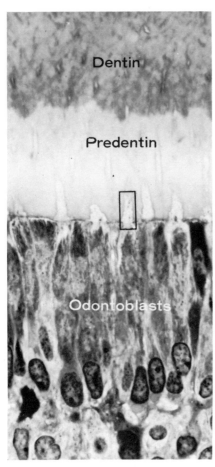

Figure 24–15. Photomicrograph from growing end of rat incisor, showing the relationship of the odontoblasts to the predentin and dentin. Notice the basal nuclei and the apical processes projecting into the predentin. An area such as that enclosed in the rectangle is shown at higher magnification in Figure 24–16. (From Weinstock, M., and C. P. Leblond. J. Cell Biol. *60*:92, 1974.)

matrix. It is deposited layer by layer onto the surface of the calcifying dentin (Fig. 24–14). On the slopes of the papilla the height of the ameloblasts decreases, and at the base of the papilla they continue into the cuboidal outer enamel epithelium.

As the mass of enamel increases, the ameloblasts recede. Light microscopists believed that the enamel matrix was a specialization of the apical cytoplasm of the ameloblast and therefore intracellular, and that the calcified enamel prisms were essentially prolongations of the columnar cells. This interpretation has now been discarded, since a distinct cell membrane has now been observed in electron micrographs between the cytoplasm and the calcified matrix. The ameloblasts are tall columnar cells with their elliptical nuclei located

near the base (Fig. 24–18). They exhibit an unusual segregation of organelles in that most of the mitochondria are clustered between the nucleus and the cell base. A long cylindrical Golgi apparatus is situated in the

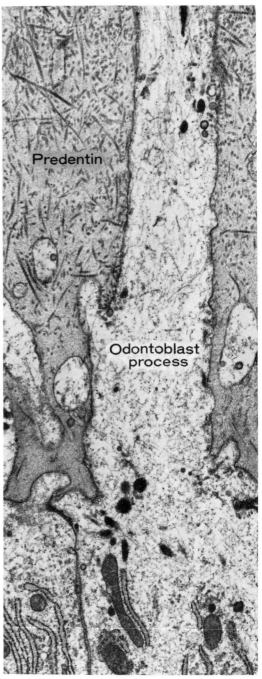

Figure 24–16. Electron micrograph of apical region of an odontoblast, showing the appearance of the odontoblast process and the fibrillar and amorphous components of the surrounding matrix of the predentin. (From Weinstock, M., and C. P. Leblond. J. Cell Biol. *60*:92, 1974.)

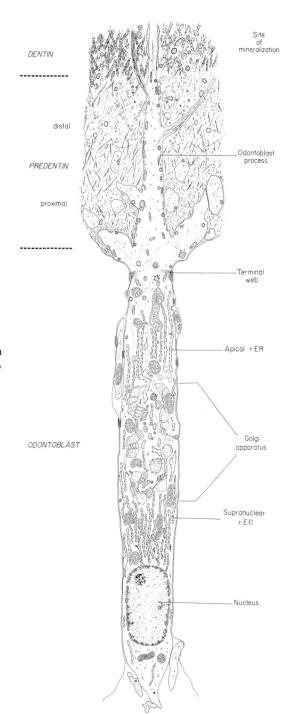

DENTIN

distal

PREDENTIN

proximal

ODONTOBLAST

Site
of
mineralization

Odontoblast
process

Terminal
web

Apical r ER

Golgi
apparatus

Supranuclear
r ER

Nucleus

Figure 24–17. Drawing depicting the ultrastructure of a typical odontoblast from rat incisor. (From Weinstock, M., and C. P. Leblond. J. Cell Biol. *60*:92, 1974.)

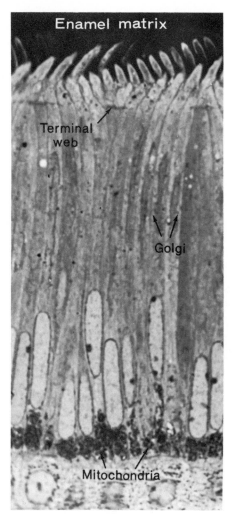

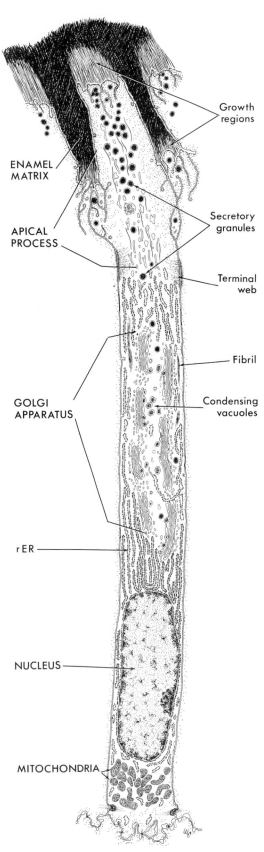

Figure 24–18. Photomicrograph of secretory ameloblasts in a region of enamel matrix secretion in rat maxillary incisor. Notice the clustering of mitochondria at the cell base, the basal location of the nuclei, and the apical processes extending into the enamel matrix. (From Weinstock, A., and C. P. Leblond. J. Cell Biol. *51*:26, 1971.)

Figure 24–19. Diagrammatic representation of the ultrastructure of a secretory ameloblast from rat maxillary incisor. (From Weinstock, A., and C. P. Leblond. J. Cell Biol. *51*:26, 1971.)

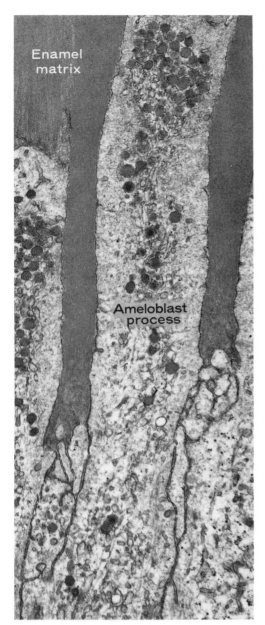

Figure 24–20. Electron micrograph of apical processes (Tomes' processes) of the ameloblasts and associated enamel matrix from rat incisor. (From Weinstock, A., and C. P. Leblond. J. Cell Biol. *51*:26, 1971.)

membrane-limited secretory granules are found in the Golgi region, the apical cytoplasm, and the proximal portion of the apical cell process (Figs. 24–19, 24–20). The secretory granules contain glycoprotein constituents of the enamel matrix. They are formed in the Golgi, transported to the cell process, and released there.

Calcification of the enamel matrix starts at the periphery of each enamel prism and proceeds toward its interior. When the organic matrix has fully calcified, so little organic material remains that the enamel is completely dissolved when teeth are decalcified. That the calcification is seldom absolutely uniform has been mentioned. The rate of deposition of enamel has been studied using sodium fluoride, and of dentin, with vital injections of alizarin. The daily thickening of dentin in the developing tooth is about 4 μm, and unusual increments (*neonatal lines*) appear in the enamel and dentin formed in the deciduous teeth at the time of birth.

When the definitive thickness and linear extent of the enamel are reached in the neck region of the tooth, the ameloblasts become small cuboidal cells and then atrophy. Before they disappear, they elaborate the enamel cuticle, which covers the external surface of the enamel of recently erupted teeth. At the deep end of the enamel organ, the outer and inner enamel epithelium form a fold, the *epithelial sheath of Hertwig.*

The development of the root begins shortly before the eruption of the tooth, continues after the crown has emerged from within the mucous membrane, and is not completed until much later. The epithelial sheath of Hertwig disappears when the root is completely developed, but as mentioned previously, remnants of this epithelial sheath are found in cementum and in the periodontal ligament.

When the germ of the permanent tooth begins to develop, its growth pressure causes resorption of the bony partition between the two teeth, then of the root, and eventually even of a part of the enamel of the deciduous tooth. Osteoclasts are prominent in this process of tooth destruction just as in the resorption of bone. The crown of the permanent tooth moving upward gradually expels and takes the place of the crown of the former deciduous tooth.

supranuclear region, and numerous cisternae of rough endoplasmic reticulum are found in the supranuclear and apical regions of the cytoplasm (Fig. 24–19). There is a diffuse terminal web, and distal to this is a broad apical process, *Tomes' process,* embedded in the enamel matrix. Numerous spherical

REFERENCES

GENERAL

Miles, A. E. W.: Structural and Chemical Organization of Teeth. Vols I & II. New York, Academic Press, 1967.

Schour, I., ed.: Noyes' Oral Histology and Embryology. 8th ed. Philadelphia, Lea & Febiger, 1960.

Sicher, H., ed.: Orban's Oral Histology and Embryology. 6th ed. St. Louis, C. V. Mosby Co., 1971.

DENTIN

Bernard, G. W.: Ultrastructural observations of initial calcification in dentin and enamel. J. Ultrastruct. Res. *41*:1, 1972.

Garant, P. R., G. Szabo, and J. Nalbandian: Fine structure of the mouse odontoblast. Arch. Oral Biol. *13*:857, 1968.

Josephsen, K., and H. Warshawsky: Radioautography of rat incisor dentin as a continuous record of the incorporation of a single dose of H³-labelled proline and tyrosine. Am. J. Anat. *164*:45, 1982.

Munhoz, C. O. G., and C. P. Leblond: Deposition of calcium phosphate into dentin and enamel as shown by radioautography of sections of incisor teeth following injection of 45Ca into rats. Calcif. Tissue Res. *15*:221, 1974.

Reith, E. J.: Collagen formation in developing molar teeth of rats. J. Ultrastruct. Res. *21*:383, 1968.

Weinstock, A., and C. P. Leblond: Synthesis migration and release of precursor collagen by odontoblasts as visualized by radioautography after (³H) proline administration. J. Cell Biol. *60*:92, 1974.

ENAMEL

Frank, R. M.: Tooth enamel: current state of the art. J. Dent. Res. *58(B)*:684, 1979.

Glimcher, M. J., L. C. Bonar, and E. J. Daniel: The molecular structure of the protein matrix of bovine dental enamel. J. Mol. Biol. *5*:541, 1961.

Glimcher, M. J., P. T. Levine, and L. C. Bonar: Mor-phological and biochemical considerations in structural studies of the organic matrix of enamel. J. Ultrastruct. Res. *13*:281, 1965.

Kallenbach, E.: Fine structure of differentiating amelo-blasts in the kitten. Am. J. Anat. *145*:283, 1976.

Katz, E. P., J. Seyer, P. T. Levine, and M. J. Glimcher: The comparative biochemistry of the organic matrix of developing enamel. Arch. Oral Biol. *14*:533, 1969.

Kerebel, B., G. Daculsi, and L. M. Kerebel: Ultrastructural studies of enamel crystallites. J. Dent. Res. *58(B)*:844, 1979.

Leblond, C. P., and H. Warshawsky: Dynamics of enamel formation in the rat incisor tooth. J. Dent. Res. *58(B)*:950, 1979.

Matthiessen, M. E., and P. Romert: Fine structure of the human secretory ameloblast. Scand. J. Dent. Res. *86*:67, 1978.

Smith, C. E.: Ameloblasts: secretory and resorptive functions. J. Dent. Res. *(B)*:695, 1979.

Warshawsky, H.: The fine structure of secretory ameloblasts in rat incisors. Anat. Rec. *161*:121, 1968.

Weinstock, A., and C. P. Leblond: Elaboration of the matrix glycoprotein of enamel by the secretory ameloblasts of the rat incisor as revealed by radioautography after galactose ³H injection. J. Cell Biol. *51*:26, 1971.

PERIODONTAL TISSUES

Beertsen, W., M. Brekelmans, and V. Everts: The site of collagen resorption in the periodontal ligament of the rodent molar. Anat. Rec. *192*:305, 1978.

Listgarten, M. A.: The ultrastructure of the human gingival epithelium. Am. J. Anat. *114*:49, 1964.

Smuckler, H., and C. J. Dreyer: Principal fibers of the periodontium. J. Periodont. Res. *4*:19, 1969.

Stern, L. B.: An electron microscopic study of the cementum: Sharpey's fibers and periodontal ligament in the rat incisor. Am. J. Anat. *115*:377, 1964.

Susi, F. R.: Anchoring fibrils in the attachment of epithelium to connective tissue in oral mucous membrane. J. Dent. Res. *48*:144, 1969.

25

THE ESOPHAGUS AND STOMACH

ESOPHAGUS

The *esophagus* is a muscular tube 25 cm in length that conveys food rapidly from the pharynx to the stomach. The greater part of its length is intrathoracic but the terminal 2 to 4 cm are below the diaphragm. Its wall includes all the layers characteristic of the digestive tube in general (Fig. 25–1). The *mucosa* is 500 to 800 μm thick. The stratified squamous epithelium (Figs. 25–2, 25–3) continues from the pharynx into the esophagus. At the junction of the esophagus with the cardia of the stomach, there is an abrupt transition from stratified squamous to simple columnar epithelium (see Fig. 25–5). On macroscopic examination, the boundary line between the smooth, white mucous membrane of the esophagus and the pink surface of the gastric mucosa appears as a jagged line.

In humans the flattened cells of the superficial layers of the epithelium contain a small number of keratohyalin granules but do not undergo true cornification. The lamina propria consists of loose connective tissue with relatively thin collagenous fibers and networks of fine elastic fibers. In addition to the usual connective tissue cells, numerous lymphocytes are scattered throughout the tissue. Small lymphatic nodules are found around the ducts of the esophageal mucous glands.

At the level of the cricoid cartilage of the larynx the elastic layer of the pharynx gives way to the *muscularis mucosae,* which consists of longitudinal smooth muscle fibers and thin elastic networks. Near the stomach the muscularis mucosae attains a thickness of 200 to 400 μm.

The dense connective tissue of the *submucosa* consists of collagenous and elastic fibers and small infiltrations of lymphocytes about the glands. The submucous layer, together with the muscularis mucosae, forms numerous longitudinal folds, which result in an irregular outline of the lumen in cross section. During the swallowing of food these folds are smoothed out. This is made possible by the elasticity of the connective tissue that forms the submucous layer.

The *muscularis* of the human esophagus is 0.5 to 2.2 mm thick. In the upper quarter of the esophagus, both its outer and inner layers consist of striated muscle. In the second quarter, bundles of smooth muscle begin gradually to replace the striated muscle, and in the lower third only smooth muscle is found. The relations between the two types of muscular tissue are subject to individual variations. The two layers of the muscularis are not as regularly circular and longitudinal, respectively, as they are elsewhere in the alimentary tract. In the inner layer there are many spiral or oblique bundles. The longitudinal muscular bundles of the outer layer are also irregularly arranged in many places.

The outer surface of the esophagus is connected with the surrounding parts by a layer of loose connective tissue constituting the *tunica adventitia.*

GLANDS OF THE ESOPHAGUS

Two kinds of small glands occur in the esophagus: *esophageal glands proper* and *esophageal cardiac glands.* The esophageal glands proper are small, compound glands with richly branched tubuloalveolar secretory portions containing only mucous cells (Fig. 25–4). They are unevenly distributed in the submucous layer and can just be recognized with the naked eye as elongated white spots. The branches of the smallest ducts are short and fuse into a cystically dilated main duct, which pierces the muscularis mucosae and opens

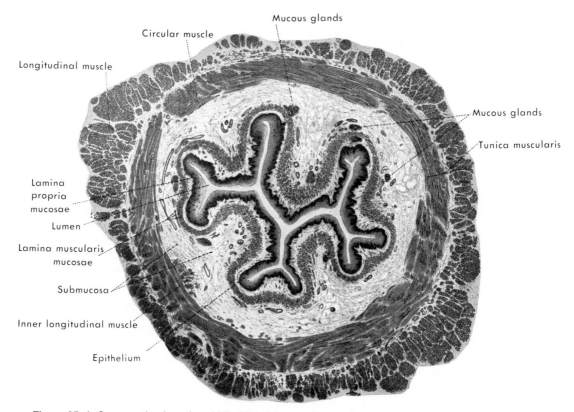

Figure 25–1. Cross section from the middle third of the esophagus of a 28-year-old man. × 8. (After Sobotta.)

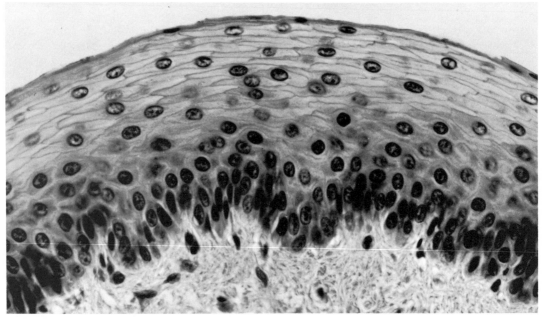

Figure 25–2. Esophageal stratified epithelium of a rhesus monkey.

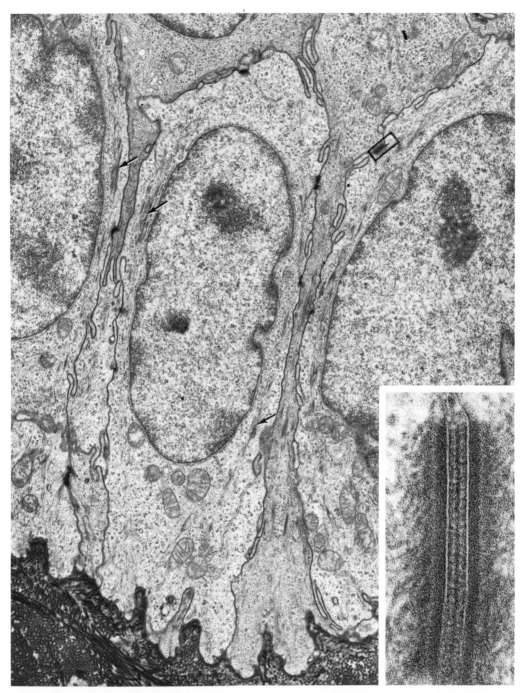

Figure 25–3. Electron micrograph of cells of the basal layer of rodent esophageal epithelium. Division of these cells is responsible for continual renewal of the epithelium. They have abundant free ribosomes and occasional fascicles of cytoplasmic filaments *(at arrows)*. They are attached by well-developed desmosomes. One enclosed in rectangle at upper right is shown at high magnification in the inset. Notice the prominent intermediate line in the interspace between the two membranes. (Micrograph courtesy of S. McNutt.)

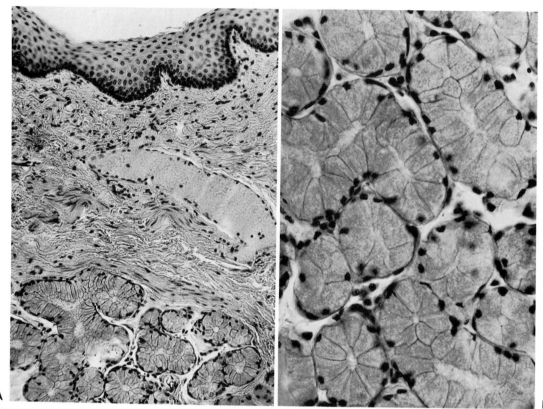

A

B

Figure 25–4. *A,* Photomicrograph of esophageal wall, showing the lumen and lining epithelium and the esophageal glands in the submucosa. × 120. *B,* Esophageal glands at higher magnification, illustrating the dark pyknotic-appearing nuclei displaced to the base of the cell by the accumulated mucigen in the apical region. × 300.

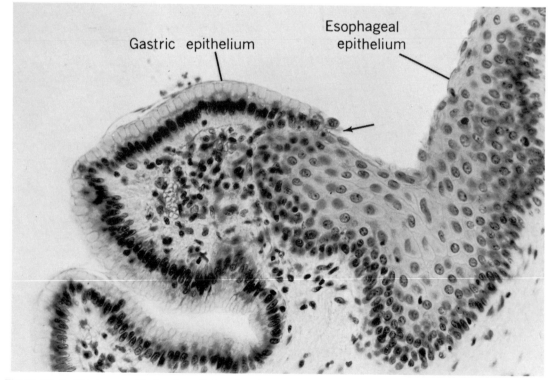

Gastric epithelium

Esophageal epithelium

Figure 25–5. Esophagogastric junction. Notice the abrupt transition from stratified squamous to simple columnar epithelium *(at arrow).* Hematoxylin and eosin. × 375.

through a small orifice. The epithelium in the smallest ducts is low columnar, whereas that in the enlarged main duct is stratified squamous epithelium. The mucous glands may give rise to cysts of the mucous membrane.

The *esophageal cardiac glands* closely resemble the cardiac glands of the stomach. Two groups of them can be distinguished. One is in the upper part of the esophagus at the level between the cricoid cartilage and the fifth tracheal cartilage; the other is in the lower part of the esophagus near the cardia. They show great individual variation and sometimes are entirely absent.

Unlike the esophageal glands proper, they are always confined to the lamina propria mucosae. Their terminal portions are branched and convoluted tubules lined by columnar or cuboidal cells with a pale granular cytoplasm, which sometimes gives a staining reaction for mucin. The smallest ducts drain into a larger duct that is sometimes cystically dilated and always opens on the tip of a small papilla. Its columnar epithelium often gives a staining reaction for mucin and resembles the mucous epithelium of the gastric foveolae.

In the regions of esophageal mucous membrane that contain the upper and lower groups of cardiac glands, the stratified squamous epithelium may be supplanted in places by a simple columnar epithelium resembling that in the gastric pits of the stomach mucosa. Seen with the naked eye, such patches may be mistaken for erosions—that is, places denuded of epithelium. Sometimes these patches lined with mucous epithelium are of considerable size and exhibit pitlike invaginations and tubular glands like those of the stomach; they may even contain typical zymogenic and parietal cells.

The number and development of the esophageal cardiac glands, as well as of the islands of gastric mucosa in the esophagus, are subject to great individual variation. According to some investigators, the presence of this ectopic gastric epithelium is of some importance in relation to the origin of cysts, ulcers, and carcinomas of the esophagus.

In many mammals, especially those that consume coarse vegetable food (rodents, ruminants, and equids), the stratified squamous epithelium of the esophagus undergoes keratinization. The esophageal glands are present in most of the mammals, but instead of being purely mucous, as in the human, they have a mixed character. No esophageal glands are found in rodents, horses, and cats.

HISTOPHYSIOLOGY OF THE ESOPHAGUS

At the junction of the pharynx and esophagus is a region of higher muscular tone referred to as the pharyngoesophageal sphincter, Similarly, the terminal few centimeters of the esophagus serve as a gastroesophageal sphincter normally maintaining an intraluminal pressure slightly higher than intragastric pressure. There is no anatomical thickening or local change in orientation of the musculature in these regions. Thus, they are physiological rather than anatomical sphincters. Nevertheless, the gastroesophageal sphincter is normally quite efficient in preventing reflux of gastric contents. However, the esophageal hiatus in the diaphragm not infrequently fails to close completely around the esophagus during embryonic development, resulting in a *hiatus hernia* through which a portion of the stomach may project into the thoracic cavity. This often interferes with the normal sphincteric function of the terminal esophagus, permitting reflux of gastric contents. The esophageal epithelium is poorly equipped to resist the acidity of gastric secretions, and the resulting inflammatory response may cause difficulty in swallowing and lead ultimately to development of fibrosis and stricture of the lower esophagus.

In swallowing, the tongue propels the food back into the pharynx. This sets in motion a train of coordinated voluntary and involuntary movements by pharyngeal and esophageal musculature. These involve closure of the glottis, elevation of the larynx, constriction of the pharynx, and reflex relaxation of the pharyngeoesophageal sphincter. When the bolus of food enters the esophagus, the local stimulus of distention initiates a peristaltic wave of contraction that is propagated toward the stomach at a rate of 4 to 6 cm per second. The gastroesophageal sphincter relaxes transiently in anticipation of the arrival of the peristaltic wave, allowing the food to pass into the stomach.

The nerves to the esophagus are derived from the vagus and the cervical and thoracic sympathetic trunks. They form a plexus of fibers and clusters of cell bodies between the two layers of the muscular coat and a second plexus in the submucosa. They are important for coordination of movements involved in swallowing. Disturbances of the neuromuscular apparatus are fairly common in older persons and individuals of nervous temperament, and may result in muscle spasm, difficulty in swallowing, and severe substernal pain.

STOMACH

The stomach is an organ specialized for storage and processing of food for subsequent absorption in the intestine. Its storage function is minimal in the human and is best exemplified in the multichambered stomach of ruminants, where food taken in during grazing or browsing is temporarily stored in the *rumen* and later returned to the oral cavity for further mastication. It is then swallowed again and proceeds successively through the *reticulum, omasum,* and *abomasum.* In other mammals having a relatively simple, single-chambered stomach, there is little or no storage, but the wall of the stomach is capable of considerable expansion during feeding without significant increase in internal pressure. In the human, it can accommodate up to 1 liter.

In the stomach, the semisolid material resulting from mastication is reduced to a fluid by contractions of the muscular wall of the organ and admixture with the acid and enzymes secreted by its glandular mucosa. The content of the upper portion of the stomach may remain semisolid for some time after a meal, while that of the most distal portion is reduced to a pulplike fluid mass referred to as the *chyme.* When it has attained the necessary softness, it is passed on in small portions to the duodenum. Thus, the digestive function of the stomach is in part mechanical and in part chemical.

The area immediately surrounding the opening from the esophagus into the stomach is called the *cardia.* To the left of the cardia a dome-shaped bulge above the level of the esophageogastric junction is called the *fundus.* The capacious central portion is the *corpus* or body, and the more distal region of transition to the duodenum is the *pylorus* (Fig. 25–6). Gastroenterologists often incorporate the fundus and corpus together under the term *fundic region.* The convex left and concave right margins are called respectively the

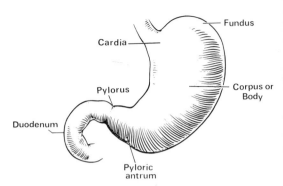

Figure 25–6. Drawing of the human stomach presenting the terminology of its various regions.

greater and *lesser* curvatures. The stomach wall consists of the layers previously defined as characteristic of the entire digestive tract: *mucosa, submucosa, muscularis,* and *serosa.*

THE GASTRIC MUCOSA

The mucosa of the living stomach is a grayish pink in color with paler zones at the cardia and pylorus. In the empty contracted stomach, the mucosa forms numerous longitudinal folds or *rugae.* This plication is permitted by the loose consistency of the submucosa and results from contraction of the muscularis mucosae. In the full stomach, the rugae flatten out and the mucosa is smooth contoured to the naked eye. On closer inspection, a pattern of low elevations is created by shallow furrows that demarcate slightly bulging areas 2 to 6 mm in diameter (Fig. 25–7). At low magnification, the surface of each area is further subdivided by a system of intercommunicating shallow furrows, the *gastric pits* or *foveolae.* This convoluted pattern of ridges and foveolae is seen most clearly in scanning electron micrographs of gastric mucosa (Fig. 25–8). At this magnification, the convex apical surfaces of the individual epithelial cells can also be identified. In histological sections of the mucosa, the foveolae appear as funnel-shaped invaginations of the surface epithelium continuous at their base with numerous tubular gastric glands (Fig. 25–9). The columnar epithelium that covers the ridges and lines the foveolae is of uniform cellular composition throughout the gastric mucosa, but there are regional differences in the cell populations comprising the gastric glands, and this is reflected in significant regional differences in the nature of the gastric secretions.

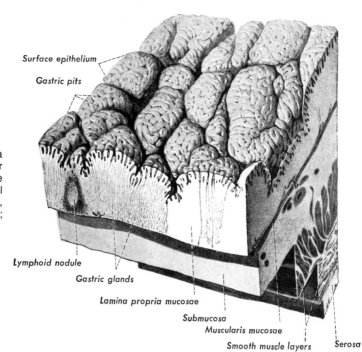

Figure 25–7. Surface of gastric mucosa of a man; drawing based on binocular microscope view. The cut surfaces are slightly diagrammatic. At left, the normal distribution of the gastric glands; to right, only a few are indicated. Glands, gray; gastric pits, black. × 17. (After Braus.)

Surface epithelium

Gastric pits

Lymphoid nodule

Gastric glands

Lamina propria mucosae

Submucosa

Muscularis mucosae

Smooth muscle layers

Serosa

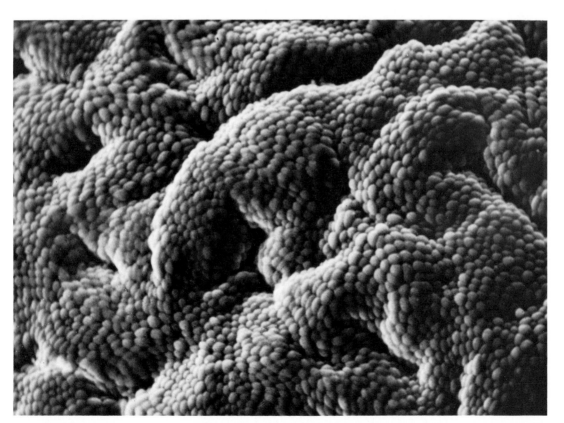

Figure 25–8. Scanning electron micrograph of the luminal surface of the gastric mucosa. The cells are all the same type—surface mucous cells. The convex apical surfaces of the individual epithelial cells are clearly seen. The convoluted pattern of ridges and gastric pits, or foveolae, is also evident. (Micrograph courtesy of J. Riddell.)

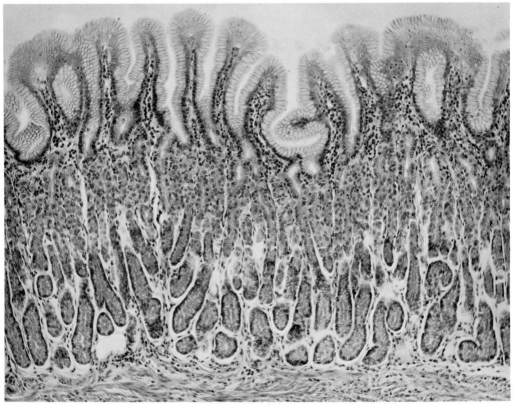

Figure 25–9. Photomicrograph of the gastric mucosa of a macaque, showing the gastric glands opening into the gastric pits, or foveolae. Hematoxylin and eosin. × 120.

Surface Epithelium

The gastric pits and the ridges between them are lined by a tall columnar epithelium that begins abruptly at the cardia under an overlying margin of the stratified squamous epithelium of the esophagus (Fig. 25–5). The apical portion of the cells of the surface epithelium is occupied by mucigen, the intracellular precursor of mucus. In routine histological sections this portion of the cell may be unstained, but after the periodic acid–Schiff (PAS) reaction for carbohydrates it stains intensely. Although there is no obvious morphological difference among surface mucous cells, the characteristics of the mucus exhibit regional variations when studied histochemically. The interfoveolar cells contain neutral mucosubstance, while the cells deep in the foveolae contain acidic carbohydrates. Cells on the surface also contain more mucous granules than those deeper in the pits or isthmus of the glands. The mucus secreted plays an essential role in lubricating the surface epithelium and forming a barrier layer, protecting it from injury by ingested substances and the potentially damaging acid and enzymes of the gastric secretions.

At the electron microscopic level, there are numerous microvilli with a prominent glycocalyx on the luminal surface, underlain by a narrow zone of cytoplasm rich in filaments forming a terminal web. Below this are mucous granules closely packed with little intervening cytoplasm (Fig. 25–10). The granules are spherical, ovoid, or discoid and vary in density from pale to completely electron-opaque. In some species, they have dense cores and a peripheral zone of lower density. Material with a texture similar to that of the granules may be found in cisternae of the supranuclear Golgi complex. The paranuclear and basal cytoplasm contains cisternal profiles of endoplasmic reticulum, numerous mitochondria, and limited numbers of microtubules and filaments. The nucleus is often irregular in outline.

Adjacent cells are held together by juxtaluminal zonulae occludentes and adherentes, and desmosomes and gap junctions are sparsely distributed on the lateral cell boundaries. Toward the base of the epithelium, the

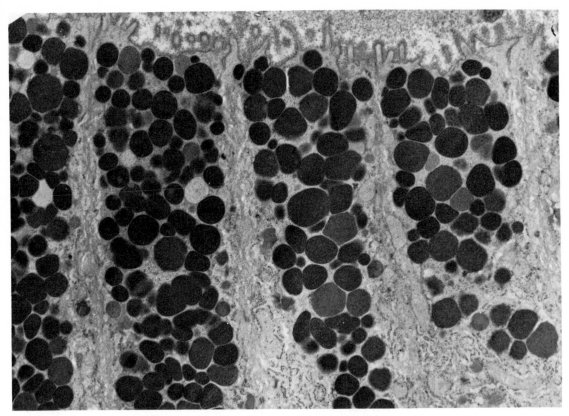

Figure 25–10. Electron micrograph of the apical portion of several surface mucous cells. The short microvilli have a prominent glycocalyx and the surface of the epithelium is covered by a layer of mucus. (Courtesy of S. Ito.)

membranes often diverge, forming a conspicuous intercellular cleft into which slender folds project from lateral surfaces of the cells.

Surface mucous cells are continuously desquamated into the lumen, and the entire population is renewed about every three days. Evidence of regeneration is seen only in the depths of the foveolae and necks of the gastric glands where mitoses are frequent in relatively undifferentiated cells that contain few mucigen granules. The newly formed cells are slowly displaced upward to replace cells lost at the surface.

Cardiac Glands

In a narrow zone of the cardia around the esophageogastric junction, the foveolae are relatively shallow, and each is continuous below with several tortuous tubular *cardiac glands*. Unlike the glands in other segments of the stomach, these consist mainly of mucous cells, with smaller numbers of undifferentiated cells and scattered endocrine cells. The endocrine cells are believed to secrete the hormone *gastrin*. The area occupied by cardiac glands varies from 5 to 30 mm in width in the human to as much as a third of the stomach in pigs.

Gastric Glands (Oxyntic Glands)

This glandular type is characteristic of the mucosa throughout the fundus and corpus of the stomach, and makes the greatest contribution to secretion of the gastric juice. The *oxyntic glands* (also called *gastric glands* or *fundic glands*) are closely packed together and extend through the entire thickness of the mucosa (0.3–1.5 mm). From one to seven open through slightly constricted necks into the bottom of each foveola. They are 30 to 50 μm in diameter with a very narrow lumen. Their blind distal ends are slightly expanded and coiled and may divide into two or three terminal branches. There are estimated to be 15 million oxyntic glands associated with 3.5 million gastric foveolae.

The oxyntic glands are composed of four cell types: (1) *mucous neck cells* (2) *chief cells* (also called *zymogenic cells*) (3) *oxyntic* or *parietal cells* and (4) *endocrine cells* (Fig. 25–13). For

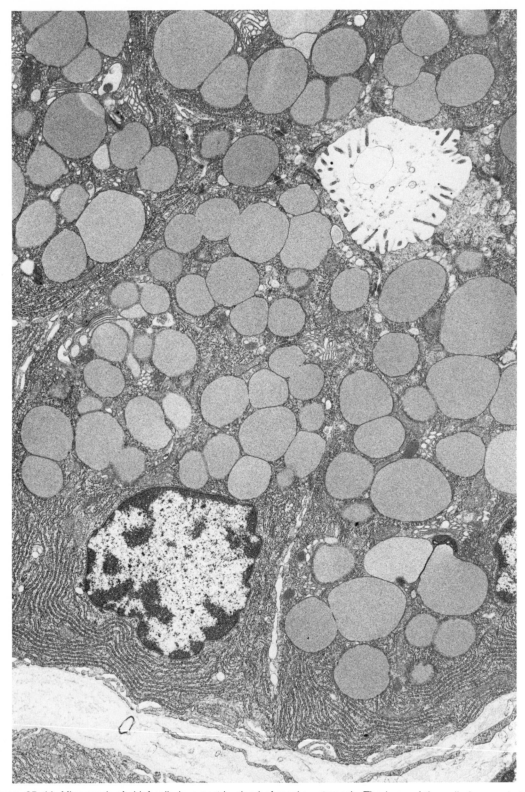

Figure 25–11. Micrograph of chief cells in a gastric gland of monkey stomach. The base of the cells is occupied by closely spaced cisternae of rough endoplasmic reticulum, and the apex crowded with pale secretory granules containing pepsinogen. (Courtesy of S. Ito.)

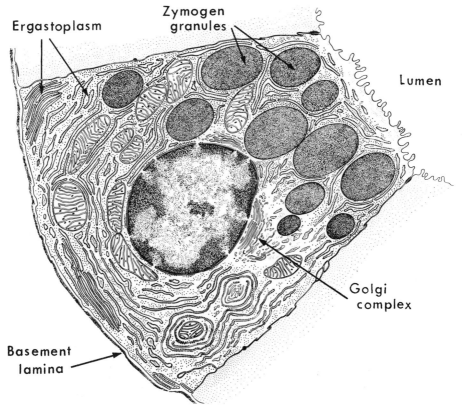

Ergastoplasm

Zymogen granules

Lumen

Golgi complex

Basement lamina

Figure 25–12. Drawing of the chief or zymogenic cell as seen with the electron microscope. (From Ito, S., and R. J. Winchester. J. Cell Biol. *16*:541, 1963.)

descriptive purposes, the gland is customarily divided into three regions. At its confluence with the foveola is the *isthmus,* containing surface mucous cells and oxyntic cells; followed by the *neck,* consisting mainly of mucous neck cells and oxyntic cells; and the *base* or *fundus,* where chief cells are the predominant cell type, with smaller numbers of oxyntic and mucous neck cells. Scattered endocrine cells may be found in any segment of the gland. Mitotic activity is largely confined to the neck of the glands and it is probable that the chief, oxyntic, and other cell types develop from a small population of relatively undifferentiated cells in this region.

Mucous Neck Cells. These cells are relatively few in number and are lodged between the parietal cells in the neck of the glands where the latter open into the gastric pits. Deeper in the glands, they are abruptly succeeded by the zymogenic cells. In fresh, unstained preparations they are filled with pale, transparent granules. These cells are easily overlooked or mistaken for zymogenic cells in preparations in which mucus either is not preserved or is unstained. In sections stained

with the PAS reaction, mucicarmine, or mucihematein, the granules that fill the apical cytoplasm are deeply colored, whereas those of the chief cells are unstained. There is evidence that the mucus secreted by these cells is somewhat different from that of the surface mucous cells.

The mucous neck cells are deformed by neighboring cells and therefore tend to be quite irregular in shape; some have a wide base and narrow apex, others a broad apex and narrow base. The nuclei are at the bases of the cells and are often somewhat flattened.

Where the necks of the glands open into the bottoms of the foveolae, a series of transitional forms between mucous neck cells and surface mucous cells can be identified. New cells arise by transformation of the relatively undifferentiated cells found in the depths of the foveolae and in the necks of the glands. In some gastric glands, mucous neck cells extend deeper into the gland and may be found scattered singly among the zymogenic cells. This is especially prominent in glands near the pyloric region. According to some, the glands of a narrow intermediate zone

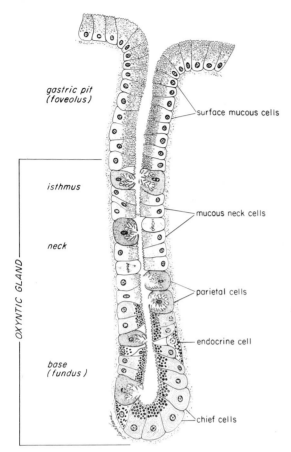

Figure 25–13. Diagram of an oxyntic gland from the corpus of a mammalian stomach. (From Ito, S. *In* Johnson, L. R., ed.: Physiology of the Gastrointestinal Tract. New York, Raven Press, 1981.)

gland (Fig. 25–14). Their cytoplasm stains intensely with eosin and phloxine. Their most unusual feature is the presence of a meandering canalicular invagination of the apical surface that may encircle the nucleus and extend nearly to the basal lamina (Figs. 25–15, 25–16). This was called the "intracellular canaliculus" by light microscopists—a somewhat misleading term. Although this channel makes a deep incursion into the cell body, its limiting membrane is continuous with the plasmalemma at the cell apex where it opens into the lumen of the gland. Thus, it is not a closed intracellular canal within the cytoplasm as the name implies, and the term *secretory canaliculus* is probably preferable. Like the apical surface of the cell, the canaliculus is lined by microvilli whose number and length vary with the state of the cell's secretory activity.

may contain only mucous neck and parietal cells, and may be devoid of zymogenic cells.

Under the electron microscope, the luminal surfaces of the columnar mucous neck cells are studded with short microvilli that have a fuzzy glycocalyx. The lateral surfaces of neighboring cells are interdigitated, particularly toward the base of the cell. The apical region of the cell contains numerous dense granules of spheroid, ovoid, or discoid form. Rod-shaped mitochondria of the usual internal structure are scattered through the cytoplasm. There is a sizable supranuclear Golgi complex. Membranous profiles of endoplasmic reticulum are present in small numbers.

Oxyntic Cells (Parietal Cells). The most conspicuous and distinctive cell type in the gastric mucosa is the *oxyntic* or *parietal cell.* These large pyramidal cells up to 25 μm in diameter have broad rounded bases that often bulge outward at the periphery of the

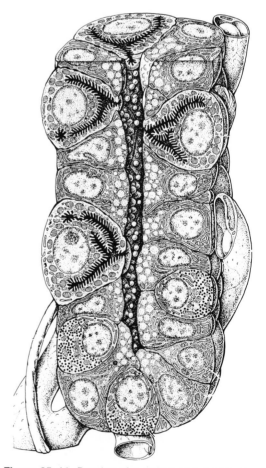

Figure 25–14. Drawing of a portion of a gastric gland, showing the parietal cells bulging outward, zymogenic cells, and endocrine cells with small basal granules. (From Krstic, R. V. Die Gewebe des Menschen und Säugetiere. Berlin, Springer-Verlag, 1978.)

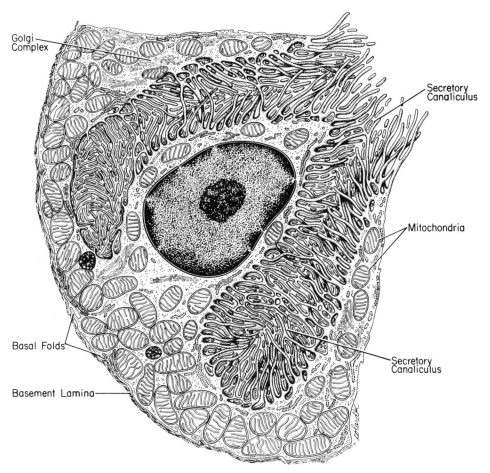

Figure 25–15. Drawing of the ultrastructure of the gastric parietal cell or oxyntic cell. It is a large cell with very abundant large mitochondria and an intracellular canaliculus lined with microvilli. (Drawing courtesy of S. Ito.)

Secretory granules are lacking and the Golgi complex, located in a paranuclear or basal position, is less well developed than in other glandular cells. The cytoplasm is crowded with large mitochondria that occupy up to 40 per cent of the cytoplasmic volume. The large number of mitochondria and the amplification of their internal surface by numerous cristae are consistent with the very high energy requirement of their secretory function. Isolated parietal cells have a rate of oxygen consumption five times that of the neighboring mucous cells.

Another unique ultrastructural feature of the cell is the presence in the cytoplasm of an extensive system of membrane-limited tubules that do not have the properties typical of the endoplasmic reticulum of other cells. Whether in the living cell these profiles are predominantly tubular or vesicular, continuous or discontinuous, and whether they are closed or open to the lumen of the secretory

canaliculus are subjects of continuing controversy among electron microscopists. It is clear that the appearance of this system varies greatly, depending on the state of activity of the cell and the method of specimen preparation. The descriptive term *tubulovesicular system,* now widely used, represents a compromise among conflicting interpretations. Recent application of the technique of rapid-freezing with liquid helium and freeze substitution strongly suggests that the system is predominantly tubular in the living state (Fig. 25–17).

Hydrochloric acid is first detected in the fetal stomach at a time coinciding with the differentiation of parietal cells, and the amount of acid produced is positively correlated with the number of these cells in the gastric mucosa. This and other indirect evidence have led to general agreement that it is the parietal cells that are responsible for the stomach's remarkable capacity to secrete

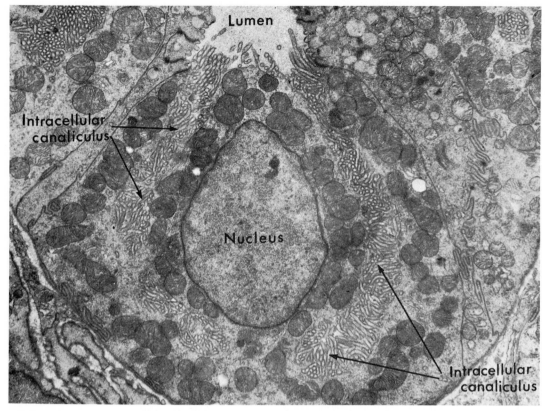

Figure 25–16. Electron micrograph of a parietal cell of bat gastric mucosa. The extensive secretory canaliculus within the limits of the cell is filled by large numbers of irregularly oriented microvilli. × 10,000. (Courtesy of S. Ito.)

hydrochloric acid. It is this function that is implied in the alternative term "oxyntic" cell. This cell type also secretes *gastric intrinsic factor,* a substance required for absorption of vitamin B_{12} in the ileum.

The internal organization of the oxyntic cell undergoes striking changes in different phases of secretory activity. In the nonsecreting cell, microvilli on the surface and in the secretory canaliculus are short and sparse, and the tubulovesicular system is extremely developed. After stimulation of acid secretion, there is a rapid increase in length and number of microvilli, resulting in a fivefold increment in surface area. A concomitant and equally dramatic reduction in the tubulovesicular membranes of the cytoplasm has fostered the belief that the tubulovesicular membranes may fuse with the plasmalemma and, by exteriorization, contribute to the rapid increase in microvillar surface area. Freezefracture studies demonstrate a similarity in pattern of intramembrane particles consistent with the hypothesis that tubulovesicular membranes fuse with the plasmalemma at the onset of induced acid secretion, but com-

pelling morphological evidence for such a translocation of preformed membrane is still lacking. When active secretion ceases, the oxyntic cells revert to their resting state and an extensive tubulovesicular system is reconstituted.

Chief Cells (Zymogenic Cells). The chief cells form a cuboidal epithelium lining the lower third or half of the gastric glands in the corpus of the stomach. They are absent from cardiac glands, sparse in the glands of the fundus, and rare in the pylorus. Chief cells are difficult to preserve adequately in routine histological preparations. When properly fixed, they contain numerous apical secretory granules and a strongly basophilic cytoplasm as in other protein-secreting zymogenic cells. They synthesize and secrete *pepsinogen* which is activated to form the digestive enzyme *pepsin.*

In electron micrographs, the chief cells have the ultrastructure characteristic of protein-secreting glandular cells such as those of the pancreas—a well-developed supranuclear Golgi complex; abundant rough endoplasmic reticulum concentrated in the basal cyto-

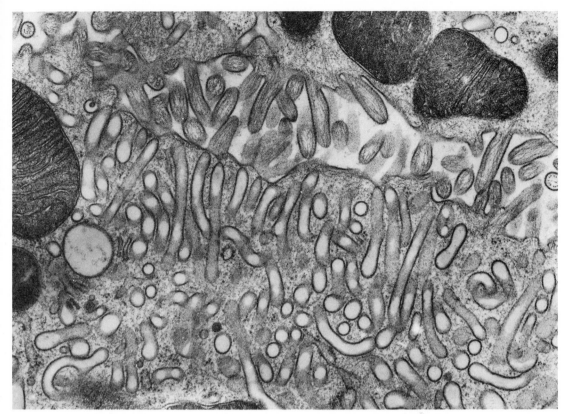

Figure 25–17. Electron micrograph of a portion of a parietal cell including a segment of the secretory canaliculus. Notice the numerous elements of the tubulovesicular system. Specimen rapidly frozen with liquid helium and further processed by freeze substitution in osmium tetroxide and acetone. (Courtesy of N. Sugai and A. Ichikawa.)

plasm; and numerous moderately dense, spherical secretory granules in the apical cytoplasm. In the chief cells of humans, dense bodies, apparently lysosomes, are commonly found among the pepsinogen granules. The luminal surface bears sparse microvilli limited by a plasma membrane with a thin glycocalyx.

Although the chief cells are the main source of gastric pepsin, studies with fluorescent-labeled antibodies to pepsinogen also localize small amounts in the mucous neck cells of the gastric glands, but not in mucous cells of the pyloric region.

Endocrine Cells. Small granulated cells scattered individually among the epithelial cells of the gastric glands have been recognized for more than a century. They can be stained selectively with silver or chromium salts and therefore were long referred to as *argentaffin* or *enterochromaffin cells*. Although these methods permitted recognition of two or more categories of silver-reducing cells, they shed no light upon the chemical nature of their granules or their physiological significance.

In the past 20 years, advances in biochemical extraction methods and radioimmunoassay procedures have led to the identification and purification of a large number of peptide hormones and biogenic amines. By using labeled antibodies to these substances, many of them have been localized to specific single cells widely scattered throughout the gastrointestinal tract. Whereas the silver-staining cells were formerly divided into two categories, immunocytochemical methods have now identified nine different endocrine or paracrine cell types in the stomach, and the list continues to grow. All are small pyramidal or ovoid cells lodged between the bases of the neighboring exocrine cells of the epithelium. The narrow apex of some extends to the lumen; others are confined to the base of the epithelium. All possess small, membrane-limited granules usually concentrated in their basal cytoplasm. Some types are readily identifiable in electron micrographs on the basis of differences in size or substructure of their granules. Those containing monoamines exhibit a characteristic fluorescence. The most reliable means of identification of the peptide-secreting cells involves use of labeled specific antibody to their respective secretory products.

Collectively these cells are now referred to as the *enteroendocrine cells.* They are found throughout the enteric tract. The terminology of cell types, the morphological criteria for their identification, and the nature of their secretions will be considered in greater detail in the chapter on the intestines (Chapter 26). Three of the enteroendocrine cell types are largely confined to the gastric mucosa: the *EC cell,* secreting serotonin; the *ECL cell,* believed to release histamine; and the *G cell,* which secretes the hormone gastrin. The *EC cells* contain small (~ 300 nm) oval or crescentic granules with a dense core, and have an apical extension of their cytoplasm to the lumen. The *ECL cell* contains larger granules (up to 450 nm) with an eccentric dense core of varying shape. It is found exclusively in the gastric mucosa.

Of particular importance in gastric physi-ology is the *G cell* or *gastrin cell.* Its hormone is a potent stimulator of acid secretion by the oxyntic cells, and is also thought to stimulate mucosal cell proliferation. The cell is pyramidal in form, with a narrow apex extending to the lumen, and possessing a tuft of long microvilli. The granules are quite heterogeneous, varying in size from 150 to 400 nm. Some appear to be vesicles with little content, others have dense cores, and still others are of intermediate density (Figs. 25–18, 25–19). Granules are concentrated at the cell base and release their product into the lamina propria by exocytosis.

Although the enteroendocrine cells appear in tissue sections to be few and widely scattered, the aggregate number in the gastric mucosa is quite large. Gastrin cells alone are estimated to number 5×10^5 per square centimeter of mucosa in dog, cat, and rat. The presence of food distending the stomach causes release of gastrin, which diffuses into the blood and is distributed to the glands of

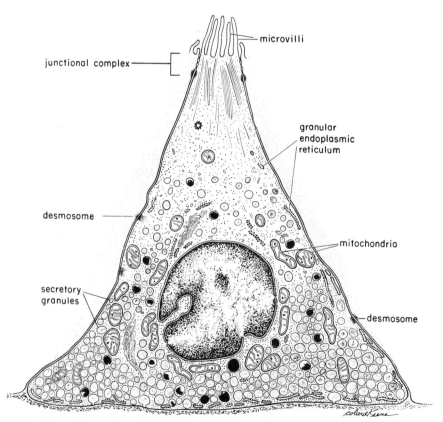

Figure 25–18. Schematic representation of the ultrastructure of the gastric cell (G cell). As in other endocrine cells, the secretory granules are concentrated at the vascular pole. (From Ito, S. *In* Johnson, L. R., ed.: Physiology of the Gastrointestinal Tract. New York, Raven Press, 1981.)

the gastric mucosa, where it stimulates the oxyntic cells and to a lesser extent the chief cells. In response, the oxyntic cells increase their rate of hydrochloric acid secretion as much as eightfold.

Pyloric Glands

The pyloric glands are found in the distal 4 to 5 cm of the stomach. In this region, the foveolae are deeper than elsewhere in the stomach, extending down into the mucous membrane for half its thickness. The glands here are also of the simple, branched tubular type, but they branch more extensively, the lumen is larger, and the tubules are coiled, so that in perpendicular sections they are seldom seen as continuous longitudinal structures (Fig. 25–20). The principal cell type of the pyloric glands has a pale cytoplasm with an indistinct granulation. Secretory capillaries have been described between the cells. The nucleus is often flattened against the base of the cell. In sections stained with hematoxylin and eosin, they are difficult to distinguish from mucous neck cells or the cells of the glands of Brunner in the duodenum. Some investigators believe that the pyloric glandular cells are identical with the mucous neck cells, for both give similar staining reactions for mucus. Cresyl violet and the Giemsa mixture of dyes, however, seem to stain them in a specific way. In the human stomach, the pyloric glands in the region of the sphincter may contain parietal cells. Gastrin cells are also described in the pyloric glands.

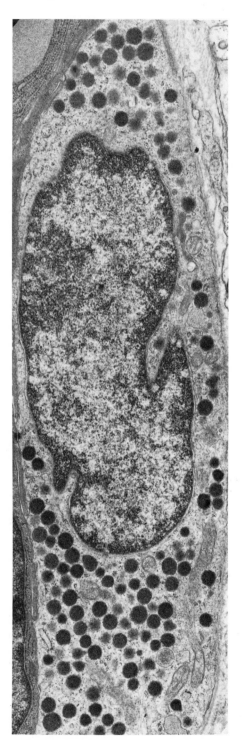

Figure 25–19. Electron micrograph of one of the types of granular argentaffin or endocrine cells. This kind is believed to secrete the hormone gastrin. (Micrograph by S. Ito.)

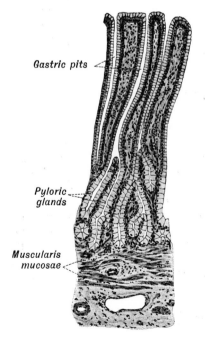

Gastric pits

Pyloric glands

Muscularis mucosae

Figure 25–20. Pyloric glands from human stomach. Slightly diagrammatic. × 75. (After Braus.)

Lamina Propria

Connective tissue of the lamina propria occupies the narrow spaces between the glands and between their bases and the underlying muscularis mucosae. It forms larger accumulations only between the necks of the glands and between the foveolae. It consists of a delicate network of collagenous and reticular fibrils and is almost devoid of elastic elements. In addition to oval pale nuclei, which seem to belong to fibroblasts, the meshes of the fibrous network contain numerous lymphocytes and some plasma cells, eosinophils, and mast cells. Lymphoid cells with coarsely granular acidophilic inclusions, called Russell's bodies, may be found between the epithelial cells of the glands. These may develop under physiological conditions but are more common in pathological states. In the lamina propria, especially in the pyloric region, strands of smooth muscle may be found and small accumulations of lymphoid tissue occur normally.

Muscularis Mucosae

Underlying the gastric glands is the *muscularis mucosae*, consisting of an inner circular and outer longitudinal layer of smooth muscle fibers. In some regions there may be an additional outer circular layer. Thin strands of smooth muscle cells extend from the inner circular layer toward the surface in the lamina propria between the glands. Their contraction compresses the mucous membrane and may facilitate discharge of secretion from the glands.

SUBMUCOSA

The connective tissue layer peripheral to the muscularis mucosae is called the *submucosa*. It is denser than the lamina propria with more abundant collagenous fibers and numerous lymphocytes, eosinophils, and mast cells. This layer contains the arterioles supplying capillaries to the mucosa and a venous plexus that receives venules descending from the mucosa. There is also a submucous network of lymphatics. Occasional adipose cells are found in this layer.

MUSCULARIS EXTERNA

The musculature of the stomach wall is called the *muscularis externa* to distinguish it from the muscularis mucosae. It consists of three layers of smooth muscle fibers: longitudinal, circular, and oblique, but these are not as clearly defined as in the muscularis of the intestine and their relationships are not easily described. The longitudinal fibers, directly beneath the serosa, are continuous with the longitudinal fibers of the esophageal wall. They radiate from the cardia, are best developed along the greater and lesser curvatures of the stomach, and do not extend to the pylorus. This layer is incomplete, and longitudinal fibers cannot be found in some areas of the dorsal and ventral surface of the corpus.

The circular fibers form a complete, uniform layer over the whole stomach deep to the longitudinal fibers. The circular muscle is continuous with the corresponding layer in the esophageal wall. It is thickest in the pylorus, where it forms an annular *pyloric sphincter.*

The oblique fibers are deep to the circular fibers and again do not form a complete layer. They are most abundant at the cardia, and sweep downward in broad bands parallel to the lesser curvature, many of their number diverging toward the greater curvature and intermingling with the fibers of the circular muscle layer. Oblique fibers are generally lacking along the lesser curvature of the stomach.

The work of the muscular components of the stomach wall is regulated with great precision by autonomic nerve plexuses between its layers. By varying smooth muscle tonus, the stomach wall adapts itself to changes in the volume of its contents with little or no alteration of the pressure in its cavity. Emptying of the stomach depends on intermittent peristaltic waves of contraction that sweep from the cardia toward the pylorus.

SEROSA

The outermost component of the stomach wall is a thin layer of loose connective tissue overlying the muscularis externa and covered on its outer aspect with mesothelium. It is continuous with the serous covering of the greater and lesser omentum.

BLOOD SUPPLY

The arterial supply to the mucosa originates from arterioles in the submucosa. These give rise to numerous vessels of capil-

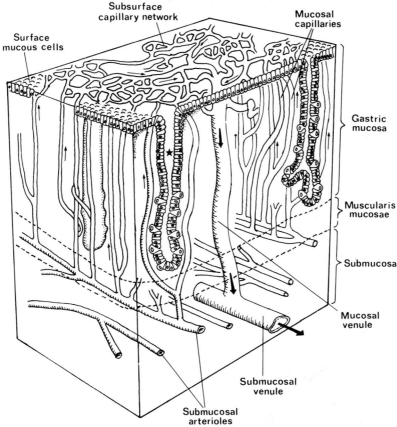

Figure 25–21. Diagramatic representation of the blood vascular supply of human gastric mucosa. The vascular relationships of the gastric gland, marked with an asterisk, are shown in greater detail in Figure 25–22. (Redrawn after Gannon, B. J., J. Browning, and J. E. McGuigan. Gastroenterology 86:866, 1984.)

lary size that ascend in the lamina propria between the gastric glands (Fig. 25–21). These capillaries are fenestrated and pass in close proximity to the parietal cells in the depths of the glands. They continue upward, forming a rich capillary network immediately underlying the surface epithelium. This superficial capillary bed is drained by venules that descend directly to a submucous venous plexus. There appear to be no arteriovenous anastomoses in the gastric mucosa.

The flow of blood upward to the subsurface capillary plexus past the parietal cells in the gastric glands encourages the speculation that bicarbonate ion generated by actively secreting parietal cells would diffuse into the fenestrated ascending capillaries and be transported rapidly to the capillary bed lying beneath the surface epithelial cells (Fig. 25–22). There it would be favorably distributed to neutralize any back-diffusing hydrogen ions from the lumen. It is tempting to believe that the microvascular architecture of the stomach is arranged to provide maximal mu-

cosal defense against potential damage by the acid content of the gastric lumen.

CELL RENEWAL AND REPAIR

The superficial portion of the gastric mucosa has a very rapid rate of cell renewal. Studies carried out in laboratory rodents using radiolabeled thymidine to identify dividing cells have shown that the surface mucous cells are completely renewed in about three days. The rate of renewal of the surface epithelium in human gastric mucosa is probably somewhat slower than in small laboratory animals. Mitotic activity is largely confined to cells in the depths of the gastric foveolae and the mucous neck cells in the isthmus of the gastric glands (Fig. 25–23). Epithelial cells exfoliated at the surface are replaced by upward migration of cells from this region of mitotic activity. The parietal cells and chief cells can be replaced by differentiation of mucous neck cells, but auto-

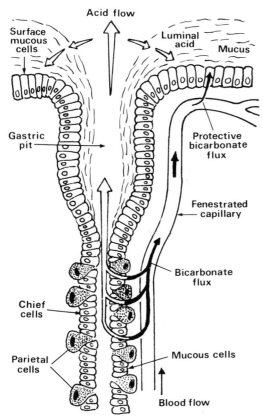

Figure 25–22. Diagram illustrating the postulated vascular transfer of bicarbonate ions, generated by active parietal cells, to the subsurface capillary network where it may protect the epithelium by neutralizing any back-diffusing hydrogen ions from the lumen. (Redrawn after Gannon, B. J., J. Browning, and J. E. McGuigan. Gastroenterology *86*:866, 1984.)

radiographic studies indicate that the cells in the glands are relatively long-lived and are renewed only very slowly.

In addition to the continual renewal of its surface mucous cells, the gastric mucosa has a remarkable capacity for reestablishment of epithelial continuity after superficial injury. In humans, the stomach is frequently insulted by aspirin (Fig. 25–24), strong alcoholic beverages, and other toxic substances that cause superficial erosion of the mucosa. Although extensive, irreversible damage and exfoliation of the surface epithelium results, there is rapid restoration of epithelial continuity by migration of viable cells from the depths of the foveolae. In experiments on rodent gastric mucosa exposed to 20 mM aspirin or 40 per cent ethanol (80 proof), the resulting injury to the surface epithelium is scarcely detectable after 30 minutes. The time course of this repair is too short to involve cell proliferation. Instead, the un-

damaged epithelium in the lower third of the gastric pits is stimulated to migrate over the vacated basal lamina of the superficial epithelium. Within 15 to 30 minutes, it is covered with a continuous sheet of squamous or low cuboidal cells, which then increase in height and soon resume their secretory activity. This capacity for epithelial migration provides a rapid defense mechanism for prompt coverage after chemical, thermal, and hyperosmolar injuries that do not extensively damage the basal lamina. Very low pH in the gastric lumen may destroy the basal lamina and completely inhibit or greatly retard restoration of epithelial continuity. Bicarbonate or other antacids favor reconstitution by neutralizing luminal acid.

HISTOPHYSIOLOGY OF THE STOMACH

The mechanical functions of storage, mixing of stomach contents, and emptying depend on the muscular wall. Peristaltic waves

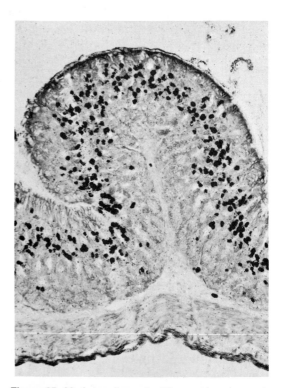

Figure 25–23. Autoradiograph of the gastric mucosa of a mouse given three injections of tritiated thymidine over a 12-hour period preceding fixation of the tissue. The distribution of the black deposits of silver demonstrates that the principal site of mitoses is in the neck region of the gastric glands. × 110. (Courtesy of A. J. Ladman.)

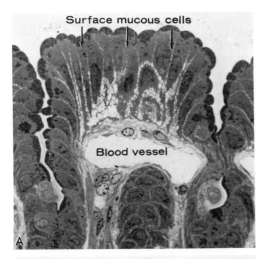

Surface mucous cells

Blood vessel

A

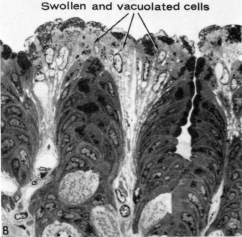

Swollen and vacuolated cells

B

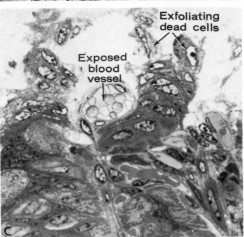

Exfoliating
dead cells

Exposed
blood
vessel

C

Figure 25–24. The protective permeability barrier that protects the stomach wall from damage by the acidity of the gastric contents is broken down by aspirin or alcohol. *A,* Normal surface mucous cells of mouse gastric mucosa. *B,* Mucosa 8 minutes after oral administration of a solution of 20 mM aspirin. The superficial cells are pale, their cytoplasm vacuolated, the chromatin marginated. *C,* Mucosa 8 minutes after 20 mM aspirin and 1 mM HCl. Damaged surface cells have exfoliated, exposing blood vessels of the lamina propria. (From Hingson, R., and S. Ito. Gastroenterology *61*:156, 1971.)

originate in the fundus and pass downward over the stomach to the pylorus. Ten to 15 ml of gastric chyme enter the duodenum with each peristaltic wave.

In species that are intermittent feeders, the capacity of the stomach as a distensible reservoir for accumulation of food is considerable. Although the luminal volume of the empty stomach is only 50 to 75 ml, nearly 1000 ml can be swallowed before the intraluminal pressure begins to rise. Distention stimulates peristalsis.

The stimulation of gastric secretion is in part neural and in part hormonal. Neural stimulation of secretion travels via the vagus nerves to the intrinsic nerve plexus, which in turn innervates the gastric glands and mucus-secreting glands. In addition the gastrin cells (G cells) in the antral mucosa respond to vagal stimulation by releasing the gastrointestinal hormone gastrin. This hormone promotes pepsinogen secretion, stimulates gastric motility, and binds to receptors on the oxyntic cells, stimulating acid secretion. Local reflexes activated by distention of the stomach with food also result in gastrin release. Substances ingested in the food, caffeine, and low concentrations of alcohol act as secretogogues favoring the release of gastrin. The activity of gastrin resides in four amino acids at its C-terminal end. This tetrapeptide has been synthesized and is used clinically to stimulate acid secretion. Release of gastrin is controlled by a feedback mechanism. When the pH of the stomach contents reaches 2, the stimulation of secretion by gastrin ceases, and when the pH rises significantly above this level, gastrin is secreted again.

The secretory activity of the stomach is considerable. The daily secretion of gastric juice in a fasting human is from 500 to 1500 ml. At each meal, several hundred milliliters of gastric juice is secreted. This clear, colorless fluid contains mucus, water, and electrolytes and the proteolytic enzyme pepsin, which is active only at the low pH that results from hydrochloric acid secretion by the parietal cells. The chief cells secrete pepsinogen, 42,500 M.W., which upon exposure to hydrochloric acid is converted to active *pepsin,* M.W. 35,000. The enzyme is optimally active at pH 2, cleaving peptide bonds and facilitating gastric digestion of proteins.

The oxyntic or parietal cells secrete the glycoprotein *gastric intrinsic factor,* which is essential for the absorption of vitamin B_{12} in the ileum. Failure of absorption of vitamin B_{12} leads to impairment of maturation of erythrocytes in the bone marrow, and results in *pernicious anemia*. Patients with this disorder show atrophy of the oxyntic cells in their gastric glands and achlorhydria (deficiency of HCl secretion).

The capacity to elaborate a secretion with a pH ranging from 2 to as low as 0.9 is perhaps the most remarkable property of the gastric mucosa. The concentration of hydrogen ions may reach a level 2 million times greater than that of the blood. This is accomplished by the parietal cells. The precise mechanism is still a subject of some disagreement, but it is the prevailing view that chloride ions are actively transported into the secretory canaliculus and that this in turn results in passive diffusion of potassium from the cytoplasm into the lumen. Hydrogen and hydroxyl ions are dissociated in the cytoplasm from water, and hydroxyl ions are actively secreted into the canaliculus in exchange for potassium, thus recovering most of the potassium ions secreted with chloride. Hydrogen ions diffuse into the canaliculus, replacing the reabsorbed potassium. Water passes through the cell along an osmotic gradient so that the content of the canaliculus is a solution of hydrochloric acid and potassium chloride. In an essential concurrent reaction in the parietal cell cytoplasm, carbonic anhydrase catalyzes the combination of carbon dioxide and water to form carbonic acid, which dissociates to hydrogen and bicarbonate ions. Bicarbonate ion diffuses from the abluminal surface of the cell into the blood. The junctional complexes between the surface mucosal cells normally provide an effective barrier preventing acid in the lumen of the stomach from diffusing back through the epithelium. However, the "alkaline tide" of bicarbonate released into the lamina propria of the actively secreting gastric mucosa is believed to be beneficial in neutralizing any back-diffusing hydrogen ions. This may be especially important when the efficiency of the barrier is greatly reduced by damage to the epithelium from imbibition of alcohol or other noxious substances.

REFERENCES

ESOPHAGUS

Edwards, D. A. W. The esophagus. Gut *12*:984, 1971.
Hapwood, D., K. R. Logan, and I. A. D. Bouchier: The electron microscopy of normal human esophageal epithelium. Virchows Archiv. [Cell Pathol.] *26*:345, 1978.
Parakkal, P.: An electron microscopic study of the esophageal epithelium in the newborn and adult mouse. Am. J. Anat. *121*:175, 1967.

STOMACH

Adair, H. M.: Epithelial repair in chronic gastric ulcers. Br. J. Exp. Pathol. *59*:229, 1978.
Bensley, R. R.: The gastric glands. *In* Cowdry, E. V., ed.: Special Cytology. Vol. 1. 2nd ed. New York, Paul Hoeber, 1932.
Forssmann, W. G., L. Orci, R. Pictet, A. E. Renold, and C. Rouiller: The endocrine cells in the epithelium of the gastrointestinal mucosa of the rat. J. Cell Biol. *40*:692, 1969.
Gannon, B. J., J. Browning, and P. O'Brien: The microvascular architecture of the glandular mucosa of rat stomach. J. Anat. *133*:677, 1982.
Gannon, B. J., J. Browning, and P. O'Brien: Mucosal microvascular architecture of the fundus and body of human stomach. Gastroenterology *86*:866, 1984.
Goldstein, A. M. B., M. R. Brothers, and E. A. Davis: Architecture of the superficial layer of the gastric mucosa. J. Anat. *104*:539, 1969.
Greider, M. H., V. Steinberg, and J. E. McGuigan; Electron microscopic identification of the gastrin cell of the human antral mucosa by means of immunocytochemistry. Gastroenterology *63*:572, 1972.
Grossman, M. I.: Gastrin and its activities. Nature *228*:1147, 1970.
Helander, H. F.: Ultrastructure of fundus glands of the mouse gastric mucosa. J. Ultrastruct Res. (Suppl.) *4*:1, 1962.
Hingson, D. J., and S. Ito: Effect of aspirin and related compounds on the fine structure of mouse gastric mucosa. Gastroenterology *61*:156, 1971.
Hoedemaeker, P. J., J. Abels, J. J. Wachters, A. Arends, and N.O. Nieweg: Investigations about the site of production of Castle's gastric intrinsic factor. Lab. Invest. *13*:1394, 1964.
Ito, S., and E. R. Lacy: Morphology of gastric mucosal damage, defenses and restitution in the presence of luminal ethanol. Gastroenterology *88*:250, 1985.
Ito, S., and R. J. Winchester: The fine structure of the gastric mucosa in the bat. J. Cell Biol. *16*:541, 1963.
Leblond, C. P., and B. E. Walker: Renewal of cell populations. Physiol. Rev. *36*:255, 1956.
Lillibridge, C. B.: The fine structure of normal human gastric mucosa. Gastroenterology *47*:269, 1964.
Lipkin, M., P. Sherlock, and B. Bell: Cell proliferation kinetics in the gastrointestinal tract of man. II. Cell renewal in stomach, ileum, colon, and rectum. Gastroenterology *47*:721, 1963.
Samloff, I. M.: Pepsinogens, pepsins and pepsin inhibitors. Gastroenterology *60*:586, 1971.
Siten, W., and S. Ito: Mechanisms for rapid epithelialization of the gastric mucosal surface. Annu. Rev. Physiol. *47*:217, 1985.
Stevens, C. E., and C. P. Leblond: Renewal of the mucous cells in the gastric mucosa of the rat. Anat. Rec. *115*:231, 1953.

26

INTESTINES

THE SMALL INTESTINE

The digestive process initiated in the stomach is continued in the small intestine by the secretions of its intrinsic glands and those of its accessory glands—the liver and pancreas. In the stomach, there is little or no absorption of nutrient materials released by digestion. Absorption is the principal function of the small intestine and this takes place mainly in its initial segments.

The small intestine is the portion of the alimentary tract between the stomach and the large intestine. It is a tubular viscus 4 to 8 m in length grossly divisible into three segments—the *duodenum, jejunum,* and *ileum.* The duodenum is about 25 cm in length and is largely retroperitoneal, being firmly attached to the dorsal body wall. The remainder of the small intestine is suspended from the dorsal wall by a mesentery and is freely movable. The proximal part of the free portion of the intestine is the jejunum, which normally occupies the upper left portion of the abdominal cavity. The distal portion, the ileum, is situated in the lower abdomen. Although there are minor gross and microscopic differences between the three segments, they have the same basic organization.

As in other parts of the gastrointestinal tract, the wall of the small intestine is made up of four concentric layers—the *serosa,* the *muscularis,* the *submucosa,* and the *mucosa.* Of these, the mucosa is the most important in relation to the digestive and absorptive functions.

THE INTESTINAL MUCOSA

To augment the efficiency of this physiologically important layer, there are a number of structural specializations that serve to increase the area of surface exposed to the lumen. The *plicae circulares* (valves of Kerckring) are grossly visible crescentic folds that extend half to two thirds of the way around the lumen (Fig. 26–1). They are permanent structures involving both the mucosa and the submucosa (Fig. 26–2). The larger plicae are some 8 to 10 mm in height, 3 to 4 mm in

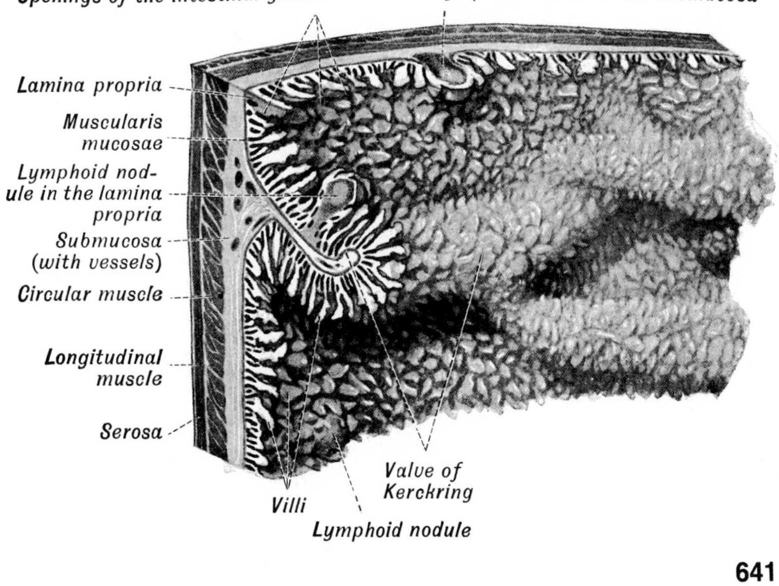

Figure 26–1. Portion of small intestine; drawn from sections using a binocular microscope. × 17. (After Braus.)

Openings of the intestinal glands

Lymphoid nodule in the submucosa

Lamina propria

Muscularis mucosae

Lymphoid nodule in the lamina propria

Submucosa (with vessels)

Circular muscle

Longitudinal muscle

Serosa

Villi

Valve of Kerckring

Lymphoid nodule

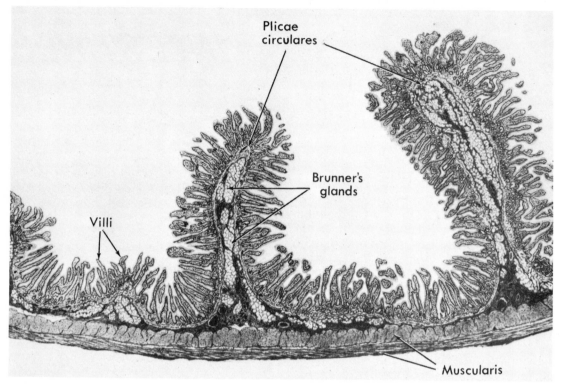

Figure 26–2. Drawing of a longitudinal section through the wall of the duodenum of an adult human, showing the plicae circulares (valves of Kerckring), the villi, and submucosal glands of Brunner. (From Bargmann, W. Histologie und Mikroskopische Anatomie des Menschen. 6th ed. Stuttgart, Georg Thieme Verlag, 1962.)

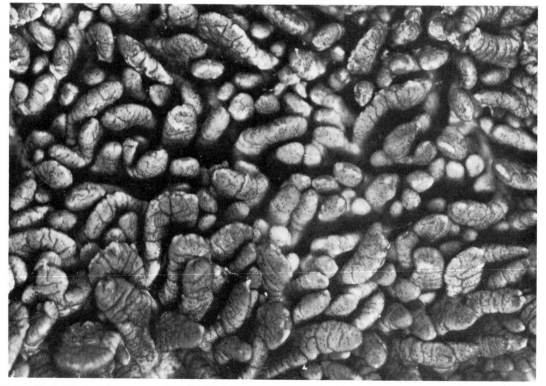

Figure 26–3. Whole mount of a human jejunal biopsy stained with PAS–Alcian blue, showing intestinal villi of both finger-like and foliate form. × 37. (Photomicrograph from Poulsen, S. Scand. J. Gastroenterol. *12*:235, 1977.)

thickness, and up to 5 cm in length. They are absent from the first portion of the duodenum, but begin about 5 cm distal to the pylorus and reach their greatest development in the last part of the duodenum and proximal portion of the jejunum. From there onward, they gradually diminish in size and number and are seldom found beyond the middle of the ileum.

A second and more effective means of augmenting the surface area of the mucosa is the presence of enormous numbers of *intestinal villi* (Figs. 26–3, 26–4). These are minute, fingerlike projections of the mucosa having a length of 0.5 to 1.5 mm, depending on the degree of distention of the intestinal wall and the state of contraction of smooth muscle fibers in their own interior. They cover the entire surface of the mucosa and give it a characteristic velvety appearance in the fresh condition. Their number varies from 10 to 40 per square millimeter. They are most numerous in the duodenum and proximal jejunum.

The surface of the epithelium is increased not only by villi, but also by invagination to form tubular glands between the bases of the villi, called *crypts of Lieberkühn* (Fig. 26–5). These are simple tubular glands 320 to 450 μm long, which extend downward nearly to the thin layer of smooth muscle comprising the *muscularis mucosae*. The spaces between the intestinal glands are occupied by the loose connective tissue constituting the *lamina propria*.

Intestinal Epithelium

The free surface of the mucosa is covered by a simple columnar epithelium in which

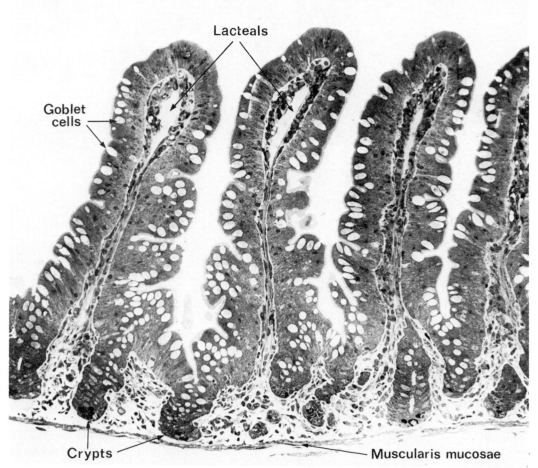

Figure 26–4. Thin section of monkey jejunal mucosa, showing the long villi and relatively short crypts. Visible in the core of each villus is the lacteal, a blind-ending lymphatic capillary through which absorbed lipid and other nutrients are transported to a submucosal lymphatic plexus, and thence via mesenteric lymphatic vessels and the thoracic duct to the bloodstream. (Courtesy of Madera, J., from Neutra, M. *In* Weiss, L., and Greep, R. O., eds.: Histology. 5th ed. New York, Elsevier, 1982.)

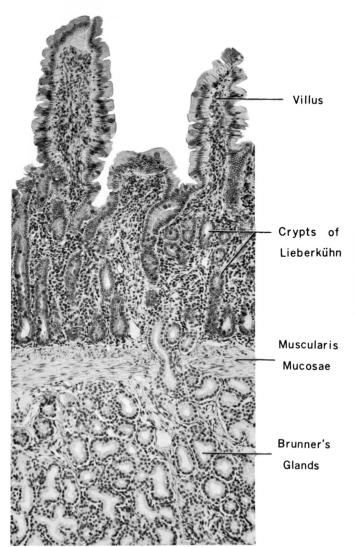

Villus

Crypts of Lieberkühn

Figure 26–5. Photomicrograph of a histological section of the duodenum of a macaque. The villi, crypts of Lieberkühn, and Brunner's glands are shown. A duct of Brunner's gland can be seen penetrating the muscularis mucosae to empty into one of the crypts. Hematoxylin and eosin. × 110.

Muscularis Mucosae

Brunner's Glands

three types of cells can be distinguished—*absorptive cells, goblet cells,* and *endocrine cells* (argentaffin cells).

Absorptive Cells. The absorptive cells are columnar in form and 20 to 26 μm in height, with an ovoid nucleus situated in the lower part of the cell. As seen with the light microscope, the free surface has a prominent striated border (Fig. 26–7) and beneath this is a clear zone usually devoid of organelles but occupied by the *terminal web.* This may exhibit birefringence when examined with the polarizing microscope and it can be selectively stained by a method that employs tannic acid, phosphomolybdic acid, and the dye amido black. The cytoplasm below the terminal web is rich in mitochondria and there is a well-developed supranuclear Golgi apparatus.

In electron micrographs, the striated or brush border of the absorptive cells is made up of large numbers of closely packed parallel microvilli that amplify the surface exposed to the lumen about 30-fold. The microvilli are 1 to 1.4 μm in length, and about 80 nm in diameter (Figs. 26–7, 26–8). The plasmalemma enclosing the microvilli has the usual unit membrane structure but is unusual in having a nap of delicate branching filaments that radiate from its outer leaflet, giving the membrane a fuzzy appearance. These filaments are longer and more numerous at the tips of the villi than on their sides (Fig. 26–9). The intermingling of the filamentous excrescences of the microvillus tips forms a continuous *surface coat* on the striated border that varies from 0.1 to 0.5 μm in thickness, depending on the species (Fig. 26–8). This

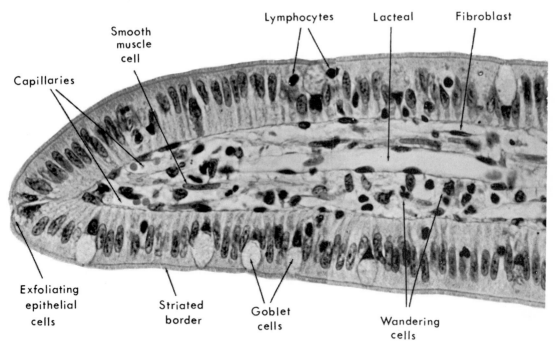

Figure 26–6. Longitudinal section of a villus from cat jejunum. Hematoxylin and eosin. × 600.

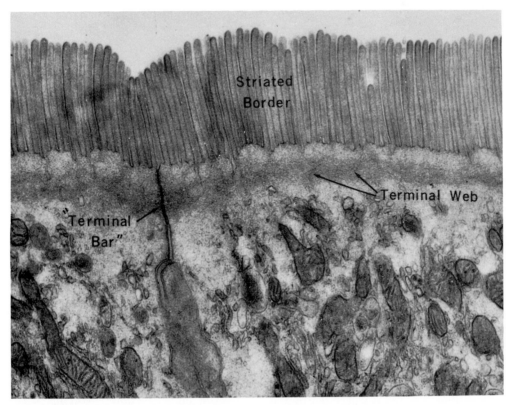

Figure 26–7. Electron micrograph of portions of two intestinal epithelial cells of the hamster, showing the striated border, the terminal web, and the junctional complex, which corresponds to the terminal bar seen with the light microscope. × 25,000. (Courtesy of E. Strauss.)

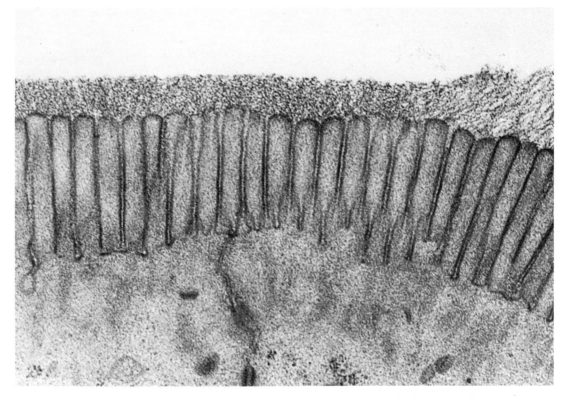

Figure 26–8. The plasma membrane on the microvilli of the intestinal brush border has a prominent surface coat consisting of polysaccharide chains of integral glycoproteins. (Micrograph courtesy of S. Ito.)

surface coat is well developed in the human. It is regarded as an integral part of the cell surface. It is glycoprotein in nature and is extremely resistant to both proteolytic and mucolytic agents. It is believed to have a protective role, but it is likely that it also participates actively in the digestive process. Intraluminal digestive enzymes such as pancreatic amylase and proteases are believed to be adsorbed onto the very large surface presented by the filaments of the surface coat. Thus, some of the digestive processes previously thought to occur only in the lumen may also take place on the microvillous surface. Isolated intestinal striated borders hydrolyze disaccharides and polypeptides to monosaccharides and amino acids. Therefore, the disaccharidases and peptidases involved in the terminal digestion of carbohydrates and proteins are believed to be localized in the membrane of the microvilli. In addition to its enzymatic activities, it has been suggested that the surface coat of the jejunum may have specific receptors or binding sites for substances that are selectively absorbed in this portion of the intestine and not in other regions. Thus, the membrane of the brush

border and its surface coat, which were not resolved with the light microscope, have now been shown to be of great physiological importance in the digestive and absorptive function of the small intestine.

In the interior of each microvillus is a bundle of thin straight filaments that run longitudinally in an otherwise homogeneous fine-textured cytoplasmic matrix (Fig. 26–10). The filaments extend downward from the microvilli into the terminal web, which is resolved in electron micrographs as a feltwork of exceedingly fine filaments oriented (Fig. 26–11), for the most part, parallel to the brush border. At the sides of the cell, the filaments of the terminal web merge with those associated with the zonula adherens. The filaments in the core of the microvilli have been shown to form arrowhead complexes with heavy meromyosin and are therefore identified as actin. There are about 20 actin filaments in each microvillus of the brush border, and these filament bundles, together with the intermediate filaments, myosin, and associated proteins of the terminal web, form one of the most highly organized cytoskeletal apparatuses thus far

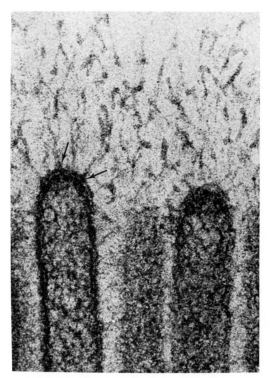

Figure 26–9. Electron micrograph of the tips of several microvilli from cat ileum, showing the branching protein-polysaccharide (mucopolysaccharide) filaments attached at one end to the outer leaflet of the unit membrane *(at arrows).* × 120,000. (Courtesy of S. Ito, after Fawcett, D. W. J. Histochem. Cytochem. *13*:75, 1965.)

ular endoplasmic reticulum are also found in the supranuclear cytoplasm but they are more abundant toward the base. The Golgi complex has the usual arrays of parallel cisternae and associated vesicles. It shows no morphological evidences of activity except during lipid absorption.

The lateral surfaces of the absorptive cells are in close apposition in the upper part of the epithelium and may have occasional slender interdigitating processes. In phases of active absorption the lateral cell membranes of neighboring cells diverge toward the base of the epithelium, and *chylomicra* may accumulate in these widened intercellular clefts. A juxtaluminal junctional complex bars access to the intercellular cleft from the lumen. The presence of occluding junctions completely encircling each cell near the lumen ensures that material being absorbed from the lumen must traverse the plasma membrane of the brush border, the apical cytoplasm, and the lateral cell membrane to gain access to the intercellular spaces of the epithelium.

described. Until recently it was thought that the actin filaments of the microvillous cores interacted with myosin in the terminal web, resulting in shortening of the microvilli. It is generally agreed that isolated brush borders contract in vitro in the presence of Ca^{++} ions and ATP; it is now believed, however, that lateral contraction of the terminal web increases the convexity of the cell apex and tends to spread the tips of the microvilli apart, but the microvilli do not shorten. What role, if any, this contractility of the cytoskeleton plays in intestinal absorption is not known.

Below the terminal web, the cytoplasm contains occasional lysosomes and numerous elongate mitochondria of orthodox internal structure. Branching profiles of smooth endoplasmic reticulum are plentiful in this region. The membranes of this organelle contain enzymes essential for synthesis of triglycerides from fatty acids and monoglycerides. The smooth endoplasmic reticulum therefore plays an important role in intestinal absorption of fat. Cisternal profiles of gran-

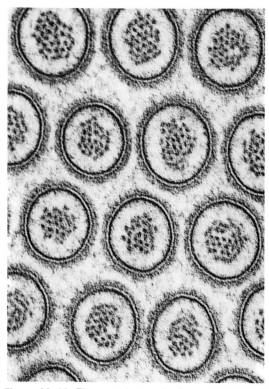

Figure 26–10. Electron micrograph of cross sections of microvilli from the brush border of an intestinal epithelial cell. The bundle of actin filaments in the core of the microvillus is clearly shown. Prepared by quick freezing in liquid helium and freeze substitution. (Micrograph courtesy of A. Ichikawa.)

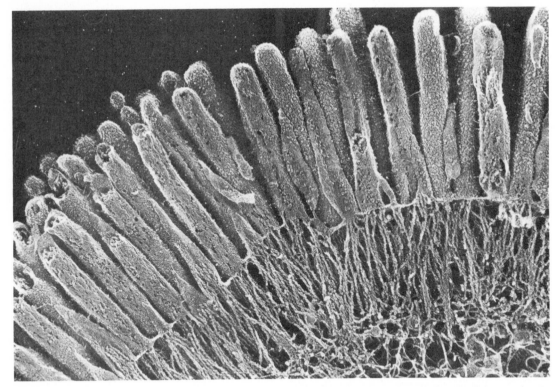

Figure 26–11. Brush border of an intestinal absorptive cell prepared by quick-freezing, deep-etching, and rotary shadowing. Bundles of actin filaments can be seen extending from the cores of the microvilli downward into the meshwork of filaments making up the terminal web. (Micrograph courtesy of N. Hirokawa and J. Heuser.)

The plasma membrane at the cell base is closely applied to a continuous basal lamina that extends across the intercellular spaces at the base of the epithelium. Absorbed material accumulating between cells must traverse this barrier to reach the capillaries and lymphatics of the intestinal villus.

Goblet Cell. The *goblet cells* are irregularly scattered among the absorptive cells (Fig. 26–6). They are described in some detail in Chapter 3, as examples of unicellular glands. Their name derives from their fancied resemblance to a wine glass. Their apical region, called the *theca*, is distended with mucigen droplets, while the base of the cell is relatively free of secretory material and forms a slender stem or stalk. The nucleus tends to be flattened and the surrounding cytoplasm strongly basophilic. The organelles are difficult to study with the light microscope in the mature goblet cell because of their close crowding.

In electron micrographs, cisternae of granular endoplasmic reticulum are arranged more or less parallel to the base and the lateral surfaces of the cell. A few cisternae may continue upward into the thin layer of cytoplasm around the theca. A highly developed Golgi complex is situated between the nucleus and the mucigen droplets in the theca. The individual droplets appear to originate in the Golgi complex and move up into the theca. Each is enveloped by a delicate membrane, which is often disrupted in preparation of the specimen. The basal and lateral plasma membranes are smooth-contoured except for a few lateral interdigitations. The goblet cells are attached to the neighboring absorptive cells by juxtaluminal junctional complexes. Sparse microvilli may be present on the free surface. Their length and number is influenced by the degree of distention of the theca with mucigen. The tendency of mucigen droplets to swell in specimen preparation has made it difficult to study the mechanism of their release, but the membranes of the droplets appear to fuse with each other and with the plasmalemma, permitting the mucus to flow out while maintaining the integrity of the cell surface.

The secretory product of the goblet cell, *mucus*, is a viscous material with the consistency of raw egg white. It serves to lubricate and protect the surface of the epithelium.

Chemical analyses indicate that goblet cell mucus is a very large glycoprotein of molecular weight 2×10^6, which is acidic owing to the presence on the molecule of both terminal sialic acid residues and sulfate esters such as N-acetylglucosamine-6-sulfate. It stains brilliantly with the periodic acid–Schiff (PAS) reaction for carbohydrates, with Alcian blue, toluidine blue, and other thiazine dyes that stain acidic glycoproteins. There appear to be minor qualitative differences between the mucus in the crypts and that on the villi, and also differences along the length of the intestine. The content of acidic carbohydrate side chains is generally higher in the goblet cells of the colon than in those of the small intestine.

The synthetic activities of goblet cells include the synthesis of protein from amino acid precursors; the formation of polysaccharides from mono- and disaccharides; the linking of oligo- and polysaccharides to proteins; and the incorporation of sulfate into acid polysaccharides. Autoradiographic studies show that protein synthesis is associated with the abundant granular endoplasmic reticulum at the cell base, whereas synthesis of polysaccharide and its sulfation take place in the Golgi complex.

Enteroendocrine Cells (Basal Granular Cells). More than a century ago, Heidenhain (1870) described small cells near the base of the gastrointestinal epithelium that possessed staining reactions similar to those of the chromaffin cells in the adrenal medulla. These later came to be called the *enterochromaffin cells.* Their basal location in the epithelium and the presence of secretory granules concentrated between the nucleus and the basal lamina suggested that they were endocrine cells liberating their secretion into the lamina propria, rather than into the intestinal lumen.

They occur singly and are widely scattered throughout the epithelial lining of the gastrointestinal tract. They are present in moderate numbers in the stomach, are common in the duodenum, and are more sparse in the jejunum and ileum, where they occur both on the villi and in the crypts. They are present in limited numbers throughout the colon and are also found in the biliary tract and the ducts of the pancreas.

In addition to their ability to bind alkaline bichromates (chromaffinity), many of these cells also precipitate silver salts in the absence of a reducing agent (argentaffinity). For many years, they were also called argentaffin cells. It was subsequently found that if tissue sections were treated with a reducing agent before being exposed to silver nitrate, a greater number of these basal granular cells could be demonstrated. Cells stainable by this method were termed *argyrophilic cells.* The differences in number of argyrophil and argentaffin cells, and the fact that some granulated cells exhibited fluorescence in ultraviolet light while others did not, gradually led to the realization that not all the enteroendocrine cells were the same. Although they have a number of morphological features in common, they have proved to be a highly heterogeneous cell population. In recent years, correlation of electron microscopic observations with immunocytochemical staining has produced a surge of new information about their secretory products and their probable function. More than 16 different endocrine cell types have now been described in the gastrointestinal tract (Fig. 26–12).

For students to learn the identifying characteristics of all the enteroendocrine cell types would be beyond the call of duty, but they should be familiar with the structural features these cells have in common and should be aware of the range of hormones secreted by the enteroendocrine cells as a group.

At the light microscope level, they are ovoid or pyramidal in the stomach and intestinal crypts, and more columnar on the epithelium of the villi. The bulk of the cell body is in the lower half of the epithelium, but a narrow apical region usually extends to the lumen and has a brush border. The nucleus is round and generally poor in heterochromatin. The cytoplasm is pale in relation to the surrounding cells. The secretory granules vary in size in the different cell types and are concentrated in the basal cytoplasm.

In electron micrographs, the microvilli of the enteroendocrine cells are often longer and thicker than those of adjacent absorptive cells—a finding that has suggested their possible function as chemoreceptors. The cytoplasm is relatively electron lucent. The cytoplasmic organelles do not differ significantly in size or form compared with those of other epithelial cells. The rough endoplasmic reticulum varies somewhat in amount from one cell type to another, but in no case is it highly developed. A few lysosomes are usually present. Morphological identification of the several types of enteroendocrine cells depends

CELL TYPE	SECRETION GRANULES	LOCALIZATION			PRODUCT
		Pancreas	Stomach	Intestines	
A	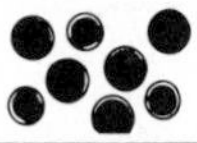 250 nm	Islets			Glucagon, Glicentin
B	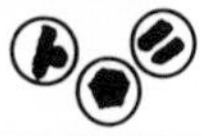 350	Islets			Insulin
D	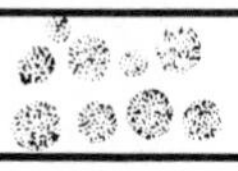 350	Islets	Fundic Pyloric	Jejunum Ileum Colon	Somatostatin
D₁	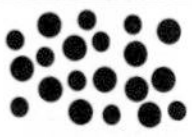 160	Islets	Fundic Pyloric	Jejunum Ileum Colon	Unknown
EC	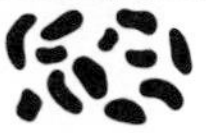 300	Islets	Fundic Pyloric	Jejunum Ileum Colon	Serotonin Various peptides
ECL	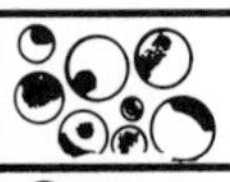 450		Fundic		Histamine
G	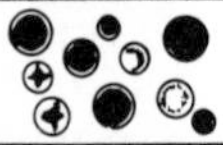 300		Pyloric	Duodenum	Gastrin
I	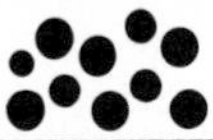 250			Jejunum Ileum	Cholecystokinin
K	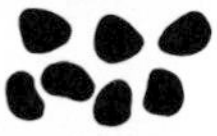 350			Jejunum Ileum	Gastric inhibitory peptide
L	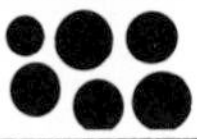 400			Jejunum Ileum Colon	Glucagon–like immunoreactivity
Mo				Jejunum Ileum	Motilin
N	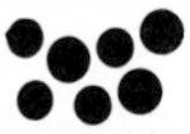 300			Ileum	Neurotensin
P	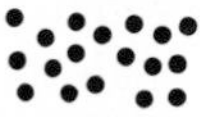 120		Fundic Pyloric	Jejunum	Unknown
PP	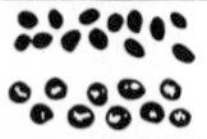 180	Islets	Fundic Pyloric	Colon	Pancreatic polypeptide
S	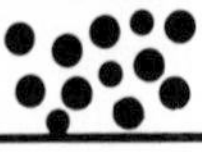 200			Jejunum Ileum	Secretin
TG				Jejunum	C–terminal gastrin immunoreactivity
X	300		Fundic Pyloric		Unknown

Figure 26–12. Summary of the enteroendocrine cell types thus far described, including their nomenclature, their distribution, the ultrastructure of their granules, and their amine or peptide products. (Modified after Grube, H., and G. Forssmann. Horm. Metab. Res. *11*:603, 1979.)

mainly on differences in size, shape, electron density, and substructure of their secretory granules complemented by immunocytochemical staining of the granules with fluorescein-labeled antibodies specific for their amine or polypeptide products.

A majority of the cells traditionally described as argentaffin cells by histologists are now called *EC cells.* They are found in the fundic and antral regions of the stomach and in the intestinal epithelium of all species so far studied. Their cytoplasmic granules have elongated cores of high electron density. In general, those in the stomach are smaller (200 nm) than those in the intestine (300–350 nm). They synthesize and secrete serotonin (5-hydroxytryptamine).

A second category of enteroendocrine cells found in the fundus and antrum of the stomach is the *D cell,* so named because of its resemblance to the delta cell of the endocrine pancreas. Its round granules (350 nm) have a core of finely granular texture and medium electron density. They secrete *somatostatin.* A subtype of similar distribution, designated D_1, has smaller granules (160 nm) and is believed to produce *vasoactive intestinal polypeptide.*

In the human duodenal mucosa and in the stomach of other species are the *A cells,* so called because of their resemblance to the alpha cells of the pancreatic islets. Their granules (250 nm) have a core of high electron density surrounded by a narrow clear space beneath their limiting membrane. They are the source of enteric *glucagon.*

Occurring in large numbers in the gastric antrum of all species studied are the G cells. Their granules (200–250 nm) are round or slightly angular with cores of variable density and heterogeneous texture. They secrete the hormone *gastrin.*

The *L cells,* generally confined to the intestinal mucosa, have quite large secretory granules (400 nm) with round or slightly angular cores of high electron density closely surrounded by the limiting membrane. Their product is still a subject of debate.

S cells are restricted to the intestinal mucosa. Their granules are among the smallest found in enteroendocrine cells (200 nm) with round cores of medium to high electron density. There is general agreement that they produce the hormone *secretin. I cells* occur in the duodenal mucosa and have granules (250 nm) intermediate in size between the L and S cells. They are probably the source of *cholecystokinin.*

The enteroendocrine cells have thus been shown to be the source of the classical gastrointestinal hormones long studied by physiologists (gastrin, secretin, and cholecystokinin-pancreozymin), and several other biologically active peptides and monoamines with less well-established functions. Rather puzzling is the fact that several polypeptide hormones found in the endocrine cells of the gut (gastrin, cholecystokinin-pancreozymin, vasoactive intestinal peptide, and motilin) have also been localized in certain cells of the central nervous system. And conversely, some polypeptide hormones originally isolated from the central nervous system (substance P, somatostatin, neurotensin) have also been found to occur in enteric or pancreatic endocrine cells. The physiological or ontogenetic significance of such a diffuse distribution of isolated endocrine cells in organ systems of such disparate function awaits clarification.

The majority of enteroendocrine cell types can take up and decarboxylate precursors of biogenic monoamines and therefore are included as members of the so-called APUD cell series. They are also components of the diffuse neuroendocrine system (see Chapter 3).

Crypts of Lieberkühn

The epithelium covering the villi continues into the intestinal glands or crypts of Lieberkühn (Fig. 26–5). The upper halves of the walls of the crypts are lined with low columnar epithelium containing absorptive cells, goblet cells, and a few basal granular cells. In the lower halves of the crypts the cells are less clearly differentiated and there are numerous mitoses. It is here that new cells are formed to continually replace those that are exfoliated at the tips of the villi. If tritiated thymidine is given to an animal, it can be shown by biopsies at later time intervals that the label incorporated into nuclei of dividing cells in the bottom of the crypts of Lieberkühn gradually moves upward onto the villi. About a day after administration of thymidine the labeled cells are on the sides of the villi, and by the fifth day they are being exfoliated at the villus tips. Thus, billions of cells are being shed every day from the human gastrointestinal tract and are being replaced by upward displacement of cells from localized regions of cell proliferation. In the small intestine, the proliferative activity is confined to the crypts of Lieberkühn.

Discovery of this rapid turnover of cells in the lining of the intestine has altered our interpretations of the physiology of some of the cell types. For example, it was formerly thought that goblet cells might accumulate secretions, discharge, and then refill, and that this cycle was repeated many times. It is now realized that the life span of intestinal goblet cells is only three or four days—the time taken for them to differentiate in the crypts, move up onto the villi, and be exfoliated at the tip. Thus, it is probable that goblet cells secrete continuously and normally pass through only one secretory cycle. This consists of an initial phase in the crypts when rate of synthesis of mucus exceeds discharge and mucin accumulates; an intermediate phase when the cells are in the upper part of the crypts and lower half of the villi, synthesis and discharge are approximately in equilibrium, and the cells appear engorged with mucus; and a final phase when rate of discharge exceeds synthesis as the cells approach the tips of the villi and appear depleted. Although this is the normal course of events, it can be modified by irritants that cause expulsion of mucus. If mustard oil is administered locally to experimental animals, the goblet cells expel nearly all of their mucus stores. Under these conditions, they then are found to initiate a new cycle of accumulation.

The discovery of the continual upward migration of epithelial cells immediately posed a number of puzzling morphogenetic problems. Do the cells move with respect to a relatively stationary basal lamina, or does the epithelium as a whole move with respect to the underlying lamina propria? The answers to these questions remain in doubt, but valuable new insight into the problem has been gained from autoradiographic studies that reveal that there is also a continuous renewal and upward migration of the pericryptal fibroblasts. Much of the relevant experimental work has been carried out on the crypts of the colon but the findings are believed to apply also to those of the small intestine and other parts of the alimentary mucosa.

The crypts are surrounded by a sheath of flattened fibroblasts closely applied to the base of the epithelium and by a highly ordered reticulum laid down with the majority of its small bundles of unit fibers of collagen arranged circumferentially around the crypt. The *pericryptal fibroblasts* are flattened squamous elements that present fusiform profiles in both longitudinal and transverse sections of the glands. At early time intervals after administration of tritiated thymidine, labeled fibroblasts are found in autoradiographs around the lower third of the crypts. At longer time intervals, these labeled cells are localized around the necks of the glands. If the changing distribution of the labeled epithelial cells and labeled pericryptal cells are compared, it is evident that the two cell types migrate in synchrony. Electron micrographs show that there is a progressive increase in degree of cytological differentiation of the fibroblasts as they move upward. The continuous renewal and upward migration of pericryptal cells constitutes an exception to the generalization that fibroblasts in the adult are a relatively stable population proliferating only in response to injury.

Paneth Cell. In addition to the cell types already described, there is a type of cell occurring in small groups only in the depths of the crypts of Lieberkühn—the *Paneth cells* (Fig. 26–13). They are pyramidal in form, with a round or oval nucleus situated near the base, and conspicuous secretory granules in the apical cytoplasm. They have the cytological characteristics of cells actively secreting protein. The cytoplasm at the base is basophilic, and in electron micrographs contains parallel arrays of cisternae of rough

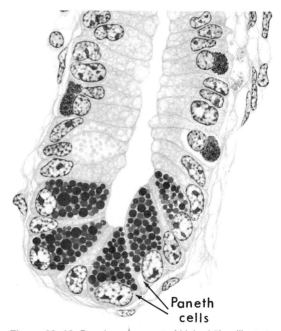

Figure 26–13. Drawing of a crypt of Lieberkühn, illustrating the Paneth cells at the base of the crypt. Higher up in the crypt are four argentaffin cells. Hematoxylin and eosin.

endoplasmic reticulum. The lumen of the cisternae not infrequently has a dense content, which may occasionally be precipitated in crystalline form. The Golgi complex is prominent, as in other active glandular cells, and often contains the formative stages of secretory granules. The granules are homogeneous in density in humans and in a number of other species. In the mouse, they have a dense core and lighter peripheral zone (Fig. 26–14). The periphery consists of an acid glycoprotein, whereas the core appears to be a neutral glycoprotein. The granules usually stain with acid dyes such as eosin or orange G.

Paneth cells are a stable population with little or no turnover. They do not incorporate tritiated thymidine and they are not observed in mitosis. They are abundant in humans, monkeys, mice, rats, guinea pigs, and ruminants, but are absent from the intestines of dogs, cats, pigs, and raccoons. They are extraordinarily abundant in the intestinal glands of the South American anteater—a finding that encouraged the speculation that in this species they might be involved in digestion of the chitinous exoskeleton of the ingested ants, but there is no solid evidence for this.

Paneth cells evidently secrete continuously, but the rate of secretion is enhanced by feeding or by administration of pilocarpine. Despite decades of study, the functional role of Paneth cells is still not known. Research on the chemical nature of the secretory product of Paneth cells has been hampered by inability to obtain their secretion free of contamination by constituents of other cell types. Immunocytochemical studies have revealed the presence of lysozyme in their well-developed phagolysosomal system. Lysozyme is a highly charged cationic protein capable of digesting the cell walls of certain bacteria. Under some circumstances Paneth cells have been observed to phagocytose and digest certain intestinal flagellates and spirilliform microorganisms commonly found in the crypts of Lieberkühn of rats. This has led to the suggestion that they may play a role in regulating the microbial flora of the intestinal glands. This leaves unexplained their obvious structural specialization as secretory cells, and

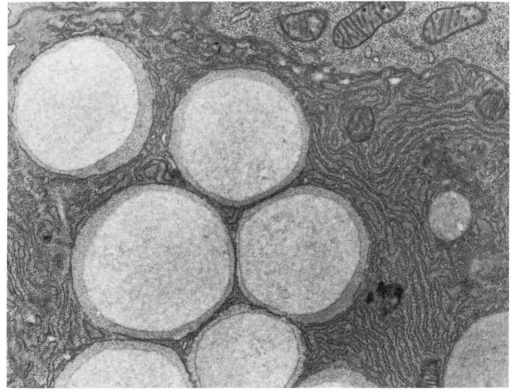

Figure 26–14. Electron micrograph of an area of cytoplasm from a Paneth cell, showing the abundance of granular reticulum and the heterogeneity of the secretory granules. (Micrograph from Staley, M., and J. Trier. Am. J. Anat. *117*:365, 1965.)

it is clear that the principal function of the Paneth cells is yet to be discovered.

Cell Turnover and Renewal

The epithelial lining of the intestinal tract is continuously being renewed by proliferation of undifferentiated cells in the crypts, migration upward onto the villi, and exfoliation of effete or dying cells at the villus tips. This whole process of cell renewal is referred to as the *cell turnover* of the epithelium, and its duration is the *cell turnover time*. The mucosa of the jejunum has the fastest rate of turnover of any tissue in the body.

The cells at the base of the crypts of Lieberkühn have high activities of the enzymes involved in nucleic acid synthesis and do not have the long interphase (G_0) characteristic of more slowly proliferating tissues. Synthesis of DNA occurs in a period of six to 11 hours (S). The premitotic (G_2) and postmitotic (G_1) stages of the mitotic cycle are brief and the mitotic phase (M) takes about one hour. The complete cell cycle occupies 10 to 17 hours in rodents and about 24 hours in humans. The intestinal epithelium is completely replaced in two to three days in laboratory rodents and three to six days in humans.

In the colon, villi are lacking but the pattern of renewal is similar. The proliferative zone in the crypts is somewhat more extensive, and cells are extruded at the mucosal surface between crypts. Cell division and migration are slightly slower, resulting in a turnover time of four to eight days in humans.

The intestine has a remarkable capacity to adapt to changing conditions of alimentation and to surgical removal of large segments. Starvation or protein deficiency results in atrophy of both muscular and mucosal components of the small intestine. The mitotic cycle in the crypts is prolonged and migration is slowed. These changes are reversed by feeding. Food intake above normal levels results in hypertrophy of the villi and increased absorption of nutrients. After surgical excision of a segment of bowel, there is a compensatory increase in the height of the villi and depth of the crypts in the remaining small intestine. This is accompanied by growth in the muscularis and in the length of the bowel. The hyperplastic response is proportional to the length of intestine resected. Much less is known about the capacity of the colon to adapt.

Lamina Propria

The *lamina propria* of the intestinal mucosa consists of loose areolar tissue that occupies the spaces between the crypts of Lieberkühn and forms the cores of the intestinal villi (Figs. 26–4, 26–5). It contains many free cells enmeshed in a stroma of argyrophilic fibers. Associated with the fibers are fixed cells resembling the reticular cells of lymphoid organs. The fine collagen fibrils of the stroma are more concentrated adjacent to the basal lamina of the epithelium. In addition there are delicate networks of elastic fibers surrounding the crypts and extending into the villi. Thin strands of smooth muscle extend from the muscularis mucosae into the core of each villus where they are oriented parallel to the central *lacteal*—a minute terminal branch of the submucous lymphatic plexus that ends blindly near the tip of each villus and provides an important channel for the transport of absorbed lipid. Periodic contractions of the smooth muscle in the villus core empty the lacteal, and propel lymph and absorbed nutrients toward the mesenteric lymph nodes and thoracic duct.

Large numbers of lymphocytes, plasma cells, eosinophils, and macrophages are found in the lamina propria. The most numerous are the lymphocytes, a reserve of immunocompetent cells of which many are capable of differentiating into antibody-producing plasma cells. Lymphocytes also penetrate into the intercellular clefts of the epithelium. The concentration of intraepithelial lymphocytes increases along the intestinal tract and reaches its highest in the large intestine. It was formerly thought that lymphocytes by the millions migrated through the epithelium into the lumen and were lost in the elimination of the intestinal contents. Radioautographic studies with tritiated thymidine provide no support for this concept. Over 95 per cent of the labeled lymphocytes are located in the basal third of the epithelium and there is no convincing evidence that they enter the lumen.

Lymphoid Nodules

In addition to the large population of wandering lymphocytes, the lamina propria of the small intestine contains numerous *solitary lymphoid nodules,* varying in diameter from 0.4 to 3 mm (Fig. 26–15). These dense aggregations of lymphocytes are scattered all

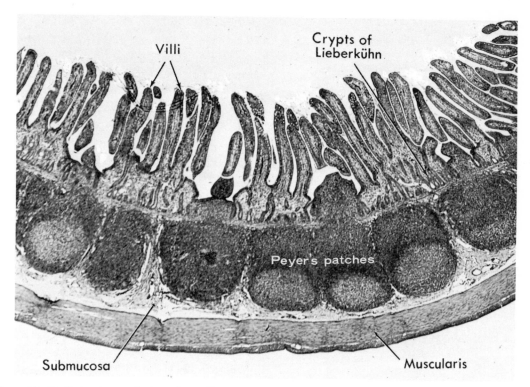

Figure 26–15. Photomicrograph of cat ileum, illustrating intestinal villi. Crypts of Lieberkühn and submucosal lymphoid nodules, or Peyer's patches, are shown.

along the small intestine but are more abundant and larger in its distal part. In the ileum, they may be found in the plicae circulares or between them. The smaller nodules occupy only that portion of the mucosa above the muscularis mucosae. The larger ones occupy the whole thickness of the mucosa, bulging at the surface and extending down through the muscularis mucosae into the submucosa. They are visible to the naked eye as bulging round or oval areas devoid of overlying villi. In sections, crypts are also lacking in the attenuated epithelium overlying the nodules. With scanning electron microscopy, a distinctive cell type (M cell) has been identified in the epithelium over large lymphoid nodules. These cells stretched over the dome of the nodule are squamous, and their microvilli are coarser and more widely separated than those in the brush border of the neighboring absorptive cells (Figs. 26–16, 26–17).

Groups of nodules massed together are called *aggregated nodules* or *Peyer's patches.* As a rule they occur in the ileum, but occasionally they may be encountered elsewhere. From 30 to 40 can usually be found scattered along the ileum. They are always located on the intestinal wall opposite the line of attach-

ment of the mesentery and are recognizable grossly as elongated thickened areas. Their long diameter is 12 to 20 mm, and the short 8 to 12 mm. In sections, they consist of dense lymphatic tissue with large germinal centers in their interior. Their periphery is demarcated by a thin layer of reticular fibers. In the vicinity of aggregated nodules, the lamina propria and submucosa are always heavily infiltrated with lymphocytes. In old age, the solitary nodules and Peyer's patches undergo considerable involution.

Secretory Immune System of the Intestine

We swallow thousands of strains of bacteria and viruses. Indeed, a large fraction of the intestinal contents consists of bacteria. Fortunately, only a small percentage of those taken in are pathogenic. The mucosal surface of the intestinal tract nevertheless presents an enormous area to be protected against invasion. A very important component of its defense is the so-called *secretory immune system,* which produces a special class of antibodies that restrain bacterial proliferation, neutralize viruses, and prevent penetration of enter-

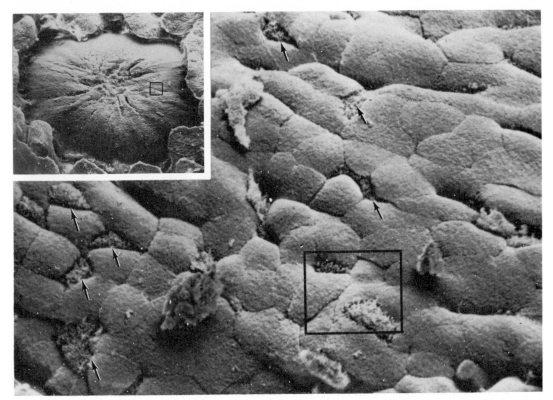

Figure 26–16. Inset presents for orientation a low-power scanning micrograph of a lymphoid nodule in rat intestine covered by an attenuated layer of epithelium and surrounded by villi. The area in the small square is shown at higher magnification in the main figure. The polygonal outlines of the flattened cells is evident and certain of them have a surface texture different from the majority *(at arrows)*. This difference is seen more clearly in Figure 26–17 (a higher magnification of area enclosed in rectangle). (Micrograph from Owen, R., and A. Jones. Gastroenterology *66*:189, 1974.)

otoxins through the epithelium. The synthesis of these antibodies and their delivery to the surface of the mucosa involves the cooperation of the lymphocytes, plasma cells, and macrophages of the lamina propria with the epithelium.

As noted in earlier chapters, there are five or more classes of immune globulins in the human of which the most abundant and best understood is IgG, the antibody mediating general humoral immunity. A second important class is IgA, the so-called *secretory immunoglobulin* found in the serum and in the secretions of the parotid, submandibular, mammary, and lacrimal glands and the tracheobronchial glands, as well as those of the gastrointestinal tract. When the cells of the lamina propria are surveyed with fluorescein-labeled antisera specifically reacting with IgG and with IgA, the great majority of the plasma cells are found to be producing IgA. The mean population density of IgA reactive plasma cells is reported to be 180,000 per mm^3 as against 18,000 for IgG.

Attention has been drawn to the frequent juxtaposition of macrophages to lymphocytes and plasma cells in the lamina propria. Macrophages are now believed to process antigens in some way that increases their effectiveness in inducing an immune response (see Chapter 13). Weak antigens may be hundreds of times more immunogenic when associated with macrophages than they are in the free state. Although macrophages may phagocytize and destroy antigen, it is postulated that some persists on their surface and is liberated and presented to neighboring immunocompetent lymphocytes in a more effective form. Thus, macrophages actively promote the immune response by priming the host for a secondary reaction to the antigen.

Antigens from the intestinal lumen that cross the mucosal barrier interact with cells in the lymphoid nodules of the lamina propria, which are precommitted to IgA production. The M cells overlying lymphoid nodules are believed to be specialized for uptake and transcellular movement of antigen. When the underlying lymphoblasts have

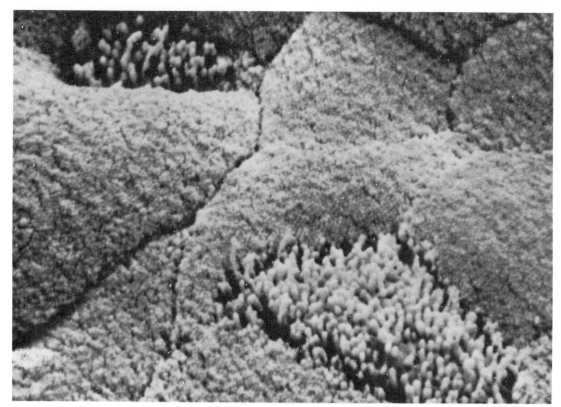

Figure 26–17. Scanning micrograph of the area shown in Figure 26–16. Two of the cells bear loosely packed microvilli that are very much broader than those composing the brush border of the surrounding cells. (Micrograph from Owen, R., and A. Jones. Gastroenterology 66:189, 1974.)

interacted with the antigen, they migrate to the mesenteric lymph nodes, and after further maturation there, they enter the systemic circulation. From the circulation, they "home" back to the intestine and become widely distributed as free cells in the lamina propria (Fig. 26–18). There they differentiate into plasma cells and produce specific IgA antibody to the absorbed antigen. The IgA that they produce is transported through the overlying epithelium bound to a special glycoprotein carrier called the *secretory component*. The secretory component contributed by the epithelium not only serves as a carrier, but is believed to protect the IgA against the cells' lysosomal system and against subsequent destruction by other enzymes on the intestinal surface. This remarkable cooperation of IgA-producing plasma cells with epithelial cells producing secretory component appears to have evolved to ensure formation of antibody molecules capable of coexisting with the proteolytic enzymes in the intestinal lumen. The secretory antibodies released at the free surface are retained in the glycocalyx of the epithelium where they are strategically

situated to interact with antigens, enterotoxins, and bacteria to prevent their attachment to the cell membrane—an effect termed *immune exclusion*.

The mystery that long enshrouded the function of the free cells and aggregations of lymphoid tissue in the lamina propria has now been largely stripped away by advances in immunology, which have provided compelling evidence that they constitute an efficient local immune system with the primary function of supporting the epithelium in its role as a barrier to the penetration of pathogenic organisms and toxins from the external environment.

It is interesting to note that in the continuing "arms race" between microbes and higher organisms, a few species of bacteria, including *Neisseria gonorrhoeae*, have evolved a counter weapon, *IgA proteases*—enzymes that readily cleave IgA immunoglobulin. No other substrate for their activity has yet been identified. These proteases may play an important part in the pathogenesis of certain human diseases by interfering with the immunological defenses mediated by IgA.

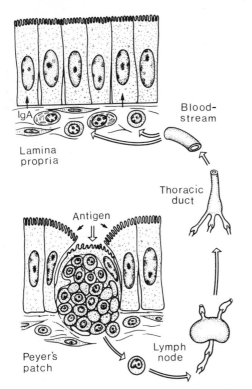

Figure 26–18. Schematic representation of the pathways involved in the secretory immune system. Lymphocytes in Peyer's patches exposed to antigens from the gut lumen migrate to regional lymph nodes and thence to the bloodstream. Circulating in the blood they home into the lamina propria of the gut and there develop into plasma cells secreting IgA, which acquires a secretory piece in the epithelium and is released into the gut lumen. (Redrawn after Walker, W. A., and K. J. Isselbacher. N. Engl. J. Med. 297:767, 1977.)

Muscularis Mucosae

The muscularis mucosae averages 38 μm in thickness, and consists of networks of elastic fibers and thin inner circular and outer longitudinal layers of smooth muscle. Its contraction increases the height of folds in the mucosa. It is usually contracted in fixed specimens exaggerating the irregularity in the outline of the lumen. It is conceivable that such changes in the surface topography of the mucosa occurring in vivo may play an ancillary role in mixing the content of the gut.

Submucosa

The submucosa consists of moderately dense connective tissue rich in elastic fibers. It may also contain occasional clusters of adipose cells. In the duodenum, but not elsewhere, it is largely occupied by the *glands of Brunner.*

Duodenal Glands (Submucosal Glands of Brunner)

Brunner's glands are usually encountered first in the region of the pyloric sphincter, but in the human they may extend a few centimeters into the pyloric antrum. They diminish in size and number along the duodenum and usually terminate in its distal third. In rare instances they may extend into the proximal part of the jejunum. Brunner's glands tend to occupy the submucosa in the plicae circulares and are separated from one another by short, gland-free intervals (Figs. 26–2, 26–19).

The terminal secretory portions of the glands consist of richly branched and coiled tubules arranged in lobules 0.5 to 1.0 mm in diameter (Fig. 26–5). The ducts ascend through the muscularis mucosae to open into a crypt of Lieberkühn.

Examined with the electron microscope, the secretory cells of the submucosal glands share the ultrastructural features of zymogenic and mucus-secreting cells. They have numerous mitochondria and abundant granular reticulum at the cell base. Their dense secretory granules bear a superficial resemblance to those of pancreatic zymogen cells. The Golgi complex is unusually large and is believed to be the site of synthesis of the carbohydrate moiety of the secretory product and of its conjugation with the protein moiety synthesized in the granular endoplasmic reticulum.

The secretion is a clear, viscous, and distinctly alkaline fluid (pH 8.2 to 9.3). Its principal function is to protect the duodenal mucosa against the erosive effects of the acid gastric juice. Its mucoid nature, its alkalinity, and possibly the buffering capacity of its bicarbonate content make it well suited to this role.

Another possible function has recently been suggested. *Urogastrone,* a polypeptide excreted in human urine, is a powerful inhibitor of gastric acid secretion, and also stimulates epithelial proliferation. The cells of origin, storage, and secretion of urogastrone have long eluded detection. Applying fluorescein-labeled antiurogastrone antibody to a large variety of human tissues, specific staining was observed only in the cells of Brunner's glands and in the duct cells of the submandibular salivary gland. It is now speculated that in addition to their other secretory functions, Brunner's glands may release urogastrone into the intestinal lumen, where its growth-stimulating properties may play an

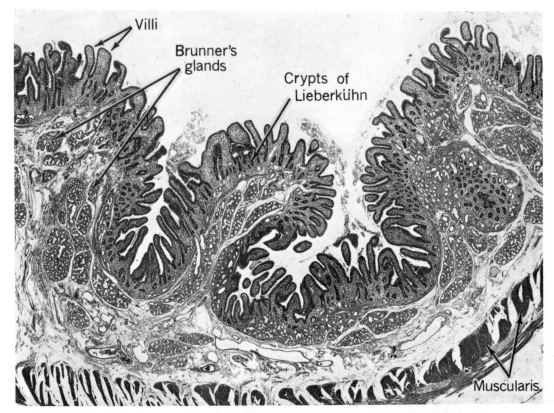

Villi

Brunner's glands

Crypts of Lieberkühn

Muscularis

Figure 26–19. Photomicrograph of duodenum from a man who had committed suicide by drinking formalin. The mucosa is unusually well preserved; the muscularis shows considerable shrinkage. × 20. (Courtesy of H. Mizoguchi.)

important role in the rapid turnover of the epithelial cells lining the intestine. A relationship between urogastrone and the acid inhibitory hormone *enterogastrone,* said to be liberated by the duodenum, remains to be established.

Muscularis

The muscular coat of the small intestine consists of an outer longitudinal and inner circular layer of smooth muscle. Between these layers is the sympathetic *myenteric nerve plexus.* Some strands of smooth muscle cells pass from one layer into the other. The smooth muscle cells have usually been regarded as a static cell population, but autoradiographic studies have now demonstrated a slow rate of cell replication distributed throughout the external muscle layer. There are differences in rate of replication in different portions of the alimentary tract.

The muscularis is responsible for *peristalsis,* a wavelike contraction that travels along the intestine at the rate of a few centimeters a second and propels the luminal contents on-

ward. The peristaltic waves are propagated for short distances along the intestine and then die out, to be followed a few minutes later by another wave. Several waves may be in progress at the same time in successive segments of the small intestine but it is rare for a single peristaltic wave to pass along its entire length. In addition to these traveling waves of contraction, there are *segmental movements,* consisting of alternate constriction and relaxation of short segments. These do not advance the contents toward the large intestine but result in to-and-fro movement that serves to agitate and mix the material in the lumen.

In the terminal portion of the ileum the muscularis is somewhat thickened, forming an *ileocecal sphincter.* It remains partially contracted, delaying emptying of the contents into the cecum. After a meal there is a reflex activation of ileal peristalsis and a relaxation of the ileocecal sphincter, permitting advance of its contents into the large intestine. At the ileocecal orifice, folds of mucosa project into the cecum. These act as a bicuspid valve, closing when the cecum fills and preventing reflux into the ileum.

Serosa

The outermost layer of the gut wall, called the *serosa,* consists of a continuous sheet of squamous epithelial cells, the *mesothelium,* separated from the underlying muscularis by a very thin layer of loose connective tissue. Most of the gastrointestinal tract is suspended from the dorsal wall of the abdomen by mesenteries. Along the site of attachment of the mesentery the serosa of the intestine is continuous with the two apposed leaves of the mesentery, and at its base these, in turn, are continuous with the serous lining of the abdominal cavity. Thus, the inner aspect of the abdominal wall and the surface of the organs suspended from it are covered by a continuous layer of mesothelium, usually referred to as the *peritoneum.* That portion lining the cavity is called the *parietal peritoneum* and that covering the organs is the *visceral peritoneum.* The transudation of fluid from underlying capillaries moistens the smooth, serous surfaces and facilitates friction-free sliding of the loops of the intestine over one another during peristalsis. Bacterial contamination of the abdominal cavity due to perforating lesions of the gut wall results in *peritonitis,* a severe inflammatory process that is often fatal.

THE LARGE INTESTINE

The large intestine includes in succession the *cecum*; the *ascending, transverse,* and *descending colon*; the *sigmoid colon*; the *rectum*; and the *anus.* The cecum is a blind-ending pouch continuous above with the ascending colon. At the junction between the two, the ileum enters its medial side. The *appendix* is a vermiform tubular appendage projecting from the cecum posteromedial to the ileocecal valve.

THE APPENDIX

The appendix arises from the blind end of the cecum and ranges in length from 2 to 18 cm. Its wall has all of the layers typical of the intestine but it is thickened by an extensive development of lymphoid tissue, which forms an almost continuous layer of large and small lymphatic nodules (Fig. 26–20). The small lumen has an angular outline in cross section and often contains masses of dead cells and acellular detritus. It is difficult to make a clear distinction between the normal structure and certain pathological conditions in this organ. Villi are absent. The crypts of Lieberkühn radiating from the lumen have an irregular shape and variable length and are largely embedded in the lymphoid tissue. The epithelium of the glands contains only a few goblet cells and consists mostly of columnar cells with a striated border. The zone of mitotically active undifferentiated cells in the crypts is shorter than in the small intestine. In addition to occasional Paneth cells, enteroendocrine cells are regularly present in the depths of the crypts and in smaller numbers in the upper parts of the glands. They are much more plentiful than in the small intestine, and may number five to ten in a single gland in section.

The lymphatic tissue of the appendix, like that of the tonsils, often shows chronic inflammatory changes. The muscularis mucosae of the appendix is poorly developed. The submucosa forms a thick layer with blood vessels and nerves and occasional fat lobules. The muscularis externa is reduced in thickness, but the two usual layers are always identifiable. The serous coat is similar to that covering the rest of the intestines.

THE CECUM AND COLON

The mucosa of the large intestine does not form folds comparable with the plicae circulares, and villi cease beyond the ileocecal valve. The interior of the colon therefore has a smooth surface when examined with the naked eye, but may be somewhat irregular in outline in sections due to contraction of the muscularis (Fig. 26–21). At low magnification one can see the openings of innumerable crypts or glands of Lieberkühn (Fig. 26–22). In histological sections these are straight tubular glands about 0.5 mm in length, somewhat longer than their counterparts in the small intestine. In the rectum they attain a length of 0.7 mm. They differ from the glands of the small intestine in the absence of Paneth cells and in the greater abundance of goblet cells (Figs. 26–23, 26–24). Enteroendocrine cells are present in small numbers. Although the goblet cells are the most conspicuous element, the majority of the cells in the middle and upper portions of the crypts are columnar absorptive cells, and these represent the principal cell type in the epithelium at the surface of the mucosa. As in the

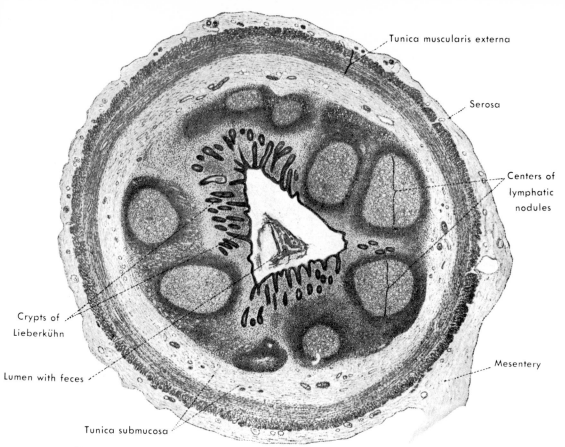

Figure 26–20. Cross section of appendix from a 23-year-old man. × 22. (After Sobotta.)

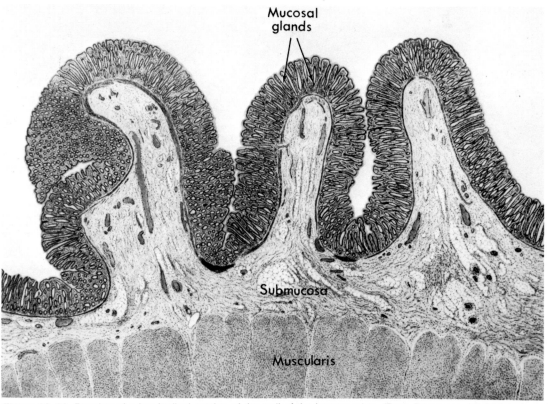

Figure 26–21. Drawing of a longitudinal section of the wall of the human colon. (From Bargmann, W. Histologie und Mikroskopische Anatomie des Menschen. 6th ed. Stuttgart, Georg Thieme Verlag, 1962.)

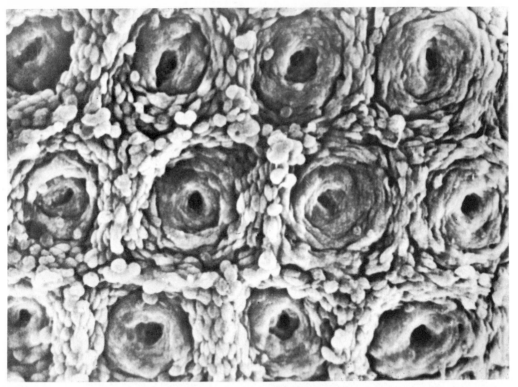

Figure 26–22. Scanning electron micrograph of the surface of the descending colon of a monkey *(Macaca mulatta)* showing the regular array of openings of the crypts. (From Specian, R., and M. R. Neutra, Am. J. Anat. *160*:461, 1981).

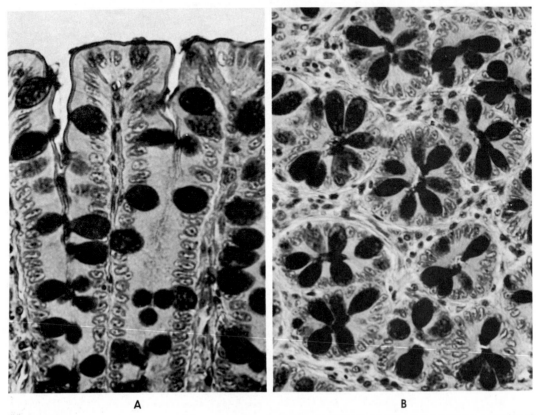

A   B

Figure 26–23. Sections of the crypts of the colon of a macaque. *A,* Vertical section of the mucosa, showing the columnar cells and goblet cells. × 550. *B,* Horizontal section of the crypts, showing the radial disposition of goblet cells around the lumen and the cellular lamina propria between crypts. Periodic acid–Schiff reaction and hematoxylin. Photomicrograph. × 425.

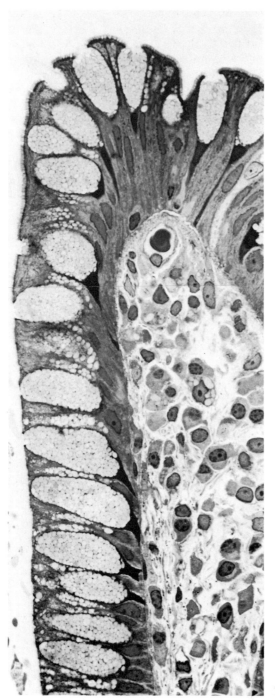

Figure 26–24 Photomicrograph of the junction of the upper portion of a crypt with the surface epithelium of human rectal mucosa. In the goblet cells at the surface the theca is smaller and the "stem" longer than in those of the upper crypt. (Photomicrograph from Neutra, M. Lab. Invest. *36*:535, 1977.)

the crypt and onto the surface. There, they slough off into the lumen from extrusion zones situated about midway between the openings of neighboring crypts. The life span of most of the cell population is about six days, but the endocrine cells appear to be exceptional, having a life span measured in weeks rather than days. This implies that they must migrate independently and at a different rate from that of the surrounding cells. Little is known about the mechanism of epithelial migration—whether they move over the basal lamina or whether it also moves. It is clear from autoradiographic studies that the subepithelial fibroblasts that ensheath the intestinal crypts proliferate at the base and move upward with the epithelial cells.

The lamina propria of the colon is similar in structure to that of the small intestine. Scattered lymphoid nodules are always present and may extend deep into the submucosa. The muscularis mucosae is well developed, consists of longitudinal and circular fibers, and may send slender fascicles of muscle cells toward the surface mucosa. The submucosa presents no unusual features.

The muscularis of the large intestine differs in its organization from that of the small intestine. Instead of forming a continuous layer of uniform thickness, the longitudinal fibers are aggregated into three evenly spaced longitudinal bands, called the *taenia coli*. Between the taenia, longitudinal smooth muscle fibers form a very thin, and often discontinuous, layer. The inner circular layer of the muscularis is similar to that of the small intestine. In the living the taenia are in a state of partial contraction, which causes the intervening portions of the wall to bulge outward, forming sacculations termed *haustrae*. These are conspicuous in the ascending, transverse, and descending colon and sigmoid flexure, but in the rectum the muscularis externa again becomes a continuous layer of uniform thickness.

The serosa of the colon is unusual in having local accumulations of adipose cells beneath the mesothelium that form pendulous protuberances called the *appendices epiploicae*.

THE RECTUM AND ANUS

The rectum is about 12 cm long and extends from the sigmoid colon to the pelvic diaphragm. It is slightly dilated in its lower portion to form the *rectal ampulla*. There are two or three transversely oriented crescentic

small intestine, the epithelium is constantly being renewed. Undifferentiated cells in depths of the crypts divide and their progeny differentiate into columnar, goblet, and enteroendocrine cells, which slowly move up folds of the mucosa above the rectal ampulla. The mucosa in the rectum is similar to that of the colon but its crypts are somewhat longer (0.7 mm).

The rectum narrows rather abruptly at the lower end of the ampulla and continues as the *anal canal,* about 4 cm in length. The mucosa here exhibits longitudinal folds, the *rectal columns of Morgagni.* The crypts of Lieberkühn in this region suddenly become short and then disappear along an irregular line about 2 cm above the anal opening, and there is an abrupt transition from simple columnar to stratified squamous epithelium. Here, at the level of the external muscular sphincter of the anus, the lining of the canal has the histological appearance of skin with typical sebaceous glands and special, large, circumanal apocrine glands. The lamina propria here contains a plexus of large veins that, when abnormally distended and varicose, protrude at the anus as hemorrhoids.

The circular layer of smooth muscle of the anal canal is considerably thickened, forming the *internal anal sphincter.* Distal to this is a circumferential annulus of striated muscle, the *external anal sphincter.*

HISTOPHYSIOLOGY OF THE INTESTINE

The function of the intestinal tract and its accessory glands, the liver and pancreas, is to digest food, reducing the carbohydrates, fats, and protein to molecules that can be absorbed by the mucosa. Each day some 8 or 9 liters of water; 100 g of fat; 50 to 100 g of amino acids; and several hundred grams of carbohydrate are absorbed from the small intestine.

Most physiologically important processes in living organisms take place at cell surfaces and at interfaces between membrane-limited intracellular compartments. The rate of metabolic activity per unit area of surface probably cannot be increased above a certain limit. Therefore, at all levels of organization there are architectural devices for increasing surface area without increasing the overall size of the organism. This principle of design is dramatically exemplified in the structure of the alimentary tract (Fig. 26–25). The absorptive surface is increased first by elongation and convolution of the tubular intestine. The mucosal surface is increased by plication to form the plicae circulares. At higher magnification, the surface is found to be amplified further by about 40 intestinal villi per square millimeter. At the level of the electron microscope, the surface of every absorptive cell in the epithelium covering the villi is augmented another 20-fold by several hundred microvilli. At the molecular level, the polysaccharide chains of membrane glycoproteins forming the surface coat are highly branched filaments, adding further to the enormous surface exposed to the intes-

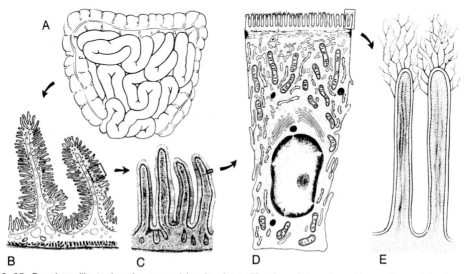

Figure 26–25. Drawings illustrating the several levels of amplification of the absorptive surface of the intestine. *A,* Lengthening and convolution of the gut. *B,* Plicae circulares. *C,* Villi. *D,* Microvilli on the cells. *E,* Polysaccharides of the integral glycoproteins of the microvillar membrane. (From Fawcett, D. The Cell. 2nd ed. Philadelphia, W. B. Saunders Co. 1981.)

tinal contents. Within the cell, convolution is again seen in the configuration of the endoplasmic reticulum, and plication to increase the surface is evident in the cristae of the mitochondria. And these are but a few of Nature's stratagems for increasing the efficiency of the metabolic machinery with minimal increase in body mass.

The secretions of the liver and pancreas that are delivered into the duodenum at the ampulla of Vater are essential to the digestion of the chyme in the small intestine. The bile from the liver and gallbladder, together with the mechanical mixing action of peristalsis, reduces ingested fat to a fine emulsion of triglycerides. The pancreatic juice contributes lipolytic, proteolytic, and carbohydrate splitting enzymes. The intestinal mucosa itself contributes intestinal juice, or *succus entericus*.

The secretion of the crypts of Lieberkühn was formerly believed to contain several digestive enzymes, but it has become clear from biochemical studies on isolated brush borders that some of the enzymes believed to be secreted into the lumen are instead incorporated in the membrane of the brush border of the absorptive cells. Among these are *leucine aminopeptidase*, and the enzymes that hydrolyze disaccharides—*sucrase*, which cleaves sucrose to glucose and fructose; *lactase*, cleaving lactose to glucose and galactose; and *maltase*, that hydrolyzes maltose, derived from starch, to glucose. These enzymes residing in the membrane and surface coat of the microvilli reduce dietary carbohydrates in the gut lumen to hexoses that are actively transported, together with sodium ions, into the absorptive cells by carrier protein present in the brush border. Thus, the brush border is not only a device for increasing surface area for absorption but also the site of the enzymes involved in the terminal steps in digestion of carbohydrates and proteins, and it possesses the carriers necessary for active transport of glucose and amino acids into the cell.

A genetic defect resulting in absence of one of the enzymes in the brush border is the basis for an uncommon disease that previously was poorly understood. Some infants cannot tolerate milk, and feeding results in bloating and copious diarrhea. These symptoms have been traced to congenital absence of the single enzyme lactase from the intestinal brush border. If lactose is eliminated from the diet, these infants do very well.

Intraluminal digestion of most food reduces it to units of molecular size whose path of absorption through the intestinal mucosa cannot be followed by microscopy. Fat lends itself best to morphological study because lipid can be preserved in the tissue and intensely stained by fixatives containing os-

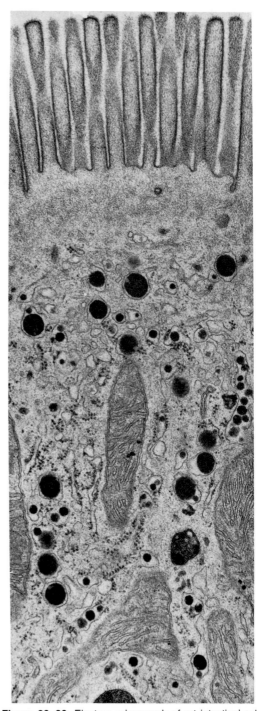

Figure 26–26. Electron micrograph of rat intestinal cell. Lipid accumulates in sizable droplets within the smooth reticulum, but very little is seen in inpocketings of the cell surface or in vesicles traversing the terminal web. Although pinocytosis undoubtedly occurs to some extent it is not the principal mechanism for absorption of lipid. (Courtesy of S. L. Palay and J. P. Revel.)

mium tetroxide (Figs. 26–26, 26–27). Dietary fat, consisting mainly of triglycerides, is hydrolyzed by pancreatic lipase in the intestinal lumen to free fatty acids and monoglycerides. These products combine with bile salts to form minute micelles about 2 nm in diameter (Fig. 26–28). When myriads of these come into contact with the microvilli of the intestinal absorptive cells, the fatty acids and monoglycerides diffuse across the plasma membrane and accumulate in the apical cytoplasm. The membranes of the smooth endoplasmic reticulum located there contain the enzymes for resynthesis of triglycerides from fatty acids and monoglycerides. During lipid absorption, the resynthesized triglycer-

ide forms numerous visible droplets in the lumen of the reticulum in the apical portion of the cell (Fig. 26–26). From there the lipid appears to be transported to the Golgi complex for further processing that converts it into *chylomicra*, the complex glycolipoprotein droplets that are transported via the lacteals and intestinal lymphatics to the bloodstream. The precise role of the Golgi complex in lipid absorption has not been established, but it seems likely that the carbohydrate moiety of the chylomicra is added there to the triglyceride synthesized in the smooth reticulum. The chylomicron also acquires in its passage through the Golgi complex a membranous investment with properties that enable it to

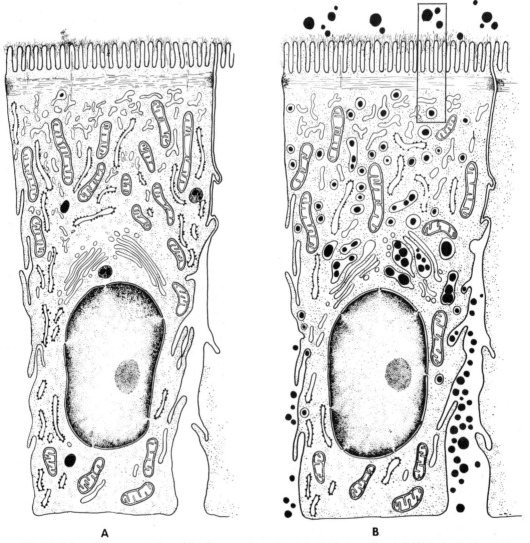

A

B

Figure 26–27. Schematic representation of the fine structure of an intestinal absorptive cell *(A)* in the fasting state and *(B)* after a lipid-rich meal. Area in rectangle is depicted at higher magnification in Figure 26–27. (Redrawn after Cardell, R., S. Badenhausen, and K. R. Porter. J. Cell Biol. *34*:123, 1967.)

coalesce with the lateral plasma membrane of the columnar cell. Vesicles of Golgi origin thus discharge chylomicra into the intercellular cleft between adjacent absorptive cells (Figs. 26–29, 26–30). From there they move across the basal lamina of the epithelium and into the lymphatic capillaries in the lamina propria of the intestinal villi.

The absorptive cells of the intestine are able to respond rapidly and to modify their internal structure to adapt it to the requirements of lipid absorption. In the fasting state, there are some profiles of granular endoplasmic reticulum and a limited amount of smooth reticulum in the apical cytoplasm, and a relatively quiescent supranuclear Golgi complex. Ingestion of lipid stimulates the formation of a more extensive smooth reticulum to provide for resynthesis of triglyceride and its transport to the Golgi complex. The rapid turnover of Golgi membranes during lipid absorption and transport also requires accelerated synthesis of new membrane to replace that lost to the cell surface in discharge of chylomicra. If protein synthesis is blocked by administration of puromycin, membrane replacement in smooth reticulum and Golgi complex is prevented, as is synthesis of protein constituents of the chylomicra. Lipid transport is therefore inhibited and large amounts of lipid accumulate in the cytoplasm of the absorptive cells.

An important part of the absorptive mechanism is the active movement of the intestinal villi. These can be observed in a living animal if a loop of intestine is split open and the surface of the mucosa is observed with a binocular microscope. A villus is seen to suddenly shorten to about half its length with an appreciable increase in its thickness, and it slowly extends again to its original length. Each villus contracts about six times a minute. During the contraction, its volume is reduced and the contents of the central lacteal are forwarded to the submucous lymphatic plexus. Contraction occurs as a result of shortening of the longitudinally oriented strands of smooth muscle in the core of the villus. The contraction of the villi is believed to be under the nervous control of Meissner's submucous plexus. Direct mechanical stimulation of the base of a villus with a bristle also calls forth a contraction, and the stimulus radiates from the affected villus to the surrounding villi.

In addition to the absorption of water and nutrients, the small intestine has an essential

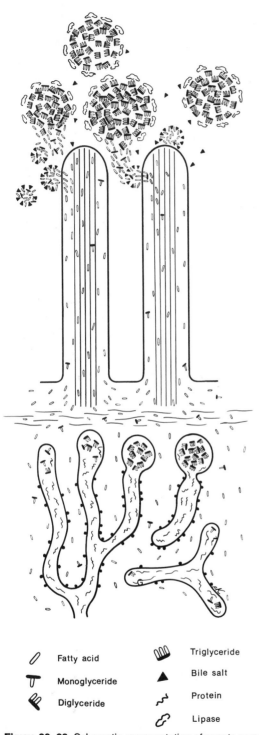

	Fatty acid		Triglyceride
	Monoglyceride	▲	Bile salt
	Diglyceride		Protein
			Lipase

Figure 26–28. Schematic representation of events occurring in a small area of the apex of an intestinal absorptive cell (see Fig. 26–27). An emulsion of fine droplets of lipid in the lumen is broken down by pancreatic lipase to fatty acids and monoglycerides. These diffuse into the microvilli and apical cytoplasm, where they are esterified to form triglycerides in the smooth endoplasmic reticulum. (Redrawn after Cardell, R., S. Badenhausen, and K. R. Porter. J. Cell Biol. *34:*123, 1967.)

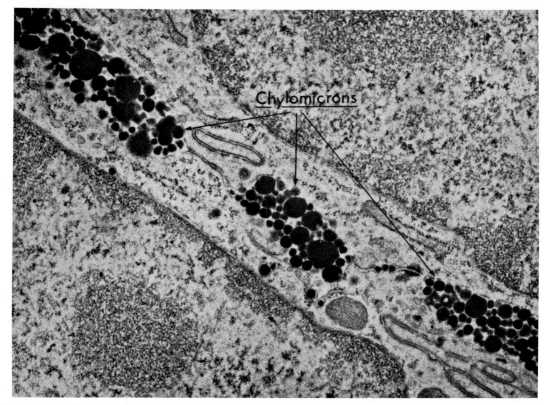

Figure 26–29. Electron micrograph of the boundary between two rat intestinal epithelial cells during lipid absorption. The absorbed lipid has been discharged through the lateral cell surfaces and is seen to have accumulated here as aggregations of chylomicrons in the intercellular spaces. × 30,000. (Courtesy of S. L. Palay and J. P. Revel.)

function in absorption and conservation of ions. About 6 g of sodium is taken in daily in the diet and 20 to 30 g are secreted into the lumen in the succus entericus, but little or none is normally lost in feces. Sodium is constantly reabsorbed in the intestine. It diffuses through the apical membrane of the absorptive cells and is actively transported through the lateral membranes, creating a standing gradient in the intercellular clefts that draws water through the epithelium and into the capillaries of the villi. Chloride ions diffuse along the electrochemical gradient following the sodium. The importance of this reabsorption of ions becomes evident in cholera and other forms of severe diarrhea in which the sodium reserves of the body can be reduced to lethal levels within several hours.

Absorption of water and electrolytes continues in the colon. About 1 liter of chyme passes through the ileocecal valve daily, but normally less than 100 ml is lost in the feces. The bulk of the feces consists of dead bacteria and undigestible fibrous constituents of in-

gested vegetable matter. The bacterial flora of the intestine in humans digest only small amounts of cellulose, but in herbivorous mammals cellulose is an important source of nutrients whose digestion depends on the bacteria of the gastrointestinal tract. In humans the major contribution of the intestinal flora is the production of vitamin B_{12}, needed for hemopoiesis, and vitamin K, which is essential for maintenance of the clotting mechanism of the blood.

BLOOD VESSELS OF THE GASTROINTESTINAL TRACT

The arrangements of the blood and lymph vessels in the wall of the stomach and in the wall of the intestine are basically similar. Because the important differences depend mainly on the presence of villi, the small intestine shows significant peculiarities.

In the stomach, the arteries arise from the two arterial arches along the lesser and

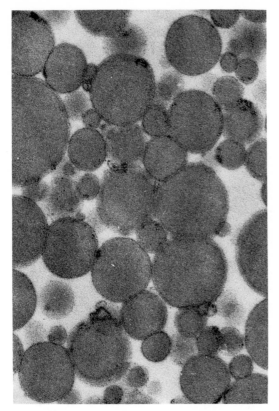

Figure 26–30. Electron micrograph of chylomicrons fixed in osmium tetroxide, embedded and sectioned. They range from 110 mm to 700 mm. (From Jones, A., and M. Price. J. Histochem. Cytochem. *16*:366, 1968. By permission of the Histochemical Society, Inc.)

greater curvatures and are distributed to the ventral and dorsal surfaces. In the intestine, the arteries reach one side in the mesentery. They run in the serosa and break up into large branches that penetrate the muscularis externa and enter the submucosal layer, where they form a large plexus (Fig. 26–31). In the stomach and colon the plexus gives off branches directed toward the surface. Some of these break up into capillaries supplying the muscularis mucosae; others form capillary networks throughout the mucosa and surrounding the glands. The capillary net is especially prominent around the foveolae of the gastric mucosa.

From the superficial, periglandular capillary networks, veins of considerable caliber arise. They form a venous plexus between the bottoms of the glands and the muscularis mucosae. From this plexus, branches run into the submucosa and form a venous plexus. From this submucosal plexus, the large veins follow the arteries and pass through the mus-

cularis externa into the serosa. In the stomach the veins of the submucosal plexus are provided with valves and a relatively thick muscular coat.

In the small intestine, the submucous arterial plexus gives off two kinds of branches that run toward the mucosa. Some of these arteries ramify on the inner surface of the muscularis mucosae and break up into capillary networks that surround the crypts of Lieberkühn in the same way they surround the glands of the stomach. Other arteries are especially destined for the villi, each villus receiving one or sometimes several such small arteries. These vessels enter the base of the villus and form a dense capillary network immediately under its epithelium (Fig. 26–32). Near the tip of the villus, one or two small veins arise from the superficial capillary network and run downward, to anastomose with the glandular venous plexus, and then pass on into the submucosa, where they join the veins of the submucosal plexus. These veins in the intestine have no valves. However, their continuations, which pass through the muscularis externa with the arteries, are provided with valves. Valves disappear again in the collecting veins of the mesentery.

LYMPH VESSELS OF THE GASTROINTESTINAL TRACT

In the stomach, the lymphatics begin as an extensive system of large lymphatic capillaries in the superficial layer of the mucosa between the glands. They are always situated more deeply than the blood capillaries. They anastomose everywhere throughout the mucosa. They surround the glandular tubules and take a downward course to the inner surface of the mucosa, where they form a plexus of fine lymphatic vessels. Branches of the plexus pierce the muscularis mucosae and form, in the submucosa, a plexus of lymphatics that is provided with valves. From the submucosal plexus, larger lymphatics run through the muscularis externa. Here they receive numerous tributaries from the lymphatic plexus in the muscular coat and then follow the blood vessels into the retroperitoneal tissues. In the wall of the colon the lymphatics show a similar arrangement.

The lymphatic vessels are important in the absorption of fat from the small intestine. During digestion, all their ramifications be-

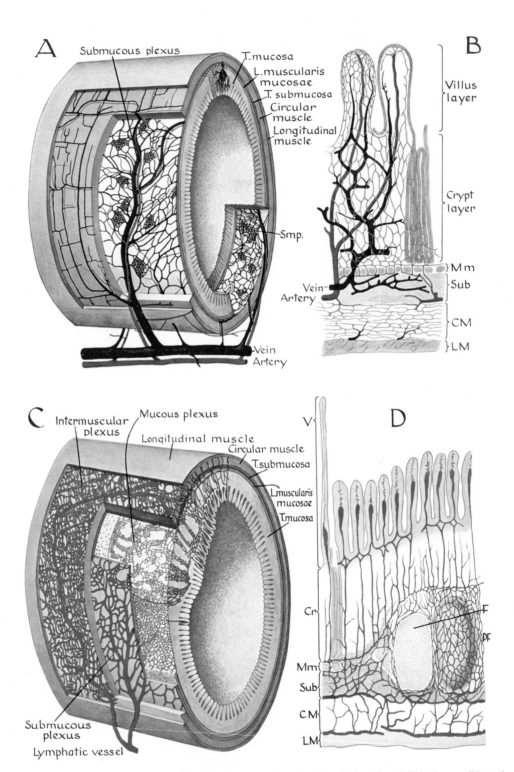

Figure 26–31. Diagrams of distribution of blood vessels (A and B) and of lymphatics (C and D) in the small intestine of the dog. B and D are drawn on a larger scale to show details. CM, Circular muscle; Cr, crypt; F, follicle; LM, longitudinal muscle; Mm, lamina muscularis mucosae; PF, perifollicular plexus; Smp, submucous plexus; Sub, tunica submucosa; V, villus. (Redrawn and slightly modified from Mall.)

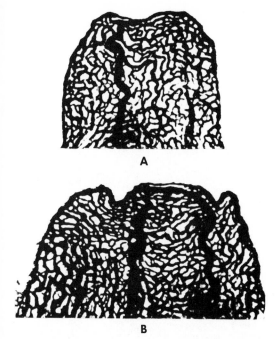

A

B

Figure 26–32. Two villi of rat intestine injected with India ink in gelatin. The villi in this species are thin, leaflike structures whose broad surface is presented in this figure. In the duodenum *(B)* they are larger and more richly vascularized than they are farther along in the jejunum *(A)*. The large surface area presented by the villi and their rich network of capillaries favors absorption of nutrients. × 100.

come filled with milky white lymph—a fine emulsion of neutral fats. This white lymph, drained from the intestine, is called *chyle,* and the lymphatics that carry it away from the epithelium are called *lacteals.*

In the small intestine the most conspicuous parts of the lymphatic system are the central lacteals in the core of the villi. Each conical villus has one lacteal, which occupies an axial position and ends blindly near the tip. The broader villi of the duodenum may contain two or perhaps more lacteals that intercommunicate. The lumen of these lacteals, when distended, is considerably larger than that of the blood capillaries. The wall consists of thin endothelial cells and is everywhere connected with the argyrophilic reticulum and surrounded by thin, longitudinal strands of smooth muscle.

The central lacteals at the base of the villi anastomose with the lymphatic capillaries between the glands. They also form a plexus on the inner surface of the muscularis mucosae. Branches of this plexus, provided with valves, pierce the muscularis mucosae and form, in the submucosa, a loose plexus of

larger lymphatics. The latter also receives tributaries from the dense network of large, thin-walled lymphatic capillaries, which closely surround the surface of the solitary and aggregated follicles. The large lymphatics that run from the submucosal plexus through the muscularis externa into the mesentery receive additional branches from a dense, tangential plexus located between the circular and longitudinal layers of the muscularis externa.

NERVES OF THE INTESTINAL TRACT

The gastrointestinal tract is innervated by the autonomic nervous system, which consists of three subdivisions: sympathetic, parasympathetic, and enteric. All three play a role in regulating intestinal activity but the enteric is the most important. The sympathetic and parasympathetic nerves to the gastrointestinal tract constitute its *extrinsic* nerve supply and exert their influence on digestive function through the *intrinsic* enteric nervous system, which consists of nerve cell bodies and their processes located within the wall of the tract. The extrinsic nerves are preganglionic fibers from the vagus nerve and postganglionic sympathetic fibers that arise mainly in the celiac ganglion. They are distributed to the intestine with the blood vessels via the mesentery. The enteric nervous system consists of ganglia and interconnecting bundles of nerve fibers that form extensive plexuses in various layers of the digestive tube and extend throughout its length from the lower esophagus to the internal anal sphincter. The enteric system contains 10^7 to 10^8 neurons including sensory neurons, interneurons, and motor neurons, which form reflex pathways that are intrinsic to the digestive tract. Unlike other subdivisions of the autonomic nervous system, the enteric system is largely autonomous and can carry out many of its functions without input from the central nervous system. Although the sympathetic and parasympathetic nerves do have some effect upon the digestive tract, cutting the extrinsic nerves results in surprisingly little impairment of digestive function. If the intestine is detached from the mesentery and immersed in warm physiological salt solution, it will show normal peristaltic movements when the mucosa is stimulated by introduction of ma-

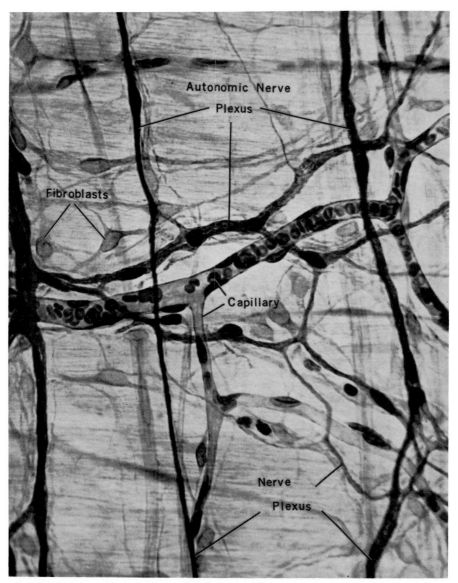

Figure 26–33. Photomicrograph of a whole mount of the longitudinal muscle coat of rabbit intestine impregnated with silver to show the nerve bundles of Auerbach's plexus. × 300. (After Richardson, K. C. J. Anat. *94*:451, 1960. Labeling added.)

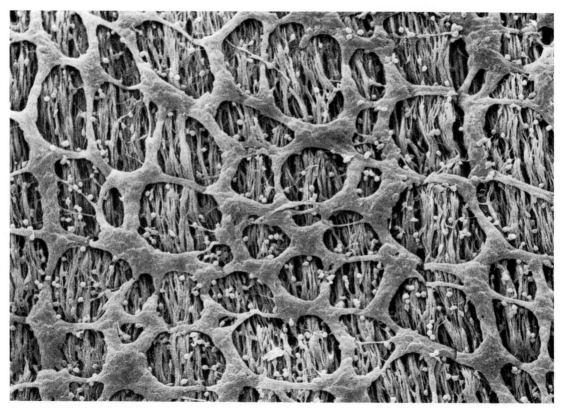

Figure 26–34. Scanning electron micrograph of the myenteric plexus of rat intestine. The overlying longitudinal muscle and connective tissue has been removed by dissection and enzymatic digestion. (Micrograph from Fujiwara, T., and Y. Uehara. J. Electron Microsc. *29:*397, 1980.)

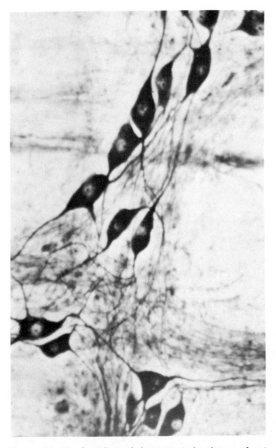

Figure 26–35. Ganglion of the myenteric plexus of cat jejunum containing bipolar and multipolar neurons. Modified Bielschowsky stain. (Photomicrograph courtesy of G. Schofield.)

terial into the lumen. Thus, intestinal movements are determined by local neuromuscular mechanisms that are modulated only by input through the extrinsic nerves.

The most superficial neural elements in the gut wall form a *subserous* plexus, which generally lacks ganglia and consists of a loose network of fine nerve fibers that connect the extrinsic nerves with the more deeply situated intrinsic plexuses. The majority of the nerves coursing from the mesentery to the deeper enteric plexuses traverse the longitudinal muscle layer near the mesenteric attachment.

The most conspicuous enteric plexus is found between the longitudinal and circular layers of the muscularis (Figs. 26–33, 26–34). This *myenteric plexus* (Auerbach's plexus) (plexus entericus externa) consists of ganglia containing three to 50 or more nerve cell bodies and bundles of unmyelinated axons that connect the ganglia to form a continuous network (Fig. 26–34). The cells of the ganglia are of two principal morphological types. One is a multipolar cell (Figs. 26–35, 26–36) with short dendrites in contact with the bodies of similar cells in the same ganglion, while the axon can be traced for a considerable distance to sites of synaptic contact with cells of the second type in neighboring ganglia. Cells of the second type are far more numerous and more variable in form. The dendrites are diffuse receptive endings related to cells of the first type, or the same type, in the same or in other ganglia. The axon enters one of the fiber bundles associated with the ganglion, and its branches terminate in the circular or longitudinal muscle layers. Thus, cells of the first type appear to be associative while those of the second type are motor. A third cell type, termed the interstitial cell, has short branching processes that intermingle with those of the other cell types. It does not contain demonstrable neurofibrils and may be a form of glial cell.

Most of the unmyelinated fibers in the ganglia and in the internodal strands of the plexus are processes of enteric neurons. The remainder are axons of extrinsic vagal or sympathetic origins. The vagal fibers terminate as perikaryal arborizations on ganglion cells of the second type. The sympathetic fibers do not seem to have synaptic relationships with the nerve cells of the ganglia, but are thought to terminate in the muscularis and on blood vessels.

A *deep muscular plexus (plexus muscularis profundus)* is situated on the mucosal aspect of the circular muscle layer. It is devoid of ganglia and consists of thin anastomosing nerve bundles with their prevailing orientation parallel to the muscle fibers. Branches from this plexus penetrate into the muscle layer and some are connected with the myenteric plexus.

The *submucous plexus (Meissner's plexus) (plexus entericus interna)* is a network of ganglia and interconnecting nerve bundles within the connective tissue of the submucosa. Its fibers innervate the muscularis mucosae and smooth muscle strands in the cores of the intestinal villi. Fibers from the submucous plexus also form a *mucosal plexus* situated in the lamina propria and extending components between the intestinal glands and into the villi.

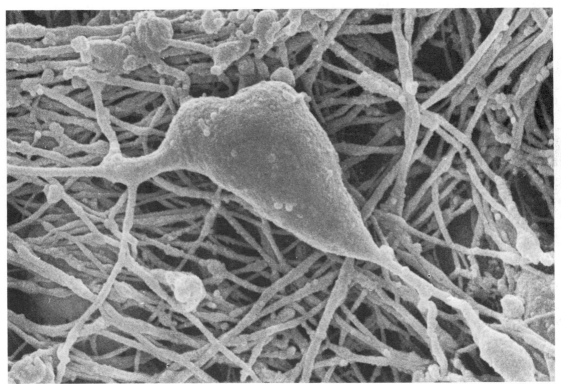

Figure 26–36. Scanning micrograph of a multipolar neuron in the myenteric plexus of a newborn rat. (Micrograph courtesy of T. Komuro and Y. Uehara.)

Although these several plexuses are distinguished on the basis of their architecture and their topographical location in the intestinal wall, they do not function independently. Connections can be traced from the subserous to the myenteric plexus; from the myenteric plexus to the submucous plexus; and from the latter to the mucosal plexus and to paravascular nerves along the submucosal arteries.

Detailed investigation of the "wiring diagram" of the enteric nervous system using traditional neuroanatomical methods is difficult, and our information is far from complete. Recent investigations have focused on histochemical and pharmacological definition of cell types on the basis of the neurotransmitters and neuromodulators that mediate their functions, and it is evident that there are many more functionally distinct cell types than have been identified to date on purely morphological criteria.

Cholinergic neurons in the intestine are the only intrinsic nerves for which both the transmitter and the functions are known. The cholinergic neurons of the enteric plexuses supply both longitudinal and circular muscle and are of prime importance in the active component of the peristaltic reflex. Another class of neurons is responsible for relaxation of intestinal smooth muscle. These are noncholinergic and non-noradrenergic inhibitory neurons. The nature of their transmitter is a subject of debate. Some workers insist that they release adenosine-5-triphosphate and refer to them as *"purinergic"* neurons. Others favor a *vasoactive intestinal polypeptide* as the more likely transmitter. These enteric nerves are believed to be responsible for inhibitory reflexes that relax smooth muscle in advance of a wave of peristaltic contraction, thus facilitating passage of intestinal contents along the tract.

The presence of other excitatory and inhibitory nerves has been postulated on the basis of neurophysiological and pharmacological experiments, but their location in the enteric plexus and the nature of their transmitters have yet to be established. Recent immunohistochemical studies have localized a variety of biologically active peptides in nerve cells of the enteric plexus. These include *substance P, somatostatin, enkephalins, vasoactive intestinal polypeptide, bombesin*, and *neurotensin*. It is not known whether these serve as neurotransmitters or neuromodulators.

REFERENCES

ABSORPTIVE CELLS

Bretscher, A., and K. Weber: Localization of actin and microfilament-associated proteins in the microvilli and terminal web of the intestinal brush border by immunofluorescence microscopy. J. Cell Biol. 79:839, 1978.

Brunser, O., and J. H. Luft: Fine structure of the apex of absorptive cells from rat small intestine. J. Ultrastruct. Res. 31:291, 1970.

Isselbacher, K. J.: The intestinal cell surface: properties of normal, undifferentiated, and malignant cells. Harvey Lect. 69:197, 1973–1974.

Ito, S.: Form and function of the glycocalyx on free cell surfaces. Philos. Trans. R. Soc. Lond. [Biol.] 268:55, 1974.

Madara, J. L., J. S. Trier, and M. R. Neutra: Structural changes in the plasma membrane accompanying differentiation of epithelial cells in human and monkey small intestine. Gastroenterology 78:963, 1980.

Mooseker, M. S., E. M. Bonder, B. G. Grimwade, C. L. Howe, T. C. Keller III, R. H. Wasserman, and K. A. Wharton: Regulation of contractility, cytoskeletal structure, and filament assembly in the brush border of intestinal epithelial cells. Cold Spring Harbor Symp. Quant. Biol. 46:855, 1982.

Mooseker, M. S., and L. G. Tilney: Organization of an actin filament-membrane complex. Filament polarity and membrane attachment in the microvilli of intestinal epithelial cells. J. Cell Biol. 67:725, 1975.

Trier, J. S.: Morphology of the epithelium of the small intestine. In Code, C. F., and W. Heidel, eds.: Handbook of Physiology. Vol. 3, Sect. 6. Washington, DC, American Physiological Society, 1968, Chapter 63.

PANETH CELLS

Behnke, O., and H. Moe: An electron microscopic study of mature and differentiating Paneth cells in the rat. J. Cell Biol. 22:633, 1964.

Erlandsen, S. L., and D. G. Chase: Paneth cell function: phagocytosis and intracellular digestion of microorganisms. J. Ultrastruct. Res. 41:296, 1972.

Erlandsen, S. L., J. A. Parsons, and T. D. Taylor: Ultrastructural immunocytochemical localization of lysozyme in the Paneth cells of man. J. Histochem. Cytochem. 22:401, 1974.

Erlandsen, S. L., C. B. Rodning, C. Montero, J. A. Parsons, C. A. Lewis, and I. D. Wilson: Immunocytochemical identification and localization of immunoglobulin A within Paneth cells of the rat small intestine. J. Histochem. Cytochem. 24:1085, 1976.

ENTEROENDOCRINE CELLS

Fujita, T. S.: Concept of paraneurons. Arch. Histol. Jpn. 40:Suppl. 1, 1977.

Fujita, T. S., and S. Kobayashi: The structure and function of gut endocrine cells. Int. Rev. Cytol. (Suppl.) 6:187, 1977.

Grube, D., and W. G. Forssmann: Morphology and function of the entero-endocrine cells. Horm. Metab. Res. 11:603, 1979.

Helmstaedter, V., G. E. Feurle, W. G. Forssmann: Ultrastructural identification of a new cell type—the N-cell as the source of neurotensin in the gut mucosa. Cell Tissue Res. 184:445, 1977.

Johnson, L. R.: The trophic action of gastrointestinal hormones. Gastroenterology 70:278, 1976.

Makhlouf, G. M.: The neuroendocrine design of the gut. The play of chemicals in a chemical background. Gastroenterology 67:159, 1974.

Pearse, A. G. E., J. M. Polak, and S. R. Bloom: The newer gut hormones. Cellular sources, physiology, pathology, and clinical aspects. Gastroenterology 72:746, 1977.

INTESTINAL IMMUNE SYSTEM

Brandtzaeg, P., and K. Baklein: Intestinal secretion of IgA and IgM: a hypothetical model. In Immunology of the Gut. Elsevier, Amsterdam, Ciba Foundation Symposium 46 (new series), 1977, p. 77.

Owen, R. L.: Sequential uptake of horseradish peroxidase by lymphoid follicle epithelium of Peyer's patches in the normal unobstructed mouse intestine: an ultrastructural study. Gastroenterology 72:440, 1977.

Owen, R. L., and A. L. Jones: Epithelial cell specialization with human Peyer's patches: an ultrastructural study of intestinal lymphoid follicles. Gastroenterology 66:189, 1974.

Owen, R. L., and P. Nemanic: Antigen processing structures of the mammalian intestinal tract: an SEM study of lymphoepithelial organs. In Scanning Electron Microscopy. Vol. II, AMF O'Hare, IL, SEM Inc., 1978, p. 367.

Plaut, A.: Microbial IgA proteases. N. Engl. J. Med. 298:1459, 1978.

Walker, W. A., and K. J. Isselbacher: Intestinal antibodies. N. Engl. J. Med. 297:767, 1977.

SUBMUCOSAL GLANDS OF BRUNNER

Elder, J. B., G. Williams, E. Lacey, and H. Gregory: Cellular localization of human urogastrone/epidermal growth factor. Nature 271:466, 1978.

Friend, D. S.: The fine structure of Brunner's glands in the mouse. J. Cell Biol. 25:563, 1965.

Moe, H.: The ultrastructure of Brunner's glands of the cat. J. Ultrastruct. Res. 4:58, 1960.

INTESTINAL ABSORPTION

Cardell, R. R., S. Badenhausen, and K. R. Porter: Intestinal absorption in the rat. An electron microscopical study. J. Cell Biol. 34:123, 1967.

Crane, R. K.: Intestinal absorption of sugars. Physiol. Rev. 40:789, 1960.

Crane, R. K.: Hypothesis for mechanism of intestinal active transport of sugars. Fed. Proc. 21:891, 1962.

Crane, R. K.: A digestive-absorptive surface as illustrated by the intestinal cell brush border. Trans. Am. Microsc. Soc. 94:529, 1975.

Johnston, T. M.: Mechanism of fat absorption. In Field, J., ed.: Handbook of Physiology. Sect. 6, Vol. III. Washington, DC, American Physiological Society, 1968, p. 1353.

Ockner, R. K., and K. J. Isselbacher: Recent concepts of intestinal fat absorption. Rev. Physiol. Biochem. Pharmacol. 71:107, 1974.

Palay, S. L., and L. J. Karlin: An electron microscope study of the intestinal villus. I. The fasting animal. II. The pathway of fat absorption. J. Biophys. Biochem. Cytol. 5:363, 373, 1959.

Palay, S. L., and J. P. Revel: The morphology of fat absorption. In Meng. H. C., ed.: Lipid Transport. Springfield, IL, Charles C Thomas, 1964, pp. 1–11.

Schonfeld, G., E. Bell, and D. H. Alpers: Intestinal apoproteins during fat absorption. J. Clin. Invest. 61:1539, 1978.

Strauss, E. W.: Electron microscopic study of intestinal fat absorption in vitro from mixed micelles containing linolenic acid, monoolein, and bile salt. J. Lipid Res. 7:307, 1966.

CELL TURNOVER AND RENEWAL

Chang, W. W. L., and C. P. Leblond: Renewal of the epithelium in the descending colon of the mouse. Parts I, II, and III. Am. J. Anat. 131:73, 101, 111, 1971.

Cheng, H., and C. P. Leblond: Origin, differentiation and renewal of the four main epithelial cell types in the mouse small intestine. Parts I to V. Am. J. Anat. 141:461–562, 1974.

Eastwood, G. L.: Gastrointestinal epithelial renewal. Gastroenterology 72:962, 1977.

Leblond, C. P.: Life history of cells in renewing systems. Am. J. Anat. 160:113, 1981.

Leblond, C. P., and B. Messier: Renewal of chief cells and goblet cells in the small intestine as shown by radioautography after injection of thymidine-H^3 into mice. Anat. Rec. 132:247, 1958.

Lipkin, M.: Cell replication in the gastrointestinal tract of man. Gastroenterology 48:616, 1965.

Parker, F. G., E. N. Barnes, and G. I. Kaye: The pericryptal fibroblast sheath. IV. Replication, migration and differentiation of the subepithelial fibroblasts of the crypts and villus of rabbit jejunum. Gastroenterology 67:607, 1974.

Pascal, R. R., G. I. Kaye, and N. Lane: Colonic pericryptal fibroblast sheath: replication, migration, and cytodifferentiation of a mesenchymal cell system in adult tissue. I. Autoradiographic studies of normal rabbit colon. Castroenterology 54:835, 1968.

Tsubouchi, S., and C. P. Leblond: Migration and turnover of entero-endocrine cells in the epithelium of the descending colon, as shown by radioautography after continuous infusion of ^{3}H-thymidine into mice. Am. J. Anat. 156:431, 1979.

Williamson, R. C. N.: Intestinal adaptation. N. Engl. J. Med. 298:1393, 1978.

LARGE INTESTINE

Essner, E., J. Schreiber, and R. A. Griewski: Localization of carbohydrate components in rat colon with fluoresceinated lectins. J. Histochem. Cytochem. 26:452, 1978.

Garry, R. C.: The movements of the large intestine. Physiol. Rev. 14:103, 1934.

Kaye, G. I., N. Lane, and R. R. Pascal: Colonic pericryptal fibroblast sheath: replication, migration, and cytodifferentiation of a mesenchymal cell system in adult tissue. II. Fine structural aspects of normal rabbit and human colon. Gastroenterology 54:852, 1968.

Lane, N., L. Caro, L. R. Otero-Vilardebo, and G. C. Godman: On the site of sulfation in colonic goblet cells. J. Cell Biol. 21:339, 1964.

Lineback, P. E.: Studies on the musculature of the human colon, with special reference to the taeniae. Am. J. Anat. 36:357, 1925.

Lorenzonn, V., and J. S. Trier: The fine structure of human rectal mucosa. The epithelial lining at the base of the crypt. Gastroenterology 55:88, 1968.

Martin, B. F.: The goblet cell pattern of the large intestine. Anat. Rec. 140:1, 1961.

Neutra, M. R., R. J. Grand, and J. S. Trier: Glycoprotein synthesis, transport and secretion by epithelial cells of human rectal mucosa: normal and cystic fibrosis. Lab. Invest. *36*:535, 1977.

Neutra, M. R., and C. P. Leblond: Synthesis of the carbohydrate of mucus in the Golgi complex as shown by electron microscope radioautography of goblet cells from rats injected with glucose-H^3. J. Cell Biol. *30*:119, 1966.

INNERVATION

Burnstock, G.: Purinergic nerves. Pharmacol. Rev. *24*:509, 1972.

Fujiwara, T., and Y. Uehara: Scanning electron microscopy of myenteric plexus: a preliminary communication. J. Electron Microsc. *29*:397, 1980.

Furness, J. B., and M. Costa: Types of nerves in the enteric nervous system. Neuroscience *5*:1, 1980.

Richardson, K. C.: Electronmicroscopic observations on Auerbach's plexus in the rabbit with special reference to the problem of smooth muscle innervation. Am. J. Anat. *103*:99, 1958.

Richardson, K. C.: Studies on the structure of the autonomic nerves in the small intestine, correlating the silver-impregnated image in light microscopy with the permanganate-fixed ultrastructure in electronmicroscopy. J. Anat. (Lond.) *94*:457, 1960.

Schofield, G. C.: Anatomy of muscular and neural tissues in the alimentary canal. *In* Code, C. F., and M. I. Grossman, eds.: Handbook of Physiology, Sect. 6. Washington, DC American Physiological Society, 1967–1968.

27

THE LIVER AND GALLBLADDER

LIVER

The liver is the largest gland in the body, weighing about 1500 g in the adult. It functions both as an *exocrine gland*, secreting bile through a system of bile ducts into the duodenum, and as an *endocrine gland*, synthesizing a variety of substances that are released directly into the bloodstream. To appreciate the importance of the liver and to correlate its structure with its functions requires an understanding of its blood supply and its strategic location in the circulation. It receives a large volume of venous blood from the intestinal tract via the *portal vein* and a small volume of arterial blood via the *hepatic artery*. It is drained by the *hepatic veins* into the inferior vena cava near the heart. The liver is thus interposed between the intestinal tract and the general circulation. It therefore receives, in the portal blood, all of the material absorbed from the intestinal tract except the bulk of the lipid, which is transported in the *chyle* via the mesenteric lymphatics to the thoracic duct. The absorbed products of digestion are taken up and metabolized in the liver or are transformed there and returned to the blood for storage or utilization elsewhere. The liver may also receive toxic substances from the intestine or from the general circulation, and is capable of degrading them by oxidation or hydroxylation or detoxifying them by conjugation. The products of their degradation or their harmless conjugates are then excreted in the *bile*. The bile is a complex fluid that can be regarded as a secretion in that it plays an important role in digestion, but it can also be regarded as a vehicle for excretion to the extent that it carries detoxified waste and potentially harmful materials to the intestine for ultimate elimination.

The liver also synthesizes several important protein components of the blood plasma, and it exercises an important degree of control over the general metabolism by virtue of its capacity to store carbohydrates as glycogen and to release glucose to maintain the normal concentration of glucose in the blood.

HISTOLOGICAL ORGANIZATION OF THE LIVER

The liver is composed of epithelial cells arranged in plates or laminae that are interconnected to form a continuous tridimensional lattice. The laminae are disposed radially with respect to terminal branches of the hepatic veins, which traditionally have been designated as *central veins* because of their location in the centers of prismatic units of liver parenchyma that constitute the liver *lobules* (Figs. 27–1, 27–2). The radially disposed plates of liver cells are exposed on either side to the blood flowing in a parallel system of vascular channels, the *hepatic sinusoids*. The radially oriented sinusoids closely conform to the broad surfaces of the cellular laminae and intercommunicate through fenestrations in them to form a labyrinthine system of thin-walled vessels intimately related to a very large surface area of liver parenchyma.

The Liver Lobule

In the pig and a few other species, a well-defined layer of connective tissue clearly demarcates the lobules. However, in most mammals, including the human, there is no boundary between the lobules, the hepatic parenchyma appearing quite continuous. The radial pattern of the cellular plates and sinusoids is such that one can, nevertheless, recognize the units of structure and assign imaginary boundaries to the lobule by relying

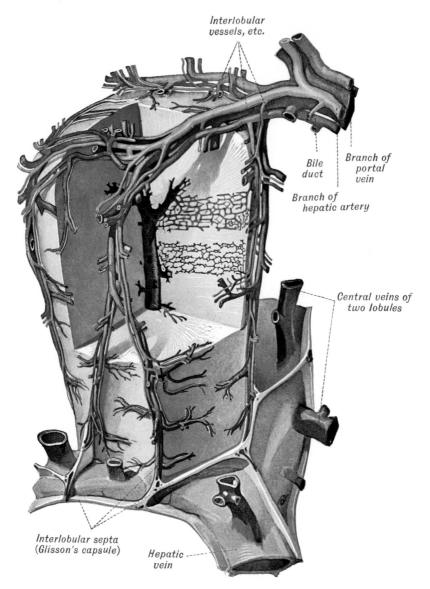

Interlobular
vessels, etc.

Bile
duct

Branch of
portal
vein

Branch of
hepatic artery

Central veins of
two lobules

Interlobular septa
(Glisson's capsule)

Hepatic
vein

Figure 27–1. Wax reconstruction (by A. Vierling) of a lobule of the liver of a pig. A portion of the lobule has been cut away to show the bile capillaries and sinusoids. × 400. (After Braus.)

upon the regularly distributed central veins and portal canals as landmarks (Fig. 27–2).

The lobules in sections are typically hexagonal, with the corners of the polygon each occupied by a *portal canal.* This latter structure consists of a small branch of the portal vein and one of the hepatic artery, as well as a bile ductule, enclosed in a common investment of connective tissue (Fig. 27–3). Blood enters the hepatic sinusoids from small branches of the hepatic artery and portal vein, flows through the lobule centripetally, and leaves via the central vein (Figs. 27–4, 27–5).

The traditional lobule as defined above is not comparable with the lobules of most glands, which are centered on the ducts that drain them. The liver lobule as just presented is conceptually convenient, however, for as a result of differential deposition of glycogen or fat, the hepatic tissue of which it is composed frequently exhibits microscopically distinguishable zones, concentric around the central vein. Moreover, in pathological conditions, necrosis may selectively involve the central or the peripheral zone, depending upon the nature of the disease process.

The lobular pattern appears to develop as

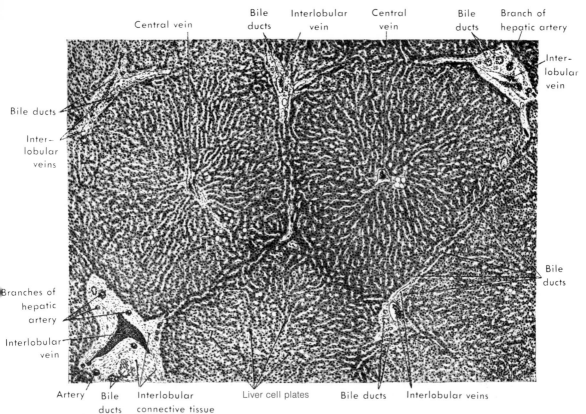

Central vein   Bile ducts   Interlobular vein   Central vein   Bile ducts   Branch of hepatic artery

Interlobular vein

Bile ducts

Interlobular veins

Branches of hepatic artery

Interlobular vein

Artery   Bile ducts   Interlobular connective tissue   Liver cell plates   Bile ducts   Interlobular veins

Bile ducts

Figure 27–2. Portion of liver from a 22-year-old man. Two complete lobules are surrounded by portions of other lobules. × 70. (After Sobotta.)

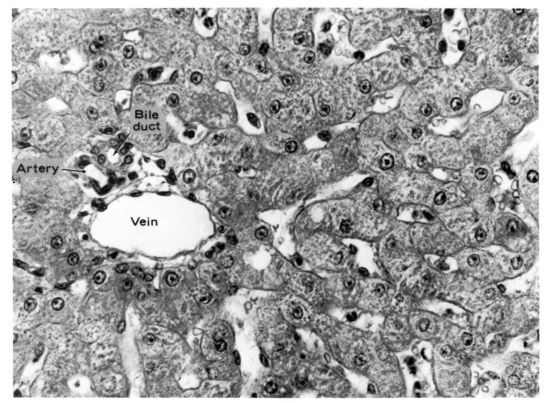

Bile duct

Artery

Vein

Figure 27–3. Photomicrograph of liver parenchyma at the periphery of a traditional lobule, showing a typical portal triad, consisting of branches of the hepatic artery and portal vein, and a small bile duct.

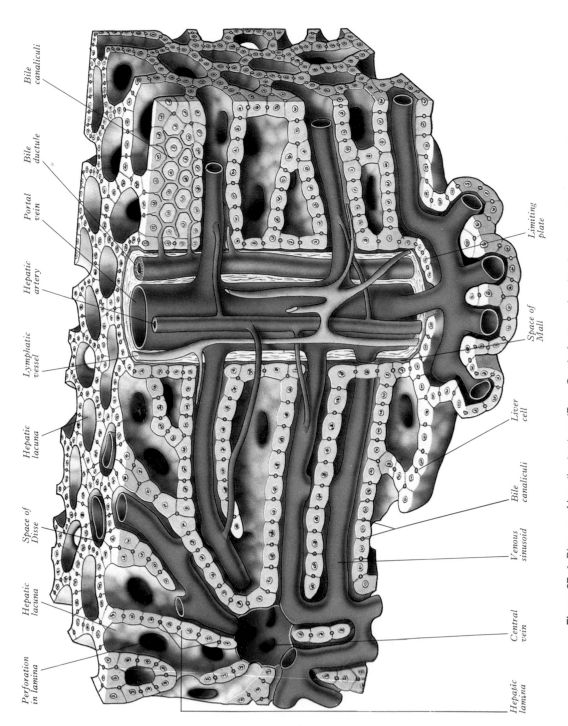

Bile canaliculi

Bile ductule

Portal vein

Hepatic artery

Lymphatic vessel

Hepatic lacuna

Space of Disse

Hepatic lacuna

Perforation in lamina

Limiting plate

Space of Mall

Liver cell

Bile canaliculi

Venous sinusoid

Central vein

Hepatic lamina

Figure 27–4. Diagram of hepatic structure. (From Gray's Anatomy. London, Longman. After Prof. H. Elias.)

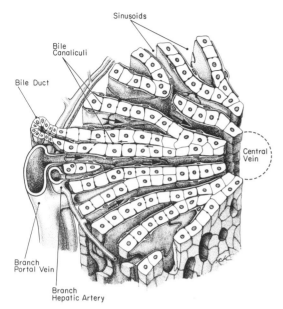

Figure 27–5. Diagrammatic representation of the radial disposition of the liver cell plates and sinusoids around the terminal hepatic venule or central vein, showing the centripetal flow of blood from branches of the hepatic artery and portal vein, and the centrifugal flow of bile *(small arrows)* to the small bile duct in the portal space. (Redrawn and modified from Ham, A. W.: Textbook of Histology. 5th ed. Philadelphia, J. B. Lippincott Co., 1965.)

center of the lobule, and the branches of the hepatic vein were said to be situated around its periphery. The lobule defined in this way is called a *portal lobule.* In such a lobule, the bile would drain toward a duct located with the vascular supply in the center of the lobule, as is the case in most other glands.

In some respects this is a more satisfactory way of interpreting the architecture of the liver than the *classical lobule,* but it has been argued that the portal lobule is not the smallest unit of functional organization of the liver. A variant of the portal lobule has been proposed by Rappaport and his colleagues, who consider the functional unit to be a mass of parenchymal tissue associated with the fine terminal branches of the portal vein, hepatic artery, and bile duct. These branches leave the portal canals at intervals, coursing perpendicular to the canals and to the central vein, and run along the side of the hexagon that forms the section of the classical lobule. The associated mass of hepatic tissue is smaller than either of the lobules proposed earlier and is composed of parts of two adjacent classical lobules (Fig. 27–6). It is called

a consequence of the hydrodynamics of the blood flow through the liver. From this point of view the liver may be considered as a tough sac filled with fluid, in which is suspended a plastic spongework of liver tissue. In the flow of fluid through the liver, the terminal branches of the portal vein are sources and the radicles of the hepatic vein are sinks (Figs. 27–4, 27–5). The flow from the one to the other is thought to determine the radial pattern of the sinusoids characteristic of the lobule. It follows also that the cells nearest the branches of the portal vein receive blood first and therefore have first call upon the nutrient and oxygen content of the portal blood. As the latter diminish in the passage of the blood from the periphery toward the center of the lobule, a gradient of metabolic activity is established, which is expressed in the morphologically detectable zonation of the lobule.

Some histologists have objected to the classical definition of the liver lobule because it is inconsistent with the lobular organization typical of other exocrine glands. In an effort to make the liver conform to the same general plan, Mall proposed an alternative concept of liver lobulation according to which the portal canal was considered to be the

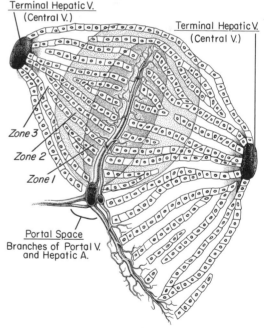

Figure 27–6. Diagram illustrating the functional unit of liver parenchyma (the acinus) according to Rappaport et al. It consists of the parenchyma centered around the terminal branches of the hepatic artery and portal vein. It should be noted that the cells in Zone 1 nearest these vessels have first call upon the incoming oxygen and nutrients, while the cells of Zone 2 are less favored and those of Zone 3 near the terminal hepatic venules are least favorably situated. (Redrawn after Rappaport, A. M., A. J. Borowy, W. M. Lougheed, and W. N. Lolto. Anat. Rec. *119*:11, 1954.)

a *liver acinus* and is defined as the tissue supplied by a terminal branch of the portal vein and of the hepatic artery and drained by a terminal branch of the bile duct. The limits of the acinus are not defined by any recognizable anatomical landmarks but extend outward to the terminal branches of the hepatic veins and to the imaginary outer limits of acini associated with neighboring portal canals. The parenchyma is continuous from one acinus to the next, and indeed from one classical lobule to the next. Therefore, if the supply and drainage of one unit should fail, it would still be supplied and drained by others. This concept of liver structure, although still not universally accepted, has proved useful in the understanding of some aspects of liver physiology and in accounting for some manifestations of liver pathology, especially that following bile duct occlusion and that found in cirrhosis of the liver.

The *classical lobule*, the *portal lobule*, and the *acinus* should not be considered as conflicting concepts of liver structure but as complementary ones. Because of the complexity of the function of the liver, it is sometimes useful to think in terms of one and at other times in terms of another. It is noteworthy that the traditional lobulation is not present in the lower vertebrates nor in the mammalian embryo.

The Blood Supply

Most organs receive their afferent blood supply from one or more arteries. The liver is exceptional in that its principal afferent blood supply is the *portal vein* carrying blood from the intestinal tract and spleen. About 75 per cent of the blood to the liver is brought to it by the portal vein and only 25 per cent by the relatively small *hepatic artery*. The portal vein entering the porta of the liver branches into *interlobar veins* and these in turn into *conducting veins* 400 μm or more in diameter. Their walls are thinner and have less adventitial connective tissue than veins of comparable size elsewhere. The conducting veins branch to give rise to *interlobular veins*, which possess few longitudinal smooth muscle cells in their walls. The *terminal portal venules* that arise from the interlobular veins are 280 μm or less in diameter and very thin walled. These, accompanied by a terminal branch of the hepatic artery and a small bile duct, are the axial structures of the smallest portal canals. Small lateral branches given off at short intervals from these terminal venules pass through fenestrations in the limiting plate of hepatic cells to become continuous with the sinosoids of the neighboring liver lobules.

The *hepatic artery* on entering the porta branches into *interlobar* and then into *intralobular arteries*. The great majority of the flow from these vessels is distributed to capillaries in the connective tissue stroma of the liver. Only a small volume continues into the *terminal hepatic arterioles* of the smallest portal canals (Fig. 27–7). These give off collateral branches to the hepatic sinusoids and numerous small branches to a dense capillary network that surrounds the bile ductules. This *peribiliary* or *periductal plexus* was formerly thought to drain into the portal venules. Vascular casts studied by scanning electron microscopy have now clearly shown that efferent vessels are given off to the hepatic sinusoids (Fig. 27–8). Thus, much of the arterial blood reaches the sinusoids indirectly via the peribiliary plexus. The extraordinarily rich vascularity of the small bile ducts suggests the possibility that some constituents of the bile may be reabsorbed in passage through the intrahepatic bile ducts.

The primary function of the hepatic circulation is carried out in the sinusoids. These form an exceedingly elaborate three-dimensional plexus presenting an enormous surface for interchange of metabolites with the hepatic parenchyma. Every liver cell in the radially arranged cellular plates of the lobule is exposed on at least one, and usually two, sides to blood circulating in the sinusoids. Corrosion preparations of vascular casts viewed with the scanning microscope illustrate dramatically the richness of the microvasculature of the liver (Fig. 27–7). The blood leaves the lobule through a terminal radicle of the hepatic vein, the *central vein* of the classical lobule. Its wall is penetrated by innumerable openings through which blood flows from the surrounding sinusoids into its lumen (Fig. 27–9). The central veins drain into *intercalated veins* (*sublobular veins*). Several of these unite to form collecting veins and these in turn join to form hepatic veins, which pursue a course through the liver independent of the portal venous system. Two or more large hepatic veins enter the inferior vena cava.

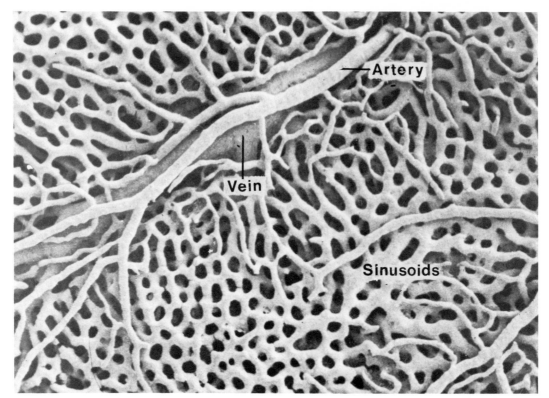

Figure 27–7. Scanning micrograph of a vascular cast of monkey liver illustrating the extraordinarily rich network of hepatic sinusoids. Crossing the figure diagonally is a terminal branch of the hepatic artery and its associated vein. (Micrograph courtesy of T. Murikami, from Johari, O., and I. Corvin, eds.: Scanning Electron Microscopy 1978. Part II. Chicago, SEM Inc. AMF O'Hare, 1978.)

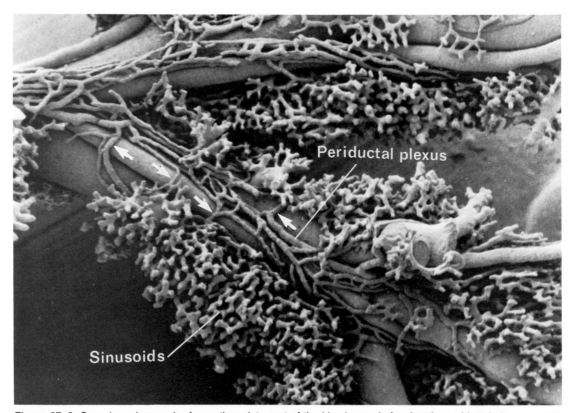

Figure 27–8. Scanning micrograph of a methacrylate cast of the blood vessels forming the periductal plexus, and its communications with the sinusoids *(at arrows)*. (Micrograph from Murikami, T. Arch. Histol. Jpn. *37*:245, 1974.)

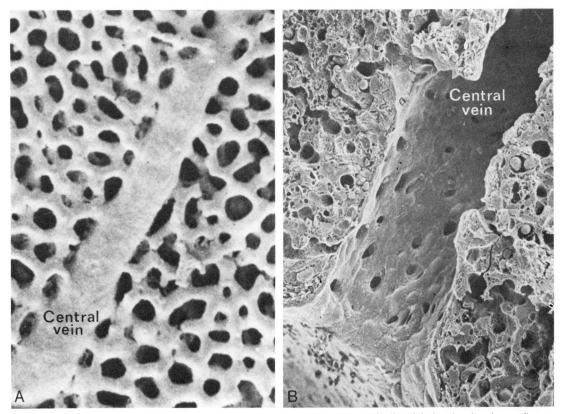

Figure 27–9. *A,* Scanning micrograph of a vascular cast of the central portion of a liver lobule, showing the confluence of numerous sinusoids with the central vein. *B,* A comparable scanning micrograph of this region of the lobule cut longitudinally through the central vein, showing the openings of sinusoids into its lumen. (*A,* Courtesy of T. Murikami. *B,* From Mota, P. M., M. Muto, and T. Fujita. The Liver. Tokyo, Igaku, Shoin, 1978.)

Hepatic Sinusoids

The hepatic sinusoids are larger than capillaries and are more irregular in shape, and their lining cells are directly apposed to the epithelial cells of the parenchyma with essentially no intervening connective tissue. The lining of the sinusoids consists of a thin layer of cells that differ from typical capillary endothelium in two respects: (1) some of the lining cells are actively phagocytic (Fig. 27–10) and (2) the cell boundaries do not blacken with silver nitrate. This latter property led some early investigators to suggest that the lining was a syncytium. Various cytological and experimental studies carried out in the era of light microscopy cast doubt upon this interpretation, and subsequent studies with the electron microscope have established beyond doubt that the endothelium is made up of individual cells.

Whether the lining is composed of one or two types of cells was long a subject of dispute. Those who distinguished two identified one as a typical endothelial cell and considered the other to be a form of tissue macrophage called the *cell of Kupffer.* Other investigators observed that, upon repeated injection of colloidal particulate matter into experimental animals, the phagocytic cells of the sinusoids became larger and more numerous; they thought they could recognize forms intermediate between endothelial cells and Kupffer cells. Therefore, it was thought that the endothelial cells could transform into phagocytic cells when the need arose and that the different appearance of the lining cells simply represented different functional states of a single cell type. The application of electron microscopy and radiolabeling techniques has now resolved the controversy in favor of distinct populations having different origins and functions. In electron micrographs of liver fixed by perfusion, it is now possible to identify three cell types associated with the sinusoids—*endothelial cells, Kupffer cells,* and perisinusoidal *fat-storing cells.*

Endothelial Cells. These flattened cells

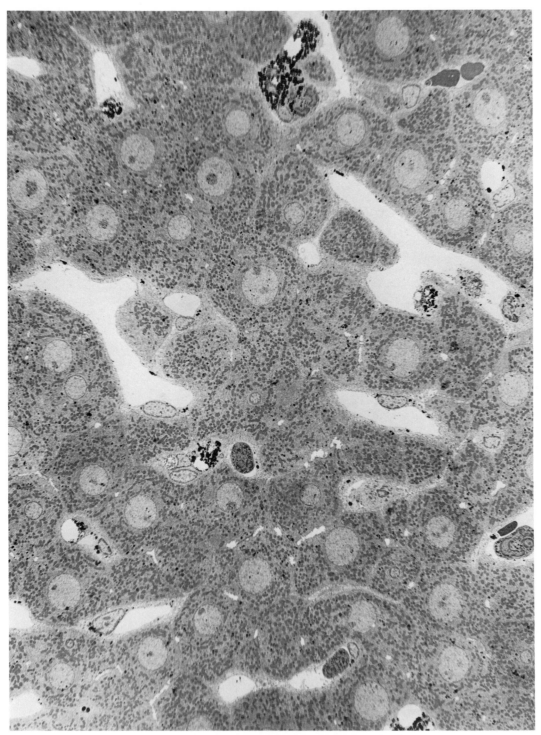

Figure 27–10. Low-magnification micrograph of rat liver, illustrating the intimate relationship of the cell plates to the sinusoids. Kupffer cells in some of the sinusoids contain dense phagocytosed material. (Micrograph courtesy of E. Wisse.)

form the greater part of the extremely thin lining layer of the sinusoids. They are not significantly phagocytic to colloidal vital dyes, although some pinocytotic activity is suggested by electron micrographs in which small plasmalemmal vesicles are seen associated with both the adluminal and the abluminal surfaces of the cell.

Whether the sinusoidal lining was continuous or discontinuous was a question long debated. Physiological observations on rates of clearance of substances from the blood during its transit through the liver and observations on the size of the molecules and colloidal particles that readily passed through the wall of the sinusoid made it seem probable that there were openings in it that permitted the blood plasma, but not the blood cells, to gain direct access to the surface of the hepatic cells. The electron microscope has provided visual confirmation of this interpretation. In the common laboratory species the endothelial cells have typical overlapping junctions in some places, but in others the attenuated margins of neighboring cells may

be separated by intercellular openings 0.1 to 0.5 μm across. In addition, it can be seen in electron micrographs that the thin peripheral portions of the endothelial cells are fenestrated, presenting a sievelike appearance (Fig. 27–11). These openings are considerably larger and more variable in size and shape than the pores in fenestrated capillaries. Thus, it appears that there are sizable transcellular fenestrations as well as small discontinuities between adjacent cells. It can be shown that in as short a time as 30 seconds after injection of colloidal thorium dioxide into the portal vein, the dense particles can be found on both sides of the endothelium and on the surface of the underlying hepatic cells. Since the endothelium of the hepatic sinusoids also lacks a basal lamina in many species, the particulate tracer evidently encounters no barrier to passage through the fenestrations.

Openings in the walls of the blood vessels are rare in the circulatory system of vertebrates, but it is now generally accepted that the wall of the sinusoids is discontinuous in

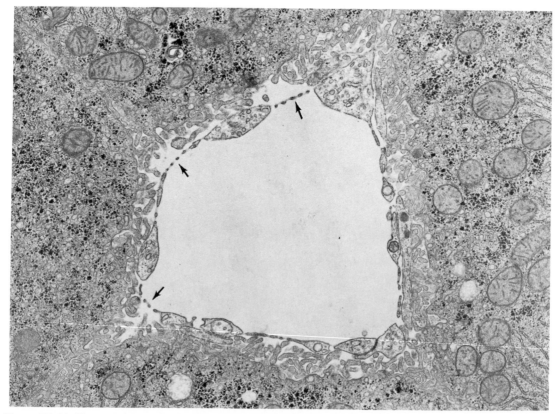

Figure 27–11. Electron micrograph of a sinusoid in rat liver fixed by vascular perfusion. The endothelium is extremely attenuated in some areas where there are fenestrations that give it a sievelike structure *(see arrows)*. (Micrograph from Wisse, E. J. Ultrastruct Res. *31*:125, 1970.)

most mammals, including the human. There are, however, significant species differences in the degree of endothelial discontinuity. The hepatic sinusoids of sheep, goats, and calves are reported to have a distinct basal lamina and an endothelium with few fenestrae. In those species with a discontinuous sinusoidal endothelium and no basal lamina, there is no filtration barrier for macromolecules or particles up to 0.5 μm in diameter. Chylomicra and very-low-density lipoprotein particles can freely traverse inter- or transcellular fenestrations.

Kupffer Cells. These stellate cells were described by Kupffer in 1898 in liver stained by a gold-chloride impregnation method. They were depicted with their processes traversing the sinusoids. Thus, they were thought to lie within the sinusoid but fixed to the endothelium. They frequently contain engulfed erythrocytes in various stages of disintegration, and deposits of iron-containing pigment. They actively phagocytize particulate matter injected into the bloodstream (Fig. 27–10) and therefore are stained intensely with such vital dyes as lithium carmine or trypan blue. They also take up injected electron-opaque particles of carbon or of thorium dioxide (Fig. 27–12). The Kupffer cells are therefore components of the diffuse mononuclear phagocyte system. They may retain for long periods phagocytosed material that cannot be digested by lysosomes.

Electron microscopic studies of Kupffer cells in livers fixed by perfusion have done much to clarify their cytological characteristics and their relations to other cells associated with the sinusoids. They are usually situated on the endothelium with processes extending between the underlying endothelial cells. Their highly variable shape suggests that their form and relations to the endothelium may change continually. They do not form desmosomes or other enduring specializations for attachment to the endothelial cells. The greater part of their irregular cell surface is exposed to the blood in the lumen of the sinusoid. A thin glycocalyx can be demonstrated. In addition to surface folds and slender villous projections, there are peculiar sinuous invaginations of the plasma membrane into the peripheral cytoplasm. These have a central dense line between parallel membranes and a faint transverse striation, resulting in a highly characteristic appearance in thin sections that has led to their description as "vermiform bodies." These are never seen in endothelial

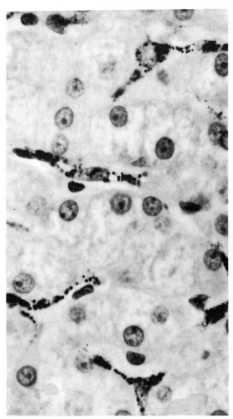

Figure 27–12. Liver of dog injected with India ink, showing uptake of carbon by the lining cells. × 675. (Courtesy of A. J. Ladman.)

cells but have been reported in macrophages of other organs and in the Langerhans cells of the epidermis.

The cytoplasm of Kupffer cells is richer in organelles and more heterogeneous in appearance than that of endothelial cells. Clear vacuoles of varying size and dense bodies presumed to be lysosomes are usually present. There is a juxtanuclear centrosome and associated Golgi complex. Short cisternal profiles of granular endoplasmic reticulum are scattered throughout the cytoplasm. These are demonstrated with unusual clarity in preparations reacted for peroxidase activity (Fig. 27–13). Peroxidase is present in the perinuclear cistern, in the lumen of the endoplasmic reticulum, and in the occasional annulate lamellae of Kupffer cells. This reaction serves clearly to distinguish them from endothelial cells, which have no peroxidase activity.

It was formerly thought that increase in the numbers of Kupffer cells after experimental stimulation of the reticuloendothelial system was due either to division of the

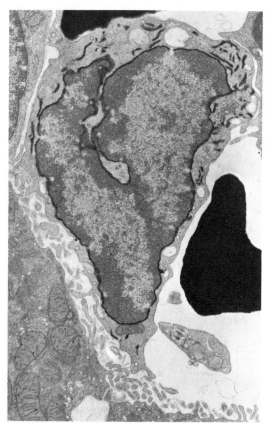

Figure 27–13. Electron micrograph of a Kupffer cell, showing a positive reaction for peroxidase in the nuclear envelope and in cisternae of the endoplasmic reticulum. This reaction serves to distinguish Kupffer cells from endothelial cells. (Micrograph from Fahimi, D. J. Cell Biol. 47:247, 1970.)

stimulated, the dividing Kupffer cells could be shown to have originated from the bone marrow of the donor. Similarly, when pairs of unirradiated histocompatible mice were maintained in parabiosis for several months, karyotypic analysis of Kupffer cells revealed limited numbers of partner-derived cells in every instance. These experiments have led to the conclusion that the Kupffer cells are derived from a precursor in the bone marrow, as are the free mononuclear phagocytes of other organs. They are now considered to be members of the mononuclear phagocyte system.

Fat-Storing Cells. Cells that contain multiple lipid droplets are found outside of the sinuses, often occupying recesses between the parenchymal cells but extending long processes that are in contact with the endothelium. These cells have been described under a variety of names: *interstitial cells, lipocytes, fat-storing cells,* and *stellate cells.* They can be stained with gold chloride (Figs. 27–14, 27–15), and it is possible that some of the stellate cells described by Kupffer were, in fact, fat-

preexisting cells of this type or to acquisition of phagocytic capacity by endothelial cells transforming into Kupffer cells. This latter source is of course excluded since it is now known that these are ontogenetically distinct populations. The experimental stimulation of phagocytic cells does result in a substantial increase in the number of Kupffer cells incorporating H³-thymidine. Thus, there seems no doubt of their ability to increase by mitosis. There is also compelling evidence that Kupffer cells are replaced and are augmented by recruitment of monocytes from the blood, which are transformed into Kupffer cells. In the relevant experiments, mice were given sufficient whole body x-irradiation to suppress division of their own cells. They then received an intravenous injection of bone marrow cells from another animal of the same strain whose cells carried a chromosomal marker. When the reticuloendothelial systems of the recipient mice were

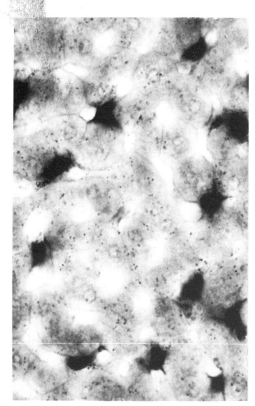

Figure 27–14. Photomicrograph of normal rabbit liver stained by Kupffer's original gold impregnation method. The perisinusoidal stellate or fat-storing cells are stained. × 600. (Photograph by Wake, K. Am. J. Anat. 132:429, 1971.)

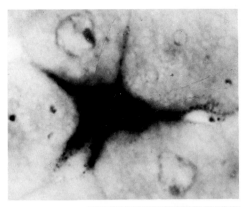

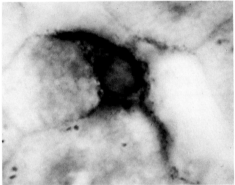

Figure 27–15. Fat-storing cells of rabbit liver after use of Kupffer's gold impregnation method. × 1800. (Photomicrographs from Wake, K. Am. J. Anat. *132:429*, 1971.)

storing cells and not exclusively the phagocytic cells that now bear his name.

These stellate perisinusoidal cells have some of the cytological characteristics of fibroblasts. They tend to be more numerous in intermediate and peripheral portions of the hepatic lobule than they are in the central zone. Their origin and functional significance are poorly understood. When exogenous vitamin A is administered it accumulates preferentially in the lipid droplets of the stellate fat-storing cells.

Pit Cells. A fourth cell type associated with the sinusoids has recently been described. The *pit cell* is also located in the perisinusoidal space and attached to the endothelium. It possesses numerous short pseudopodia but is nonphagocytic. Its most characteristic feature is the presence in its cytoplasm of small dense granules resembling those of the endocrine cells of the gastrointestinal epithelium. Pit cells are present in small numbers in rat liver but have not yet been described in human liver. Their origin and function remain unknown.

Perisinusoidal Space (Space of Disse)

The relationship of the sinusoid lining to the underlying liver cells has been settled by the electron microscope. Formerly a controversy stemmed from the fact that in histological sections of human postmortem material, a space, called the *space of Disse,* could be seen between the sinusoid lining and the liver cells. This was not apparent in biopsy material nor in the usual sections of livers of laboratory animals used in research. It was therefore regarded by many histologists as a consequence of agonal or postmortem change in the liver. In electron micrographs of well-fixed material, the endothelium of the sinusoids is not closely applied to a smooth parenchymal cell surface, as was previously thought to be the case, but instead rests lightly on the tips of a large number of irregularly oriented microvilli on the surface of the liver cell (Figs. 27–16, 27–17). There is therefore a true perivascular space in the normal liver into which the microvilli project. The space of Disse described by pathologists was evidently the result of an edematous expansion of this space. The term has now come to be applied freely to the narrow perivascular space revealed by the electron microscope in the normal liver.

Occasional unmyelinated nerve axons are encountered in the space of Disse (Fig. 27–18) and small bundles of collagen fibrils forming the argyrophilic reticulum described by light microscopists (Fig. 27–19), but the space contains no true ground substance, and plasma can apparently move freely through it. Although its content is plasma rather than interstitial fluid, it must be considered an interstitial space and not a lymphatic space, because it is not lined by lymphatic endothelium. The space of Disse may, nevertheless, be important in the formation of the abundant liver lymph.

It is evident that direct access of the plasma to the surface of the liver cell is a structural feature of great functional importance in the active exchange of metabolites between the liver and the bloodstream. The efficiency of this exchange is further promoted by the increase in surface achieved by the microvilli. From measurement of electron micrographs, it is estimated that the length of the plasma membrane covering the microvilli and lining the clefts between them is six times greater than the linear extent of cell surface measured across the bases of the microvilli.

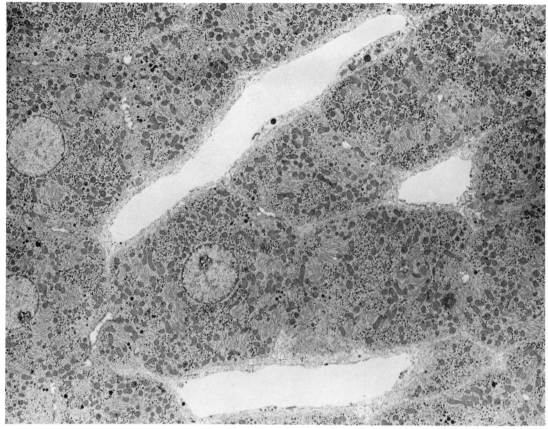

Figure 27–16. Electron micrograph of plates of liver cells and intervening sinusoids. (Micrograph by E. Wisse.)

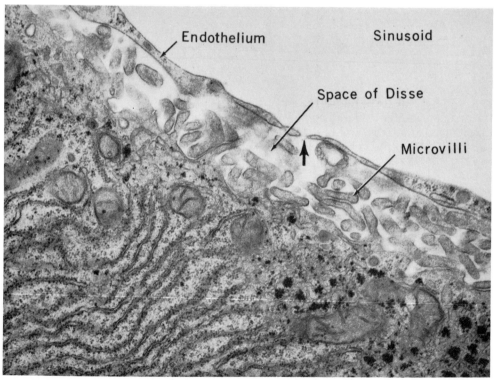

Figure 27–17. Electron micrograph of part of the surface of a rat liver cell bordering on a sinusoid. Numerous irregularly oriented microvilli project into a narrow space between the hepatic cell and the endothelium lining the sinusoid. The perivascular space is often called the space of Disse. Notice the small discontinuity in the lining of the sinusoid *(at heavy arrow).* × 18,000. (Courtesy of K. R. Porter and G. Millonig; labeling added.)

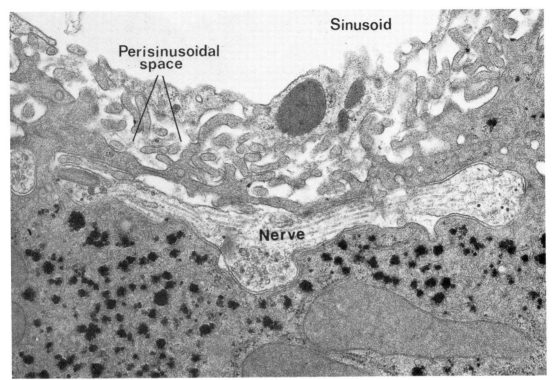

Figure 27–18. In some species, nerve axons are found occasionally in the perisinusoidal space in apparent synaptic contact with the hepatocytes. (Micrograph courtesy of E. Weihe and G. Metz.)

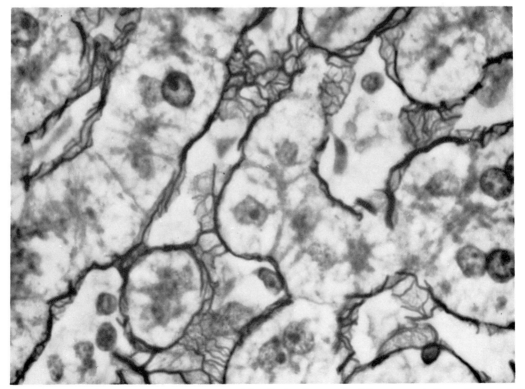

Figure 27–19. Photomicrograph of rat liver prepared by Pap's silver method for demonstrating reticulum. A fine meshwork of argyrophilic fibers is situated between the hepatic cells and the cells lining the sinusoids. × 1250.

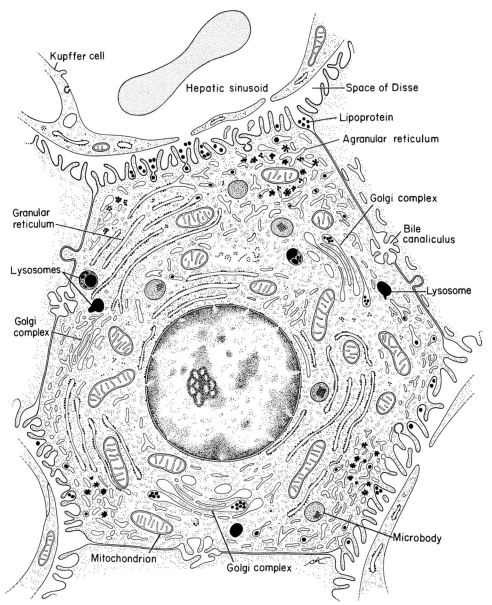

Figure 27–20. Drawing depicting the relationship of the liver cells to each other and to the sinusoids, and showing the principal components of the hepatic cell as seen in electron micrographs. (Drawing by Sylvia Colard Keene.)

The Cytology of the Hepatic Parenchymal Cells

The liver cells are polyhedral, with six or more surfaces. The surfaces are of three sorts: those exposed to the perisinusoidal space; those exposed to the lumen of the bile canaliculus; and those in contact with adjacent liver cells (Fig. 27–20). The nuclei are large and round, with a smooth surface, but may vary in size from cell to cell. The variation in size has been shown to be an expression of polyploidy. Most cells have a single nucleus, but as many as 25 per cent are binucleate; 70 per cent or more of the nuclei are tetraploid, and 1 to 2 per cent are octaploid. The nucleus is typically vesicular, with a few scattered chromatin clumps and one or more prominent nucleoli. In electron micrographs the liver cell nucleus has few features that distinguish it from the nuclei of other cells. The chromatin is represented by ill-defined aggregations of filaments that appear granular in section. Somewhat larger granules 30 nm in diameter, called perichromatin granules, are located near the masses of chromatin. These are usually surrounded by a clear zone about 25 nm wide. These granules stain with uranyl acetate and indium and are therefore believed to contain nucleic acids. The nucleoli consist of fine fibrils (6 nm) and dense granules (15 nm), and both of these components are present in the anastomosing strands that constitute the nucleolonema. As in other cell types, the nuclear envelope consists of two parallel membranes bounding a perinuclear cisterna. The conspicuous basophilic bodies seen in the cytoplasm with the light microscope (Fig. 27–21) are found in electron micrographs to be aggregations of cisternae of an extensive rough endoplasmic reticulum (Fig. 27–22). The cisternae are spaced somewhat farther apart and are less precisely parallel than the cisternae in the pancreas and other protein-secreting cell types. The cisternae are studded with numerous ribosomes, but the ends of their profiles are apt to be slightly expanded and free of granules. In addition to the ribosomes associated with the cytoplasmic membranes, there are numerous polyribosomes free in the cytoplasmic matrix.

The liver cell also contains a moderately extensive smooth endoplasmic reticulum that takes the form of a close-meshed plexus of branching and anastomosing tubules, somewhat variable in caliber (Fig. 27–23). Owing to the thinness of the sections, however, the continuity of the system is not always evident, and it may appear as a congeries of separate profiles of irregular outline. Sites of continuity between the rough- and smooth-surfaced reticulum are frequently observed (Fig. 27–24). Small globules about 30 to 40 nm in diameter are often seen in the lumen of the smooth reticulum (Fig. 27–23). These represent the very-low-density serum lipoprotein (VLDL), which is synthesized in the liver and released into the blood.

In histological sections the cytoplasm of the liver cell presents an extremely variable appearance, which reflects to some extent the functional state of the cell. The principal source of variation is in the content of the stored material—glycogen and fat. In the preparation of histological sections, both fat and glycogen have been removed, but the presence of glycogen is indicated by irregular empty spaces, and the presence of lipid is represented by round vacuoles. By appropri-

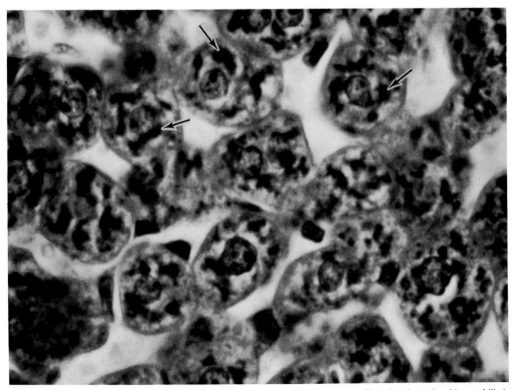

Figure 27–21. Photomicrograph of rat liver stained with eosin and methylene blue. The deeply stained basophilic bodies *(at arrows)* in the cytoplasm correspond to the aggregations of granular endoplasmic reticulum seen in electron micrographs. × 1250.

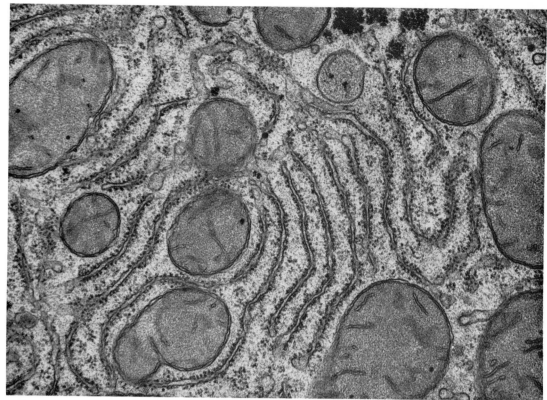

Figure 27–22. Electron micrograph showing an area of granular endoplasmic reticulum from hamster liver, corresponding to one of the basophilic bodies seen with the light microscope. The mitochondria and the granular reticulum are often in close topographical relation to one another. × 34,000. (After Jones, A. L., and D. W. Fawcett. J. Histochem. Cytochem. *14*:215, 1966.)

ate methods of fixation, both fat and glycogen can be preserved and stained. The content of these materials in the liver may vary greatly with the diet or the time after feeding (Fig. 27–25).

When adequately preserved, glycogen appears in electron micrographs of liver cells as dense aggregates or rosettes up to 0.1 μm in diameter (alpha particles) composed of beta particles 20 to 30 nm in diameter. Glycogen is not uniformly distributed in the cytoplasm but tends to be closely associated with the areas of smooth endoplasmic reticulum (Fig. 27–26).

Lipid occurs in the form of osmiophilic droplets of varying size. These are few in number in the normal liver, but may be dramatically increased after consumption of alcohol or other hepatotoxic substances. The lipid droplets are not limited by a membrane. They may occur anywhere in the cytoplasm and have no special topographical relation to any of the organelles other than mitochondria, which may be closely applied to the surface of the droplet.

Mitochondria cannot be seen in the usual histological preparation but can be revealed by special cytological techniques. They are numerous and for the most part filamentous, but they vary somewhat in size and shape in different parts of the lobule and in different physiological conditions. The mitochondria are in no way unusual in their fine structure. Lamellar or tubular cristae project into a matrix of relatively low density. A number of matrix granules are usually seen in each mitochondrial profile.

The Golgi system of the cell consists of several parts, each situated near a bile canaliculus (Fig. 27–27). Each complex is made up of three to five flat saccules or cisternae in close parallel array. The ends of the cisternae are often dilated and contain numerous moderately dense granules 30 to 60 nm in diameter. These are identical to the low-density lipoprotein particles observed in the smooth reticulum. Associated with each of the Golgi complexes are several membrane-limited dense bodies 0.2 to 0.5 μm in diameter. These peribiliary dense bodies contain

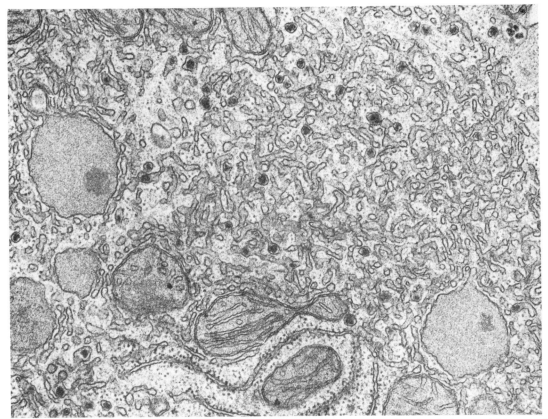

Figure 27–23. Electron micrograph of hepatocyte cytoplasm showing smooth-surfaced reticulum containing small, spherical dense particles representing newly synthesized, very-low-density serum lipoprotein. Also present are two microbodies or peroxisomes with eccentrically placed nucleoids. (Micrograph by R. Bolender.)

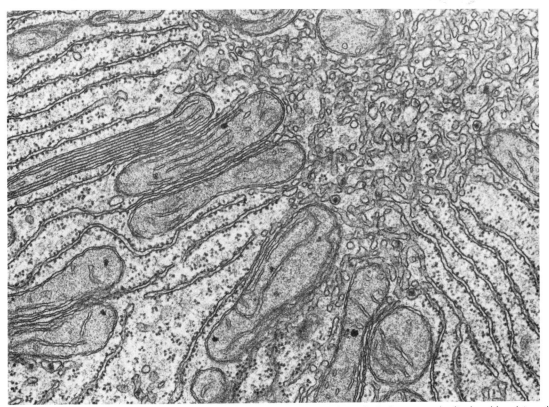

Figure 27–24. Electron micrograph of a small area of hepatocyte cytoplasm including several mitochondria, cisternal profiles of granular endoplasmic reticulum, and *(at upper right)* a close-meshed plexus of agranular reticulum. (Micrograph by R. Bolender.)

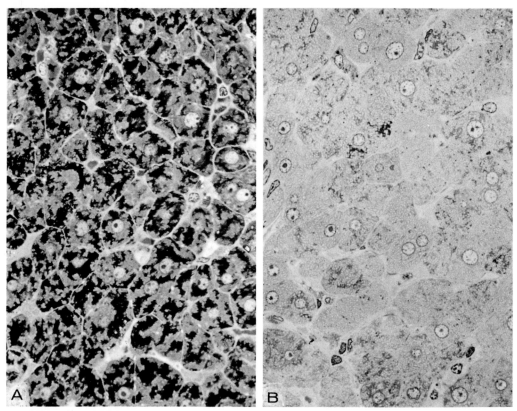

Figure 27–25. Dietary differences in amount of stored glycogen are clearly illustrated by comparison of these photomicrographs of rat liver. *A,* Liver of an animal fasted for 2 hours, containing 8.2 per cent glycogen. *B,* Liver of an animal fasted for 21 hours, containing 0.9 per cent glycogen. (From Cardell, R., J. Larner, and M. B. Babcock: Anat. Rec., *177*:23, 1973.)

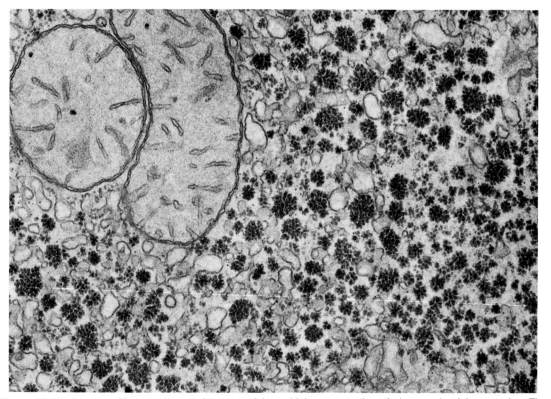

Figure 27–26. An area of hepatocyte cytoplasm containing a high concentration of glycogen in alpha granules. The glycogen is always closely associated with profiles of smooth endoplasmic reticulum.

histochemically demonstrable acid hydrolases and therefore correspond to the lysosomes isolated from homogenates of liver.

Scattered throughout the cytoplasm of the hepatocyte are *peroxisomes* (Figs. 27–28, 27–29). These are spherical bodies 0.2 to 0.8 μm in diameter enclosed by a membrane. In the laboratory rodents they contain a crystalline *nucleoid* eccentrically placed in a moderately dense, finely granular matrix. The nucleoids have been isolated and found to contain *uricase*. This component is lacking in peroxisomes of the human. The positive staining of peroxisomes with the histochemical reaction for peroxidase is attributed to the enzyme *catalase,* which is present in the matrix. Peroxisomes are respiratory organelles that contain hydrogen peroxide generating oxidases and catalase. They are involved in plasmalogen synthesis and oxidation of very-long-chain fatty acids, but their significance in liver cell metabolism is still poorly understood.

Zonation Within the Liver Lobule

In organs with multiple functions, it is often possible to demonstrate cytological differences between cells performing different functions. In the liver, despite its diverse activities, the cells are all very similar in appearance. All the parenchymal cells are probably capable of carrying out all the functions of the liver. However, cytologists have long believed that the degree of their activity under normal conditions depends primarily on their location within the lobule. The classical lobule can be divided into concentric zones on the basis of the cytological evidences of activity of the cells. A zone of varying width around the periphery of the lobule has been designated the "zone of permanent function." Next there is an intermediate "zone of varying activity" and finally a narrow zone around the central vein that is called the "zone of permanent repose." These zones correspond respectively to the portions of the lobule where the liver cells are most favorably situated, are intermediate, and are least favorably situated with respect to the sequence in which oxygen and nutrients reach them in the blood entering the sinusoids from the terminal branches of the hepatic artery and portal vein at the periphery of the lobule (at the center of the functional unit of Rappaport). This zonation is quite striking in some species but less obvious in others.

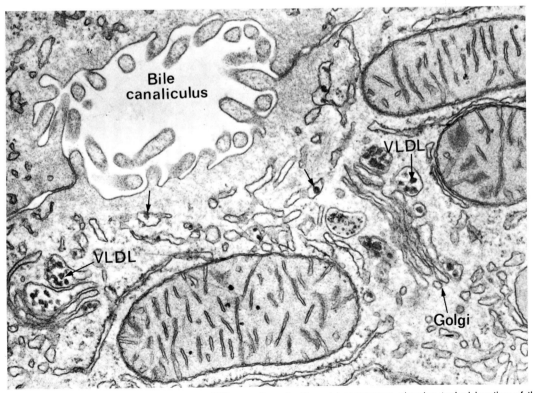

Figure 27–27. Electron micrograph of the peribiliary region of adjacent hepatocytes, showing typical location of the Golgi complex. Low-density lipoprotein (VLDL) is seen in distended cisternae of the Golgi and in the lumen of the smooth endoplasmic reticulum *(at arrows).* (Micrograph courtesy of R. Bolender.)

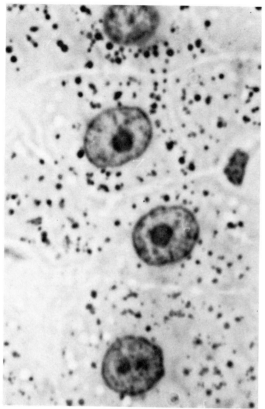

Figure 27–28. Photomicrograph of rat liver stained by a histochemical reaction for demonstration of peroxidase activity. The distribution of reactive granules corresponds to that of the microbodies or peroxisomes identifiable in electron micrographs. (Micrograph from Fahimi, D. J. Cell Biol. *43*:275, 1969.)

Typically, after the feeding of a large meal, glycogen is deposited first in the zone of permanent function at the periphery of the lobule. During active digestion, glycogen fills cells progressively farther into the intermediate zone until, in extreme cases, all but the cells immediately adjacent to the central vein may be filled with it. With the conclusion of digestion, carbohydrate is returned to the blood, as needed, by removal of the glycogen, beginning at the most centrally located deposits. If the fast is prolonged, glycogen may ultimately disappear completely at the periphery. Thus, in an animal such as the mouse, which normally feeds at night, there is a diurnal tide of glycogen within the lobule, which may be spectacularly accentuated by restricting the feeding time to one hour, with the animal fasting the rest of the day.

Accompanying this tide is a corresponding change in the mitochondria. Those in the central zone are thin, elongated, and sparse,

staining so lightly that they are frequently seen only with difficulty in mitochondrial preparations. In the peripheral zone, however, they are large, deeply staining spheres or short rods that may crowd the cytoplasm. In the intermediate zone, the rods become progressively elongated until, as one approaches the central zone, they are slender filaments. The width of the intermediate zone varies with the state of the diurnal tide of alimentation. In other species, including man, such changes are not demonstrable.

Under certain conditions, both pathological and physiological, fat may accumulate in the liver. Usually it appears first in the cells of the central zone as small spherical droplets; these become progressively larger by coalescence as well as by further accumulation, until the cell may be distended by a single large drop. In certain conditions, notably some sustained dietary deficiencies, fat is deposited in the peripheral rather than in the central zone. In both cases, fat disappears when the condition responsible is corrected.

Position in the lobule may not be the only determining factor in the relative activity of liver cells. Application of the fluorescent antibody technique to localize the sites of production of plasma albumin has shown marked differences among liver cells immediately adjacent to one another, and the distribution of synthetically active cells in this case appears to bear little relation to the zonation within the lobule.

Bile Canaliculi

Minute canals run between liver cells throughout the parenchyma. As a rule, a single canaliculus is found between each adjacent pair of cells. Thus, in a plate of liver cells one cell thick, these *bile canaliculi* form a network having hexagonal meshes with a single cell in each mesh. Because the laminae of parenchymal cells branch and anastomose, the canaliculi form an extensive three-dimensional net with polyhedral meshes (Fig. 27–30). In amphibians, there are small branches that extend between cells from a core canaliculus and end blindly. It is now generally agreed that there are no such blind branches in the mammalian liver. Instead the canaliculi form a continuous network without interruption from lobule to lobule throughout the parenchyma. The membrane lining the canaliculi is a site of adenosine triphosphatase activity, and histochemical reactions for this

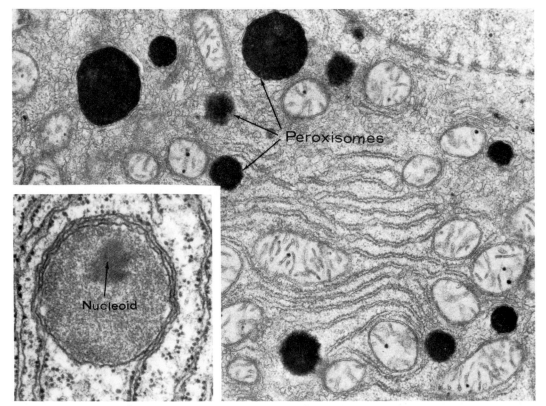

Figure 27–29. Microbodies or peroxisomes of rodent liver are limited by a single membrane and contain a "nucleoid" consisting of a paracrystalline array of tubular subunits. (Micrograph by R. Wood.) When stained for peroxidase activity, the matrix of the microbodies reacts intensely but the nucleoid remains unstained. (From Fahimi, D. J. Cell Biol. *43*:275, 1969.)

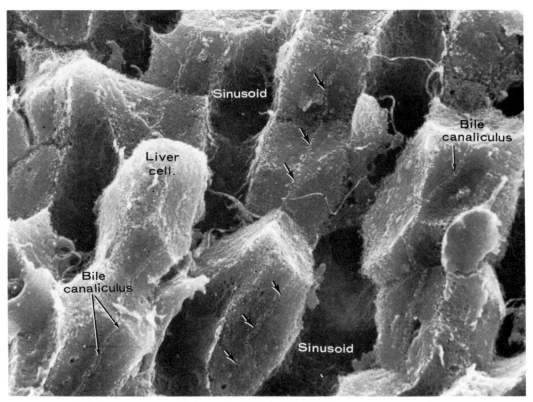

Figure 27–30. Scanning electron micrograph of rat liver fixed by perfusion and then broken open to reveal its internal architecture. The micrograph affords a three-dimensional view of the plates of polygonal hepatic cells alternating with sinusoids. Where the liver plates have been broken, the bile canaliculi can be identified on the contact surfaces of the hepatic cells *(at arrows)*. (Micrograph courtesy of M. Karnovsky.)

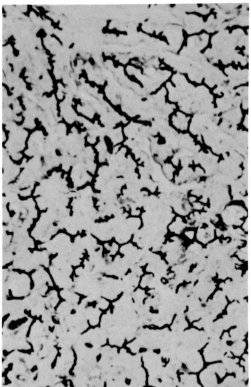

Figure 27–31. Photomicrograph of rat liver, showing the branching pattern of bile canaliculi, which are demonstrated here by their positive histochemical staining reaction for adenosine triphosphatase. × 200. (Courtesy of A. Novikoff.)

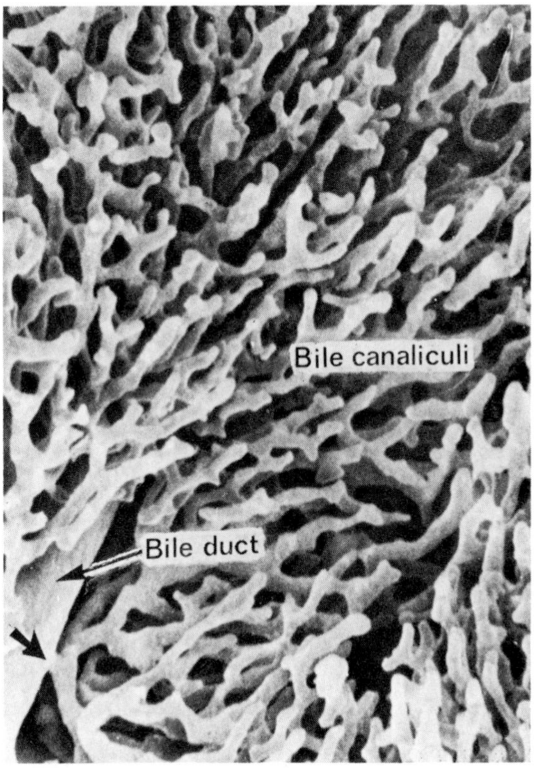

Figure 27–32. Scanning micrograph of a cast of a branch of the biliary tree, showing the arborizing pattern of bile canaliculi. At the arrow is a canal of Herring communicating with the duct of a portal triad. (Micrograph from Murikami, T. Dig. Dis. Sci. 25:609, 1980.)

enzyme provide a useful method for selectively staining this system of minute intercellular canals (Figs. 27–31, 27–32).

From observations with the light microscope, it seemed reasonable to assume that the bile canaliculi were distinct entities having walls of their own. Indeed, it was suggested that their hexagonal network around the hepatic cells contributed significantly to the structural stability of the liver. This erroneous interpretation was abandoned when the electron microscope revealed that the lumen of the bile canaliculus is merely an expansion of the intercellular space and that its wall is simply a local specialization of the surfaces of adjoining hepatic cells (Fig. 27–27). Over most of their length, the apposed membranes of the two cells are relatively straight and separated by an intercellular cleft about 15 nm wide. At the site of the bile canaliculus they diverge to form a canalicular intercellular space 0.5 to 1 μm in diameter. The portion of the cell membrane bordering on this space bears short microvilli that project into its lumen. Along the margins of the canaliculus the membranes of the opposing cells come into close contact and form an occluding junction comparable with the zonula occludens of other epithelia. These two bands of tight junction evidently seal the commissures of the canaliculus and prevent its contents from escaping into the intercellular cleft on either side. A narrow zone of cytoplasm immediately adjacent to the canaliculus is free of organelles and has the finely fibrillar structure characteristic of a gelated ectoplasmic layer.

In addition to the zonulae occludentes adjacent to the canaliculus, a number of gap junctions are found on the boundaries between adjoining hepatic cells. These sites of low electrical resistance permit communication between cells and provide for coordination of their physiological activities. These junctional specializations are visible in electron micrographs of thin sections, but they are studied to best advantage in freeze-fracture preparations (Fig. 27–33).

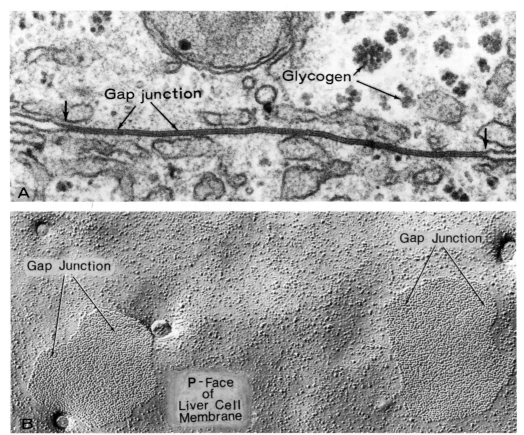

Figure 27–33. *A,* Electron micrograph of a portion of the boundary between two liver cells in thin section, showing the cell membranes converging at the arrows and coming into close apposition to form a nexus or gap junction between the arrows. (Micrograph courtesy of R. Wood.) *B,* Surface replica of an area of liver cell membrane freeze-fractured to expose its P-face. In addition to the population of randomly distributed intramembranous particles, there are two gap junctions exhibiting closely packed particles of uniform diameter. (Micrograph courtesy of A. Yee.)

The bile canaliculi vary in diameter, becoming somewhat distended with active secretion and more or less collapsed with decreasing activity. When distended, the microvilli are more widely scattered and appear to be shorter, and when the canaliculi are collapsed, the microvilli may pack the lumen so completely that it is virtually occluded. This may explain why the canaliculi are hard to see with the light microscope.

The junction of the bile canaliculus with the bile duct system is not easily demonstrated. The fine terminal branches of the bile duct leave the portal canal with the terminal branch of the portal vein and penetrate the parenchyma between two lobules (i.e., in the core of a functional unit of Rappaport.) They are so small and have such thin walls that they are recognized only with difficulty. These channels are quite different in appearance from the smallest bile ducts and are called bile ductules or *cholangioles.*

They have small diverticula that expand against the adjacent parenchyma and are applied tightly to it. The bile capillaries continue between the hepatic cells to empty into the lumen of the diverticula. The structure of this transitional region of the duct system is well demonstrated if the cholangioles and bile canaliculi are distended, as they are following occlusion of the bile duct.

Connective Tissue Stroma

For an organ of its size, the liver has remarkably little stroma. A small amount of dense connective tissue forms a thin layer *(Glisson's capsule)* underlying the organ's investment of peritoneal mesothelium. It extends into the organ in the portal canals and follows them to their finest terminals ensheathing the branches of the portal vein, hepatic artery, and bile duct. It also contains the network of lymphatics that drains lymph from the liver. In these sites it is typical connective tissue with dense collagenous fibers and occasional fibroblasts. Within the lobule, the only stromal structure is a network of reticular fibers between the sinusoid lining and the hepatic cell plates (Fig. 27–19). This can be demonstrated by various techniques, but especially well by some of the silver impregnation methods. At the periphery of the lobule, where terminal branches of the portal veins enter the sinusoids, the collagenous fibers of the portal canals are continuous with the network of reticular fibers surrounding the sinusoids. This reticulum is the only supporting tissue of the liver parenchyma. It contains no associated fibroblasts, the fibers apparently being formed by the sinusoid lining cells.

Lymph Spaces

The liver produces a large amount of lymph. From one quarter to one half of the total volume of the thoracic duct lymph comes from the liver, less from the intestine via the mesenteric lymphatics, and still less from the other organs of the posterior part of the body. The hepatic lymph differs from the rest of the lymph in that it contains a large amount of plasma protein, with the ratio of albumin to globulin a little higher than in the plasma. The network of lymphatics follows the portal vein to its finest terminal branches. Here it ends in the connective tissue of the portal canals. No lymphatics have been demonstrated within the liver lobules. It is believed that plasma traversing the discontinuities in the sinusoid lining and entering the space of Disse moves along toward the periphery of the lobule, bathing the microvilli of the hepatic cells as it goes. It then percolates into the extracellular spaces around the interlobular twigs of the bile duct and the portal vein. It thus becomes the tissue fluid of portal canals, and the liver lymph is drained by the lymphatic capillaries that accompany ducts and blood vessels.

REGENERATION

The liver parenchyma, compared with that of many other organs, is a fairly stable population of cells that rarely need to be replaced in a normal adult. It is, however, capable of spectacular regeneration. In the rat, two

thirds of the liver can be removed and in a few days most of this tissue will be replaced. Similarly, after administration of hepatotoxic agents, notably the chlorinated hydrocarbons, a substantial part of each lobule may be destroyed, and in this case too the lost tissue is rapidly replaced.

Regeneration after partial hepatectomy results from cell division occurring throughout the remaining liver mass. Therefore, the original pattern of liver lobes is not restored. Most of the research on regeneration has been done on the rat and the mouse, in which the amount restored is usually as great as the amount removed. In other animals, the amount regenerated may be considerably less, in inverse ratio to the size of the animal.

Central necrosis after a toxic dose of carbon tetrachloride may involve as much as one third to one half of each lobule and is remarkably uniform throughout the liver. Only the parenchymal cells are killed, leaving the sinusoid linings intact, so that the circulation through the lobule is maintained. The necrotic cells are removed by autolysis, while the cells in the remaining part of the lobule divide rapidly by mitosis. The mass of normal liver tissue increases until in five or six days the original lobular architecture of the liver is completely restored. If the dose of carbon tetrachloride is repeated at regular intervals when regeneration is still in progress, thus repeatedly producing new injury before the old has been repaired, fibrosis occurs, and if it is continued long enough, *cirrhosis of the liver* ensues.

If the cellular injury is at the periphery of the lobule, as it is after bile duct occlusion or after treatment with other hepatotoxic agents, cell division occurs throughout the remaining tissue, but there is also considerable mitotic activity in the epithelium of the bile ductules and smaller bile ducts, with a corresponding increase in their number. The ductules penetrate into the injured peripheral part of the lobule, to reestablish the pathway for bile drainage interrupted by the death of the peripheral cells and dissolution of their bile canaliculi. If the injury continues, the increase in ductules and ducts may develop into a spectacular proliferation of the bile ducts. If it does not continue, the normal architecture of the liver is rapidly restored, with removal of the excess of the new ducts and ductules. It is not clear whether the duct cells atrophy and disappear or transform into parenchymal cells. In repair after severe injury, the occurrence of cells of intermediate cytological appearance gives credence to the latter possibility.

The mechanism of initiation of mitosis in a normally quiescent tissue and of its cessation when the lost tissue has been replaced has been extensively investigated. Partial hepatectomy with the ensuing regeneration has been a favored system in which to study this and a variety of related problems.

HISTOPHYSIOLOGY OF THE LIVER

The liver is a highly vascular organ receiving about 100 ml of blood from the portal vein and 400 ml from the hepatic artery each minute. In flowing through the sinusoids the blood is exposed to about 1.2×10^7 phagocytic Kupffer cells per gram of liver. These remove cellular debris and foreign particulate matter. The liver therefore has an important *blood-filtering* function.

The hepatic sinusoids normally present a very low resistance to blood flow. However, in heart failure pressure may increase in the veins draining the liver and the sinusoids may then become distended with as much as 400 ml more blood than they normally contain. Under these conditions the liver enlarges markedly. Conversely, after blood loss from hemorrhage a substantial volume of blood may be contributed by the liver to the general circulation to offset the blood loss. The liver thus serves as an important site of *blood storage*.

In the disease *cirrhosis*, fibrosis greatly increases the resistance to blood flow through the liver. Back pressure in the portal system results in *ascites*—transudation and accumulation of protein-rich fluid in the peritoneal cavity.

Because of the remarkable range of its biochemical functions in intermediary metabolism and its strategic location in the circulation, the liver is a vital organ for processing nutrients absorbed from the gastrointestinal tract and for transforming them into materials needed by the other specialized tissues of the body. One of its most important functions is maintenance of the normal blood glucose concentration. Liver cells take up glucose from the blood and by means of a series of enzymatic reactions polymerize it to form glycogen, the storage form of carbohydrate. Simpler compounds, such as lactic acid, glycerol, and pyruvic acid, can be converted in the liver into glucose and then to glycogen. As the need arises, glycogen is broken down to glucose again in a process catalyzed by the enzyme phosphorylase. This enzyme usually occurs in an inactive form but is specifically activated by the hormones epinephrine and glucagon, which act upon the liver and cause it to release glucose into the blood.

Many of the enzymes involved in glycogenesis and glycogenolysis are free in the cytoplasmic matrix. These functions, therefore, cannot be attributed to any particular cell organelle. However, in electron micrographs, the glycogen is usually localized in areas of cytoplasm rich in smooth endoplasmic reticulum. The exact significance of this close topographical relationship is not yet clear, but the enzyme glucose-6-phosphatase, which is known to reside in these membranes, may participate in some way in the release of glucose to the blood.

The liver also plays a major role in the metabolism and transport of lipids and in the maintenance of normal lipid levels in the circulating blood. The lipids in the blood plasma are derived from ingested food, from mobilization of fat reserves in adipose tissue, or from synthesis from carbohydrate or protein in the liver. The main vehicle for the transport of lipids is the *plasma lipoprotein,* and it is in the liver that the transformation of lipids into serum lipoprotein takes place. Small spherical particles 30 to 100 nm in diameter are seen in electron micrographs of liver in agranular terminal expansions of the granular reticulum, in tubular elements of the smooth reticulum, in exocytotic vesicles at the cell surface, and in the space of Disse. These particles contain a triglyceride lipid core surrounded by a more water-soluble, polar surface coat of protein, phospholipid, and cholesterol. In the isolated perfused liver, the number of these particles is strikingly increased when fatty acids are added to the perfusate. They represent *very-low-density lipoproteins* (VLDL) being formed in the liver and released into the space of Disse. Triglycerides are formed in the smooth reticulum from fatty acids, and these are combined there with protein synthesized in the granular reticulum to form lipoprotein particles (Figs. 27–23, 27–34). There is also good evidence that the reticulum, particularly the smooth form, plays an important part in the synthesis of cholesterol in the liver. An experimentally induced increase in the abun-

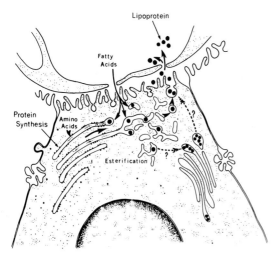

Figure 27–34. Diagram illustrating intracellular pathway of synthesis and release of very-low-density serum lipoprotein (VLDL). Fatty acids from the blood are esterified in the smooth reticulum to form triglycerides. These are combined with protein synthesized on ribosomes associated with the rough reticulum. The particles are released into the space of Disse and enter the blood in the sinusoids.

dance of smooth reticulum is accompanied by an enhanced capacity to synthesize cholesterol from acetate.

The liver is the site of synthesis of plasma proteins, and the rate of their production is quite substantial. Studies on the isolated perfused organ indicate that the liver of an adult rat synthesizes in excess of 13 mg of albumin per day. It is likely that the organelle principally involved is the granular endoplasmic reticulum. A fine flocculent substance is sometimes observed in the lumen of the cisternae, and protein with the properties of albumin has been identified in liver microsomes, but the entire secretory pathway of plasma proteins has not been worked out.

The liver also synthesizes many of the substances involved in blood clotting—fibrinogen, prothrombin, Factor III, and several others. The concentrations of these substances in the blood can be used clinically as a measure of liver cell function. Liver disease may result in impaired synthesis of clotting factors and a tendency to bleed excessively from minor injuries.

In addition to its many functions in nutritional metabolism and bile secretion, the liver takes up and either catabolizes or secretes some 20 proteins and glycoproteins that circulate in the blood. These include immunoglobulins, albumin, transferrin, insulin, α_2-macroglobulin, and epidermal growth factor.

The hepatocytes have specific membrane receptors for several of these proteins that are taken up by receptor-mediated endocytosis, moved through the cytoplasm by a vesicular transport system, and secreted into the bile canaliculi. Other plasma proteins, for which there are no plasmalemmal receptors, are taken up by nonselective fluid-phase endocytosis and are similarly transported. Using radioactively labeled compounds, the transcellular movements of the transport vesicles can be traced autoradiographically. *Direct* and *indirect pathways* are described (Fig. 27–35). In the former, the endocytic vesicles form at the sinusoidal surface, traverse the cell, and fuse with the membrane of the bile canaliculus, discharging their ligands intact. In the indirect pathway, the vesicles fuse en route with small primary lysosomes that modify or degrade the vesicle contents. The catabolic products are then released into the bile.

This function of the hepatocytes is of special interest in relation to the secretory immune system of the intestine. As stated in the foregoing chapter, immunoglobulin A synthesized by plasma cells in the lamina propria of the gut is complexed with a secretory component in the intestinal epithelium and is released into the lumen to serve in the immunological defense of the gut. However, only a small fraction of the antibody produced in the lamina propria takes this direct route to the lumen. The remainder is carried in the lymph to the thoracic duct and thence into the general circulation. Much of the IgA in the plasma is destined to reach the intestinal lumen via the hepatobiliary pathway described above. Immunoglobulin A is present in the bile at five times its concentration in the plasma. If the bile duct is surgically occluded in animal experiments, the level of secretory IgA in the blood plasma rises markedly while its level in the gut falls to one tenth its normal concentration. Thus, biliary IgA makes a very major contribution to the supply of antibodies in the intestinal lumen. The secretory component synthesized in the hepatocytes is inserted as a transmembrane protein in the plasmalemma at the sinusoidal surface of the cell, and its exposed portion serves as the receptor for plasma IgA that is taken up by endocytosis and transported to the bile.

The liver is responsible for the metabolism of a large variety of lipid-soluble drugs, including the barbiturates commonly used as sedatives. The enzymes responsible for the

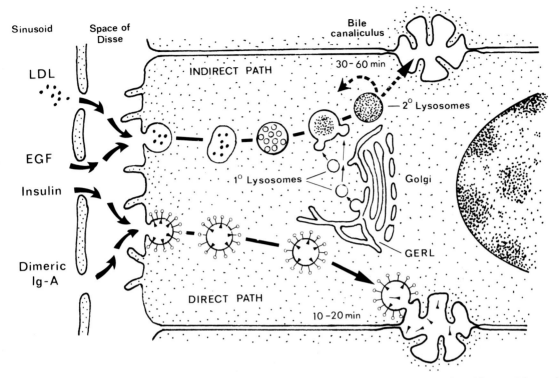

Figure 27–35. Schematic representation of the uptake, intracellular transport, and biliary secretion of four proteins and glycoproteins of the plasma. Low-density lipoproteins (LDL) and epidermal growth factor (EGF) are taken up mainly by fluid-phase endocytosis and are modified in transit by lysosomes. Insulin and immunoglobulin A take the direct path. Taken up in vesicles by receptor-mediated endocytosis, they are released into the bile canaliculi unchanged. (Redrawn and modified after Jones, A. L. K., R. H. Reston, and S. V. Burwen. *In* Popper, H., and F. Schaffner, eds.: Progress in Liver Disease. Vol. 7. New York, Grune & Stratton, 1982.)

degradation of these compounds are localized mainly in the smooth-surfaced microsome fraction of liver homogenates and hence reside in the smooth reticulum of the intact liver cell. Moreover, administration of such drugs induces a marked increase in the smooth-surfaced membranes of the cytoplasm and this morphological change is accompanied by a concomitant increase in the drug-metabolizing enzymes. These changes do not represent toxic effects of the drug but rather an adaptive response of the liver cell, which enhances its efficiency in eliminating the inducing drug. These morphological and biochemical changes thus appear to be the basis of *drug tolerance*—the progressive loss of effectiveness of a drug with continued use. Certain of the steps in the metabolism of steroid hormones in the liver also take place in the endoplasmic reticulum and probably depend on some of the same hydroxylating enzymes that are involved in the metabolism of exogenous drugs.

An important excretory function of the liver is the uptake and excretion of the pigment *bilirubin*, which originates from the breakdown of aged red blood cells being eliminated from the circulation by Kupffer cells and phagocytes of the spleen. This substance, carried in the blood, is conjugated with glucuronide in the liver by enzymes in the endoplasmic reticulum. The conjugate, bilirubin glucuronide, is excreted into the bile. In the intestine, it is reduced by the action of bacteria into a group of compounds collectively referred to as *urobilinogens*. While most of these are eliminated in the feces, some are reabsorbed and reexcreted in the bile. When bilirubin accumulates in the blood (hyperbilirubinemia), a person becomes jaundiced. This may result from (1) increased production of bilirubin beyond the capacity of the liver to excrete it—e.g., in hemolytic jaundice; (2) decreased uptake of bilirubin by the liver; (3) disturbance in conjugation of bilirubin in the liver—e.g., in jaundice of the newborn; (4) interference with excretion due to obstruction of the bile duct system. Determination of the relative amounts of conjugated and unconjugated bilirubin in the blood is therefore an important means of evaluating liver function and of distinguishing among the several causes of jaundice in patients.

A major function of hepatic cells is the secretion of *bile*—a complex fluid consisting of cholesterol, lecithin, fatty acids, electrolytes, and bile salts. Bile salts, the most important component, are synthesized from cholesterol by conversion to cholic and chemodeoxycholic acids, which then combine with glycine or taurine to form the corresponding conjugated acids. Their salts are secreted in the bile in the amount of about 0.5 g/day. The cell organelles involved in the biosynthetic pathway of bile acids are still poorly understood. The bile salts have a detergent or emulsifying action on ingested fat. They form micelles with fatty acids and monoglycerides, facilitating their absorption by the intestinal epithelium. In the absence of bile secretion, much of the fat in the diet is not absorbed and passes out in the feces.

BILE DUCTS

The constituents of the bile are emptied into the bile canaliculi, which communicate with the interlobular bile ducts by the canals of Hering. The finest radicles of the bile ducts are 15 to 20 μm in diameter and have a small lumen surrounded by cuboidal epithelial cells. They do not have a striated border. The cells show occasional mitoses.

The interlobular bile ducts form a richly anastomosing network that closely surrounds the branches of the portal vein. Closer to the porta, the lumen of the ducts of the second order gradually becomes larger, while the epithelium becomes taller and has an accumulation of mitochondria at the base and another near the free border. These cells commonly contain fat droplets. Lymphocytes are frequently seen migrating through the epithelium into the lumen. As the ducts become larger, the surrounding layer of collagenous connective tissue becomes thicker and contains many elastic fibers. At the transverse fossa of the liver, the main ducts from the different lobes of the liver fuse to form the *hepatic duct*, which, after receiving the *cystic duct*, continues from the gallbladder to the duodenum as the *common bile duct (ductus choledochus)*. The epithelium of the extrahepatic ducts is tall columnar. The mucosa is thrown into many folds and is said to secrete an atypical variety of mucus. The scanty subepithelial connective tissue contains large numbers of elastic fibers and some lymphoid cells. Many of these migrate through the epithelium and pass into the lumen. Scattered bundles of smooth muscles first appear in the common bile duct. They run in the longitudinal and oblique directions, and form an incomplete layer around the wall of the duct. As it nears the duodenum, the smooth muscle layer of the ductus choledochus becomes more prominent, and at the duodenum its intramural portion functions as a sort of sphincter, regulating the flow of bile.

THE GALLBLADDER

The gallbladder is a pear-shaped, hollow viscus occupying a shallow fossa on the inferior surface of the liver. It consists of a fundus, a body, and a neck that continues into the cystic duct. Normally it measures approximately 10 by 4 cm in the human, and has a capacity of 40 to 70 ml. It shows marked variations in shape and size and is frequently the seat of pathological processes that change its size and the thickness of its wall. The function of the gallbladder is to store, concentrate, and release into the duodenum the 600 to 1000 ml of bile secreted each day by the liver.

The gallbladder is covered over all but its hepatic surface by a serosa continuous with that of the liver. Its wall consists of a subserosal connective tissue layer overlying a layer of smooth muscle. Deep to this is the mucosa composed of the epithelium and its highly vascular lamina propria. The mucosa is plicated into numerous convoluted folds of varying height that demarcate narrow bays or clefts. In sections of the contracted gallbladder these mucosal folds are tall and close together. When the organ is distended they are short and some distance apart. The changes in topography occurring in different states of filling and contraction are most dramatically illustrated in surface views of the mucosa with the scanning electron microscope. In the contracted gallbladder each highly sinuous fold follows a course generally parallel to that of neighboring folds (Fig. 27–36). In the distended condition the folds are reduced to low ridges and it is apparent that they branch and anastomose to form a net-

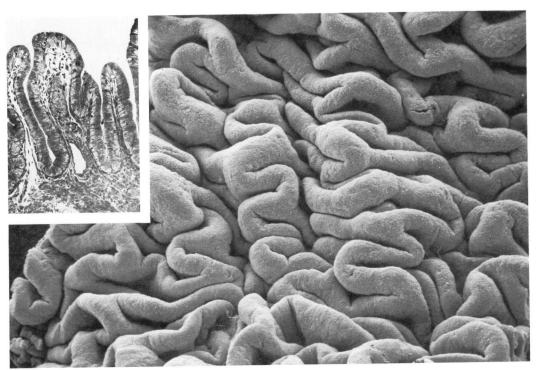

Figure 27–36. Scanning micrograph of the contracted gallbladder. The mucosa is thrown up into highly convoluted folds. A histological section through these has the appearance shown in the inset. Compare with Figure 27–37. (Micrographs from Castellucci, M. J. Submicrosc. Cytol. *12*:375, 1980.)

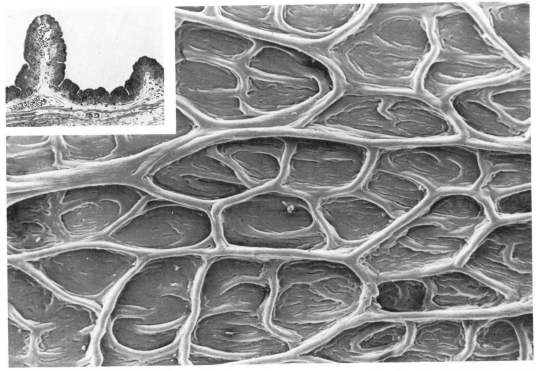

Figure 27–37. Scanning micrograph of the mucosal surface of a normally distended gallbladder. Relatively low mucosal folds have the pattern of a network with polygonal meshes. A histological section of the gallbladder in this state has the appearance shown in the inset. Compare with Figure 27–36. (Micrographs from Castellucci, M. J. Submicrosc. Cytol. *12*:375, 1980.)

work outlining shallow polygonal recesses (Fig. 27–37). The loose organization of elastic and reticular fibers of the lamina propria provides the flexibility to accommodate these marked changes in mucosal topography.

The epithelium consists of a single layer of tall columnar cells, with oval nuclei (Fig. 27–38). The cytoplasm stains faintly with eosin. An inconspicuous striated border is seen in histological sections, and with the electron microscope the apical surface of the columnar cells is found to have numerous microvilli (Fig. 27–39). These are somewhat shorter and less regular in their orientation than are those of the striated border of the intestinal epithelium. At the tips of the microvilli the membrane bears minute filiform appendages similar to those making up the glycocalyx on intestinal mucosa and on various other epithelia.

The lateral cell boundaries are relatively straight at the apical portion of the epithelium, but from the level of the nucleus to the basal lamina there is a complex plication and interdigitation of the cell surface. The intercellular space in the upper portion of the epithelium is 15 to 20 nm wide and is sealed near the lumen by a typical zonula occludens. Toward the base, the intercellular space may be narrow or greatly widened. The width of the intercellular clefts at the base depends on the functional state of the gallbladder epithelium (see below).

In the lamina propria and in the perimuscular layer near the neck of the gallbladder there are simple tubuloalveolar glands. Their epithelium is cuboidal and clear, and the dark nuclei are compressed at the base of the cell. They thus stand out sharply against the darker, tall columnar epithelium of the gallbladder. These glands are said to secrete mucus.

Outpocketings of the mucosa in this region have sometimes been confused with glands. These are lined by and are continuous with the surface epithelium and extend through the lamina propria and the muscular layer. They are called *Rokitansky-Aschoff sinuses* and probably are indicators of a pathological change in the wall of the organ that permits an evagination of the mucosa through enlarged meshes of the submucosal network of

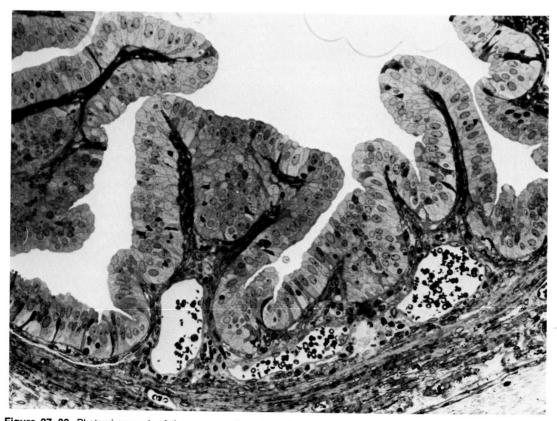

Figure 27–38. Photomicrograph of the mucosa of contracted rabbit gallbladder. (Micrograph from Castellucci, M. J. Submicrosc. Cytol. *12*:375, 1980.)

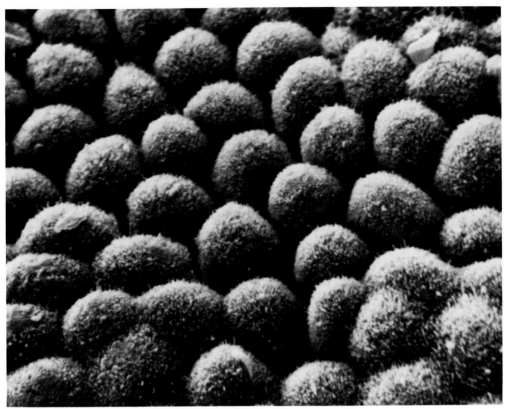

Figure 27–39. Scanning electron micrograph of the luminal surface of gallbladder epithelium. The convex apical ends of the cells are covered with short microvilli. (Micrograph from Mueller, J. C., A. L. Jones, and J. A. Long. Gastroenterology *63*:856, 1972. © 1972 The Williams & Wilkins Co., Baltimore.)

smooth muscle. They are not found in the fetal gallbladder and apparently are acquired in adult life.

The smooth muscle beneath the epithelium is an irregular network of longitudinal, transverse, and oblique fibers, with an associated network of elastic fibers. The spaces between the bundles of muscle fibers are occupied by collagenous, reticular, and elastic fibers, and occasional fibroblasts.

A fairly dense connective tissue layer external to the muscularis completely surrounds the gallbladder and is in places continuous with the interlobular connective tissue of the liver. It contains many collagenous and a few elastic fibers, scattered fibroblasts, macrophages and lymphoid cells, and small lobules of fat cells. The blood vessels, nerves, and lymphatics supplying the organ run in this layer and send branches into and through the muscular layer to the mucosa.

Not infrequently, particularly on the hepatic surface of the gallbladder and near its neck, peculiar ductlike structures may be seen. They can be traced for considerable distances in this connective tissue layer, and

some of them connect with the bile ducts. They never connect with the lumen of the gallbladder and are probably aberrant bile ducts laid down during the embryonic development of the biliary system. They have been called *Luschka ducts*, to distinguish them from the epithelial outpouchings described above.

The *cystic duct* continues from the neck of the gallbladder for a distance of 3 to 4 cm and joins the hepatic duct to form the *common bile duct (ductus choledochus)*. Coursing downward behind the head of the pancreas, it approaches the *pancreatic duct (ductus pancreaticus)*. The two pass together through an opening in the muscularis of the descending portion of the duodenum. In their oblique course through the submucosa, the two ducts unite to form the *hepatopancreatic ampulla (ampulla of Vater)*, which opens into the duodenal lumen at the tip of a small papilla. In the wall of the duodenum, the bile and pancreatic ducts and ampulla are encircled by a common annular band of smooth muscle called the *sphincter of Oddi*. This muscle complex is described as consisting of four parts: (1) a strong band of circular smooth muscle, the *sphincter choledochus*, around the terminal portion of the bile duct; (2) a corresponding *sphincter pancreaticus* around the pancreatic duct; (3) longitudinal bundles of muscle fibers, the *fasciculus longitudinalis*, which span the space between the ducts; and (4) a meshwork of muscle fibers around the ampulla, the *sphincter ampullae.*

The degree of development of these components of the sphincter of Oddi is subject to great individual variation. Normally, contraction of the sphincter choledochus stops the flow of bile. The longitudinal fasciculi shorten the intramural portion of the ducts and probably facilitate flow of bile into the duodenum. When the sphincter ampullae is well developed, its contraction may have the undesirable effect of causing reflux of bile into the pancreatic duct, resulting in pancreatitis.

Blood Vessels, Lymphatics, and Nerves

The gallbladder is supplied with blood by the cystic artery. The venous blood is collected by veins that empty primarily into small veins of the liver and only secondarily into the cystic branch of the portal vein.

A prominent feature of the gallbladder is its rich supply of lymphatic vessels, of which there are two main plexuses, one in the lamina propria and the other in the connective tissue layer. The latter plexus receives tributaries from the liver, thus affording a pathway that accounts for hepatogenous cholecystitis. These plexuses are collected into larger lymphatics, which pass through the lymph node or nodes at the neck of the gallbladder and then accompany the cystic and common bile ducts. They pass through several lymph nodes near the duodenum and finally join the cisterna chyli. The nerves are branches of the splanchnic sympathetic and the vagus nerves. Study of the effects of stimulation of these nerves has given rise to contradictory reports by different investigators. It is probable that both excitatory and inhibitory fibers are contained in each of them. Of greater clinical importance are the sensory nerve endings, because overdistention or spasms of the extrahepatic biliary tract may inhibit respiration and set up reflex disturbances in the gut.

Histophysiology of the Gallbladder

The gallbladder serves as a site of concentration and storage of bile, which is secreted continuously by the liver. The bile does not normally enter the intestine until a specific stimulus causes the gallbladder to contract. The stimulus is usually the presence of lipid in the small intestine. Ingestion of fat automatically causes discharge of the contents of the gallbladder. After a test meal of egg yolks or cream, three fourths of its content are expelled within 40 minutes.

When fat enters the small intestine, it causes release of a hormone, *cholecystokinin,* from the mucosa. This is carried via the blood to the gallbladder, inducing rhythmic contractions. In the peristalsis of the duodenum, as waves of relaxation of its smooth muscle pass by the ampulla of Vater, the tonic contraction of the sphincter of Oddi relaxes, permitting intermittent outflow of bile. Thus, the emptying of the gallbladder results from the combined action of cholecystokinin on the musculature of the gallbladder and peristalsis in the duodenum.

Of special clinical importance is the concentrating function of the gallbladder. Its mucosa reabsorbs water and ions from the bile. Experimental studies suggest the mechanism. In gallbladders known to be trans-

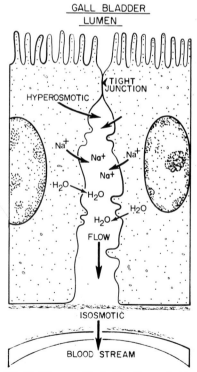

Figure 27–40. Diagram illustrating the probable mechanism of concentration of the bile. Sodium is actively pumped into the intercellular cleft below the occluding junction, creating a standing gradient that moves water from the lumen to the blood vessels in the wall of the gallbladder.

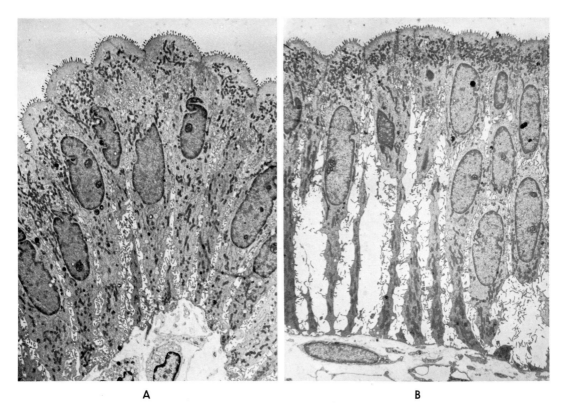

A   B

Figure 27–41. Photomicrograph of rabbit gallbladder epithelium. *A,* With a hyperosmotic solution in the lumen, the net water flux is very low and the intercellular spaces at the base of the epithelium are relatively inconspicuous. *B,* In a gallbladder actively transporting fluid in vitro, the intercellular spaces are greatly distended. × 1400. (From Kaye, G. J. Cell Biol. *30:*237, 1966.)

porting fluid, the intercellular spaces at the base of the epithelium are always distended and the subepithelial capillaries are dilated. In experiments carried out in vitro, if either sodium or calcium is omitted from the medium, there is no fluid transport and the intercellular spaces are narrow. If either ion is replaced, fluid transport is restored and the intercellular spaces again appear distended. It is believed that during concentration of bile, active transport of solute (Na^+) across the lateral cell membrane increases the concentration of solute in the intercellular space (Figs. 27–40, 27–41). Because of the resulting osmotic gradient, water moves into and through the cell to the intercellular space, causing its distention. Development of hydrostatic pressure in this space drives the solution across the basal lamina into the submucosa.

The functional capacity of the gallbladder is assessed clinically by observing its capacity to concentrate halogen salts of phenolphthalein, which are opaque to x-rays (Graham-Cole test). Failure to visualize the gallbladder after this test indicates that the organ is diseased. If the mucosa is damaged, it may lose its concentrating power. Undoubtedly,

absorption of bile salts under such conditions is an important factor in the precipitation of gallstones. After obstruction of the cystic duct the bile may be resorbed in toto or replaced by a colorless fluid consisting largely of exudate and mucus. A small amount of mucus is added to the bile as it passes down the larger bile ducts, and mucus-secreting glands are fairly numerous in the gallbladder neck. In some mammalian species, no gallbladder is present. Its surgical removal in man is often followed by a marked dilatation of the biliary passages.

REFERENCES

LIVER

Babcock, M. B., and R. R. Cardell: Hepatic glycogen patterns in fasted and fed rats. Am J. Anal. *140:*229, 1974.

Brauer, R. W.: Liver circulation and function. Physiol. Rev. *43:*115, 1963.

Brown, T. A., M. W. Russell, and J. Mestecky: Elimination of intestinally absorbed antigen into the bile by IgA. J. Immunol. *132:*780, 1984.

Bruni, C., and K. R. Porter: The fine structure of the parenchymal cell of the normal rat liver. I. General observations. Am. J. Pathol. *46:*691, 1965.

Bucher, N. L. R.: Experimental aspects of hepatic cell regeneration. N. Engl. J. Med. *277*:686, 1967.

Burkel, W. E.: The fine structure of the terminal branches of the hepatic arterial system of the rat. Anat. Rec. *167*:329, 1970.

Cardell, R. R., Jr., J. Larner, and M. B. Babcock: Correlation between structure and glycogen content of livers from rats on a controlled feeding schedule. Anat. Rec. *177*:23, 1973.

Crofton, R. W., M. M. Diesselhoff-den Dulk, and R. van Furth: The origin, kinetics, and characteristics of Kupffer cells in the normal steady state. J. Exp. Med. *148*:1, 1978.

Daems, W. Th.: The micro-anatomy of the smallest biliary pathways in mouse liver tissue. Acta Anat. *46*:1, 1961.

Deane, H. W.: A cytological study of the diurnal cycle of the liver of the mouse in relation to storage and secretion. Anat. Rec. *88*:39, 1944.

Elias, H.: A re-examination of the structure of the mammalian liver. I. Parenchymal architecture. II. The hepatic lobule and its relation to the vascular and biliary systems. Am. J. Anat. *84*:311 and *85*:379, 1949.

Fahimi, H. D.: Cytochemical localization of peroxidatic activity of catalase in rat hepatic microbodies (peroxisomes). J. Cell Biol. *43*:275, 1969.

Fahimi, H. D.: The fine structural localization of endogenous and exogenous peroxidase activity in Kupffer cells of rat liver. J. Cell Biol. *47*:247, 1970.

Fawcett, D. W.: Observations on the cytology and electron microscopy of hepatic cells. J. Natl. Cancer Inst. *15*:(Suppl.) 1475, 1955.

Fisher, M. M., H. Bazin, B. Nagy, and B. J. Underdown: Biliary transport of IgA: role of secretory component. Proc. Natl. Acad. Sci. U.S.A., *76*:2008, 1979.

Forker, E. L.: Mechanisms of hepatic bile formation. Annu. Rev. Physiol. *39*:323, 1977.

Fouts, J. R.: Factors influencing the metabolism of drugs in liver microsomes. Ann. N. Y. Acad. Sci. *104*:875, 1963.

Greenway, C. V., and R. D. Stark: Hepatic vascular bed. Physiol. Rev. *51*:23, 1971.

Hamashima, Y., J. G. Harter, and A. H. Coons: The localization of albumin and fibrinogen in human liver cells. J. Cell Biol. *20*:271, 1964.

Harkness, R. D.: Regeneration of liver. Br. Med. Bull. *13*:87, 1957.

Howard, J. G.: The origin and immunological significance of Kupffer cells. *In* van Furth, R., ed.: Mononuclear Phagocytes. Oxford, Blackwell Scientific Publications, 1970, pp. 178–199.

Ito, T.: Cytological studies on stellate cells of Kupffer and fat-storing cells in the capillary wall of the human liver. Acta Anat. Nippon. *26*:2, 1951.

Ito, T., and S. Shibasaki: Electron microscopic study on the hepatic sinusoidal wall and the fat-storing cells in the normal human liver. Arch. Histol. Jpn. *29*:137, 1968.

Jones, A. L., and D. W. Fawcett: Hypertrophy of the agranular endoplasmic reticulum in hamster liver induced by phenobarbital (with a review of the functions of this organelle in liver.) J. Histochem. Cytochem. *14*:215, 1966.

Jones, A. L., R. H. Renston, and S. J. Burwen: Uptake and intracellular disposition of plasma-derived proteins and aproteins by hepatocytes. Prog. Liver Dis. *7*:51, 1982.

Jones, A. L., N. B. Ruderman, and M. G. Herrera: Electron microscopic and biochemical study of lipoprotein synthesis in the isolated perfused rat liver. J. Lipid Res. *8*:429, 1967.

Jones, A. L., and D. L. Schmucker: Current concept of liver structure as related to function. Gastroenterology *73*:833, 1977.

Jones, A. L., D. L. Schmucker, R. H. Renston, and T. Murakami: The architecture of bile secretion. A morphological perspective of physiology. Dig. Dis. Sci. *25*:609, 1980.

von Kupffer, C.: Über Sternzellen der Leber. Arch. Mikr. Anat. *12*:353, 1876.

von Kupffer, C.: Über die sogenannten Sternzellen der Saugthierleber. Arch. Mikr. Anat. *54*:254, 1899.

Lee, F. C.: On the lymph-vessels of the liver. Carnegie Contrib. Embryol. *15*:63, 1923.

Magari, S., K. Fujikawa, and A. Nishi: Form, distribution, fine structure and function of hepatic lymphatics with special reference to blood vessels and bile ducts. Asian Med. J. *24*:254, 1981.

Mostov, K. E., J. P. Kraehenbuhl, and G. Blobel: Receptor mediated transcellular transport of immunoglobulin: synthesis of secretory component as multiple and larger transmembrane forms. Proc. Natl. Acad. Sci. U.S.A. *77*:7257, 1980.

Murikami, T., T. Itoshima, and Y. Shimada: Peribiliary portal system in the monkey liver as evidenced by the injection replica scanning method. Arch. Histol. Jpn. *37*:245, 1974.

Noel, R.: Recherches histo-physiologiques sur la cellule héparique des mammifères. Arch. Anat. Micr. *19*:1, 1923.

Novikoff, P. M., and A. Yam: Sites of lipoprotein particles in normal rat hepatocytes. J. Cell Biol. *76*:1, 1978.

Orrenius, S., J. L. E. Ericksson, and L. Ernster: Phenobarbital induced synthesis of microsomal drug metabolizing enzyme system and its relationship to the proliferation of endoplasmic membranes. J. Cell Biol. *25*:627, 1965.

Peters, T., B. Fleischer, and S. Fleischer: The biosynthesis of rat serum albumin. IV. Apparent passage of albumin through the Golgi apparatus during secretion. J. Biol. Chem. *246*:240, 1971.

Rappaport, A. M., Z. J. Borowy, W. M. Lougheed, and W. N. Lotto: Subdivision of hexagonal liver lobules into a structural and functional unit; role in hepatic physiology and pathology. Anat. Rec. *119*:11, 1954.

Remmer, H., and H. J. Merker: Effect of drugs on the formation of smooth endoplasmic reticulum and drug metabolizing enzymes. Ann. N. Y. Acad. Sci. *123*:79, 1965.

Sztyl, E. S., K. E. Howell, and G. E. Palade: Intracellular and transcellular transport of secretory component and albumin in rat hepatocytes. J. Cell Biol. *97*:1582, 1983.

Wake, K.: "Sternzellen" in the liver; perisinusoidal cells with special reference to storage of vitamin A. Am J. Anat. *132*:429, 1971.

Wake, K.: Perisinusoidal stellate cells (fat storing cells, interstitial cells, lipocytes), their related structure in and around the liver sinusoids, and vitamin A storing cells in extrahepatic organs. Int. Rev. Cytol. *66*:303, 1980.

Wisse, E.: An electron microscopic study of the fenestrated endothelial lining of rat liver sinusoids. J. Ultrastruct. Rev. *31*:125, 1970.

Wisse, E., and W. Th. Daems: Fine structural study on the sinusoidal lining cells of rat liver. *In* van Furth, R., (ed.): Mononuclear Phagocytes. Oxford, Blackwell Scientific Publications, 1970, pp. 200–211.

Wisse, E., and D. L. Knook: Investigation of sinusoidal cells: a new approach to the study of liver function. Prog. Liver Res. *6*:153, 1982.

GALLBLADDER AND BILE DUCTS

Banfield, W. J.: Physiology of the gallbladder. Gastroenterology *69*:770, 1975.

Boyden, E. A.: The anatomy of the choledochoduodenal junction in man. Surg. Gynecol. Obstet. *104*:641, 1957.

Castellucci, M., and A. Caggiati: Surface aspects of rabbit gallbladder mucosa and their functional implications. J. Submicrosc. Cytol. *12*:375, 1980.

Chapman, G. B., A. J. Chiardo, R. J. Coffey, and K. Weineke: The fine structure of the human gall bladder. Anat. Rec. *154*:579, 1966.

Diamond, J. M.: Transport of salt and water in rabbit and guinea pig gall bladder. J. Gen. Physiol. *48*:1, 1964.

Evett, R. D., J. A. Higgins, and A. L. Brown, Jr.: The fine structure of normal mucosa in the human gall bladder. Gastroenterology *47*:49, 1964.

Hayward, A. F.: Electron microscopic observations on absorption in the epithelium of the guinea-pig gall bladder. Zeitschr. Zellforsch. *56*:197, 1962.

Hayward, A. F.: The structure of gall bladder epithelium. Int. Rev. Gen. Exp. Zool. *3*:205, 1968.

Kaye, G. I., H. O. Wheeler, R. T. Whitlock, and N. Lane: Fluid transport in rabbit gall bladder. A combined physiological and electron microscope study. J. Cell Biol. *30*:237, 1966.

Mueller, J. C., A. L. Jones, and J. A. Long: Topographical and subcellular anatomy of the guinea-pig gall bladder. Gastroenterology *63*:856, 1972.

Schwegler, R. A., Jr., and E. A. Boyden: The development of the pars intestinalis of the common bile duct in the human fetus, with special reference to the origin of the ampulla of Vater and the sphincter of Oddi. I. The involution of the ampulla. II. The early development of the musculus proprius. III. The composition of the musculus proprius. Anat. Rec. *67*:441, *68*:17, and *68*:193, 1937.

28

PANCREAS

The pancreas is the second largest gland associated with the alimentary tract. It consists of an *exocrine portion*, which secretes daily about 1200 ml of digestive juice essential for the digestion of carbohydrates, fats, and proteins of the diet; and an *endocrine portion* secreting hormones essential for the control of carbohydrate metabolism.

The pancreas is a pinkish white organ lying retroperitoneally at the level of the second and third lumbar vertebrae (Fig. 28–1). On the right its head is adherent to the middle portion of the duodenum, and its body and tail extend transversely across the posterior wall of the abdomen to the spleen. In the adult it measures from 20 to 25 cm in length and varies in weight from 65 to 160 g. It is covered by a thin layer of connective tissue, which does not, however, form a definite fibrous capsule. It is finely lobulated, and the outlines of the larger lobules can be seen with the naked eye.

THE EXOCRINE PANCREAS

Acinar Tissue

The pancreas is a compound acinous gland organized in many small lobules that are bound together by a loose connective tissue stroma through which run the blood vessels, nerves, lymphatics, and interlobular ducts. The acini of the exocrine pancreas are round or elongate (Fig. 28–2). They consist of 40 to 50 pyramidal cells in a single row around a narrow lumen. The size of the lumen varies with the physiological state of the organ, being small when the gland is at rest and becoming somewhat larger during active secretion. Between the acinar cells are short secretory canaliculi that open into the lumen (Fig. 28–2).

Examined in the living state with a dissecting microscope, the basal portion of the acinar cells is homogeneous, while the apical

portion is filled with highly refractile secretory granules. In histological sections stained with basic dyes, the base of the cells is intensely colored owing to the presence of a high concentration of ribonucleoprotein in this region (Fig. 28–3). There is a paler-staining supranuclear Golgi region that varies in size in different phases of the secretory cycle. The apical cytoplasm is crowded with secretory granules, usually called *zymogen granules* because they contain the precursors of the enzyme-rich pancreatic juice. They are most numerous in fasting and are relatively few after the massive release of secretion induced by a meal. After depletion of the zymogen granules, the Golgi complex enlarges as new secretory granules are being formed.

The pancreatic acinar cell has been a highly favored example of a protein-secreting cell and its ultrastructure and biochemistry have probably been more intensively studied than any other glandular cell. The participation of the various cytoplasmic organelles in the biosynthetic pathway and the mode of discharge of the secretory product were described in some detail in Chapter 3 on Glands and Secretion, and need only be reviewed here.

The basal half of the cell is crowded with parallel arrays of cisternae of rough endoplasmic reticulum. The intervening cytoplasmic matrix is rich in free polyribosomes, and contains long mitochondria with well-developed cristae and numerous matrix granules (Fig. 28–4). The endoplasmic reticulum is the site of synthesis of the secretory proteins and is therefore unusually extensive. Morphometric studies have shown that this organelle occupies some 20 per cent of the cell volume and presents a membrane surface of about 800 μm^2 per cell. The supranuclear Golgi complex consists of several curved stacks of parallel cisternae and numerous small vesicles associated mainly with its convex *cis-face*. At the concave *trans-face* of the Golgi are one or more condensing vacuoles

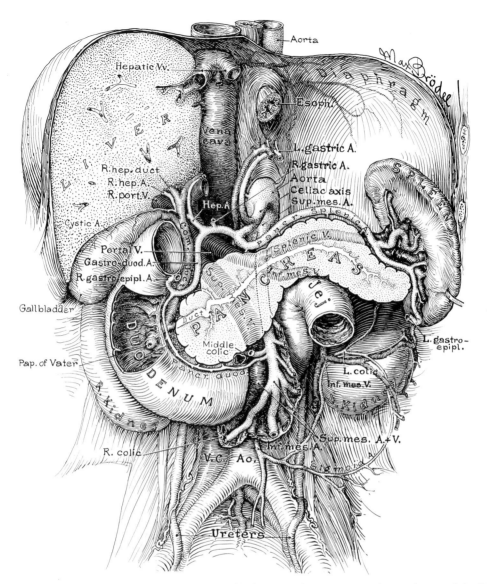

Figure 28–1. Drawing of the upper abdominal viscera with the stomach, transverse colon, and most of the liver cut away to show the location and relationships of the pancreas. (Drawing by M. Brödel, from Trimble, I. R., J. W. Parsons, and C. P. Sherman. Surg. Gynecol. Obstet. 73:711, 1941. By permission of Surgery, Gynecology & Obstetrics.)

with a homogeneous content of relatively low density representing formative stages of new secretory granules. Occasional lipid droplets and lysosomes may also be found in this region.

The apical pole of the cell is the site of accumulation and storage of the product and between meals is packed with large, dense zymogen granules (Fig. 28–5). The narrow free surface of the acinar cell usually has sparse, irregularly oriented microvilli.

In actively secreting glands, zymogen granules may be found in the process of discharging their content into the lumen. Although it is customary to call the stored products zy-

mogen "granules," implying a semisolid consistency, it is evident from electron micrographs of exocytosis that their content is fluid at the time of its release, for it appears to flow out through the opening formed by local fusion of its limiting membrane with the plasmalemma (Fig. 28–6). The secreted zymogen is not in the form of granules but is a moderately dense homogeneous material distributed throughout the lumen. Normally the zymogen granules or droplets in the apex of the cell remain discrete even though closely crowded together. In cells that are very actively secreting, however, one whose membrane has become continuous with the

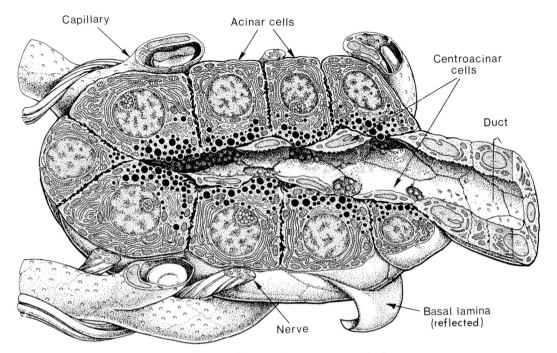

Figure 28–2. Drawing of an acinus of the exocrine pancreas and its associated capillaries and nerves. Notice the intercellular secretory canaliculi and the extension of the centroacinar cells into the acinus. (Reproduced from Krstić, R. V. Die Gewebe des Menschen und Säugetiere. Berlin, Heidelberg, Springer-Verlag, 1978.)

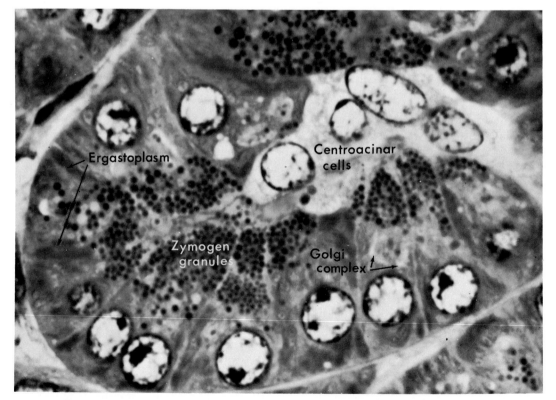

Figure 28–3. Photomicrograph of human pancreas, showing an acinus and its centroacinar cells. The ergastoplasm, Golgi complex, and zymogen granules of the acinar cells are clearly identifiable. The fixation of the nuclei is less than ideal, but adequate preservation of pancreas from postmortem material is difficult. (Courtesy of S. Ito.)

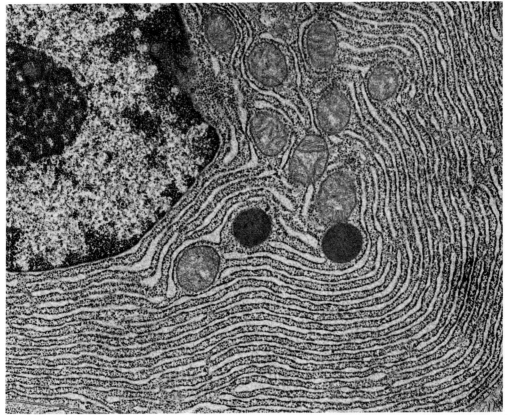

Figure 28–4. Electron micrograph of the basal region of a human pancreatic acinar cell, showing a portion of the nucleus and the extensive development of cisternae of granular endoplasmic reticulum. (Micrograph courtesy of A. Like and S. Ito.)

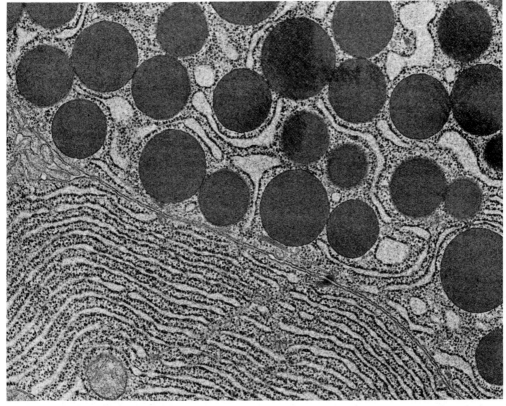

Figure 28–5. A portion of two neighboring human pancreatic acinar cells. Below is the endoplasmic reticulum of the paranuclear region of one cell, and above is the apical region of the adjacent cell filled with zymogen granules and tubular elements of reticulum. (Micrograph courtesy of A. Like and S. Ito.)

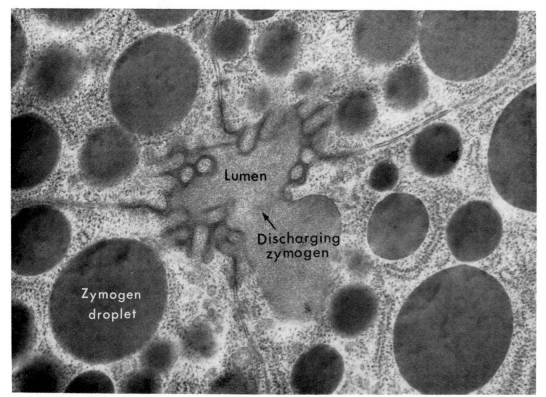

Figure 28–6. Electron micrograph of the lumen of an acinus and the apical portions of four acinar cells. Large, dense zymogen droplets or granules are found in the cell apex. The limiting membrane of one of these has fused with the cell membrane and its zymogen is being discharged into the lumen. The free surface of the acinar cells bears short microvilli.

plasma membrane may be joined by a second fusing with it and this one in turn by a third. In this way, a series of interconnected zymogen granules may come to extend for some distance downward into the apical cytoplasm (Fig. 28–7).

The digestive enzymes of the pancreas are synthesized in the basal cytoplasm of the acinar cells, where they accumulate in the lumen of the endoplasmic reticulum. Through it, they are channeled into the Golgi region, where they are segregated in vesicular elements of Golgi complex origin and concentrated into typical zymogen granules. In most species it is only after the product has undergone this concentration that it is sufficiently insoluble to resist extraction during specimen preparation. Consequently, zymogen granules are visible in the Golgi region and apex of the cell, but their precursors in the endoplasmic reticulum are extracted, and its lumen usually appears empty. Nevertheless, the presence of the digestive enzymes within the reticulum has been established in biochemical studies of the microsome fraction. In the guinea pig, and occasionally in

the bat and the dog, electron micrographs of stimulated glands reveal, in the lumen of the reticulum, dense spherical bodies that resemble small zymogen granules. In these species, at least, concentration of the product evidently can occur in the reticulum as well as in the Golgi apparatus.

HISTOPHYSIOLOGY OF THE EXOCRINE PANCREAS

The exocrine secretory function of the pancreas has a rhythmic cycle with a low basal rate of continuous secretion, periodically greatly increased by nervous and hormonal stimulation associated with ingestion of food. Concurrently with the initiation of gastric secretion, nerve impulses carried by the vagus nerve cause release of acetylcholine at the periphery of the pancreatic acini. This induces some release of enzymes into their lumen but no significant flow in the duct system. Hormonal control of secretion appears to be more important. The presence of food in the gastric antrum and the passage

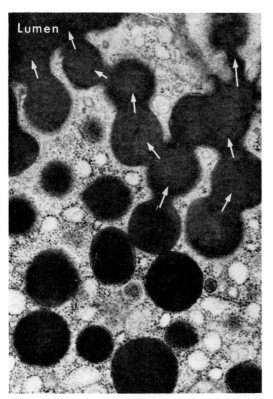

Lumen

Figure 28–7. Electron micrograph of the apical portion of an acinar cell from a dog pancreas. A zymogen granule or droplet opening onto the lumen may be joined to a second and this to a third, so that zymogen may be discharged through several intercommunicating membrane-limited vacuoles. × 24,500. (After Ichikawa, A. J. Cell Biol. 24:369, 1965.)

of the acidic products of gastric digestion into the duodenum stimulates release of two intestinal hormones, *secretin* and *cholecystokinin*.

Secretin is a polypeptide hormone of 27 amino acid residues. Carried in the blood to the pancreas, it causes secretion of a large volume of fluid containing a high concentration of bicarbonate. It does not stimulate the acinar cells, and the secretion induced has little or no enzymatic activity. This copious alkaline juice serves to neutralize the acidic chyme entering the intestine from the stomach and creates the neutral or alkaline pH required for optimal activity of the pancreatic enzymes.

Cholecystokinin is a polypeptide hormone of 33 amino acids secreted by the duodenum and upper jejunum. Carried in the blood to the pancreas, it causes secretion of large quantities of digestive enzymes. Acting alone it does not significantly increase the volume of outflow from the pancreatic ducts, but the coordinated action of secretin and cholecystokinin results in a copious secretion of enzyme-rich pancreatic juice. Cholecystokinin also activates contraction of the gallbladder, adding bile to the duodenal contents.

Pancreatic juice contains enzymes for digestion of the three major classes of nutrients: carbohydrates, fats, and protein. Starches and glycogen are broken down by *pancreatic amylase*. Fat is hydrolyzed to glycerol and fatty acids by *pancreatic lipase*. The proteolytic enzymes include *trypsin, chymotrypsin, carboxypeptidase, ribonuclease*, and *deoxyribonuclease*. These enzymes are released from the acinar cells as inactive proenzymes or zymogens and are activated by enzymes in the lumen of the intestine. These powerful proteases, if activated prematurely, would digest the pancreas. Induced in the pathological condition *acute pancreatitis*, this occurs with rapid destruction of much of the gland. To minimize this danger, the acini also synthesize *trypsin inhibitor* secreted with the enzymes to prevent their premature activation within the cells or the duct system. Under some circumstances this intrinsic safeguard is overwhelmed and acute pancreatitis rapidly progresses, often with fatal outcome.

THE ENDOCRINE PANCREAS

Islets of Langerhans

The endocrine function of the pancreas is segregated in small masses of endocrine cells forming the *islets of Langerhans*, which are scattered throughout the gland (Fig. 28–8). They are not distinguishable with the naked eye, but if the gland is perfused with a dilute solution of neutral red, the islets are selectively stained and their number and distribution can then be studied. In the pancreas of the adult human there are over a million islets, but owing to their small size they constitute only 1 to 2 per cent of the volume of the gland. They are somewhat more numerous in the tail than in the body and head.

The islets are demarcated from the surrounding acinar tissue by a thin layer of reticular fibers, but there is very little reticulum within the islet other than the delicate fibrils associated with the capillaries. The islets are often described as composed of anastomosing cords or plates of epithelial cells, but this conveys a misleading impression of their organization. Reconstruction

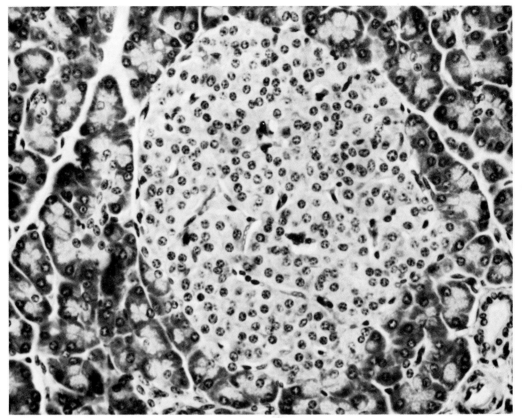

Figure 28–8. Photomicrograph of an islet of Langerhans and surrounding acinar tissue in guinea pig pancreas. Hematoxylin and eosin. × 500.

from serial sections reveals that each islet is a compact mass of epithelial cells permeated by a labyrinthine network of capillaries. No cords or plates are evident in such reconstructions.

The islets contain three principal types of cells, each secreting a different hormone: *alpha cells* (A_2 cells) secreting *glucagon; beta cells* (B cells) producing *insulin*; and *delta cells* (*D cells*, A_1 cells) secreting *somatostatin*. In histological sections prepared using the routine hematoxylin and eosin method, these cell types cannot be distinguished and the islets simply appear as rounded masses of cells staining less intensely than the surrounding acinar tissue (Fig. 28–8). However, techniques have been devised for selective staining of each cell type. In islets stained using the aldehyde-fuchsin trichrome method, the secretory granules of the B cells are deeply colored (Fig. 28–9). With the Grimelius silver impregnation technique, the A cells are blackened (Fig. 28–10A), and with the Hellerström-Hellman silver method the

D cells are selectively impregnated (Fig. 28–10B). Fluorescein-conjugated antibodies to the three hormones are now commonly used for definitive immunocytochemical identification of the islet cells.

In humans the A cells tend to be located mainly at the periphery of the islet, but some are scattered along the capillaries in its interior. The B cells are the predominant cell type distributed throughout the islet, making up about 60 per cent of its mass. The D cells are least abundant. They are quite variable in shape, are often greatly elongated, and may occur anywhere in the islet. All the cell types are polarized with their secretory granules toward the capillaries.

Additional cells have been reported in some but not all species, and their physiological significance is obscure. *C cells* found in the guinea pig pancreas are devoid of secretory granules and may be undifferentiated endocrine cells. *E cells* are described in opossum islets, and *F cells* in the uncinate process of the canine pancreas and in several other

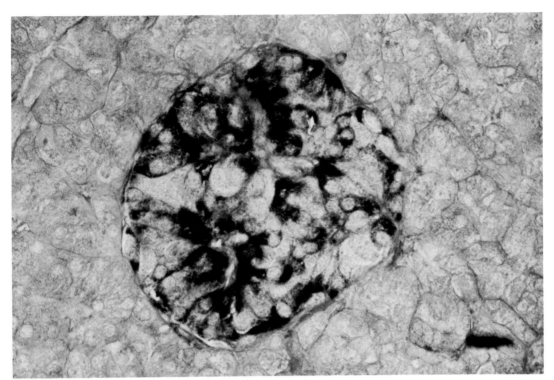

Figure 28–9. Photomicrograph of an islet of Langerhans in the human pancreas stained with aldehyde-fuchsin, which specifically colors secretory granules in the cytoplasm of insulin-producing B cells. The secretory material is often polarized toward capillaries. × 500. (Micrograph from Hellerström, C. Acta Paediatr. Scand. Suppl. 270:7, 1977.)

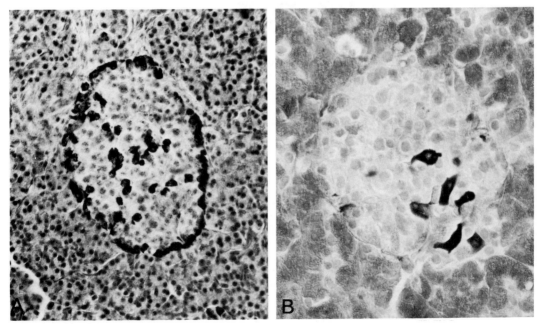

Figure 28–10. *A,* Photomicrograph of a human pancreatic islet stained with the Grimelius silver technique for demonstrating glucagon-producing A cells (A$_2$ cells). The A cells are preferentially localized at the periphery of the islet or along islet capillaries. × 250. *B,* Human pancreatic islet stained with the Hellerström-Hellman silver technique for demonstration of somatostatin-producing D cells (A$_1$ cells). The cells are few in number and irregular in shape. × 400. (Photomicrographs from Hellerström, C. Acta Paediatr. Scand. Suppl. 270:7, 1977.)

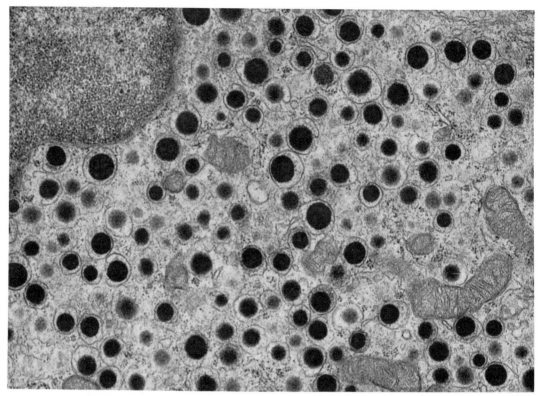

Figure 28–11. Electron micrograph of a juxtanuclear area of an alpha cell in a human islet of Langerhans. The alpha granules have a very dense spherical core and a less dense outer region bounded by a membrane. × 24,000. (Courtesy of A. Like.)

species. A cell type recently described and designated the *PP cell* is believed to secrete *pancreatic polypeptide*. It occurs not only in the islets but also scattered among the acini of the exocrine pancreas.

It has been assumed that the islets throughout the pancreas were similar in their content of endocrine cells. This has now been challenged on the basis of immunofluorescent staining of successive serial sections from the rat pancreas. Marked differences are found in the number of cells containing glucagon and pancreatic polypeptide in different regions of the gland. The pancreas develops from two primordia, and these receive their blood supply from different arteries. In the dorsal region supplied by the celiac artery, the islets are found to be glucagon rich and pancreatic polypeptide poor. In the ventral region irrigated by the superior mesenteric artery, they are pancreatic polypeptide rich and glucagon poor. The question as to whether this distinction of two types of islets of Langerhans applies to other species has not been explored.

The ultrastructural characteristics of the principal cell types has been studied in considerable detail. The A cells contain large numbers of distinctive secretory granules, which, after aldehyde fixation, have spherical cores of high electron density and homogeneous texture surrounded by a narrow zone of lower density (Fig. 28–11). After primary osmium fixation the outer zone is extracted, leaving a clear space between the dense core and the limiting membrane of the granule. The cytoplasm contains a few cisternae of rough endoplasmic reticulum and a juxtanuclear Golgi region that may contain nascent secretory granules. The mitochondria are of varying length and orthodox internal structure.

In the B cells the mitochondria are somewhat larger and the Golgi complex more prominent. The endoplasmic reticulum is not extensive. The ultrastructure of the B-cell granules shows marked species differences. Pale and dark categories of granules have been described. In some species the granules are homogeneous and distinguishable from those of A cells only by their slightly lower density and larger size. In the human, cat, and dog they have a very distinctive appearance, containing one or more dense crystals in a matrix of low electron density (Fig. 28–12). In the human the crystals are rectangular or polygonal in section, and at high magnification they have a very regular internal periodic structure. The surrounding matrix is often extracted in specimen preparation and the crystals stand out in sharp contrast against the clear background enclosed in a loosely fitting membrane (Fig. 28–12).

D cells are unusually heterogeneous in the size, shape, and density of their granules. Their identity as a separate cell type was formerly a subject of dispute, some investigators considering them to be immature or degenerating A cells. Their existence in many, if not all, mammalian species is no longer in doubt. Their granules are larger and considerably less dense than those of the A cell (Fig. 28–13). The cytological features that suggested that they were degenerative forms may have been attributable to their inadequate preservation. Occasional cells bearing a superficial resemblance to D cells are immunoreactive for *gastrin* and are called G cells. Rare islet cell tumors of humans produce large amounts of gastrin, resulting in hypersecretion of acid and severe gastric ulcers.

All the cells of the islets are polarized toward the capillaries, which are of the fenestrated type as in other endocrine glands.

HISTOPHYSIOLOGY OF THE ENDOCRINE PANCREAS

The hormones secreted by the three principal cell types of the islets of Langerhans are all involved in controlling the level of circulating glucose. When the blood glucose falls below an optimal level, the A cells secrete glucagon, which raises blood glucose. When the glucose level rises too high, the B cells release insulin, which lowers its level. The role of somatostatin produced by the D cells is less completely worked out but it is capable of suppressing secretion of either insulin or glucagon and is assumed to modulate the activity of the α and β cells to maintain normal glucose levels.

Insulin is a polypeptide hormone composed of 51 amino acids in two chains, designated A and B, linked by disulfide bonds. It is a very important hormone directly or

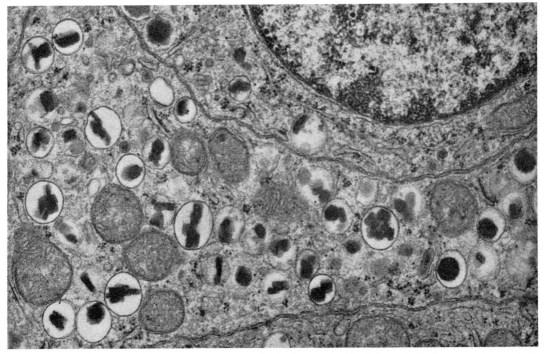

Figure 28–12. Electron micrograph of portions of two adjoining beta cells. The beta granules in man and several other species are membrane-bounded spherical vesicles containing dense crystals of varying configuration. (Courtesy of A. Like.)

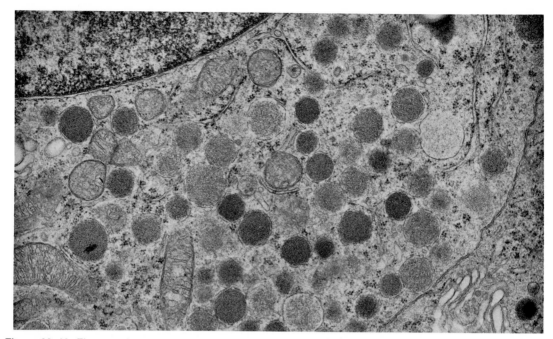

Figure 28–13. Electron micrograph of a portion of a delta cell. The granules are homogeneous and tend to fill their limiting membrane, but they vary considerably in density. It is not clear whether these cells represent a distinct type or are altered alpha cells. (Courtesy of A. Like.)

indirectly affecting the function of nearly every organ in the body. Its most general effect is to facilitate the movement of glucose through cell membranes, especially those of liver, muscle, and adipose tissue. Insulin binds to specific receptors in the cell membrane but the mechanism by which it augments glucose entry is still poorly understood. Brain, muscle, and many other organs are heavily dependent on glucose as an energy source, and the facilitation of its entry into cells is essential for normal metabolism. Glucose is rapidly phosphorylated within the cells and in this form cannot diffuse out. Thus, insulin results in a trapping of glucose in cells and a consequent lowering of its concentration in the circulating blood. In addition to its effect on transport, insulin also influences glucose utilization by enhancing the activity of glucokinase and glycogen synthetase. In adipose tissue, insulin promotes accumulation of lipid by facilitating entry of glucose and its conversion to fatty acids and triglycerides, and by inhibiting release of fatty acids from adipose cells to the blood.

In *diabetes*, glucose cannot enter cells and be utilized owing to a deficiency in insulin production. The resulting excess of glucose in the blood (hyperglycemia) leads to excretion of an abnormal volume of urine (poly-

urea), which in turn causes dehydration and excessive thirst (polydipsia). Failure of insulin to affect the cells in the hypothalamus that control appetite leads to eating in excess (polyphagia). To generate the energy needed in the absence of glucose utilization, fat and muscle protein are metabolized and body weight is rapidly lost despite increased food intake. Increased mobilization of fat results in accumulation of ketones in the blood plasma and their excretion in the urine (ketonuria). The loss of sodium in excreting ketone salts alters the buffering capacity of the blood, which becomes excessively acid (acidosis). Without exogenous insulin, the diabetic is at risk of becoming comatose and dying from dehydration and metabolic acidosis.

Insulin is synthesized in the B cells in the form of *proinsulin*, a single polypeptide chain of about 73 amino acid residues that undergoes post-translational processing involving removal of a 22-amino acid segment generating *insulin* consisting of two polypeptide chains linked by two disulfide bonds. Until now, insulin used in the treatment of diabetics has been extracted from the pancreas of cattle and swine slaughtered for meat. This source may not long continue to meet the needs of the increasing number of diabetics in the population. Fortunately the gene for human insulin has now been isolated and introduced into *E. coli* bacteria, which then synthesize human insulin. With this recombinant DNA technology it will soon be possible to produce insulin in unlimited quantity.

Histological examination of the pancreas of diabetic humans reveals hyalinization or fibrosis of the islets of Langerhans with destruction of a large portion of the B cells. Much less common than diabetes is the occurrence of tumors of islet cells, either benign or metastasizing. The increased volume of B cells results in *hyperinsulinism* and puts the patient at risk of insulin shock. As the blood glucose level falls during massive release of insulin, the central nervous system becomes hyperactive; there is extreme agitation, tremor, and sweating, which may be followed by convulsions and ultimately coma. A similar train of events occurs if a diabetic accidentally takes an overdose of insulin. Timely intravenous administration of glucose will arrest progression of insulin shock and even restore comatose patients to consciousness.

THE DUCT SYSTEM

The lumen of each acinus is continuous with the lumen of a small duct bounded by the *centroacinar cells*, so named because they are surrounded by and appear to extend into the center of the acinus (Fig. 28–14). The centroacinar cells are easily distinguished by their pale staining in histological sections and by the very low density of their cytoplasm and the paucity of their organelles in electron micrographs. Near the termination of the duct system, part of the wall may be made up of centroacinar cells and part by acinar cells (Fig. 28–14). The terminal portion of the duct system drains proximally into the *intralobular* or *intercalated ducts*. These are lined by cells similar to the centroacinar cells that form a low columnar epithelium. These ducts are tributaries of larger *interlobular ducts* (Fig. 28–15) lined by a low columnar epithelium in which goblet cells and occasional argentaffin cells are interspersed. Small mucous glands may bulge slightly from the duc-

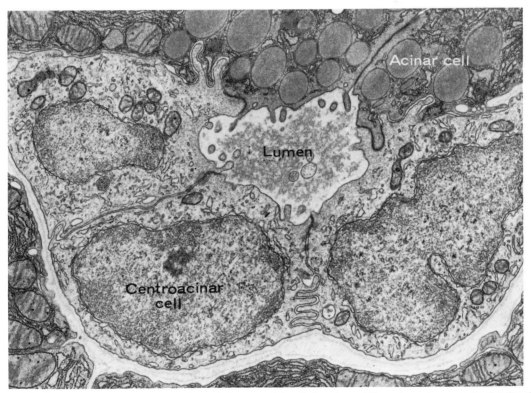

Figure 28–14. Electron micrograph of a terminal segment of the duct system of the guinea pig pancreas showing the lumen bounded on one side by acinar cells and on the other by centroacinar cells. (From Bolender, R. P. J. Cell Biol. *61*:269, 1974.)

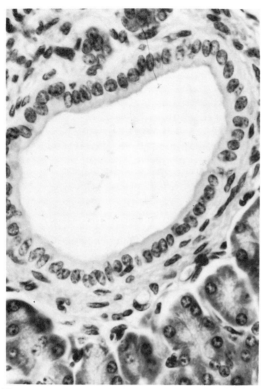

Figure 28–15. Photomicrograph of a small interlobular pancreatic duct.

tal epithelium. The interlobular ducts join the main pancreatic ducts, of which there are two. The larger, or *duct of Wirsung*, begins in the tail and runs through the substance of the gland, receiving throughout its course numerous branches, so that it gradually increases in size as it nears the duodenum. In the head of the pancreas, it runs parallel with the ductus choledochus, with which it may have a common opening in the *ampulla of Vater*. The opening and closing of these ducts are controlled by the *sphincter of Oddi*. The accessory *duct of Santorini* is about 6 cm long. It is nearly always present and lies cranial to the duct of Wirsung. These larger ducts have around the epithelium a moderately thick layer of dense connective tissue containing some elastic fibers.

In addition to the system of ducts just described, the pancreas is said to contain a system of anastomosing small tubules that arise from the large ducts and run in the connective tissue surrounding them. These tubes have a diameter of 12 to 27 μm; they are connected with the islets of Langerhans and only occasionally with the acini. These structures, although studied most extensively in the guinea pig, are said to be also present in the human. Their epithelium is of a low, irregularly cuboidal type. They show occasional mitoses. Occasional goblet cells may be found. Some of the projections from these tubules consist of islet cells, singly or in groups, but the most striking feature of the tubules is their connection, by one or more short stalks, with large islets of Langerhans. It has long been thought that these ductules are composed of undifferentiated epithelium from which new islets can arise after destruction of the endocrine pancreas by disease or injury. This interpretation is now less widely accepted, for it has been shown that the islet cells themselves can divide mitotically and have considerable regenerative capacity.

BLOOD VESSELS, LYMPHATICS, AND NERVES

The arterial supply of the pancreas is from branches of the celiac and superior mesenteric arteries. From the celiac it receives branches through the pancreaticoduodenal and splenic arteries; it also receives small branches from the hepatic artery. The inferior pancreaticoduodenal artery is a branch of the superior mesenteric. The vessels run in the interlobular connective tissue and give off fine branches that enter the lobules. Veins accompany the arteries throughout and lead the blood either directly into the portal vein or indirectly through the splenic vein.

The lymphatic supply of the gland has not been worked out in detail. The lymphatic drainage is principally into the celiac nodes about the celiac artery.

The nerve supply is mainly by unmyelinated fibers arising from the celiac plexus. These fibers accompany the arteries into the gland and end around the acini. There are also many sympathetic ganglion cells in the interlobular connective tissues. The organ also receives myelinated fibers from the vagus nerves.

In electron micrographs, axons are seen penetrating the basal lamina to end in intimate contact with the base of the acinar cells (Fig. 28–16). These nerve terminals often contain numerous synaptic vesicles. The source of these nerves is not clear, but it is likely that they are the terminations of branches from the vagus and may be involved somehow in regulation of secretion.

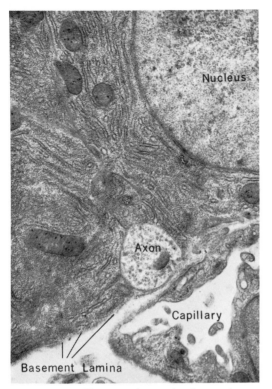

Figure 28–16. Electron micrograph of a nerve axon between the bases of two neighboring pancreatic acinar cells from the bat. The axon contains synaptic vesicles and lies within the basal lamina of the acini.

The presence of unmyelinated nerves in the islets of Langerhans has also been reported, and some of these end on the endocrine cells. The axons are lodged between islet cells or in deep recesses in their bases inside the basal lamina. Two types of endings are distinguishable. Those presumed to be cholinergic contain small, empty-appearing synaptic vesicles, whereas in those endings believed to be adrenergic, many of the vesicles contain dense cores or granules of irregular shape. Both kinds of endings have been found in intimate relation to both alpha and beta cells.

It is generally believed that the regulation of secretion in the exocrine pancreas depends largely on gastrointestinal hormones. There is strong evidence for this in the observation that grafted or denervated pancreas secretes zymogen in response to the hormones *secretin* and *cholecystokinin*, and releases insulin in response to elevated blood sugar. The physiological evidence concerning the role of nerves is contradictory, but the morphological evidence for innervation of the cells is indisputable. If the nerves to the pancreatic islets and acinar cells do not directly activate the secretory mechanism, it is possible that they may modulate the permeability of the cell membranes or the sensitivity of the cells to hormones.

REFERENCES

EXOCRINE PANCREAS

Caro, L. G., and G. E. Palade: Protein synthesis, storage and discharge in the pancreatic exocrine cell: an autoradiographic study. J. Cell Biol. *20:*4, 1964.

Grossman, M. I.: Nervous and hormonal regulation of pancreatic secretion. *In* de Reuch, A. V., and M. P. Cameron, eds.: The Exocrine Pancreas. Ciba Foundation Symposium. Boston, Little, Brown & Co., 1961.

Herzog, V., and M. G. Farquhar: Luminal membrane retrieved after exocytosis reaches most Golgi cisternae. Proc. Natl. Acad. Sci. U.S.A. *74:*5073, 1977.

Herzog, V., and H. Reggio: Pathways of endocytosis from luminal plasma membrane in rat exocrine pancreas. Eur. J. Cell Biol. *21:*141, 1980.

Ichikawa, A.: Fine structural changes in response to hormonal stimulation in the perfused canine pancreas. J. Cell Biol. *24:*369, 1965.

Jamieson, J. D., and G. E. Palade: Condensing vacuole conversion and zymogen granule discharge in pancreatic exocrine cells: metabolic studies. J. Cell Biol. *48:*503, 1971.

Jamieson, J. D., and G. E. Palade: Production of secretory proteins in animal cells. *In* Brinkley, R. B., and K. R. Porter, eds.: International Cell Biology. New York, Rockefeller University Press, 1976–1977, p. 308.

Janawitz, H. D.: Pancreatic secretion of fluid and electrolytes. *In*: Code, C. F., and M. I. Grossman, eds.: Handbook of Physiology. Sect. 6. Washington, DC, American Physiological Society, 1967–1968.

Palade, G. E., P. Siekevitz, and L. G. Caro: Structure, chemistry, and function of the pancreatic exocrine cell. *In* de Reuch, A. V. S., and M. P. Cameron, eds.: The Exocrine Pancreas. Ciba Foundation Symposium. Boston, Little, Brown & Co., 1962.

Rothman, S. G.: The digestive enzymes of the pancreas: a mixture of inconstant proportions. Annu. Rev. Physiol. *39:*373, 1977.

Sarles, H.: The exocrine pancreas. Int. Rev. Physiol. *12:*173, 1977.

Stroud, R. M., Kossiakoff, A. A., and Chambers, J. L.: Mechanisms of zymogen activation. Annu. Rev. Biophys. Bioeng. *6:*177, 1977.

ENDOCRINE PANCREAS

Baetens, D., J. De Mey, and W. Gepts: Immunohistochemical and ultrastructural identification of the pancreatic polypeptide producing (PP-CELL) in the human pancreas. Cell Tissue Res. *185:*239, 1977.

Baetens, D., F. Maisse-Lagae, A. Perrelet, and L. Oorci: Endocrine pancreas: three-dimensional reconstruction shows two types of islets of Langerhans. Science *206:*1323, 1979.

Banting, F. G., J. B. Best, W. R. Campbell, and A. A. Fletcher: Pancreatic extracts in the treatment of diabetes mellitus. Can. Med. Assoc. J. *12:*141, 1922.

Baum, J. B., R. H. Simmons, R. H. Unger, and L. L. Madison: Localization of glucagon in the alpha cells in the pancreatic islet by immunofluorescent techniques. Diabetes *11*:371, 1962.

Bensley, R. R.: Studies on the pancreas of the guinea-pig. Am. J. Anat *12*:297, 1911.

Bjorkman, N., C. Hellerstrom, B. Hellman, and B. Petersson: The cell types in the endocrine pancreas of the human fetus. Zeitschr. Zellforsch. *72*:425, 1966.

Bloom, W.: A new type of granular cell in the islets of Langerhans of man. Anat. Rec. *49*:363, 1931.

Cooperstein, G. J., and D. T. Walkins, eds.: The Islets of Langerhans. New York, Academic Press, 1981.

Dubois, M.P.: Immunoreactive somatostatin is present in discrete cells of endocrine pancreas. Proc. Natl. Acad. Sci. U.S.A. *72*:1340, 1975.

Erlandsen, G. L.: Types of pancreatic islet cells and their immunocytochemical identification. Int. Acad. Pathol. *21*:140, 1980.

Gerick, J. E., S. Raptis, and J. Rosenthal, eds.: Somatostatin symposium. Metabolism *25* (Suppl. 1):1129, 1978.

Lacy, P. E.: Endocrine secretory mechanisms. J. Pathol. *79*:170, 1975.

Larson, L. I., F. Sundler, and R. Hakansson: Pancreatic polypeptide. A postulated new hormone: identification of its storage site by light and electron immunocytochemistry. Diabetologia *12*:211, 1976.

Like, A. A.: Ultrastructure of the secretory cells of the islets of Langerhans in man. Lab. Invest. *16*:937, 1967.

Unger, R. H., R. E. Dobbs, and L. Orci: Insulin, glucagon, and somatostatin secretion in the regulation of metabolism. Annu. Rev. Physiol. *40*:307, 1978.

29

RESPIRATORY SYSTEM

All higher animals require oxygen to maintain their metabolic processes. The respiratory system provides for the intake of oxygen in the inspired air and the elimination of carbon dioxide produced in cell metabolism throughout the body. Oxygen is carried to, and carbon dioxide from, the cells by the circulatory system.

The respiratory tract can be thought of as having a *conducting portion* proximally, which connects the exterior of the body with a *respiratory portion,* distally, where the exchange of gases between the blood and air takes place. The conducting portion includes the passages of the *nose,* the *pharynx,* the *larynx,* the *trachea,* and a branching system of *bronchi* of progressively diminishing caliber. The smallest branches, the *bronchioles,* are continuous with the respiratory portion of the lungs. This consists of *respiratory bronchioles, alveolar ducts,* and *alveoli,* which together make up the greater part of the volume of the lungs.

THE NOSE

The nose is composed of bone, cartilage, muscle, and connective tissue. Its skin is provided with very fine hairs and unusually large sebaceous glands. The integument continues through the anterior nares into the vestibule of the nose. The stratified squamous epithelium here bears large stiff hairs that project into the airway and are believed to help in excluding particles of dust from the inspired air. The remainder of the nasal cavity is lined with mucus-secreting, pseudostratified ciliated epithelium. Dust particles trapped in the layer of mucus on the surface of the epithelium are continually transported by ciliary action toward the pharynx, where they are disposed of by swallowing.

The ciliated columnar epithelium contains abundant goblet cells, and rests on a basal lamina that separates it from an underlying connective tissue layer that contains mucous glands (Fig. 29–1). The mucus from these glands keeps the lining of the nasal cavity moist. Beneath the epithelium on the lower nasal conchae are rich venous plexuses that serve to warm the air as it passes through the nose. The tissue containing these venous plexuses is capable of considerable engorgement, and in this respect bears a superficial resemblance to erectile tissue, but differs from it in the absence of septa containing smooth muscle. This region is a common site of "nose bleed." Collections of lymphoid tissue beneath the epithelium are a characteristic feature of the mucous membrane of the nose, especially near the nasopharynx.

The Olfactory Epithelium

The receptors for the sense of smell are located in a specialized region of the nasal epithelium that occupies the roof of the nasal cavity and extends downward 8 to 10 μm on each side of the septum and onto the surface of the upper nasal conchae. The olfactory area is irregular in outline and has a total surface area on both sides of about 500 sq mm.

The *olfactory epithelium* is a tall, pseudostratified columnar epithelium about 60 μm thick (Fig. 29–2). It consists of three kinds of cells: *supporting cells, basal cells,* and *olfactory cells.*

The *supporting cells* were traditionally described as tall slender elements with an axial bundle of tonofibrils and a prominent "cuticular plate" immediately beneath the free surface, inserting at either side into a prominent "terminal bar." In electron micrographs the cuticular plate is found to be a typical terminal web associated on either side with the zonula adherens of well-developed junctional complexes that attach the supporting cells to the adjacent sensory cells. The free surface of the cell bears numerous long slender microvilli that project into the overlying blanket

Lamina propria   Periosteum   Bone

Opening
of duct

Blood
vessel

Glands

Blood
vessels

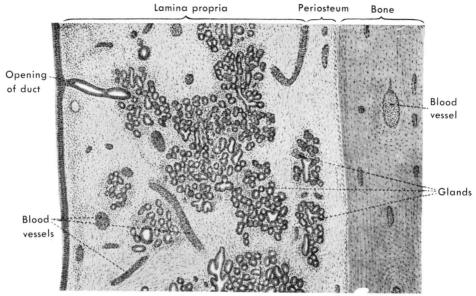

Figure 29–1. Section of the mucosa of the osseous portion of the nose of a 22-year-old man. (After Sobotta.)

of mucus (Fig. 29–4). There is a small Golgi complex in the apical cytoplasm, and pigment granules that are responsible for the brown color of the olfactory area. In some species the supporting cells are secretory and contain numerous mucigen granules in the apical cytoplasm.

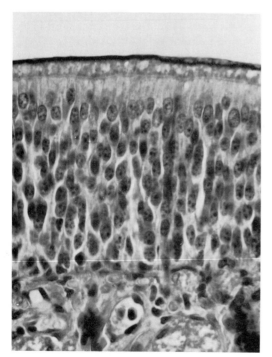

Figure 29–2. Photomicrograph of a celloidin-embedded section of mammalian olfactory epithelium. Masson stain.

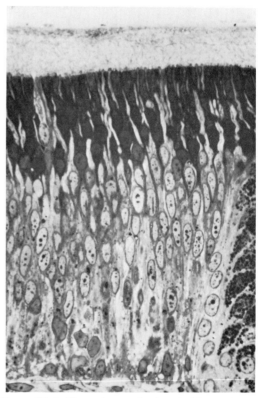

Figure 29–3. Photomicrograph of an Araldite-embedded section of olfactory epithelium from a frog. The slender, lighter-staining cells that extend to the surface of the epithelium are the olfactory rods of the bipolar receptor cells. The darker cells making up the bulk of the upper third of the pseudostratified epithelium are sustentacular cells. At lower right is a portion of a gland of Bowman. Toluidine blue stain. (After Reese, T. J. Cell Biol. 25:209, 1965.)

Between the bases of the supporting cells, the *basal cells* form a single layer of small conical elements with dark nuclei and branching processes.

The *olfactory cells*, evenly distributed among the supporting cells, are bipolar nerve cells. Their round nuclei occupy a zone between the nuclei of the supporting cells and the connective tissue. The apical portion of the cell is a modified dendrite and extends as a cylindrical process from the nucleus to the surface of the epithelium (Fig. 29–4). The basal portion of the cell tapers into a thin, smooth process about 1 μm thick. This is an axon—one of the fibers of the olfactory nerve. It passes into the subepithelial connective tissue and there, with similar fibers, forms small nerve bundles. These assemble into about 20 macroscopically visible *fila olfactoria*.

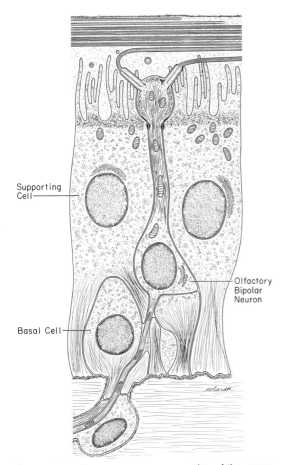

Figure 29–4. Diagrammatic representation of the essential features of the olfactory epithelium based on electron microscopic studies. The height of the epithelium has been foreshortened. The vertical lines in the rod or dendrite of the olfactory bipolar neuron represent microtubules.

The cytoplasm of the olfactory cell contains a network of neurofibrils, which are especially conspicuous around the nucleus. The cell may be slightly constricted at the level of its junctional complexes with the neighboring supporting cells. Distal to this constriction, the bulbous head of the olfactory cell dendrite projects above the general surface of the epithelium. This protruding portion is sometimes inappropriately called the *olfactory vesicle*. Radiating from its surface are six to eight *olfactory cilia* originating from basal bodies embedded in a superficial ectoplasmic layer of cytoplasm having the character of a terminal web. These olfactory cilia are for the most part nonmotile and extremely long. In the frog, in which they have been studied in some detail with the electron microscope, they attain lengths of 150 to 200 μm. They have an atypical structure. The proximal segment of the ciliary shaft is about 250 nm in diameter and contains the usual 9 + 2 arrangement of longitudinal microtubules. A few micrometers from their base there is an abrupt narrowing of the shaft to about 150 nm. This slender portion of the shaft continues to the tip of the cilium, constituting some 80 per cent of its overall length. In this segment, the axoneme consists of 11 single microtubules instead of the usual two singlets and nine doublets. The slender distal segments of the olfactory cilia course parallel to the surface of the epithelium embedded within a thick layer of mucus, but with their tips near its surface. On the basis of the anatomical and physiological evidence now available, these specialized cilia appear to be the component of the sense organ that is excited by contact with odorous substances.

The unmyelinated fibers of the olfactory nerve are enmeshed in a delicate connective tissue rich in macrophages. The fila olfactoria pass through openings of the cribriform plate of the ethmoid bone and enter the olfactory bulb of the brain, where the primary olfactory center is located. The olfactory mucosa is also provided with myelinated nerve fibers originating from the trigeminal nerve. After losing their myelin sheaths, the fibers enter the epithelium and end in fine arborizations between the supporting cells. These endings are receptors for stimuli other than odors.

The lamina propria of the olfactory mucosa is continuous with the dense connective tissue forming the periosteum of the cribriform plate. In it are numerous pigment cells and some lymphoid cells. The lamina propria contains a rich plexus of blood capillaries. In its deeper layers it includes a plexus of large veins and dense networks of lymphatic capillaries. The latter continue into large lymphatics, which course toward the lymph nodes on either side of the head. If a colored material is injected into the subarachnoid spaces of the brain, it can penetrate into the lymph capillaries of the olfactory region as well as into the sheaths of the fila olfactoria. This demonstrates a possible pathway for infections to spread from the nasal mucosa to the meninges.

The lamina propria in the olfactory area also contains the branched, tubuloalveolar *olfactory glands of Bowman.* The secretory portions are oriented mainly parallel to the surface, whereas the narrow ducts assume a perpendicular course and open onto the surface. Immediately under the epithelium the duct is often considerably enlarged. The low pyramidal cells of the secretory portion of the glands are serous and contain obvious secretory granules.

Olfactory stimuli are of chemical nature. The secretion of the glands of Bowman keeps the surface of the olfactory epithelium moist and furnishes the necessary solvent. As most odoriferous substances are much more soluble in lipids than in water, and as the membranes and other constituents of olfactory cells and their cilia contain lipids, odoriferous substances, even if present in extreme dilution, presumably become concentrated in these structures. The continuous stream of the secretion of the olfactory glands, by removing the remains of the stimulating substances, keeps the receptors ready for new stimuli. In this respect, the olfactory glands doubtless have a function similar to that of the glands associated with the taste buds.

PARANASAL SINUSES

Connected with the nasal cavity, and forming cavities in the respective bones, are the frontal, ethmoidal, sphenoidal, and maxillary sinuses—the *accessory sinuses of the nose.* These are lined with ciliated epithelium similar to that of the nasal cavity but containing fewer and smaller glands. The cilia beat so as to move a blanket of mucus toward the nasal cavity. The mucosa of all the sinuses is thin and the lamina propria cannot be differentiated as a separate layer from the periosteum of the bones, to which is is tightly adherent.

The paranasal sinuses are often a site of painful inflammation, *sinusitis,* and occasionally require surgical drainage.

THE LARYNX

The larynx is an elongated structure of irregular shape, whose walls contain hyaline and elastic cartilage, connective tissue, striated muscles, and a mucosa with associated glands. It serves to connect the pharynx with the trachea. As a result of changes resulting from the contraction of its muscles, it produces variations in the width of the opening between the vocal cords. The size of this opening and the degree of muscular tension exerted upon the cords determine the pitch of the sounds made by the passage of air through the larynx.

The framework of the larynx is made up of several cartilages. Of these, the thyroid and cricoid cartilages and the epiglottis are unpaired, whereas the arytenoid, corniculate, and cuneiform cartilages are paired. The thyroid and cricoid and the lower parts of the arytenoids are hyaline cartilage. The *extrinsic muscles* of the larynx support and connect it with surrounding muscles and ligaments and their contraction raises it during deglutition. The *intrinsic muscles* join together the cartilages of the larynx. By their contraction they give different shapes to the laryngeal cavity and thus play a role in phonation.

The anterior surface of the *epiglottis,* the upper half of its posterior surface (the *aryepiglottic folds*), and the *vocal cords* are all covered with stratified squamous epithelium. In the adult, ciliated epithelium usually begins at the base of the epiglottis and extends down the larynx, trachea, and bronchi.

The cilia, which are 3.5 to 5 μm long, beat toward the mouth, and thus move foreign particles, bacteria, and mucus from the lungs toward the exterior of the body.

Goblet cells are scattered among the cylindrical cells of the laryngeal epithelium in varying numbers. The glands of the larynx are of the tubuloacinous, mixed mucous variety. The acini secrete mucus and may have serous crescents. A few taste buds are scattered on the undersurface of the epiglottis.

The *true vocal cords* contain the vocal or inferior thyroarytenoid ligaments. Each of these (one on each side of the midline) consists of a band of elastic tissue bordered on its lateral side by the thyroarytenoid muscle and covered medially by a thin mucous membrane consisting of stratified squamous epithelium (Fig. 29–5). The anteroposterior dimension of the space between the vocal cords is said to be about 23 mm in men and 18 mm in women. The shape of this opening between the vocal cords undergoes great variations in the different phases of respiration and in the production of various sounds in talking and singing. Contraction of the thyroarytenoid muscle approximates the arytenoid and thyroid cartilages, and this relaxes the vocal cords.

The larynx is supplied by the upper, middle, and lower laryngeal arteries, which in turn arise from the superior and inferior thyroid arteries. The veins from the larynx empty into the thyroid veins. The larynx contains several rich plexuses of lymphatics, which lead into the upper cervical lymph nodes and to those about the trachea. The superior laryngeal nerve carries sensory nerves to the mucous membrane, and the inferior laryngeal nerve sends motor nerves to the muscles of the larynx.

CONDUCTING PORTION OF THE RESPIRATORY TRACT

The *airway* or *conducting portion* of the respiratory tract is an arborescent system of tubules that begins with the trachea and continues through 16 generations of dichotomous branching to end in the terminal bronchioles. This pattern of branching results in a progressive decrease in the diameter of the channels, and a concurrent increase in their number and in the total cross-sectional area of the system, as shown in Figure 29–6. It is customary to refer to the branches distal to the trachea as *bronchi, bronchioles*, and *terminal bronchioles*, but it should be borne in mind that there are several generations of branching within the first two categories, so that at the level of terminal bronchioles the number has reached about 65,000, each with a diameter of about 0.2 mm. The channels throughout the bronchial tree serve simply to conduct the inspired and expired air to and from the *respiratory portion* of the lung where the gaseous exchange with the blood takes place.

The Trachea

The trachea is a flexible tube about 11 cm long and 2 cm in diameter. It is lined by ciliated, pseudostratified columnar epithelium with an unusually thick basal lamina. Many goblet cells are scattered throughout the epithelium.

In electron micrographs, the *ciliated cells* have a microvillous border through which the cilia project into the lumen (Fig. 29–7). The apical cytoplasm contains a small Golgi apparatus and numerous mitochondria. The endoplasmic reticulum is not extensive and the cytoplasmic matrix contains only a moderate number of ribosomes. The *goblet cells* are similar to those of the gastrointestinal tract. Their expanded apical region is occupied by closely packed mucinogen granules of low electron density and a somewhat compressed supranuclear Golgi apparatus. Their narrow basal region is rich in cisternae of rough endoplasmic reticulum.

Small pyramidal *basal cells* are intercalated

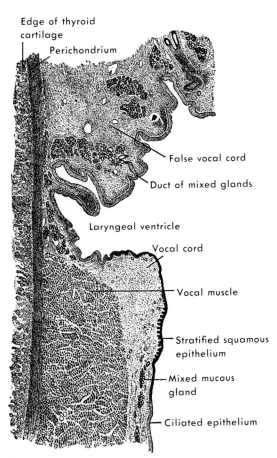

Edge of thyroid cartilage

Perichondrium

False vocal cord

Duct of mixed glands

Laryngeal ventricle

Vocal cord

Vocal muscle

Stratified squamous epithelium

Mixed mucous gland

Ciliated epithelium

Figure 29–5. Frontal section through the middle of the glottis of a 9-year-old boy. (After von Ebner.)

Generation of branching	Name	Diameter (cm)	Cross section (cm²)	Number
CONDUCTING PORTION				
0	Trachea	2	3	1
1	Mainstem bronchi	1.3	1.35	2
2	Lobar bronchi	0.9	0.70	4
3	Segmental bronchi	0.7	0.38	8
4	Subsegmental bronchi	0.5	0.20	16
12	Bronchiole	0.05	0.0021	4,096
13	Bronchiole	0.04	0.0012	8,192
16	Terminal bronchiole	0.018	0.00024	65,536
RESPIRATORY PORTION				
17	Respiratory bronchiole 1	0.015	0.00015	131,072
18	Respiratory bronchiole 2	0.012	0.00011	262,144
19	Respiratory bronchiole 3	0.011	0.00010	524,288
20	Alveolar duct 1	0.010	0.00008	1,048,576
21	Alveolar duct 2	0.010	0.00008	2,097,152
22	Alveolar duct 3	0.010	0.00008	4,194,304
23	Alveoli	0.005	0.00002	8,388,608

Figure 29–6. Table showing the numbers and average dimensions of the successive orders of dichotomous branching of the bronchial tree and the respiratory portion of the human lung inflated to three-fourths capacity. (Modified after Weibel, E.R. Morphometry of the Human Lung. New York, Academic Press, 1963.)

between the bases of the columnar cells. The alignment of their nuclei below those of the ciliated columnar cells gives the epithelium its characteristic "pseudostratified" appearance. They have few organelles and are evidently a reserve of relatively undifferentiated cells capable of replacing other cellular elements of the epithelium.

A less common cell type is the so-called *brush cell*—a slender columnar cell with a microvillous luminal border and a well-developed smooth endoplasmic reticulum, but no secretory granules. Small aggregations of glycogen particles may be scattered through the cytoplasm. The function of the brush cells and their relationship to other cells of

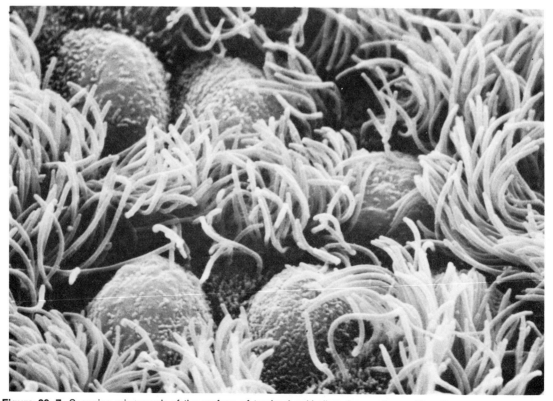

Figure 29–7. Scanning micrograph of the surface of tracheal epithelium from a horse. The dome-shaped apices of goblet cells bearing short microvilli can be seen among the tufts of cilia on the ciliated epithelial cells. (Micrograph courtesy of P. Gehr.)

the epithelium remain to be clarified. They have been variously interpreted as depleted goblet cells or as intermediate stages in the differentiation of basal cells to replace exfoliated columnar cells. The occasional observation of synapses with intraepithelial nerve fibers has led to the speculation that some brush cells may function as sensory receptors, but physiological validation of this suggestion is lacking.

Sparsely distributed in the tracheobronchial epithelium are cells resembling the argentaffin cells of the gastrointestinal tract. Viewed in electron micrographs, these cells contain numerous small, dense, secretory granules often concentrated near the basal lamina. There may be more than one category of such cells. Some do not reach the lumen, and have the staining properties and fluorescence characteristic of cells that store catecholamines. Others are columnar and resemble the peptide hormone–secreting cells of the enteroendocrine system. To date, the small granule-containing cells of the respiratory tract have received less investigative attention than those of the gut epithelium.

The lamina propria of the tracheal epithelium is a loose connective tissue, unusually rich in elastic fibers. It contains many *submucous glands* consisting of tubular acini radiating from a duct that opens onto the surface of the epithelium (Fig. 29–1). The cells lining the duct are rich in mitochondria but devoid of secretory granules. The elongate acini are lined, in their proximal portion, by mucus-secreting cells, and their terminal portion consists of serous cells. The granules of the serous cells are discrete and electron dense, while those of the mucous cells are electron lucent and tend to be confluent. The secretory product of both is glycoprotein, but its composition is quite different in each.

The secretion of a blanket of mucus onto the epithelium of the airway has an important role in trapping inhaled dust and other particulate matter, and in protecting the conducting and respiratory portions of the lungs against potentially damaging toxic fumes. The blanket of mucus is constantly moved by ciliary action toward the pharynx, where it is swallowed with the saliva. When the airway is exposed to tobacco smoke or other irritants, the submucous glands increase in size, and the goblet cells of the tracheal and bronchial epithelium increase in number. The composition of the glycoprotein secreted also undergoes some modification. After removal of the irritant, these changes are reversed in a few months.

A characteristic feature of the trachea is its supporting framework of 16 to 20 C-shaped hyaline cartilages that encircle it on its ventral and lateral aspects (Fig. 29–8). These successive incomplete cartilaginous rings are separated by interspaces that are bridged by fibroelastic connective tissue. Because of this arrangement, the trachea has much more pliability than it would have if enveloped in a continuous layer of cartilage. The tracheal cartilages reinforce the wall and keep its lumen open by resisting external forces that otherwise might constrict the airway. Outside of the cartilages, there is a layer of dense connective tissue containing many elastic fibers.

The posterior wall of the trachea adjacent to the esophagus is devoid of cartilages (Fig. 29–8). In their place is a thick band of bundles of smooth muscle, which, in the main, run transversely. At their ends, they are inserted among the dense elastic and collagenous fiber bundles making up the layer of dense connective tissue peripheral to the tracheal cartilages. The smooth muscle is also joined to the mucosa by loose connective tissue continuous with the lamina propria.

A delicate network of lymphatics is found beneath the tracheal epithelium. These communicate with a much coarser plexus in the

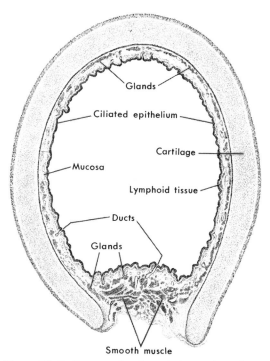

Figure 29–8. Cross section through the trachea of a 9-year-old boy. × 6. (Redrawn and modified from Kölliker-von Ebner.)

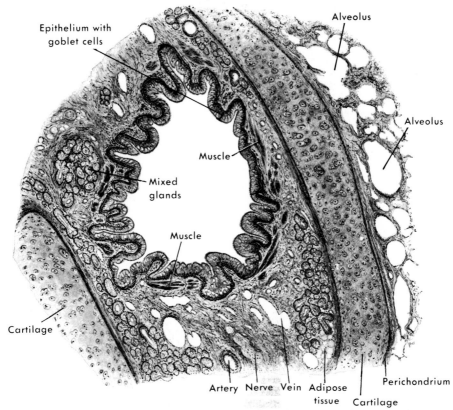

Figure 29–9. Cross section through a small bronchus of a man. × 30. (After Schaffer.)

submucosa, which drains into lymph nodes associated with the trachea along its entire length. The blood supply comes mainly from the inferior thyroid artery. The nerves to the trachea arise from the recurrent branch of the vagus and from the sympathetic chain. The autonomic nerves of the trachea have small ganglia from which fibers lead to the smooth muscle in its posterior wall. Sensory nerves are also associated with the mucosa and are afferent pathways of the cough reflex.

The Bronchi

The trachea divides into two branches called *primary bronchi* or *main stem bronchi*. These enter the right and left lung at its hilus. Coursing downward and outward, they divide into *lobar bronchi*. The left lung has upper and lower lobes; the right has upper, middle, and lower lobes. Correspondingly, there are two lobar bronchi in the left and three in the right lung. The lobar bronchi in turn divide into *segmental bronchi* to the several bronchopulmonary segments in each lung. There are three segments in the right

upper lobe, two in the middle lobe, and five in the lower lobe. In the left lung, there are five in the upper and five in the lower lobe. The segmental bronchi branch into *subsegmental bronchi*. The blood supply to the lung follows the same pattern of branching as the bronchi. The parallel course of the bronchi and blood vessels is of great importance to the thoracic surgeon because it makes lobectomy or segmental resection of part of a lobe technically feasible.

The structure of the primary bronchi is very similar to that of the trachea up to the point where they enter the lungs. Thereafter, the cartilage rings disappear and are replaced by cartilage plates of irregular outline, distributed around the circumference of the tube (Fig. 29–9). Thus, the intrapulmonary bronchi are cylindrical and not flattened on one side as are the trachea and extrapulmonary bronchi. Farther along the airway, the intramural cartilage plates become reduced in size and number and disappear altogether in subsegmental bronchi about 1 mm in diameter.

As the cartilage in the wall of the bronchial tree diminishes, the smooth muscle becomes more prominent. It is organized in interlacing bundles, some of which have a prevailing circular or spiral course. In the larger intrapulmonary bronchi, the bundles are packed closely enough to form a more or less continuous layer. In sections, the bronchial mucosa exhibits longitudinal folds, presumably owing to agonal contraction of the smooth muscle layer (Fig. 29–9). In more distal portions of the bronchial tree, the smooth muscle is more attenuated and loosely organized. It is present, however, throughout the conducting portion of the respiratory tract.

The bronchial epithelium is ciliated columnar with goblet cells and associated submucosal glands. The latter diminish in number, and end at the level of the bronchioles. The height of the epithelium gradually decreases along the tract, becoming cuboidal in the bronchioles and sparsely ciliated, low cuboidal in terminal bronchioles. The lamina propria, which is set off from the epithelium by a prominent basal lamina, is loose connective tissue rich in reticular and elastic fibers. In addition to fibroblasts, it contains lymphocytes, mast cells, and occasional eosinophils.

Bronchioles

The bronchioles, representing the 12th to 15th generations of branching of the bronchial tree, are about 0.3 to 0.5 mm in diameter. There are no glands or cartilaginous plates in their walls, and the muscularis does not form a continuous circumferential layer, but is represented by discrete bundles of varying orientation that join to form a loose network with loose connective tissue filling in the meshes. The smooth muscle is innervated by parasympathetic nerve fibers. Although not a conspicuous feature of the bronchiolar wall in sections, contraction of the smooth muscle very effectively constricts the lumen. It is said to relax during inspiration and contract at the end of expiration. When contraction is abnormally persistent, as in asthma attacks, the constriction of the airway at this level makes emptying of the lungs during exhalation quite difficult.

The epithelium lining the bronchioles lacks goblet cells and consists mainly of ciliated cells and *Clara cells*. Except for their reduction in height, the ciliated cells are very similar in their ultrastructure to those more proximally situated in the airway. The Clara cells are confined to the bronchiolar epithelium. Their smooth-contoured, rounded apices or "domes" project into the lumen above the level of the surrounding ciliated cells. Their most characteristic feature is the presence of numerous electron-dense secretory granules in their apical cytoplasm. The chemical nature of the granule contents has not been definitely established. It is not mucin, is resistant to lipid solvents, and seems to consist mainly of protein. In the rat, the granules have a crystalline substructure not evident in other species. The granules are discharged by exocytosis. An extracellular material of similar density is seen in electron micrographs between the microvilli and around the bases of the cilia. It is believed that the secretory product of the Clara cells forms a surface coating, lining the bronchioles in much the same way that mucus lines the larger bronchial tubes. A mucus lining would not be suitable for such small passages because of its stickiness. The walls of the bronchioles come into contact late in expiration and it is speculated that a nonsticky, proteinaceous lining layer of low-surface tension may be required here to ensure their reopening on inspiration. Thus, the secretion of the Clara cells may play a role analogous to that of the surfactant lining the alveoli of the lung.

Another ultrastructural feature of the Clara cells in some species that has aroused considerable speculation is an unusually extensive smooth endoplasmic reticulum in the supranuclear cytoplasm. This organelle is well developed in cells engaged in lipid metabolism or in cholesterol and steroid secretion, whereas rough endoplasmic reticulum is expected in cells synthesizing products rich in protein. In the liver, the smooth reticulum is rich in cytochrome P-450 and mixed-function oxidases involved in the metabolism of drugs. It has been suggested that this organelle in the Clara cells might metabolize toxins in the inspired air, but to date this is purely conjectural.

RESPIRATORY PORTION OF THE LUNGS

Respiratory Bronchioles

The bifurcation of the terminal bronchioles gives rise to *respiratory bronchioles*, short tubes 0.15 to 2.0 mm in diameter. In the human, there are three successive generations of respiratory bronchioles, constituting the transition from the conducting to the

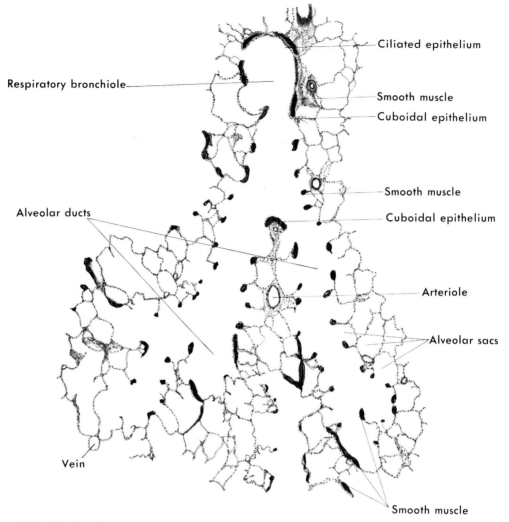

Ciliated epithelium

Respiratory bronchiole

Smooth muscle

Cuboidal epithelium

Smooth muscle

Cuboidal epithelium

Alveolar ducts

Arteriole

Alveolar sacs

Vein

Smooth muscle

Figure 29–10. Drawing of a section through a respiratory bronchiole and two alveolar ducts of human lung. Note the smooth muscle in the walls of the alveolar ducts. (Slightly modified from Baltisberger.)

respiratory portion of the lung. Their lining epithelium is cuboidal at this level, becoming low cuboidal and nonciliated in the subsequent branches. They differ from other bronchioles in that their walls are interrupted at intervals by thin saccular outpocketings, *alveoli*. Gas exchange can take place in these thin-walled appendages, hence the name "respiratory" bronchioles. The number of alveoli increases with each branching so that much of the bronchiolar wall is replaced by openings into alveoli.

Alveolar Ducts

The respiratory bronchioles are continuous with the *alveolar ducts*. Here the alveoli are so numerous and closely spaced that the limits of the duct are discernible in sections only by the alignment of the free edges of thin connective tissue septa between the adjacent alveoli (Fig. 29–10). The thickened adluminal ends of these interalveolar septa are covered by a few bronchiolar epithelial cells overlying delicate strands of smooth muscle in the septal connective tissue.

After two or three branchings, each alveolar duct ends in a minute space. This is simply the terminal portion of the alveolar duct with no distinguishing histological features. Although it is often called the *atrium*, it is debatable whether it deserves a separate designation (Figs. 29–11, 29–12). It is merely a common lumen or vestibule into which clusters of four or more alveoli open.

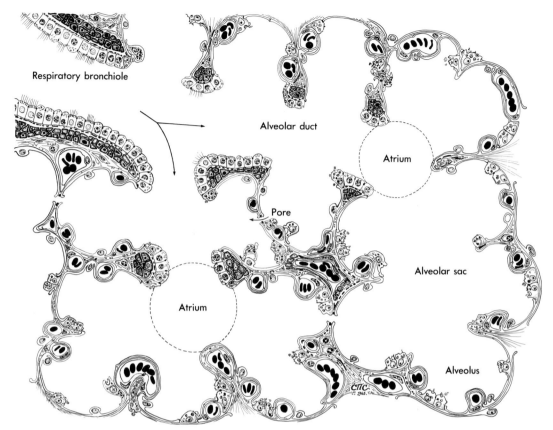

Respiratory bronchiole

Alveolar duct

Atrium

Pore

Atrium

Alveolar sac

Alveolus

Figure 29–11. Schematic representation of the respiratory unit of the lung: respiratory bronchiole, alveolar ducts, alveolar sacs, and alveoli. The atria indicated by the circles are spaces bounded on one side by the termination of the alveolar duct and on the other by the openings of the alveolar sacs. (Slightly modified after Sorokin, S. *In* Greep, R. O., ed.: Histology. 2nd ed. New York, McGraw-Hill Book Co., 1966.)

Alveoli

Physiologically the most important components of the lung are the thin-walled, terminal saccular compartments, the *pulmonary alveoli* (Figs. 29–13, 29–14). Their number in the human lung is estimated to be 300 million, presenting a surface of about 143 sq m, which is available for gaseous exchange between the inspired air and the blood.

The alveolar epithelium consists of two cell types, the *Type I alveolar cell* (Type I pneumonocyte) and the *Type II alveolar cell* (also called Type II pneumonocyte, granular pneumonocyte, and great alveolar cell). The Type I alveolar cells are highly specialized squamous cells covering a large area, but they are less than 0.2 μm in thickness except where they are locally thickened to accommodate the nucleus (Fig. 29–15). The free surface of these cells is usually smooth contoured. They are attached to each other and

to the Type II alveolar cells by occluding junctions.

The Type II alveolar cell is rounded and its margins are partially overlain by the neighboring squamous cells of the epithelium. The free surface has a limited number of short microvilli, especially at the periphery (Fig. 29–16). The rounded basal surface of the cell bulges into the connective tissue of the alveolar septa. These cells are most commonly found in niches in the alveolar wall along the junctions of the alveolar septa. Although the thinly spread Type I alveolar cells are quite inconspicuous in sections of the alveoli, their cytoplasmic volume is twice that of the thicker Type II cells and their surface area exposed to the lumen is 50 times greater. Both cell types rest on a thin basal lamina.

The Type II alveolar cell is a secretory cell that is the source of the thin layer of surface active phospholipid, *pulmonary surfactant*, that

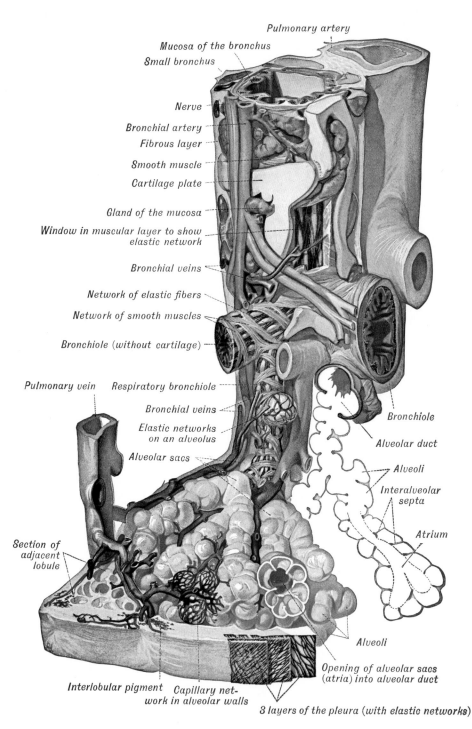

Pulmonary artery

Mucosa of the bronchus

Small bronchus

Nerve

Bronchial artery

Fibrous layer

Smooth muscle

Cartilage plate

Gland of the mucosa

Window in muscular layer to show
elastic network

Bronchial veins

Network of elastic fibers

Network of smooth muscles

Bronchiole (without cartilage)

Pulmonary vein   Respiratory bronchiole

Bronchial veins

Elastic networks
on an alveolus

Alveolar sacs

Section of
adjacent
lobule

Bronchiole

Alveolar duct

Alveoli

Interalveolar
septa

Atrium

Alveoli

Opening of alveolar sacs
(atria) into alveolar duct

Interlobular pigment   Capillary network in alveolar walls

3 layers of the pleura (with elastic networks)

Figure 29–12. Portion of a pulmonary lobule from the lung of a young man. Free reconstruction by Vierling, somewhat foreshortened. Mucosa and glands, green; cartilage, light blue; muscles and bronchial artery, orange; elastic fibers, blue-black; pulmonary artery, red; pulmonary and bronchial veins, dark blue. (After Braus.)

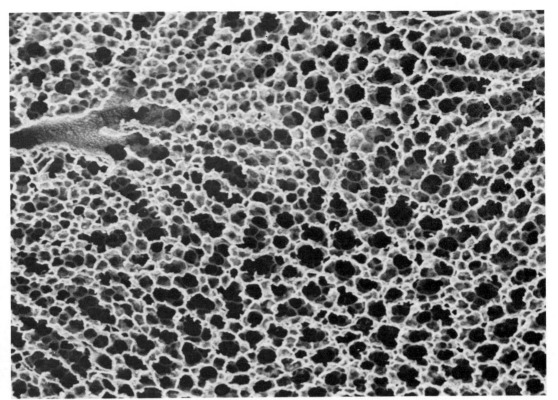

Figure 29–13. Scanning micrograph of lung from a gazelle, prepared by instillation of the fixative to prevent collapse of the alveoli and terminal segments of the bronchial tree. (Micrograph courtesy of P. Gehr.)

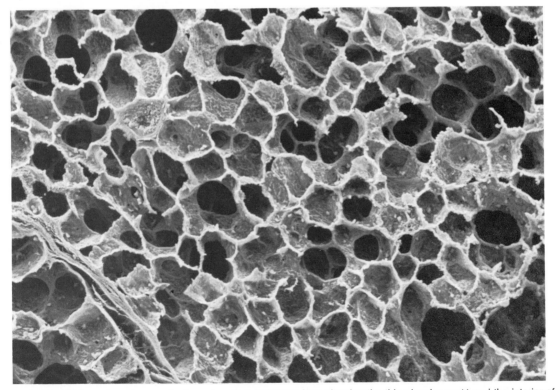

Figure 29–14. Scanning micrograph of a cut surface of human lung showing the thin alveolar septa and the interior of numerous alveoli. × 68. (Micrograph courtesy of P. Gehr.)

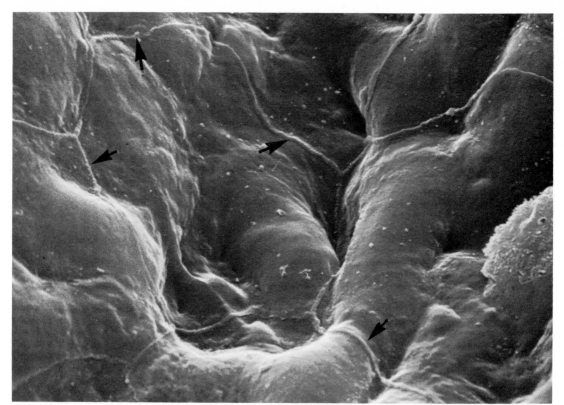

Figure 29–15. High-magnification scanning micrograph of the interior of an alveolus from bovine lung. The extremely thin Type I alveolar cells conform to the rounded contours of the underlying capillaries. The boundaries of adjacent polygonal cells appear as linear ridges *(at arrows)*. (Micrograph courtesy of P. Gehr.)

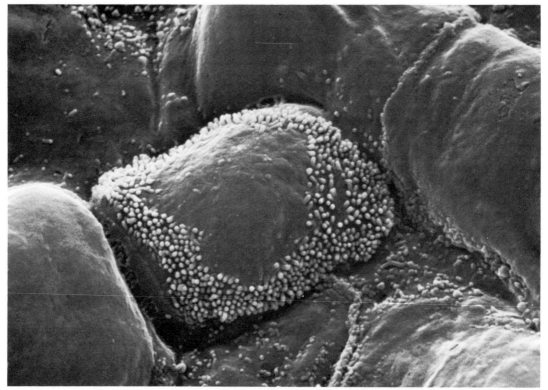

Figure 29–16. Scanning micrograph of the interior of human pulmonary alveolus, showing a Type II alveolar cell with its short microvilli located mainly at the periphery of its bulging free surface. × 7600. (Micrograph courtesy of P. Gehr.)

coats the epithelial lining of the alveoli. In addition to the usual cytoplasmic organelles, they have conspicuous dense secretory granules usually located in the supranuclear region (Fig. 29–17). These secretory granules contain the precursors of pulmonary surfactant and have a characteristic lamellar substructure in electron micrographs. Their content is very rich in phospholipid, the phospholipid: protein ratio varying from 3:1 to 6:1. In freeze-fracture preparations, the lamellae within the granules are straight and stacked with a very regular periodicity. It is reported, however, that when rapidly frozen with liquid helium without prior aldehyde fixation, no lamellar structure is seen. The formation of the lamellae may therefore be induced during fixation and may not accurately reflect their structure in the living state. Nonetheless the lamellar substructure of the granules in routine preparations is a useful identifying feature of Type II alveolar cells. The granules are discharged by exocytosis (Fig. 29–18). The recently released surfactant often forms patterns resembling myelin forms of hydrated phospholipid, but it ulti-

mately spreads to form a monomolecular film over the alveolar surface (Fig. 29–19).

The interstitium of the alveolar septa is the tissue between the two layers of pulmonary epithelium lining adjacent alveoli. It includes a very close-meshed network of capillaries, pericytes, septal cells (interstitial fibroblasts), mast cells, monocytes, and occasional lymphocytes (Fig. 29–20). The most numerous of the cellular elements of the interstitium are the septal cells. They are considered by some to be a form of fibroblast and to function in maintenance and repair of the connective tissue of the lung. Strips of peripheral lung tissue contract in vitro in response to hypoxia. Actin and myosin have been found in the septal cells by immunocytochemical methods, and it is speculated that contraction of these cells may decrease alveolar size and decrease capillary perfusion under certain physiological conditions. There is also some experimental evidence that they participate in resynthesis of elastin after enzymatic induction of emphysema.

In sections, capillaries occupy most of the thickness of the alveolar septa, and where

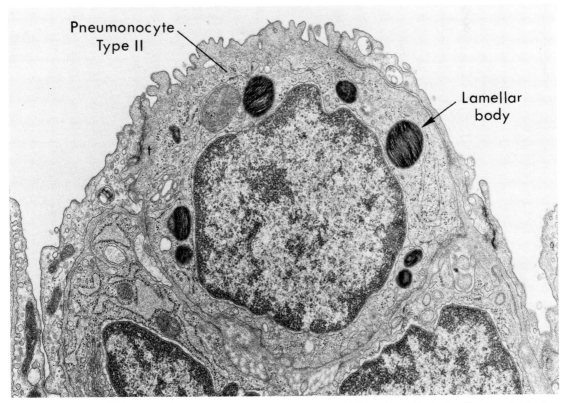

Figure 29–17. Electron micrograph of a Type II alveolar cell from fetal rat lung, illustrating the lamellar bodies. (Micrograph courtesy of M. C. Williams.)

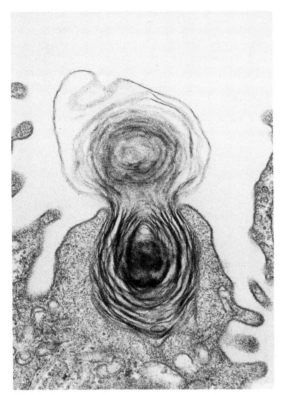

Figure 29–18. Micrograph of a lamellar body being extruded from an alveolar cell in a 21-day fetal rat lung. (Micrograph courtesy of M. C. Williams.)

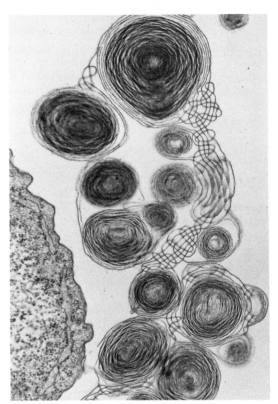

Figure 29–19. After release from the Type II epithelial cell, the phospholipid of the lamellar bodies forms complex myelin figures in the alveolar lumen, as shown in this micrograph from fetal rat lung near term. The surfactant ultimately spreads over the lining of the alveoli in a monomolecular film. (Micrograph courtesy of M. C. Williams. Reproduced from The Journal of Cell Biology 72:260, 1977 by copyright permission of The Rockefeller University Press.)

the pulmonary epithelium overlies the capillaries, the interstitial space is reduced to an exceedingly thin layer between the basal lamina of the epithelium and that of the capillary endothelium. The barrier to diffusion between the alveolar air and the blood thus consists of (1) a layer of fluid and surfactant, (2) the attenuated epithelium, (3) its basal lamina, (4) a thin interstitial space, (5) the basal lamina of the capillary, and (6) the capillary endothelium. The total thickness of these six components may be as little as 0.2 μm but averages about 0.5 μm (Fig. 29–21).

Between the neighboring capillaries, the interstitium is somewhat thicker, and it is in these areas that the septal cells reside together with a delicate network of elastic fibers. In the early phase of various forms of pulmonary pathology, there is a leakage of fluid from the capillaries, resulting in interstitial edema and accumulation of fluid in the alveoli.

Small openings, *alveolar pores* (pores of Kohn), traverse the thin wall between adjacent alveoli. These minute apertures are only 7 to 9 μm in diameter and are located in the spaces between the capillaries of the alveolar wall (Fig. 29–22). From one to six may be found and larger numbers have been reported. Their significance is not entirely clear but it is thought that they may provide for a collateral air circulation that would tend to prevent alveolar collapse (*atelectasis*) when peripheral branches of the bronchial tree become obstructed. They may also be disadvantageous in that they provide pathways for the spread of bacteria from alveolus to alveolus in pneumonia.

The interstitial tissue near the mouths of the alveoli is rich in elastic fibers and contains a wreath of wavy bundles of collagen fibers. These fibers are continuous with those encircling the mouths of neighboring alveoli and thus tend to give some substance to the wall of the alveolar duct. The wavy collagen fibers probably straighten out as the alveoli expand during inspiration. The extensive network of

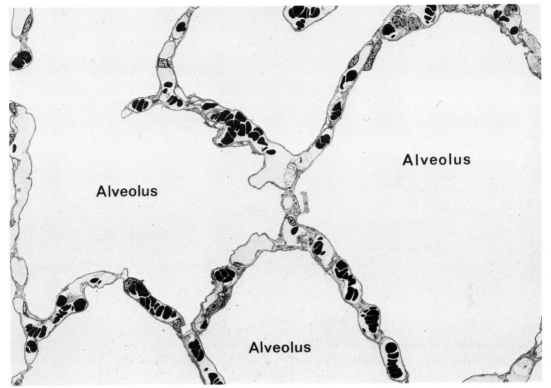

Figure 29–20. Micrograph of equine lung, showing erythrocyte-filled capillaries in the thin septa between alveoli. × 640. (Micrograph courtesy of P. Gehr.)

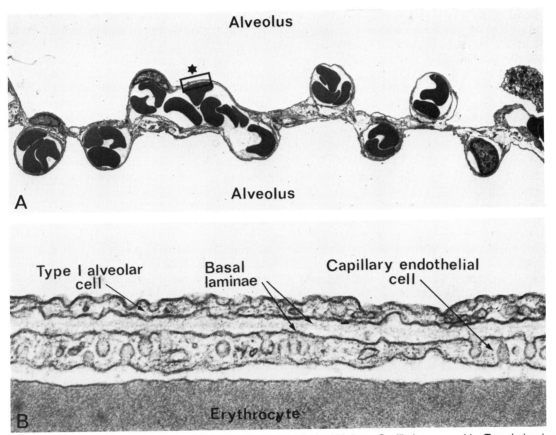

Figure 29–21. *A,* Micrograph of the septum between two alveoli of rabbit lung. Capillaries covered by Type I alveolar cells bulge into the lumen, exposing a large surface to the inspired air. *B,* Higher magnification of an area such as that enclosed in the rectangle (*) in *A,* showing the layers making up the diffusion barrier for gaseous metabolites. (Micrographs courtesy of P. Gehr.)

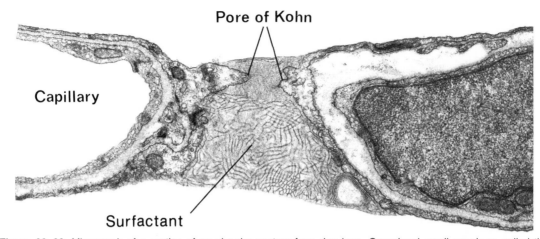

Pore of Kohn

Capillary

Surfactant

Figure 29–22. Micrograph of a section of an alveolar septum from dog lung. Occasional small openings, called the pores of Kohn, traverse the thin wall between adjacent alveoli. The opening here is partially obscured by an accumulation of surfactant. (Micrograph courtesy of P. Gehr.)

septal reticular fibers is continuous with the collagen bundles that encircle the mouths of the alveolar sacs. These latter in turn merge with collagen fibers in the walls of the bronchioles and small arteries and veins.

Alveolar Macrophages. The *pulmonary alveolar macrophage* is the principal mononuclear phagocyte of the lungs. It is not a part of the alveolar wall, but a free cell resting on its surface. In this location, it is directly exposed to inhaled dust, environmental toxins, and bacteria and serves as the primary defense against such particulate matter.

Alveolar macrophages vary in size from 15 to 40 μm in diameter and have an irregularly shaped nucleus with a prominent nucleolus. The cytoplasm contains numerous vacuoles and may appear "foamy" with the light microscope owing to its high degree of vacuolization. In electron micrographs, the cytoplasmic organelles include a prominent Golgi apparatus and a few mitochondria. The endoplasmic reticulum is not extensive. Free ribosomes and β particles of glycogen are present in moderate numbers in the cytoplasmic matrix. The most striking ultrastructural feature of the cell is the large number and heterogeneity of its membrane-bounded inclusions (Fig. 29–23). Many of these are primary lysosomes, 0.5 μm or less in diameter and round or oblong in shape. These contain a large number of hydrolytic enzymes. The specific activities of acid phosphatase, β-glucuronidase, and lysozyme are reported to be substantially higher in alveolar macrophages than they are in comparable phagocytes from the peritoneal cavity.

In cigarette smokers, the cytoplasm of these cells is crowded with large, irregularly shaped masses of pigment representing undigestible residues of phagocytized material (Fig. 29–24). These heterogeneous inclusions have electron-dense and electron-lucent areas, and contain lipid, myelin figures, and occasionally crystals of unknown provenance. In persons with heart disease attended by pulmonary congestion, the alveolar macrophages contain many vacuoles filled with *hemosiderin* resulting from phagocytosis of extravasated erythrocytes and degradation of their hemoglobin.

The origin of alveolar macrophages was a subject of disagreement, some workers believing that they arose by exfoliation of alveolar lining cells, others insisting that they were derived from fixed macrophages present in the alveolar septa. This controversy now seems to have been resolved by use of DNA-labeling techniques and chromosomal markers for identifying cells and tracing their origins. It is now widely accepted that pulmonary macrophages are part of the general mononuclear phagocyte system of the body (see Chapter 5). They originate from stem cells in the bone marrow and are transported in the blood as monocytes that enter the interstitium of the lung, where they undergo certain maturational changes. The mature cells then migrate to the surface of the alveoli. Most of the proliferative activity giving rise to pulmonary macrophages takes place in the bone marrow, but the maturing monocytes in the interstitium of the lung also have a limited capacity for division.

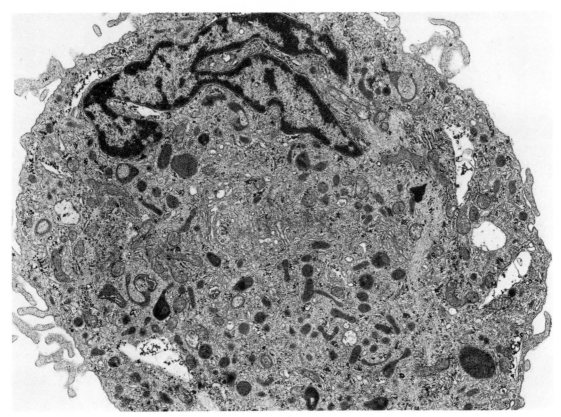

Figure 29–23. Electron micrograph of a human alveolar macrophage from a nonsmoker. Numerous small lysosomes are present but relatively few heterophagic vacuoles are seen. (Micrograph courtesy of S. Pratt and A. J. Ladman.)

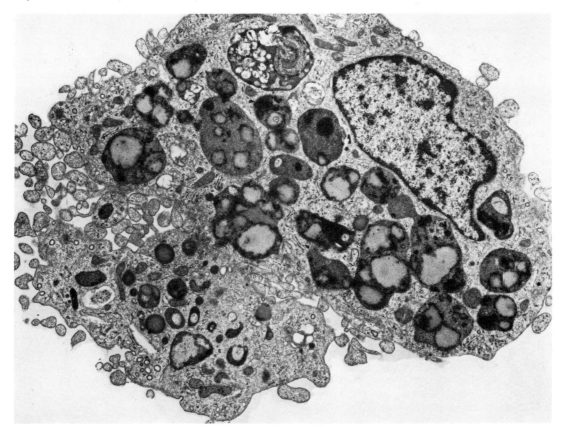

Figure 29–24. Electron micrograph of an alveolar macrophage from an 18-year-old cigarette smoker. The cytoplasm is crowded with pigment masses representing undigestible residues of material phagocytized from the alveoli. (Micrograph courtesy of S. Pratt and A. J. Ladman.)

In common with other phagocytes, the alveolar macrophages have receptors on their surface for IgG and the C3b component of complement. Their ability to ingest bacteria is enhanced in the presence of specific antibody. Intracellular destruction of bacteria is carried out by their phagolysosomal system supplemented by the generation of superoxide ion.

The alveolar macrophages form the first line of defense of the lungs and are remarkably efficient. Although large numbers of infectious organisms are continually carried into the lungs in the inspired air, the alveolar surface is usually sterile. Alveolar macrophages greatly outnumber all other cell types in the lung and are constantly being eliminated and replaced. They migrate or are passively transported from the alveolar surface to the bronchioles, and then are carried by ciliary action through the upper airways to the pharynx, where they mingle with salivary secretions and are swallowed. The mechanism of their directed movement to the bronchioles is not entirely clear, but the continuous production of surfactant and the transudation of fluid from the capillaries may form a moving surface film for transport of the macrophages. The number cleared from the lungs each day is astronomical. On the basis of counts of mononuclear cells in the respiratory fluid of cats with tracheal cannula, it has been estimated that the clearance rate is about 2×10^6 alveolar macrophages per hour. Comparable measurements for humans would no doubt give much higher numbers.

THE PLEURA

The cavities containing the lungs are lined by a serous membrane, the *pleura,* which consists of a thin layer of collagenous tissue containing some fibroblasts and macrophages and several prominent layers of elastic fibers. It is covered by a layer of mesothelial cells like those of the peritoneum. The layer lining the wall of the thoracic cavity is called the *parietal pleura;* that reflected over the surface of the lungs is the *visceral pleura.* A prominent feature of the pleura is the great number of blood capillaries and lymphatic vessels distributed in it. The few nerves of the parietal pleura are branches of the phrenic and intercostal nerves. The nerves to the visceral pleura are believed to be branches of the vagus and the sympathetic nerves supplying the bronchi.

INNERVATION OF THE LUNGS

The lung is innervated by parasympathetic nerves via the vagus nerve and by sympathetic nerves arising from the second to fourth thoracic sympathetic ganglia. These nerves form plexuses around the hilus of the lung and give rise to intrapulmonary nerves that accompany the ramifications of the bronchial tree and its associated blood vessels. Parasympathetic and sympathetic nerves to the lung contain both afferent and efferent fibers. The bronchoconstrictor fibers are from the vagus, and the bronchodilator fibers are sympathetic.

Both sensory and motor nerves have been identified extending as far peripherally as the terminal bronchioles. Light microscopic observations based on methylene blue and silver stains left some doubt as to whether the innervation of the lung extended beyond the respiratory bronchioles. Electron microscopic studies have now shown nerve endings in the alveolar ducts and alveolar walls of laboratory rodents and they probably also occur in humans. These endings are of two types. One located in the interstitium, and containing many small mitochondria, is considered to be sensory. It may possibly correspond to the juxtacapillary (J-type) receptor postulated by physiologists and believed to be stimulated by an increase in pulmonary capillary pressure. The second type of ending is of less common occurrence and contains many dense-cored vesicles. It is found in close association with Type II pneumonocytes and it is speculated that it may be the morphological basis for the reported effect of the nervous system on the secretion of pulmonary surfactant.

Neuroepithelial Bodies

Physiologists have long postulated the existence of chemoreceptors in the lung sensitive to the composition of the inhaled air. A morphological basis for this function has only recently been identified. Isolated groups of specialized cells are found throughout the epithelium lining the airways. These cells are selectively stained by silver salts (argentaffin reaction) and emit fluorescence at the wavelength characteristic of serotonin (5-hydroxytryptamine). These aggregations of cells have been called *neuroepithelial bodies*. They occur in the epithelium of bronchi, and distally to the terminal bronchioles, and seem to be preferentially located at or near sites of bifurcation. The groups of cells forming these bodies have the general shape of a truncated cone, 15 μm high with a rounded base 30 to 45 μm wide. The apex projects slightly above the surface of the surrounding bronchiolar epithelium.

In histological sections, the neuroepithelial bodies consist of two cell types—modified Clara cells that serve as supporting elements and 10 to 15 neurosecretory cells containing small granules in their basal cytoplasm. In electron micrographs, the apical pole of the secretory cells extends to the lumen, and bears numerous slender microvilli and occasionally a solitary cilium. The nucleus is large and indented, with the clumps of chromatin situated mainly at the periphery. The Golgi complex is supranuclear, and most mitochondria are in the apical cytoplasm. Granular endoplasmic reticulum is moderately extensive in the apical and paranuclear regions. Free ribosomes are abundant in the cytoplasmic matrix and there are a few granules of glycogen.

The most characteristic feature of the cells is the presence of small, dense-cored vesicles or granules throughout the cytoplasm, but most concentrated near the base. Their fluorescence, positive chromaffin reaction, and argentaffin staining leave little doubt that these granules contain serotonin. There is suggestive evidence that these cells may also synthesize or store other biologically active peptides, some of which may cause contraction of bronchiolar smooth muscle. The granules are released by exocytosis in response to hypoxia and hypercapnia. It is probably significant that the capillaries associated with the neuroepithelial bodies are fenestrated, while those elsewhere in the lamina propria of the bronchial tree are not.

It is believed that the neuroepithelial bodies are directly responsive to diminished oxygen content in the inspired air, releasing serotonin and possibly other mediators into the blood, thereby regulating alveolar capillary circulation and affecting the ventilation: perfusion ratio. The bodies appear to have a special innervation with unmyelinated afferent and efferent fibers ending among the neuroendocrine cells, as in other chemoreceptors such as the carotid body. The response of the neuroepithelial bodies may therefore be modulated by the central nervous system.

BLOOD SUPPLY

The lungs receive most of their blood from the pulmonary arteries. These are of large caliber and of elastic type. The branches of these arteries accompany the bronchi and their branches as far as the respiratory bronchioles. The arterial paths in the lung, however, are subject to considerable variation. From the respiratory bronchioles they divide, and a branch passes to each alveolar duct and is distributed in a capillary network over all the alveoli that communicate with this duct. The venules arise from the capillaries of the pleura and from the capillaries of the alveolar septa and portions of the alveolar ducts. They run in the intersegmental connective tissue, independently of the arteries, and join to form the pulmonary veins. In passing through the lung, the pulmonary artery is usually above and behind its accompanying bronchial tube, whereas the vein is below and in front of it. The bronchial arteries and veins are much smaller than the pulmonary vessels. These arteries arise from the aorta or the intercostal arteries and follow the bronchi. They are distributed to the walls of the bronchi, their glands, and the interlobular connective tissue beneath the pleura. Most of the blood carried by the bronchial arteries is brought back by the pulmonary veins. In the alveoli that arise from the respiratory bronchioles, there are capillary anastomoses between the terminations of the pulmonary and the bronchial arteries.

LYMPHATICS

There are two main divisions of the lymphatics of the lungs. One set is in the pleura and the other in the pulmonary tissue. They communicate infrequently. Both drain into the lymph nodes at the hilus of the lung. The lymphatics of the pleura form a dense network with large and small polygonal meshes. The large meshes are formed by large vessels and demarcate the lobules; the small meshwork is formed of smaller vessels that mark out the anatomical units. There are many valves in these lymphatics that control the flow of lymph so that it passes toward the hilus and not into the pulmonary tissue. These pleural lymphatics join to form several main trunks, which drain into the lymph nodes at the hilus.

The pulmonary lymphatics may be divided into several groups, which include those of the bronchi, of the pulmonary artery, and of the pulmonary vein. The lymphatics accompanying the bronchi extend peripherally as far as the alveolar ducts, and their end branches join the lymphatic radicles of the plexuses about the pulmonary artery and vein. There are no lymphatic vessels beyond the alveolar ducts. The pulmonary artery is accompanied by two or three main lymphatic trunks. The lymphatics associated with the pulmonary vein begin with its radicles in the alveolar ducts and in the pleura. All the lymphatics of the pulmonary tissue drain toward the hilar nodes. Efferent trunks from the hilar nodes anastomose to form the right lymphatic duct, which is the principal channel of lymph drainage from both the right and left lungs. There are no valves in the intrapulmonic lymphatics except in a few vessels, in the interlobular connective tissue near the pleura, which accompany the branches of the pulmonary veins. These lymphatic vessels connect the pulmonary and pleural lymphatic plexuses. As their valves point only toward the pleura, they provide a mechanism whereby lymph can flow from the pulmonary tissue into the pleural lymphatics if the normal flow of lymph from the pulmonary tissue toward the hilus is interrupted.

As mentioned, the mucosa of the bronchi is infiltrated with lymphocytes and often contains germinal centers. There are other accumulations of lymphatic tissue in the adventitia of the pulmonary arteries and veins.

HISTOPHYSIOLOGY OF THE RESPIRATORY TRACT

The functions of the nasal passages in warming, humidification, and filtration of the inspired air are often not fully appreciated. The mucous membrane lining the nasopharynx and covering the turbinates is richly vascularized and presents a large surface area. Air flowing over it is warmed and moistened before it reaches the trachea and lungs. The importance of the partial saturation of the air with water vapor during its passage through the nose is evident in patients with a tracheotomy who are obliged to take air directly into the trachea. Under these conditions, excessive drying of the mucosa may lead to encrustation, interference with clearance of the upper airway, and ultimately to serious infection. Similarly, if one nostril of a dog is surgically closed, the increased ventilation of the other side of the nasal cavity exceeds its humidifying capacity, and the drying effect may result in transformation of the ciliated columnar epithelium into stratified squamous epithelium—a phenomenon called *squamous metaplasia*.

The filtration of the inspired air during its passage through the nose is also important. Large particles are excluded by the coarse hairs in the external nares, while the smaller ones tend to be entrapped in the layer of mucus in the lining epithelium, which is continually moved by ciliary action toward the pharynx, where it is swallowed.

The clearing of the respiratory passages by coordinated beating of cilia on the lining epithelium also takes place in the paranasal sinuses and throughout the trachea and bronchi. The secretion of goblet cells and submucosal glands forms a coherent sheet of mucus covering the surface of the mucosa. Cilia constantly beating at about 14 cycles a second beneath it move this blanket of mucus at a speed of as much as 1 cm per minute, carrying adherent dust particles, bacteria, cellular debris, and adsorbed chemical pollutants toward the pharynx, where they are disposed of by swallowing. The physiological importance of ciliary activity is clearly demonstrated in those rare individuals who have the inherited condition known as *Kartagener's disease* or *immotile cilia syndrome*. Their genetic defect results in failure to synthesize dynein, the ATPase-containing protein that forms the "arms" on the microtubules of ciliary and flagellar axonemes (see Chapter 2). Since dynein is essential for conversion of the chemical energy in ATP to the mechanical work of microtubule sliding, males with this deficit have immotile spermatozoa and are infertile, and individuals of both sexes suffer from chronic sinusitis, chronic bronchitis, and bronchiectasis owing to the absence of motile cilia to clear their respiratory passages.

Another essential device for removal of particulate matter and irritant chemicals from the airway is the *cough reflex*. This depends on the presence of sensory nerve endings in the lining epithelium. Afferent impulses pass from these to the medulla in the central nervous system, triggering an automatic sequence of events that involves deep inspiration; closure of the epiglottis and vocal cords; and forceful contraction of abdominal and internal intercostal muscles that raises pressure on the air entrapped in the lungs. The epiglottis and larynx are then suddenly opened and the air under pressure bursts out, attaining velocities as high as 100 mph. The rush of air carries with it the irritant foreign matter, removing it from the trachea and bronchi. The *sneeze reflex* involves a similar train of events that results in clearance of the nasal passages.

The primary function of the lungs is, of course, to provide for assimilation of oxygen from the air and removal of carbon dioxide from the body. In inspiration, contraction of the diaphragm lowers intra-alveolar pressure, drawing air into the lungs. The network of blood capillaries in the walls of the alveoli is separated from the air by a very thin moist sheet of alveolar epithelium that permits rapid diffusion of oxygen into, and carbon dioxide out of, the blood. The exchange of gases takes place by passive diffusion, but the liberation of carbon dioxide from carbonic acid is accelerated about 5000-fold by the enzyme *carbonic anhydrase*, which resides in the red blood cells. In addition to gas exchange, there is a loss of approximately 800 ml of water a day in the expired air. Ether, other volatile anesthetics, and alcohol in the blood may also be eliminated via the lungs.

Expiration results from relaxation and elevation of the diaphragm, diminishing the size of the thorax. A significant component of expiration is attributable, however, to the inherent elastic properties of the lung. The parenchyma of the lung is rich in delicate extracellular elastic fibers that stretch during inspiration and recoil during expiration. In addition, intermolecular forces within the thin film of fluid on the alveolar lining maintain a surface tension that tends to reduce the surface area of the alveoli. Surface tension is responsible for about two thirds of the recoil of the lungs, and elastic fibers account for the rest. The resistance to alveolar expansion imposed by surface tension would be very much greater were it not for the secretion of surfactant by the Type II epithelial cells, which lowers surface tension and facilitates expansion. Deficiency of surfactant secretion occurs occasionally in the newborn, resulting in *respiratory distress syndrome* (*hyaline membrane disease*), a condition that often results in the death of the infant because of inadequate pulmonary ventilation.

Destruction of elastic fibers and diminished elastic recoil are prominent features of the pathophysiology of *emphysema*, a condition characterized by destructive changes in the alveolar walls, resulting in great enlargement of the air spaces distal to the terminal bronchioles and progressive inefficiency of gaseous exchange. A number of environmental factors, including cigarette smoking and air pollution, may contribute to the development of the disease. However, it may occur in certain susceptible individuals in the absence of these factors. Susceptible persons lack normal blood levels of α_1-antitrypsin, a versatile inhibitor of various proteases, including elastase. Such individuals may be unable to control the effects of hydrolytic enzymes released from the lysosomes of macrophages and granulocytes that accumulate in chronic pulmonary infections, and enzymatic destruction of the connective tissue framework of the alveolar wall then follows.

The lungs also have important nonrespiratory functions. Since the entire output of the heart passes through the lungs, the endothelium of the pulmonary vessels is favorably situated to metabolize or transform various substances that circulate in the blood. Although the endothelium of these vessels is morphologically identical to that of capillaries elsewhere in the body, it possesses distinctive enzymatic properties. It contains monoamine oxidase, which enables it to break down serotonin that is released into the blood by other organs. Enzymes that transform the vasoactive substance angiotensin I to angiotensin II, and enzymes that inactivate bradykinin, also have been demonstrated in pulmonary endothelium. These and other biologically active substances are metabolized almost completely in a single passage through the vascular bed of the lungs.

The lung can also be considered to have an endocrine function. In response to certain stimuli, it releases into the blood prostaglandins, histamine, slow-reactive substance of anaphylaxis, and other mediators. Thus, the lung is not merely concerned with exchange of gaseous metabolites, but also plays a significant role in control of the blood levels of many biologically active substances.

REFERENCES

GENERAL

Bertalanffy, F. D.: Respiratory tissue: Structure, histophysiology and cytodynamics. Int. Rev. Cytol. *16*:233, 1964.

Bryant, C.: The Biology of Respiration. Baltimore, University Park Press, 1979.

Comroe, J. H., Jr.: Physiology of Respiration. Chicago, Year Book Medical Publishers, 1974.

Heinemann, H. O., and A. P. Fishman: Nonrespiratory Functions of mammalian lung. Physiol. Rev. *49*:1, 1969.

Murray, J. F.: The Normal Lung. Philadelphia, W. B. Saunders Co., 1976.

Nagaishi, C.: Functional Anatomy and Histology of the Lung. Baltimore, University Park Press, 1973.

Thurlbeck, W. M. Structure of the lungs. Int. Rev. Physiol. *14*:1, 1977.

NOSE, PHARYNX, AND LARYNX

Allison, A. C.: The morphology of the olfactory system in the vertebrates. Biol. Rev. *28*:195, 1953.

Baker, M. A.: A brain-cooling system in mammals. Sci. Am. *240/5*:130, 1976.

Bojsen-Moller, F.: Glandulae nasales anteriores in the human nose. Ann. Otol. Rhinol. Laryngol. *74*:363, 1965.

Cauna, N.: Blood and nerve supply of the nasal lining p.45. *In* Procter, B. F., and I. Anderson, eds. The Nose: Upper Airway Physiology and the Atmospheric Environment. New York, Elsevier Biomedical Press, 1982.

Cauna, N., and K. H. Hinderer: Fine structure of the blood vessels of the human nasal respiratory mucosa. Ann. Otol. *78*:865, 1969.

Dovek, E.: The Sense of Smell and its Abnormalities. New York, Churchill Livingstone, 1974.

Fink, B. R.: The Human Larynx. A Functional Study. New York, Raven Books, Abelard-Schuman Ltd., 1975.

Reese, T. G.: Olfactory cilia in the frog. J. Cell Biol. *25*:209, 1965.

Swindle, P. F.: The architecture of the blood vascular networks in the erectile and secretory lining of the nasal passages. Ann. Otol. Rhinol. Laryngol. *144*:913, 1935.

TRACHEA, BRONCHI, AND BRONCHIOLES

Boyd, M. R.: Evidence for the Clara cell as a site of cytochrome P450-dependent mixed function oxidase activity in lung. Nature (Lond.) *269*:713, 1977.

Foliguet, B., and J. L. Cordonnier: Pulmonary neuroepithelial bodies. Bull. Europ. Physiopathol. Respir. *17*:113, 1981.

Hoyt, R. F., Jr., S. P. Sorokin, and H. Feldman: Number, subtypes, and distribution of small granule neuroendocrine cells in the infracardiac lobe of hamster lung. Exp. Lung Res. *3*:273, 1983.

Hung, K. S., M. S. Hertwick, J. D. Hardy, and C. L. Loosli: Ultrastructure of nerves and associated cells in bronchiolar epithelium of the mouse lung. J. Ultrastruct. Res. *43*:426, 1973.

Jeffery, P. K., and L. Reid: New observations of rat airway epithelium: a quantitative and electron microscopic study. J. Anat. *120*:295, 1975.

Lauweryns, J. M., and M. Cokelaere: Hypoxia-sensitive neuro-epithelial bodies. Intrapulmonary secretory neuro-receptors modulated by the CNS. Z. Zellforsch. *145*:521, 1973.

Lauweryns, J. M., M. Cokelaere, P. Theunynck, and M. Delearsnyder: Neuroepithelial bodies in mammalian

respiratory mucosa: light optical, histochemical and ultrastructural studies. Chest *65*:(Suppl) 22S, 1974.

Meyrick, B., J. M. Sturgess, and L. Reid: A reconstruction of the duct system and secretory tubules of human bronchial submucosal glands. Thorax *24*:729, 1969.

RESPIRATORY PORTION OF THE LUNG

Boyden, E. A.: The terminal air sacs and their blood supply in a 37-day infant lung. Am. J. Anat. *116*:413, 1965.

Boyden, E. A.: The structure of a pulmonary acinus in a child of 6 years. Anat. Rec. *169*:282, 1971.

Bradley, K. H., O. Kawanami, V. J. Ferrons, and R. G. Crystal: The fibroblast of human lung alveolar structures: a differentiated cell with a major role in lung structure and function. Methods Cell Biol. *21A*:38, 1980.

Gehr, P., M. Bachofen, and E. R. Weibel: The normal human lung: ultrastructure and morphometric estimation of diffusion capacity. Respir. Physiol. *32*:121, 1978.

Gehr, P., B. Siegwart, and E. R. Weibel: Allometric analysis of the morphometric pulmonary diffusing capacity in dogs. J. Morphol. *168*:5, 1981.

Gil, J.: Organization of the micro-circulation in the lung. Annu. Rev. Physiol. *42*:177, 1980.

Horsfield, K.: The relation between structure and function in the airways of the lung. Br. J. Dis. Chest *68*:145, 1974.

Hung, K. S., M. S. Hertwick, J. D. Hardy, and C. G. Loosli: Innervation of pulmonary alveoli of the mouse lung: an electron microscopic study. Am. J. Anat. *135*:477, 1972.

Ryan, U. S., J. W. Ryan, and D. S. Smith: Alveolar Type II cells: studies on the mode of release of lamellar bodies. Tissue Cell *7*:587, 1975.

Sorokin, S. P.: A morphologic and cytochemical study of the great alveolar cell. J. Histochem. Cytochem. *14*:884, 1967.

Tenny, S. M., and J. E. Remmers: Comparative quantitative morphology of the mammalian lung: diffusing area. Nature (Lond.) *197*:54, 1963.

Thurlbeck, W. M.: Structure of the lungs. Int. Rev. Physiol. *14*:1, 1977.

Weibel, E. R. Morphological basis of alveolar-capillary gas exchange. Physiol. Rev. *53*:419, 1973.

Weibel, E. R., P. Gehr, D. Haies, and J. Gil: The cell population of the normal lung. *In* Bouhuys, A., ed.: Lung Cells in Disease. Elsevier/North Holland Biomedical Press, 1976.

Williams, M. C.: Conversion of lamellar body membranes to tubular myelin in alveoli of fetal rat lung. J. Cell Biol. *72*:260, 1977.

PULMONARY MACROPHAGES AND MAST CELLS

Brain, J. D., J. J. Godleski, and S. P. Sorokin. Quantification, origin and fate of pulmonary macrophages. *In* Brain, J. D., D. F. Proctor, and L. Reid, eds.: Respiratory Disease Mechanisms. New York, Marcel Dekker, 1977, p. 849.

Hocking, W. G., and D. W. Golde: The pulmonary-alveolar macrophage. N. Engl. J. Med. *301*:580, 639, 1979.

Sorokin, G.: Phagocytes in the lungs: incidence, general behavior, and phylogeny. *In* Brain, J. D., D. F. Proctor, and L. Reid, eds.: Respiratory Disease Mechanisms. New York, Marcel Dekker, 1977, p. 711.

Wasserman, G. I.: The lung mast cell: its physiology and potential relevance to defense of the lung. Environ. Health Perspect. *35*:153, 1980.

30

THE URINARY SYSTEM

The urinary system consists of the kidneys, ureters, urinary bladder, and urethra. The system functions to clear the blood of the waste products of metabolism and to regulate the concentration of many constituents of the body fluids. In addition to their excretory function, the kidneys have an endocrine function—producing and releasing into the bloodstream a humoral agent that affects blood formation (erythropoietin) and another that influences blood pressure (renin). In the male, the urethra not only conveys the urine to the outside but also serves the reproductive system as the pathway for the discharge of semen.

KIDNEYS

The human kidneys are paired organs situated retroperitoneally on the posterior wall of the abdominal cavity on either side of the vertebral column. They are roughly bean-shaped, 10 to 12 cm in length, 5 to 6 cm in width, and 3 to 4 cm in thickness. A concavity, the *hilus,* is found on the medial border. The large excretory duct, the *ureter,* emerges from the hilus and courses downward to the urinary bladder, which is situated in the pelvis directly behind the pubis. The kidney is closely invested by a thin but strong capsule of dense collagenous fibers. The parenchyma of the kidney surrounds a large cavity, the *renal sinus,* that extends inward from the hilus and contains the *renal pelvis.* The remainder of the sinus around the renal pelvis is occupied by loose connective tissue and adipose tissue, through which the blood vessels and nerves pass into the renal tissue.

The renal pelvis is a funnel-shaped expansion of the upper end of the ureter, which sends into the substance of the kidney two or three sizable outpocketings called *major calyces.* These in turn have a number of smaller branches called *minor calyces* (Fig. 30–1).

When the cut surface of the hemisected kidney is viewed with the naked eye, a darker reddish brown *cortex* is readily distinguishable from a lighter *medulla.* The medulla is made up of 5 to 11 conical subdivisions called *renal pyramids,* each having its base toward the cortex and its apex or *papilla* projecting into the lumen of a minor calyx. The lateral boundaries of each pyramid are defined by inward extensions of the darker cortical tissue forming the *renal columns* (of Bertin). A renal pyramid together with the cortical tissue overlying its base and covering its sides constitutes a *renal lobe.* Each lobe of the human kidney corresponds to the entire unipyramidal kidney of common laboratory rodents. During embryonic development, each lobe arises in association with a different minor calyx, and during fetal life the several lobes are recognizable as distinct convexities on the surface of the organ, but later in development they fuse into a continuous smooth-contoured cortex.

The gray substance of each pyramid is radially striated with brownish lines that converge toward the apex of the papilla. These striations are a reflection of the orientation of the straight portions of the microscopic uriniferous tubules and of the blood vessels that course parallel to them. The tip of each papilla, called the *area cribrosa,* is perforated by about 25 small openings, where the terminal segments of the uriniferous tubules open into a minor calyx.

The myriad renal tubules that constitute the parenchyma of the kidney are specialized along their length for different functions, and each of the specialized segments tends to be located at a particular level. This consistency in distribution of corresponding segments is reflected in grossly distinguishable zones in the medulla, which differ slightly in color or pattern. There is an *inner* and *outer zone* of the medulla, and the outer zone is sometimes further subdivided into a darker and thicker *inner band* or *stripe* and a lighter and thinner *outer band.*

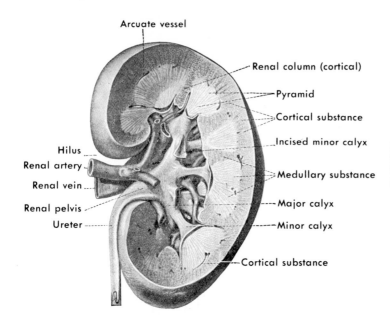

Arcuate vessel

Renal column (cortical)

Pyramid

Cortical substance

Incised minor calyx

Medullary substance

Major calyx

Minor calyx

Cortical substance

Hilus

Renal artery

Renal vein

Renal pelvis

Ureter

Figure 30–1. Human kidney, seen from behind, after removal of part of the organ. Three fifths natural size. (After Braus.)

From the bases of the medullary pyramids, thin, radially directed striations extend into the cortical substance. These bear some resemblance to the striations in the pyramid but do not extend through the entire thickness of the cortex. These markings are called the *medullary rays* (of Ferrein) and represent continuations of bundles of tubules from the pyramid into the cortex (Figs. 30–2, 30–3). Each medullary ray and its immediately associated cortical tissue are referred to as a *renal lobule,* although they are not separated from one another by connective tissue septa, as is often the case in lobules of other glands. The structural basis of the patterns that are visible on the cut surface of the normal kidney will be better understood after the description of the uriniferous tubules. It is sufficient here to note that recognition of these gross markings is not only an aid to understanding of the complex microscopic organization of this organ, but is also of practical value to the pathologist to the extent that loss or distortion of the normal pattern is associated with particular disease entities.

URINIFEROUS TUBULES

The tubules composing the kidney have two principal portions. The first portion, the *nephron,* corresponding to the secretory elements of other glands, is concerned with the formation of urine; the second portion, the *collecting tubule,* carries out a final concentration of urinary solutes to form a hypertonic

urine, and serves as the excretory duct conveying the urine to the renal pelvis. These two components arise in the embryo from separate primordia that become connected secondarily. This is in contrast to the devel-

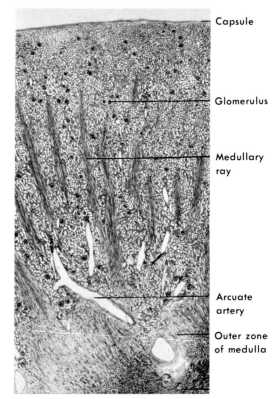

Capsule

Glomerulus

Medullary ray

Arcuate artery

Outer zone of medulla

Figure 30–2. Section of kidney of *Macacus rhesus.* Fixation by vascular perfusion—hence the empty blood vessels. Photomicrograph (slightly retouched). × 13.

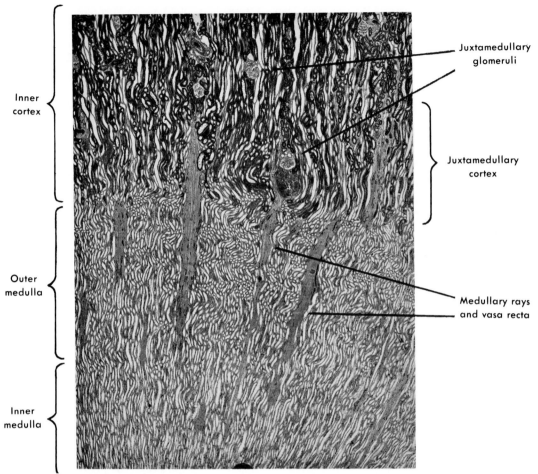

Figure 30–3. Section of dog kidney, showing medullary rays and vasa recta extending from juxtamedullary glomeruli to the border of the inner medulla. Mallory stain. × 30. (After Thorburn, W., et al. Circulation Res. *13*:290, 1963.)

opment of other glands, in which the ducts and secretory portions arise from a single primordium that branches dichotomously and becomes secretory in the distal part of its arborescent pattern.

The Nephron

The nephron is the tubular functional unit of this organ. There is estimated to be about two million in each kidney, and the output of urine represents a summation of the functions of this very large number of units. Along the length of the nephron are several morphologically distinct segments, each having a characteristic configuration and occupying a definite position in the cortex or medulla. Each segment is lined with a specific type of epithelium specialized for a particular role in the formation of urine.

At the proximal end of each is a thin-walled expansion called *Bowman's capsule,*

which is deeply indented by a globular tuft of capillaries, the *glomerulus* (Fig. 30–4). This mass of capillaries and its surrounding chalice-shaped epithelial capsule together constitute the *renal corpuscle*. It has a *vascular pole* where the afferent and efferent vessels enter and leave the glomerulus, and a *urinary pole* where the slitlike cavity within the capsule of Bowman is continuous with the lumen of the next segment of the nephron, the *proximal tubule* (Fig. 30–5). This segment consists of a convoluted and straight portion. The latter is followed by a *thin segment,* and this in turn by the straight and convoluted portions of the *distal tubule*. The convoluted portion of the proximal tubule *(proximal convoluted tubule)* and the convoluted portion of the distal tubule *(distal convoluted tubule)* are both located in the cortex close to the renal corpuscle. The portion of nephron between the two convoluted segments (namely, the straight portion of the proximal tubule, the thin seg-

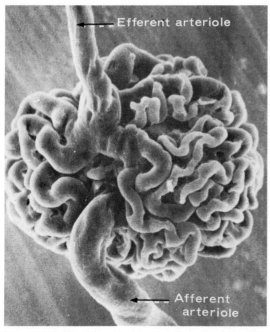
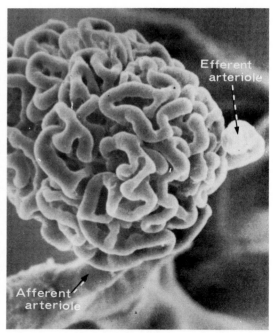

Figure 30–4. Scanning micrographs of plastic casts of two glomeruli. *Left,* viewed at the vascular pole; *right,* from the capsular side. Observe in both that the caliber of the efferent arteriole is smaller than that of the afferent arteriole. This no doubt ensures an adequate filtration pressure in the capillaries. (Micrographs from Takizawa, J., et al. Lab. Invest. *40*:519, 1979.)

ment, and the straight portion of the distal tubule) forms a loop, the *loop of Henle,* extending from the cortex for a variable distance into the medulla. The radially oriented descending and ascending limbs of the loop run parallel to each other and are connected by a sharp bend (Fig. 30–5). These several segments are represented in the same sequence in all nephrons, but the length of the loop and the proportions of the segments of which it is formed vary with the position of the glomerulus in the cortex. Nephrons whose glomeruli are in the outer or subcapsular portion of the cortex have short loops of Henle with abbreviated thin segments, and these loops extend only a very short distance into the outer zone of the medulla. Nephrons whose glomeruli are situated in the deep or juxtamedullary region of the cortex form a loop with long descending and ascending limbs and an extensive thin segment, which penetrates deep into the inner zone of the medulla. Nephrons with glomeruli midway in the cortex have intermediate characteristics. In addition, there are significant differences in the vascular supply to these three categories of nephrons. These will be described later. The distal convoluted tubules are joined to the collecting duct system by a short connecting segment, often referred to as the *arched collecting tubule* to distinguish it

from the radially oriented *straight collecting tubules.* The latter are continuous with the *papillary ducts,* which deliver urine to the minor calyces.

The tortuous convoluted tubules of neighboring nephrons in the cortex intermingle so extensively that the identity and shape of the individual units cannot be ascertained from study of histological sections. What is known of their three-dimensional configuration has been established by their reconstruction from serial sections or by maceration of the tissue and teasing out the individual nephrons by time-consuming micromanipulation. It has also been possible by micropuncture to penetrate individual glomerular capsules and to observe directly the progress of injected contrast media through the lumen of a single nephron.

The renal corpuscles have evolved as efficient ultrafiltering devices for clearing the blood of wastes. About 1200 ml of blood flows through the kidneys per minute and about one fifth of the plasma volume is filtered off in the renal corpuscles. Thus, about 120 ml of a fluid, called the *glomerular filtrate,* enters the renal tubules each minute. As this fluid passes through the various segments of the nephron, its composition is modified by secretion of certain substances into it and reabsorption of water and other constituents

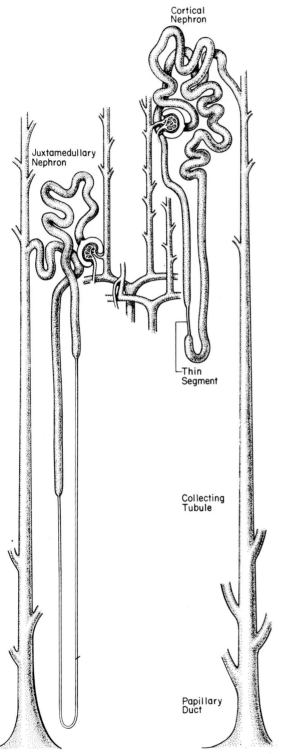

from it. The final product, *urine*, is drained through the collecting ducts into the renal pelvis.

Renal Corpuscle. The capsule of Bowman around the tuft of glomerular capillaries is a double-walled cup composed of squamous epithelium. Although not strictly true, it is conceptually useful to consider that in the embryonic development of the renal corpuscle, the glomerulus is pushed into, and deeply indents, a blind terminal expansion of the uriniferous tubule like a fist thrust into a balloon. From this mode of development it would follow that there is a *visceral layer* of epithelium (the *glomerular epithelium*) applied to the capillaries, as well as a *parietal layer* (the *capsular epithelium*). Between these is a narrow chalice-shaped cavity, the *capsular space* (Bowman's space). At the vascular pole of the renal corpuscle, the visceral layer is reflected off the afferent and efferent glomerular vessels to become continuous with the epithelium of the parietal layer. At the urinary pole, the squamous capsular epithelium is continuous with the cuboidal epithelium in the neck of the proximal convoluted tubule (Fig. 30–6).

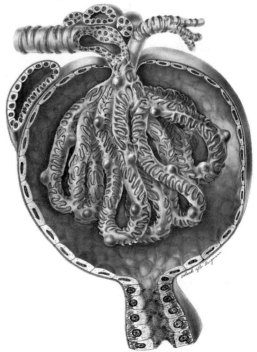

Figure 30–5. Highly schematic drawing of a cortical nephron and a juxtamedullary nephron, comparing the renal corpuscles, proximal convoluted tubules, straight descending portions of proximal tubule, thin segments, straight ascending portions of the distal tubule, distal convoluted tubules and collecting tubules. The cortical nephrons have a short loop of Henle with a very short thin segment, whereas these structures are long and extend deep into the medulla in juxtamedullary nephrons.

Figure 30–6. Highly schematic representation of the renal corpuscle. The parietal layer of Bowman's capsule is depicted considerably thicker than it actually is, and the visceral layer overlying the capillaries of the glomerulus is greatly simplified, with only the major processes of the podocytes depicted. Although earlier described as a cluster of simple loops, the capillaries are now believed to branch and anastomose to form a network. (Redrawn and modified after Bargmann.)

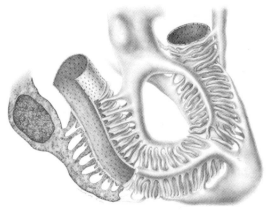

Figure 30–7. Highly schematic representation of the interdigitating pattern of secondary processes (foot processes or pedicels) of the podocytes on the outer surface of a glomerular capillary loop. This arrangement provides a very large area of slender filtration slits or slit pores between adjacent processes. (Redrawn and modified after Gordon. *In* Ham, A. W.: Histology. 5th ed. Philadelphia, J. B. Lippincott Co., 1965.)

In the development of the renal corpuscle, the parietal layer remains a typical squamous epithelium of flat polygonal cells, but the cells of the visceral layer become so extensively modified that, in the adult, they bear little resemblance to any other epithelial cells. These cells, called *podocytes*, are closely applied to the capillaries and are basically stellate, with several radiating *primary processes* that embrace the vessels in a manner reminiscent of the pericytes of other capillaries (Fig. 30–7). The primary processes give rise to very numerous *secondary processes*, also called *foot processes* or *pedicels*. These interdigitate with corresponding elements of neighboring podocytes to create an extraordinarily elaborate system of intercellular clefts, called *filtration slits* (Figs. 30–8, 30–9).

In thin sections examined with the electron microscope, the cell bodies of the podocytes are rarely found in extensive contact with the basal lamina. Instead, they stand off 1 or 2 μm and are attached to it via their primary and secondary processes, which ramify over the surface of the basal lamina. The cell body and major processes of one podocyte may arch over undermining primary processes of neighboring podocytes (Fig. 30–9). As a consequence of these relationships, the greater

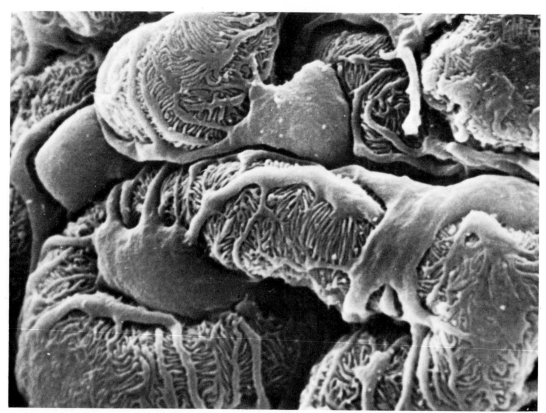

Figure 30–8. Scanning electron micrograph of a small area of the glomerulus, showing the visceral epithelium, consisting of podocytes with their interdigitating processes forming an elaborate filigree around the cylindrical capillaries. (Micrograph courtesy of F. Spinelli, Ciba-Geigy Ltd. Research Laboratories, Basle, Switzerland.)

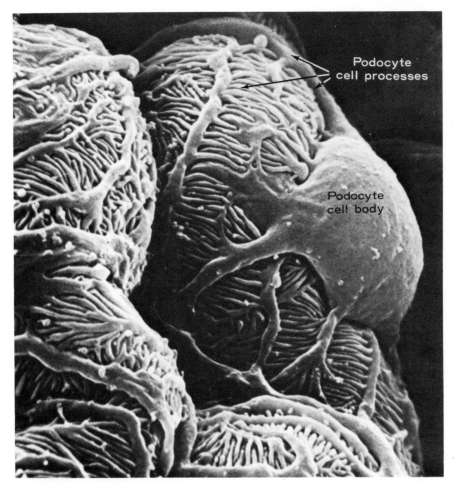

Figure 30–9. Scanning micrograph of two adjacent capillary loops of rat glomerulus, illustrating the remarkable complexity of the primary and secondary processes of the podocytes, whose ramification and interdigitation leaves an enormous area of filtration slits through which the glomerular filtrate passes into the capsular space. (Micrograph courtesy of F. Spinelli, Ciba-Geigy Ltd. Research Laboratories, Basle, Switzerland.)

part of the capsular surface of the glomerular capillaries is carpeted by interdigitating foot processes, thus providing a maximal area of slit pores for filtration. By laborious study of thin sections with the transmission electron microscope and imaginative reconstruction, students of renal cytology have ventured to depict the three-dimensional configuration of the podocytes, as shown in Figures 30–6 and 30–7. With the scanning elecron microscope, it is now possible to obtain three dimensional images of the cellular topography of this remarkably specialized epithelium. Its actual complexity (Figs. 30–8, 30–9) far exceeds the most daring earlier interpretations of its structure based on conventional light and electron microscopy.

Demonstration of the cytology of the podocytes and the finer details of the filtration barrier requires the higher resolution available in transmission electron micrographs. The podocytes have nuclei of complex form, often deeply infolded. Their cytoplasm contains a well-developed Golgi complex, cisternal profiles of granular endoplasmic reticulum and abundant free ribosomes. Cytoplasmic filaments and microtubules are plentiful, both in the cell body and in the primary and secondary processes. The foot processes are aligned upon the outer surface of a thick basal lamina, which they share with the endothelium of the underlying glomerular capillary (Fig. 30–12). Adjacent processes are not in contact but are separated by filtration slits about 25 nm wide. The plasma membrane of the foot processes has a prominent surface coat, or glycocalyx, that stains intensely with ruthenium red and osmium

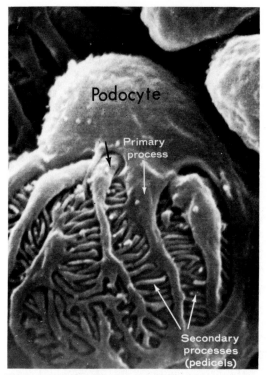

Figure 30–10. Scanning micrograph showing the relationship of primary processes and small secondary processes of the podocytes, called pedicels. Notice that the cell body of the podocyte may be elevated from the capillary surface, and processes of a neighboring podocyte may extend under it *(at arrow)* to interdigitate with its own pedicels. (Micrograph courtesy of F. Spinelli, Ciba-Geigy Ltd. Research Laboratories, Basle, Switzerland.)

tetroxide owing to its sialic acid content. In the living state, the 1- to 2.5-nm filamentous molecules forming the surface coat of adjacent foot processes largely fill the filtration slits. At the outer edge of the basal lamina, the slits are bridged by a thin *slit diaphragm* 4 to 6 nm in thickness (Fig. 30–13) extending between the membranes of adjacent foot processes.

The basal lamina is 0.1 to 0.15 μm in thickness and consists of three zones of differing electron density: the *lamina rara externa,* adjacent to the epithelium; the *lamina rara interna,* adjacent to the capillary endothelium; and a denser central zone, the *lamina densa.* In routine electron micrographs, the basal lamina shows little resolvable substructure, but when it is stained with ruthenium red or exposed to cationized ferritin, a pattern of regularly spaced densities is observed in the laminae externa and interna, and the density of the lamina densa is en-

hanced. Fine filaments appear to connect the densities to the membranes of the epithelium and endothelium, respectively. Similar discrete binding sites for cationic molecules are seen between other epithelia and endothelia and their basal lamina. It is speculated that these sites may play a role in attachment of the cells to the meshwork of macromolecules of Type IV collagen and proteoglycans that make up the basal lamina. A major glycosaminoglycan of the glomerulus is heparan sulfate, which contributes to the strongly anionic properties of its basal laminae, together with the carboxyl groups of collagenous and noncollagenous glycoproteins.

The endothelium of glomerular capillaries is quite thin and is perforated by pores or fenestrae 70 to 90 nm in diameter. In other fenestrated endothelia, the pores have a thin-pore diaphragm. This is not present in glomerular endothelium. The abundance and distribution of endothelial pores are best seen in the extended *en face* views provided by the freeze-fracture method of specimen preparation (Fig. 30–14). The thicker portions of the endothelial cells containing the nucleus are usually on the side of the capillary away from the capsular space.

The intercapillary spaces of the glomerulus that radiate from its hilus are occupied by the *mesangium,* consisting of *mesangial cells* and an extracellular matrix resembling the material of basal laminae. The mesangial cells are stellate in form and have a number of cytological characeristics in common with the pericytes of other capillaries, but these cells are phagocytic. It is believed that they are involved in maintenance of the basal lamina of the glomerular capillaries, removing and disposing of residues of filtration. They probably also participate in its turnover by removal of the older deep portions of the basal lamina as it is renewed at the epithelial surface.

The ultrafiltration of blood plasma in the renal glomeruli is of fundamental importance in the control of the extracellular fluid volume, plasma volume, cardiac output, and systemic blood pressure. The structural components of the *filtration barrier* between blood flowing through the glomerular capillaries and the capsular space consist of (1) the fenestrated endothelium, (2) the basal lamina, and (3) the filtration slits between the interdigitating foot processes of the podocytes (Fig. 30–13). Which of these components is the primary filter serving to retain

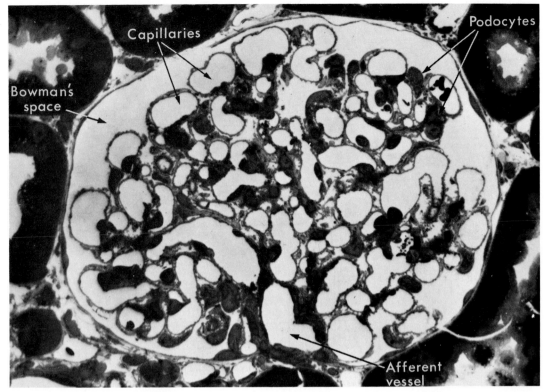

Figure 30–11. A thin plastic section of a renal corpuscle from a rat kidney fixed by perfusion and showing the open lumens of the capillaries. The irregularity of their outer surface is due to the sections of podocyte processes on their exterior. × 700. (Courtesy of A. Aoki.)

plasma proteins in the circulation has been a subject of debate. Experiments using electron-dense particulate tracers of differing molecular weight led some investigators to conclude that the basal lamina was only a course prefilter and that the filtration slits were the most significant barrier. Others regarded the basal lamina as the critical barrier. Additional experimental evidence using particulate tracers has provided strong support for the basal lamina as the main barrier to passage of molecules in the same size range as plasma proteins (32,000 to 125,000 M.W.). The filtration depends not only on the size and shape of the molecules retained but on their charge, with cationic molecules binding firmly to anionic binding sites in the basal lamina. The prevailing view of the functions of the structural components of the glomerulus is that the basal lamina is the main filter; the endothelial fenestrae act only as a coarse sieve holding back the formed elements of the blood and controlling access of its macromolecular constituents to the filter; and the mesangium serves to unclog and recondition the filter by phagocytosing and disposing of filtration residues that accumulate against it.

The Proximal Tubule. At the urinary pole of the renal corpuscle, the squamous parietal epithelium of Bowman's capsule is continuous with the cuboidal epithelium of the proximal tubule (Fig. 30–6). This segment of the nephron is about 14 mm long and 60 μm in diameter. The proximal convoluted tubules make up the bulk of the renal cortex. Each is composed of a convoluted portion (*pars convoluta*) and a straight portion (*pars recta*). In addition to many small loops, the convoluted portion usually forms a large loop directed toward the kidney capsule. The recurrent limb of this loop returns to the vicinity of the renal corpuscle and then courses toward the nearest medullary ray, where it straightens out to become the pars recta, running inward toward the medulla.

The epithelium of the proximal convoluted tubule consists of a single layer of cells with a conspicuous brush border on their luminal surface. In kidney tissue fixed by routine methods, the lumen of the proximal tubule is often occluded by the apposition of the

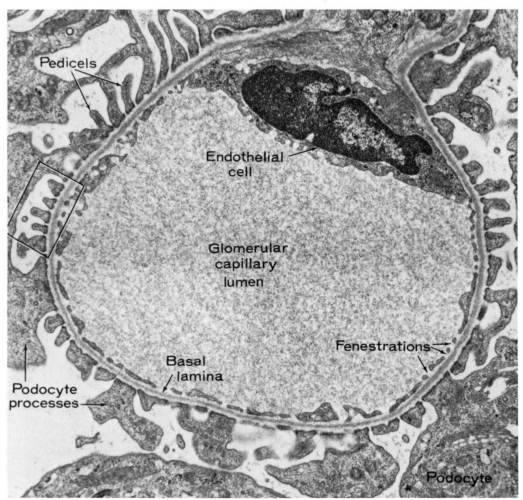

Figure 30–12. Transmission electron micrograph of a transverse section of a glomerular capillary, showing its basal lamina interposed between the fenestrated capillary endothelium on the inside and the slit pores between pedicels of the visceral epithelium on the outside. An area comparable with that in the rectangle is shown at higher magnification in Figure 30–13. (Micrograph from Tyson, G., and R. Bulger. Anat. Rec. *172*:669, 1972).

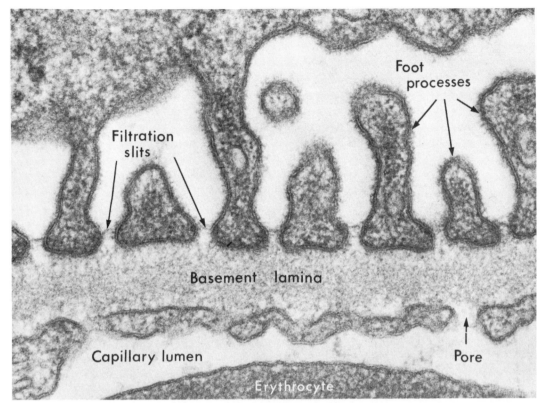

Figure 30–13. Electron micrograph of a portion of the wall of a glomerular capillary, showing pores in the extremely attenuated endothelium. On the outer surface of the basal (basement) lamina are the foot processes of the podocytes, with the narrow filtration slits between them. × 70,000. (Courtesy of D. Friend.)

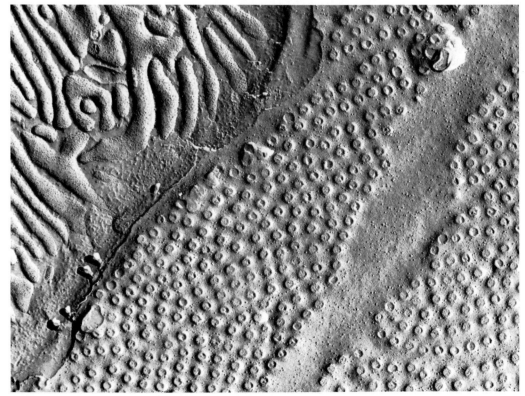

Figure 30–14. Freeze-cleaving preparation of rat kidney glomerulus. At right, the membrane of the endothelium of a capillary has been cleaved, showing the very uniform size and regular distribution of the endothelial pores. At upper left, the membranes of a number of pedicels on the outer aspect of the capillary have been cleaved. (Micrograph courtesy of D. Goodenough.)

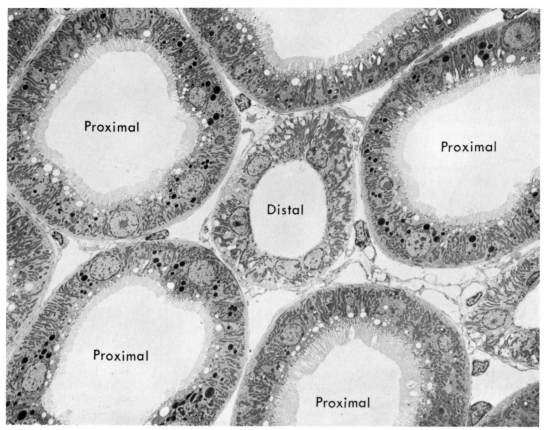

Figure 30–15. Low-magnification electron micrograph from the cortex of rat kidney fixed by vascular perfusion. The field includes five proximal convoluted tubules in transverse section, showing their open lumen and prominent brush border. Two distinct segments of the proximal convolution can be recognized. The first portion has a deeper brush border (section at *lower right*). The second portion has a thinner brush border and prominent dense bodies in the cytoplasm (other three labeled sections). × 2000. (After Maunsbach, A. J. Ultrastruct. Res. *15*:252, 1966.)

brush borders of the surrounding cells. It was formerly thought that this was the normal condition, and that the glomerular filtrate might percolate through the interstices among the microvilli of the brush borders. It is now known that this constriction of the tubules and obliteration of the lumen is an artifact. If the fixative is dripped onto the surface of the living kidney, or if the organ is perfused under conditions that involve no agonal fall of blood pressure, all the proximal tubules will have a wide open lumen (Figs. 30–15, 30–16). Each proximal tubule cell contains a single spherical nucleus in an eosinophilic cytoplasm. In cytological preparations, the Golgi apparatus forms a crown around the upper pole of the nucleus, and long rodlike mitochondria in the basal half of the cell tend to be oriented parallel to the cell axis. In well-preserved tissues, this orientation of the mitochondria may result in a faint vertical striation of the cell base, even without special staining of the mitochondria. The lateral limits of the cells are rarely resolved with the light microscope because their sides are elaborately fluted and deeply interdigitated with complementary ridges and grooves on the neighboring cells. In favorable preparations, affording surface views of the epithelium, some of the major interdigitations of the cell surfaces can be seen, but the true complexity of the shape of these cells can only be appreciated by careful study of electron micrographs. There are columnar lateral ridges that extend the full height of the cell. An even greater number of slender lateral processes near the cell base extend under adjacent cells (Fig. 30–17). The resulting compartmentation of the base of the epithelium seen in micrographs of thin sections was originally attributed to a simple infolding of the basal plasma membrane. However, most of the membrane-bounded basal compartments seen in micrographs are

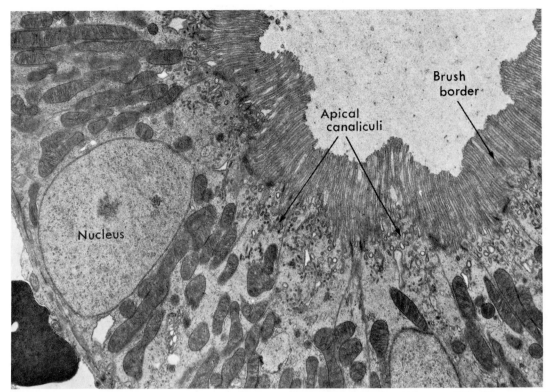

Figure 30–16. Electron micrograph of a sector of the wall of a proximal tubule of rat kidney. × 6000. (Courtesy of R. Bulger.)

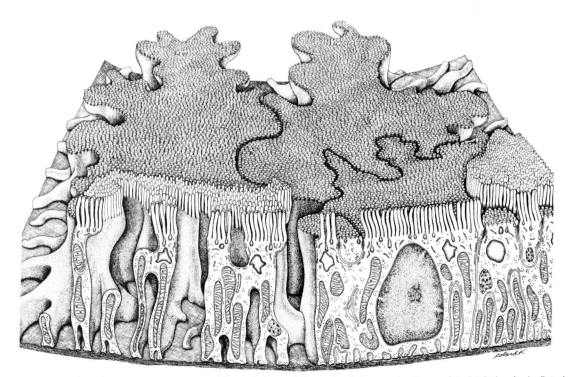

Figure 30–17. Drawing of the shapes and interrelations of the cells of the proximal convoluted tubule. As in fluted columns, some of the interdigitated lateral processes extend the full height of the cell; others are confined to the base and extend beneath adjacent cells. (After Bulger, R. Am. J. Anat. *116*:237, 1965.)

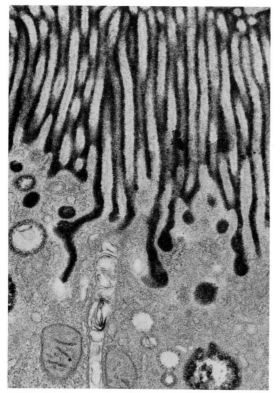

Figure 30–18. Electron micrograph of a portion of the brush border of the proximal convoluted tubule a few seconds after intravenous injection of myoglobin. The myoglobin has passed into the glomerular filtrate and appears between the microvilli and in the apical canaliculi. It is also present in vacuoles in the apical cytoplasm. (Micrograph courtesy of W. Anderson.)

cytoplasm are numerous tubular invaginations called *apical canaliculi* (Fig. 30–18). The membrane lining them has a conspicuous surface coat and short spiny projections into the cytoplasm as on the membrane of coated vesicles in other cell types. Vacuoles are also found in the apical cytoplasm, often in close relationship to the ends of the apical canaliculi. Some of these have a content of appreciable density and stain with histochemical reactions for acid phosphatase, indicating that they are secondary lysosomes. It is well established that albumen and other small proteins that are not retained by the glomerular filter are absorbed by the proximal convoluted tubule. The apical canaliculi and associated vacuoles are involved in endocytotic uptake of protein and its transport to lysosomes for intracellular digestion. When uptake of protein in the proximal convoluted tubules is experimentally suppressed by administration of certain positively charged dibasic amino acids (lysine, arginine), there is a marked increase in the protein content of the urine.

A very rapid degradation of small peptides to amino acids has also been demonstrated in the proximal tubule. This is not attributable to endocytosis and lysosomal hydrolysis, but probably occurs at the luminal surface through the action of peptidases in the membrane of the brush border. This mechanism is thought to be important in (1) conservation of amino acids, (2) inactivation of toxic peptides, and (3) regulation of circulating levels of small peptide hormones.

In addition to uptake of proteins and amino acids, the proximal tubule reabsorbs nearly all the glucose in the glomerular filtrate and certain essential vitamins, while allowing waste products and substances of no nutritional value to be excreted in the urine.

Although the entire length of the proximal tubule seems to have much the same structure in ordinary histological preparations and has customarily been divided, on the basis of macroscopic criteria, into the convoluted portion and the straight portion, these designations do not adequately express the structural and functional heterogeneity found along the length of this portion of the tubule. Three ultrastructurally distinct segments (S_1, S_2, and S_3) are identifiable in the proximal tubule of all the mammals studied to date, and their distribution does not consistently conform to the division into pars convoluta and pars recta. Cells in S_1 are taller than in the other two segments, and the basal and lateral inter-

not open at any point to the cytoplasm of the overlying cell. It is clear, therefore, that many of them are, in fact, sections of undermining basal processes of neighboring cells. In addition to the basal processes, there are smaller lateral processes that are confined to the juxtaluminal region of the epithelium.

The elaborate interdigitation of the lateral and basal portions of the cells greatly amplifies the area of the cell surface exposed to a labyrinthine system of intercellular clefts. This region of the cell membrane is rich in $Na^+ + K^+ - ATPase$ and is the site of active pumping of sodium out of the cell to create the electrochemical gradient responsible for movement of water and solute from the tubule lumen to the peritubular capillaries.

At the cell apex, the thousands of microvilli forming the brush border are long, regularly oriented and closely packed, increasing the surface area exposed to lumen more than 20-fold. Arising from the clefts between the microvilli and extending downward into the digitation of adjacent cells is extensive. The apical canaliculi and endocytosis vesicles are more conspicuous and the number of mitochondria and compartmentation of the base of the epithelium are greater than in succeeding segments. In S_2, the cell height is lower, mitochondrial length and number are lower, and interdigitation with adjacent cells is less. The cells of S_3 are cuboidal and have only a few small basal interdigitations, and the mitochondria are fewer and randomly oriented. All three segments have a prominent brush border, but the microvilli are noticeably longer in S_3.

The Thin Segment. The *loop of Henle* consists of the straight portion of the proximal tubule, the thin segment, and the ascending straight portion of the distal tubule. In the outer zone of the medulla, the descending portion of the proximal tubule abruptly narrows from a width of about 60 μm to continue as the *thin segment,* about 15 μm in diameter (Fig. 30–19). The epithelium changes from cuboidal to squamous, with a height of only 0.5 to 2 μm. There is a sudden termination of the brush border, which gives

way to very sparse, irregularly oriented, short microvilli on the luminal surface of the thin segment. The nuclei cause the central portions of the cells to bulge into the lumen. Owing to the small caliber of the tubule, its thin wall, and the bulging of the perikaryon into the lumen, the thin segment of Henle's loop in cross section bears a superficial resemblance to a capillary or venule (Fig. 30–20).

The mammalian kidney usually contains short-looped nephrons and long-looped nephrons (Figs. 30–5, 30–21). The short loop of Henle has a *descending thin limb* that is continuous at the flexure with the ascending straight portion of the distal tubule, but has no ascending thin limb. The long loop consists of a descending thin limb and an *ascending thin limb.* The thin limbs of the loop are lined by epithelium that exhibits marked regional differentiations in its ultrastructure. Four structurally distinct segments are recognizable (Fig. 30–21). Type I, characteristic of the abbreviated thin limb of the short loop, is a very simple flat epithelium with no interdigitation of neighboring cells. Its zonulae occludentes consist of two to four anas-

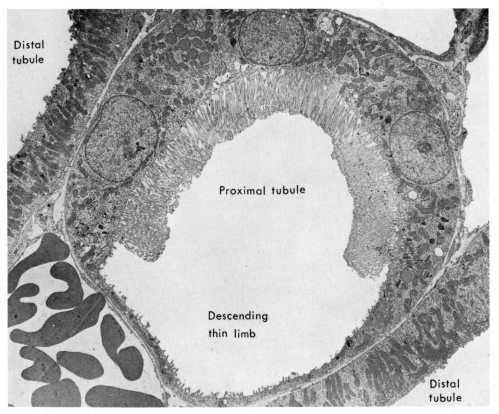

Figure 30–19. Electron micrograph of the abrupt junction of the straight portion of the proximal tubule with the thin limb of the loop of Henle. Slightly oblique section through the junction. The brush border stops suddenly and the epithelium becomes very thin. × 4200. (After Osvaldo and Latta. J. Ultrastruct. Res. *15:*144, 1966.)

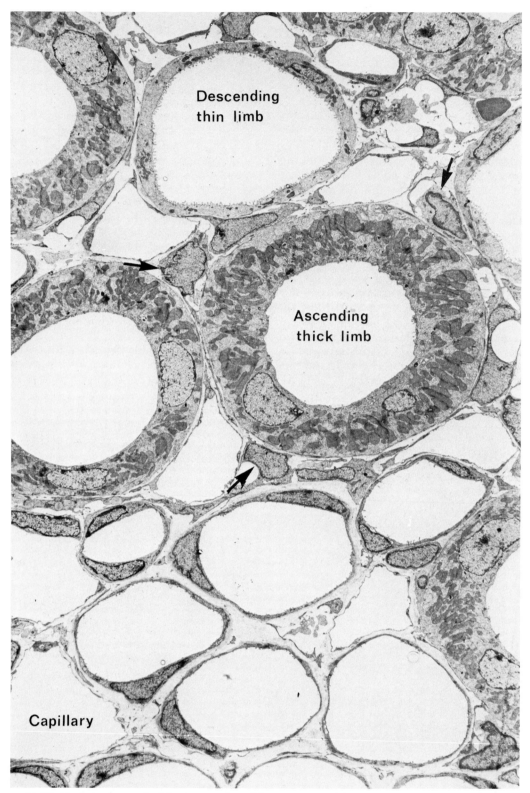

Figure 30–20. Electron micrograph of the inner portion of the outer zone of the medulla in rat kidney. Descending thin and ascending thick limbs of the loop of Henle are seen above, and capillaries of the vascular bundle below. Note that the endothelium in the descending arterial limb of the capillary loops is continuous, while that of the ascending venous limb is fenestrated. Interstitial cells are indicated by arrows. (Micrograph from Bohman, S.-O. J. Ultrastruct. Res. 47:329, 1974.)

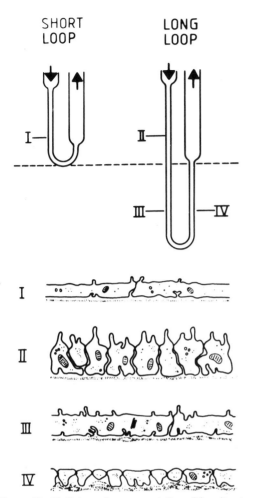

SHORT LOOP

LONG LOOP

I

II

III — IV

I

II

III

IV

Figure 30–21. Schematic representation of the ultrastructural features of the epithelium of the thin limb of the loop of Henle in its several segments. Nuclear region of the cells is not drawn. (Modified after Kriz, W., et al. *In* Maunbach, A. L., et al., eds.: Functional Ultrastructure of the Kidney. London, Academic Press, 1980.)

tional strands in freeze-fracture preparations.

There is a gradual simplification of the epithelium as the loop descends to the inner portion of the medullary pyramid. There the Type III epithelium is again composed of flat, noninterdigitating cells with several strands in their occluding junctions. In the ascending thin limb, Type IV epithelium is thin and again has elaborately interdigitated cell processes and very few microvilli. The shallow junctions consist of only one or two strands.

The segmental differentiation of the thin region of the loop of Henle is as described above in the common laboratory rodents, but differs significantly in lagomorphs and felidae. It has been studied in less detail in the human, but comparable differences are found in the height of the epithelium and the degree of interdigitation of the cells in the descending and ascending portions of the long loops.

In rats and certain other species whose kidneys have a single pyramid, the corresponding segments of the loops tend to be in register. As mentioned earlier, this regularity of arrangement is reflected in a zonation within the medulla that is detectable on naked eye inspection of the cut surface. An *outer* and *inner zone of the medulla* can be recognized, and an *inner* and *outer band* or *stripe* are distinguishable within the outer zone of the medulla. In these species, the boundary between the outer and inner band of the outer medulla is at the junctions of the straight portion of the proximal tubules with the descending thin limbs of Henle's loops. The transition between the inner and outer medulla is at the junctions of the ascending thin limbs with the ascending straight portion of the distal tubule. The inner medulla therefore contains collecting tubules, thin limbs of the loop of Henle, and blood vessels (Figs. 30–22*B*, 30–23).

In the human, a similar zonation of the medulla is detectable, though less easily, because the loops of Henle are of different lengths, depending on the position of their renal corpuscle in the cortex and the length of their thin segment (Fig. 30–5). The short loops are associated with the renal corpuscles located nearer the surface of the kidney. Loops of this type are about seven times as numerous as the long ones. Their bend, which is distal to the thin segment, is located in the outer part of the medulla and is formed by the thick ascending limb. The thin

tomosing junctional strands. In the outer portion of the descending thin limb of long loops, the Type II epithelium is somewhat higher and has numerous microvilli on its luminal surface. In micrographs of thin sections, typical cellular units containing a nucleus make up only a small portion of the wall. Most of the wall is composed of small membrane-bounded profiles 1 to 3 μm across, separated from one another by intermembranous clefts extending from the basal lamina to the lumen. These short anucleate units of the epithelium are sections through deeply interdigitating processes of adjacent cells. Some contain one or two mitochondria; others are largely devoid of organelles. They are attached to one another by juxtaluminal zonulae occludentes having one or two junc-

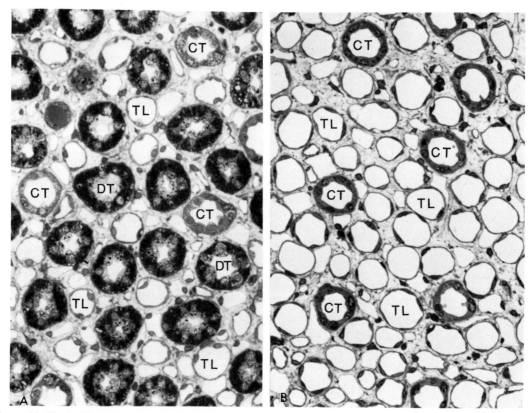

Figure 30–22. *A*, Photomicrograph of a transverse section through the outer medulla, which is composed of thin segments (TL) ascending straight portions of distal tubules (DT), and collecting tubules (CT). *B*, Transverse section through the inner medulla, composed of thin limb (TL) of the loop of Henle and collecting tubules (CT).

segment is in the descending limb of the loop and may be very short or in some instances may even be absent. In the latter event, the straight descending portion of the proximal tubule continues directly into the thick ascending limb. In the longer loops, which are associated with the deeper-lying juxtamedullary renal corpuscles, the bend is formed by the thin limb. These long loops may extend nearly to the apex of the papilla. In this event, the length of the thin limb may be 10 mm or even more.

The junction of the outer and inner zones of the medulla is marked by the transition of the thin limb to the ascending thick limb of the long loops of Henle. The boundary between the outer and inner bands of the outer medulla in the human kidney is somewhat obscured by the prevalence in this region of short loops having the junctions between their successive segments at different levels.

The Distal Tubule. The distal tubule is shorter and somewhat thinner than the prox-imal tubule and is composed of three parts: the straight portion *(pars recta);* the portion adjacent to the renal corpuscle, containing the macula densa *(pars maculata);* and the convoluted portion *(pars convoluta).* The straight portion begins in the inner band of the outer zone of the medulla and constitutes the ascending thick limb of the loop of Henle. The transition from the thin segment to the ascending limb of the distal tubule is abrupt. The epithelium is cuboidal, but the lumen is generally wider than that of the proximal tubule. A typical brush border is lacking. Some cells have numerous microvilli, while others have a smooth luminal surface except near the cell margins, where a few microvilli are found. These smooth-surfaced cells predominate in the medullary segment of the distal tubule. The apical vesicles and canaliculi characteristic of the proximal tubule are absent in the distal tubule. The base of the epithelium is elaborately compartmentalized by infoldings of the basal membrane that

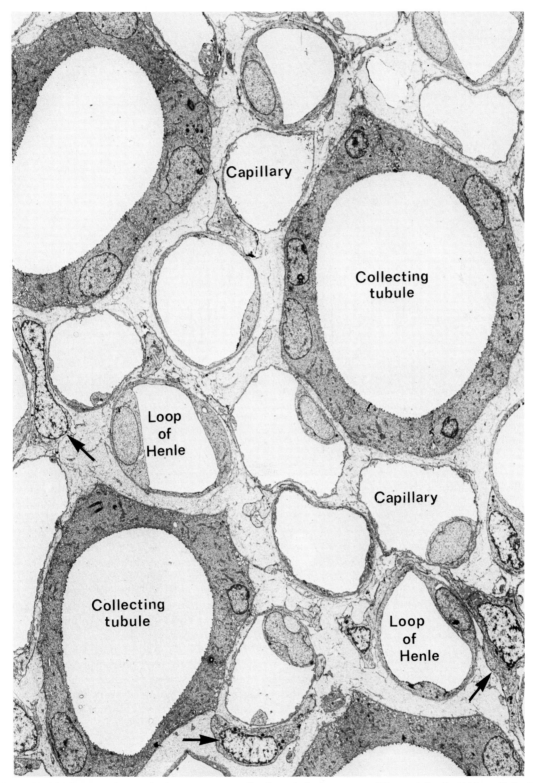

Figure 30–23. Electron micrograph of a transverse section through the inner zone of the medulla of rat kidney. Collecting tubules, loops of Henle, and capillaries are seen in cross section surrounded by an interstitium with a homogeneous extracellular matrix of low electron density. (Micrograph from Bohman, S.-O. J. Ultrastruct. Res. *47*:329, 1974.)

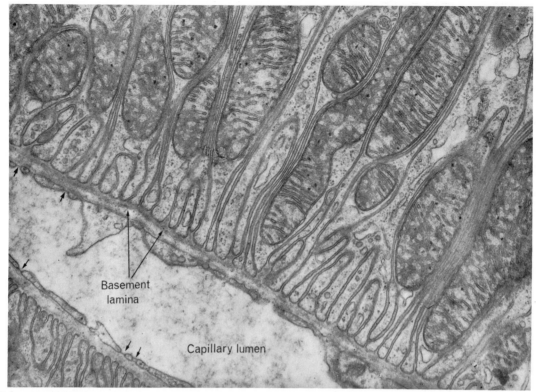

Basement
lamina

Capillary lumen

Figure 30–24. Electron micrograph of a portion of the base of a distal convoluted tubule of guinea pig kidney, illustrating the small and large basal compartments. The latter contain long mitochondria oriented perpendicular to the cell base. Notice that the peritubular capillary is of the fenestrated type with several of its pores indicated by arrows. (Courtesy of A. Ichikawa.)

make deep incursions into the cell (Fig. 30–24). In addition, there are undermining basal processes of neighboring cells comparable with those described for the proximal tubule. Long mitochondria are lodged in these basal compartments, and their orientation parallel to the axis of the cell results in the prominent striation of the basal cytoplasm observed with the light microscope. The mitochondria have many cristae and numerous matrix granules. The Golgi complex is small and forms a crown around the upper pole of the nucleus. There are a few cisternal profiles of granular endoplasmic reticulum and a moderate number of free ribosomes. A pair of centrioles is located in the apical cytoplasm, and from one of these a single flagellum projects into the lumen.

The junctional complexes between cells are shallow and permeable to lanthanum. This finding, together with the relatively low transepithelial electrical resistance, suggests that there is a functional paracellular pathway for solute and water movement across the epithelium in addition to the high-resistance transcellular pathway.

The thick ascending limb of Henle's loop or straight portion of the distal tubule enters the cortical tissue, returns to the renal corpuscle of the same nephron, and attaches to its vascular pole, particularly to the afferent arteriole. The side of the tubule in contact with the afferent arteriole forms an elliptical disc of taller cells measuring 40 by 70 μm in the human kidney. This area, called the *macula densa* has been reported to have some function in the hemodynamics of the kidney, but its precise role has not been defined. From here the straight portion continues as the convoluted portion of the distal tubule. This portion of the tubule has many short loops and irregular contortions. It usually courses toward the surface above the corresponding renal corpuscle.

Collecting Ducts

The connections of the nephrons with the collecting tubules are located in the cortex of the kidney along medullary rays. The distal tubules are continuous with *arched collecting tubules*, which are tributaries of straight collecting tubules located in the medullary rays. The collecting tubules pass inward in the medullary ray, through the outer zone of the medulla. When they reach the inner zone, they join at acute angles with other, similar tubules. There are about seven such convergences in the medulla near the pelvis, and they result in the formation of large, straight tubules called *papillary ducts* (of Bellini). These have a lumen 100 to 200 μm in diameter and open on the area cribrosa at the apex of each papilla.

The system of the intrarenal excretory ducts has an epithelium quite different from that of the various parts of the nephron. In the smallest collecting tubules, the cells are cuboidal and very distinctly outlined; they contain a darkly staining round nucleus, and most of the cells have a clear pale cytoplasm. There are a few mitochondria and, near the surface, a pair of centrioles with a central single flagellum.

In addition to the *principal* or *light cells,* which have a relatively smooth convex apical surface, there are small numbers of *intercalated* or *dark cells* with more abundant organelles, a denser cytoplasm, and an apical surface bearing longer microvilli. The dark cells are rarely found in the inner medullary segment. The principal cells gradually increase in height from low cuboidal in the outer part of the medulla to cuboidal, and finally to low columnar in the papillary ducts. They are always arranged in a single layer, with all the nuclei at one level and with the free surfaces bulging slightly into the lumen of the tubule. The cytoplasm keeps its pale appearance. The centrioles remain at the bulging free surface. In the area cribrosa, the simple columnar epithelium of the ducts continues onto the surface of the papilla.

It was formerly believed that the collecting ducts were merely inert conduits conveying fluid from the distal tubule to the renal pelvis. This is now known to be untrue. The cortical collecting ducts respond to vasopressin by swelling and dilatation of the lateral intercellular clefts, and the medullary collecting ducts play a major role in the countercurrent mechanism for urine concentration in the mammalian kidney.

THE RENAL INTERSTITIUM

The interstitium is usually defined as the space outside both the basal laminae of the renal tubules and the blood and lymph vessels. In the cortex, it constitutes about 7 per cent of the tissue volume, while the vasculature occupies an additional 6 per cent. The relative volume of the interstitium increases considerably toward the inner region of the medulla and in the papilla. The interstitial tissue of the kidney attracted little investigative interest until it was discovered that the concentration of solutes in the intertubular spaces of the medulla has an important role in concentration of the urine by reabsorption of water.

Two types of interstitial cells have been described in the cortex, one bearing a superficial resemblance to fibroblasts and the other a lymphocyte-like cell. The fibroblast-like cells are of irregular shape, with long tapering processes often in contact with processes of neighboring cells of the same type. The endoplasmic reticulum is well developed and its cisternae may be somewhat distended by a flocculent material. The cortical cytoplasm is rich in actin filaments and microtubules. Occasional lipid droplets are present in the cytoplasm. The lymphocyte-like cells have a nucleus with abundant heterochromatin, and their sparse cytoplasm is rich in free ribosomes. The function of cortical interstitial cells is not firmly established, but it seems likely that the fibroblast-like cells produce collagen and glycosaminoglycans of the extracellular matrix of the interstitium. The small round cells may be blood-derived lymphocytes or early cells of the monocyte-phagocyte series.

In the renal medulla, three types of interstitial cells have been described. Type I is a highly pleomorphic cell containing multiple small lipid droplets. Type II is lymphocyte-like, and Type III is a pericyte associated with the descending vasa recta. The medullary interstitial cells, Type I, have been most thoroughly studied owing to the suggestion that they may have an endocrine function. They are distributed at regular intervals between the parallel tubules and vessels (Fig. 30–25). They are variable in form and their processes are often in close apposition to the basal lamina of thin limbs of the loop of Henle and to the capillaries (Fig. 30–20). Gap junctions occur at sites of contact between processes of neighboring Type I cells. The endoplasmic reticulum resembles that of the comparable cells in the cortex and is generally more extensively developed in cells of the outer zone of the medulla. The mitochondria and Golgi apparatus are unremark-

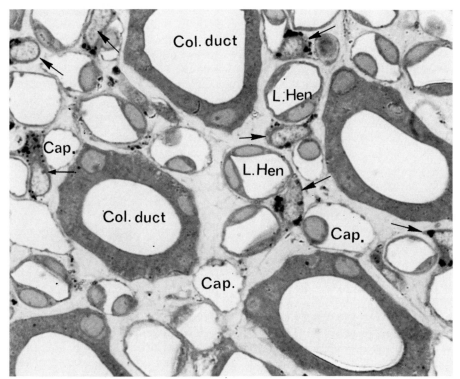

Figure 30–25. Photomicrograph of the renal medulla showing the location *(at arrows)* of the interstitial cells. (Photomicrograph from Bohman, S.-O. Cell Tissue Res. *189*:1, 1978.)

able. A few lysosomes are present, as well as peculiar inclusions called "cylindrical bodies." These consist of bundles of 5 to 50 parallel cylinders ~ 0.15 μm in diameter and up to 11 μm in length. These are believed to be derivatives of the endoplasmic reticulum. Their function is unknown.

A characteristic feature of these cells are lipid droplets about 0.5 μm in diameter and generally exhibiting little osmiophilia (Fig. 30–26). The number of lipid droplets increases in salt depletion and water loading, and decreases in water deprivation and in hypertension. The isolated lipid droplets have been found to consist of triglycerides unusually rich in long-chain polyunsaturated fatty acids. There is no evidence that the droplets are released from the cells, but they may contain precursors of some secretory product.

A number of functions have been suggested for the Type I interstitial cell, but with little supporting evidence. The renal medulla is known to be unusually rich in prostaglandin, and prostaglandin synthesis can be stimulated by antidiuretic hormone. These observations led to the suggestion that the Type I interstitial cells were specialized prostaglan-

din-producing cells. This hypothesis has now been abandoned for lack of direct evidence. The most attractive possibility is that they are endocrine cells involved in regulation of blood pressure. The belief that the medullary interstitial cells may secrete a hormone rests mainly upon experiments in which medullary tissue was transplanted subcutaneously in animals with high blood pressure. The transplants developed into nodules consisting of cells identified as proliferating interstitial cells, and the blood pressure fell. Upon removal of the nodule, the pressure rose again to hypertensive levels. These observations strongly suggest secretion by interstitial cells of a hormone with antihypertensive activity. The postulated hormone has not been isolated.

JUXTAGLOMERULAR COMPLEX

In addition to their function in excretion, the kidneys have a role in the regulation of blood pressure. There is a clear association between certain types of kidney disease and high blood pressure (hypertension). The kidney produces and releases into the blood a

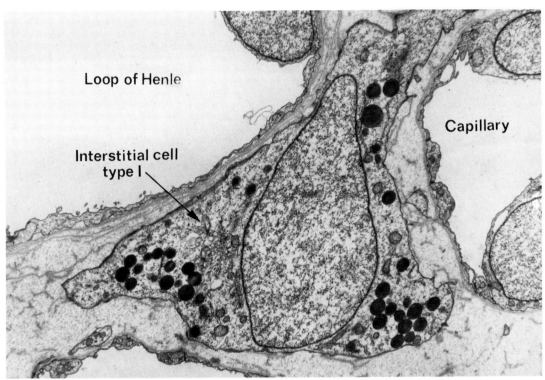

Loop of Henle

Capillary

Interstitial cell
type I

Figure 30–26. A type I interstitial cell in the renal papilla in close relationship to a capillary and a loop of Henle. The cytoplasm contains numerous small lipid droplets. (Micrograph from Bohman, S.-O. J. Ultrastruct. Res. *38*:225, 1972.)

substance called *renin*. This has no vasomotor effect itself but is an enzyme that acts upon a plasma globulin, *angiotensinogen,* to split off a decapeptide, *angiotensin I.* A converting enzyme in the blood plasma then acts upon this to split off two more amino acids, converting it to *angiotensin II*—the most potent vasoconstrictor known. Renin is synthesized in the juxtaglomerular region of the nephron, where the ascending straight portion of the distal tubule returns to the renal corpuscle and comes into intimate relation with its vascular pole (Fig. 30–27).

Among the smooth muscle cells in the wall of the afferent arteriole just proximal to its entrance into the glomerulus are cells that contain conspicuous cytoplasmic granules. These granular *juxtaglomerular cells* are in contact with the intima of the arteriole on the one side, and on the other side they are intimately related to the base of the epithelial cells making up the *macula densa* in the wall of the distal tubule (Fig. 30–28). Also associated with the granular cells are a few nongranular ones and a group of pale-staining extraglomerular mesangial cells (also called lacis cells, polkissen, or polar cushion) located in the angle between the afferent and effer-

ent arterioles at the vascular pole of the glomerulus. The interrelations of the granular juxtaglomerular cells, the macula densa, and the extraglomerular mesangial cells are poorly understood. They are believed to have related functions, however, and together they constitute the *juxtaglomerular apparatus* or *complex.* The juxtaglomerular cells are described as "myoepithelioid" because they appear to be highly modified smooth muscle cells. They have a slightly basophilic cytoplasm and their specific granules are most clearly demonstrated by the Bowie stain, the PAS reaction, or the fluorochrome dye thioflavine T. In electron micrographs they have a moderately abundant granular endoplasmic reticulum and a well-developed Golgi complex. The granules appear to arise in the cisternae of the Golgi complex, as in other glandular cells. When first formed the granules are of variable shape, and have a crystalline internal structure with a periodicity of 5 to 10 nm. Coalescence of these elements gives rise to mature granules, which are irregularly shaped conglomerates that may retain evidences of crystalline order but more often appear homogeneous.

The secretory nature of these granules was

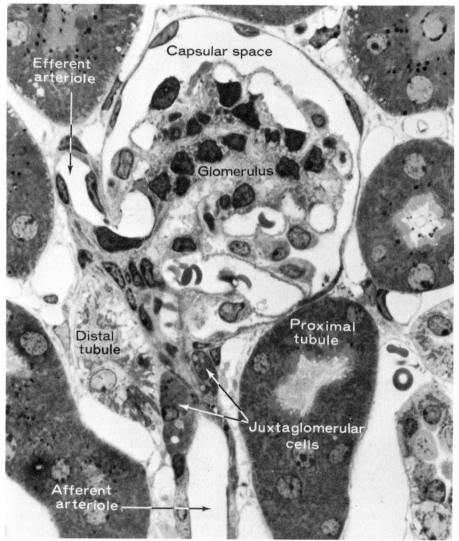

Figure 30–27. Photomicrograph of a thin plastic section of rat kidney, showing a glomerulus and clusters of juxtaglomerular cells in the wall of its afferent arteriole. (Micrograph courtesy of R. Bolender.)

established in experimental studies that demonstrated changes in granule content of the juxtaglomerular cells secondary to renal ischemia or to experimental alteration of salt intake. These studies led to the hypothesis that these cells are the site of production of renin. Support for this thesis has come from the finding that the solubility characteristics of renin and of the granules of the juxtaglomerular cells are similar, and that there is a direct correlation between the level of renin determined by bioassay and the degree of granulation of the juxtaglomerular cells. Microdissection methods have localized the renin to the immediate vicinity of the renal corpuscle, and application of the immuno-

fluorescence technique using antibody to highly purified antigen localizes renin exclusively in the granules of myoepithelial cells in the juxtaglomerular apparatus, and not in the macula densa.

The kidney is apparently not the only site of renin production. In the mouse and other species that exhibit sexual dimorphism of the submaxillary gland, renins that cross-react with that of the kidney are localized by immunofluorescence in certain segments of the gland.

The bases of the cells of the macula densa are in very close relation to the juxtaglomerular cells, and the basal lamina between them is exceedingly thin. This close topographical

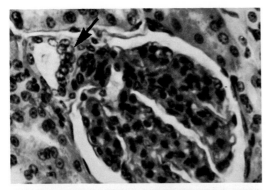

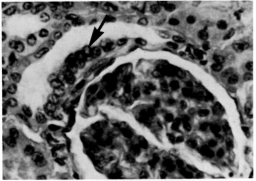

Figure 30–28. Photomicrograph of two renal corpuscles from macaque kidney, showing *(at arrows)* two typical examples of the macula densa, an area of the wall of the distal tubule where the cells are thicker and the nuclei are crowded together and superimposed. × 175.

relationship has been interpreted as suggesting some interchange of substances between the macula densa and the juxtaglomerular cells. Consistent with such a relationship is the report that the polarity of the Golgi complex in the cells of the macula densa is toward the juxtaglomerular cells, whereas in the remainder of the circumference of the distal tubule, it is toward the lumen.

The finding that the cells of the macula densa show changes in their histochemically demonstrable enzymatic activities when the rate of secretion of the juxtaglomerular cells is altered provides further indication that the two structures are functionally related. The juxtaglomerular complex also has an important function in regulation of tissue hydration and blood volume. Any condition that reduces blood or extracellular fluid volume seems to be sensed by the afferent arteriole acting as a baroreceptor or by the macula densa as a sensor of sodium concentration. The juxtaglomerular cells are stimulated to synthesize and release renin. The resulting angiotensin II in the blood directly stimulates

the zona glomerulosa of the adrenal cortex to release *aldosterone;* this acts in turn upon the collecting ducts of the kidney to induce sodium and water retention, which tends to correct the reduction of plasma and interstitial tissue fluid volume.

BLOOD SUPPLY

Because the kidneys serve to clear the blood of accumulated waste products of metabolism, they have a very large blood flow, averaging about 1200 ml/min through both kidneys. A knowledge of the blood supply of the kidney is essential to an understanding of its function.

The *renal artery* enters the hilus of the kidney and divides into two main sets of branches directed toward the dorsal and ventral aspects of the organ. In the adipose tissue surrounding the pelvis, these branches in turn divide into smaller *interlobar arteries* that enter the substance of the kidney and course peripherally in the renal columns between the pyramids or lobes of the kidney. At the level of the base of the medullary pyramids, the interlobar arteries arch over to run parallel to the surface of the organ as the *arcuate arteries* at the corticomedullary junction. Small *interlobular arteries*, given off from the arcuate arteries at regular intervals, course radially toward the kidney surface (Fig. 30–29).

The interlobular arteries running radially in the cortex give off numerous *afferent arterioles* to the glomeruli. The blood is carried from the glomeruli via *efferent arterioles*. The efferent vessels of glomeruli situated in the outer part of the cortex are of small diameter and break up to form the cortical intertubular capillary network. The efferent vessels of the more deeply situated juxtamedullary glomeruli are of larger caliber and pass downward into the medulla, breaking up into bundles of thin-walled vessels somewhat larger than ordinary capillaries, called *vasa recta* (Fig. 30–30). The efferent vessels of the juxtamedullary glomeruli and the vasa recta both contribute branches to an intertubular capillary network in the medulla.

The vasa recta form hairpin loops at various levels in the medulla, turning back toward the cortex and running close to and parallel with the vessels from which they recur. The descending vessels penetrate the outer medulla to different depths before

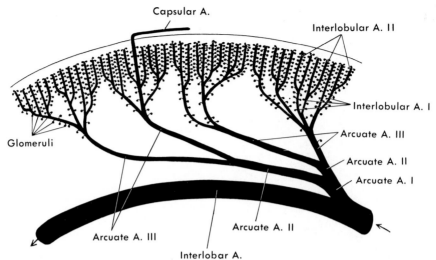

Figure 30–29. Schematic representation of the finer arterial branching in dog kidney. (After Kügelgen, A., and K. J. Otto. *In* Zwanglose Abhandlungen aus dem Gebiet der normalen und pathologischen Anatomie. Vol. 5. Stuttgart, Georg Thieme, 1959.)

turning back. The descending and ascending limbs of these loops form a countercurrent system of vessels referred to as a *vascular bundle* or *rete mirabile*. As more vessels turn back, the vascular bundles taper down as they approach the inner medulla. The descending vessels forming the arterial limbs of the vascular bundle or rete are slightly smaller than the recurrent vessels that constitute the venous limbs (Fig. 30–31). The fine structure of the vessel walls also differs, the arterial component having a continuous endothelium, whereas the venous component has a thin fenestrated endothelium. The proximity of the vessels in the vascular bundles and the large surface they present to one another facilitate rapid movement of diffusible substances between the ascending and descending limbs of the loops. The vasa recta thus serve as efficient countercurrent exchangers for diffusible substances.

The capillaries of the outermost layers of the cortex are drained toward the surface by radially arranged branches, the *superficial cortical veins*, which join veins of characteristic configuration on the surface of the kidney, called *stellate veins*. This outer mantle of venous channels is drained by a relatively small number of *interlobular veins* into the *arcuate veins* that accompany the arteries of the same name. The capillaries in the deeper part of the cortex empty into radially oriented *deep cortical veins*, of which there are some 400 per square centimeter running parallel to a cor-

responding number of interlobular arteries. The blood in these flows inward to the arcuate veins and thence to the *interlobar* veins, which finally become confluent in the hilus to form the *renal vein*.

The hemodynamics of the renal circulation are such that the flows to various zones of the kidney are very different. Measurements of blood flow distribution in the unanesthetized dog give values of 472 ml/100 g/min in the cortex, 132 ml/100 g/min in the outer medulla, and 17 ml/100 g/min in the inner medulla. Although the cortical flow is normally very rapid, strong stimulation of sympathetic nerves may diminish it almost to zero. Under various stressful circumstances, the cortex of the kidney becomes pale, and red blood may appear in the renal vein. Evidently, under these conditions, the renal cortex is relatively ischemic and the bulk of the blood that would normally pass through the cortical glomeruli for filtration is bypassed through the juxtamedullary glomeruli and the vasa recta into the interlobular veins, and thence to the renal vein.

LYMPHATICS

The distribution of lymphatics in the kidney has been a subject of controversy. A number of investigators have contended that intrarenal lymphatics are found only in association with the larger blood vessels and

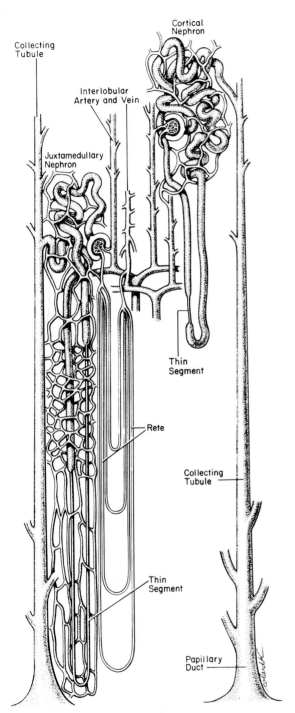

Collecting
Tubule

Cortical
Nephron

Interlobular
Artery and Vein

Juxtamedullary
Nephron

Thin
Segment

Rete

Collecting
Tubule

Thin
Segment

Papillary
Duct

Figure 30–30. Schematic drawing of the blood supply associated with cortical and juxtamedullary nephrons. In the latter, the efferent arteriole runs downward into the medulla, where it gives rise to a bundle of vasa recta. These, together with their recurrent venules, form long bundles of parallel vessels called retia mirabilia. Here the arterial and venous elements have been separated to illustrate their continuity in long loops. In life, the arterial and venous limbs of the loops intermingle, as shown in Figure 30–31.

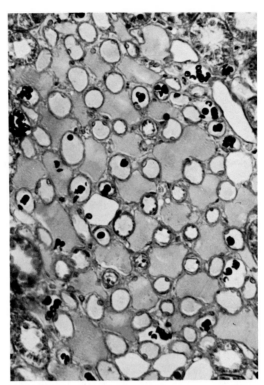

Figure 30–31. Photomicrograph of a rete mirabile from dog kidney. Notice that the vessels are of two morphological types: the descending arterial limbs are capillaries with a round cross section and walls of appreciable thickness; the ascending venous limbs are larger, are more irregular in outline, and have exceedingly thin walls. The latter are filled here with gray precipitate of plasma, while the former appear empty or contain a few erythrocytes. × 250.

extending peripherally only as far as the interlobular vasculature. Others have reported that the initial lymphatic capillaries are tributaries of interlobular lymphatics and are found among the tubular elements making up the parenchyma of the renal lobules. The latter interpretation has now been strongly supported by combined light and electron microscopic studies employing improved methods for identification and delineation of lymphatics. In addition to the generally accepted association of lymphatics with the larger arterial vessels, lymphatic capillaries are present within the parenchyma of the renal cortex. Morphometric analysis has shown that, in the dog, as many as one third of the cortical lymphatics are intralobular. These drain mainly to interlobular lymphatics and thence to lymphatic plexuses in the hilus of the kidney. Some in the outer cortex drain to a capsular lymphatic plexus. The volume of lymph in the cortex is estimated to be about 1 per cent of the volume of blood in peritubular capillaries.

NERVES

Macroscopic dissection shows that the sympathetic celiac plexus sends many nerve fibers into the kidney. Their distribution inside the organ has not been worked out satisfactorily. It is relatively easy to follow nonmyelinated and myelinated fibers along the course of the larger blood vessels. They provide the adventitia with sensory nerve endings and the muscular coat with motor endings. Along with the afferent arterioles, nerve fibers may reach the renal corpuscles, and some of them seem to end on their surfaces. A nerve supply of the uriniferous tubules, however, has not been convincingly demonstrated. Some investigators describe plexuses of fine nerve fibers that surround and seem to penetrate the basal lamina. On its inner surface they are said to form another plexus, from which terminal branches arise to end between the epithelial cells. There is a good possibility that the silver stains on which these descriptions are based were impregnating reticulum and not axons. The finer innervation of the kidneys has not been systematically studied at the electron microscope level, where the fine nerve fibers can be identified with greater certainty.

HISTOPHYSIOLOGY OF THE KIDNEYS

In forming urine, the kidneys do not produce new material in significant amounts, but eliminate water and some of the waste products of metabolism that are carried in solution in the blood. In addition to their *excretory function*, in which they dispose of waste and foreign substances, the kidneys have equally important *conservative functions*, by which they retain the amounts of water, electrolytes, and other substances needed by the body, while eliminating excesses of these substances. They therefore play an important role in the maintenance of the organism. The kidney carries out its functions by a combination of filtration, passive diffusion, active secretion, and selective absorption. The form, topographical relations, and microscopic organization of its components represent structural adaptations favoring these processes.

The blood circulates through the glomerular capillaries with a *hydrostatic pressure* of about 70 mm Hg. This tends to press the fluid constituents of the blood through the pores and intercellular spaces of the endothelium, across the basal lamina, through the filtration slits between foot processes of the podocytes, and into Bowman's capsule. The hydrostatic pressure in the capillaries is opposed by an average *colloid osmotic pressure* of about 32 mm Hg and a *capsular pressure* of about 20 mm Hg. The net *filtration pressure* is thus about 18 mm Hg. With some 1300 ml of blood flowing through the glomeruli of both kidneys each minute, approximately 125 ml of glomerular filtrate is produced. Analysis of fluid aspirated from Bowman's capsule by micropuncture has established that it is an ultrafiltrate of blood plasma with nearly the same composition as the interstitial fluid. It contains small molecules such as phosphates, creatine, uric acid, and urea, and small amounts of albumin, but is free of larger protein molecules and substances combined with them. Molecules of molecular weight 100,000 and larger are arrested in the basal lamina. However, the capillary wall not only is a size-selective barrier in the filtration of macromolecules, but also exhibits selectivity based on charge. Anionic molecules are more limited in their passage across the glomerular filter than are neutral molecules of the same size. The filter thus serves to retain albumin and other anionic proteins in the circulation. The negatively charged sites responsible for this selectivity are located on the surface of the capillary endothelium; on the surface coat of the podocyte foot processes; and within the basal lamina of the glomerulus (Fig. 30–32). The polyanion of the podocyte surface coat is a 140,000-M.W. sialoprotein, which has been isolated and called *podocalyxin*. The basal lamina contains Type IV collagen, which possesses acidic amino acids with free carboxyl groups and a heteropolysaccharide region that includes sialic acid. In addition to these the basal lamina contains a proteoglycan, rich in heparan sulfate. This highly charged anionic macromolecule occurs in a more or less regular lattice in the laminae interna and externa (Fig. 30–32).

Of the 125 ml of filtrate formed per minute in the glomeruli, 124 ml are reabsorbed as the fluid passes through the various segments of the nephrons and the collecting ducts, leaving a volume of only 1 ml to be excreted as urine. This small remainder is not simply derived by absorption of water; its contents

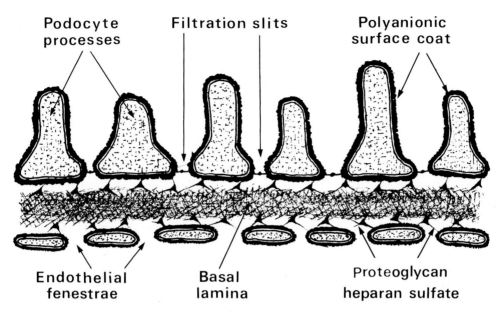

Podocyte processes **Filtration slits** **Polyanionic surface coat**

Endothelial fenestrae **Basal lamina** **Proteoglycan heparan sulfate**

Figure 30–32. Diagrammatic representation of the glomerular filtration barrier. The anionic sites reside in the surface coat of the endothelium and of the podocyte processes, and in proteoglycan macromolecules, rich in heparan sulfate, that form a network of angular particles in the lamina rara externa and interna of the basal lamina. (From Farquhar, M. G. Reproduced from The Journal of Cell Biology 81:137, 1979 by copyright permission of The Rockefeller University Press.)

are modified in its passage along the tubules by (1) diffusion of some substances back into the blood, (2) absorption of some by osmotic work, and (3) excretion of others into the lumen.

The transport of certain substances into and out of the nephron can be fairly precisely measured in healthy humans and is the basis of a variety of clinical measurements of kidney function. *Inulin* is a nonmetabolized carbohydrate that, when injected intravenously, rapidly appears in the glomerular filtrate but is not secreted or absorbed by the tubules. It can be used, therefore, as a means of measuring the amount of plasma filtered by all the glomeruli of both kidneys. This calculation is based on the concentrations of inulin in the urine and in the plasma during the experiment. The volume of plasma containing the same amount of inulin as that found in the urine is the amount of plasma that has been "cleared" of this substance by filtration during the period of the test. The *inulin clearance* furnishes a standard from which it is possible to estimate what proportions of other substances are reabsorbed or excreted by cells in various parts of the tubule.

Much of our knowledge of the functions of renal tubules has been derived from studies on amphibian species, in which it is possible to puncture the glomerular capsule and the tubules at different levels in living animals and carry out microchemical analyses

on the fluid aspirated. The change in the composition of the filtrate as it passes along the nephron can thus be studied directly. Similarly, fluid of known composition can be perfused through a segment of tubule between two pipettes, and the substances added to or subtracted from it can be determined. By these and other methods, it has been shown that 85 per cent or more of the sodium chloride and water of the glomerular filtrate is reabsorbed in the proximal tubule. In this process, the cells actively transport sodium from the lumen, and the water and chloride passively follow it to maintain osmotic equilibrium.

The remarkable functional efficiency of the proximal convoluted tubule is attributable in large part to the configuration of its cells, which are specialized to maximize the surface area of the physiologically important regions of their plasma membrane. In the current interpretation of proximal tubule function, water and solutes may pass from the tubule lumen via a paracellular route through the juxtaluminal intercellular junctions, or via a transcellular route that involves flux across the luminal surface and then across the lateral membranes into the intercellular clefts below the junctions. The passive movement of water along this path is due to an osmotic gradient generated by active transport of solute across the lateral cell membranes. Stereological morphometric studies of proximal convoluted tubule have shown that the microvilli of the brush border increase the apical surface 36 times, and the amplification of the lateral surfaces by processes interdigitating with adjacent cells gives them an area equal to that of the brush border, and both are 20 times greater than the area of the cell base. In the straight portion of the proximal tubule, the luminal surface is amplified only 15 times by its less well-developed brush border, and the luminal and lateral surfaces are only 10 times greater than the cell base. These configurational differences in the cells of the two segments of the proximal tubule are reflected in quantitative differences in resorption of water from the glomerular filtrate.

Normally, all the glucose in the filtrate is also reabsorbed in the proximal convoluted tubule and it is calculated that nearly half a pound of glucose and more than three pounds of sodium chloride are recovered per day from the glomerular filtrate of man. If the level of glucose in the blood is raised experimentally above a certain level, the glucose is not completely absorbed and appears in the urine. This *tubular maximum for reabsorption of glucose* (glucose Tm) is a useful index of the reabsorptive capacity of the kidney tubules.

Other metabolically important substances that are reabsorbed in the proximal tubule are amino acids, protein, acetoacetic acid, and ascorbic acid. On leaving the proximal tubules, the fluid contains essentially none of these substances. The absorption of proteins in the proximal tubule has been followed morphologically by intravenous administration of peroxidase and its subsequent detection by a histochemical method. Similar studies have been carried out by administration of ferritin and ^{125}I-labeled albumin by micropuncture, followed by direct or autoradiographic visualization of the tracer substance. The results of these studies are in close agreement, all showing uptake in the apical invaginations and apical vacuoles of the proximal tubule within a very few minutes. In 30 to 60 minutes, the label is localized in dense granules containing acid phosphatase, interpreted as secondary lysosomes. It is assumed that absorbed albumin is degraded by the lysosomes and is not returned to the bloodstream.

Thus, useful substances are conserved by reabsorption. On the other hand, the end products of metabolism, *urea, uric acid,* and *creatinine,* which are of little or no use to the body, are not completely reabsorbed but are allowed to remain in the urine and are eliminated from the body. While some 99 per cent of the water of the glomerular filtrate is conserved, only 40 per cent of the urea and none of the creatinine is reabsorbed.

In addition to its capacity for active reabsorption, the proximal tubule has the capacity to secrete creatinine, para-aminohippuric acid, the organic iodine compound Diodrast, and sulfonic dyes such as phenol red. The secretory capacity of the proximal tubule does not have the physiological importance in man that it does in some lower animals, particularly those fish that have aglomerular kidneys. However, the substances that are secreted are useful in the clinical evaluation of kidney function and renal blood flow. When introduced into the blood in moderate concentrations, Diodrast and para-aminohippuric acid are entirely removed during a single passage of blood through the kidneys. Since it is impossible to remove by filtration all the substances dissolved in the blood and have any fluid plasma left, the complete removal of a substance in one passage of blood through the kidney must occur in part by filtration and in part by excretory work. Knowledge of the concentration of such a substance in the blood and the amount found in the urine produced in a given time makes it possible to calculate the blood flow through the kidney. The blood flow is equal to the plasma flow plus the cell volume found by hematocrit. From the values for Diodrast clearance and for inulin clearance, one can determine the fraction of renal plasma flow that is filtered by the glomeruli. If one then raises the concentration of Diodrast in the blood, a point is reached at which the kidney fails to remove all the material from the blood. The maximal concentration that is completely cleared is taken as a measure of the *excretory capacity of the tubule (Tm,* or *tubular maximum).* If the values are known for renal plasma flow and inulin clearance, the measurement of other substances (such as urea, uric acid, and phosphate and bicarbonate buffers) in the blood and urine can be related to the activities of the total number of nephrons with regard to these substances. In this way it has been determined which substances are secreted, which are reabsorbed, and which diffuse passively from the glomerular filtrate. The localizations of these specific events in various portions of the tubule are less well known.

The loop of Henle is essential for the

production of hypertonic urine. Only those birds and mammals that have a thin segment in the loop excrete urine that is hypertonic to the blood plasma. The length of this segment, and of the renal papilla where it is located, are correlated with the degree to which the species can concentrate the glomerular filtrate. Mammals such as beaver living in an aqueous environment have little need to conserve water, and the osmolarity of their urine is only about twice that of plasma. Animals living in the desert, on the other hand, have a long renal papilla and very long loops of Henle, and can concentrate urine to over 20 times the osmolarity of plasma. The maximal concentration achieved by humans is about fivefold.

Fluid in the outer renal cortex is approximately isosmotic with plasma, but from the corticomedullary junction to the tip of the papilla, there is a continuous increase in osmolarity of the interstitial fluid. The main-

tenance of this gradient depends on the arrangement of the vascular supply and loop of Henle, and on the permeability properties of its various segments (Fig. 30–33, 30–34). The thin descending limb is highly permeable to water but not to NaCl. The thin ascending limb is impermeable to water but permeable to salt. The thick ascending limb, which continues into the cortex as the distal tubule, is impermeable to diffusion of salt and water but has considerable capacity for active transport of salt from the glomerular filtrate to the interstitial fluid. This active salt transport creates hypertonicity in the outer medulla and inner cortex. Water diffuses from the descending limb of the loop, which is relatively impermeable to salt and urea. Diffusion of water into the interstitium creates an increased intratubular concentration of solute, mainly salt. After the fluid rounds the bend of the loop, the permeability of the thin ascending limb allows salt to diffuse out

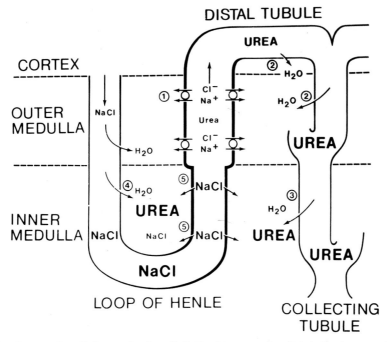

Figure 30–33. Countercurrent multiplier mechanism. Both the thin ascending limb in the inner medulla and the thick ascending limb in the outer medulla, as well as the first part of the distal tubule, are impermeable to water, as indicated by the thickened lining. In the thick ascending limb, active chloride reabsorption, accompanied by passive sodium movement (1), renders the tubule fluid dilute and the outer medullary interstitium hyperosmotic. In the last part of the distal tubule and in the collecting tubule in the cortex and outer medulla, water is reabsorbed down its osmotic gradient (2), increasing the concentration of urea that remains behind. In the inner medulla both water and urea are reabsorbed from the collecting duct (3). Some urea reenters the loop of Henle *(not shown)*. This medullary recycling of urea, in addition to trapping of urea by countercurrent exchange in the vasa recta *(not shown)*, causes urea to accumulate in large quantities in the medullary interstitium (indicated by the larger type), where it osmotically extracts water from the descending limb (4) and thereby concentrates sodium chloride in descending-limb fluid. When the fluid rich in sodium chloride enters the sodium chloride–permeable (but water-impermeable) thin ascending limb, sodium chloride moves passively down its concentration gradient (5), rendering the tubule fluid relatively hypo-osmotic to the surrounding interstitium. (From Jamieson, R. L., and R. H. Maffly. N. Engl. J. Med. *295*:1059, 1976.)

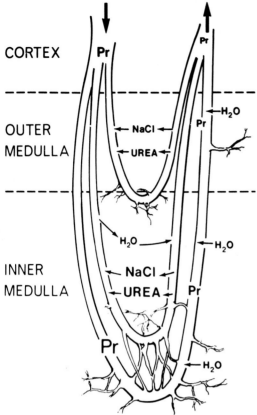

CORTEX

OUTER MEDULLA

INNER MEDULLA

Figure 30–34. Countercurrent exchange by the vasa recta. The medullary circulation, unlike the loops of Henle, consists of a network of channels with main thoroughfares (the vasa recta) and branch connections. Pr denotes plasma protein. The size of type indicates the relative concentrations of each solute with respect to its location in the medulla but not necessarily with respect to other solutes. The progressive rise in the concentration of sodium chloride and urea in the medullary interstitium is due to the loop of Henle and collecting tubule. Since the capillaries are permeable to sodium chloride and urea, these solutes enter descending vasa recta and leave ascending vasa recta. This transcapillary exchange helps "trap" the solutes in the medulla. Conversely, water leaves the descending vasa recta, causing the plasma protein concentration to increase. In the ascending vasa recta, the sum of oncotic (that due to plasma protein) and osmotic (that due to nonprotein solutes) pressures results in capillary fluid uptake. Thus, water reabsorbed from the collecting tubule and Henle's descending limb is removed from the medulla and returned to the general circulation. Vasa recta function in a dual capacity, trapping solute and removing water, to preserve the hyperosmolality of the renal medulla. (From Jamieson, R. L., and R. H. Maffly. N. Engl. J. Med. *295*:1059, 1976.)

of the tubule down its own concentration gradient, resulting in dilution of the ascending-limb fluid. The thin ascending limb thus passively contributes to maintenance of high interstitial osmolarity in the inner medulla.

The thick ascending limb, distal tubule, and cortical and outer medullary portions of the collecting duct can be thought of as a second loop. These segments are permeable to water but impermeable to salt and urea. In this loop, tubular fluid diluted by active transport of salt in the thick ascending limb and distal tubule continues to lose some water, and the concentration of urea in the collecting duct increases. In the inner medulla, the collecting duct is permeable to water and urea. Urea leaves the tubule fluid down its concentration gradient, contributing to the high osmolarity of the interstitial fluid, and water diffuses out of the collecting duct to achieve the final concentration of the urine.

Maintenance of the osmotic gradient that drives this passive countercurrent multiplier thus involves two solutes: (1) salt, which diffuses from the thin ascending limb and is actively transported in the thick limb; and (2) urea, which diffuses from the collecting duct in its passage through the inner medulla.

The classical countercurrent multiplier mechanism advanced by physiologists in the 1960s to account for concentration of the urine assumed active sodium transport by the entire ascending limb of the loop of Henle, and assigned no significant role to urea in maintenance of the gradient. Electron micrographs of the thin ascending limb revealed a very simple structure incompatible with active transport. Subsequent development of a technique for perfusion of isolated segments of tubules in vitro showed that the descending and ascending thin limbs were quite different in their permeability properties, and neither had a mechanism for active sodium transport. The new *passive countercurrent multiplier mechanism* described above is now consistent with these observations and with the ultrastructure of these segments of the nephron.

The water permeability of collecting ducts is controlled by antidiuretic hormone (ADH) from the posterior lobe of the hypophysis. In the presence of this hormone, fluid within the duct can come to osmotic equilibrium with the interstitial fluid surrounding the duct. In the absence of the hormone, the duct is relatively impermeable to water, and the urine passing through the medulla remains dilute in spite of the concentration gradient in the surrounding interstitium.

The efficiency of reabsorption of sodium ions is also under hormonal control. Aldosterone secreted by the zona glomerulosa of the adrenal cortex acts specifically upon the renal tubules to increase their rate of sodium transport to the interstitium. In the absence of aldosterone, there is a serious loss of sodium via the urine. When the hormone is present in normal amount, some 1200 g of sodium are reabsorbed each day and only a few hundred milligrams escape in the urine.

PASSAGES FOR THE EXCRETION OF URINE

The excretory passages convey urine from the parenchyma of the kidney to the outside. Their walls are provided with a well-developed coat of smooth muscle. Its contractions move the urine forward.

The calyces, the pelvis, the ureter, and the bladder all have a similar structure, but the thickness of the wall gradually increases from the upper to the lower part of the urinary tract. The inner surface is lined with a mucous membrane. There is no distinct sub-mucosa, and the lamina propria of the mucosa blends with the smooth muscle coat, which in turn is covered by an adventitial layer of connective tissue.

All the excretory passages of the urinary tract are lined with transitional epithelium. In the calyces, it is two or three cells thick, and in the ureter, four or five. When the wall of the bladder is contracted, the epithelium is six to eight cells thick and its superficial cells are rounded or even club-shaped (Fig. 30–35). When the bladder is distended, the epithelium is thin and the cells are greatly flattened and stretched.

Electron micrographs of transitional epithelium reveal fine structural features peculiar to this tissue. The free surface of the cells at the lumen has a characteristic scalloped appearance. Segments of membrane of varying length are quite straight and seemingly stiff (Fig. 30–36). Neighboring straight segments may be so oriented as to produce angular surface contours not seen on other cells. There is a superficial ectoplasmic layer of cytoplasm rich in fine filaments, and bundles of filaments course through the deeper

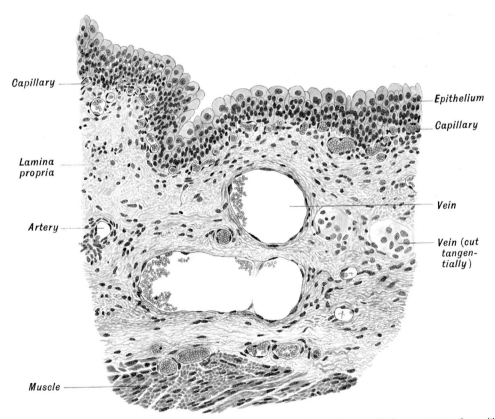

Figure 30–35. Section of wall of human urinary bladder in contracted condition; capillaries penetrate the epithelium. × 150. (After A. A. Maximow.)

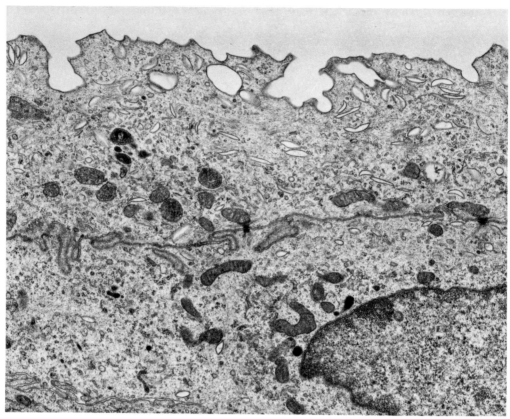

Figure 30–36. Electron micrograph of portions of two transitional epithelial cells from the bladder. Notice the flattened elliptical vesicles in the cytoplasm of the upper cell and the peculiar angular appearance of the luminal surface. This apparently results from insertion of relatively stiff segments of membrane into the surface when the lenticular vesicles fuse with the plasma membrane. (Micrograph from Hicks, M., and B. Ketterer, J. Cell Biol. *45*:542, 1970.)

cytoplasm as well. Flattened, elliptical, or lenticular vesicles are present in the superficial cytoplasm, and these are bounded by thick membranes of the same character as that on the luminal surface. Vesicles of this kind are peculiar to the cells of transitional epithelium. It is speculated that they may be formed within the cell and may be added to the surface membrane, providing for its replacement or for its rapid expansion in distention of the bladder.

The luminal plasma membrane of the superficial cells of bladder epithelium has a unique ultrastructure and unusual physiological properties. It is thicker (12 nm) than most cell membranes and asymmetrical in sections, with the outer dense line of the unit membrane significantly thicker than the inner dense line. When this membrane is isolated and examined by negative staining and optical diffraction, it is found to have a highly ordered substructure consisting of hexagonally arranged subunits. Each subunit seems to be a hexamer composed of twelve smaller subunits arranged in a stellate configuration (Fig. 30–37). The significance of this lattice structure in relation to the function of the bladder epithelium is by no means clear. It is known, however, that in man the tonicity of the bladder urine may be two to four times higher than that of the plasma in the capillaries of the lamina propria. If the transitional epithelium were to act as a semipermeable membrane, water would pass from blood to urine, and the latter would become diluted. This does not occur, and it seems evident therefore that the epithelium possesses an effective barrier preventing water loss. The barrier function is diminished or lost if the thick surface membrane is chemically altered or mechanically damaged. The barrier is believed to reside in occluding junctions between the superficial cells that close the intercellular spaces, and in the special properties of their thick luminal membrane.

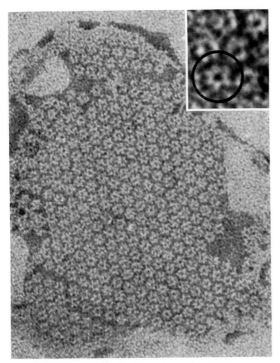

Figure 30–37. Electron micrograph of a negatively stained portion of the cell membrane at the free surface of transitional epithelium. This membrane has a unique substructure *(see inset)* consisting of hexagonally arranged subunits. This structure may be related to the unusual permeability properties of the bladder epithelium. (Micrograph from Hicks, M., and B. Ketterer. J. Cell Biol. 45:542, 1970.)

No true glands are present in the calyces, the pelvis, or the ureter, but glands may be simulated here by small, solid nests of epithelial cells within the thickness of the epithelial sheet. In the urinary bladder, however, and in the vicinity of the internal urethral orifice, small invaginations of the epithelium into the subjacent connective tissue can be found. They contain numerous clear, mucus-secreting cells and are similar to the glands of Littré in the urethra.

There is a thin basal lamina between the epithelium and the lamina propria. The connective tissue of the latter forms thin folds that may penetrate deep into the epithelium. The connective tissue underlying the mucosa is abundant and contains elastic fiber networks and sometimes small lymphatic nodules. Its deeper layers have a loose arrangement. The mucous membrane in the empty ureter, therefore, is thrown into several longitudinal folds, which in cross section give a festooned appearance to the margin of the lumen (Fig. 30–38). In the bladder, the deep,

looser layer of connective tissue is especially abundant so that in the contracted condition of the organ, the mucous membrane forms numerous thick folds.

The muscular coat of the urinary passages, in contrast to that of the intestine, does not form clearly defined separable layers. Instead, it occurs as loose anastomosing strands of smooth muscle separated by abundant collagenous connective tissue. In general, the muscular coat consists of an inner longitudinal and an outer circular layer, but their limits are ill defined. Beginning in the lower third of the ureter, a third external longitudinal layer is added. This is especially prominent in the bladder.

In the small calyces capping the papillae of the pyramids, the strands of the inner longitudinal muscle layer end at the attachment of the calyx to the papilla. The outer circular strands reach higher up and form a muscular ring around the papilla. The calyces show periodic contractions. This muscular activity is believed to assist in moving the urine out of the papillary ducts into the calyces. The muscular coat of the ureter also performs slow peristaltic movements. The waves of contraction proceed from the pelvis toward the bladder.

Because the ureters pierce the wall of the bladder obliquely, their openings are usually closed by the pressure of the contents of the bladder and are open only when the urine is forced through them. A fold of the mucous membrane of the bladder extending over the ureteral orifice and acting as a valve usually prevents the backflow of the urine. In the intramural part of the ureters, the circular muscular strands of their wall disappear, and the connective tissue of the mucous membrane contains longitudinal muscular strands whose contraction opens the lumen of the ureter.

The muscular coat of the bladder is very strong. Its thick strands of smooth muscle cells form three layers, which intermingle at their margins and cannot be separated from one another. The outer longitudinal layer is developed best on the dorsal and ventral surfaces of the viscus, while in other places its strands may be wide apart. The middle circular or spiral layer is the thickest of all. The inner layer in the body of the bladder consists of relatively sparse longitudinal or oblique strands. In the region of the trigone, thin dense bundles of smooth muscle form a circular mass around the internal opening of

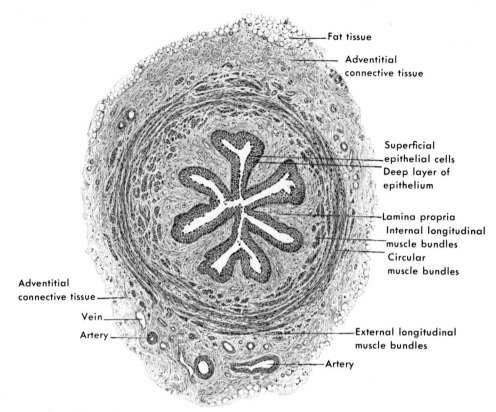

Figure 30–38. Cross section of markedly contracted human ureter. × 30. (After Schaffer.)

the urethra, forming the *internal sphincter* of the bladder.

Blood Vessels, Lymphatics, and Nerves

The blood vessels of the excretory passages penetrate first through the muscular coat and provide it with capillaries. They then form a plexus in the deeper layers of the mucous membrane. From here, small arteries pass toward the surface and form a rich capillary plexus immediately under the epithelium.

The deeper layers of the mucosa and the muscularis in the renal pelvis and the ureters also contain a well-developed network of lymph capillaries. In the bladder, lymph vessels are said to be present only in the muscularis.

Nerve plexuses, small ganglia, and scattered nerve cells can be found in the adventitial and muscular coats of the ureter. Most of the fibers supply the muscle, but some fibers apparently of efferent nature have been traced into the mucosa and the epithelium.

A sympathetic nerve plexus in the adventitial coat of the bladder, the *plexus vesicalis,* is formed in part by the pelvic nerves, which originate from the sacral nerves, and in part by the branches of the hypogastric plexus. The vesical plexus sends numerous nerves into the muscular coat. A continuation of the nerve plexus, but seemingly without nerve cells, is found in the connective tissue of the mucosa. Here the sensory nerve endings are located. Many fibers penetrate into the epithelium between the cells, forming varicose free endings.

URETHRA

Male Urethra

The male urethra has a length of 18 to 20 cm. Three parts can be distinguished. The short proximal segment surrounded by the prostate is the *pars prostatica (prostatic urethra).* Here the posterior wall of the urethra forms an elevation, the *colliculus seminalis (verumontanum).* On its surface in the midline is the

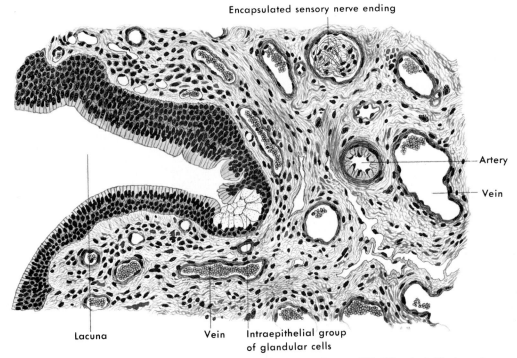

Encapsulated sensory nerve ending

Artery

Vein

Lacuna   Vein   Intraepithelial group
                                 of glandular cells

Figure 30–39. Section of cavernous part of male human urethra. × 165. (After A. A. Maximow.)

opening of the *utriculus prostaticus*, the rudimentary homologue of the uterus in the male. Located to the right and to the left of this are the two slitlike openings of the *ductus ejaculatorius (ejaculatory duct)* and the numerous openings of the ducts of the prostate gland. The second, very short segment of the urethra (18 mm long), the *pars membranacea (membranous urethra)*, extends from the lower pole of the prostate to the bulb of the corpus spongiosum of the penis. The third portion, *pars spongiosa (penile urethra)*, which is about 15 cm long, passes longitudinally through the corpus spongiosum of the penis.

The prostatic part is lined with the same transitional type of epithelium as the bladder. The pars membranacea and the pars spongiosa are lined with a stratified or pseudostratified columnar epithelium (Figs. 30–39, 30–40). Patches of stratified squamous epithelium are common in the pars spongiosa. In the terminal enlarged part of the canal, the *fossa navicularis*, stratified squamous epithelium occurs as a rule. In the surface epithelium, occasional mucous goblet cells may be found. Intraepithelial cysts containing a colloid-like substance are common.

The lamina propria of the mucosa is a loose connective tissue with abundant elastic

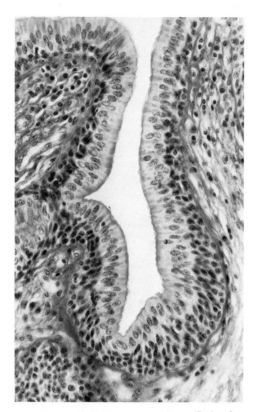

Figure 30–40. Photomicrograph of stratified columnar epithelium of human urethra.

Stratified columnar epithelium | Epithelium with clear cells | Outpocketings of clear mucous cells | Blood vessel

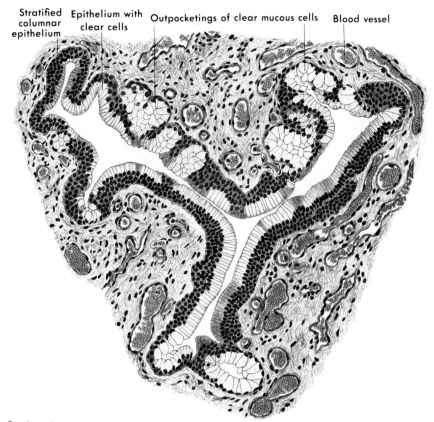

Figure 30–41. Section of urethral gland (gland of Littré) from cavernous part of male human urethra. × 165. (After A. A. Maximow.)

networks. No separate submucous layer can be distinguished. This connective tissue contains numerous scattered bundles of smooth muscle, mainly oriented longitudinally. In the outer layers, however, circular bundles are also present. The lamina propria has no distinct papillae extending into the epithelium; these appear only in the fossa navicularis. The membranous portion of the urethra is surrounded by a mass of striated muscle, a part of the urogenital diaphragm.

The surface of the mucous membrane of the urethra shows many recesses, the *lacunae of Morgagni*. These outpocketings continue into deeper, branching tubules, the *glands of Littré* (Fig. 30–41). The larger ones among them are found especially on the dorsal surface of the pars spongiosa of the urethra. They run obliquely in the lamina propria and are directed with their blind end toward the root of the penis. They sometimes penetrate far into the corpus spongiosum. The glands of Littré are lined with the same epithelium as the surface of the mucous membrane, but in many places this epithelium is transformed into compact intraepithelial nests of clear cells, which have the staining reactions of mucus. In old age some of the recesses of the urethral mucosa may contain concretions similar to those of the prostate.

Female Urethra

The female urethra is 25 to 30 mm long. Its mucosa forms longitudinal folds and is lined with stratified squamous epithelium. In many cases, however, pseudostratified columnar epithelium can be found. Numerous invaginations are formed by the epithelium (Fig. 30–42). The outpocketings in their wall are lined in many places with clear mucous cells, as in the glands of Littré of the male urethra. The glands may accumulate colloid material in their cavities or may even contain concretions. The lamina propria, devoid of papillae, is a loose connective tissue with abundant elastic fibers. It is provided with a highly developed system of venous plexuses and has, therefore, a character resembling

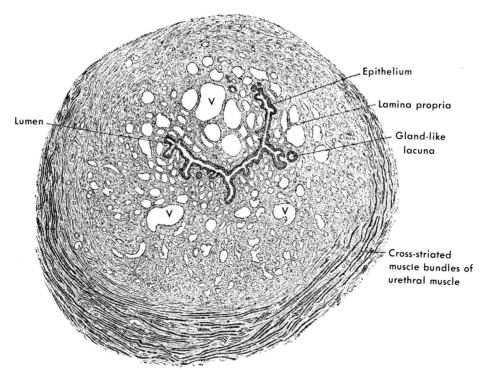

Figure 30–42. Cross section through female human urethra. The darker portions of the lamina propria are smooth muscle bundles. × 10. (After von Ebner.)

the corpus spongiosum of the male. The mucous membrane with its veins is surrounded by a thick mass of smooth muscles; the inner layers of the latter have a longitudinal, the outer layers a circular, arrangement. Distally, the smooth muscles are strengthened by a sphincter of striated muscle.

REFERENCES

GENERAL

Rouiller, C.: General anatomy and histology of the kidney. *In* Rouiller, C., and A. F. Muller, eds.: The Kidney. Vol. 1. New York, Academic Press, 1969.

Smith, H. W.: The Kidney. New York, Oxford University Press, 1969.

Smith, H. W.: Principles of Renal Physiology. New York, Oxford University Press, 1956.

RENAL CORPUSCLE

Blau, E. B., and J. E. Haas: Glomerular sialic acid and proteinuria in human renal disease. Lab. Invest. *28*:477, 1973.

Caulfield, J. P., and M. G. Farquhar: The permeability of glomerular capillaries to graded dextrans. J. Cell Biol. *63*:883, 1974.

Courtoy, P. J., Y. S. Kanwar, R. O. Hynes, and M. G. Farquhar: Fibronectin localization in the rat glomerulus. J. Cell Biol. *87*:691, 1980.

Elema, J. D., J. R. Hoyer, and R. L. Vernier: The glomerular mesangium: uptake of intravenously injected colloidal carbon. Kidney Int. *9*:35, 1976.

Farquhar, M. G.: The primary glomerular filtration barrier—basement membrane or epithelial slits? Kidney Int. *8*:197, 1975.

Farquhar, M. G., and Y. S. Kanwar: Characterization of anionic sites in the glomerular basement membranes of normal and nephrotic rats. *In* Leaf, A., et al., eds.: Penile Pathophysiology. New York, Raven Press, 1980, pp. 57–74.

Farquhar, M. G., and G. E. Palade: Functional evidence for the existence of a third cell type in the renal glomerulus. Phagocytosis of filtration residues by a distinctive "third" cell. J. Cell Biol. *13*:55, 1962.

Kerjaschki, D., D. J. Sharkey, and M. G. Farquhar: Identification and characterization of podocalyxin—the major sialoprotein of the renal glomerular epithelial cell. J. Cell Biol. *98*:1591, 1984.

Kanwar, Y. S., and M. G. Farquhar: Presence of heparan sulfate in the glomerular basement membrane. Proc. Natl. Acad. Sci. U.S.A. *76*:1303, 1979.

Kurtz, S. M., and J. D. Feldman: Experimental studies on the formation of the glomerular basement membrane. J. Ultrastruct. Res. *6*:19, 1962.

Latta, H. W., W. H. Johnston, and T. M. Stanley: Sialoglycoproteins and filtration barriers in the glomerular capillary wall. J. Ultrastruct. Res. *51*:354, 1975.

RENAL TUBULES

Bulger, R. E.: The shape of rat kidney tubule cells. Am. J. Anat. *116*:237, 1965.

Bulger, R. E., and B. F. Trump: Fine structure of the rat renal papillae. Am. J. Anat. *118*:685, 1966.

Ericsson, J. L. E., A. Bergstrand, G. Andres, H. Bucht, and G. Cinotti: Morphology of the renal tubular epithelium in young healthy humans. Acta Pathol. Microbiol. Scand. *63*:361, 1965.

Kokko, J. P., and F. C. Rector: Countercurrent multiplication system without active transport in the inner medulla. Kidney Int. *2*:214, 1972.

Kriz, W., and H. Koepsell: The structural organization of the mouse kidney. Z. Anat. Enwicklungsgesch. *144*:137, 1974.

Kriz, W., A. Schiller, B. Kairsling, and R. Taughner: Comparative and functional aspects of thin loop ultrastructure. *In* Maunsbach, A. B., T. S. Olsen, and E. I. Christensen, eds.: Functional Ultrastructure of the Kidney. London, Academic Press 1980.

Maunsbach, A. B.: Observations on the segmentation of the proximal tubule of the rat kidney. J. Ultrastruct. Res. *16*:239, 1966.

Maunsbach, A. B.: Absorption of I^{125} labelled homologous albumin by rat kidney proximal tubule cells. J. Ultrastruct. Res. *15*:197, 1966.

Meyers, C. E., R. E. Bulger, C. C. Tischer, and B. F. Trump: Human renal ultrastructure. IV. Collecting duct of healthy individuals. Lab. Invest. *15*:1921, 1966.

Neustein, H. B., and A. B. Maunsbach: Hemoglobin absorption by proximal tubule cells of rabbit kidney. A study by electron microscopic autoradiography. J. Ultrastruct. Res. *16*:141, 1966.

Oswaldo, L., and H. Latta: The thin limb of the loop of Henle. J. Ultrastruct. Res. *15*:144, 1966.

Pricam, C., F. Humbert, A. Perrelet, and L. Orci: A freeze etch study of the tight junctions of the rat kidney tubules. Lab. Invest. *30*:286, 1974.

Schwartz, M. M., and M. A. Venkatachalam: Structural differences in thin limbs of Henle. Physiological implications. Kidney Int. *6*:193, 1974.

Tisher, C. C.: Morphology of the ascending thick limb of Henle. Kidney Int. *9*:8, 1976.

Tisher, C. C., R. E. Bulger, and B. F. Trump: Human renal ultrastructure. I. Proximal tubule of healthy individuals. Lab. Invest. *15*:1357, 1966.

Tisher, C. C., R. E. Bulger, B. F. Trump: Human renal ultrastructure. III. The distal tubule in healthy individuals. Lab. Invest. *18*:655, 1968.

Welling, L. W., and D. J. Welling: Surface areas of brush border and lateral cell walls in the rabbit proximal nephron. Kidney Int. *8*:343, 1975.

Welling, L. W., and D. J. Welling: Shape of epithelial cells and intercellular channels in the rabbit proximal nephron. Kidney Int. *9*:385, 1976.

INTERSTITIUM

Bohman, S. O.: The interstitial cells of the renal medulla. Thesis, University of Aarhus, Denmark, 1979.

Bohman, S. O.: The ultrastructure of the renal medulla and the interstitial cells. *In* A. K. Mandal, and S. O. Bohman, eds.: The Renal Papilla and Hypertension. New York, Plenum Publishing Corp., 1980.

Bulger, R. E., and R. B. Nagle: The ultrastructure of the interstitium in the rabbit kidney. Am. J. Anat. *136*:183, 1973.

Johnson, F. R., and S. J. Darnton: Ultrastructural observations on the renal papilla of the rabbit. Z. Zellforsch. *81*:390, 1967.

Muirhead, E. F., G. S. Germain, F. B. Armstrong, B. Brooks, B. E. Leach, L. W. Byers, J. A. Pitcock, and P. Brown: Endocrine-type antihypertensive function of renomedullary interstitial cells. Kidney Int. *8*:271, 1975.

Schifferli, J., A. Grandcamp, and F. Chatelanat: Ultrastructure of the interstitial cells of the rat renal papilla. Kidney Int. *7*:366, 1975.

JUXTAGLOMERULAR APPARATUS

Barajas, L.: The ultrastructure of the juxtaglomerular apparatus as disclosed by three dimensional reconstructions from serial sections. J. Ultrastruct. Res. *33*:116, 1970.

Barajas, L., and H. Latta: Structure of the juxtaglomerular apparatus. Circ. Res. *20,21* (Suppl. II):15, 1967.

Edelman, R., and P. M. Hartroft: Localization of renin in the juxtaglomerular cells of the rabbit and dog by the fluorescent antibody technique. Circ. Res. *9*:1069, 1961.

Goormaghtigh, N.: Existence of an endocrine gland in the media of renal arterioles. Proc. Soc. Exp. Biol. Med.. *42*:688, 1939.

Hartroft, P. M.: Juxtaglomerular cells. Circ. Res. *12*:525, 1963.

Tanaka, T., E. W. Gresek, A. M. Michelakis, and T. Barka: Immunocytochemical localization of renin in kidneys and submandibular gland of SWR/J and C57BL/6J mice. J. Histochem. Cytochem. *28*:1113, 1980.

Tobian, L.: Relationship of juxtaglomerular apparatus to renin and angiotensin. Circulation *25*:189, 1962.

BLOOD VESSELS

Beeuwkes, R.: The vascular organization of the kidney. Annu. Rev. Physiol. *42*:531, 1980.

Beeuwkes, R.: Tubular organization and vascular-tubular relations in dog kidney. Am. J. Physiol. *229*:695, 1975.

Brenner, B. M., and R. Beeuwkes: The renal circulations. Hosp. Pract. *13(7)*:35, 1978.

LYMPHATICS

Albertine, K. H., and C. C. O'Morchoe: Distribution and density of the canine renal cortical lymphatic system. Kidney Int. *16*:470, 1979.

Bell, R. D., M. J. Kayl, F. R. Shrader, E. W. Jones, and L. P. Henry. Renal lymphatics: the internal distribution. Nephron *5*:454, 1968.

Pierce, E. C.: Renal lymphatics. Anat. Rec. *90*:315, 1944.

Rojo-Ortega J. M., E. Yeghiayan, and J. Genest: Lymphatic capillaries in the renal cortex of the rat. Lab. Invest. *29*:336, 1973.

HISTOPHYSIOLOGY

Beeuwkes, R.: Renal countercurrent mechanisms or how to get something for almost nothing. *In* Taylor, C. R., K. Johansen, and L. Bolis, eds.: A Companion to Animal Physiology. New York, Cambridge University Press, 1982.

Brenner, B. M., J. L. Troy, and T. M. Daugharty: The dynamics of glomerular ultrafiltration in the rat. J. Clin. Invest. *50*:1776, 1971.

Gottschalk, C. W.: Micropuncture studies of tubular function in the mammalian kidney. Physiologist *4*:35, 1961.

Jamieson, R. L., and R. H. Maffly: Urine concentrating mechanism. N. Engl. J. Med. *295*:1059, 1976.

Levinsky, N. G., and R. W. Berliner: The role of urea in the urine concentrating mechanism. J. Clin. Invest. *38*:741, 1959.

Stephensen, J. L.: Countercurrent transport in the kidney. Annu. Rev. Biophys. Bioeng. 7:315, 1978.

URINARY BLADDER

Hicks, R. M.: The fine structure of transitional epithelium of the rat ureter. J. Cell Biol. *26*:25, 1965.

Hicks, R. M.: The permeability of rat transitional epithelium, keratinization and the permeability to water. J. Cell Biol. *28*:21, 1966.

Hicks, R. M., and B. Katterer: Isolation of the plasma membrane of the luminal surface of epithelium, and the occurrence of a hexagonal lattice of subunits both in negatively stained whole mounts and in sectional membranes. J. Cell Biol. *45*:542, 1970.

Koss, L. G.: The asymmetric unit membranes of the epithelium of the urinary bladder of rat. Lab. Invest. *21*:154, 1969.

Warren, R. C., and R. M. Hicks: Structure of the subunit in the thick luminal membrane of rat urinary bladder. Nature *227*:280, 1970.

31

MALE REPRODUCTIVE SYSTEM

The male reproductive system includes the gonads, two *testes* and their duct system (the *ductuli efferentes, ductuli epididymides, ductus deferens,* and *ejaculatory ducts)* together with associated accessory glands—the *seminal vesicles, prostate,* and *bulbourethral glands* (Cowper's glands) (Figs. 31–1, 31–2).

TESTIS

The testis is a compound tubular gland enclosed in a thick fibrous capsule, the *tunica albuginea.* On the posterior aspect of the organ, a thickening of the connective tissue capsule projects into the gland as the *mediastinum testis.* Thin fibrous septa, called the *septula testis,* extend radially from the mediastinum to the tunica albuginea, dividing the organ into about 250 pyramidal compartments, the *lobuli testis.* The septula may be incomplete toward the periphery, so that the lobules intercommunicate, but where their apices converge upon the mediastinum they are more completely separated.

Each lobule is composed of one to four highly convoluted *seminiferous tubules.* These are 150 to 250 μm in diameter, 30 to 70 cm long, and extremely tortuous (Fig. 31–3). The seminiferous tubules constitute the exocrine portion of the testis, which is in essence a cytogenous gland whose holocrine secretory product is whole cells, the *spermatozoa.* The tubules are usually highly convoluted loops, but they may also branch or end blindly. At the apex of each lobule its seminiferous tubules pass abruptly into the *tubuli recti,* the first segment of the system of excretory ducts. They in turn are confluent with the *rete testis,* a plexiform system of epithelium-lined spaces in the connective tissue of the mediastinum.

On the inner aspect of the tunica albuginea, dense connective tissue gives way to a looser layer provided with numerous blood vessels, the *tunica vasculosa testis.* A loose connective tissue of similar character extends inward from this layer to fill all of the interstices among the seminiferous tubules. It contains fibroblasts, macrophages, mast cells, and perivascular mesenchymal cells. In addition, there are clusters of epithelioid *interstitial cells,* also called *Leydig cells.* These constitute the endocrine tissue of the testis.

Each testis is suspended in the scrotum at the end of a long vascular pedicle, *the spermatic cord,* which consists of the excretory duct of the testis, the *ductus deferens,* and the blood vessels and nerves supplying the testis on that side. The *epididymis,* an organ closely applied to the posterior surface of the testis, is made up of the convoluted proximal part of the excretory duct system (Figs. 31–2, 31–3). Each testis and epididymis is surrounded on its anterior and lateral surfaces by a cleftlike serous cavity that arises late in embryonic development as a detached portion of the peritoneal cavity.

The testes develop early in embryonic life in the dorsal wall of the abdominal cavity and later descend into the scrotum, each carrying with it an outpocketing of the peritoneum, the *tunica vaginalis propria testis,* which forms the serous cavity around the testis. It consists of an outer *parietal* and an inner *visceral* layer that is closely applied to the tunica albuginea of the testis on its anterior and lateral surfaces. On the posterior aspect of the testis, where the blood vessels and nerves enter the organ, the visceral layer is reflected from its surface and is continuous with the parietal layer. After removal of the parietal layer, the visceral coat covering the testis appears as a glistening, smooth surface covered with mesothelium, which is the rem-

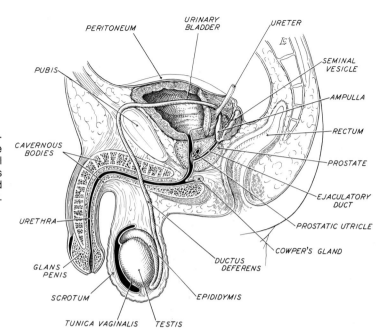

Figure 31–1. Diagrammatic representation of the male genital system. The midline structures are shown in sagittal section; bilateral structures, such as testis, epididymis, vas deferens, and seminal vesicle, are depicted intact. (After C. D. Turner.)

nant of the coelomic epithelium that covered the primordium of the gonad in the embryo. The tunica vaginalis enables the testis, which is sensitive to pressure, to glide freely in its envelopes.

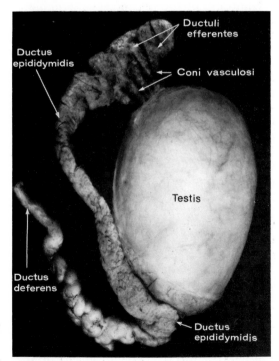

Figure 31–2. Photomicrograph of human testis, epididymis, and ductus deferens. The epididymis has been dissected free and drawn away from the testis to reveal more clearly the coni vasculosi. (Photograph courtesy of A. F. Holstein.)

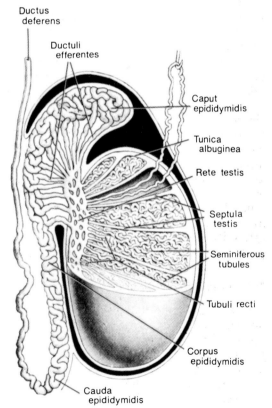

Figure 31–3. Cutaway diagram of the architecture of the testis and excurrent duct system. The septula divide the organ into a number of compartments occupied by highly convoluted seminiferous tubules. One has been unraveled and drawn out to show its length and the fact that it is a loop terminating in the rete testis. (Drawing modified from Hamilton, W. J. Textbook of Human Anatomy. London, Macmillan & Co., 1957.)

SEMINIFEROUS TUBULES

The Lamina Propria or Boundary Tissue

The seminiferous tubules are enclosed by one or more layers of adventitial cells derived from primitive connective tissue elements of the interstitium. The organization of this boundary tissue varies from species to species. In the common laboratory rodents, there is a single layer of flattened polygonal cells that meet edge to edge to form a continuous epithelioid sheet surrounding the tubule. In their ultrastructure, these cells have the cytological characteristics of smooth muscle and are contractile. They cannot be called true smooth muscle cells because of their atypical shape and epithelioid organization, and therefore are referred to as *myoid cells* or *peritubular contractile cells*. They are believed to be responsible for the rhythmic shallow contractions that can be observed in the seminiferous tubules of these species. The contractions seem to be intrinsically generated, since no nerves have been observed in or near this layer.

In larger species, such as ram, boar, and bull, there are multiple layers of adventitial cells. In these, only the innermost layer is muscle-like, the next layer has some of the characteristics of smooth muscle, and outer layers have the appearance of fibroblasts. In monkey and man there are also multiple layers of cells, but these are not epithelioid and the cells do not resemble smooth muscle as much as in other species. Contractility of seminiferous tubules has not been observed in primates. In many cases of human male infertility, the boundary tissue becomes greatly thickened.

The Seminiferous Epithelium

In the adult, the seminiferous tubules are lined by a complex stratified epithelium composed of two major categories of cells: *supporting cells* and *spermatogenic cells*. The supporting elements are of a single kind, the *Sertoli cells*, whereas the spermatogenic cells include several morphologically distinguishable types: *spermatogonia, primary spermatocytes, secondary spermatocytes, spermatids,* and *spermatozoa* (Figs. 31–4 to 31–8). These germ cells are not ontogenetically distinct cell types but are successive stages in a continuous process of differentiation of the male germ cells.

Sertoli Cells. The three-dimensional configuration of the Sertoli cell is extraordinarily complex, but it can be thought of as basically columnar, resting upon the basal lamina and extending upward through the full thickness of the epithelium to its free surface. From the columnar portion of these cells an elaborate system of thin processes radiate laterally to surround the spermatogenic cells and occupy all of the interstices among them. The earliest of the germ cells, the spermatogonia, also rest upon the basal lamina, while the more advanced stages of the germ cell line are found at successively higher levels in the epithelium (Figs. 31–7, 31–8). The proliferative activity in the epithelium is confined to the spermatogonia and spermatocytes near the base. The continual formation of new generations of cells in this region displaces the more advanced cells to higher levels until, as mature sperm, they come to border directly upon the lumen. To understand spermatogenesis, it is important to bear in mind that the seminiferous epithelium consists of (1) a fixed population of nonproliferating supporting cells and (2) a proliferating and differentiating population of germ cells that move slowly upward along the sides of the Sertoli cells to the free surface. This dynamic relationship of the cells makes the lining of the seminiferous tubules unique among epithelia.

Owing to the elaborate shape of the Sertoli cells and the limitations of resolution of the light microscope, their outlines cannot be seen distinctly. Earlier, this gave rise to the widespread belief that they constituted a syncytium, but this interpretation is now known to be erroneous. In sections parallel to the basal lamina of the epithelium, the bases of the Sertoli cells can be seen with the light microscope as distinctly outlined polygonal areas. Electron micrographs clearly show pairs of apposed membranes at the boundary between adjacent Sertoli cells and between the latter and the germ cells. Therefore, the spermatogenic cells are not embedded in a "Sertolian syncytium," but instead occupy deep recesses of conforming shape in the lateral and apical surfaces of the Sertoli cells. The elaborate shape of these cells (Fig. 31–9) is probably attributable to their close coaptation to the highly irregular and changing contours of the differentiating germ cells that they surround.

The nucleus of the Sertoli cell is generally ovoid in outline but may have one or more

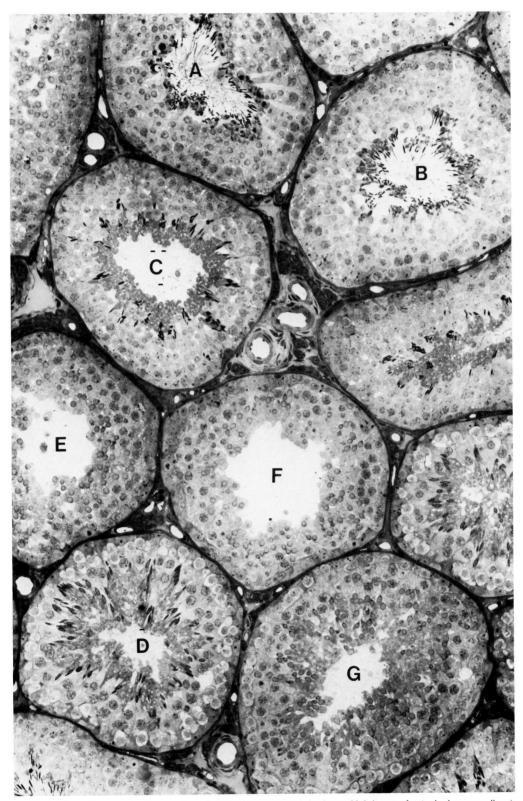

Figure 31–4. Photomicrograph of several seminiferous tubules and the interstitial tissue of a typical mammalian testis. Notice that the plane of section transects neighboring tubules in different stages of the spermatogenic cycle. Tubules A and B contain nearly mature sperm about to be released; in C and D, elongating spermatids are the most advanced germ cells; in E, F, and G, spermatogenesis has proceeded only to the round spermatid stage.

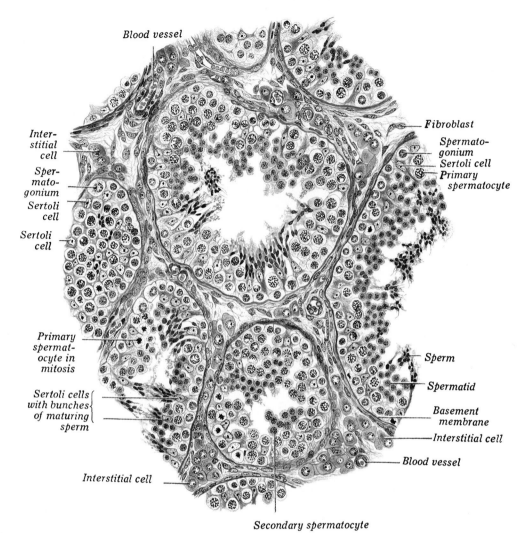

Figure 31–5. Section of human testis (obtained at operation). The transected tubules show various stages of spermatogenesis. × 170. (After A. A. Maximow.)

deep infoldings of its surface. It is about 9 by 12 μm in average size, with a relatively homogeneous nucleoplasm, except for a large and highly characteristic nucleolus, consisting of a round or oval central body flanked by two rounded basophilic masses. In electron micrographs, the tripartite structure of this complex is confirmed. The central element consists of a typical nucleolonema organized around a homogeneous central area of relatively low density. The two adjacent darker masses of finely granular material appear to be nucleolus-associated chromatin.

The cytoplasm contains numerous slender elongated mitochondria often oriented parallel to the long axis of the cell. Numerous

lipid droplets and occasional lipofuscin pigment granules are found near the cell base. The granular endoplasmic reticulum is sparse but the agranular reticulum is well developed, especially near the cell base. It usually occurs in the form of a network of smooth-surfaced tubules, but in some species it may form concentric systems of membranes around lipid droplets. The presence of a well-developed smooth endoplasmic reticulum at the cell base has been interpreted by some as evidence for secretion or modification of steroid hormones, but such a function has yet to be clearly established for the Sertoli cell. In certain stages of the spermatogenic cycle, close aggregations of smooth reticulum are found in the cytoplasm immediately adjacent to the developing acrosomal cap of each associated spermatid (Fig. 31–9). The significance of this striking localization remains unexplained, but may be an expression of the "nurse cell" function of Sertoli cells.

The Golgi complex is extensive but shows no morphological indication of involvement in secretory activity. The slender mitochondria have the usual foliate internal membrane structure and are remarkable only for their length. The lysosomal system of the cell exhibits a diversity of components, ranging from membrane-limited, spherical primary lysosomes to pleomorphic, dense, secondary

lysosomes, and to large irregular conglomerates of lipochrome pigment with a very heterogeneous content of globular and granular components of varying density. Although the lysosomal digestive system of these cells is well developed, the amount of accumulated pigment is not large when one considers that they are responsible for degradation and disposal of the residual cytoplasm of generation after generation of spermatids.

The filamentous component of the cytoplasmic matrix of Sertoli cells is more abundant than in many other cell types. A feltwork

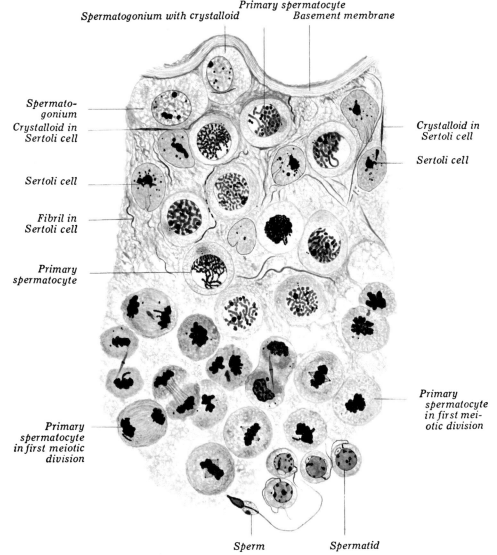

Figure 31–6. Section of same testis as in Figure 31–5; seminiferous epithelium with primary spermatocytes in first meiotic division. Iron-hematoxylin stain. × 750. (After A. A. Maximow.)

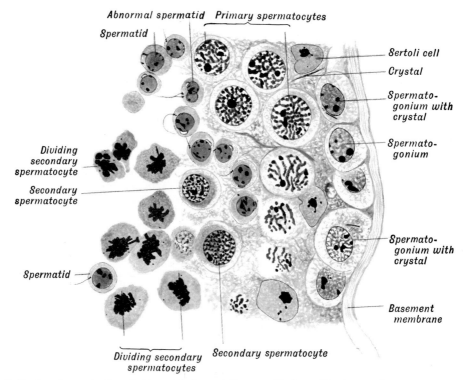

Abnormal spermatid Primary spermatocytes

Spermatid

Sertoli cell

Crystal

*Spermato-
gonium with
crystal*

*Spermato-
gonium*

*Dividing
secondary
spermatocyte*

*Secondary
spermatocyte*

*Spermato-
gonium with
crystal*

Spermatid

*Basement
membrane*

*Dividing secondary
spermatocytes* *Secondary spermatocyte*

Figure 31–7. Section of same testis as in Figure 31–5; seminiferous epithelium with mitoses of secondary spermatocytes in second meiotic division. The loosening of the spermatocytes and spermatids from their normal attachment to the Sertoli cells is an artifact of specimen preparation. × 750. (After A. A. Maximow.)

of 8- to 10-nm filaments excludes organelles and inclusions and results in a thin clear zone surrounding the nucleus. Filaments in lower concentrations are randomly dispersed in the cytoplasm. Occasionally they associate laterally to form fascicles parallel to the long axis of the cell. At certain stages of the spermatogenic cycle, microtubules are also abundant in the supranuclear columnar portion of the Sertoli cell. They are very uniformly spaced and oriented parallel to the cell axis. The escalation of the germ cells in the epithelium and the release of spermatozoa probably depend upon active changes in shape of the supporting cells. The filaments and microtubules of the Sertoli cells are very probably the agents of these cytoplasmic movements.

Inclusions peculiar to the human Sertoli cell are the *crystalloids of Charcot-Böttcher* (Fig. 31–8). These are slender, fusiform structures 10 to 25 μm long, often visible with the light microscope. In electron micrographs, they consist of dense straight filaments 15 nm in diameter. These subunits are generally parallel or converge toward the end of the crys-

talloid. They are often rather poorly ordered and there may be irregular defects in the interior of these crystalloids, occupied by cytoplasmic matrix. Their chemical nature and physiological significance are unknown.

The Sertoli cells provide mechanical support and protection for the developing germ cells, and they participate in their nutrition. They also seem to play an active role in the release of the mature spermatozoa. The Sertoli cells are never observed in division in the mature testis. They are resistant to heat, ionizing radiation, and various toxic agents that destroy the more sensitive spermatogenic cells.

THE SPERMATOZOON

It will facilitate the student's understanding of the complex cytological changes that take place in the germ cells of the seminiferous epithelium if the structure of the end product—the spermatozoon—is described first.

The mature spermatozoon is an actively motile, free-swimming cell consisting of a

Fibrils in Sertoli cell   *Sertoli cell*

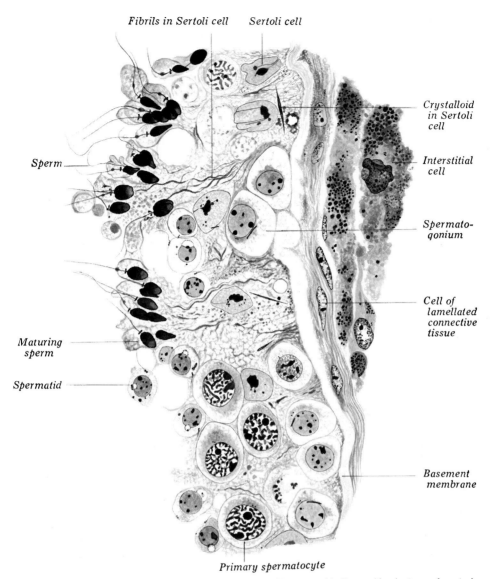

Sperm

Maturing sperm

Spermatid

Crystalloid in Sertoli cell

Interstitial cell

Spermato-gonium

Cell of lamellated connective tissue

Basement membrane

Primary spermatocyte

Figure 31–8. Section of same testis as in Figure 31–5; seminiferous epithelium with clusters of maturing sperm, connected with Sertoli cells. Iron-hematoxylin stain. × 750. (After A. A. Maximow.)

head, which contains a nucleus endowed with all the genetic traits a father can transmit to his offspring, and a *tail* or flagellum, which provides the motility that assists in transport of the sperm to the site of fertilization and ensures that it is appropriately oriented for penetration of the coatings of the ovum (Figs. 31–10 to 31–12).

The human sperm head is ovoid in outline in frontal view and pyriform when seen on edge, being thicker near the base and tapering toward the tip. The head is 4 to 5 μm in length and 2.5 to 3.5 μm in width. The greater part of its bulk consists of the nucleus, whose chromatin has become greatly condensed to diminish its volume for greater mobility and to protect its genome from damage in transit to the egg. The anterior two thirds of the nucleus is covered by the *acrosomal cap*—an organelle containing enzymes that have an important role in sperm penetration during fertilization (Figs. 31–11, 31–13). The mammalian sperm head varies greatly in size and shape from species to species.

The sperm tail is about 55 μm long and

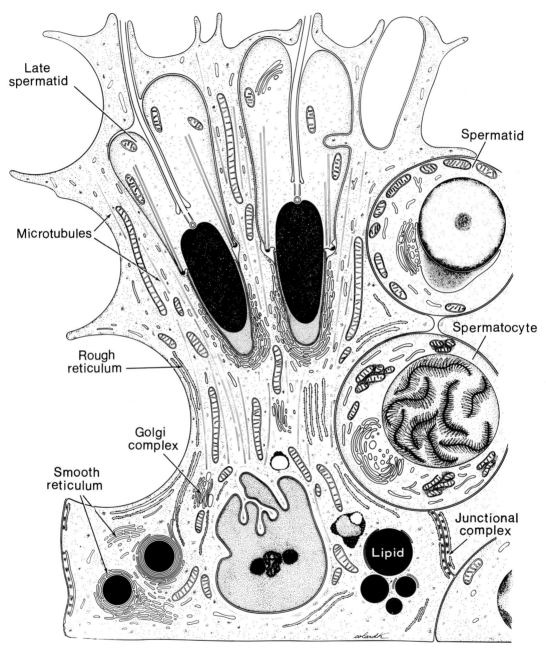

Figure 31–9. Drawing illustrating the ultrastructure of the Sertoli cell and its relationship to the germ cells. The spermatocytes and early spermatids occupy niches in the sides of the columnar supporting cell, while late spermatids reside in deep recesses in its apex. (After Fawcett, D. W., *In* Male Fertility and Sterility. Serono Symposium, 1973.)

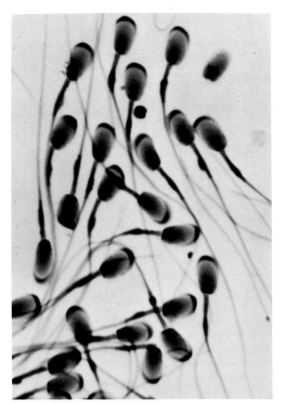

Figure 31–10. Photomicrograph of chinchilla sperm stained by the Feulgen reaction and counterstained with light green. The crescentic apical segment of the acrosome can be seen at the leading edge of the sperm head. × 3000.

varies in thickness from about 1 μm near the base to 0.1 μm near its tip. It presents four segments along its length recognizable with the light microscope by slight differences in thickness and in the nature of their sheaths. From proximal to distal, these regions are the *neck*, the *middle piece*, the *principal piece*, and the *end piece* (Fig. 31–11). There are significant differences in the internal structure of these segments. These cannot be clearly resolved in fresh preparations but require special cytological techniques, or electron microscopy, for their demonstration. The description of spermatozoon structure that follows is based largely on electron microscopic studies.

Sperm Head. The acrosome is a caplike, membrane-limited organelle that closely conforms to the contours of the tapering anterior portion of the sperm nucleus. The inner acrosomal membrane, which is adherent to the nuclear envelope, is continuous at the posterior margin of the cap with the outer

acrosomal membrane. The two membranes run parallel throughout most of their course and enclose a narrow cavity occupied by a homogeneous amorphous material—the enzyme-rich acrosomal contents. In the human spermatozoon, the acrosome is relatively small and does not extend anteriorly much beyond the leading edge of the nucleus. In many other mammalian species, however, there is a conspicuous thickening of the cap that extends well beyond the nucleus and may exhibit a species-specific shape. It is useful to designate this region as the *apical segment* of the acrosomal cap. The main por-

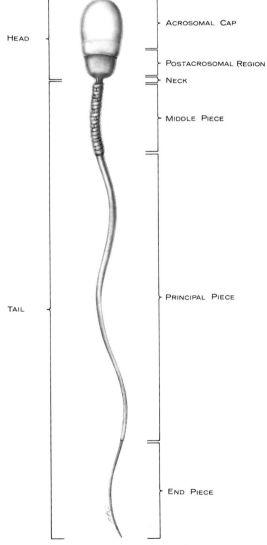

Figure 31–11. Drawing of a mammalian spermatozoon as seen with the light microscope, presenting the terms used in describing its various regions.

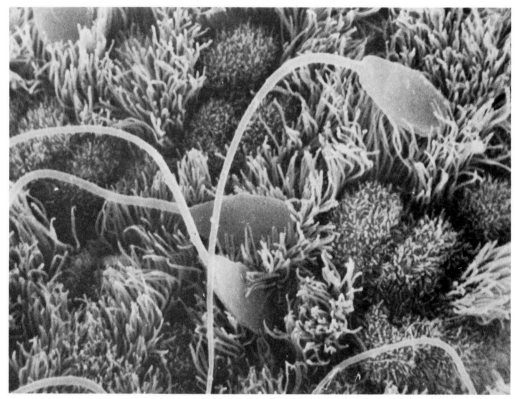

Figure 31–12. Scanning micrograph of rabbit sperm migrating over the surface of the uterine endometrium. (Micrograph courtesy of P. Motta.)

tion of the acrosome is then called the *principal segment*. In addition, in all mammalian species, there is a specialized caudal region where there is an abrupt narrowing of the cap and a slight condensation of its contents. With special staining techniques, this region was visible to light microscopists as a band around the middle of the head and was therefore called the *equatorial segment* (Fig. 31–13). The functional significance of this specialization has yet to be discovered.

The acrosome of mammalian spermatozoa stains with the periodic acid–Schiff reaction and hence contains appreciable amounts of carbohydrate. In addition, it is known to contain several enzymes of lysosomal nature. Among those identified to date are hyaluronidase, neuraminidase, acid phosphatase, β-*N*-acetylglucosamidase, and aryl sulfatase. There is also a proteolytic enzyme called *acrosin*, remarkably similar to trypsin in its substrate specificity, pH optimum, and range of inhibitors. The precise role of these enzymes in fertilization is still unclear, but extracts of sperm acrosomes will disperse the adhering cells of the corona radiata and will digest the zona pellucida from recently ovulated eggs. Sperm in the vicinity of ova in the oviduct undergo a sequence of structural changes called the *acrosome reaction*: the outer membrane of the acrosome fuses at multiple points with the overlying plasma membrane of the sperm head to create numerous openings through which the enzyme-rich contents of the acrosome are liberated in a process not unlike the release of secretory products from a glandular cell. The release of the enzymes is believed to facilitate sperm entry.

The nucleus of the mature mammalian spermatozoon is usually dense and homogeneous in electron micrographs (Figs. 31–13, 31–14). Human spermatozoa are subject to considerably more variation in size, in shape, and in texture of their chromatin than are those of other species. In ejaculates of fertile men, the chromatin in a certain proportion of the sperm nuclei is not homogeneous but is a dense conglomerate of closely packed coarse granular subunits. In these, the process of chromatin condensation during sper-

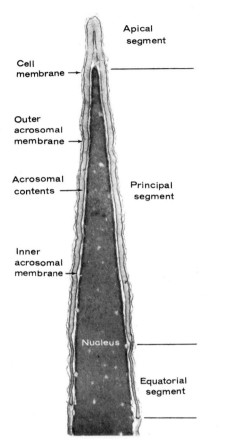

Cell membrane

Outer acrosomal membrane

Acrosomal contents

Inner acrosomal membrane

Apical segment

Principal segment

Nucleus

Equatorial segment

Figure 31–13. Electron micrograph of a monkey spermatozoon, illustrating the relationship of the acrosomal cap to the condensed nucleus and to the cell membrane.

miogenesis does not seem to have progressed to completion. Another peculiarity of human sperm nuclei is the frequent occurrence of irregularly shaped clear spaces of varying size in the chromatin. These are commonly referred to as *nuclear vacuoles*, although they are not membrane bounded. They seem to result from randomly occurring defects in condensation of the chromatin, and there is no evidence at present that they interfere with fertilizing capacity. Despite the absence of resolvable order in the fine structure of the nucleoplasm, there are indications that the chromosomes retain their identity and have a consistent arrangement within the nucleus. For example, quinacrine mustards have been found to stain the Y chromosome of man more or less selectively. When this method is applied to human sperm, a yellow fluorescent spot is located in approximately the same position in the heads of all of the male determining sperm.

Caudal to the acrosome, a specialized dense layer is found between the plasma membrane and the nuclear envelope (Fig. 31–14) that exhibits a characteristic pattern of fine structure that differs from species to species. It seems more closely adherent to the inner aspect of the cell membrane than to the underlying nucleus. This component corresponds to the "postnuclear cap" of classical light microscopy. However, inasmuch as it is not continuous over the posterior surface of the nucleus but is simply a broad band encircling the postacrosomal region, the term postacrosomal cap is no longer appropriate. Although the chemical nature and functional significance of this layer are not known, it is thought to be an important structure, for it is specifically in this region that the membrane of the sperm first fuses with that of the egg during fertilization.

The plasma membrane is firmly adherent to the nuclear envelope along a line, called the *posterior ring,* which encircles the sperm head at the caudal edge of the postacrosomal dense layer (Fig. 31–14). Behind this line or groove the membrane diverges somewhat from the underlying structures of the nucleus. The nuclear envelope, which is generally closely applied to the condensed chromatin, diverges from it caudal to this line of membrane adherence and forms a fold of variable size extending back into the neck region. Pores and annuli that are absent from the nuclear envelope over the condensed nucleus are abundant in this fold or scroll that extends back into the neck. This portion of the envelope is interpreted as a redundancy resulting from the diminution in volume of the nucleus associated with nuclear condensation during spermiogenesis. The nuclear envelope over the caudal surface of the head is again devoid of pores, and its membranes are in close apposition. The nuclear envelope lines the shallow *implantation fossa* where the tail attaches to the head. In this area there are regular periodic densities bridging the 10-nm interspace between the leaves of the nuclear envelope. These may help strengthen this region of attachment of tail to head.

The Neck. Immediately behind the head is a *connecting piece* that has a dense *capitulum* conforming in shape to the implantation fossa to which it attaches (Fig. 31–27). Extending backward from this capitulum are nine segmented columns 1 to 1.5 μm long

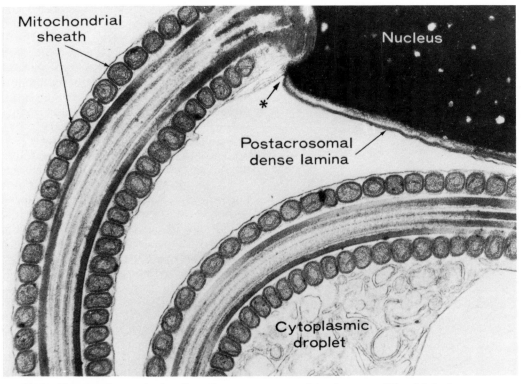

Figure 31–14. Electron micrograph of portions of two spermatozoa of the dormouse *(Glis glis)*. In the postacrosomal region, the membrane is reinforced by a dense lamina. This specialization may be important for fertilization, for it is this region that first fuses with the egg membrane. The asterisk indicates the site of the posterior ring, a circumferential line of fusion of the plasmalemma and the outer and inner membranes of the nuclear envelope. (Micrograph by D. Phillips, from Fawcett, D. W. Biol. Reprod. 2:Suppl. 2, 1970.)

that are continuous at their caudal ends with nine *outer dense fibers* of the sperm flagellum. In the interior of the connecting piece immediately subjacent to the articular surface of the capitulum is a transversely oriented *proximal centriole* (Fig. 31–27). The triplet microtubules of the centriole wall are embedded to varying degrees in the dense material composing the articular surface and segmented columns of the connecting piece. A *distal centriole* oriented in the axis of the sperm flagellum is usually absent from the mature spermatozoon, but vestiges of its nine triplets may be associated with the inner aspect of the segmented columns. The central pair of microtubules of the flagellar axoneme may extend anteriorly in the interior of the connecting piece as far as the proximal centriole.

One or two longitudinally oriented mitochondria may be found in the neck region outside the connecting piece, and these may have processes that extend between the segmented columns into its interior. In the human sperm, a sizable mass of residual cytoplasm may surround the neck, but in most mammals this *cytoplasmic droplet* is either absent from mature sperm or located at the caudal end of the middle piece.

The Middle Piece. In the core of the sperm flagellum is the *axoneme* consisting of two central singlet microtubules surrounded by nine evenly spaced doublets, an arrangement commonly described by the formula (9 + 2). This microtubule complex extends without significant change in structure throughout the length of the tail from the neck to near the tip of the end piece. The sperm flagellum differs from other flagella in that the axoneme is surrounded by nine *outer dense fibers* (9 + 9 + 2). Each dense fiber is continuous anteriorly with one of the segmented columns of the connecting piece, and each courses longitudinally in close relation to one of the nine doublets of the axoneme. The axoneme is considered to be the motor component, and the outer dense fibers to be resilient stiffening structures of the tail.

Three regions of the sperm tail are defined by the nature and extent of the sheaths that surround the 9 + 9 + 2 core complex (Fig. 31–20). The *middle piece* is characterized by a sheath of circumferentially oriented mitochondria arranged end to end in a tight helix (Figs. 31–14, 31–15, 31–20). These mitochondria generate the energy for sperm motility. The structural organization of the mid-

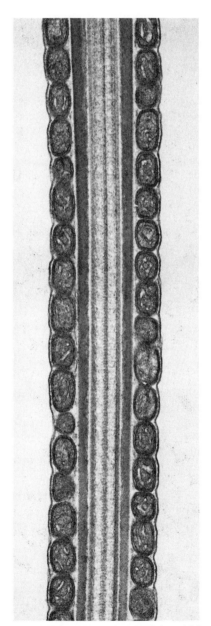

Figure 31–15. Electron micrograph of the midpiece of a spermatozoon in longitudinal section, showing the close apposition of the mitochondrial sheath to the outer dense fibers of the flagellum.

dle piece is basically similar in all mammalian spermatozoa, but the length of the mitochondrial helix varies from about 15 gyres in primates to over 300 in some rodents. In the human, the middle piece is from 5 to 7 μm long and somewhat more than 1 μm thick.

Immediately caudal to the last turn of the mitochondrial sheath is the *annulus*, a ring of dense material to which the flagellar membrane is firmly adherent (Fig. 31–16). The annulus and its attachment to the membrane are presumed to prevent caudal displacement of the mitochondria during the tail movements.

The Principal Piece. The principal piece of the spermatozoon is about 45 μm long and about 0.5 μm thick at the base, gradually tapering toward the end piece. It has a highly characteristic *fibrous sheath* (Figs. 31–17 to 31–20). Studied by electron microscopy, the latter is seen to consist of continuous dorsal and ventral longitudinal columns connected by regularly spaced circumferential ribs that extend halfway around the sheath and are continuous at their ends with the longitudinal

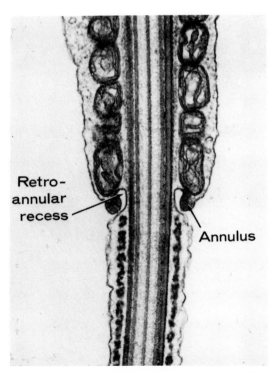

Figure 31–16. Electron micrograph of the junction of the midpiece and principal piece of a rodent spermatozoon. This is the site of the annulus, a dense ring fused to the plasma membrane. In some species, the cell membrane forms a deep groove or recess immediately behind the annulus. In others, the membrane is relatively smooth.

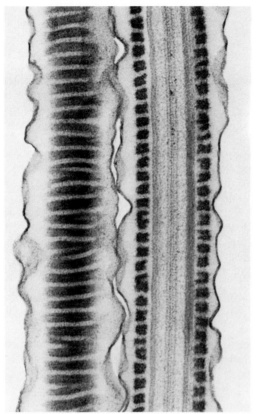

Figure 31–17. Longitudinal sections of two adjacent sperm tails. One has been cut tangentially to the fibrous sheath and shows some of its ribs in surface view; the other is a midline section and therefore shows the circumferential ribs of the sheath in cross section.

columns (Fig. 31–18). In cross sections of the principal piece, it is apparent that outer dense fibers 3 and 8 terminate a short distance beyond the annulus (Fig. 31–18). Distal to their termination, the tapering inner edges of the dorsal and ventral columns of the sheath extend into the position of these fibers and are attached to a short flange projecting radially from doublets 3 and 8 of the axoneme (Fig. 31–18). A plane through the longitudinal columns of the fibrous sheath coincides approximately with the plane through the centers of the central pair of microtubules of the axoneme. This plane divides the cross section of the tail asymmetrically (Fig. 31–18). On one side is a *minor compartment* containing three outer dense fibers, and on the other is a *major compartment* containing four. The asymmetry in the distribution of these fibers in the cross section is believed to be reflected in the movements

of the sperm tail. The principal plane of bending appears to be perpendicular to the dorsoventral axis of the tail, and the more rapid "power stroke" observed in the proximal portion of the tail is assumed to be toward the side having four outer dense fibers, two of which (numbers 5 and 6) are especially large. The details of the mechanism of sperm tail movement have yet to be worked out. It is now believed that the microtubules of the axoneme produce bending by a sliding mechanism comparable with that of skeletal muscle (See Cilia, Chapter 2.)

The End Piece. The fibrous sheath ends abruptly 5 to 7 μm from the tip of the flagellum. The terminal portion, distal to this point, consisting of the axoneme covered only by the flagellar membrane, is called the *end piece* (Fig. 31–20). Its structure is essentially identical to that of a simple flagellum or cilium. The manner in which the axoneme ends varies somewhat from species to species. In some, the doublets terminate at different levels in the tapering tip, but in primates, the nine doublets dissociate into 18 single microtubules. Thus, including the central pair, cross sections through the terminal half micrometer may show 20 closely spaced single microtubules.

SPERMATOGENESIS

Spermatogenesis comprises the entire sequence of events by which spermatogonia are transformed into spermatozoa. For convenience of description it may be divided into three principal phases. In the first, called *spermatocytogenesis*, the most primitive spermatogonia (Type A) proliferate by mitotic division to replace themselves and to give rise to several successive generations of spermatogonia, each somewhat more differentiated than the preceding one. Division of the last generation of spermatogonia (Type B) yields preleptotene spermatocytes. In the second phase, *meiosis*, the spermatocytes undergo two maturation divisions, which reduce the chromosome number by half and produce a cluster of spermatids. In the third phase, called *spermiogenesis*, the spermatids undergo a remarkable series of cytological transformations leading to the formation of spermatozoa.

For spermatogenesis to continue without exhausting the supply of stem cells, the sper-

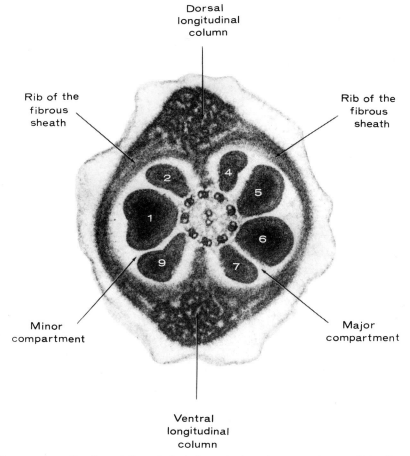

Figure 31–18. Transverse section through the principal piece of a hamster spermatozoon. Outer fibers 3 and 8 have terminated and their place is filled by inward extensions of the dorsal and ventral longitudinal columns of the fibrous sheath. The cross section is asymmetrical, with a major compartment containing four dense fibers and a minor compartment containing three.

matogonia must perpetuate themselves and also produce generation after generation of spermatocytes. In human testicular tissue preserved in Zenker-formol fixative, at least two types of spermatogonia (*A* and *B*) can be distinguished with little difficulty. The *Type A spermatogonium* has a spherical or ellipsoid nucleus with very fine chromatin granules and one or two irregularly shaped nucleoli attached to the inner aspect of the nuclear envelope. The cytoplasm is homogeneous and pale-staining. In some spermatogonia of this type, the nucleoplasm is dark, and a large, pale-staining nuclear vacuole is present. These cells in the human and monkey are designated as dark Type A spermatogonia, to distinguish them from the others with paler nucleoplasm and no nuclear vacuole. The *Type B spermatogonium* has a spher-

ical nucleus containing chromatin granules of varying size, many of which are distributed along the nuclear envelope. The single nucleolus is centrally located and often has granules of chromatin associated with it. The cytoplasm is not significantly different from that of the Type A spermatogonium.

The Type A spermatogonium undergoes a series of divisions that give rise to other Type A spermatogonia. Of these progeny, certain ones serve as stem cells for future cycles of spermatogonial renewal and spermatocytogenesis. Others proceed to differentiate through recognizable intermediates into Type B spermatogonia. The division of Type B spermatogonia then gives rise to primary spermatocytes.

In somatic cells, chromosomes are present in pairs. These cells are conventionally de-

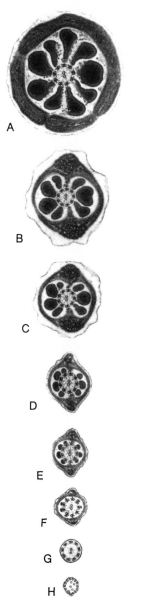

Figure 31–19. Cross sections at successive intervals along the length of the Chinese hamster sperm tail, illustrating the reduction in diameter of the outer dense fibers and the tapering of the tail as a whole. *A* is a section at the level of the midpiece. *B–F*, Successive levels in the principal piece. *G* and *H* are through the end piece. (Micrographs courtesy of D. Phillips.)

fertilization the spermatozoon and ovum each contribute a haploid set of chromosomes to the zygote, reestablishing the diploid chromosome number. The special type of nuclear division that results in formation of the haploid gametes is called *meiosis* (See also Chapter 1). In spermatogenesis it occurs in the spermatocytes.

The *primary spermatocytes* at first resemble in size and cytological characteristics the spermatogonia from which they arise, but as they move away from the basal lamina of the germinal epithelium, they accumulate more cytoplasm and become distinctly larger. Almost immediately after their formation, the spermatocytes enter prophase of the first maturation division. Their chromatin becomes reorganized into thin threadlike chromosomes characteristic of the *leptotene* stage of meiosis. The homologous chromosomes, which have duplicated themselves during the preceding interphase, undergo intimate pairing during the *zygotene* stage through formation of *synaptonemal complexes*. Because of the greater thickness and deeper staining of the paired chromosomes at this stage, they show up more clearly than those of the leptotene stage. When the pairing of the chromosomes to form *bivalents* or *tetrads* is complete, they continue the process of coiling and shortening to form the much coarser and more obvious chromosomal strands typical of the *pachytene* stage. At this stage, the duplicated chromosomes can be identified as *dyads* or *sister chromatids* held together at their *centromeres*. Each pachytene element consists of four chromatids. It is also at this period that *crossing over* occurs, in which corresponding regions of the chromatids of the paired chromosomes are exchanged. During the ensuing *diplotene* stage the chromosomes complete their process of shortening and the synaptonemal complexes disappear.

These stages of meiotic prophase are extremely prolonged, extending over about 22 days. For this reason, a great many spermatocytes in different stages of prophase can be seen in cross sections of seminiferous tubules.

At the end of prophase, the nuclear membrane disappears. The tetrads, or bivalents, arrange themselves at the equatorial plate in *metaphase I*. At *anaphase I* the centromeres of each homologous pair move to opposite poles of the spermatocyte taking both chromatids (dyads) along with them. This is in contrast to mitosis, during which the duplicated chro-

scribed as *diploid* in chromosome number, while the gametes that contain only one chromosome of each pair are *haploid*. The reduction in chromosome number of the gametes to half the somatic number is part of an orderly process that maintains a constant number of chromosomes for each species. At mosomes line up on the equatorial plate and the centromeres divide, sending copies of each chromosome to the opposite poles. The chromosomes that separate in meiosis are also unique in that they may differ from both maternal and paternal chromosomes because of exchanges that have taken place during crossing over. Anaphase I and *telophase I* are

quickly completed, resulting in the formation of secondary spermatocytes carrying only half the number of chromosomes originally present. Since the chromosomes have already been duplicated, the secondary spermatocytes remain in interphase only briefly and are therefore encountered only infrequently in sections of seminiferous tubules. The sec-

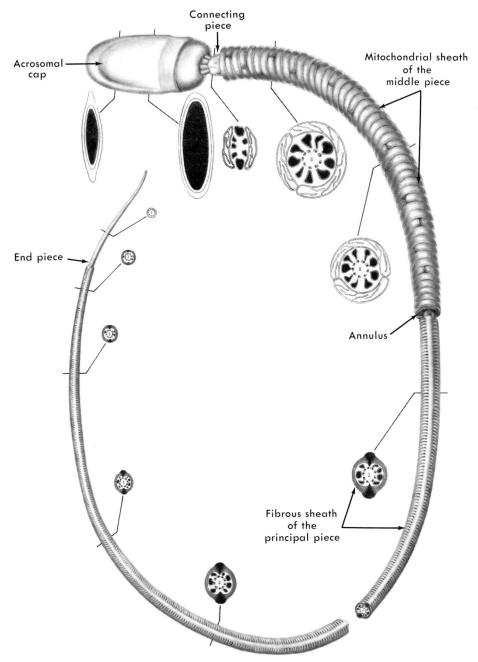

Figure 31–20. Generalized diagram of the structure of a mammalian spermatozoon as revealed by electron microscopy.

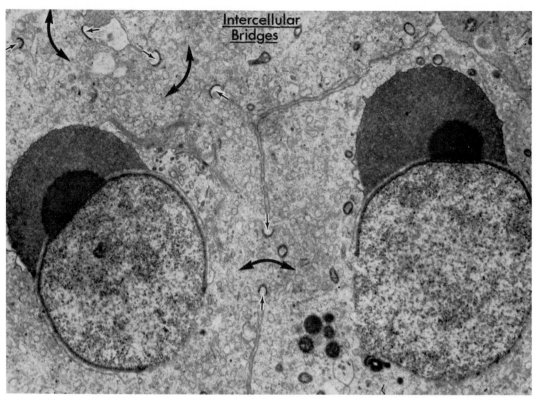

Figure 31–21. Electron micrograph showing two guinea pig spermatids and the intercellular bridges by which they are joined to each other and to two other spermatids of the same cluster. The small arrows indicate the local thickening of the cell membrane encircling the bridges. The large arrows passing through the bridges indicate the sites of continuity of the cytoplasm from cell to cell. × 9000.

ondary spermatocytes quickly complete the second phase of the meiotic division with a brief *prophase II* followed by *metaphase II* with the chromosomes aligned on the equatorial plate. *Anaphase II* differs from anaphase I in that the centromeres divide as in mitosis, permitting the sister chromatids to move to opposite poles. Upon completion of meiosis at *telophase II*, spermatids are formed that have a haploid set of chromosomes.

In the human spermatogonium there are 46 chromosomes, consisting of 22 pairs of *autosomes* and one pair of *sex chromosomes* (XX or XY). The different pairs of autosomes vary in size and in the location of the kinetochore, but the two members of any given pair of autosomes are morphologically identical. The sex chromosomes in the female (XX) are also identical, but those of the male (XY) differ markedly in size. At the end of the first maturation division in spermatogenesis, each bivalent, including the XY pair, separates into its two constituent chromosomes along the line of their previous con-

jugation. Therefore of any two secondary spermatocytes resulting from the first maturation division, one will contain 22 autosomes and an X chromosome, while the other will contain 22 autosomes and a Y chromosome. Since all the eggs produced by the female are the same, containing 22 autosomes plus X, those sperm developing from spermatocytes containing X will be *female determining,* because fertilization will result in a zygote containing 44 + XX (female), whereas sperm developing from secondary spermatocytes containing a Y chromosome will be *male determining,* for the zygote will contain 44 + XY (male).

Electron microscopic studies have shown that the division of all male germ cells, except the most undifferentiated spermatogonia, differ from somatic cell divisions in another important respect. Following division of the nucleus *(karyokinesis),* division of the cell body *(cytokinesis)* is incomplete, and the daughter cells remain connected by protoplasmic bridges at the site where the constricting cleavage furrow encounters the spindle remnant. Such spindle bridges occur as transient structures in mitosis of somatic cells, but in the seminiferous epithelium they remain, after dispersal of the spindle, as sizable communications between the daughter cells (Fig. 31–21). They persist to a late stage in the differentiation of the spermatids into spermatozoa. It has been the traditional view that each spermatogonium divided and the daughter cells each developed into a primary spermatocyte; this ultimately divided into two secondaries, and these in turn divided to form four individual spermatids. This interpretation is now known to be incorrect. In all but the earliest spermatogonial division,

cytokinesis is incomplete, resulting in groups of conjoined spermatogonia and larger syncytial clusters of primary spermatocytes. These produce double the number of interconnected secondary spermatocytes. Their division in turn produces very large numbers of conjoined spermatids (Fig. 31–22). The progeny of a single spermatogonium thus form a cluster of germ cells that remain in protoplasmic continuity throughout their differentiation. This arrangement is probably responsible for the synchrony of development of large numbers of germ cells in any one area of the seminiferous tubule. Individual sperm are separated from the syncytia at the moment of their release from the epithe-

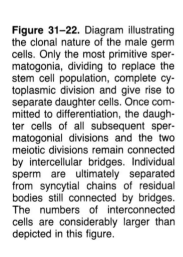

Figure 31–22. Diagram illustrating the clonal nature of the male germ cells. Only the most primitive spermatogonia, dividing to replace the stem cell population, complete cytoplasmic division and give rise to separate daughter cells. Once committed to differentiation, the daughter cells of all subsequent spermatogonial divisions and the two meiotic divisions remain connected by intercellular bridges. Individual sperm are ultimately separated from syncytial chains of residual bodies still connected by bridges. The numbers of interconnected cells are considerably larger than depicted in this figure.

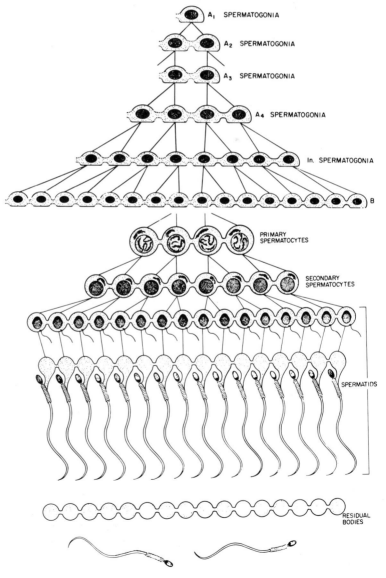

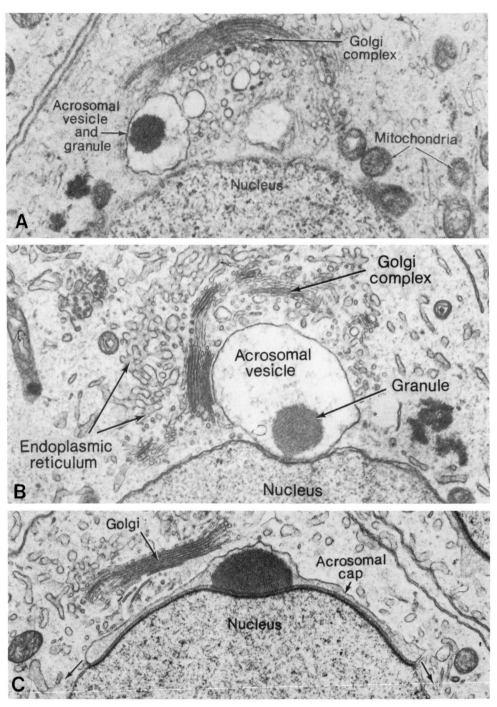

Figure 31–23. Electron micrographs of the juxtanuclear region of macaque spermatids, illustrating successive stages in formation of the acrosome. *A*, The initial event is the appearance of an acrosome vesicle and granule at the transface of the Golgi complex. *B*, The vesicle and granule are enlarged by further contributions from the Golgi complex and become closely adherent to the nuclear envelope. *C*, The acrosomal vesicle then spreads over the anterior hemisphere of the nucleus to form the acrosomal cap. The substance of the granule subsequently spreads laterally to occupy the entire interior of the acrosomal cap. (Micrographs courtesy of M. Dym.)

lium. Partial failures of this process may account for the frequency of abnormal double spermatozoa in the ejaculate.

Spermiogenesis

The term *spermiogenesis* describes the sequence of developmental events by which spermatids are transformed into spermatozoa. Each of the relatively small spherical or polygonal spermatids resulting from division of the secondary spermatocytes has a nucleus 5 to 6 μm in diameter with pale-staining finely granular chromatin. A small Golgi apparatus can be seen in the juxtanuclear cytoplasm. The first sign of differentiation of a specific component of the spermatozoon is the appearance of one or more small granules within the Golgi apparatus (Fig. 31–23A). In some species these are first observed in the spermatocytes; in others they are not seen until the spermatid stage. These *proacrosomal granules* are rich in carbohydrate and are most clearly demonstrated in specimens stained for light microscopy by the periodic acid–Schiff reaction. In electron micrographs, each is found to be enclosed within a membrane-limited vesicle associated with the Golgi apparatus. Although the general features of spermiogenesis can be followed with the light microscope, the finer details described here can be visualized only with the electron microscope. As development progresses, the several separate granules in the Golgi region coalesce into a single large globule, the *acrosomal granule,* contained within a membrane-bounded *acrosomal vesicle* or vacuole. This becomes adherent to the outer aspect of the nuclear envelope (Fig. 31–23B). The point of its adherence marks the future anterior tip of the sperm nucleus. The Golgi apparatus remains closely associated with the surface of the acrosomal vesicle, and it continues to form smaller vesicles that coalesce with the membrane of the acrosomal vesicle, contributing their contents to its enlargement.

It is convenient to divide spermiogenesis into four phases. That period from the appearance of the proacrosomal granules to the development of a hemispherical acrosomal granule fixed to the nuclear envelope is referred to as the *Golgi phase.* In the second or *cap phase,* the limiting membrane of the acrosomal vesicle increases its area of adherence to the nuclear envelope, forming a thin fold that spreads over the pole of the nucleus,

ultimately to cover its entire anterior hemisphere as a membranous *head cap.* The acrosomal granule meanwhile remains localized at the pole of the nucleus.

In the third or *acrosomal phase* of spermiogenesis, there is redistribution of the acrosomal substance, a condensation of the nucleoplasm, and an elongation of the spermatid (Fig. 31–24). The bulk of the acrosome remains localized at the anterior pole of the nucleus, but during this phase of spermiogenesis its substance gradually spreads in a thin layer into the fold of membrane composing the head cap until the acrosome and head cap are coextensive and constitute the *acrosomal cap* (often simply called the *acrosome*). In its definitive form it is a caplike structure, limited by a membrane and containing a substance rich in carbohydrate and hydrolytic enzymes. It varies in size and shape in different species but is present on the sperm of all mammals. The spermatid nucleus becomes elongated and flattened during this period. Its uniformly dispersed, finely granular nucleoplasm becomes transformed into thin strands or filaments that subsequently shorten and thicken into coarse dense granules.

During the fourth or *maturation phase* of spermiogenesis, there is little further change in the simple acrosome of primate sperm, but in other species it continues to undergo further alterations and gradually takes on the shape characteristic of the species.

The dense granules in the condensing nucleus become coarser, increasing in size at the expense of the intervening spaces until they finally coalesce and the nucleus is transformed into a homogeneous dense mass devoid of visible substructure. By the time this condition has been reached, the nucleus has attained the flattened pyriform shape characteristic of the human sperm head. Defects in the condensation of the nucleoplasm often leave one or more clear areas of variable shape and size, recognized with the light microscope as nuclear "vacuoles." These are large and of frequent occurrence in the human sperm but are small and relatively uncommon in the spermatozoa of other species.

While the early stages of acrosome formation are in progress at the anterior pole of the nucleus, the centrioles migrate to the opposite end of the spermatid. There the distal centriole becomes oriented perpendicular to the cell surface and gives rise to a slender flagellum that grows out into the

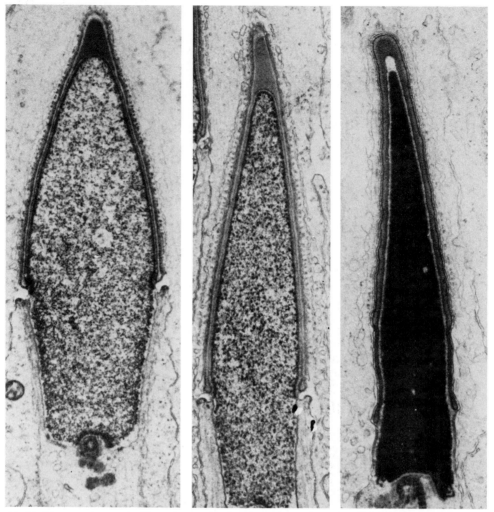

Figure 31–24. Electron micrographs illustrating successive stages in condensation of the chromatin and shaping of the nucleus of the spermatid late in spermiogenesis. (Micrographs courtesy of M. Dym.)

narrow extracellular cleft between the spermatid and the surrounding Sertoli cell (Fig. 31–25). As the nucleus begins to elongate and condense, the pair of centrioles and the base of the flagellum recede from the surface and take up a position at the caudal pole of the nucleus (Fig. 31–26). At about the same time, cytoplasmic microtubules arise and become laterally associated to form a roughly cylindrical structure, called the *manchette,* which extends caudally from a ringlike specialization of the cell membrane located at the posterior margin of the acrosomal cap (Fig. 31–28). Concurrently with the appearance of the manchette, there is a marked elongation of the spermatid, so that the bulk of the cytoplasm is displaced well behind the caudal pole of the nucleus, where it surrounds the proximal part of the flagellum (Fig. 31–28C,D,E).

The flagellum at this time consists only of the axial filament complex or *axoneme,* with two central fibrils and nine peripheral doublets. The latter are continuous with the wall of the distal centriole. The centriole is encircled by a ring of moderately dense filamentous or granular material. This annular structure was called the "ring centriole" by classical cytologists in the belief that it arose by unequal division of one of the centrioles. Electron microscopic studies provide no evidence in support of this interpretation. Instead, the ring appears to be a derivative of the *chromatoid body* (Fig. 31–27A). This loose ring is intimately associated with another small dense ring that arises as a local specialization on the inner aspect of the plasma membrane, where the latter is reflected from the cell body onto the flagellum.

In the further differentiation of the tail,

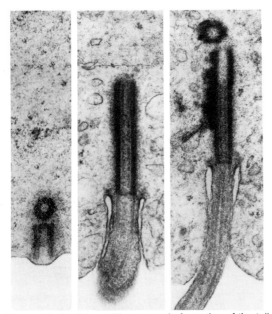

Figure 31–25. The earliest events in formation of the tail consist of migration of the centrioles to the cell surface in the postnuclear region, and polymerization of microtubule protein on the template provided by the distal centriole. A typical 9 + 2 axoneme is formed and the simple flagellum elongates by accretion of microtubule subunits to its distal end.

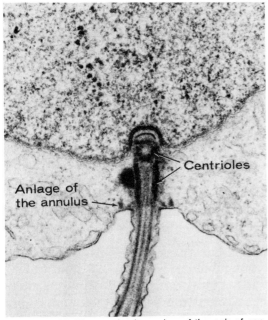

Figure 31–26. The proximal member of the pair of centrioles comes to occupy a shallow groove, the implantation fossa, in the caudal pole of the nucleus. The anlage of the future annulus then appears as a ringlike density adjacent to the membrane at its site of reflection onto the flagellum.

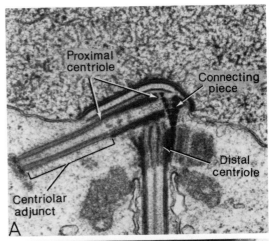

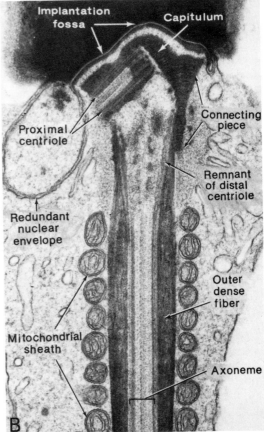

Figure 31–27. A, After establishing contact with the implantation fossa, the proximal or juxtanuclear centriole forms, at its distal end, the centriolar extension or adjunct. The segmented connecting piece begins to form around the distal centriole. B, Later in development, the centriolar adjunct disappears and the distal centriole disintegrates, leaving the proximal centriole in a vault or niche in the connecting piece that joins the nucleus to the outer dense fibers of the tail.

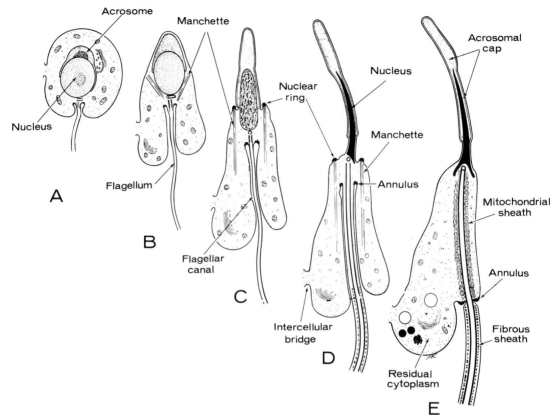

Figure 31–28. Diagram of successive stages in guinea pig spermatid differentiation, including nuclear condensation, appearance of the manchette, elongation of the cell, appearance of the fibrous sheath, caudal migration of the annulus, and formation of the mitochondrial sheath. (From Fawcett, D. W., W. A. Anderson, and D. M. Phillips. Dev. Biol. *26*:220, 1971.)

nine longitudinally oriented segmented columns arise around the centrioles. These are joined to each other proximally and to the base of the nucleus to constitute the connecting piece. Distally the nine structural elements forming the connecting piece are joined to nine longitudinal dense fibers that develop just peripheral to the doublets of the axoneme. The distal centriole and the large ring that earlier encircled it gradually disappear as the connecting piece and outer fibers of the tail develop. The smaller dense ring fixed to the flagellar membrane persists, and in the further elongation of the tail, it is carried distally several micrometers. As it moves back, the manchette disappears and mitochondria gather around the segment of flagellum between the annulus and the nucleus and become disposed helically around it to complete the differentiation of the middle piece (Fig. 31–28*C,D,E*).

While these developmental events are in progress, a succession of circumferentially oriented ribs or hoops are deposited around the tail distal to the annulus to form the fibrous sheath of the principal piece.

Spermiation

With the completion of differentiation of the tail, the spermatozoon is separated from the excess cytoplasm, which remains in the epithelium (Fig. 31–29) as a membrane-limited anucleate mass called the *residual body (of Regnaud)*, consisting of fine granules, lipid droplets, and degenerating excess organelles not used in formation of the spermatozoon.

The Cycle of the Seminiferous Epithelium

Spermatogenesis has been most thoroughly studied in the common laboratory rodents, where it displays a degree of order and regularity that facilitates a systematic analysis of the process. As stated earlier, several steps

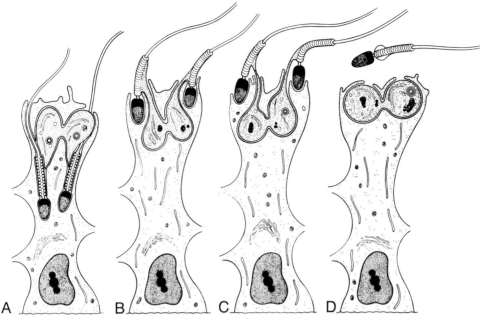

Figure 31–29. Diagrammatic representation of successive stages in sperm release. The axial components of the sperm are gradually extruded while the syncytial mass of spermatid cell bodies is retained in the epithelium. The attenuated stalk connecting the sperm to the residual cytoplasm finally gives way, freeing the spermatozoon. (From Fawcett, D. W. *In* Segal, S. J., et al., eds.: The Regulation of Mammalian Reproduction. Springfield, IL, Charles C Thomas, 1973.)

of germ cell development are found at different levels in the germinal epithelium, with the stem cells found at the base and the more differentiated cells located at successively higher levels (Fig. 31–30). The development of any one generation of germ cells goes on concurrently with the development of earlier and later generations at other levels in the epithelium. The cells in different phases of development are not randomly distributed within the epithelium but occur in a number of well-defined and easily recognized combinations or associations. The number of distinguishable cell associations varies with the species. In the guinea pig, for example, 12 such cellular associations or *stages of spermatogenesis* are identified. These are illustrated in the 12 vertical columns of Figure 31–31 and are designated by the Roman numerals at the bottom of each column. In any histological section of guinea pig testis, the cross sections of neighboring seminiferous tubules will vary in their appearance because of the different cell associations they contain (compare Figs. 31–32 and 31–33). If enough tubules are examined, all 12 cell associations or stages will be found, corresponding to the vertical columns in Figure 31–31. In studying this figure, it should be realized that a spermatogonium, in the course of its differentia-

tion into a spermatozoon, passes through all the cell types encountered by starting at the bottom of column I in this figure and reading from left to right along the horizontal rows from the bottom to the top row.

Spermatids at different phases of differentiation are always associated with spermatocytes and spermatogonia at their specific phases of development. The particular association of cells found at any point along the length of a seminiferous tubule changes with time, passing successively through all 12 stages and then repeating the sequence. The *cycle of the seminiferous epithelium* is defined as the series of changes occurring in a given area of the epithelium between two successive appearances of the same cellular association. The duration of the cycle has not been determined for the guinea pig, but it is about 12 days in the rat, and a spermatogonium takes about four cycles or 48 days to complete its differentiation and be released as a mature spermatozoon.

The various cell associations also occur in a numerically orderly sequence along the length of the seminiferous tubule. Thus, instead of considering the changes at a given point in the tubule, one can look at it from a different point of view, namely, as a series of successive cell associations found along the

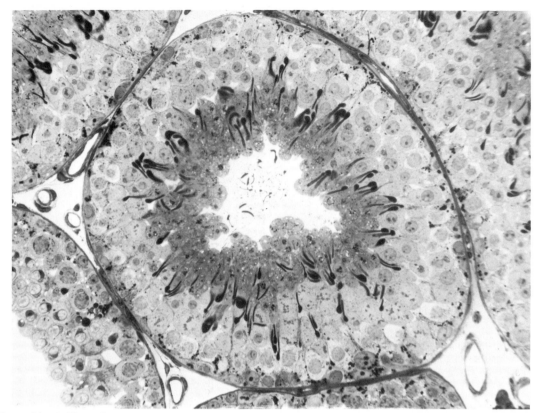

Figure 31–30. Photomicrograph of a guinea pig seminiferous tubule and portions of adjacent tubules. Notice that the epithelium in these four tubules exhibits different associations of cell types, representing different stages of spermatogenesis.

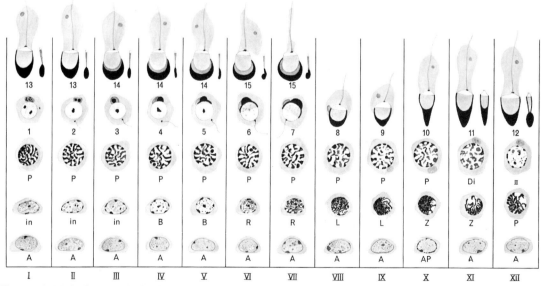

Figure 31–31. In these vertical columns, all 12 different cell associations or stages found in guinea pig seminiferous tubules have been assembled in their correct temporal sequence. Reading from lower left to right and from bottom to top, one follows the morphogenetic events from spermatogonium to release of spermatozoa. The time from the appearance of any one of these cell associations at a given point along the tubule until the reappearance of the same cell association is defined as one cycle of the seminiferous epithelium. (From Clermont, Y. Fertil. Steril. 6:563, 1960.)

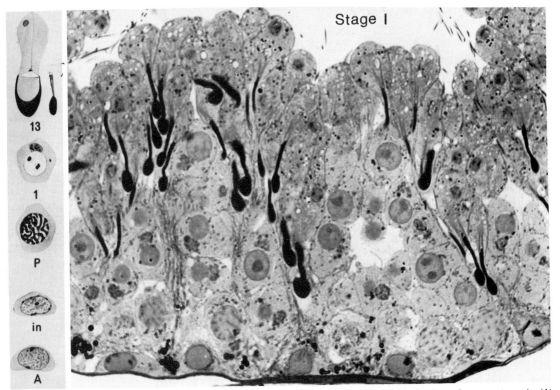

Figure 31–32. Photomicrograph of Stage I of guinea pig spermatogenesis, which includes type A spermatogonia *(A)*, intermediate spermatogonia *(in)*, pachytene spermatocytes *(P)*, spermatids at the beginning of acrosome formation *(1)*, and a more advanced generation of elongated spermatids with flattened, condensed nuclei *(13)*. (Inset from Clermont, Y. Fertil. Steril. 6:563, 1960.)

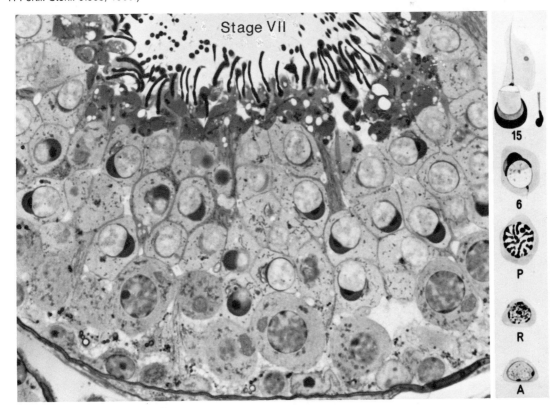

Figure 31–33. Photomicrograph of Stage VII of guinea pig spermatogenesis, characterized by the presence of spermatogonia *(A)*; large pachytene spermatocytes *(P)*; spermatids in the cap phase of acrosome formation *(6)*; nearly mature spermatids projecting into the lumen *(15)*; and residual bodies with dense cytoplasm forming a layer adjacent to the lumen.

length of the same tubule. The *wave of the seminiferous epithelium* is then the distance between two successive identical cell associations. That portion of the length of a wave occupied by one cell association is referred to as a *segment*.

The sequence of pictures along a wave is similar to the sequence of events taking place in one given area during a cycle of the seminiferous epithelium. In the rat there are said to be about 12 waves along the length of each tubule. The length of each segment in the wave corresponds roughly to the relative duration of that particular cell association or stage of the cycle.

In contrast to the very regular ordering of germinal elements in rodents, the appearance of the seminiferous epithelium in histological sections of the human testis at first suggests a haphazard arrangement of its cell types. Because of this apparent disorder, it was formerly believed that no synchronicity of germ cell development comparable with that found in rodents existed in man, and that no "cycle of the seminiferous epithelium" could be defined.

This has now been found to be erroneous. Six well-defined stages can be recognized, but instead of each occupying the entire cross section of the seminiferous tubule, as in ro-

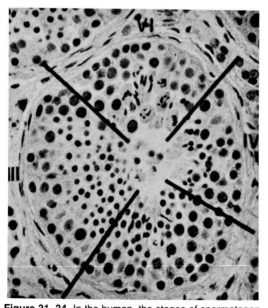

Figure 31–34. In the human, the stages of spermatogenesis do not occupy the whole circumference of a tubule as in other species. In this photomicrograph, for example, four different associations of cells are found in the same cross section. (From Clermont, Y. *Am. J. Anat.* 112:50, 1963.)

dents, the recognizable stages or cell associations in man occupy small wedge-shaped areas in the tubular epithelium (Fig. 31–34).

The human germinal epithelium is therefore a mosaic of irregularly shaped areas made up of the six different cell associations. Three or more stages of the cycle may be seen in a single cross section of a tubule. The situation is further complicated by the fact that the cells at the borders of these areas may intermingle to give atypical or heterogeneous associations of cells. The six typical associations are depicted in Figure 31–35.

The duration of the cycle of the human seminiferous epithelium has been determined by autoradiographic analyses of testicular biopsies from volunteers. Within one hour of local injection of tritiated thymidine, the label was found in nuclei of preleptotene spermatocytes in Stage III, but not in the pachytene spermatocytes of that stage nor in any other cells more advanced in their development. With the passage of time these labeled cells would be expected to pass through leptotene, zygotene, and early pachytene stages of meiotic prophase and reappear at the end of the cycle in a Stage III cell association as midpachytene spermatocytes. Serial biopsies revealed that the midpachytene spermatocytes of Stage III first showed that label 16 days after the initial injection of thymidine. It was thus established that the duration of one cycle is 16 days. As expected, labeled spermatids in Stage III were found at 32 days (two cycles). Assuming one cycle for the cells to develop from spermatogonia to preleptotene spermatocytes, and one to advance from spermatids to release of spermatozoa, the total duration of spermatogenesis in man is estimated to be four consecutive cycles or 64 days.

Degenerative and Regenerative Phenomena

In seasonally breeding mammals, active spermatogenesis, beginning at puberty, is discontinued and reinitiated periodically for the rest of the life of the animal. Each time, it continues only during the period of rut, at the end of which most of the spermatogenic cells are eliminated by degeneration or maturation depletion. Concomitantly, the seminiferous tubules shrink and gradually come to contain only Sertoli cells and some spermatogonia. In this condition, they resemble the tubules of a prepubertal testis. At the

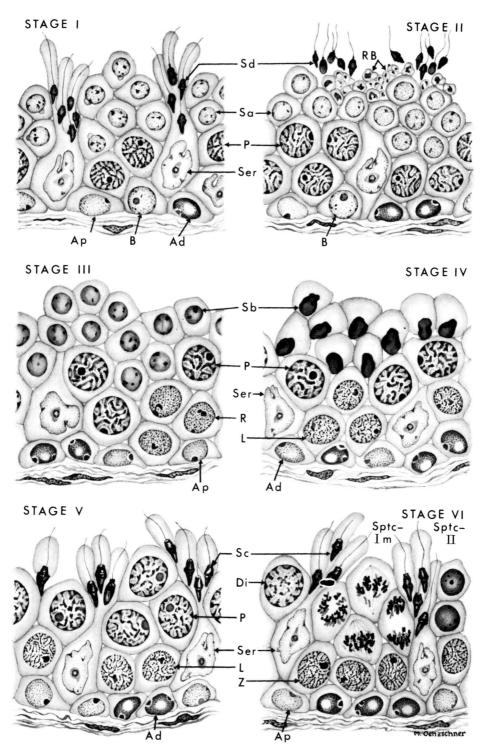

Figure 31–35. Diagram of the six recognizable cell associations or stages of the cycle of the human seminiferous epithelium. *Ser*, Sertoli cell; *Ad* and *Ap*, dark and pale type A spermatogonia; *B*, type B spermatogonia; *R*, resting primary spermatocyte; *L*, leptotene spermatocyte; *Z*, zygotene spermatocyte; *P*, pachytene spermatocyte; *Di*, diplotene spermatocyte; *Sptc-lm*, primary spermatocyte in division; *Sptc-II*, secondary spermatocyte in interphase; *Sa, Sb, Sc, Sd*, spermatids in various stages of differentiation; *RB*, residual bodies of Regnaud. (From Clermont, Y. Am. J. Anat. *112*:35, 1963.)

beginning of a new period of sexual activity, spermatogonia multiply and rapidly regenerate the various generations of spermatogenic cells. In the lower vertebrates, these seasonal changes of the testis are even more prominent.

In man and other mammals that are not seasonal breeders, spermatogenesis is continuous. Nevertheless, in an active human testis the tubules contain scattered degenerating spermatogenic cells in the seminiferous epithelium. This is not pathological unless it exceeds certain limits. The degenerating cells are seen in segments of the tubule in which the seminiferous epithelium is active and normal spermatogenesis is in full progress. The significance of the normal degeneration of a certain number of germ cells is not known.

Abnormal spermatogenic cells can often be found. In spermatogonia and spermatocytes, giant forms, as well as cells with two nuclei, are not uncommon. Multinucleated giant spermatids likewise are not infrequent. These abnormalities appear to be a consequence of the peculiar mode of cytokinesis in the dividing germinal cells, which normally leaves them connected by intercellular bridges. Failure of initial constriction between the daughter cells or a subsequent opening up of the bridges between two or more cells may lead to the formation of multinucleated spermatocytes or spermatids. Spermatids with two nuclei may continue to develop; thus, monstrous sperm with two tails or with one tail and two heads, may arise. These abnormal sperm are carried with the normal mature sperm into the epididymis, where some degenerate, but others persist and are also found in ejaculated semen.

The germ cells of the seminiferous epithelium are sensitive to noxious agents. In pathological conditions of general (infectious diseases, alcoholism, dietary deficiencies) or local (inflammation) character, degenerative changes, especially the formation of multinucleated giant cells by the coalescing spermatids, may become prominent. Exposure of the testis to a sufficient dose of x-rays causes an extensive degeneration of spermatogenic cells and may result in sterility. These cells are also sensitive to high temperature. Even the normal internal temperature of the body is incompatible with spermatogenesis. In the majority of adult mammals, the testes are therefore lodged in a scrotum, which has a temperature a few degrees lower than the rest of the body. Testes that fail to descend into the scrotum during development and remain in the abdomen never produce mature sperm. They show atrophic tubules containing only Sertoli cells and scattered spermatogonia. Failure of descent of the testis is called *cryptorchidism.* In experimentally produced cryptorchidism, the testis soon decreases in size and comes to contain only Sertoli cells and spermatogonia. The seminiferous tubules also atrophy in experimental animals fed a diet lacking vitamin E; they also undergo regression in vitamin A deficiency.

In all such cases, the Sertoli cells are more resistant than spermatogenic cells. Some spermatogonia frequently remain. Thus, under favorable conditions, when the noxious factor is removed or the vitamin deficiency corrected, a more or less complete regeneration of the seminiferous epithelium may take place. In mammals with a short life span, spermatogenesis continues undiminished until death. Although spermatogenesis continues far into senility in man, the seminiferous tubules do undergo gradual involution with advancing age. A testis of a man older than 35 usually shows scattered atrophic tubules; in the remainder of the organ, however, spermatogenesis may continue without visible alterations. In very old men, all the tubules may be depleted of spermatogenic cells.

INTERSTITIAL TISSUE

The endocrine component of the testis, the Leydig cells, are located in the angular interstices between the convoluted seminiferous tubules. The blood vessels form peritubular plexuses in the intertubular spaces. The organization of the interstitial tissue varies considerably from species to species. In the human the extravascular interstitial tissue is a loose connective tissue exceptionally rich in extracellular fluid (Fig. 31–36). In addition to small clusters of Leydig cells, there are infrequent fibroblasts, a few macrophages, occasional mast cells, and some relatively undifferentiated cells of mesenchymal origin that are capable of developing into Leydig cells in response to gonadotropic stimulation. In other species, especially in the pig, horse, and opossum (Fig. 31–37), Leydig cells are very abundant, occupying most of the intertubular space.

The interstitial cells of Leydig occur in

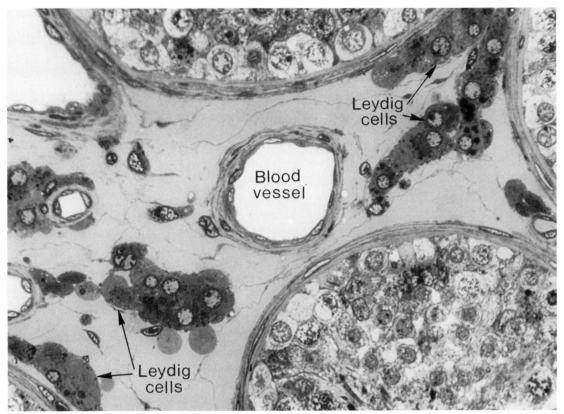

Figure 31–36. Photomicrograph of the interstitium between seminiferous tubules of human testis, showing several clusters of Leydig cells. Most of the extravascular space is occupied by a protein-rich interstitial fluid, which appears a uniform gray in this figure. There is little collagen in the interstitial tissue of the normal human testis. (Photomicrograph courtesy of W. Neaves.)

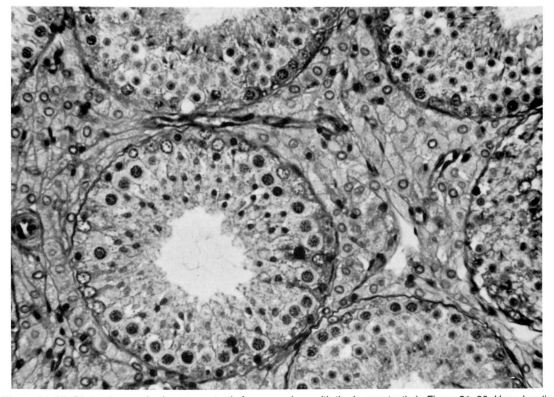

Figure 31–37. Photomicrograph of opposum testis for comparison with the human testis in Figure 31–36. Here, Leydig cells occupy nearly all the interstitial space.

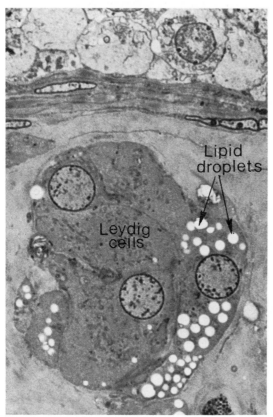

Lipid droplets

Leydig cells

Figure 31–38. Photomicrograph of a group of Leydig cells in human testis. These cells often contain numerous lipid inclusions, which are extracted in specimen preparation and appear as clear vacuoles. (Photomicrograph courtesy of W. Neaves.)

clusters of varying size, sometimes closely associated with blood vessels. They are usually irregularly polyhedral, 14 to 20 μm across, where they are closely packed, but at the periphery of the clusters or where occurring individually they may be elongated or spindle shaped. The large spherical nucleus contains a small amount of peripherally disposed heterochromatin and one or two prominent nucleoli. Binucleate cells are common. Adjacent to the nucleus is a large clear area that is found in electron micrographs to be occupied by a well-developed Golgi apparatus. Although the Golgi complex is prominent and responds to gonadotropic stmulation by enlargement, the role of this organelle in the biosynthetic and secretory processes of this cell type is not known. There is no visual evidence of accumulation of a product in secretory granules in the Golgi region, and at present we have little understanding of the mechanism of release of steroid hormones by these cells. Mitochondria are abundant and quite variable in size and shape. In electron micrographs, their cristae

tend to be tubular instead of lamellar, but this is not true in all mammalian species. The cytoplasm is acidophilic in routine preparations and may contain a number of vacuoles where lipid droplets have been extracted (Fig. 31–38). In common with other steroid-secreting endocrine cells, the most striking ultrastructural feature of the interstitial cell is its extensive smooth endoplasmic reticulum (Figs. 31–39, 31–40). Cisternal profiles of the granular reticulum are also present, but the bulk of the cytoplasm is filled with a branching and anastomosing system of smooth-surfaced tubules. These membranes contain the enzymes necessary for several of the steps in the biosynthesis of androgenic steroids. Peroxisomes and lysosomes are found in abundance, but their function in the economy of these cells is not understood. Golden-brown deposits of lipochrome pigment occur in the Leydig cells in men of all ages, but they become increasingly prominent with advancing age (Fig. 31–39).

A feature peculiar to the human Leydig cell is the presence of conspicuous cytoplasmic crystals 3 μm or more in thickness and up to 20 μm in length. These *crystals of Reinke* are highly variable in size and shape; they may be rounded or pointed at the ends (Fig. 31–41). They have little affinity for the common histological stains and appear nearly colorless in routine preparations. They can, nevertheless, be recognized in negative image in ordinary preparations and, if desired, they can be stained by azocarmine. They are isotropic in polarized light and have the solubility properties of protein. In electron micrographs they present a highly ordered structure that differs in its pattern, depending on the plane of section. The crystal consists of filamentous molecules about 5 mm thick. The crystals occur in the testes of most men from puberty to senility, but their abundance is subject to considerable variation. They are found in no other mammalian species and their significance is unknown.

BLOOD VESSELS AND LYMPHATICS OF THE TESTIS

The blood supply of the human testis is from a branch of the abdominal aorta called the *internal spermatic* or *testicular artery*. It divides either before reaching the testis or on its surface, giving rise to several main branches that penetrate the organ. These in turn give rise to *centripetal branches* that course toward the rete testis. Major branches of

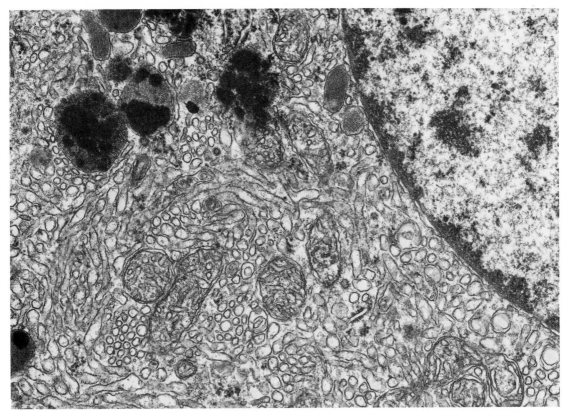

Figure 31–39. Electron micrograph of a portion of a human Leydig cell. As in other steroid-secreting cells, its most striking ultrastructural feature is the very extensive smooth endoplasmic reticulum. The dense bodies at the top of the figure are deposits of lipofuscin pigment that accumulate with age. (Micrograph courtesy of W. Neaves.)

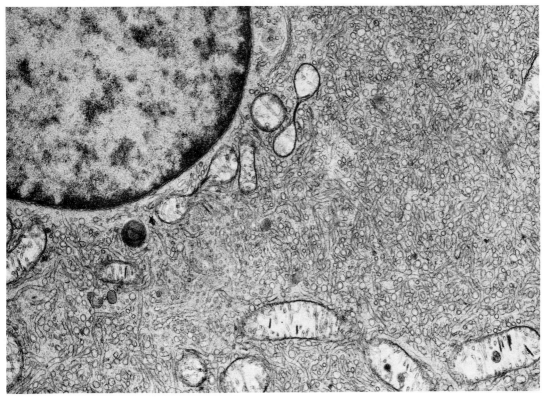

Figure 31–40. Interstitial cells in some species contain abundant droplets of lipid, whereas others are virtually devoid of lipid. The electron micrograph of opossum interstitial cell shown here is free of lipid. The cytoplasm is occupied by a very extensive agranular endoplasmic reticulum. × 10,000. (After Christensen, A., and D. W. Fawcett. J. Biophys. Biochem. Cytol. *9*:653, 1961.)

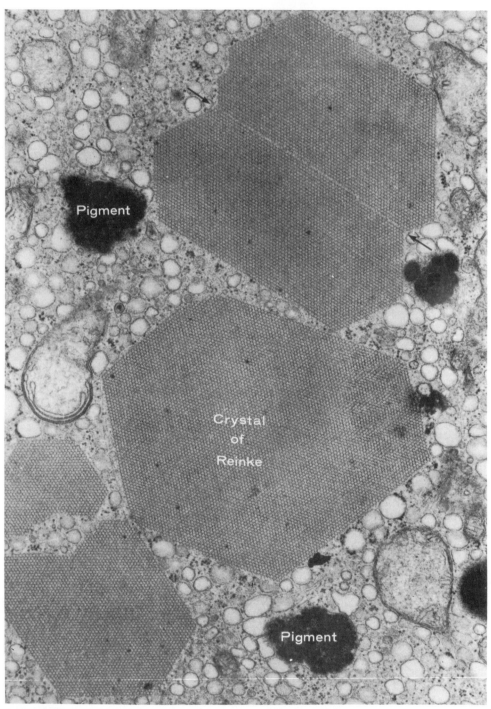

Figure 31–41. Electron micrograph of Leydig cell cytoplasm from human testis showing lipochrome pigment deposits, vesicular elements of smooth reticulum, and several crystals of Reinke. (Micrograph from Nagano, T., and I. Ohtsuki. J. Cell Biol. *51*:148, 1971.)

these vessels run in the opposite direction as *centrifugal branches.* The branching of the centripetal and centrifugal arteries gives rise to many *intertubular arterioles* located in the angular columns of interstitial tissue between the seminiferous tubules. The *intertubular capillaries* derived from these form networks in the interstitial tissue. The capillaries in neighboring interstitial columns are connected by ladder-like, circumferentially oriented *peritubular capillaries* (Fig. 31–42).

Postcapillary venules join to form collecting venules, and the confluence of these in turn forms veins that course toward the tunica albuginea (*centrifugal veins*) or toward the rete testis (*centripetal veins*). The former drain into veins of the tunica; the latter, running in the septula testis, converge upon a venous plexus associated with the rete testis. Upon reaching the surface, these veins join those of the tunica in forming the *pampiniform plexus* of veins in the spermatic cord. The right pampiniform plexus drains directly into the inferior vena cava via the *internal spermatic vein.*

The corresponding vein on the left joins the left renal vein. This evidently results in some slight impairment of venous return, so that the left pampiniform plexus is often more distended than the right, and the left testis is generally lower. The veins of the left pampiniform plexus are sometimes varicose, a condition described as *varicocele.*

In many animal species and possibly in man, the arrangement of blood vessels in the spermatic cord (the internal spermatic artery surrounded by the pampiniform plexus) constitutes a countercurrent heat exchange system that allows the arterial blood to lose heat to the cooler venous blood in the pampiniform plexus. This precooling of the arterial blood helps maintain the temperature of the testis a few degrees below deep body temperature. This lower temperature is essential for continued spermatogenesis.

The intertubular areas of the human testis also contain thin-walled lymphatic vessels that drain into larger lymphatics in the septula testis and tunica albuginea, and thence up-

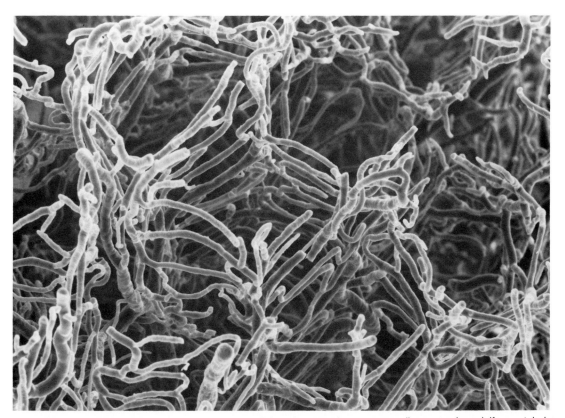

Figure 31–42. Scanning micrograph of a resin cast of the microvasculature surrounding several seminiferous tubules that have been dissolved out of the preparation. Intertubular vessels coursing parallel to the tubules are interconnected by closely spaced peritubular capillaries to form a circumferentially oriented ladder-like pattern. (Micrograph from Suzuki, F. Am. J. Anat. *163*:309, 1982.)

ward in lymph vessels of the cord to para-aortic lymph nodes and nodes associated with the renal blood vessels.

The lymphatics show considerable variation in pattern from species to species. In the common laboratory rodents, they form very extensive peritublar sinusoids. The aggregations of Leydig cells in these species are centrally located and closely associated with the walls of the blood vessels. They are surrounded by sinusoidal lymphatics. The steroid-secreting cells are thus interposed between the blood vascular elements on the one side and the lymphatic sinusoids on the other, and release their hormone into both. In larger species—ram, bull, and man—the lymphatics are not sinusoidal but form thin-walled vessels more or less centrally located in the intertubular areas. The Leydig cells are not intimately related to either the blood vessels or the lymphatics, but evidently they release androgen into the abundant extracellular fluid of the interstitial tissue, whence it diffuses to the tubules for its local effect on spermatogenesis, and to the vessels for its effect on distant target organs.

HISTOPHYSIOLOGY OF THE TESTIS

Endocrine Function

The endocrine function of the testis resides mainly in the interstitial cells of Leydig. These synthesize and release the male sex hormone *testosterone,* which is required in high local concentration to sustain spermatogenesis in the seminiferous tubules. In addition to its local action, testosterone circulating in the blood is essential for maintenance of function in the accessory glands of the male reproductive tract—the seminal vesicles, prostate, and bulbourethral glands. Testosterone is also responsible for development and maintenance of the male secondary sex characteristics—male pattern of pubic hair; growth of beard; low-pitched voice; and muscular body-build.

Production of testosterone by the Leydig cells depends primarily on the hypophyseal *luteinizing hormone* (LH), formerly referred to as *interstitial cell stimulating hormone* (ICSH). The action of LH on the Leydig cells involves binding to specific receptors in their plasma membrane. This, in turn, induces cyclic AMP

formation and activation of protein kinases. Cholesterol esterase liberates free cholesterol from cholesterol esters in lipid droplets of the Leydig cells. Mitochondrial enzymes cleave off the side chain of cholesterol to form pregnenolone and enzymes in the smooth endoplasmic reticulum, then carry out the several biosynthetic steps in transformation of this molecule to testosterone.

Although the Leydig cells constitute only a small percentage of the total volume of the testis, their steroidogenic potential is impressive. In the rat, where they make up only 1 per cent of the testis volume, there is estimated to be 22 million Leydig cells per gram of testis. The smooth endoplasmic reticulum, which contains the steroidogenic enzymes, has an estimated surface area of $10,500 \ \mu m^2$, and the mitochondria number about 600 per cell. From this morphometric data it is calculated that an average Leydig cell can produce about 10,000 molecules of testosterone per second. Testosterone appears to be produced as needed, and not stored in secretory granules for release on demand as in many other glandular cells. Detailed stereological analysis of the human testis has not been carried out, but it is likely that Leydig cells occupy less than 3 per cent of the total volume of the organ.

The hypophyseal control of Leydig cell function has proved to be more complex than was formerly thought. The release of LH from the pituitary gonadotropes is now known to be a discontinuous process, occurring mainly during the night in pulses at intervals of about 90 minutes. Moreover, hormones other than LH have been found to influence testosterone production. Prolactin binds to specific receptors on Leydig cells, affecting the number of their LH receptors and impairing their capacity to store cholesterol esters as precursors of testosterone. LH-releasing hormone (LHRH) not only affects pituitary gonadotropes but is reported to act directly upon Leydig cells, affecting their LH binding and their steroidogenic responsiveness.

There is increasing evidence that the seminiferous tubules also exert a local regulatory effect on the ultrastructure and function of the Leydig cells. An LHRH-like peptide, thought to be produced by the Sertoli cells, is inhibitory to Leydig cells. Local damage to seminiferous tubules appears to remove this inhibition and results in hypertrophy of the neighboring Leydig cells.

Exocrine Function

The spermatozoa can be thought of as a secretory product of the seminiferous tubules. The numbers of sperm produced are astronomical. Improved methods for estimating daily sperm production in the human yield a mean value of 94.6×10^6 per testis or 5.6×10^6 per gram of testicular tissue. Although this seems a very large number, it is low compared with other species. Daily sperm production per gram of testis in the rat is at least 20×10^6; in the rabbit, 25×10^6; and in the boar, 23×10^6. Taking into account the weight of the testis in the boar, the daily production of the two testes would amount to about 16.2×10^9 spermatozoa.

In the human, a normal ejaculate is 2 to 5 ml in volume and contains 40 to 100 million sperm per milliliter. This represents only a fraction of the number stored in the epididymis. Men with counts below 20 million per milliliter are usually infertile. The production of such large numbers of spermatozoa is less surprising if one considers that the two testes contain 800 to 1200 seminiferous tubules, each 30 to 70 cm long, which, in the aggregate, add up to one third of a mile of continuously proliferating seminiferous epithelium.

Spermatogenesis depends on testosterone produced by the Leydig cells in response to stimulation by LH and on follicle stimulating hormone (FSH), which acts upon the seminiferous tubules, binding specifically to the Sertoli cells. FSH is believed to be necessary for completion of spermatogenesis, but its mode of action remains controversial. It is known that FSH increases Sertoli cell synthesis of an *androgen-binding protein* that is required to maintain a high concentration of testosterone within the seminiferous epithelium. It may also promote synthesis of other products involved in the nurse-cell function of the Sertoli cells. Androgen-binding protein is secreted into the lumen of the tubules and transports testosterone downstream to maintain normal function of the epithelium lining the ductuli efferentes and epididymis.

The release of LH by the hypophysis is regulated by a negative feedback mechanism. Elevated levels of circulating testosterone suppress the release of LH, and abnormally low levels of testosterone result in increased LH release. The feedback regulation of FSH is less well understood. It is thought to involve a nonsteroidal factor called *inhibin*, probably produced by the Sertoli cells. In the presence of a normal complement of germ cells in the seminiferous epithelium, inhibin is believed to be continuously released and to act upon the hypophysis to suppress FSH production. Depletion of germ cells results in an increase in circulating levels of FSH. The FSH-inhibiting substance, inhibin, has yet to be completely characterized and its physiological importance remains a subject of controversy.

The secretory function of the seminiferous epithelium thus includes the synthesis and release of androgen-binding protein; an LHRH-like peptide; and possibly inhibin. It also elaborates a considerable volume of fluid that serves as a vehicle for transport of the spermatozoa to the rete testis and epididymis. This fluid is rich in potassium and other ions, in glutamate, and in inositol. These constituents are probably important for maintenance of the spermatozoa in their transit through the excretory duct system.

Blood-Testis Permeability Barrier

It has been known for several decades that vital dyes and many other substances introduced into the blood stream readily leave the vessels and enter the extracellular spaces of most of the tissues and organs except the brain. This vital organ is protected by a *blood-brain barrier* that resides in the endothelial junctions of the brain capillaries. More recently a *blood-testis barrier* has been described. The permeability barrier in this case is not in the walls of the blood vessels, which are in fact unusually permeable in the interstitial tissue. Instead, the exclusion of dyes and other large molecules from the seminiferous tubules is due to the presence of special junctional complexes between adjacent Sertoli cells near the base of the seminiferous epithelium. These consist of many parallel lines of fusion of the apposed membranes, which effectively prevent entry of substances into the system of intercellular clefts in the upper parts of the epithelium. These occluding junctions are situated at the interface between overarching Sertoli cell processes just above the spermatogonia (Fig. 31–43). Thus, they divide the epithelium into a *basal compartment*, containing the spermatogonia and preleptotene spermatocytes and an *adluminal compartment*, containing the more advanced stages of germ cell differentiation. Substances in the extracellular spaces of the interstitium have relatively unimpeded access to the basal compartment but are barred from deeper penetration into the epithelium

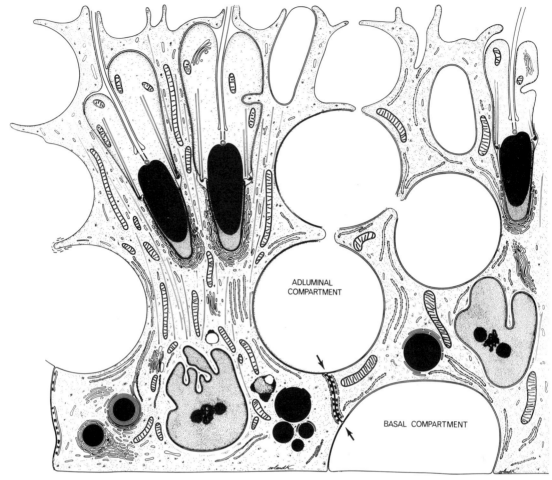

Figure 31–43. Drawing illustrating how the occluding junction *(at arrows)* between overarching processes of adjacent Sertoli cells divides the epithelium into basal and adluminal compartments. Substances diffusing from the interstitium have direct access to the spermatogonia in the basal compartment, but are excluded from the adluminal compartment by membrane fusion in the junction complexes. These then constitute the main structural basis of the blood-testis permeability barrier. (From Fawcett, D. W. *In* Handbook of Physiology. Vol. 3. Baltimore, Williams and Wilkins Co., 1975.)

by the Sertoli cell junctional specializations. At the appropriate stage of the spermatogenic cycle, spermatocytes must move from the basal compartment into the adluminal compartment. This is accomplished without disruption of the permeability barrier. Undermining processes are extended from the Sertoli cells to join beneath the spermatocytes and form new occluding junctions. The preexisting Sertoli junctions above the spermatocytes then dissociate, permitting upward movement of this cohort of conjoined germ cells.

The full significance of this arrangement is still being studied, but it is clear that a barrier near the base of the epithelium enables the Sertoli cells to maintain in the adluminal compartment a microenvironment especially favorable for germ cell differentia-

tion. Moreover, the postmeiotic germ cells are genetically different from the parent cells. The blood-testis barrier no doubt serves to prevent foreign protein from these cells from reaching the blood and inducing the formation of antibodies, which would result in autoimmune infertility.

EXCRETORY DUCTS OF THE TESTIS

The Tubuli Recti and Rete Testis

The seminiferous tubules occupy lobules or compartments within the testis that are demarcated by connective tissue septula extending inward from the tunica albuginea.

The several tubules in each lobule form convoluted loops, the ends of which converge toward a posteriorly situated region of highly vascular connective tissue described as the *mediastinum of the testis*. Within its substance is a labyrinthine plexus of epithelium-lined channels called the *rete testis* (Fig. 31–3).

Near the ends of the seminiferous tubules, the germ cells disappear from the epithelium, leaving a short terminal segment lined by Sertoli cells only. An abrupt narrowing then occurs where the seminiferous tubule is continuous with the *tubulus rectus*, a short, narrow channel connecting the seminiferous tubule to the rete testis. The tubuli recti and rete testis are lined by a simple cuboidal epithelium. The cells are relatively simple in their fine structure and do not give the appearance of being highly active. Their free surface bears a sparse covering of microvilli. Many—perhaps all—of the lining cells have a single flagellum projecting into the lumen. This is presumed to be motile, although it is not obvious what function it could serve other than some degree of agitation of the fluid contents of the rete.

In the guinea pig, the cells of the tubuli recti and the proximal portion of the rete testis store a remarkable amount of glycogen, which displaces the nucleus toward the lumen and all other organelles toward the cell periphery. This has not been reported in other species.

Ductuli Efferentes

From the posterosuperior aspect of the testis, 12 or more *ductuli efferentes* arise from the rete and emerge on the surface of the testis. Through numerous spiral windings and convolutions they form five to ten conical bodies about 10 mm in length called the *coni vasculosi*. These have their bases toward the head of the epididymis and their apices toward the mediastinum testis (Figs. 31–2, 31–3). They are held together by connective tissue and constitute part of the head of the epididymis.

The ductuli efferentes have a characteristic epithelium. The lumen has a festooned outline because it is lined by alternating groups of tall ciliated and lower nonciliated cells. The shorter cells may form small, cuplike excavations in the thickness of the epithelium. The nonciliated cells may contain granules. These were formerly interpreted as secretory material, but ultrastructural and histochemical studies now indicate that they

are lysosomes. There is no evidence that the epithelium of the ductuli efferentes is secretory. The nonciliated cells have short microvilli and canalicular invaginations of the free surface that are pathways of endocytosis. In animals injected with vital dyes, the cells accumulate dye inclusions, as a result of absorption from the lumen. The tall ciliated cells usually have a conical form, with the broad end toward the lumen. The cilia on the free surface beat toward the epididymis and move the sperm in this direction.

Outside the basal lamina of the epithelium is a thin layer of circularly arranged smooth muscle cells. In the distal portion of the ductuli forming the coni vasculosi, the muscular layer becomes more prominent.

Ductus Epididymidis

The convoluted tubules of the coni vasculosi gradually fuse with one another to form the single highly coiled *ductus epididymidis*. It forms a compact organ less than 7.6 cm long, but if the duct were uncoiled and straightened out, it would be over 6 m long. The epididymis is the site of accumulation and storage of spermatozoa. In addition, there is evidence from work on experimental animals that the spermatozoa are not physiologically mature when they leave the testis but gradually acquire the ability to fertilize and the capacity for normal motility as they slowly move through the long epididymal duct. The epithelium lining this organ may play an important role in creating a fluid environment favorable for continued maturation of the spermatozoa. The epididymis is customarily subdivided into three regions for descriptive convenience: the *caput* (head), *corpus* (body), and *cauda* (tail) (Fig. 31–3). At the distal end of the cauda, the duct gradually straightens out and continues as the *ductus deferens*.

The epididymis is lined with a pseudostratified columnar epithelium in which at least two cell types are distinguishable. The *principal cells* in the initial segment of the caput are very tall but gradually become lower in successive segments and are low columnar or cuboidal in the cauda epididymidis. The free surface of each principal cell bears a tuft of very long, nonmotile stereocilia (Figs. 31–44, 31–45). These have no basal bodies and in electron micrographs appear to be enormous microvilli. They have a bundle of fine filaments in their core that extends downward for some distance into the apical cytoplasm.

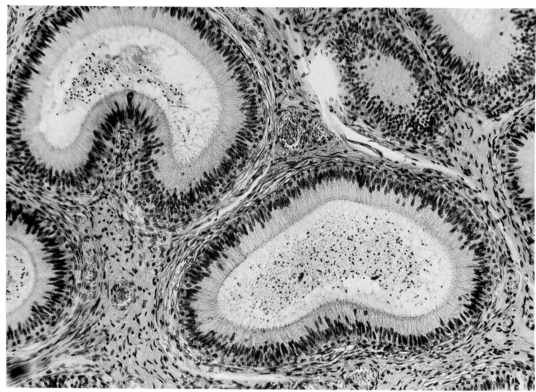

Figure 31–44. Section of ductus epididymidis from an adult man. Spermatozoa are seen in the lumen. × 180.

The cell surface between stereocilia is irregular in contour, exhibiting numerous invaginations suggestive of active pinocytosis. Large numbers of coated vesicles and large multivesicular bodies are present in the apical cytoplasm. These structural elements are believed to participate in the absorptive func-

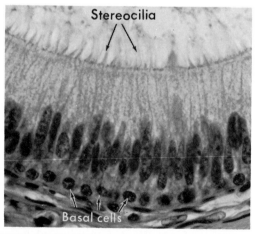

Figure 31–45. Photomicrograph of human epididymal epithelium, showing the characteristic row of basal cells and the stereocilia on the free surface.

tions of the epididymal epithelium. Over 90 per cent of the fluid leaving the testis is absorbed in the ductuli efferentes and ductus epididymidis. If horseradish peroxidase or an electron-opaque particulate marker is injected into the rete testis, it can be shown to be taken into vacuoles and ultimately into multivesicular bodies of the principal cells of the epididymal epithelium. Lysosomes are also found in these cells, and in certain segments of the epididymis of some species they are so large and numerous as to be easily visualized with the light microscope. They were interpreted as secretory granules by a number of early investigators, but this view has now been abandoned.

The principal cells have a number of cytological characteristics typical of actively synthesizing secretory cells. Their basal cytoplasm is filled with cisternae of granular endoplasmic reticulum, and the apical portion of the cell contains many profiles of smooth or sparsely granulated reticulum that are distended with a homogeneous content of low density. The supranuclear Golgi complex is remarkably large, but is not obviously involved in segregation of a secretory product. There are no secretory granules and no unambiguous indication of exocytosis. The functional significance of the high degree of differentiation of the principal cells still eludes us. The epididymal epithelium is known to produce glycerophosphorylcholine, and a sperm-coating glycoprotein.

Cells of the second type, the *basal cells,* are small round or pyramidal elements lodged between the bases of the columnar cells (Fig. 31–45). Their cytoplasm has little affinity for stains and is of low density in electron micrographs. The organelles are few and relatively simple in their structure. Lipid droplets are common in the basal cells of some species. The basal cell surface may interdigitate extensively with the neighboring principal cells. The function of the basal cells is even more obscure than that of the principal cells.

Scattered among the columnar cells at various levels in the epithelium are small cells with pale cytoplasm and dark heterochromatic nuclei. These have been termed "halo cells" by some authors, but recent electron microscopic studies identify them as intraepithelial lymphocytes.

External to the epithelium of the ductus epididymidis is its smooth musculature, which exhibits a gradual proximodistal increase in thickness. In the caput, the contractile cells are very slender, and the bundles they form are, for the most part, oriented circumferentially. In the corpus, sparse strands of longitudinally and obliquely oriented cells form an incomplete outer layer. At the transition from the corpus to the cauda, typical large smooth muscle cells are added to the smaller contractile cells characteristic of more proximal portions of the epididymis (Fig. 31–46). These progressively increase in number. In the distal portion of the cauda, the two-layered muscle coat is

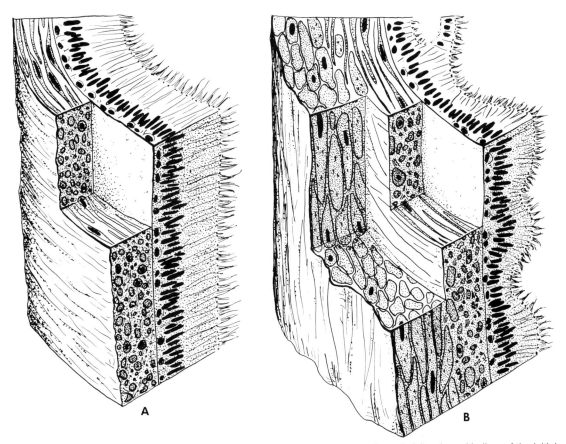

Figure 31–46. *A,* Drawing showing circumferentially oriented thin contractile cells underlying the epithelium of the initial portion of the ductus epididymidis. *B,* Corresponding illustration of the transitional zone between the corpus and the cauda. Slender contractile cells are found immediately subjacent to the epithelium, and several layers of typical large smooth muscle cells are found peripheral to these. (From Baumgarten, H., A. Holstein, and E. Rosengren. Z. Zellforsch. *120:*37, 1971.)

transformed into a three-layered coat, which continues into the ductus deferens.

The regional differences in the cytology of the musculature are associated with differences in the motility of the ductus epididymidis. In the caput and upper corpus, where slender muscle cells predominate, the duct undergoes spontaneous rhythmic peristaltic contractions that serve to transport the spermatozoa slowly along the tract. These contractions are independent of nervous stimulation and continue when the duct is excised and maintained in vitro. Contractions of this character are much reduced in the cauda, the principal site of sperm storage. The larger smooth muscle fibers that predominate in this region evidently require adrenergic sympathetic nervous stimulation. The sympathetic nerve net increases in density along the cauda and reaches a maximum in the intra-abdominal portion of the ductus deferens, which is principally involved in the powerful contractions that expel sperm during the ejaculatory reflex.

The epididymis is a highly vascular organ with the highest volume flow associated with the metabolically active initial segment of the caput (Figs. 31–47, 31–48).

Ductus Deferens

On passing into the ductus deferens, the excretory pathway acquires a larger lumen and a thicker wall. The epithelium and the lamina propria mucosae form longitudinal folds, which result in the highly irregular outline of the lumen seen in cross section (Figs. 31–49, 31–50). The pseudostratified columnar epithelium is lower than in the epididymis, and the cells usually have stereocilia. The connective tissue of the mucous membrane contains extensive elastic networks. The highly developed muscular coat forms a layer 1 mm thick. It consists of inner and outer longitudinal layers, and a powerful intermediate layer of circular muscle. Outside the muscle there is an adventitial coat of connective tissue. The firm duct is easily palpable through the thin skin of the scrotum.

The *spermatic cord* consists of the ductus deferens and its accompanying spermatic artery, pampiniform plexus of veins, and nerves of the spermatic plexus. The cord is enclosed by the *cremaster muscle*, a discontinuous layer of loose, mainly longitudinal strands of striated muscle. This layer extends

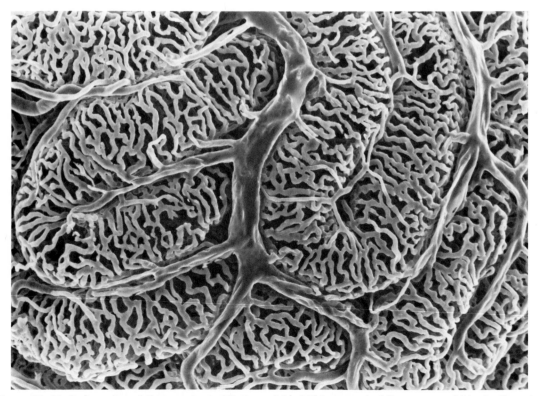

Figure 31–47. Surface view of the vascular architecture of the initial segment of the mouse epididymis. Scanning micrograph of a resin cast. (Micrograph from Suzuki, F. Am. J. Anat. *163*:309, 1982.)

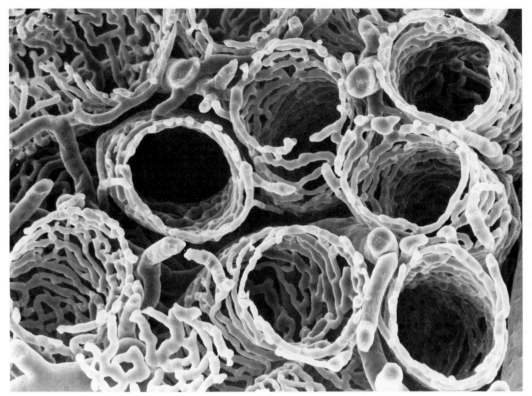

Figure 31–48. Transverse section through the initial segment of mouse epididymis, showing the extraordinarily rich periductal capillary network. (Micrograph from Suzuki, F. Am. J. Anat. *163*:309, 1982.)

Figure 31–49. Cross section of human ductus deferens. × 30. (After Schaffer.)

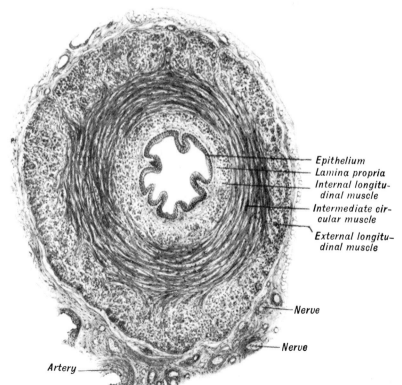

Epithelium

Lamina propria

Internal longitudinal muscle

Intermediate circular muscle

External longitudinal muscle

Nerve

Nerve

Artery

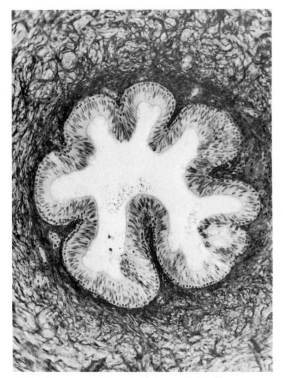

Figure 31–50. Histological section of the human ductus deferens, showing its irregular lumen, pseudostratified epithelium, lamina propria, and surrounding bundles of longitudinal smooth muscle. (Micrograph courtesy of A. Hoffer.)

downward to invest the testes and serves to raise them in response to cold, fear, and other stimuli.

The ductus deferens, after crossing the ureter in the abdominal cavity, forms a fusiform enlargement, the *ampulla*. At the distal end of the ampulla it receives the duct of a large gland, the *seminal vesicle*. Then, as the short (19-mm) straight *ejaculatory duct*, it pierces the body of the *prostate gland*, at the base of the urinary bladder. It opens by a small slit into the prostatic urethra, on a thickening of its posterior wall, called the *colliculus seminalis* or *verumontanum* (Figs. 31–51, 31–53). The openings of the ejaculatory ducts are located on either side of a blind invagination on the summit of the colliculus, the *utriculus masculinus*. This vestigial organ represents in the male the homologue of the uterus.

In the ampulla of the ductus deferens, the mucosa is thrown into numerous thin, irregularly branching folds, which in many places fuse to give the appearance in sections of a netlike system of partitions with angular meshes. The epithelium shows evidence of secretion. From the excavations between the folds, numerous tortuous branched outpocketings reach far into the surrounding muscular layer and are lined with a single layer

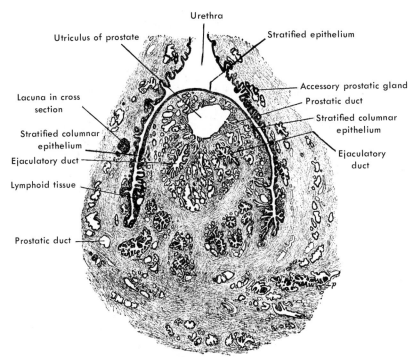

Figure 31–51. Cross section through colliculus seminalis of a young man. The urethra has been incised above. The utriculus of the prostate has prostatic ducts emptying into it. × 10. (After von Ebner, from Schaffer.)

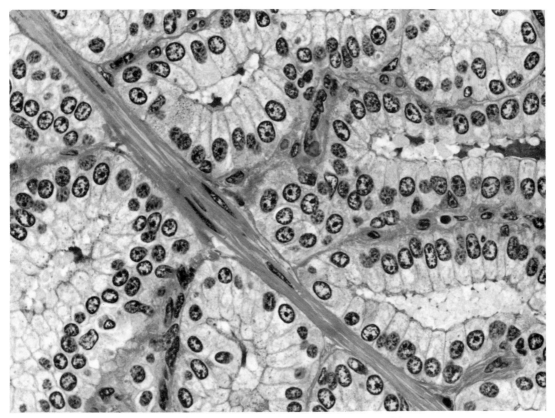

Figure 31–52. Photomicrograph of monkey seminal vesicle.

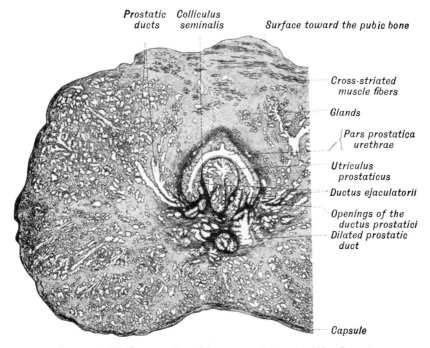

Prostatic   *Colliculus*
ducts   *seminalis*   *Surface toward the pubic bone*

Cross-striated
   muscle fibers

Glands

{Pars prostatica
* urethrae*

Utriculus
* prostaticus*

Ductus ejaculatorii

Openings of the
* ductus prostatici*
Dilated prostatic
* duct*

Capsule

Figure 31–53. Cross section of human prostate. × 4. (After Braus.)

of columnar, clear cells of glandular nature containing secretion granules. The musculature is much less regularly arranged here than in the other parts of the ductus deferens.

Ejaculatory Ducts

The epithelium lining the ejaculatory ducts is a simple or pseudostratified columnar epithelium, probably endowed with glandular functions. Its cells contain a large quantity of yellow pigment granules. Near the openings of the duct, the epithelium often assumes the structure of "transitional" epithelium. The mucosa of the ducts forms many thin folds reaching far into the lumen; its connective tissue is provided with abundant elastic networks. The dorsomedial walls of the ducts contain a series of glandular outpocketings, which may be accessory seminal vesicles. The ducts proper are surrounded only by connective tissue.

ACCESSORY GLANDS OF THE MALE REPRODUCTIVE TRACT

Seminal Vesicles

The seminal vesicles are elongated organs with numerous lateral outpocketings from an irregularly branching lumen. They arise as evaginations of the ductus deferens and are basically similar to it in structure. The wall consists of an external connective tissue layer rich in elastic fibers, a middle layer of smooth muscle thinner than in the ductus deferens, and an epithelium resting on a thin layer of loose connective tissue. The mucosa forms an intricate system of thin, primary folds, which branch into secondary and tertiary folds. These project far into the lumen and anastomose frequently. In this way, numerous cavities in different sizes are formed, separated by thin branching partitions (Fig. 31–52). All these cavities open into the larger central cavity, but in sections many of them may seem to be isolated.

The epithelium shows great individual variations, which probably depend on age and physiological conditions. As a rule, it is pseudostratified and consists of rounded basal cells lodged between larger cuboidal or low columnar cells. All basal cells have a supranuclear pair of centrioles, whereas in the

superficial cells the centrioles are located just beneath the surface and give rise to a central flagellum. The cells contain numerous granules and clumps of yellow lipochrome pigment that first appears at puberty. Similar pigment may also be found in the smooth muscles and in the connective tissue of the seminal vesicles. The epithelial cells contain secretion granules. The secretion of the seminal vesicles is a slightly yellowish, viscid liquid. In sections it appears as coagulated, netlike, deeply staining masses in the lumen. After castration, the epithelium atrophies, but it can be restored to normal by injections of testosterone.

The muscular wall of the seminal vesicles is provided with a plexus of nerve fibers and contains small sympathetic ganglia.

Prostate Gland

The prostate is the largest of the accessory glands of the male reproductive tract. Its secretion, together with that of the seminal vesicles, serves as a diluent and vehicle for transport of sperm from the male to the female. The prostate is about the size of a horse chestnut and surrounds the urethra at its origin from the urinary bladder. It is a conglomerate of 30 to 50 small, compound tubuloalveolar or tubulosaccular glands, from which 16 to 32 excretory ducts open independently into the urethra on the right and left sides of the colliculus seminalis (Fig. 31–53). The form of the glands is irregular. Large cavities, sometimes cystic, alternate with narrow branching tubules. The blind ends of the secreting portions are sometimes narrower than the excretory ducts. In many places, branching papillae and folds with a thin core of connective tissue project far into the lumen. In sections they may appear as isolated, epithelium-lined islands in the cavities. The basal lamina is indistinct, and the glandular epithelium rests on a layer of connective tissue with dense elastic networks and numerous blood capillaries. In the larger alveolar cavities the epithelium may be low cuboidal or even squamous, but in most places it is simple or pseudostratified columnar. The cytoplasm of the cells contains numerous secretory granules. The epithelial cells become smaller and lose their secretion granules after castration. Injections of testosterone restore the cells quickly to their normal appearance and activity.

Dense connective tissue forms a capsule around the organ and extends into it to constitute its abundant stroma. Thick septa of collagenous fibers and smooth muscle radiate from the colliculus seminalis toward the capsule partitioning the glandular tissue. Around the urethra, smooth muscle forms a thick ring—the internal sphincter of the bladder.

The secretion of the prostate is a thin, opalescent liquid with a slightly acid (pH 6.5) reaction. It has a rather low protein content but contains diastase, beta glucuronidase, several proteolytic enzymes, and a potent fibrinolysin. It is the main source of the citric acid and acid phosphatase of the semen. In sections, the secretion in the glandular cavities appears granular. It contains occasional desquamated cells and spherical or ellipsoid concentrically lamellated bodies—the *prostatic concretions* (Fig. 31–54). These are believed to originate through condensation of the secretions. They may become calcified, and may exceed 1 mm in diameter. The smaller concretions pass into the semen and can be found in the ejaculate. The larger ones are unable to pass out through the ducts and may remain in the gland lodged in cysts. Their number increases with age.

The prostate is abundantly provided with plexuses of nonmyelinated nerve fibers connected with small sympathetic ganglia. Sensory nerve endings of various kinds (end bulbs, genital corpuscles, and so on) are scattered in the interstitial connective tissue. Free nerve endings have been described in the epithelium.

The *utriculus prostaticus*, situated deep in the interior of the prostate gland and opening on the colliculus seminalis, may be a minor accessory gland of the male sexual apparatus. It is a blind vesicle of considerable size lined with an epithelium with many folds and glandlike invaginations. The epithelium is similar to that of the prostate. Sometimes, patches of ciliated columnar epithelium can also be found.

The prostate is of great medical interest because *benign nodular hyperplasia of the prostate* is the most common tumor in the aging male. The disease begins at about 45 years of age, and by the time the age of 80 is reached, 80 per cent of the male population is affected with varying degrees of obstruction of the bladder neck and urinary retention. Cancer of the prostate is also the most common malignant tumor in the male.

Unfortunately, the physiology of the gland

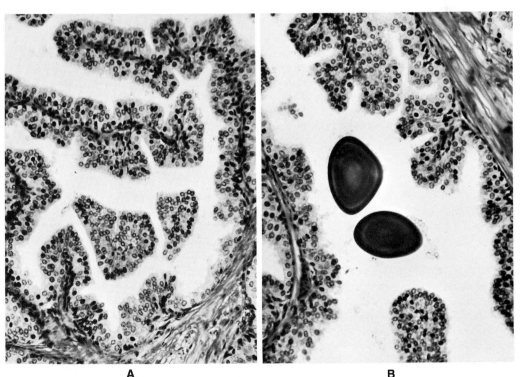

A	B

Figure 31–54. Photomicrographs of human prostate. *A*, The character of the epithelium. *B*, Typical concretions. Hematoxylin and eosin.

is not well understood, and even its morphology has been a subject of controversy and terminological confusion. On the basis of embryological studies, the prostate has traditionally been subdivided into middle, lateral, and posterior lobes, all pyramidal in form and situated respectively anterior, lateral, and posterior to the axis determined by the course of the ejaculatory ducts through the gland. These lobes merge at their boundaries as development progresses, and in the adult they have no reality. There is now a tendency to abandon these regional designations. Some authors do, however, distinguish *central* and *peripheral zones* on the basis of histological criteria. In the central zone, the stroma is denser, the branching of the duct system is more elaborate, the epithelium is more exuberant, and the sacculations are larger, with prominent intraluminal partitions. In the peripheral zone, the stroma is looser, the duct system simpler, and the sacculations smaller and less partitioned. This histological heterogeneity may well be reflected in functional differences.

For the interpretation of prostatic disease, it is probably more important to realize that in addition to the glandular tissue of the prostate proper, there are smaller glands that originate as diverticula of the urethra above the verumontanum. These extend radially into the periurethral connective tissue and the smooth muscle of the surrounding sphincter. Although surrounded by the prostate and formerly considered a part of it, these urethral glands are ontogenetically and functionally distinct. It is now widely accepted that these are the site of origin of benign "prostatic" hyperplasia (BPH). On the other hand, the prostate proper is the site of predilection for the development of cancer.

Bulbourethral Glands

The *bulbourethral glands (Cowper's glands)*, each the size of a pea, are of the compound tubuloalveolar variety. In some respects they resemble mucous glands. Their ducts enter the membranous urethra or the posterior portion of the cavernous urethra. The ducts as well as the secreting portions are of irregular size and form, and in many places they show cystlike enlargements. The terminal portions end blindly. The connective tissue partitions between the glandular lobules measure 1 to 3 mm across and contain elastic fibers and thick strands of striated and smooth muscles. The latter may penetrate with the connective tissue into the interior of the lobules.

The structure of the epithelium in the secreting portions and in the ducts is subject to great functional variations. In the enlarged alveoli the cells are usually flattened; in the other glandular spaces they are cuboidal or columnar, with the nuclei at the base (Fig. 31–55). The cytoplasm contains small mucoid secretion droplets and spindle-shaped inclusions staining with acid dyes. It has been suggested that they leave the cell body as such and then dissolve and mix with the mucin. The excretory ducts are lined with a pseudostratified epithelium resembling that of the urethra and may contain large patches of secreting cells. They are also provided with small accessory glandular outpocketings having the structure of the glands of Littré in the urethra.

After fixation, the secretion appears in the lumen of the glandular spaces and ducts as a precipitate that stains brightly with eosin. In life the secretion is a clear, viscid, mucuslike lubricant, which can be drawn out into long thin threads. Unlike true mucus, it does not form a precipitate with acetic acid. In the

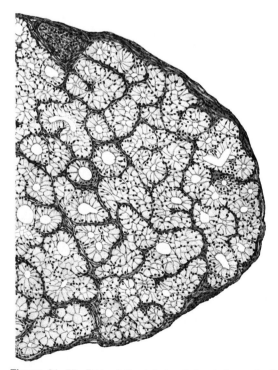

Figure 31–55. Part of the lobule of the bulbourethral gland of a 23-year-old man. Zenker. × 120. (Slightly modified from Stieve.)

boar, the secretion is extremely viscous and rubbery, and plays an important role in the gelation of the seminal plasma that takes place soon after ejaculation in this species.

THE PENIS

The penis is formed of three cylindrical bodies of cavernous or erectile tissue, the two *corpora cavernosa penis* and the unpaired *corpus cavernosum urethrae (corpus spongiosum)*. Arising from the ascending rami of the pubis on either side, the corpora cavernosa converge and join at the pubic angle. From there they run distally side by side to their conical distal ends, forming the dorsal two thirds of the shaft of the penis. On the upper surface of the penis, along the line of their junction, is a shallow longitudinal groove occupied by the dorsal artery and vein. On their lower surface the corpora cavernosa form a deep

groove occupied by the corpus cavernosum urethrae (Fig. 31–56). The latter is traversed throughout its length by the *penile urethra* and ends with an acorn-shaped enlargement, the *glans penis*, bearing on its posterior aspect a pair of concavities that cap the conical ends of the two corpora cavernosa penis.

The erectile tissue of the corpora cavernosa is a vast, spongelike system of irregular vascular spaces fed by the afferent arteries and drained by the efferent veins. In the flaccid condition of the organ, the cavernous spaces contain little blood and appear as collapsed irregular clefts. In erection they become large cavities engorged with blood under pressure. This increased inflow of blood and relative restriction of outflow causes the enlargement and rigidity of the erect penis.

The three cavernous bodies making up the shaft of the penis are surrounded by a thick, resistant, fibrous capsule, the *tunica albuginea*. In the flaccid state the tunica albuginea is 2 mm in thickness; it is reduced in erection to

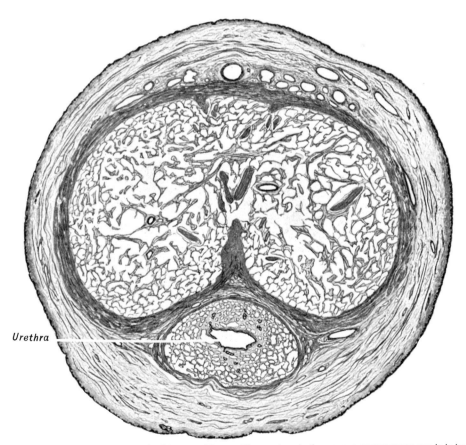

Urethra

Figure 31–56. Cross section of a penis of a 21-year-old man. The septum in the corpus cavernosum penis is incomplete, because the section is from the distal part of the organ. The penis was fixed by injection of formalin into the corpus cavernosum. (Slightly modified from Stieve.)

about 0.5 mm. Its bundles of collagenous fibers are arranged mainly longitudinally in its outer layer and circularly in its inner portion. The collagen fiber bundles have a wavy course in the flaccid state, but straighten out during erection to accommodate the considerable increase in volume of the corpora cavernosa. Elastic fibers are relatively sparse. The extensibility of the tunica is attributable very largely to the arrangement of the collagen bundles and their ability to lengthen to a fixed limit by changing from sinuous to straight. By analogy, an elastic bandage is made up of inelastic cotton fibers, but can be stretched greatly and can then return to its initial length because of the pattern in which they are woven. The few elastic fibers in the tunica albuginea may play some role in the recoil of the collagen to its resting pattern.

The tunica albuginea also forms a fibrous partition between the two corpora cavernosa. In the distal half of the shaft, this septum is fenestrated so that the cavernous spaces of the two corpora communicate. Dense fibrous trabeculae extend inward from the tunica, branching and anastomosing to form a complex framework around the cavernous spaces. This trabecular meshwork is also continuous with a dense connective tissue sheath that surrounds the deep artery, which is centrally located in each corpus. Bundles of smooth muscle fibers run longitudinally in the fibrous sheath of the central artery and along the trabecular meshwork throughout the corpora, and insert upon the inner aspect of the tunica albuginea. The abundance of smooth muscle in the organ has not been fully appreciated, but recent studies indicate that it is the predominant tissue of the parenchyma of the corpora cavernosa.

The central artery gives off helicine branches that course through the fibrous trabeculae, terminating in end arteries that open into the cavernous spaces or sinuses. These are lined by endothelium and are irregularly shaped clefts 1 mm or so across in the flaccid state, but which fill with blood and expand to several times that diameter when the corpora are engorged. The cavernous spaces are largest in the central region of the corpora and gradually diminish in size toward the cavernous venules on the inner aspect of the tunica albuginea. These in turn are continuous with larger veins that penetrate the tunica albuginea to join circumflex veins that are tributaries of the deep dorsal vein of the penis.

The tunica albuginea of the corpus cavernosum urethrae is much thinner than that of the corpora cavernosa penis and contains circularly arranged smooth muscle fibers in its inner layer. It also is provided with abundant elastic networks. The blood lacunae here, unlike those of the corpora cavernosa, are everywhere the same in size. The trabeculae between them contain more numerous elastic fibers, whereas smooth muscle fibers are relatively scarce. The cavernous spaces occupying the axis of the corpus cavernosum urethrae gradually pass into the venous plexus of the urethral mucosa.

The *glans penis* consists of dense connective tissue containing a plexus of large anastomosing veins, with circular and longitudinal smooth muscles in their thick walls. The longitudinal muscle strands often bulge into the lumen of the veins.

The skin covering the penis is thin and is provided with an abundant subcutaneous layer containing smooth muscle, but is devoid of adipose tissue. The skin on the distal part of the shaft of the penis is devoid of hair and has only sweat glands in limited numbers. The glans is covered by an encircling fold of skin, the *prepuce*. Its inner surface, adjacent to the glans, is moist and has the character of a mucous membrane. The dermis of the glans penis is fused with the deeper connective tissue of the glans. In this region there are peculiar sebaceous glands (*glands of Tyson*), which are not associated with hairs. They show great individual variations in number and distribution.

Mechanics of Erection

Erection of the penis is a vascular phenomenon controlled by complex neural pathways activated by both psychic and tactile stimuli. Reflex erection results from afferent sensory input carried via the pudendal nerve to the spinal cord where vasomotor impulses are generated in parasympathetic fibers of the nervi erigentes. These produce vasodilatation of the arteries of the penis, filling the cavernous spaces in the corpora and causing erection. In addition to this simple reflex arc, there is a thoracolumbar pathway that can be activated by psychic stimuli including memory and imagination, as well as visual and tactile input to the cerebral cortex. Higher neural centers appear to control vasodilator fibers originating in thoracic sympathetic ganglia. These can cause erection independently of reflex stimulation. An adrenergic nerve supply to the corpora from sacrococcygeal sympathetic ganglia is believed to be involved in the vasoconstriction that results in detumescence.

The hemodynamics of erection continues to be a subject of debate. It is agreed that erection involves rapid filling of the corpora following vasodilatation of the deep arteries and their helicine branches, and accompanied by relaxation of the intrinsic smooth muscle of the parenchyma. Dilatation of the arteries results in an initially greater rate of inflow than outflow. A majority of investigators believe that this is sufficient to explain erection, and experimental evidence, obtained mainly from dogs, seems to support this view. Others believe that there must also be constriction of venous outflow. Noninvasive measurement of intracavernosal pressure in man during erection indicates that it is several times higher than systolic blood pressure. It is argued that since the helicine arteries open mainly into the larger axial cavernous spaces, the expansion of these spaces compresses the smaller peripheral spaces and the thin-walled veins underlying the relatively unyielding tunica adventitia. In this way, the outflow of blood is throttled down as the blood accumulates in the corpora under increasing pressure. Contraction of the intrinsic smooth muscle is thought to contribute to the high intracavernosal pressure and rigidity of the erect penis. In further support of the concept of restriction of outflow is the observation that the walls of the circumflex veins are unusually muscular. In addition, these veins consistently exhibit unique specializations of their intima called *polsters* (Fig. 31–57). These are local accumulations of fibroblasts and smooth muscle cells beneath the endothelium that form conspicuous longitudinal thickenings or ridges that can be followed through hundreds of

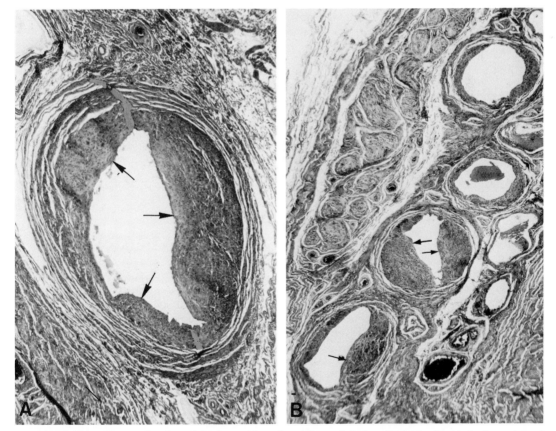

Figure 31–57. Photomicrographs of specializations of the veins of the penis believed to be involved in the hemodynamics of erection. *A,* Cross section through a circumflex vein at the proximal end of the corpora cavernosa of a 68-year-old man, showing *(at arrows)* thick muscular polsters. × 350. *B,* Sections through circumflex veins at the distal end of the corpora cavernosa. The polsters are indicated by arrows. × 40. (Photomicrographs from Goldstein, A. M. B., et al. Urology 20:259, 1982.)

serial sections. These are believed to have a role in constricting the lumen and retarding venous outflow during erection.

Superficially similar intimal thickenings have been reported in the arteries of the human penis, but these are regarded as prearteriosclerotic changes. These so-called arterial polsters are found only occasionally and are probably pathological, whereas venous polsters are a constant finding and are more likely to have physiological significance.

Lymphatics

Dense, superficial networks of lymphatic capillaries are found in the skin of the prepuce and shaft of the penis. They form a dorsal superficial lymph vessel, which runs toward the medial inguinal lymph nodes. Deep nets of lymphatic capillaries collect the lymph from the glans; they form a plexus on each side of the frenulum and continue into a dorsal subfascial lymph vessel.

Nerves

The nerves of the penis come both from the sacral plexus, via the pudendal nerve, and from the pelvic sympathetic system. The former supply the striated muscles of the penis (such as the bulbocavernosus) and also furnish the sensory nerve endings in the skin and the mucosa of the urethra. Among these sensory endings, free nerve endings can be demonstrated in the epithelium of the glans, the prepuce, and the urethra. In addition, there are free nerve endings in the subepithelial connective tissue of the skin and the urethra. Finally, numerous encapsulated corpuscles of various types are present: *corpuscles of Meissner* in the papillae of the skin of the prepuce and the glans; *genital corpuscles* in the deeper layers of the stratum papillare of the dermis of the glans and in the mucosa of the urethra; and *corpuscles of Vater-Pacini*, which occur along the dorsal vein in the subcutaneous fascia, in the deeper connective tissue of the glans, and under the albuginea in the corpora cavernosa. The sympathetic nervous plexuses are connected with the smooth muscles of the vessels and form extensive, nonmyelinated networks among the smooth muscles of the trabeculae in the corpora cavernosa.

SEMEN

As the sperm pass along the excretory ducts, the secretions of the ducts and accessory glands are added to them. The final product is the *semen*. The sperm in the seminiferous tubules are nonmotile. They are slowly forwarded into the tubuli recti and the rete testis by the fluid secreted into the tubules. The seminiferous tubules may also actively move the quiescent sperm by executing peristaltic movements. The flattened cells investing the seminiferous tubules have been shown to have many of the fine structural characteristics of smooth muscle cells. In some species, slow contractile movements of the excised seminiferous tubules have been observed. In the ductuli efferentes, the epithelium with its cilia beating toward the epididymis contributes to the transport of the sperm.

The long, winding duct of the epididymis is slowly traversed by the sperm propelled by peristaltic contractions of smooth muscle in the duct wall. They are kept here, especially in the tail, for a long time, sometimes for several weeks. In some species, the sperm acrosome undergoes continuing morphological differentiation during the passage through the epididymis, and the fertilizing capacity of the spermatozoa is known to increase progressively. As previously noted, the ductus epididymidis has an outer layer of smooth muscle that is responsible for rhythmic peristaltic movements that move the sperm along the duct. During ejaculation, contraction of the ductus deferens is of primary importance in expulsion of stored sperm.

The epididymis is the site of storage of spermatozoa. The sperm do not accumulate to any great extent in the ductus deferens. This part of the excretory system, with its heavy muscular coat, is adapted for their speedy transportation during sexual activity.

The function of the seminal vesicles is primarily glandular. Their thick secretion contributes substantially to the volume of the ejaculate. It is rich in fructose, which is the principal sugar of the semen and provides the carbohydrate substrate utilized as an energy source by motile spermatozoa of the ejaculate. The secretion contains small amounts of yellowish pigment, mainly flavins, which give the semen a strong fluorescence in ultraviolet light—a property of some medicolegal importance in the detection of semen stains.

In the process of ejaculation, the muscular tissue of the prostate also contracts and discharges its abundant liquid secretion. The semen, entering the urethra and mixing with the secretion of the glands of Cowper and Littré, is expelled by the contraction of the bulbocavernosus muscle compressing the bulbus urethrae.

The average volume of the ejaculate in man is about 3.5 ml, and of this the sperm account for less than 10 per cent, the rest being *seminal plasma*. The sperm density varies from 50 to 150 million per ml. Each ejaculate therefore contains 200 to 300 million sperm.

Under suitable conditions the sperm may remain alive outside the body for several days. They also survive for some time in the excretory ducts after death. In the uterus and the fallopian tube, living sperm have been found some days after coitus. They can now be stored in the frozen state for months or years and retain their fertilizing capacity upon thawing.

Besides the sperm, the semen contains degenerated cells, probably cast off from the epithelium of the excretory ducts and the urethra. Occasionally, columnar epithelial cells and wandering cells of connective tissue origin may also occur. There are, furthermore, round hyaline bodies of unknown origin, concretions from the prostate, and minute lipid, protein, and pigment granules. When the semen cools and begins to dry, peculiar crystals of various forms develop—the *crystals of Böttcher*. They are believed to consist of phosphate of sperimine, a polyamine compound present in considerable amounts in human semen and contributed mainly by the prostate.

It has been claimed that the different components of the semen are discharged from the urethra in a certain sequence. With the development of erection, the slippery secretion of the glands of Cowper and Littré lubricates the urethra. At the beginning of the ejaculation, the prostatic secretion is discharged first. Next, the masses of sperm accumulated in the ductus deferens and distal portion of the ductus epididymidis are expelled. The final portion of the ejaculate is mainly the thick secretion of the seminal vesicles. In some animals (e.g., mouse), the abundant secretion of the seminal vesicles is coagulated in the vagina by an enzyme contained in the prostatic juice, and thus a solid plug is formed in the vagina that temporarily occludes its lumen and prevents the escape of the semen.

REFERENCES

GENERAL

Bardin, C. W., and R. J. Scherins, eds.: Cell Biology of the Testis. Ann. N.Y. Acad. Sci. Vol. 383, 1982.

Brandes, D.: Male Accessory Sex Organs. Structure and Function in Mammals. New York, Academic Press, 1974.

Hamilton, D. W., and R. O. Greep, eds: Handbook of Physiology: Endocrinology. Vol. 5, Sec. 7, Male Reproductive System. Washington, DC, American Physiological Society, 1975.

Hamilton, D. W., and F. Naftolin: Basic Reproductive Medicine. Vol. 2. Reproductive Function in Men. Cambridge, MA, MIT Press, 1982.

Johnson, A. D., W. R. Gomes, and N. L. Vandemark, eds.: The Testis. Vol. 2. Development, Anatomy, Physiology, Biochemistry. New York, Academic Press, 1970.

Mann, T.: Biochemistry of Semen and of the Male Reproductive Tract. London, Methuen & Co., 1964.

SPERMATOZOA

Bedford, J. M.: Sperm capacitation and fertilization in mammals. Biol. Reprod. (Suppl.) *2*:128, 1970.

Bishop, D.: Sperm motility. Physiol. Rev. *42*:1, 1962.

Fawcett, D. W.: Anatomy of the mammalian spermatozoon with particular reference to the guinea pig. Zeitschr. Zellforsch. *67*:279, 1965.

Fawcett, D. W.: A comparative view of sperm ultrastructure. Biol. Reprod. (Suppl. 2) *2*:90, 1970.

Fawcett, D. W.: The mammalian spermatozoon. Dev. Biol. *44*:394, 1975.

Friend, D. S.: Organization of the spermatozoon membrane. *In* Edinin, M., and M. H. Johnson, eds.: Immunobiology of the Gametes. Oxford, England, Alden Press, 1977.

Friend, D. S., and D. W. Fawcett: Membrane differentiations in freeze-fractured mammalian sperm. J. Cell Biol. *63*:466, 1974.

Friend, D. S., L. Orci, A. Perrelet, and R. Yanagimachi: Membrane particle changes attending the acrosome reaction in guinea pig spermatozoa. J. Cell Biol. *74*:561, 1977.

Soupart, P., and L. L. Morgenstern: Human sperm capacitation and in vitro fertilization. Fertil. Steril. *24*:462, 1973.

Zamboni, L., R. Zemjanis, and M. Stefanini: The fine structure of monkey and human spermatozoa. Anat. Rec. *169*:129, 1971.

SEMINIFEROUS EPITHELIUM

Clermont, Y.: The cycle of the seminiferous epithelium in man. Am. J. Anat. *112*:35, 1963.

Clermont, Y.: Renewal of spermatogonia in man. Am. J. Anat. *118*:509, 1966.

Clermont, Y.: Kinetics of spermatogenesis in mammals.

Seminiferous epithelium cycle and spermatogonial renewal. Physiol. Rev. *52*:198, 1972.

De Kretser, D. M., J. B. Kerr, and C. A. Paulsen: Peritubular tissue in the normal and pathological human testis. Biol. Reprod. *12*:317, 1975.

Dym, M.: The fine structure of the monkey Sertoli cell and its role in maintaining the blood-testis barrier. Anat. Rec. *175*:639, 1973.

Dym, M., and D. W. Fawcett: The blood-testis barrier in the rat and the physiological compartmentation of the seminiferous epithelium. Biol. Reprod. *3*:308, 1970.

Dym, M., and D. W. Fawcett: Further observations on the numbers of spermatogonia, spermatocytes and spermatids connected by intercellular bridges in the mammalian testis. Biol. Reprod. *4*:195, 1971.

Fawcett, D. W.: The ultrastructure and functions of the Sertoli cell. *In* Handbook of Physiology: Endocrinology. Vol. 5, Sect. 7, Male Reproductive System. Washington DC, American Physiological Society, 1975.

Fawcett, D. W., and D. M. Phillips: Observations on the release of spermatozoa and on changes in the head during passage through the epididymis. J. Reprod. Fertil. (Suppl.) *6*:405, 1969.

Flickinger, C. J., and D. W. Fawcett: The junctional specializations of Sertoli cells in the seminiferous epithelium. Anat. Rec. *158*:207, 1970.

Gilula, N. B., D. W. Fawcett, and A. Aoki: The Sertoli cell occluding junctions and gap junctions in mature and developing mammalian testis. Dev. Biol. *50*:142, 1976.

Huckins, C.: The spermatogonial stem cell population in adult rats. I. Their morphology, proliferation and maturation. Anat. Rec. *169*:533, 1971.

Setchell, B. P.: The functional significance of the blood-testis barrier. J. Androl. *1*:3, 1980.

INTERSTITIAL TISSUE

Christensen, A. K.: Leydig cells. *In* Hamilton, D. W., and R. O. Greep, eds.: Handbook of Physiology: Endocrinology. Vol. 5, Sect. 7, Male Reproductive System. Washington, DC, American Physiological Society, 1975.

Christensen, A. K.: The fine structure of the testicular interstitial cells of the guinea pig. J. Cell Biol. *26*:911, 1965.

Crabo, B.: Fine structure of the interstitial cells of the rabbit. Zeitsch. Zellforsch. *61*:587, 1963.

Fawcett, D. W., W. B. Neaves, and M. N. Flores: Comparative observations on intertubular lymphatics and the organization of interstitial tissue of the mammalian testis. Biol. Reprod. *9*:500, 1973.

Johnson, L, and W. B. Neaves: Age related changes in the Leydig cell population, seminiferous tubules, and sperm production in stallions. Biol. Reprod. *24*:703, 1981.

Kaler, L. W., and W. B. Neaves: Attrition of the human Leydig cell population with advancing age. Anat. Rec. *192*:513, 1978.

Mori, H., and A. K. Christensen: Morphometric analysis of Leydig cells in the normal rat testis. J. Cell Biol. *84*:340, 1980.

BLOOD VESSELS AND LYMPHATICS

Fawcett, D. W., P. M. Heidger, and L. V. Leak: Lymph vascular system of the interstitial tissue of the testis as revealed by electron microscopy. J. Reprod. Fertil. *19*:109, 1969.

Kormano, M., and H. Suoranta: Microvascular organization of the adult human testis. Anat. Rec. *170*:31, 1971.

Setchell, B. P.: Testicular blood supply, lymphatic drainage and secretion of fluid. *In* Johnson, A. D., et al., eds.: The Testis. Vol. 1. New York, Academic Press, 1970, pp. 101–218.

Suzuki, F.: Microvasculature of the mouse testis and excretory duct system. Am. J. Anat. *163*:309, 1982.

EXCRETORY DUCTS OF THE TESTIS

Dym, M.: The mammalian rete testis—a morphological examination. Anat. Rec. *186*:493, 1976.

Hamilton, D. W.: Structure and function of the epithelium lining the ductuli efferentes, ductus epididymidis and ductus deferens in the rat. *In* Hamilton, D. W., and R. O. Greep, eds.: Handbook of Physiology: Endocrinology. Vol. 5, Sect. 7, Male Reproductive System. Washington, DC, American Physiological Society, 1975.

Hoffer, A., D. W. Hamilton, and D. W. Fawcett: The ultrastructure of the principal cells and intraepithelial leucocytes in the initial segment of rat epididymis. Anat. Rec. *175*:169, 1973.

Jones, R., D. W. Hamilton, and D. W. Fawcett: Morphology of the rete testis, ductuli efferentes and ductus epididymidis of the rabbit. Am. J. Anat. *156*:373, 1979.

Nagano, T., and F. Suzuki: Cell junctions in the seminiferous tubule and the excurrent ducts of the testis. Int. Rev. Cytol. *81*:163, 1983.

Nicander, L.: Studies on the regional histology and cytochemistry of the ductus epididymis in stallions, rams, and bulls. Acta Morphol. Neerl. Scand. *1*:337, 1958.

Orgebin-Crist, M. C.: Studies on the function of the epididymis. Biol. Reprod. (Suppl.) *1*:155, 1969.

ACCESSORY GLANDS OF MALE REPRODUCTION

Brandes, D., D. Kirchheim, and W. W. Scott: Ultrastructure of the human prostate; normal and neoplastic. Lab. Invest. *13*:1541, 1964.

Franks, L. M.: Benign nodular hyperplasia of the prostate: a review. Ann. R. Coll. Surg. Engl. *14*:92, 1954.

Harbitz, T. B., and O. A. Haugen: Histology of the prostate in elderly men. Acta Pathol. Microbiol. Scand. [Sect. A] *80*:756, 1972.

McNeal, J. E.: The prostate and prostatic urethra—a morphologic synthesis. J. Urol. *197*:1008, 1973.

PENIS

Conti, G.: L'Érection du penis humain et ses bases morphologicovasculaires. Acta Anat. *14*:217, 1952.

Goldstein, A. M., J. P. Meehan, R. Zakhary, P. A. Buckley, and F. A. Rogers: New observations on the microarchitecture of the corpora cavernosa in man and their possible relationship to the mechanism of erection. Urology *20*:259, 1982.

Meehan, J. P., and A. M. B. Goldstein: High pressure within the corpus cavernosum in man during erection. Its probable mechanism. Urology *21*:385, 1983.

Shirai, M., and N. Ishii: Hemodynamics of erection in man. Arch. Androl. *6*:27, 1981.

Weiss, H.: The physiology of human penile erection. Ann. Intern. Med. *76*:793, 1972.

32

FEMALE REPRODUCTIVE SYSTEM

The female reproductive system includes the internal organs—*ovaries, oviducts, uterus,* and *vagina*; and the external genitalia—*mons pubis, labia majora, labia minora,* and *clitoris* (Fig. 32–1). The size and microscopic structure of these organs change greatly with age. They are relatively small and functionally quiescent until *puberty,* which involves gradual breast development and other changes of body form; the appearance of axillary and pubic hair; and growth and differentiation of the internal reproductive organs. These changes culminate in *menarche,* the first menstrual flow, which occurs at about 13 years of age. Thereafter, throughout the reproductive life of the woman, the ovaries and the endometrium of the uterus undergo a regularly repeated cycle of hormonally controlled histological changes about every 28 days. Cessation of menses, or *menopause,* occurs at a mean age of 51 years as a result of depletion of ovarian follicles and consequent reduction in estrogen secretion.

OVARY

The human ovaries are slightly flattened paired organs, each measuring 2.5 to 5 cm

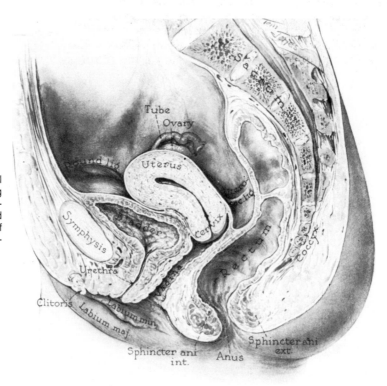

Figure 32–1. Drawing of a sagittal section of the female pelvis, showing the reproductive organs and their relationships to bladder, urethra, and rectum. (From Anson, B. J. Atlas of Human Anatomy. 2nd ed. Philadelphia, W. B. Saunders Co., 1963.)

in length, 1.5 to 3 cm in width, and 0.6 to 1.5 cm in thickness. One of the edges, the *hilus,* is attached by the *mesovarium* to the *broad ligament,* which extends from the uterus laterally to the wall of the pelvic cavity.

The ovary has a thick peripheral zone, or *cortex,* which surrounds the *medulla.* Embedded in the connective tissue of the cortex are *follicles* containing the female sex cells, *oocytes.* The follicles are present in a wide range of sizes representing various stages of their development (Fig. 32–2). When a follicle reaches maturity it ruptures at the surface of the ovary to release the ovum, which then enters the open end of the neighboring oviduct. The boundary between the ovarian cortex and medulla is poorly defined. The medulla consists mainly of loose connective tissue and a mass of contorted blood vessels that are large in proportion to the size of the ovary.

The ovary is covered by a continuous sheet of squamous or cuboidal epithelium, which was named the *germinal epithelium* in the mistaken belief that the primordial oocytes originated from it (Fig. 32–3). The term persists although the evidence now overwhelmingly favors the extragonadal origin of the primordial germ cells. Beneath the germinal epithelium is a layer of dense connective tissue, the *tunica albuginea* (Fig. 32–4).

Ovarian Follicles

Embedded in the stroma of the cortex deep to the tunica albuginea are the follicles. The younger the woman, the more numerous they are. In a normal young adult, over 400,000 have been counted in serial sections of both ovaries. Of this large number, fewer than 500 ova are released by the process of ovulation during a woman's reproductive life.

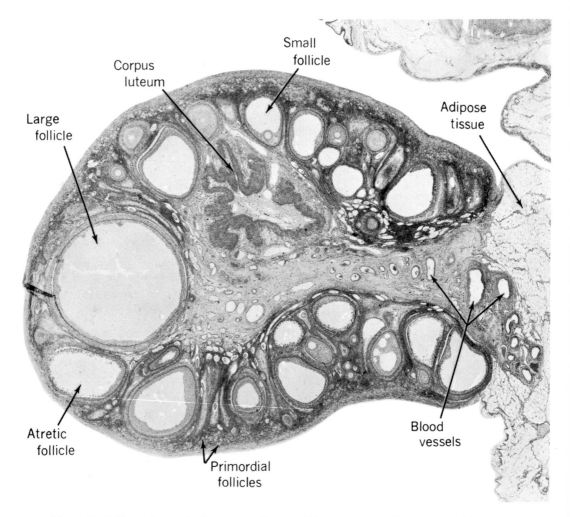

Figure 32–2. Photomicrograph of a transected ovary of *Macacus rhesus.* (Courtesy of H. Mizoguchi.)

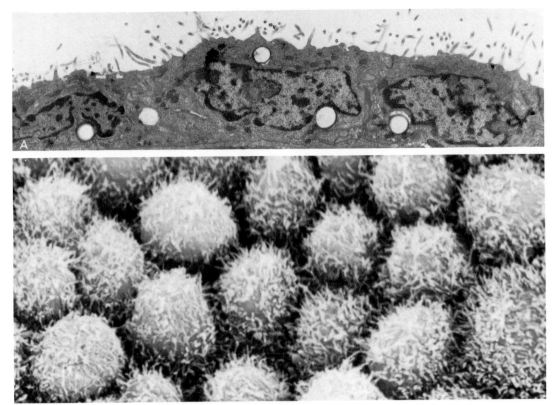

Figure 32–3. *A,* Cells of the germinal epithelium of the ovary as seen with the transmission electron microscope in a thin section. The surface bears irregularly oriented microvilli. *B,* Scanning electron micrograph of the germinal epithelium of the ovary. The bulging free surfaces have many more microvilli than one would infer from study of thin sections of this epithelium. The germinal epithelium resembles the peritoneal mesothelium covering other abdominal and pelvic organs. (Micrographs courtesy of E. Anderson.)

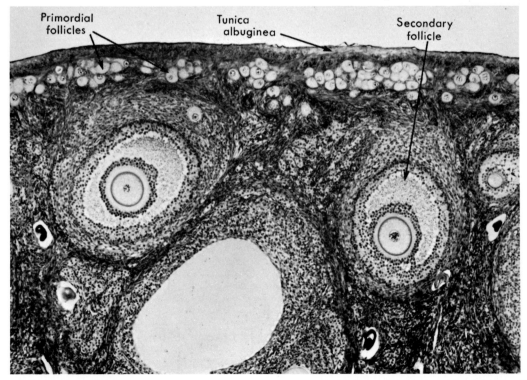

Figure 32–4. Photomicrograph of cat ovary, showing numerous primordial follicles and two secondary follicles with a well-developed antrum. × 100.

During each menstrual cycle, from five to 15 follicles begin to grow and develop, but only one of these is destined to proceed to ovulation. The others become arrested at various stages of development, and degenerate in the process called *follicular atresia*. The number of follicles decreases progressively throughout life, and at menopause follicles are hard to find, although a few may persist into old age.

The vast majority of follicles are *primordial* or *unilaminar follicles*. They are found mainly in the periphery of the cortex, immediately beneath the tunica albuginea (Figs. 32–4, 32–5). Each consists of a large round *oocyte* surrounded by a single layer of flattened *follicular cells*. Owing to the large size of the oocyte, there may be several follicular cells around its circumference in sections. Primordial follicles may contain more than one oocyte, but such polyovular follicles are quite uncommon.

Primordial Follicles (Unilaminar Follicles). The oocyte of the primordial follicle is enveloped by a single layer of flattened follicular cells. It has a large, eccentrically placed vesicular nucleus with a conspicuous nucleolus. In favorable thin sections the meiotic chromosomes can be seen (Fig. 32–6). Associated with the juxtanuclear cell center is a well-developed Golgi apparatus surrounded by numerous small mitochondria. The surfaces of the oocyte and the enveloping follicular cells at this stage are smooth and in close apposition.

In electron micrographs the prominent juxtanuclear Golgi complex consists of short parallel arrays of cisternae and large numbers of small vesicles. Similar vesicular profiles are distributed in smaller numbers throughout the ooplasm, and it is believed that these may originate in the Golgi apparatus. Annulate lamellae are often found adjacent to the nucleus or free in the neighboring ooplasm. The spherical or short plump mitochondria tend to congregate in the vicinity of the cell center. Later, when the oocyte begins to grow, they become dispersed throughout the ooplasm (Fig. 32–8). The endoplasmic reticulum in the early stages of oocyte development takes the form of vesicles or slightly elongated profiles bearing a few ribosomes. Longer cisternal profiles subsequently arise in limited numbers and finally become associated in parallel arrays. Multivesicular bodies are a common component of the ooplasm but are more numerous in later stages of development.

Primary Follicles. Development of follicles in the ovary occurs continuously from infancy to the menopause, uninterrupted by anovulatory cycles or pregnancies. The transition from a quiescent primordial follicle to a developing primary follicle involves cytological changes in the oocyte, the follicular cells, and the adjacent stromal cells. As the oocyte enlarges, the follicular cells become cuboidal or low columnar and by mitotic proliferation give rise to a stratified epithelium of *granulosa cells*, thus transforming the unilaminar primordial follicle to a multilaminar *primary follicle* (Figs. 32–7, 32–9). The stratified epithelium rests on a thick basal lamina, the *membrana limitans externa*, which separates the granulosa from the surrounding stromal cells that have become concentrated around the follicle and have differentiated to form the *theca folliculi* (Figs. 32–9, 32–10).

In the concurrent growth of the oocyte, there is a noticeable change in the distribution of its organelles. The single large juxtanuclear Golgi gives rise to multiple complexes widely dispersed in the ooplasm. The rough endoplasmic reticulum becomes more extensive, and the number of free polyribosomes increases. Mitochondria proliferate and disperse throughout the ooplasm. Small vesicles and multivesicular bodies increase in number. Between the oocyte and the surrounding granulosa cells, a space develops into which irregularly shaped microvilli project from the oolemma and from the neighboring granulosa cells (Figs. 32–8, 32–11). An amorphous material accumulates in this space around the microvilli and gradually condenses to form the *zona pellucida*, a highly refractile glycoprotein layer that stains intensely with the periodic acid–Schiff reaction. The microvilli of the oocyte and the slender processes of the neighboring granulosa cells are in contact within the substance of the zona pellucida throughout the subsequent development of the follicle. The zona pellucida, which may attain a thickness of 5 μm in the mature follicle, is usually considered to be a product of the granulosa cells, but there is some evidence that the oocyte may contribute to its formation.

As the primary follicle develops, the mitochondria, rough endoplasmic reticulum, and free ribosomes of the granulosa cells increase in abundance and the Golgi complex becomes more prominent. Lipid droplets are common in the cytoplasm in some species. Large gap junctions are found in areas of

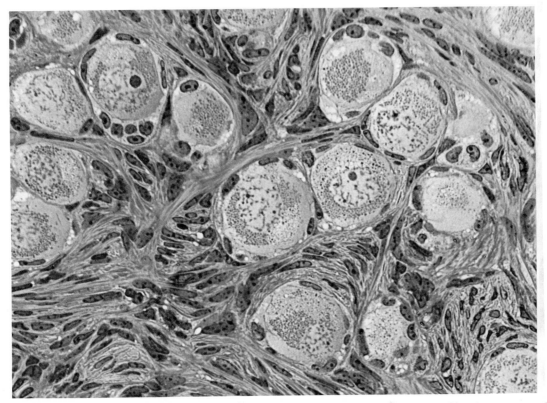

Figure 32–5. Photomicrograph of a number of primordial follicles in the cortex of monkey ovary. The chromosomes of the dictyate stage of meiosis are visible in the oocyte nuclei. The oocytes are surrounded by a single layer of flattened follicular cells.

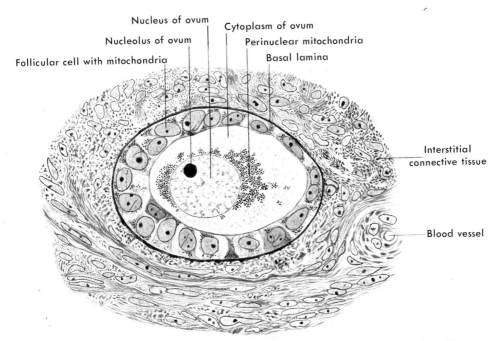

Figure 32–6. Primary unilaminar follicle in an early stage of its growth. Drawing from a preparation of human ovary by C. M. Bensley. (After A. A. Maximow.)

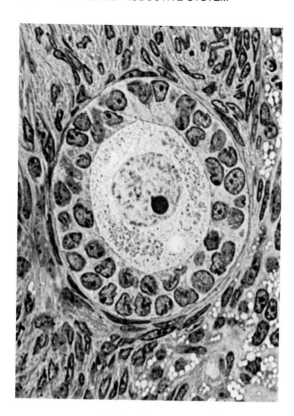

Figure 32–7. Bilaminar primary follicle from monkey ovary.

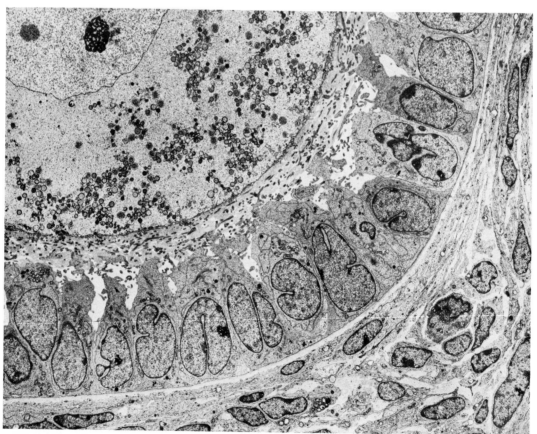

Figure 32–8. Electron micrograph of an early primary follicle. The cytoplasm of the oocyte contains numerous mitochondria. A space has appeared between the oocyte and the follicular cells, and amorphous material is accumulating in it to form the zona pellucida. (Micrograph courtesy of P. Motta.)

Blood vessel
with erythrocytes

Basal lamina   Mitosis of follicular cell

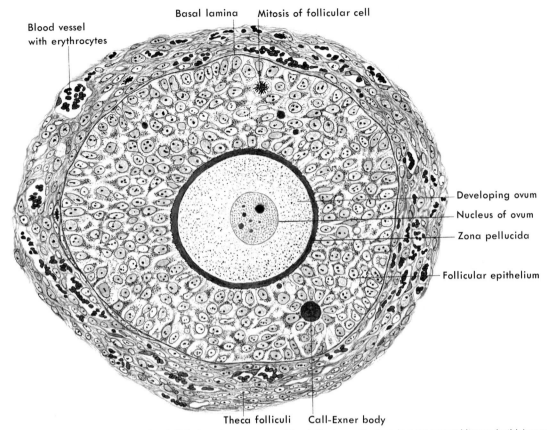

Developing ovum

Nucleus of ovum

Zona pellucida

Follicular epithelium

Theca folliculi   Call-Exner body

Figure 32–9. Drawing of a growing follicle from human ovary. The follicular epithelium is now several layers in thickness and the oocyte is considerably enlarged. (After A. A. Maximow.)

contact between adjacent granulosa cells, providing low-resistance pathways for their electrical and metabolic coupling.

As the follicles increase in size, they gradually move deeper into the cortex (Fig. 32–2). Concurrently with the proliferation of the granulosa cell layer, the sheath of stromal cells forming the *theca folliculi* becomes more prominent, and a wedge-shaped thickening extends from the follicle toward the surface of the ovary, forming the *theca cone.* The theca subsequently differentiates into a highly vascular inner layer of secretory cells, the *theca interna,* and an outer layer, the *theca externa,* composed mainly of connective tissue. Numerous small vessels penetrate the theca externa to supply a rich capillary plexus in the theca interna, but the granulosa cell layer remains avascular throughout the growth of the follicle.

The cells of the theca interna are initially fibroblast-like, fusiform cells, but they subsequently accumulate small lipid droplets and their cytoplasm takes on the ultrastructural characteristics of steroid-secreting endocrine cells (Fig. 32–15). The cells of the theca

externa do not undergo further cytological differentiation and continue to resemble fibroblasts. The boundaries between the theca interna and theca externa and between the theca externa and the surrounding stroma are indistinct.

Secondary Follicles (Antral Follicles). In the course of the continuing proliferation of the follicular cells, the enlarging follicle becomes oval in shape and the oocyte eccentric in position. When the follicle reaches a diameter of about 0.2 mm and has six to 12 layers of cells, irregular spaces filled with clear fluid appear among the granulosa cells. This fluid, called *liquor folliculi,* increases in amount as the follicle enlarges and the irregular spaces among the granulosa cells become confluent to form a single crescentic cavity, the *antrum.* Thenceforth the follicle is described as a *secondary follicle,* or *antral follicle* (Fig. 32–13). By the time the formation of the antrum begins, the oocyte has usually attained its full size, 125 to 150 μm. Although the ovum grows no more thereafter, the follicle as a whole continues to enlarge until it reaches a diameter of 10 mm or more.

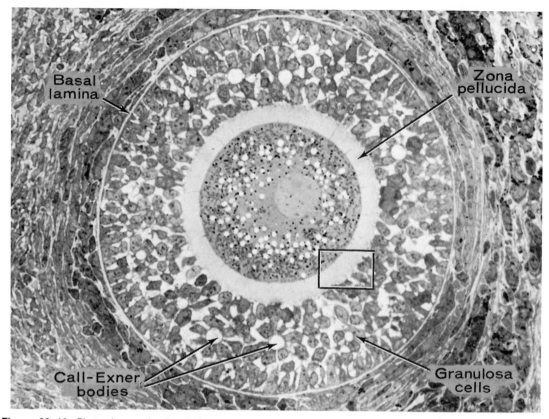

Figure 32–10. Photomicrograph of a follicle comparable with that in Figure 32–8, showing the stratified folliculi epithelium, its prominent basal lamina, and the thick zona pellucida around the oocyte. The spherical clear areas among the granulosa cells are Call-Exner bodies. An area similar to that in the rectangle is shown in an electron micrograph in Figure 32–11. (Photomicrograph courtesy of E. Anderson.)

The typical small antrum follicle is lined with a stratified epithelium of granulosa cells, which displays a local thickening on one side called the *cumulus oophorus*. This thicker region protruding into the fluid-filled cavity has the oocyte in its center (Figs. 32–13, 32–14). The oocyte is surrounded by a single layer of cuboidal follicular cells whose apical processes are firmly anchored in the zona pellucida. This cellular investment is referred to as the *corona radiata*.

Although the lining of the follicle is described as a stratified epithelium, its granulosa cells are less compact in their organization than the cells of most epithelia. They may be columnar immediately surrounding the zona pellucida, but elsewhere liquor folliculi accumulates between them, they become angular or stellate in form, and they are connected with one another by short processes. In growing follicles, small accumulations of densely staining material may appear among the granulosa cells. These are the *Call-Exner bodies* (Figs. 32–9, 32–10).

Whether they are intra- or extracellular was formerly a subject of dispute, but electron micrographs clearly show them to be extracellular (Fig. 32–12). They stain positively with the PAS reaction. Their origin and significance are unknown.

Mature Follicule (Graafian Follicle). In the human, follicles require 10 to 14 days from the beginning of the cycle to reach maturity. As they approach their maximal size, they are large vesicles that occupy the full thickness of the ovarian cortex and bulge from the free surface of the organ. The follicles appear tense, as though the liquid in the follicular cavity were under considerable pressure, but actual measurements have not borne out this impression.

In late stages of follicular growth, mitotic figures gradually decrease in number among the granulosa cells. Intercellular spaces among the cells of the inner layers of the epithelium become more prominent. The connection of the ovum and the associated granulosa cells of the cumulus oophorus with

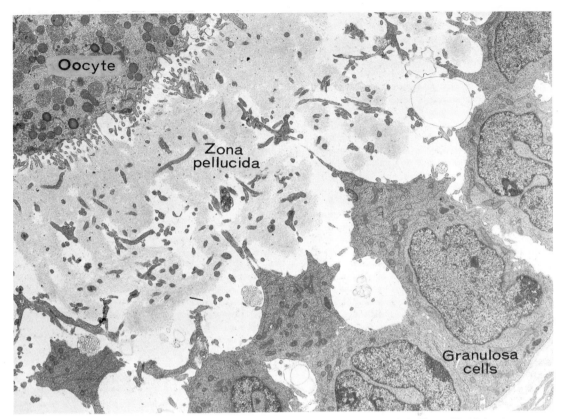

Figure 32–11. Electron micrograph of an area similar to that enclosed in the rectangle in Figure 32–10, but in a younger follicle. There are many microvilli on the oocyte and slender irregular apical processes on the follicular cells, which extend into the substance of the zona pellucida. (Micrograph courtesy of E. Anderson.)

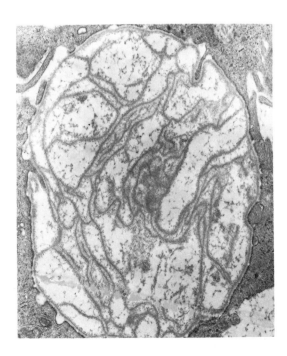

Figure 32–12. Electron micrograph of Call-Exner body. It appears to consist of a cavity lined with a distinct basal lamina and with a filigree of excess basal lamina in the interior. There is also a sparse flocculent precipitate of proteinaceous material. (Micrograph courtesy of E. Anderson.)

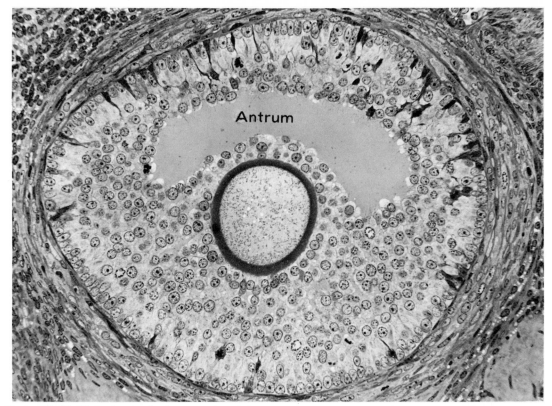

Figure 32–13. Photomicrograph of a secondary follicle from monkey ovary, showing a small antrum and cumulus oophorus. A well-developed theca is seen around the periphery of the follicle.

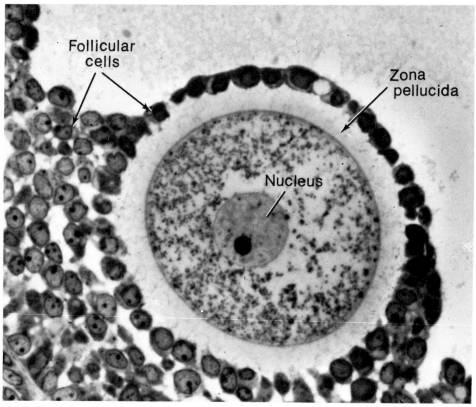

Figure 32–14. Photomicrograph of a human oocyte in an antral follicle. Where it projects into the antrum, the investment of granulosa cells is reduced to a single layer whose processes are anchored in the zona pellucida. (Photomicrograph courtesy of L. Zamboni.)

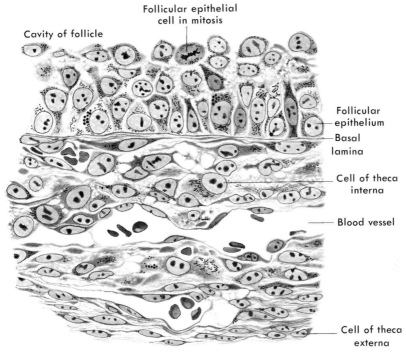

Cavity of follicle

Follicular epithelial cell in mitosis

Follicular epithelium

Basal lamina

Cell of theca interna

Blood vessel

Cell of theca externa

Figure 32–15. Section of part of wall of large follicle, illustrating the organization of the theca folliculi. (After A. A. Maximow.)

the rest of the epithelium is gradually loosened by the development of new, liquid-filled intercellular spaces. In the loosening up of the cumulus the ovum, together with its zona pellucida and corona radiata, are freed of their attachment in preparation for ovulation.

The theca folliculi reaches its greatest development in the mature follicle. The theca interna is composed of large, spindle-shaped or polyhedral cells with oval or elliptical nuclei and fine lipid droplets in their cytoplasm (Figs. 32–15, 32–16). They are enmeshed in a network of reticular fibers that are continuous with those of the theca externa and the rest of the ovarian stroma. Although they are modified stromal cells and superficially resemble fibroblasts, the cells of the theca interna in electron micrographs have cytological characteristics similar to those of cells in other steroid-secreting endocrine glands. They are principally responsible for elaboration of the steroid precursor of the female sex hormones, *estrogens.* Consistent with the endocrine function of the theca interna is its rich capillary plexus. The theca externa consists of concentrically arranged fibers and fusiform cells that do not appear to have any secretory function.

Histophysiology of the Ovarian Follicles. In addition to their role in sustenance of the oocytes, the ovarian follicles have important endocrine functions. Of the several follicles that are activated and undergo varying degrees of development in each cycle, usually only one progresses to ovulation. Nothing is known about what determines the number of primordial follicles that will begin to grow or how one among them is selected to complete its development. It is possible that those which become atretic serve some transient endocrine function unrelated to ovulation. Certainly the maturing follicle is active as an endocrine gland.

The granulosa cells of developing follicles have receptors for follicle stimulating hormone (FSH), luteinizing hormone (LH), estrogens, and testosterone. The relative number of each of these receptors is subject to modulation by the varying levels of the other hormones at successive stages of follicle development in the menstrual cycle. The primary stimulus for follicular growth is provided by FSH from the adenohypophysis. LH induces differentiation of the cells of the theca interna and stimulates their secretion of testosterone, which diffuses into the follicle where aromatizing enzymes in the gran-

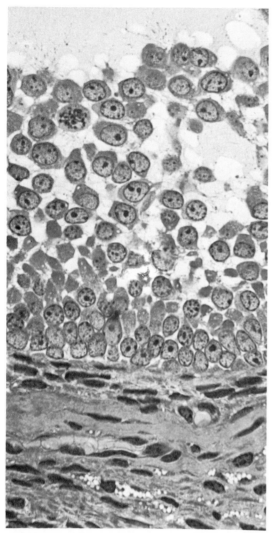

Figure 32–16. Photomicrograph of a portion of the wall of an antral follicle, illustrating the loose organization of the follicular epithelium *(above)* and the fusiform thecal cells *(below)*, with multiple lipid droplets in their cytoplasm, appearing here as clear vacuoles.

receptors in the membrane of the granulosa cells. Responding to LH, the granulosa cells then begin to secrete progesterone. At the same time, the midcycle increase in plasma LH down-regulates the number of FSH receptors on the granulosa cells, reducing their estrogen production as they shift to secretion of progesterone.

There is increasing experimental evidence that the granulosa cells also secrete a nonsteroidal hormone that acts back upon the hypothalamohypophyseal axis to suppress FSH release. This substance, detectable in follicular fluid, has yet to be isolated and fully characterized but seems to be a relatively small peptide. It has been called *folliculostatin*, but since most preparations inhibit secretion of both FSH and LH, some prefer the less specific term *gonadostatin*. Its precise role in the complex regulation of reproduction remains to be elucidated.

Ovulation

The process by which the follicle ruptures and sets free the ovum is called *ovulation*. A follicle matures at intervals of about 28 days in the human female, although variations of a week are not uncommon. Normally ovulation occurs on or about the 14th day of an ideal 28-day cycle. Usually only one ovum is released, but occasionally two, and rarely more, may be discharged. Cycles of typical duration may occur without associated ovulation. These are called *anovulatory cycles*. The stages preparatory to rupture of the follicle have been extensively studied in histological sections of ovaries, and the actual process of ovulation has been directly observed and photographed in anesthetized living animals and in humans.

The ovum and the granulosa cells immediately surrounding it are loosened from the cumulus oophorus in the last stages of follicular maturation and float free in the liquor folliculi. During this period, the follicular fluid seems to accumulate faster than the follicle grows, and the part of the follicular wall that bulges on the surface of the ovary becomes progressively thinner. The follicular fluid that forms just before ovulation contains more water than that formed earlier and appears to be secreted at a rapid rate. The first indication of impending ovulation is the appearance on the outer surface of the follicle of a small oval area, the *macula pellucida* or *stigma*. In this area the flow of blood slows and then ceases, resulting in a local change

ulosa catalyze its conversion to the estrogen, 17β estradiol. FSH acting upon the granulosa cells induces this conversion of thecal androgen to estrogen, which in turn stimulates granulosa cell proliferation and growth of the follicle. Estrogen also diffuses into the capillaries of the theca interna, raising the level of the hormone in the general circulation. The increasing level of estrogen in the blood late in the follicular phase of the cycle acts back upon the hypothalamohypophyseal system to induce the preovulatory surge of LH. Concurrently, the increasing concentration of estrogen within the follicle shortly before ovulation induces formation of LH in color and translucency of the follicular wall. The germinal epithelium overlying this area becomes discontinuous and the intervening stroma greatly thinned out. The stigma then bulges outward as a clear vesicle or cone. In the rat, in which these events have been observed in greatest detail, the formation of the stigma takes place in five minutes or less. The cone then ruptures, and in a minute or two the ovum and its adherent mass of cumulus cells pass through the orifice, followed by a gush of follicular fluid (Fig. 32–17). The fluid immediately associated with the ovum appears viscous, while that which follows is quite thin.

The turgid fronds or fimbriae of the oviduct, or fallopian tube, are closely applied to the surface of the ovary at the time of ovulation. Their active movements, and the currents created in the surface film by the cilia on their epithelial cells, are responsible for drawing the ovum into the open ostium of the oviduct.

The mechanisms involved in rupture of the follicle and extrusion of the ovum are still poorly understood. It has been suggested that collagenase and other proteases may depolymerize collagen fibrils of the extracellular matrix, contributing to the weakening of the follicular wall at the stigma, but there is no compelling evidence that enzymes are involved. Electron microscopic studies have shown that some of the fusiform cells of the theca externa have the ultrastructural features of smooth muscle cells. However, their role in ovulation is questionable. Contraction of circumferentially oriented muscle cells in

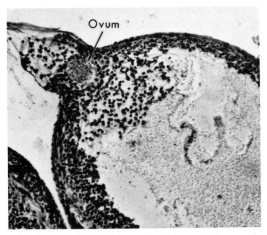

Figure 32–17. Photomicrograph of an ovulating ovarian follicle from the rat. The cumulus with the enclosed egg *(at arrow)* can be seen passing through the stigma. (Courtesy of R. J. Blandau.)

the theca externa would be expected to compress the follicular contents and raise intrafollicular pressure. Sensitive pressure recordings have failed to demonstrate any significant rise in intrafollicular pressure immediately preceding ovulation. Therefore, the smooth muscle–like cells in the theca probably do not play a role in this process. They may, however, be involved in the postovulatory collapse of the follicle that precedes formation of the corpus luteum.

At the risk of some redundancy, it may be useful to review here the endocrine control of the menstrual cycle and ovulation.

Endocrine Control of Ovulation

Ovulation depends on a complex sequence of endocrine events involving the hypothalamus, the hypophysis, and the ovary. The central control of the menstrual cycle resides in the arcuate region of the medial basal hypothalamus. Neurons in this region have an inherent rhythm of activity with a periodicity of 90 minutes in the human. Their activity results in a pulsatile release of gonadotropin releasing hormone (GnRH), which is carried in the hypophyseoportal vessels to the anterior lobe of the hypophysis. There, the hormone stimulates synthesis and release of follicle stimulating hormone (FSH) and luteinizing hormone (LH) by the gonadotropes. FSH carried to the ovary in the general circulation stimulates growth and maturation of ovarian follicles. The growing follicles, in turn, secrete progressively increasing amounts of the steroid hormone estradiol during the follicular phase of the cycle. The rising level of estradiol is believed to act back on the gonadotropes, inducing them to accumulate LH and to a lesser extent FSH. At midcycle, when the dominant follicle attains maturity, the circulating estradiol reaches a critical threshold level that exerts a positive feedback on the hypophysis, altering gonadotrope function from a phase of hormone accumulation to one of abrupt release. The resulting surge of circulating LH triggers rupture of the follicle and discharge of its ovum.

The ruptured follicle is rapidly transformed into a corpus luteum secreting increasing amounts of progesterone, which inhibits the positive feedback of the ovary on the hypophysis. If fertilization does not occur, the corpus luteum has a life span of about 14 days. With its involution, progesterone and estrogen are no longer produced in appreciable amounts, and menstruation follows. Continuing activity of the hypothalamus then initiates a new cycle.

It was formerly thought that the LH surge inducing ovulation depended on an increased release of luteinizing hormone–releasing hormone (LHRH) acting directly upon the hypophysis and that the target of the estradiol feedback was the hypothalamus. Although an effect of ovarian steroids on hypothalamic function cannot be ruled out, it is now generally accepted that the feedback of ovarian steroids acts mainly at the level of the hypophysis rather than on the hypothalamus. The inhibition of positive feedback by progesterone is the basis for the widespread contraceptive use of progesterone and its analogues to prevent ovulation.

The essential central component of the system controlling the cycle in the female is the hypothalamic pulse generator. The release of pulses of LHRH at regular intervals of 90 minutes in the human (60 minutes in the macaque) is all that is required to initiate and maintain the menstrual cycle. In prepubertal primates, pituitary function is normal in all respects except that little or no gonadotropin is secreted. Pulsatile administration of LHRH to prepubertal monkeys or humans initiates puberty and the onset of normal ovulatory cycles. In women who are amenorrheic owing to a pathologic condition in the hypothalamus, normal menstrual cycles can be induced by pulsatile administration of LHRH with a small computerized pump.

Maturation of the Oocyte

Before ovulation and fertilization, the oocyte must complete meiosis, reducing the diploid complement of chromosomes to the haploid number. In the female, meiosis begins early in fetal life. The primordial germ cells in very early embryos are located in the endoderm of the yolk sac. They subsequently migrate along the root of the mesentery and laterally into the germinal ridges that give rise to the ovaries. During their migration they proliferate by mitosis, greatly increasing their number. Mitosis continues for some time after the primordial germ cells take up residence in the developing ovaries. The resulting *primary oocytes* then enter prophase of the first meiotic division and then proceed to the diplotene stage. Meiosis is then arrested, and the oocytes remain in this state throughout the remainder of fetal life, childhood, and puberty. Thereafter, each month

throughout the reproductive life of the woman one oocyte, as a rule, undergoes maturation and completes meiosis shortly before ovulation. This long interruption in continuity of the meiotic process, lasting from 12 to 40 years, is one of the most remarkable phenomena in reproductive biology and one of the least understood. Various substances have been postulated to account for the switch of primordial germ cells from mitosis to meiosis; the acceleration of the process to diplotene; and the arrest at the diplotene stage of prophase, but the experimental evidence for the existence of these substances is scant. There is some indication that cells in the rete ovarii derived from the mesonephros are responsible for induction of meiosis by secreting a meiosis-inducing substance. The mechanism for arrest of meiosis is not understood, but the follicular fluid in small and large follicles and the supernatant of granulosa cells in culture have been shown to inhibit resumption of meiosis and maturation of large oocytes.

There has been some progress in our understanding of the factors involved in resumption of meiosis in the preovulatory follicle. The trigger for completion of meiosis appears to be a surge in the release of LH occurring near the middle of the cycle. If large follicles are removed from rat ovaries and placed in organ culture before the LH surge has occurred, the oocytes remain in the diplotene stage. However, addition of LH to the culture medium, or microinjection of dibutyryl cyclic AMP into the antrum, will induce resumption of meiosis and completion of oocyte maturation in vitro. Thus, the LH surge seems to activate the prepared oocyte, and the action of the hormone is mediated by the adenyl cyclase/cyclic AMP system.

In the resulting division of the primary oocyte, the chromosomes are divided equally between the daughter cells, but cytoplasmic division is exceptional, in that nearly all the cytoplasm remains with one daughter cell, the *secondary oocyte*. In this division the nucleus of a primary oocyte moves to a position immediately beneath the oolemma. The nuclear envelope is broken down and the condensed chromosomes assemble on the metaphase plate of a spindle that is oriented paratangential to the oolemma (Fig. 32–18*A*). The spindle then rotates to a position perpendicular to the oolemma. A small, rounded protrusion of cytoplasm appears on the surface of the oocyte at the pole of the spindle. At anaphase, half of the chromosomes are drawn into this minute bleb of cytoplasm, which is pinched off to form the *first polar body,* lying free in the perivitelline space between the secondary oocyte and the zona pellucida (Fig. 32–18*B*). The spindle of the second meiotic division forms almost immediately with the chromosomes that remain in the oocyte arranged on the metaphase plate (Fig. 32–19). From the resumption of meiosis until the attainment of this state occupies a period of about ten hours immediately preceding ovulation, and the ovum remains arrested in this condition until its fertilization in the ampulla of the oviduct.

Fertilization

At the time of ovulation the turgid fronds or fimbriae of the oviduct are closely applied

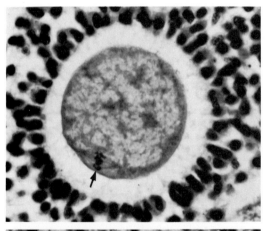

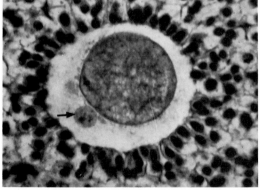

Figure 32–18. Photomicrographs of two stages in the maturation of the rat ovum. *A,* Section of a rat egg shortly before ovulation, showing the first polar spindle with diploid chromosomes on the metaphase plate *(arrow).* (Courtesy of R. J. Blandau.) *B,* Ovulated egg recovered from the ampulla of the oviduct but before sperm penetration. The first polar body lies in the perivitelline space *(arrow).* The second maturation spindle can be seen just above it. (Courtesy of R. J. Blandau.)

to the surface of the ovary. Their active sweeping movements over its surface, and the currents created in the overlying film of fluid by the cilia on its epithelial cells, are responsible for drawing the ovum into the ostium of the oviduct.

The newly ovulated tubal ovum in most mammalian species is surrounded by a corona radiata of adhering granulosa cells. With the invasion of this mass of cells by spermatozoa, their attachments to one another are loosened. The gradual dispersion of the cells of the corona radiata is attributed to a depolymerization of the intercellular substance by enzymes released from the acrosomes of the spermatozoa. Increased surface activity of the cells themselves may also be involved.

Upon reaching the zona pellucida, the sperm head gradually penetrates this layer. The details of this process are still not completely understood. The spermatozoon remains actively motile during its penetration. This movement may contribute to the process, but local lysis of the zona by enzymes of the sperm acrosome is also believed to play an important role in sperm penetration. Once within the vitelline space, the movements of the sperm cease. The membrane overlying the postacrosomal region of the sperm head fuses with the oolemma, and the sperm sinks into the ooplasm.

Fertilization proper consists of the entry of the spermatozoon into the ovum. This event somehow stimulates the ovum to complete the second meiotic division and cast off the second polar body. This is followed by fusion of the egg and sperm nuclei to restore the diploid chromosome number, and cleavage of the zygote ensues.

If the ovum is not fertilized, it gradually fragments and is absorbed or phagocytized. The length of the period during which the human ovum remains fertilizable is not precisely known, but it is probably less than 24 hours.

Formation of the Corpus Luteum

Following ovulation and discharge of the liquor folliculi, the wall of the follicle collapses, and its granulosa cell lining is thrown into folds (Fig. 32–20). The basal lamina that formerly separated the granulosa and the theca interna is depolymerized. There may be some associated extravasation of blood from the capillaries of the theca interna, resulting in the formation of a central clot. The cells of the plicated granulosa layer and those of the theca interna then undergo strik-

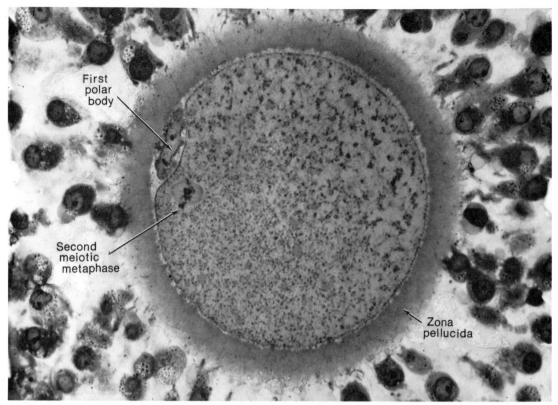

Figure 32–19. Photomicrograph of human follicular oocyte at completion of the first meiotic division. A first polar body has been extruded, and the chromosomes and spindle of the second meiotic metaphase are visible. (Photomicrograph courtesy of L. Zamboni.)

ing cytological alterations. They enlarge, accumulate lipid, and are transformed into plump, pale-staining polygonal cells—the *lutein cells*. After these postovulatory changes have taken place, the follicle is called the *corpus luteum*.

Early in the development of the corpus luteum, two kinds of lutein cells are distinguishable. Those at the periphery that are smaller and more deeply stained have been called *theca lutein cells* in the belief that they originate from cells of the theca interna. Those in the interior that make up the bulk of the lutein tissue have been called *granulosa lutein cells* (Figs. 32–21, 32–22). It is not clear whether these two types are ontogenetically distinct or are merely transitional stages in the development of a single type of lutein cell.

The lipid in the lutein cells is dissolved in routine histological preparations, leaving numerous vacuoles. Their vacuolated cytoplasm gives them an appearance reminiscent of the cells of the adrenal cortex. In electron micrographs they have mitochondria with tubular cristae and the abundant smooth endo-

plasmic reticulum characteristic of steroid-secreting cells (Figs. 32–23, 32–24). The corpus luteum secretes the steroid hormone *progesterone*.

While the cells of the collapsed follicular wall are undergoing luteinization, the capillaries of the theca interna sprout and invade the lutein tissue. Connective tissue elements also penetrate the developing corpus luteum from its periphery, forming a delicate reticulum around the lutein cells and gradually converting the resolving blood clot in the central cavity into a fibrous core.

If the ovum is not fertilized, the ruptured follicle gives rise to a *corpus luteum of menstruation*, which lasts for only about 14 days. Its rate of secretion of progesterone then drops as it undergoes histological involution. The lutein cells become loaded with lipid and ultimately degenerate. In the succeeding months the connective tissue cells become pyknotic, hyaline intercellular material accumulates, and the former corpus luteum is reduced to a white scar, the *corpus albicans* (Fig. 32–25). This slowly sinks deeper into the interior of the ovary and gradually dis-

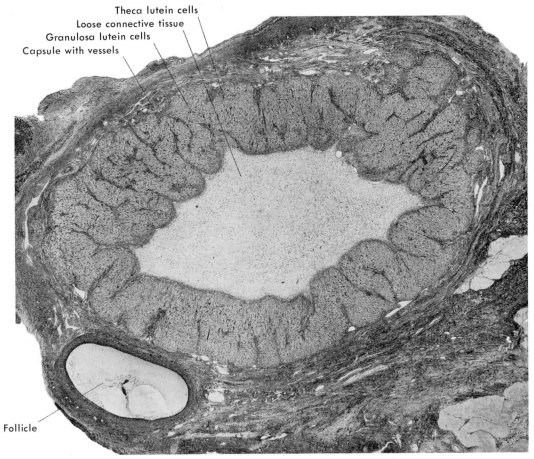

Theca lutein cells
Loose connective tissue
Granulosa lutein cells
Capsule with vessels

Follicle

Figure 32–20. Photomicrograph of section of corpus luteum from human ovary, × 11.

appears over a period of many months or years.

If ovulation is followed by fertilization, the corpus luteum enlarges further and becomes a *corpus luteum of pregnancy,* which persists for about six months and then gradually declines up to full term. After delivery its involution is accelerated and it undergoes changes leading to the formation of a scar similar to that left behind by the corpus luteum of menstruation.

The development of the corpora lutea has now been studied by electron microscopy in the human and in the rhesus monkey. In addition to vascular and connective tissue invasion of the ruptured follicular epithelium, there is hyperplasia and hypertrophy of the cells. The two populations of lutein cells identified with the light microscope are also distinguishable in electron micrographs (Figs. 32–23, 32–24). The lighter-appearing granulosa lutein cells are very large, measuring up to 30 μm in diameter, in contrast

to darker theca lutein cells, which are only about 15 μm in diameter. In the luteinization of granulosa cells there is (1) a transformation of a dense heterochromatic pattern in the nucleus to a more homogeneous nucleoplasm with a single prominent nucleolus; (2) a change in form of the mitochondria from elongate organelles with lamelliform cristae to highly pleomorphic mitochondria with a dense matrix, with tubular cristae, and often with osmiophilic inclusions; (3) an increase in lipid droplets and in the smooth membranes of the agranular reticulum, which take the form of networks of anastomosing tubules or concentric systems of cisternae; (4) evolution of a single Golgi complex of the granulosa cells to multiple small stacks of cisternae widely dispersed in the cytoplasm of the lutein cells; (5) an increase in lysosomes and lipofuscin pigment deposits; and (6) development of many microvilli on the surface of granulosa lutein cells, that project into intercellular clefts and invaginations of the cell

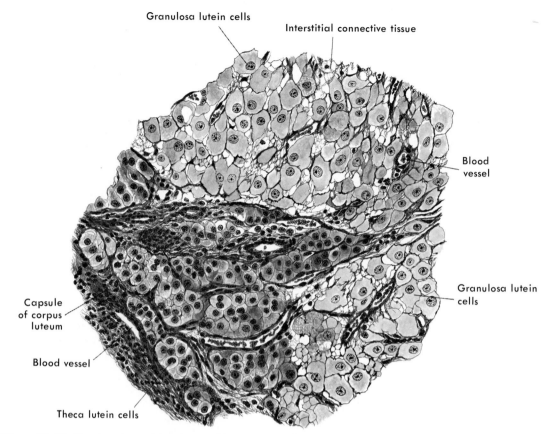

Figure 32–21. Drawing of a peripheral area of human corpus luteum of pregnancy, stained for reticular fibers by the Bielschowsky method. The smaller darker cells at lower left are theca lutein cells, the large paler cells above are granulosa lutein cells. (After A. A. Maximow.)

surface that are reminiscent of the intracellular canaliculi of gastric parietal cells. This surface amplification is less apparent on the theca lutein cells, which remain smaller and generally have a somewhat less extensive smooth endoplasmic reticulum, and more numerous lipid droplets.

The cytological changes described for luteinization *in vivo* have also been observed in tissue cultures of granulosa cells from preovulatory follicles. The acquisition of the ultrastructural characteristics of lutein cells is correlated with the synthesis of increased amounts of progesterone.

Late in pregnancy, a new population of small dense granules appears in the cytoplasm of the lutein cells. These do not contain lysosomal enzymes. They are believed to represent sites of storage of the polypeptide hormone *relaxin,* which has been localized to the corpus luteum by fluorescent antibody methods. The exact physiological role of this hormone is still poorly understood, but it is known to inhibit contractions of the myo-

metrium in pregnancy. It also promotes dilatation of the cervix, and in some species loosens the symphysis pubis, thus facilitating parturition.

Atresia of Follicles

In the human female during the early part of each cycle, a group of follicles starts to grow. Usually only one of these goes on to develop into a mature follicle, and all the others undergo a degenerative process called *follicular atresia.* Some 99 per cent of the oocytes present in the ovary at birth are destined to degenerate. This depletion of the stock of oocytes begins in intrauterine life, becomes prominent at birth and before puberty, and continues on a smaller scale throughout reproductive life. Every normal ovary, therefore, contains degenerating follicles. Why only a few follicles reach maturity and rupture, while the great majority degenerate at various stages of development, is not known. The mechanism by which a single

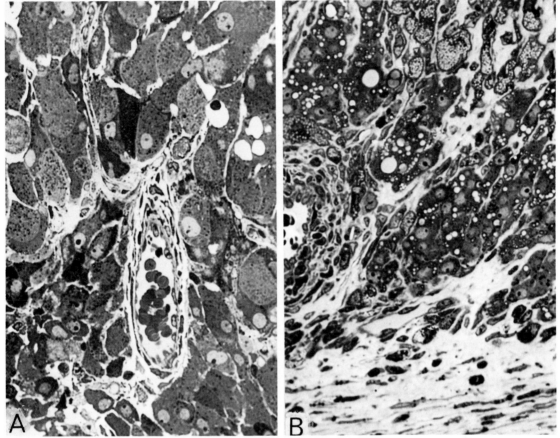

Figure 32–22. *A,* Photomicrograph of human corpus luteum at nine weeks' gestation. Larger cells above are granulosa lutein cells; smaller ones below are theca lutein cells derived from the theca interna. *B,* Corpus luteum of the human menstrual cycle about one day after ovulation. Cells of the theca interna have luteinized and are migrating into the developing corpus luteum. (Photomicrographs from Crisp, T. M., et al. Am. J. Anat. *127*:37, 1970.)

follicle is selected to complete its development is also unknown. Nor do we have any clear idea of the biological significance of this wastage of oocytes.

Atresia may begin at any stage of development of the follicle, even in ones that are apparently mature. In a primary follicle doomed to destruction, the ovum shrinks and degenerates, a process followed by the dissolution of the granulosa cells. The resulting small cavity in the stroma is closed rapidly without leaving a trace. In small secondary follicles, the earliest sign of abnormality is often the eccentric location of the egg nucleus, which goes on to develop a coarse granularity and finally becomes pyknotic. In follicles of larger size, the histological changes in atresia become somewhat more complex and variable. In the cyclic atresia of follicles in the adult human ovary, the process appears to be initiated in the follicle wall, with secondary effects upon the oocyte. One of

the earliest indications of this atretic process is the invasion of the granulosa layer and cumulus oophorus by strands of vascularized connective tissue. This is followed by a loosening and shedding of the granulosa cells into the follicular cavity and a hypertrophy of the theca interna. In follicles exhibiting these changes, the oocyte may still appear normal in routine histological preparations. As the degeneration of granulosa cells advances, the follicle collapses, its outlines become wavy, and the cavity is filled by a large number of fibroblasts. The remnants of the degenerated follicular epithelium are rapidly resorbed. The folded and collapsed zona pellucida may remain alone amid the connective tissue elements.

The theca interna also undergoes important changes. The basal lamina that separates it from the epithelium often increases in thickness and is transformed into a thick hyaline layer, the "glassy membrane," which

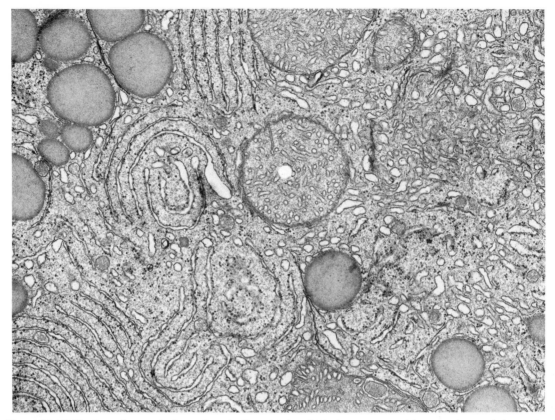

Figure 32–23. Electron micrograph of a portion of a theca lutein cell of a human corpus luteum at nine weeks' gestation. The granular and agranular endoplasmic reticulum are well developed and lipid droplets are abundant. The mitochondria are highly variable in size and have tubular cristae. (From Crisp, T. M., et al. Am. J. Anat. *127*:37, 1970.)

is characteristic of follicles in advanced atresia. The large cells of the theca interna increase further in size and are usually arranged in radial groups or strands, separated from one another by partitions of collagenous fibers and smaller fusiform cells. The cells acquire a typical epithelioid character and are filled with lipid droplets. They are very similar in appearance to the theca lutein cells but reach a higher degree of development in the atretic follicle. The cavity of the atretic follicle, containing the collapsed zona pellucida and connective tissue, is now surrounded by a broad, festooned layer of epithelioid, lipid-containing theca interna cells, arranged in radial cords and provided with a rich capillary network. The microscopic appearance of such an atretic follicle is rather similar to that of an old corpus luteum. Such structures have therefore been given the misleading name *corpora lutea atretica*. The main differences are, of course, the presence of the glassy membrane, degenerated granulosa cells, and sometimes a zona pellucida in the center.

Strands of fibrous connective tissue and blood vessels ultimately penetrate the glassy membrane, and the remains of the degenerated elements in the interior are broken down. The resulting scar with its hyaline streaks sometimes resembles a corpus albicans derived from old corpora lutea, but is usually much smaller, and sooner or later it disappears in the stroma of the ovary. The layer of hypertrophic theca interna cells surrounding the atretic follicle is broken up by the invading strands of fibrous tissue into separate cell islands of various shapes and sizes. These islands are irregularly scattered in the stroma and may persist for a time. They contribute to the so-called "interstitial gland" of the ovary.

The Interstitial Tissue of the Ovary

The stroma of the human ovarian cortex consists of spindle-shaped cells and networks of reticular fibers. Elastic fibers occur only in the walls of blood vessels. The cells bear a superficial resemblance to smooth muscle but

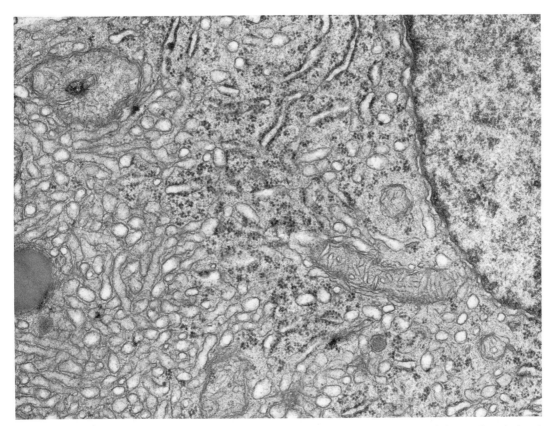

Figure 32–24. Electron micrograph of a portion of human granulosa lutein cell at nine weeks' gestation. As in other steroid-producing endocrine glands, there is an extensive development of tubular smooth reticulum, and lesser amounts of the granular form. (From Crisp, T. M., et al. Am. J. Anat. *127*:37, 1970.)

do not have myofilaments in their cytoplasm.

The endocrine function and developmental potentialities of the layer of specialized interstitial tissue composing the theca folliculi have already been described. The interstitial tissue of the ovarian cortex consists of reticular fibers and spindle-shaped cells that have potentialities distinct from those of ordinary fibroblasts. The medulla, on the other hand, is made up of more typical loose connective tissue with fibroblasts, many elastic fibers, and strands of smooth muscle cells accompanying the blood vessels.

In many mammals the ovarian stroma also contains conspicuous clusters and cords of large epithelioid interstitial cells. They are rich in lipid and strikingly resemble lutein cells. In some species they have been shown to secrete estrogen. Because of their epithelioid appearance and presumed secretory functions, these cells, dispersed in the stroma, are referred to collectively as the *interstitial gland*. In animal species that have large litters, particularly among the rodents, the development of the interstitial gland may be very extensive. Cell clumps originating from the breaking up of the hypertrophied theca interna of atretic follicles persist, enlarge, and fuse. Through the continuous addition of new cells, a large part of the organ is ultimately transformed into a diffuse mass of large, closely packed, lipid-containing interstitial cells that are almost identical in appearance to lutein cells. The follicles and the corpora lutea are embedded in this cell mass, and only a thin tunica albuginea separates it from the germinal epithelium on the surface.

The interstitial gland is less well developed in the human ovary. Interstitial cells are found in the greatest numbers during the first year of life, when atretic follicles are most numerous, and they are believed to arise from the hypertrophied theca interna of regressing follicles. The interstitial gland involutes at puberty with the onset of menstruation and the cyclic development of corpora lutea. In the adult human ovary, cells of this kind are present only in small numbers widely scattered in the stroma.

In the hilus of the ovary and in the adjacent

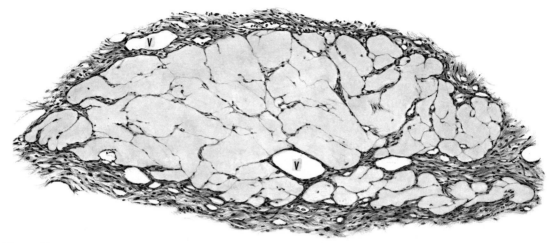

Figure 32–25. Corpus albicans of human ovary. Fixation by perfusion—hence the empty vessel *(V)*. Dense hyaline material separates the residual cells of the corpus luteum. The whole structure is surrounded by the stroma of the ovary. × 135.

mesovarium, groups of another kind of large epithelioid cell may be found closely associated with vascular spaces and unmyelinated nerve fibers. These cell clusters, now simply called *hilus cells,* were originally named the *sympathicotropic hilus gland* and were considered to be chromaffin cells. This view is now less widely accepted, since they do not always stain with chromates. Moreover, convincing evidence has been presented that they are similar to the Leydig cells of the testis. They are rich in lipid, contain cholesterol esters, and lipochrome pigment, and may even have cytoplasmic crystals apparently identical to the crystals of Reinke (see Chapter 31). They have the histochemical and cytological characteristics of actively secreting endocrine cells. They are prominent during pregnancy and at the menopause. Tumor or hyperplasia of the ovarian hilus cells is accompanied by masculinization. This clinical observation and their cytological and cytochemical resemblances to Leydig cells suggest that they secrete androgens.

In the broad ligament and in the mesovarium, the occurrence of small accumulations of "interrenal tissue" corresponding to adrenocortical tissue has also been described.

Vestigial Organs Associated with the Ovary

Certain vestigial organs are found in connection with the ovary. The most obvious of these is the *epoophoron.* It consists of several parallel or divergent tubules, running in the mesovarium from the hilus of the ovary to-

ward the oviduct and fusing with a longitudinal canal parallel to the oviduct. All of these tubules end blindly. They are lined with low cuboidal or columnar epithelium, which is sometimes ciliated, and are surrounded by a condensed connective tissue layer containing smooth muscle. The upper end of the longitudinal duct sometimes ends in a cystlike enlargement, the *hydatid of Morgagni,* while its other end may extend far toward the uterus as the so-called *duct of Gartner.* The transverse tubules and the longitudinal duct of Gartner together comprise the *epoophoron.* Between the epoophoron and the uterus in the tissue of the broad ligament is another group of irregular fragments of epithelial tubules, the *paroophoron.* The epoophoron is a rudiment of the embryonic mesonephros and is the homologue of the ductuli efferentes and epididymis of the male. The paroophoron is the remnant of the caudal part of the mesonephros and corresponds to the vestigial paradidymis of the male.

Vessels and Nerves

The principal arterial supply to the ovary is from the ovarian artery, which arises from the aorta below the level of the renal vessels and reaches the ovary through the infundibulopelvic ligament. Along the mesovarial border of the ovary this vessel anastomoses with the uterine artery, which courses upward along the lateral aspect of the uterus from the region of the cervix. Relatively large vessels from the region of anastomosis of the uterine and ovarian arteries enter the hilus of the ovary and branch profusely as they course through the medulla. Because of their tortuous course, they are called *arteriae helicinae,* or helicine arteries. These vessels, like those in the corpora cavernosa penis, may show longitudinal ridges on their intima. In the periphery of the medulla they form a plexus, from which smaller twigs penetrate radially, passing between the follicles to enter the cortex, where they break up into loose networks of capillaries. These are continuous with dense networks in the theca of the larger follicles. The veins accompany the arteries. In the medulla they are large and tortuous and form a plexus in the hilus.

Networks of lymph capillaries arise in the cortex, especially in the theca externa of the large follicles. Lymph vessels with valves are found only outside the hilus.

The nerves of the ovary are derived from the ovarian plexus and from the uterine nerves. They enter the organ through the hilus, together with the blood vessels. They consist, for the most part, of nonmyelinated fibers, but thin myelinated fibers are also present. The reported presence of sympathetic nerve cells in the ovary has not been confirmed. The majority of the nerves supply the muscular coat of blood vessels. Many

fibers penetrate into the cortex and form plexuses around the follicles and under the germinal epithelium. It seems doubtful that they penetrate through the basal lamina into the epithelium of the follicles. Sensory fibers ending in corpuscles of Pacini have been described in the ovarian stroma.

THE OVIDUCT OR FALLOPIAN TUBE

The *oviduct* or *fallopian tube* is the part of the female reproductive tract that receives the ovum, provides the appropriate environment for its fertilization, and transports it to the uterus. It is a muscular tube about 12 cm long situated in the edge of the mesosalpinx, which is the upper free margin of the broad ligament of the uterus. Its lumen communicates with the uterine cavity at one end and is open to the peritoneal cavity at the other. Several segments along its length are identified by different descriptive terms (Fig. 32–26). The part of the tube traversing the wall of the uterus is called the *pars interstitialis.* The narrow medial third near the uterine wall is the *isthmus.* The expanded intermedi-

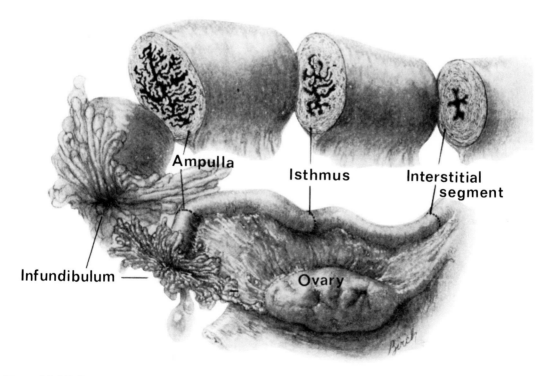

Figure 32–26. Drawing illustrating the mucosal pattern of the various segments of the human oviduct and the topographical relationship of the oviduct to the ovary. (From Eastman, M. J., and L. M. Hellman, eds.: Williams Obstetrics. 13th ed. New York, Appleton-Century-Crofts, 1961. Labeling added.)

ate segment is the *ampulla,* and the funnel-shaped abdominal opening is the *infundibulum.* The margins of the latter are drawn out into numerous tapering, fringelike processes, the *fimbriae.*

Histological Organization

The wall of the oviduct consists of a mucosa, a muscular layer, and an external serous coat. The mucosa in the ampulla is thick and forms numerous elaborately branched folds. The lumen in cross section, therefore, is a labyrinthine system of narrow spaces between profusely branching folia covered by epithelium (Figs. 32–26, 32–27C). In the isthmus the longitudinal folds are much shorter and less highly branched (Fig. 32–27B), and in the interstitial part they are reduced to low ridges (Fig. 32–27A).

The epithelium is of the simple columnar variety (Figs. 32–28, 32–29A) but may sometimes appear pseudostratified when cut obliquely. It is highest in the ampulla and diminishes in height toward the uterus. It consists of two kinds of cells. One of these, especially numerous on the fimbriae and in

the ampulla, is provided with cilia that beat toward the uterus (Fig. 32–30). The other cell type is devoid of cilia and is commonly considered to be secretory. The secretion may provide the ovum with nutritive material, and in some species, notably the rabbit, it adds to the ovum an outer albuminous envelope. In the monotremes and some marsupials, a shell, as well as an albuminous coat, is formed around the ova. The two types of epithelial cells are probably different functional states of a single cell type. In women the epithelium of the oviduct undergoes cyclic changes along with those of the uterine mucosa. True glands are absent in the oviduct.

The relative proportions of ciliated and nonciliated cells is under endocrine control. Ciliated cells are said to increase in height in the human oviduct during the follicular phase of the cycle and to decrease during the luteal phase, but they do not seem to lose their cilia completely. The cyclic changes have been most thoroughly studied in the rhesus monkey. The changes are most marked in the fimbria and upper ampulla, and diminish toward the isthmus. On the

A

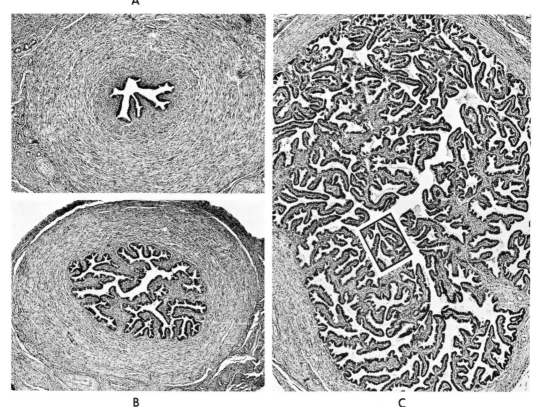

B   C

Figure 32–27. Photomicrographs of the fallopian tube of a 23-year-old woman. × 30. *A,* The pars interstitialis; *B,* the isthmus; *C,* the outer portion of the ampulla. Area enclosed in rectangle is shown at higher magnification in Figure 32–28.

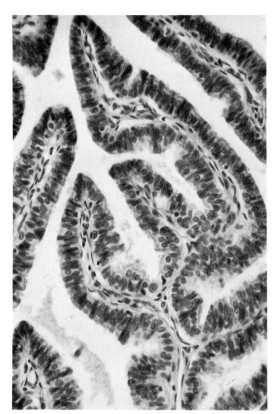

Figure 32–28. Photomicrograph of the branching folds of the mucous membrane of the human fallopian tube. × 280. For orientation, see rectangle in Figure 32–27.

other parts of the body are completely indifferent to circulating estrogens.

Steroid hormones also appear to affect the rate of ciliary beat. A significant increase has been reported 48 hours after copulation in the rabbit and after progesterone treatment of the estrogen-primed monkey oviduct. Thus, estrogen seems to prepare the ciliated surface destined to transport the ovum, and progesterone accelerates the ciliary beat at the time an ovum is available to be trans-

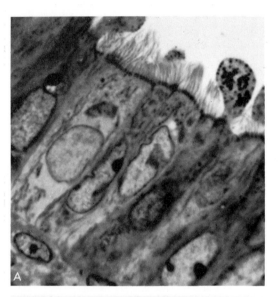

fimbria, the epithelium becomes devoid of cilia and nonsecretory in the late luteal phase of the cycle. In the early follicular phase, the cells hypertrophy and begin active ciliogenesis. There is also cytological evidence of secretory activity. These changes reach their peak at midcycle. Dedifferentiation is so complete on the fimbriae in the late luteal phase that one cannot distinguish deciliated cells from atrophic secretory cells. The degree of dedifferentiation is less marked toward the isthmus, suggesting that this segment of the oviduct is less estrogen dependent.

After ovariectomy the oviductal epithelium rapidly atrophies and dedifferentiates (Fig. 32–29*B*). Within a few weeks the fimbriae are almost completely deciliated and all the cells are structurally indistinguishable (Fig. 32–29*B*). In the ampulla some cells retain their cilia, and in the isthmus regression is still less marked. Similar dedifferentiation after ovariectomy is observed in the rabbit and in other species (Fig. 32–31). Within a week after administration of estradiol, there is a remarkable hypertrophy, with restoration of cilia and secretory activity. Ciliated epithelia in

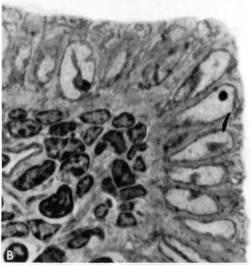

Figure 32–29. *A,* Photomicrograph of oviductal epithelium from a normal macaque in the follicular phase of the cycle. Ciliated and nonciliated cells are distinguishable. *B,* oviductal epithelium of a macaque six weeks after ovariectomy. The cells are shorter and nonciliated, and two types of cells are no longer distinguishable. (From Brenner, R. *In* Hafez, E. S., and R. J. Blandau, eds.: The Mammalian Oviduct. Chicago, University of Chicago Press, 1969.)

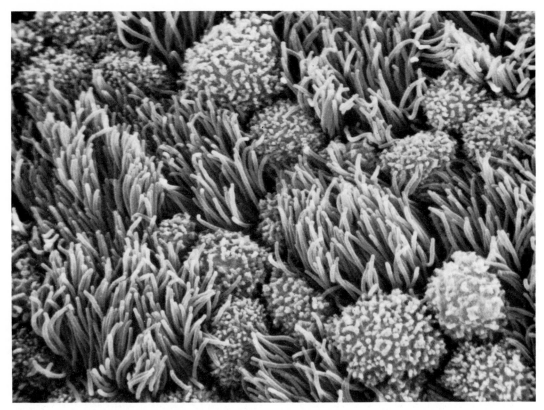

Figure 32–30. Scanning electron micrograph of the surface of the epithelium on the fimbria of rabbit oviduct in the postovulatory period, showing the dense ciliation and the convex apices of the secretory cells covered with microvilli (From Rumery, R. E., and E. M. Eddy. Anat. Rec. *178*:83, 1974.)

ported. Later in the cycle, progesterone favors the loss of cilia.

The lamina propria of the mucosa in the oviduct consists of a network of reticular fibers and of numerous fusiform cells. Lymphocytes, monocytes, and mast cells also occur in limited numbers. The fixed cells here seem to have the same developmental potentialities as those in the stroma of the uterus. In cases of tubal pregnancy, some of them are transformed into typical decidual cells.

No true muscularis mucosae can be distinguished in the oviduct. The mucosa is surrounded directly by the muscularis, which consists of two layers of smooth muscle bundles. The inner layer is circular or spiral; the outer is principally longitudinal, but there is no distinct boundary between the two. Toward the periphery, longitudinal bundles gradually appear in increasing numbers among the circular bundles. The smooth muscle bundles are embedded in an abundant, loose connective tissue, and they extend into the broad ligament. Toward the uterus the muscularis increases in thickness. The peritoneal coat of the fallopian tube has the usual serosal structure.

At the time of ovulation the oviduct exhibits active movements. The abdominal opening of the oviduct contains large blood vessels in its mucosa, especially veins, and these extend into the fimbriae. Smooth muscle bundles form a network between the blood vessels. This results, in effect, in a sort of erectile tissue. At the time of ovulation the vessels are engorged with blood, and the resulting enlargement and turgescence of the fimbriae, together with the contraction of their intrinsic muscle, brings the opening of the tubal infundibulum into contact with the surface of the ovary.

The rhythmic contractions of the oviduct are probably of primary importance in the transport of the ovum. Contraction waves pass from the infundibulum to the uterus, and the beat of the cilia on the mucosa is in the same direction.

Blood Vessels, Lymphatics, and Nerves

The mucosa and its folds, as well as the serous coat, contain abundant blood and lymph vessels. The lymph channels within

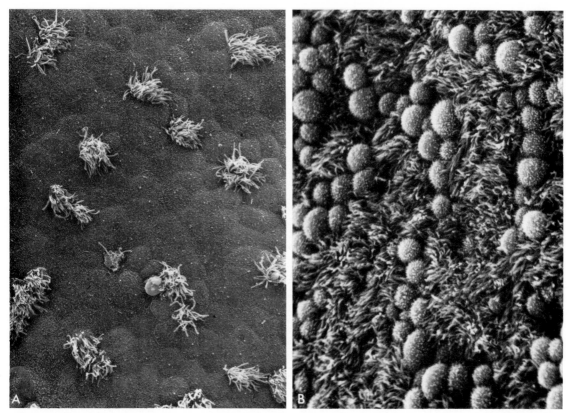

Figure 32–31. Scanning micrographs illustrating the dependence of cytological differentiation of the oviductal epithelium upon hormones. *A,* From the fimbria of a rabbit oviduct 16 months after ovariectomy. The epithelium is flat and smooth, with only occasional ciliated cells. *B,* The other oviduct of the same rabbit after receiving estrogen replacement for ten days. (From Rumery, R. E., and E. M. Eddy. Anat. Rec. *178*:83, 1974.)

the folds of the mucosa are extensive and appear in sections as long clefts that are often mistaken for artifactitious splits in the tissue, but careful inspection reveals their smooth endothelial lining. In periods of vascular engorgement, when these lymphatics are also distended with lymph, they no doubt contribute to the increased turgor of the tissue and stiffen the mucosal folds.

Larger nerve bundles are found accompanying the vessels in the serous layer and in the peripheral parts of the longitudinal muscle. The circular muscle layer contains a dense plexus of thin nerve bundles supplying the muscle fibers and penetrating into the mucosa.

UTERUS

The uterus is the portion of the reproductive tract that receives the fertilized ovum from the oviduct, provides its attachment, and establishes the vascular relations neces-

sary for sustenance of the embryo throughout its development. In the human it is a single pear-shaped organ with a thick muscular wall (Fig. 32–32). It is slightly flattened dorsoventrally and contains a corresponding flattened uterine cavity. In the nonpregnant condition, the uterus is about 6.5 cm long, 3.5 cm wide, and 2.5 cm thick. Several regions are distinguished. The expanded upper portion, constituting the bulk of the organ, is called the *body* or *corpus uteri*. The rounded upper end of the body, where the oviducts join the uterus, is often referred to as the *fundus.* The slightly constricted portion below the corpus is the *isthmus,* and the cylindrical lower part is the *cervix.* The portion of the cervix that protrudes into the vagina is the *portio vaginalis.* The slender cervical canal that passes from the uterine cavity down through the cervix opens into the vagina at the *external os.*

A serous membrane, the peritoneum, covers the fundus and much of the posterior aspect of the uterus. The peritoneum is reflected onto the bladder anteriorly and onto

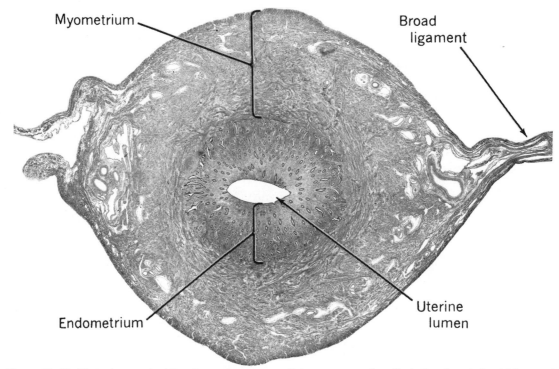

Figure 32–32. Photomicrograph of the uterus of a macaque in transverse section, illustrating the relative thickness of the myometrium and the late proliferative endometrium. ×9. (Courtesy of H. Mizoguchi.)

the rectum posteriorly, so that this layer is found only on part of the surface of the uterus. The greater part of the thickness of the uterine wall is smooth muscle, the *myometrium*. The uterus is lined by a glandular mucosa called the *endometrium*.

Myometrium

The smooth muscle fibers of the muscular layer are arranged in cylindrical or flat bundles separated by thin septa of connective tissue. Several layers can be distinguished in the myometrium according to the direction and disposition of the bundles. The layers are not sharply demarcated, however, because fiber bundles cross over from one layer into another.

Immediately beneath the mucosa is a thin layer of smooth muscle called the *stratum submucosum*. Its fibers are predominantly longitudinal, but some oblique and circular bundles may be found. This layer forms distinct muscular rings around the intramural portions of the oviducts and may have a sphincter-like action. The next layer is the thickest and is called the *stratum vasculare,* because it contains many large blood vessels that give it a spongy appearance. Circular and oblique

muscle bundles are predominant. In the succeeding *stratum supravasculare*, the fibers are mainly circular and longitudinal. Finally, the outermost *stratum subserosum* is a thin longitudinal muscle layer. The two most superficial layers send muscular bundles out into the wall of the oviduct and into the broad ligament and the round ligament.

The smooth muscle cells of the myometrium ordinarily have a length of about 50 μm. In pregnancy, when the mass of the uterus increases about 24 times, they hypertrophy to a length of more than 500 μm. Although smooth muscle hypertrophy accounts for much of the enlargement of the gravid uterus, there also appears to be an increase in the number of muscle fibers through division and possibly through transformation of persisting embryonic connective tissue cells into new muscular elements, especially in the innermost layers of the myometrium. There is also a marked increase in the amount of connective tissue as indicated by a fivefold increase in the amount of collagen. There is evidence that smooth muscle cells can synthesize collagen in response to estrogen stimulation. During return of the uterus to normal size after delivery, the muscle cells rapidly diminish in size. It is possible that some of them degenerate.

The connective tissue between the muscular bundles consists of collagenous fibers, fibroblasts, undifferentiated connective tissue cells, macrophages, and mast cells. A typical argyrophilic reticulum surrounds the smooth muscle cells and is continuous with the collagenous tissue septa between muscle bundles. Elastic networks are especially prominent in the peripheral layers of the uterine wall. From there they extend inward between the muscle bundles. The innermost layers of the myometrium contain no elastic fibers, except those in the walls of the blood vessels.

The cervix is composed mainly of dense collagenous and elastic fibers, among which are distributed fibroblasts and smooth muscle cells. The dense fibrous nature of the cervix accounts for the very firm consistency of this segment of the uterus.

Histophysiology of the Myometrium. The maintenance of normal size and cytological differentiation of uterine smooth muscle cells depends on estrogen produced by the ovary and carried to the uterus in the blood. In the absence of estrogen, uterine smooth muscle atrophies.

Contractions of the myometrium are very largely responsible for expulsion of the fetus at parturition. In the normal nonpregnant uterus, the musculature is continually undergoing shallow, intermittent myogenic contractions that are not attended by any subjective sensation. These may become exaggerated during sexual stimulation or during menstruation, resulting in cramplike pain. The factors regulating this activity are poorly understood.

When pregnancy ensues, the activity of the myometrium is greatly reduced. Experiments on animals have led to a widely held belief that the level of progesterone produced by the corpus luteum of pregnancy inhibits myometrial contractility, and that withdrawal of this inhibition at the end of gestation initiates labor. This theory is now seriously challenged. An unequivocal demonstration of an effect of progesterone on the human uterine muscle is lacking, and in several other animal species, progesterone has been shown to have no effect. Cross circulation experiments between pregnant and nonpregnant animals clearly show that some other blood-borne substance plays a more important role than progesterone. There is some reason to believe that this effect may be mediated by the hormone *relaxin*.

Uterine contractility is increased by *oxytocin*, a hormone of the neurohypophysis. The responsiveness of the uterine muscle to oxytocin increases during the last few months of pregnancy, and the rate of secretion of oxytocin by the neurohypophysis increases at the onset of labor. Thus, there is reason to believe that this hormone plays an important role in preparation of the uterus for parturition. Oxytocin is sometimes used by the obstetrician to initiate labor or to increase the effectiveness of the uterine contractions.

Another class of compounds that affect the uterine musculature is the *prostaglandins*. The fetal membranes release prostaglandins in high concentration during labor and this may increase the strength of the uterine contractions. Although the mechanism of action of prostaglandins on smooth muscle is not well understood, they are now widely used to induce abortion.

Contractility of the uterus is also increased by mechanical factors. Stretching of the wall of hollow viscera in general increases smooth muscle contractility. The greater stretching of the uterine wall is believed to account for the fact that twin pregnancies terminate, on the average, at least two weeks earlier than single pregnancies. Stretching or irritation of the cervix also appears to induce uterine contractions. Obstetricians take advantage of this when they rupture the fetal membrane to induce labor. In the absence of amniotic fluid, the fetal head irritates and stretches the endocervix, initiating reflexes that result in contraction of the body of the uterus.

Endometrium

The primary functions of the endometrium are preparation for implantation of a fertilized ovum, participation in implantation, and formation of the maternal portion of the placenta. The structural and functional changes of the endometrium are dependent on the hormones secreted by the ovaries. Upon removal of the ovaries, the endometrium atrophies. Upon administration of estrogen, there is a rapid increase in the blood flow to the uterus, the endometrium becomes edematous, its cells begin to proliferate and hypertrophy, and there is a marked increase in its metabolic activity.

Beginning with puberty at 11 to 15 years of age and continuing until *menopause* at age 45 to 50, the uterine mucosa undergoes monthly cyclic changes in its structure in response to rhythmic variations in the secretion of ovarian hormones. At the end of each cycle there is a partial degeneration and sloughing of the endometrium, accompanied by a more or less abundant extravasation of blood. The products of these destructive changes appear as a bloody vaginal discharge, the *menstrual flow*, which normally continues for three to five days.

The endometrium is approximately 5 mm in thickness at the height of its development in a normal menstrual cycle. It consists of a surface epithelium invaginated to form numerous tubular *uterine glands* that extend down into a very thick lamina propria, usually referred to as the *endometrial stroma.*

The surface epithelium is simple columnar and is composed of a mixture of ciliated and secretory cells. The epithelium of the uterine glands is similar, but the ciliated cells are fewer. The direction of ciliary beat is said to be upward in the glands and toward the vagina on the endometrial surface. The glands are, for the most part, simple tubules, but they may show some bifurcation in the zone adjacent to the myometrium. They occasionally penetrate a short distance among the muscle bundles. Under pathological conditions the myometrium may be extensively invaded in this manner, a change described by the term *adenomyosis.* In old age, the endometrium atrophies and becomes thin. The openings of the glands may become partly obliterated and they then become distended to form small cysts.

The endometrial stroma strongly resembles mesenchyme. Its irregularly stellate cells have large, ovoid nuclei. The cell processes appear to be in contact throughout the tissue and adhere to a delicate framework of reticular fibers. Elastic fibers are absent except in the walls of the arterioles. There is an extracellular matrix, which at some phases of the cycle is rich in metachromatic glycoprotein. In the interstices of the reticulum and stellate cells are lymphoid cells and granular leukocytes. Macrophages are not uncommon but, for some unknown reason, they are not mobilized to phagocytize the blood extravasated in menstruation.

A knowledge of the blood supply of the endometrium is of special importance for an understanding of the mechanisms of menstruation and of placentation. From the uterine arteries that course in the broad ligaments along the sides of the uterus, branches penetrate to the stratum vasculare of the myometrium. In this layer, circumferentially oriented *arcuate arteries* run toward the midline, where they anastomose with corresponding vessels from the other side. Branches from the arcuate arteries penetrate the deeper layers of the myometrium to reach the endometrium. Where they cross the myometrial-endometrial junction, they give off small *basal arteries* supplying the deepest portion of the endometrium, the *basalis* or *stratum basale* (the portion that is not sloughed off during menstruation). Continuing into the thicker layer commonly called the *functionalis,* the arteries are unbranched but highly contorted. These "coiled or spiral arteries" ramify into arterioles that supply a rich capillary bed in the superficial portion of the endometrium. The thin-walled veins form an irregular anastomosing network with sinusoidal enlargements at all levels of the endometrium. During most of the cycle, the coiled arteries constrict and dilate rhythmically, so that the surface is alternately blanched or suffused with blood. These vessels play an important role in initiating menstruation.

Cyclic Changes in the Endometrium

In the course of a normal menstrual cycle, the endometrium passes through a continuous sequence of morphological and functional changes, but for convenience of description the cycle is divided into three recognizable stages that are correlated with the functional activities of the ovary. These are the *proliferative,* the *secretory,* and the *menstrual* phases. The proliferative phase coincides with the period of growth of the ovarian follicles and their secretion of estrogenic hormone. The secretory phase is the period when the corpus luteum is functionally active and secreting progesterone, and the menstrual phase ensues when the hormonal stimulation of the endometrium by the ovaries rapidly declines (Fig. 32–33).

The Proliferative or Follicular Phase. During this phase, which begins at the end of the menstrual flow, there is a two- to threefold increase in thickness of the endometrium. Mitoses are numerous in the epithelium and in the stroma. The straight tubular glands increase in number and in length (Fig. 32–34). Their epithelium is columnar, and the lumen narrow. The extracellular matrix of the stroma is abundant and metachromatic. The coiled arteries are elongating but are only moderately convoluted and do not yet extend into the superficial third of the endometrium. Toward the end

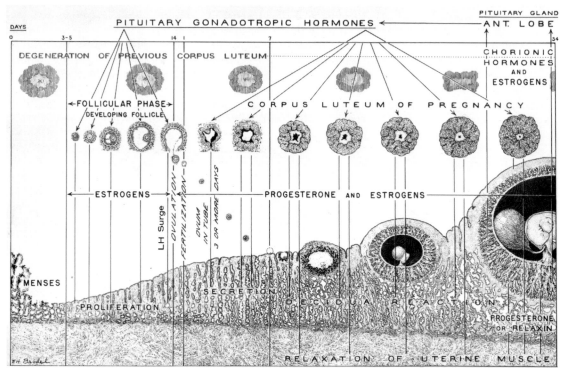

Figure 32–33. Drawing depicting the morphological changes in the ovary and the endometrium in the course of the menstrual cycle, and the hormones controlling these changes. (From Eastman, N. J., ed.: Williams Obstetrics. 11th ed. Englewood Cliffs, NJ, Appleton-Century-Crofts, 1956.)

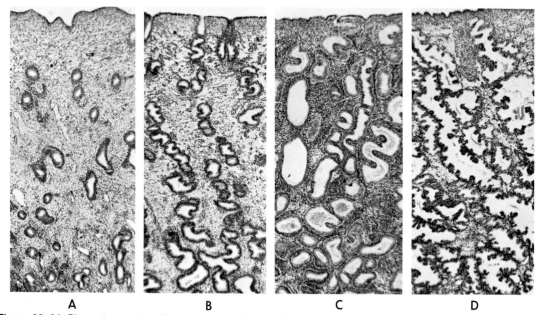

Figure 32–34. Photomicrographs of human endometrium in different days of the cycle. *A,* Proliferative endometrium of the ninth day. *B,* Early secretory endometrium, 15th day. *C,* Secretory endometrium, 19th day. *D,* Gestational hyperplasia, 12th day of pregnancy. (Courtesy of A. T. Hertig.)

of this phase, the glands become somewhat sinuous and their cells begin to accumulate glycogen (Fig. 32–34*B*).

The proliferative growth of the endometrium may continue for a day after ovulation, on about day 14 of an ideal 28-day cycle. There may be some diapedesis of erythrocytes into the stroma beneath the surface epithelium, and rarely a little blood may enter the uterine lumen and reach the vagina. Such *intermenstrual bleeding* is rare in the human, but is common in the dog.

When the endometrium has been prepared by the normal sequential action of estrogen and progesterone, it is capable of undergoing *decidualization*—a change in which its stromal cells transform into large, pale *decidual cells* rich in glycogen. The normal stimulus for this transformation is an implanting blastocyst, but electrical stimulation, intraluminal injection of oil, or simple mechanical traumatization of the endometrium will induce the same changes and result in formation of a mass of decidual cells, called a *deciduoma*. The exact function of the decidual tissue is still a subject of debate, but there is agreement that it provides a favorable milieu for nourishment of the conceptus and creates a specialized layer facilitating dehiscence of the placenta at the termination of pregnancy.

The Secretory or Luteal Phase. In this phase of the cycle, some further thickening of the endometrium occurs, but this is largely attributable to edema of the stroma and to the accumulation of secretion in the uterine glands. The glandular epithelium early in the secretory phase of the endometrium shows a characteristic displacement of the nuclei toward the free surface, owing to the accumulation of a large amount of glycogen in the basal cytoplasm. This appearance is transient and is no longer seen after active secretion is established. The glands continue to grow, becoming more tortuous and ultimately developing a marked sacculation, resulting in a relatively wide lumen of irregular outline, containing a carbohydrate-rich secretion (Fig. 32–34*C*).

The elongation and convolution of the coiled arteries continues in this phase. They extend into the superficial portion of the endometrium and become more prominent in sections because of the hypertrophy of the periarterial stromal cells.

The Menstrual Phase. About two weeks after ovulation, in a cycle in which fertilization fails to occur, the stimulation of the endometrium by ovarian hormones declines and marked vascular changes take place. The coiled arteries constrict, so that the superficial zone of the endometrium is blanched for hours at a time. The glands cease secreting; the height of the endometrium shrinks somewhat, owing to loss of interstitial fluid; and the stroma appears more cellular and stains more deeply. Many leukocytes are found in the stroma at this time. After about two days of intermittent ischemia, the coiled arteries close down, making the superficial zone ischemic, while blood continues to circulate in the basal zone. After a variable number of hours, the constricted arteries open up for a short time; the walls of the damaged vessels near the surface burst, and blood pours into the stroma and soon breaks out into the uterine lumen. Normally such blood does not clot. Subsequently, patches of blood-soaked tissue separate off, leaving the torn ends of glands, arteries, and veins open to the surface. Blood may ooze from such veins, refluxing from the intact basal circulation. The menstrual discharge thus contains (1) altered arterial and venous blood, with hemolyzed, and sometimes agglutinated erythrocytes; (2) partially intact, autolyzed epithelial and stroma cells; and (3) the secretions of the uterine and cervical glands. Sometimes there are tissue fragments in the menstrual discharge, but blood clots are considered abnormal. The average loss of blood is 35 ml. By the third or fourth day of the flow, the entire lining of the uterus presents a raw-appearing surface.

The endometrium deep to the zone of extravasation remains intact during menstruation, although it does shrink down. The deep ends of glands typical of the secretory phase are recognizable as such until the end of menstruation. Before the vaginal discharge has ceased, epithelial cells glide out from the torn ends of the glands, and the surface epithelium is quickly restored. The superficial circulation is resumed; the stroma again becomes rich in ground substance; and the proliferative activity of the follicular phase of the new cycle begins.

The typical thick secretory endometrium (Fig. 32–33) is not always attained. In some cycles, the ovary may not produce a mature follicle. In such *anovulatory cycles* the endometrial changes are minimal. The proliferative endometrium develops as usual, but since there is no ovulation and no corpus luteum is formed, the endometrium does not progress to the secretory phase but continues to be of the proliferative type until menstruation begins.

The various morphological changes in the normal menstrual cycle are so characteristic and reproducible that an experienced pathologist can establish the day of the cycle with surprising accuracy from examination of endometrial curettings or biopsies (Fig. 32–35). It is also possible from examination of biopsies in the second half of the cycle to determine whether a woman is having an ovulatory or an anovulatory cycle. Such examinations are essential in clinical investigation of the causes of infertility, or detection of dysfunction of the ovaries, or disorders of menstruation. It is therefore of practical value to be able to recognize the principal phases of the endometrial cycle. The criteria, in brief, are as follows. (1) *Proliferative or follicular phase:* endometrium 1 to 5 mm thick; straight, narrow glands becoming wavy; the epithelium tall, becoming vacuolated; many mitoses in all tissues; and no coiled arteries in the superficial third. (2) *Secretory or luteal phase:* endometrium 3 to 6 mm thick; glands sinuous and sacculated, with wide lumina; epithelial cells tall, with surface blebs; stroma edematous superficially; mitoses confined to coiled arteries, which are present near the surface. (3) *Premenstrual phase:* endometrium 3 to 4 mm thick; greatly contorted glands and arteries; dense stroma with leukocytic infiltration. (4) *Menstrual phase:* endometrium 0.5 to 3 mm thick; superficially extravasated blood; the glands and arteries appear collapsed and shortened; the stroma is dense; and the surface is denuded of epithelium.

Isthmus and Cervix

The mucosa of the corpus uteri passes over abruptly into that of the isthmus, which remains thin and shows little evidence of cyclic morphological changes. It lacks coiled arteries and usually does not bleed during menstruation.

The cervix forms the wall of the cervical canal, which is about 3 cm in length. Its mucosal lining has a thickness of 2 to 3 mm and a structure quite different from that of the corpus uteri. Its irregular surface consists of branching folds called the *plicae palmatae*. Its stroma is dense, and the glands, which are relatively sparse, are oriented obliquely to the axis of the cervical canal.

The canal is lined by a tall columnar epithelium in which the nuclei are located near the base of the cells, and the greater part of the cytoplasm is filled with mucus. The mucosa contains numerous large glands, which differ from those of the corpus and isthmus in that they are extensively branched and are lined with tall, mucus-secreting columnar cells similar to those of the surface epithelium. Occasional cells are ciliated. The cervical canal is usually filled with mucus. In the human, the ducts of some of the glands not infrequently become occluded, and accumulation of secretion then transforms these glands into cysts that may reach 5 to 6 mm in diameter. These are called *nabothian cysts*.

The outer surface of the portio vaginalis of the cervix is smooth and covered with a stratified squamous epithelium similar to that of the vagina (Fig. 32–49). The cells of this epithelium are rich in glycogen. The transition between the columnar mucus-secreting epithelium of the cervical canal and the stratified squamous epithelium of the portio vaginalis is abrupt. As a rule, the borderline is just inside the external os of the cervix. In some individuals, however, particularly after childbearing, patches of the columnar epithelium of the endocervix may extend for varying distances out onto the portio vaginalis. These are inappropriately called cervical "erosions." They are especially susceptible to inflammatory reactions and are a common cause of increased vaginal discharge, *leukorrhea*. Virtually all multiparous women have some degree of cervical inflammation. If untreated, cervical erosions and their attendant chronic inflammation may predispose to cancer of the cervix, which accounts for 10 per cent of all cancer deaths in women.

The superficial cells of the cervical epithelium are constantly being exfoliated into the vaginal fluid. These can be examined in stained "vaginal smears," and the discovery of abnormal cells may provide a very early diagnosis of cancer.

Histophysiology of the Cervix. The mucosa of the cervix does not take part in the menstrual changes that are characteristic of the endometrium. There are, however, cyclic changes in the secretory activity of its mucous glands. The gland cells are affected by the circulating levels of ovarian hormones so that the amount and properties of the mucus secreted vary at different times in the menstrual cycle. There are normally about 100 crypts or aggregations of glands in the cervix, and these secrete up to 60 mg of mucus a day throughout much of the cycle. At midcycle, there is a tenfold increase in secretion

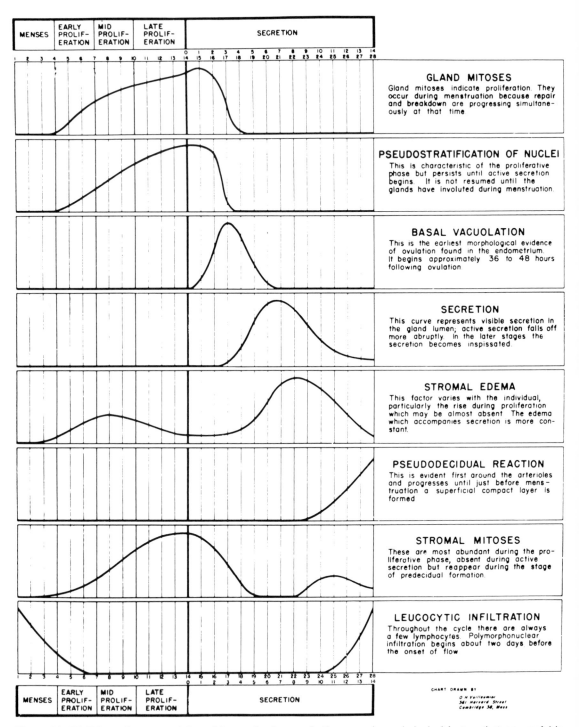

Figure 32–35. Schematic representation of the cyclic changes in the several morphological factors that are useful in dating the endometrium. (From Noyes, R. W., A. T. Hertig, and J. Rock. Fertil. Steril. *1*:3, 1950.)

rate, probably as a result of increasing estrogenic stimulation. There is also a change in the consistency of the mucus, from the highly viscous state that prevails during most of the cycle, to a less viscous, more highly hydrated condition at midcycle. These changes have significance for fertility in that the viscous cervical mucus appears to be a hostile environment and a serious impediment to progress of spermatozoa throughout much of the cycle. The changes occurring at midcycle, however, favor sperm migration.

In pregnancy, the cervical glands enlarge, proliferate, and accumulate large quantities of mucus, and the connective tissue between them is reduced to thin partitions.

The thick wall of the cervix is composed of very dense connective tissue, with smooth muscle constituting only about 15 per cent of its mass. In the portio vaginalis, smooth muscle cells are absent. In the very late stage of pregnancy, changes take place in the fibrous and amorphous components of the extracellular matrix that result in softening of the cervix, facilitating its dilatation by the advancing fetal head during labor.

ENDOCRINE REGULATION OF THE FEMALE REPRODUCTIVE SYSTEM

The histology of the female reproductive system cannot be fully understood without some overview of the interactions of the brain, the hypophysis, the ovaries, and the uterus in regulation of the cyclic changes involved in reproduction. Although some of these relations have already been presented, a brief recapitulation may promote understanding of the cyclic changes described in this chapter.

The cyclic activities of the ovary are under the control of the anterior lobe of the hypophysis. The secretion of follicle stimulating hormone (FSH) is responsible for the growth of the follicle up to the point of ovulation. Luteinizing hormone (LH), together with FSH, is required for ovulation and for the early development of the corpus luteum. The endometrium of the uterus exhibits two phases of functional activity that are correlated with the events in the ovary—a *follicular* (or *proliferative*) *phase* of endometrial growth, coinciding with maturation of the follicles and their ovulation, and a *luteal* (or *secretory*) *phase,* correlated with the development of a corpus luteum and during which the endometrium is prepared for reception of a fertilized egg.

At the end of the follicular phase in most mammals, morphological and neural changes occur that make the female receptive to the male at or near the time of ovulation. This is the period of heat or *estrus.* Although the menstrual cycle in the human female is basically similar to the estrus cycle of other species, receptivity to the male is not limited to the end of the follicular phase and there is no behavioral indication that ovulation has occurred or is imminent.

During the ensuing luteal phase of the cycle, the preparation of the endometrium for reception of a fertilized ovum is more extensive in the primates than in many other animals. If no egg reaches the uterus, the bulk of the endometrium breaks down after about two weeks. Its discharge is attended by uterine bleeding—menstruation.

In a cycle in which the ovum is fertilized, the secretion of gonadotropins by the trophoblast of the implanting ovum helps to maintain the corpus luteum beyond its usual life span, and it becomes the corpus luteum of pregnancy. The continuing function of this corpus luteum prevents the regressive and ischemic changes that lead to menstruation in an infertile cycle. Instead of regressing, the secretory endometrium persists and undergoes further hyperplasia (Fig. 32–34D), and menstruation is suppressed for the duration of pregnancy.

The temporal correlation of the events in the endometrium with those of the ovary is mediated by ovarian hormones. The developing follicle secretes the steroid hormones *estradiol* and *estrone,* collectively described as *estrogens.* These stimulate growth of the uterine endometrium. In species exhibiting estrus, the estrogens also act upon the central nervous system to bring about sexual receptivity and its associated behavioral manifestations. After ovulation, the collapsed follicle is reorganized and transformed into a corpus luteum that secretes *progesterone.* This hormone is responsible for the secretory changes in the endometrium that are characteristic of the luteal phase of the cycle.

The secretion of gonadotropins by the hypophysis is influenced by various factors. The rhythm of hypothalamic stimuli carried by the neurohumoral pathway to the adenohypophysis appears to be determined by some internal clock, but it can also be influenced by psychic factors and various external stimuli. Production of excess ovarian hormones also acts back upon the hypothalamus to diminish gonadotropin secretion. This feedback mechanism is not only operative in the regulation of the normal cycle but is also the basis for the successes in conception control, wherein orally administered analogues of ovarian steroids act upon the hypothalamus and hypophysis to suppress the surge of LH that is essential for ovulation.

IMPLANTATION

After fertilization takes place in the upper part of the oviduct, segmentation of the ovum proceeds as it passes down the oviduct (Fig. 32–36A, B). When it reaches the uterus on about the fourth day, it consists of many cells arranged in a hollow sphere called the *blastocyst* (Fig. 32–36C). The blastocyst remains free in the lumen of the uterus for a day or so and then attaches to the surface of the secretory endometrium. The blastocyst by this time has differentiated into (1) an assemblage of cells at one pole called the *inner cell mass,* which is destined to form the embryo proper; and (2) a layer of primitive *trophoblast cells* making up the rest of the wall of the blastocyst. The trophoblast cells are concerned with the attachment and implantation of the ovum and with the subsequent establishment of the *placenta,* the organ in which the physiological exchange of nutrients and waste products takes place between the embryonic and the maternal circulations. When the trophoblast makes contact with the surface of the endometrium, its cells proliferate rapidly, forming, at the interface between the ovum and the maternal tissue, a multinucleate mass of protoplasm in which no cell boundaries are discernible. This is called the *syncytial trophoblast.* This actively erosive syncytium destroys the surface epithelium and permits the blastocyst to invade the underlying stroma (Fig. 32–37A). By the 11th day the blastocyst is entirely within the endometrium; the trophoblast has formed a broad layer completely surrounding the inner cell mass; and the uterine epithelium has repaired the breach made in it by the implanting blastocyst (Figs. 32–38, 32–39). This form of implantation, in which the embryo and its associated membranes become embedded in and completely encapsulated by the endometrium, is called *interstitial implantation* and is characteristic of the human.

From the ninth to the 11th day, the expanding trophoblastic shell becomes

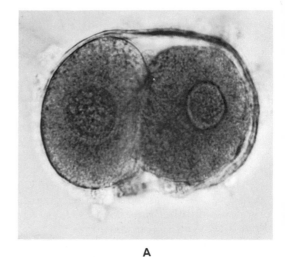

A

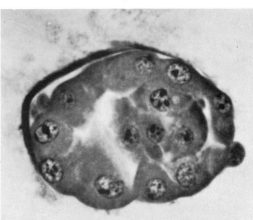

B

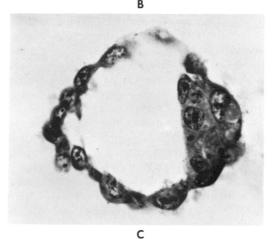

C

Figure 32–36. Photomicrographs of early human ova. *A,* Segmenting human ovum. Two-cell stage recovered from the fallopian tube. Ovulation age 1½ to 2½ days. Notice polar body between the two blastomeres. ×500. *B,* Free human blastocyst. Section of a 58-cell intrauterine blastocyst. Segmentation cavity is just beginning to form. Zona pellucida is disappearing. Ovulation age 4 days. ×600. *C,* Free human blastocyst. Section of a 107-cell blastocyst recovered from the uterine cavity. The inner cell mass is at the right. Ovulation age 4½ days. ×600. (All three micrographs from Hertig, A., J. Rock, and E. Adams. Am. J. Anat. *98:*435, 1956.)

A

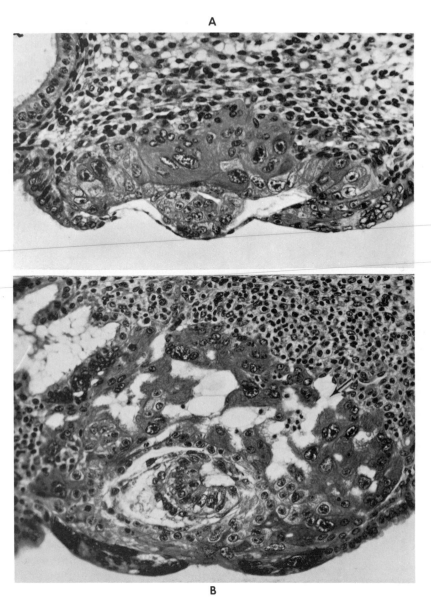

B

Figure 32–37. Photomicrographs of early human implantation sites. *A,* Human seven-day implantation. The embryo is a simple bilaminar disc. Development of an amniotic cavity is beginning. There is a solid plaque of syncytio- and cytotrophoblast. ×300. (After Hertig and Rock, 1941. Courtesy of the Carnegie Institution of Washington.) *B,* Human nine-day implantation. The embryo is a bilaminar disc. The syncytiotrophoblast now shows prominent lacunae. Notice at arrow a maternal blood space communicating with lacuna. ×25. (After Hertig and Rock, 1941. Courtesy of the Carnegie Institution of Washington.)

permeated by a labyrinthine system of inter-communicating lacunae containing blood liberated by erosion of maternal blood vessels (Fig. 32–39). This extravasated blood evidently serves as a source of nourishment for the embryo and represents the first step toward establishment of the uteroplacental circulation on which the growth of the embryo will later depend.

Two forms of trophoblast are recognizable, an inner layer of *cytotrophoblast,* composed of individual cells, and a thicker outer layer of *syncytiotrophoblast.* The cytotrophoblast is mi-

totically active and contributes to the increasing mass of the syncytiotrophoblast by forming new cells that fuse with and become part of the syncytium.

At the 11-day stage, the embryo proper consists of a bilaminar disc of epithelial cells—a thick plate of ectoderm and a thinner layer of primitive endoderm. The ectodermal plate is continuous at its margins with a thin layer of squamous cells that enclose a small *amniotic cavity.* The endoderm is similarly continuous with a thin sheet of cells forming the *yolk sac.* Surrounding these structures are

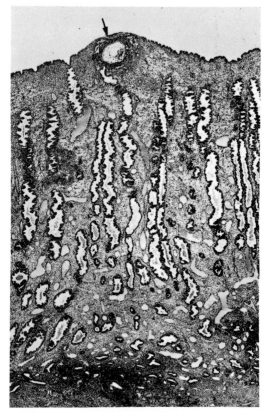

Figure 32–38. Human gestational endometrium with an 11-day implantation site *(arrow)*. The entire thickness of the endometrium is shown. The glands are secretory, the stroma is edematous, and the superficial veins are dilated. × 18. (After Hertig and Rock, 1941. Courtesy of Carnegie Institution of Washington.)

large extracellular spaces traversed by tenuous strands of extraembryonic mesenchyme (mesoblast). These spaces constitute the *exocoelom*. The surrounding broad zone of trophoblast is called the *chorion*.

PLACENTA

Formation and Structure

From the 11th to the 16th day of pregnancy the trophoblast continues to proliferate rapidly, and the implantation cavity is progressively enlarged at the expense of the surrounding maternal tissue. Invasion of the maternal blood vascular system by syncytiotrophoblast becomes extensive. The large lacunae in the syncytial labyrinth communicate at many places with venous sinuses in the endometrium. From the 15th day onward,

solid cords of trophoblast grow outward from the surface of the chorion to form the *primary chorionic villi*. These are soon invaded at their base by chorionic mesenchyme, which advances toward their growing tips, converting the primary villi into *secondary villi* (Figs. 32–40, 32–41). The secondary villi then consist of an outer layer of syncytial trophoblast, an inner layer of cytotrophoblast, and a mesenchymal core. They are bathed in maternal blood that flows sluggishly through a labyrinthine system of intercommunicating channels collectively making up the *intervillous space*.

From the ends of the secondary chorionic villi, solid cords of trophoblast, the *cytotrophoblastic cell columns*, extend across the intervillous space and, upon reaching the opposite wall, spread along it, coalescing with similar outgrowths from neighboring villi to form a more or less continuous *trophoblastic shell*, interrupted only at sites of communication of maternal vessels with the intervillous space. The trophoblastic shell consists mainly of cytotrophoblast, but some areas of syncytiotrophoblast can be found. Through its interstitial growth, the trophoblastic shell provides a mechanism for rapid circumferential expansion of the entire implantation site and for enlargement of the intervillous space. From the time of its formation throughout the remainder of pregnancy, the intervillous space is lined by trophoblast and traversed by villi that are attached to the maternal tissue via the trophoblastic shell. The villi absorb nutriments from the maternal blood in the intervillous space and excrete wastes into it. The efficiency of this process is greatly enhanced after the development of a functioning vascular system in the embryo.

Fetal blood vessels differentiate in the mesenchymal cores of the secondary villi as discontinuous endothelial-lined spaces, which later coalesce to form continuous vascular channels. These become connected with the embryonic heart via vessels that differentiate in the mesenchyme of the inner surface of the chorion and in the body stalk or umbilical cord. By the 21st to the 23rd day, fetal blood begins to circulate through the capillaries of the villi. After their vascularization, the secondary villi are called *tertiary* or *definitive placental villi* (Fig. 32–47). These radiate from the entire periphery of the chorion (Fig. 32–41). In the subsequent growth of the placenta, the villi, which extend across the intervillous space to the trophoblastic shell, develop numerous lateral branches whose

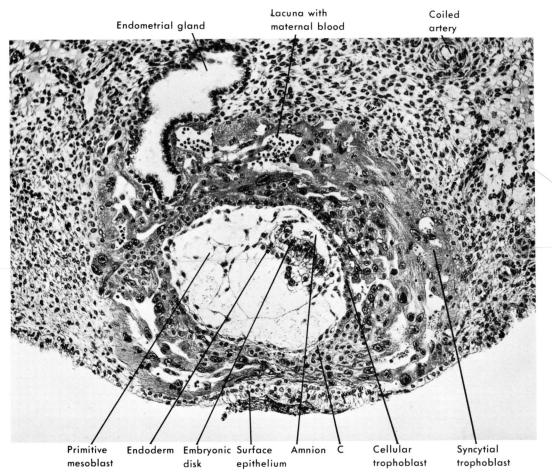

Figure 32–39. Photomicrograph from the same section as Figure 32–37, magnified 160 diameters. The bulk of the ovum consists of masses of trophoblast (syncytium) invading the endometrium. Within the syncytial trophoblast is the cellular trophoblast with obvious cell boundaries. The cells are arranged as a simple epithelium except for the clump at C. The cellular trophoblast immediately surrounds the primitive chorionic mesoblast in which the embryo is suspended. (After Hertig and Rock, 1941. Courtesy of the Carnegie Institution of Washington.)

unattached tips float free in the blood of the intervillous space.

The villi that arise from the chorionic plate are usually called *stem villi;* those branches that attach to the basal plate are *anchoring villi* (Figs. 32–44, 32–45); and those that end free in the intervillous space are the *terminal villi* (Fig. 32–46). The stem villi undergo extensive branching—as many as 15 generations of branches have been described. The terminal villi are very slender and no doubt easily moved by movement of blood in the intervillous space. They present a very large surface area for diffusion of nutrients and metabolites between the maternal and fetal circulations. The villous surface of the mature human placenta is estimated to be about 10 sq m. This is further amplified by the numerous microvilli on the syncytiotropho-

blast, bringing the total surface area to about 90 sq m—another remarkable example of the strategem of increasing efficiency by amplification of the area of physiologically important membranes.

The villi of the early placenta have capillaries with continuous unfenestrated endothelium in a stroma of loose mesenchyme. Scattered in the interstices of this stellate reticulum are large, globular *Hofbauer cells* filled with clear vacuoles. Their function remains obscure but they are believed to be macrophages whose vacuolated appearance early in pregnancy is due to uptake of extracellular fluid by pinocytosis. As pregnancy progresses, they lose much of their vacuolation and take on an appearance more typical of tissue macrophages.

The core of the villus is enclosed by two

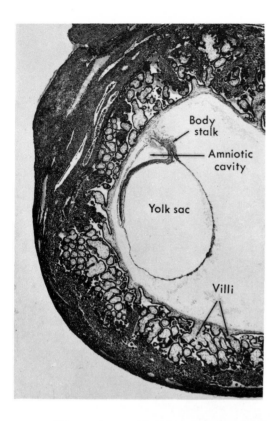

Figure 32–40. Human embryo of ovulation age 18 to 19 days. The curved embryonic disc lies between a large yolk sac and a smaller crescentic amniotic cavity. The body stalk bends back and blends with the chorionic mesoblast. Many secondary villi project into an extensive intervillous space. ×15. (Courtesy of A. T. Hertig.)

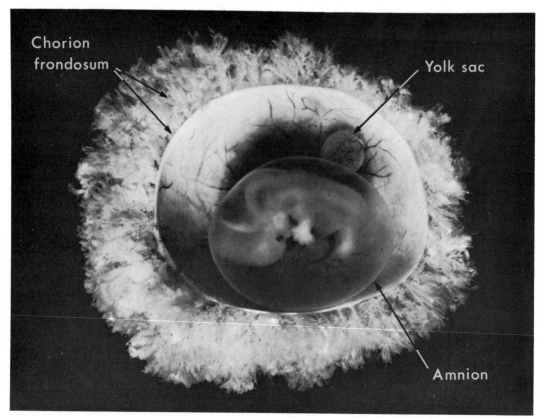

Figure 32–41. Photograph of a 40-day-old human embryo (Carnegie No. 8537), showing placental villi projecting from the entire surface of the chorion. (McKay, D. G., C. C. Roby, A. T. Hertig and M. V. Richardson. Am. J. Obstet. Gynecol. 69:735, 1955. Courtesy of the Carnegie Institution of Washington.)

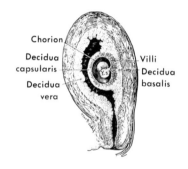

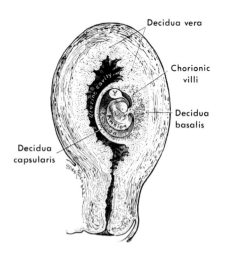

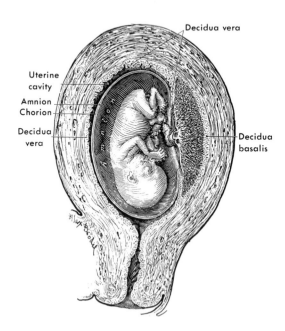

Figure 32–42. Drawings of successive stages of human pregnancy, showing the gradual obliteration of the uterine lumen, the disappearance of the decidua capsularis, and the establishment of the definitive discoid placenta. (Drawings by Brödel, M., from Williams, J. Am. J. Obstet. Gynecol. *13*:1, 1927.)

layers of trophoblast—the inner *cytotrophoblast* and the outer *syncytial trophoblast,* directly exposed to the maternal blood. The cytotrophoblastic cells have a euchromatic nucleus and a relatively pale-staining cytoplasm poor in cell organelles. They function mainly as stem cells for the overlying syncytium. Early in pregnancy they divide frequently, transform, and fuse with the expanding syncytium. Their number therefore decreases, and from the fifth month onward they are relatively few and no longer form a continuous inner layer. The thickness of the syncytium gradually comes to vary, thick areas containing clusters of nuclei alternating with thin areas devoid of nuclei. In these thin areas, dilated capillaries of the villus core are closely applied to the inner aspect of the attenuated syncytium so that the diffusion barrier between the bloodstreams is little more than 2 μm—a relationship reminiscent of the thin blood-air diffusion barrier in the lung.

In contrast to the relatively undifferentiated cytotrophoblast, the syncytial trophoblast is highly specialized for its multiple functions associated with the uptake of nutrients and synthesis, and secretion of both steroid and protein placental hormones. The free surface is irregular in contour and provided with abundant microvilli. Between the bases of the microvilli are numerous coated pits and coated vesicles involved in receptor-mediated endocytosis of macromolecules. The cytoplasm is strongly basophilic, and in electron micrographs has an extensive development of rough endoplasmic reticulum and abundant free polyribosomes. Multiple Golgi complexes are distributed at intervals in the syncytium. The numerous long mitochondria have foliate and tubular cristae. The ultrastructural appearance of the syncytium is predominantly that of cells actively synthesizing protein for export. The smooth endoplasmic reticulum that is the most conspicuous organelle in other steroid-secreting endocrine glands is not evident in the syncytium, and one must assume that enzymes of this biosynthetic pathway are incorporated in the membrane of the rough endoplasmic reticulum. The presence of numerous cholesterol-rich lipid inclusions is consistent with steroid synthesis, as are mitochondria with tubular cristae.

The products of conception occupy only a portion of the entire endometrium of pregnancy *(decidua).* Different regions are identified by separate terms descriptive of their topographical relation to the implantation

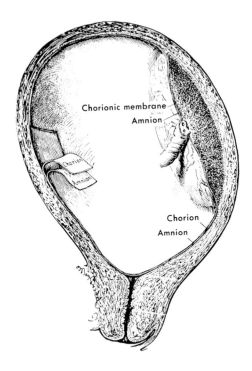

Figure 32–43. Drawing of the disposition of the fetal membranes in the later months of pregnancy. The amnion and chorion have come into contact and have become adherent to each other and to the decidua vera. (Drawings by Brödel, M., from Williams, J. Am. J. Obstet. Gynecol. *13*:1, 1927.)

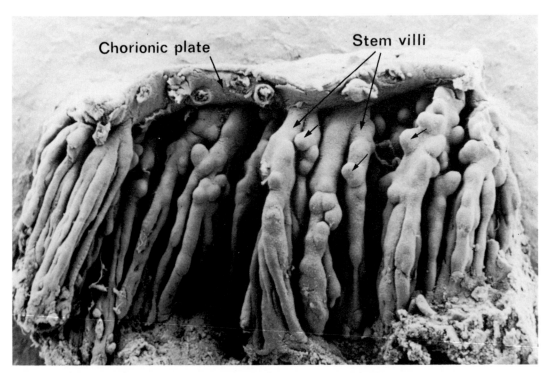

Figure 32–44. Scanning micrograph of a portion of the placental disc of a macaque at 22 days' gestation. Side branches from the stem villi are just beginning to appear *(small arrows)*. (Micrograph from King, B. Anat. Embryol. *165*:361, 1982.)

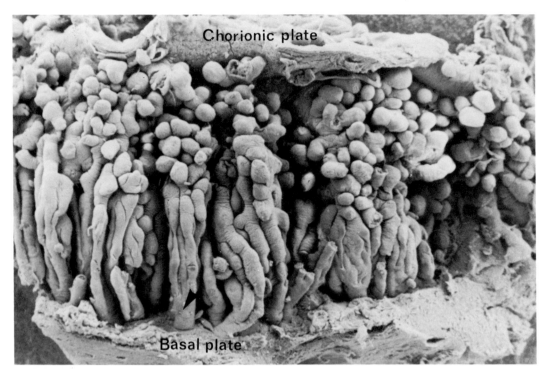

Figure 32–45. Scanning micrograph of a portion of the placental disc of a macaque at 31 days' gestation. Free villous side branches have continued to develop near the chorionic plate. Longitudinally branched central villi and cell columns appear to reunite before merging with the basal plate *(at arrowhead)*. (Micrograph from King, B. Anat. Embryol. *165*:361, 1982.)

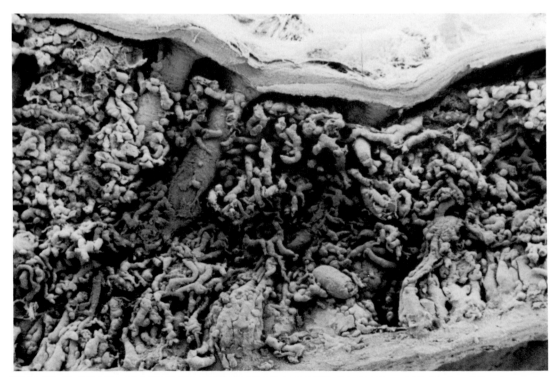

Figure 32–46. Scanning micrograph of a segment of the placental disc of a macaque at 60 days' gestation. Large-stem villi can be seen at upper left emerging from the chorionic plate. The greater part of the placenta is now made up of long, slender, branching terminal villi. (Micrograph from King, B. Anat. Embryol. *165*:361, 1982.)

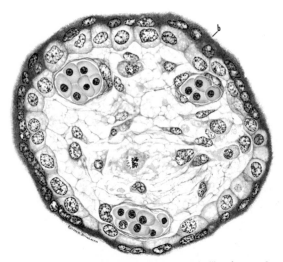

Figure 32–47. Section through placental villus from a 2-cm human embryo. The brush border *(b)* on the syncytial trophoblast is barely visible. Beneath it is the continuous layer of cellular trophoblast. The vessels in the mesenchyme are filled with primitive erythrocytes. One mesenchymal cell is in mitosis. × 450.

site. The portion that underlies the implantation site and forms the maternal component of the placenta is the *decidua basalis.* The thin superficial portion between the implantation site and the lumen is the *decidua capsularis,* and that lining the remainder of the uterus down to the internal os is the *decidua vera* (Figs. 32–42, 32–43).

Up to about the eighth week, the villi are equally numerous around the entire surface of the chorion (Fig. 32–41), but as pregnancy advances the villi adjacent to the decidua basalis enlarge and rapidly increase in number, while those facing the decidua capsularis degenerate, leaving this surface of the chorion smooth and relatively avascular after the third month. This region is thenceforth called the *chorion laeve,* while the villous portion toward the base is called the *chorion frondosum.* This latter becomes confined to a circular area that goes on to form the definitive discoid placenta.

As the volume of the conceptus increases and it bulges further into the lumen, the decidua capsularis becomes greatly attenuated. Its vascularity is jeopardized, and it degenerates. By four and a half months, the decidua capsularis has disappeared and the chorion laeve has fused with the decidua vera of the opposite wall, largely obliterating the uterine lumen (Fig. 32–43). The later development of the placenta involves a steady growth in size and length of the villi of the chorion frondosum and a concomitant expansion of the intervillous space. During the fourth and fifth months the placental disc is partitioned into 15 to 20 *cotyledons* by the formation of incomplete septa that project from the decidual plate into the intervillous space. There are also changes during this period in the histological organization of the villi.

Placental Circulation

Blood poor in oxygen is carried from the fetus to the placenta in the *umbilical arteries* of the umbilical cord. At the junction of the cord with the placenta, the umbilical arteries divide into a number of radially disposed placental arteries that branch freely in the chorionic plate. Numerous branches from these pass downward into the stem villi and ramify in the arborescent pattern of subsidiary villi down to the capillary networks of the terminal villi. The oxygen-rich venous blood is collected into thin-walled veins, which return the blood through vessels of increasing caliber that follow the course of the arteries to the chorionic plate. There they join veins that converge upon the single *umbilical vein,* which carries the blood through the umbilical cord to the ductus venosus, whence it enters the inferior vena cava near its point of confluence with the right atrium.

On the maternal side, blood from the arcuate branches of the uterine arteries is carried by the coiled arteries through openings in the basal plate of the placenta into the intervillous space. The flow from the maternal arterioles is pulsatile and is delivered at a pressure considerably higher than that prevailing in the intervillous space. It therefore spurts from the basal plate deep into the intervillous space in jets (Fig. 32–48). As its pressure is dissipated, it flows back around and over the surface of the placental villi, permitting exchange of metabolites with the fetal blood. Since the human has a *hemochorial placenta,* the trophoblast of the villi is exposed directly to maternal blood, and the diffusion barrier in the mature placenta consists only of the thin layer of syncytiotrophoblast, its basal lamina, and the wall of the subjacent fetal capillaries.

The pressure of the incoming blood and its fountain-like distribution tend to force the blood back toward the basal plate, where it is drained away through numerous communications between the intervillous space and dilated veins in the decidua basalis.

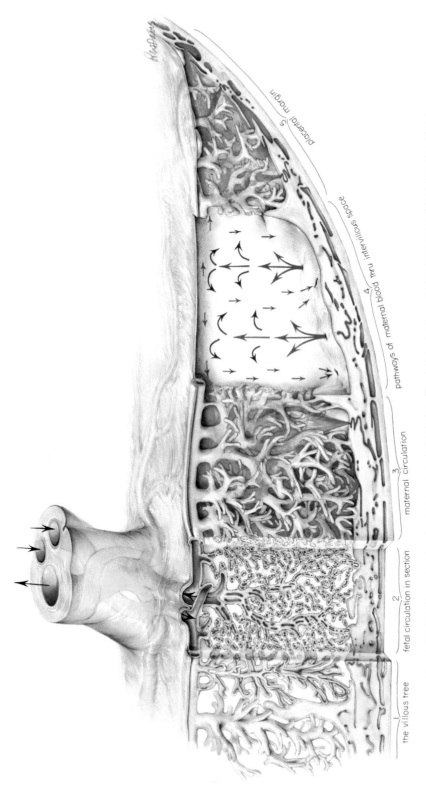

Figure 32-48. Placenta, showing structure and circulation. The head of maternal blood pressure drives entering blood toward the chorionic plate in fountain-like spurts. As the head of pressure is dissipated, lateral dispersion of blood occurs. Inflowing arterial blood pushes venous blood out into the endometrial veins. (After Ramsey, E. M., and J. W. Harris. Contributions to Embryology, No. 261, Vol. 38, 1966. Courtesy of the Carnegie Institution of Washington. Drawing by Ranice Davis Crosby.)

Histophysiology of the Placenta

The placenta is a transient organ consisting of both maternal and fetal components so structured as to bring fetal and maternal blood into close proximity to permit exchange of gaseous metabolites, nutrients, and waste products. In the early months of pregnancy it also has an important storage function, accumulating carbohydrate in the form of glycogen that can later be released as glucose. Similarly, proteins, calcium, and iron are stored for use later in pregnancy. Thus, for the fetus the placenta has some of the same functions as the lung, intestine, liver, and kidney in postnatal life.

In addition, the placenta is a major endocrine gland delivering directly into the maternal blood hormones that are essential for the continuance of pregnancy. The hormone *chorionic gonadotropin* is first secreted by the trophoblast when the blastocyst is implanting six to eight days after fertilization, and increases rapidly thereafter, declining to low levels by the fifth month. This glycoprotein hormone is very similar to luteinizing hormone in chemical structure and function. It prevents the involution of the corpus luteum of ovulation that would otherwise occur, and stimulates the corpus luteum of pregnancy to grow and secrete more progesterone.

The placenta also secretes the steroid hormones *estrogens* and *progesterone* in the latter half of pregnancy at a rate hundreds of times that of a normal cycle. The estrogen produced is predominantly *estriol*, which has relatively low estrogenic potency. Nevertheless, the total estrogenic activity of that produced is some 30 times normal. These high levels of estrogen contribute to growth of the uterus and to gestational development of the mammary glands.

The tenfold increase in the rate of progesterone secretion in the course of pregnancy stimulates differentiation and proliferation of decidual cells in the endometrium of the gravid uterus, and contributes to development of the mammary glands.

Another placental hormone was initially called *placental lactogen* because in some species it had an effect on the mammary glands similar to that of prolactin. An effect on lactation has not been demonstrated in the human and it is now commonly called *somatomammotropin*. Its chemical structure resembles that of the growth hormone somatotropin, and it has some growth-promoting action. More significant is its action upon the carbohydrate and fat metabolism of the mother, which makes more glucose available for nutrition of the fetus. The bulk of available evidence indicates that all the placental hormones are products of the syncytial trophoblast. The messenger RNA for somatomammotropin has recently been localized in the syncytium by *in situ* hybridization.

The syncytiotrophoblast is unique among absorptive epithelia in that substances cannot traverse it by a paracellular route. Owing to its syncytial nature all substances, from ions to macromolecules, entering or leaving the fetal blood must pass through it. Oxygen, carbon dioxide, fatty acids, steroids, lipid-soluble vitamins, and electrolytes can traverse it by *passive diffusion*. Sugars cross the syncytium more rapidly than expected on the basis of passive diffusion, and it is likely that a carrier molecule is involved in their *facilitated diffusion*. The fetus synthesizes its own proteins from amino acids that cross the placenta by *active transport*. Polypeptides and larger protein molecules are transported across the syncytium by coated vesicles formed by *receptor-mediated endocytosis*. The syncytium has receptors for insulin, transferrin, the Fc portion of immunoglobulin, and probably for certain other macromolecules. The vesicular transport of IgG is, in part, the basis for the passive immunization of the baby against certain pathogens.

VAGINA

The vagina is a distensible muscular tube extending from the vestibule of the female external genitalia to the cervix of the uterus. The lower end of the vagina in the virgin is marked by a transverse semicircular fold or fenestrated membrane, the *hymen*. The wall of the vagina consists of three layers: the mucosa, the muscular coat, and the adventitial connective tissue.

The adventitial coat is a thin layer of dense connective tissue, which merges into the loose connective tissue joining the vagina to the surrounding structures. In this connective tissue can be found an extensive venous plexus, nerve bundles, and small groups of nerve cells.

The interlacing smooth muscle bundles of the muscular layer are arranged circularly and longitudinally. The longitudinal bundles are far more numerous, especially in the outer half of the layer. Striated fibers of the

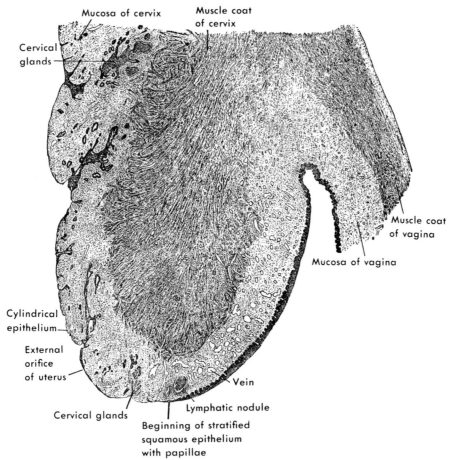

Figure 32–49. Sagittal section through posterior half of the portio vaginalis uteri and the fornix vaginae of a young woman. ×10. (After von Ebner.)

bulbocavernous muscles form a kind of sphincter around the ostium of the vagina.

The mucosa consists of a surface epithelium and an underlying lamina propria. The epithelium is a typical stratified squamous epithelium 150 to 200 μm in thickness, consisting of about 45 layers of cells during the follicular phase of the cycle and about 30 in the luteal phase. The superficial cells may contain keratohyaline granules, but they retain stainable nuclei and undergo little keratinization. Their cytoplasm is filled with glycogen, especially at midcycle. In electron micrographs the cells are joined by numerous desmosomes and occasional gap junctions. The latter are most numerous in the deeper layers, and diminish toward the surface. Tight junctions of limited extent and lamellar intercellular deposits of a lipid material have also been described near the free surface. These apparently constitute a permeability barrier for large water-soluble molecules. Electron-opaque tracers readily

infiltrate the intercellular spaces from the base of the epithelium but do not penetrate the intercellular clefts of the superficial layers.

The vagina is devoid of glands, and much of the lubricating fluid is contributed by secretion from glands of the cervix. It is generally agreed, however, that there is a true vaginal fluid that increases in abundance during sexual stimulation. This is believed to arise as a transudate from capillaries of the lamina propria and to move through intercellular channels of the epithelium to the lumen. The discrepancy between this interpretation and the demonstration of a permeability barrier to electron-opaque tracers has yet to be resolved.

The intercellular spaces of the epithelium are accessible to mononuclear leukocytes. Lymphocytes normally breach the basal lamina, open the desmosomes, and invade the enlarged intercellular channels so formed. It has recently been shown that, like the epidermis, the vaginal epithelium includes a population of Langerhans cells, which appear as scattered clear cells occupying expanded intercellular channels in its basal and intermediate layers. In the epidermis the Langerhans cells are known to participate in antigen presentation and cooperate with T lymphocytes in immunological surveillance. They no doubt play a similar role in the vagina.

Superficial cells are continually shed from the surface of the vaginal epithelium throughout the cycle, but this desquamation is greater late in the luteal phase and during menstruation. Glycogen from the exfoliated cells is a rich substrate for certain members of the bacterial flora, which break it down to lactic acid, lowering the pH of the vagina. Since the amount of glycogen in the epithelium is controlled by estrogen, the pH of the vaginal fluid is lowest at midcycle. With less estrogen being secreted in the luteal phase of the cycle, less glycogen is formed and the

pH of the vagina rises, favoring growth of the protozoan parasite *Trichomonas vaginalis*. Thus, estrogen can be administered as an adjunct to antimicrobial therapy for this and other vaginal infections.

The lamina propria is a moderately dense connective tissue. Toward the muscular layer it becomes looser, and this layer may be considered a submucosa. In the anterior wall of the vagina, papillae associated with the deep surface of the epithelium are few and small, but in the posterior wall the lamina propria sends numerous papillae far into the covering epithelium. Immediately under the epithelium there is a dense network of fine elastic fibers. From there, fine fibers run downward to the muscular layer. Accumulations of lymphocytes are numerous, and sometimes lymph nodules are present. Lymphocytes are always found migrating into the epithelium. The deeper layers of the lamina propria contain a dense plexus of small veins.

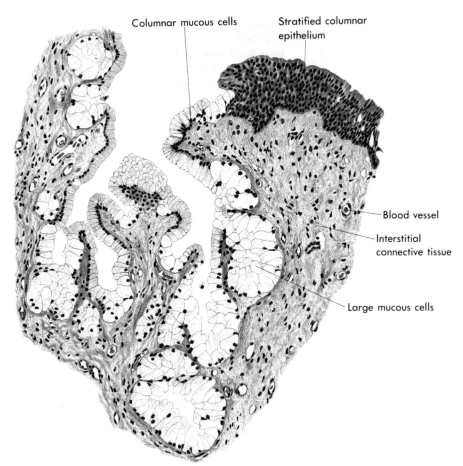

Columnar mucous cells

Stratified columnar epithelium

Blood vessel

Interstitial connective tissue

Large mucous cells

Figure 32–50. Section of gland of Bartholin. A large duct with patches of stratified columnar epithelium gives off smaller branches lined with columnar mucous cells and continuing into tubuloalveolar terminal portions, which are lined with large mucous cells. ×185. (After A. A. Maximow.)

EXTERNAL GENITALIA

The external genital organs of the female comprise the *clitoris*, the *labia majora* and *minora*, and certain glands that open into the *vestibule*, the space flanked by the labia minora.

The *clitoris* corresponds embryologically to the dorsal part of the penis. It consists of two small, erectile, corpora cavernosa ending in a rudimentary *glans clitoridis*. The vagina and the urethra open into the vestibule, which is lined with stratified squamous epithelium. Around the opening of the urethra and on the clitoris are several small *vestibular glands (glandulae vestibulares minores)*. They resemble the glands of Littré in the male urethra and contain mucous cells.

Two larger glands, the *glands of Bartholin (glandulae vestibulares majores)*, each about 1 cm in diameter, are located in the lateral walls of the vestibule and open on the inner surface of the labia minora. They are of the tubuloalveolar type, closely corresponding structurally to the bulbourethral glands of the male and secreting a similar lubricating mucus (Fig. 32–50).

The *labia minora* are covered with stratified squamous epithelium and have a core of spongy connective tissue permeated by fine elastic networks. Blood vessels are very numerous. The epithelium contains pigment in its deeper layer and has a thin keratinized layer on the surface. Numerous large sebaceous glands are found on both surfaces. There are no associated hairs.

The *labia majora* are folds of skin containing a large amount of subcutaneous adipose tissue and a thin layer of smooth muscle, corresponding to the tunica dartos of the scrotum. The outer surface is covered with hair; the inner is smooth and hairless. Sebaceous and sweat glands are numerous on both surfaces.

The outer genital organs are richly supplied with sensory nerve endings. Meissner corpuscles are scattered in the papillae of the epithelium, and genital corpuscles are present in the subpapillary layer. Pacinian corpuscles have been found in the deeper parts of the connective tissue of the labia majora and in the cavernous bodies of the clitoris.

REFERENCES

GENERAL

Austin, C. R.: The Mammalian Egg. Oxford, Blackwell Scientific Publications, 1961.

Blandau, R. J.: Biology of Eggs and Implantation. *In* Young, W. C. ed.: Sex and Internal Secretions. Vol. 2. 3rd ed. Baltimore, Williams & Wilkins Co., 1955.

Blandau, R. J., and K. Moghissi: The Biology of the Cervix. Chicago, University of Chicago Press, 1973.

Finn, C. A., and D. G. Porter: The Uterus. Handbooks of Reproductive Biology. London, Paul Elek Ltd., 1974.

Hafez, E. S. E., and R. J. Blandau: The Mammalian Oviduct. Chicago, University of Chicago Press, 1969.

Reid, L. N., ed.: Neuroendocrine Aspects of Reproduction. ORPRC Symposia on Primate Reproductive Biology. New York, Academic Press, 1983.

Yen, S. S. C., and R. B. Jaffe: Reproductive Endocrinology: Physiology, Pathophysiology and Clinical Management. 2nd ed. Philadelphia, W. B. Saunders Co., 1986.

OVARY

Anderson, E., and H. W. Beams: Cytological observations on the fine structure of the guinea pig ovary with special reference to the oogonium, primary oocyte and associated follicle cells. J. Ultrastruct. Res. *3*:432, 1960.

Baker, T. G., and L. L. Franchi: The fine structure of oogonia and oocytes in human ovary. J. Cell Sci. *2*:213, 1967.

Corner, G. W., Jr.: The histological dating of the human corpus luteum of menstruation. Am. J. Anat. *98*:337, 1956.

Crisp, T. M., and C. Channing: Fine structural events correlated with progestin secretion during luteinization of rhesus monkey granulosa cells in culture. Biol. Reprod. 7:55, 1972.

Crisp, T. M., D. A. Dessouky, and F. R. Denys: The fine structure of the human corpus luteum of early pregnancy and during the progestational phase of the menstrual cycle. Am. J. Anat. *127*:37, 1970.

Gillim, S. W., A. K. Christensen, and C. E. McLennan: Fine structure of human granulosa and theca lutein cells at the stage of maximum progesterone secretion during the menstrual cycle. Anat. Rec. *163*:189, 1969.

Greep, R. O.: Histology, histochemistry and ultrastructure of adult ovary. *In* Smith, D. E., ed.: The Ovary. Baltimore, Williams & Wilkins Co., 1962.

Hertig, A. T.: The primary human oocyte: some observations on the fine structure of Balbiani's vitelline body and the origin of the annulate lamellae. Am. J. Anat. *122*:107, 1968.

Hertig, A. T., and E. C. Adams: Studies on the human oocyte and its follicle. 1. Ultrastructural and histochemical observations on the primordial follicle stage. J. Cell Biol. *34*:647, 1957.

Long, J. A.: Corpus luteum of pregnancy in the rat—ultrastructural and cytochemical observations. Biol. Reprod. 8:87, 1973.

Mossman, M. H., M. J. Koering, and D. Ferry, Jr.: Cyclic changes of interstitial gland tissue of the human ovary. Am. J. Anat. *115*:235, 1964.

Ryan, K. J., and R. V. Short: Formation of estradiol by granulosa and theca cells of the equine ovarian follicle. Endocrinology 76:108, 1965.

Strassman, E. O.: The theca cone and its tropism toward the ovarian surface, a typical feature of growing human mammalian follicles. Am. J. Obstet. Gynecol. *41*:363, 1941.

OVULATION

Blandau, R. J.: Ovulation in the living albino rat. Fertil. Steril. 6:391, 1955.

Decker, A.: Culdoscopic observations on the tubo-ovarian mechanism of ovum reception. Fertil. Steril. 2:253, 1951.

Doyle, J. B.: Exploratory culdotomy for observation of tubo-ovarian physiology at ovulation time. Fertil. Steril. 2:474, 1951.

OVIDUCT

Brenner, R. M.: Electron microscopy of estrogen effects on ciliogenesis and secretory cell growth in rhesus monkey oviduct. Anat. Rec. 157:218, 1967.

Brenner, R. M.: The biology of oviductal cilia. In Hafez, E. S. E., and R. J. Blandau, eds.: The Mammalian Oviduct. Chicago, University of Chicago Press, 1969.

UTERUS

Bartelmez, G. W.: Histological studies on the menstruating mucous membrane of the human uterus. Carnegie Inst. Contrib. Embryol. 24:141, 1933.

Markee, J. E.: Menstruation in intraocular endometrial transplants in the Rhesus monkey. Carnegie Contrib. Embryol. 28:219, 1940.

Markee, J. E.: The morphological and endocrine basis for menstrual bleeding. Progr. Gynecol. 2:63, 1950.

Schmidt-Matthiesen, H.: The Normal Human Endometrium. New York, McGraw-Hill Book Co., 1963.

CERVIX

Blandau, R. J., and K. Moghissi: The Biology of the Cervix. Chicago, University of Chicago Press, 1973.

Danforth, D. N.: The fibrous nature of the human cervix, and its relations to the isthmic segment in gravid and non-gravid uteri. Am. J. Obstet. Gynecol. 53:541, 1947.

Flukman, C. F.: The glandular structures of the cervix uteri. Surg. Gynecol. Obstet. 106:515, 1958.

Moghissi, K. S.: The function of the cervix in fertility. Fertil. Steril. 23:295, 1972.

Vickery, B. H., and J. P. Bennett: The cervix and its secretions in mammals. Physiol. Rev. 48:135, 1968.

IMPLANTATION AND PLACENTA

Amoroso, E. C.: Placentation. In Parker, A. S., ed.: Marshall's Physiology of Reproduction. Vol. 2. 3rd ed. London, Longmans, Green & Co. Ltd., 1952.

Amoroso, E. C.: Histology of the placenta. Br. Med. Bull. 17:81, 1961.

Austin, C. R.: The Mammalian Egg. Oxford, Blackwell Scientific Publications, 1961.

Baker, T. G.: A quantitative and cytological study of oogenesis in the rhesus monkey. J. Anat. 100:761, 1966.

Dancis, J., W. L. Money, S. Springer, and M. Levitz: Transport of amino acids by placenta. Am. J. Obstet. Gynecol. 101:820, 1968.

Enders, A. C.: Formation of syncytium from cytotrophoblast in the human placenta. Obstet. Gynecol. 25:378, 1965.

Enders, A. C.: Fine structure of anchoring villi of the human placenta. Am. J. Anat. 122:419, 1968.

Enders, A. C., and A. G. Hendrickx: Morphological basis of implantation in the rhesus monkey. In Hubinont, P. O., C. A. Finn, A. Psychoyos, and F. Leroy, eds.: Blastocyst Endometrium Relationship. Basel, S. Karger, 1980.

Enders, A. C., and B. F. King: The cytology of Hofbauer cells. Anat. Rec. 167:231, 1970.

Hamilton, W. J., and J. D. Boyd: Development of the human placenta in the first three months of gestation. J. Anat. 94:297, 1960.

Hertig, A. T.: Gestational hyperplasia of the endometrium. Lab. Invest. 13:1153, 1964.

Hertig, A. T., and J. Rock: Two human ova of the previllous stage, having an ovulation age of about eleven and twelve days respectively. Carnegie Contrib. Embryol. 29:127, 1941.

Hertig, A. T., and J. Rock: Two human ova of the previllous stage, having a development age of about seven and nine days respectively. Carnegie Contrib. Embryol. 31:67, 1954.

Hertig, A. T., J. Rock, E. C. Adams, and W. J. Mulligan: On the preimplantation stages of the human ovum; a description of four normal and four abnormal specimens ranging from the second to the fifth day of development. Carnegie Contrib. Embryol. 35:199, 1954.

Johnson, L. W., and C. H. Smith: Monosaccharide transport across microvillous membrane of human placenta. Am. J. Physiol. 238 (Cell Physiol. 7):C160, 1980.

Kaufman, P., D. K. Sen, and G. Schweikhart: Classification of human placental villi. I. Histology. Cell Tissue Res. 200:409, 1979.

King, B. F.: Localization of transferrin on the surface of the human placenta by electron microscopic immunocytochemistry. Anat. Rec. 186:151, 1976.

Metcalfe, J., H. Barters, and W. Moll: Gas exchange in the pregnant uterus. Physiol. Rev. 47:782, 1967.

Nelson, M. D., A. C. Enders, and B. F. King: Cytological events involved in glycoprotein synthesis in cellular and syncytial trophoblast of human placenta. An electron microscope autoradiographic study of (³H)galactose incorporation. J. Cell Biol. 76:418, 1978.

Nelson, D. M., A. C. Enders, and B. F. King: Cytological events involved in protein synthesis in cellular and syncytial trophoblast of human placenta. An electron microscope autoradiographic study of (³H)leucine incorporation. J. Cell Biol. 76:400, 1978.

Okleford, C. D., and J. M. Clint: The uptake of IgG by human placental chorionic villi: a correlated autoradiographic and wide aperture counting. Placenta 1:91, 1980.

Schneider, H., K. H. Mohlen, and J. Dancis: Transfer of amino acids across in vitro perfused human placenta. Pediatr. Res. 13:236, 1979.

Wislocki, G. B., and H. S. Bennett: The histology and cytology of the human and monkey placenta, with special reference to the trophoblast. Am. J. Anat. 73:335, 1943.

VAGINA

Averette, H. E., G. D. Weinstein, and P. Frost: Autoradiographic analysis of cell proliferation kinetics in human genital tissues I. Normal cervix and vagina. Am. J. Obstet. Gynecol. 108:8, 1970.

Burgos, M. H., and C. E. Roig de Vargas-Linares: Cell junctions in the human vaginal epithelium. Am. J. Obstet. Gynecol. 108:565, 1970.

Burgos, M. H., and C. E. Roig de Varga-Linares: Ultrastructure of the vaginal mucosa. In Hafez, E. S. E., and T. N. Evans, eds.: Human Vagina. Amsterdam, Elsevier/North Holland Biomedical Press, 1978.

King, B. F.: Ultrastructure of the non-human primate vaginal mucosa: epithelial changes during the menstrual cycle and pregnancy. J. Ultrastruct. Res. 82:1, 1983.

King, B. F.: The permeability of non-human primate vaginal epithelium: a freeze-fracture and tracer perfusion study J. Ultrastruct. Res. 83:99, 1983.

Roig de Vargas-Linares, C. E., and M. H. Burgos: Migration of lymphocytes in the normal human vagina. Am. J. Obstet. Gynecol. 102:1094, 1968.

Roig de Vargas-Linares, C. E., and M. H. Burgos: Langerhans cells in the intercellular channels of normal human vagina. Microsc. Electron. Biol. Cell. 7:93, 1983.

33

MAMMARY GLAND

The mammary glands are specialized accessory glands of the skin that have evolved in mammals to provide for the nourishment of their offspring, which are born in a relatively immature and dependent state. They are paired glands that are laid down in the embryo along two lines called the *mammary lines*, extending from the axilla to the groin on either side of the midline on the ventral aspect of the thorax and abdomen. Mammary glands may arise anywhere along these lines. The number formed and their location vary with the species. In humans, only two normally develop, but additional accessory nipples or glandular masses are not uncommon.

In their structure and mode of development, mammary glands somewhat resemble sweat glands. Their differentiation during embryonic life is similar in the two sexes. In the male, however, little additional development occurs in postnatal life, whereas in the female the glands undergo extensive structural changes correlated with age and with the functional condition of the reproductive system. The greatest development of the female breast is reached in about the twentieth year, with atrophic changes setting in by the age of 40 and becoming marked after the menopause. In addition to these gradual changes, there are variations in the size of the breasts correlated with the menstrual cycle, and striking changes in the amount and functional activity of the glandular tissue during pregnancy and lactation.

Nipple and Areola

The nipple is surrounded by a circular pigmented area of skin called the *areola*. The base of the epidermis of the nipple and areola is invaded by unusually long dermal papillae, whose capillaries bring blood close to the surface, imparting a pinkish color to this region in immature and blonde individuals. The epidermis becomes pigmented at puberty, and the degree of pigmentation increases during pregnancy. An elaborate pattern of bundles of smooth muscle disposed longitudinally along the lactiferous ducts and circumferentially both within the nipple and around its base (Fig. 33–1) are responsible for the erection of the nipple in response to certain stimuli. At other times it is flat. In the areola are the accessory *areolar glands of Montgomery*, which are intermediate in their structure between sweat glands and true mammary glands. Along the margin of the areola are large sweat glands and sebaceous glands, which usually lack associated hairs.

The skin at the tip of the nipple is richly innervated with free nerve endings and Meissner's corpuscles in the dermal papillae. There are also superficial nerves and nerve end organs on the sides of the nipple and on the areola. The skin peripheral to the areola has neural plexuses around hair follicles, as well as nerve endings resembling Merkel's discs and Krause's end bulbs. Pacinian corpuscles may also be found deep in the dermis and in the glandular tissue. The sensory innervation of the nipple and areola are of great functional importance because their stimulation by the suckling infant initiates the train of neural and neurohumoral events that result in ejection of milk and maintenance of secretion of prolactin from the pituitary, which is essential for continued lactation.

Resting Mammary Gland

The mammary gland is a compound tubuloalveolar gland consisting of 15 to 25 irregular lobes radiating from the *mammary papilla*, or *nipple*. The lobes are separated by layers of dense connective tissue and surrounded by abundant adipose tissue. Each lobe is provided with a *lactiferous duct* 2 to 4.5 mm in diameter and lined by stratified squamous epithelium. Each duct opens on the nipple and has an irregular angular outline in cross section. Deep to the areola, each of the ducts

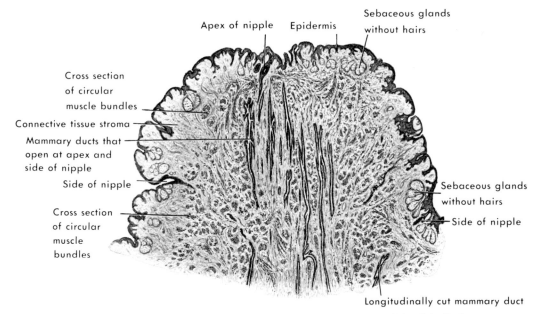

Figure 33–1. Nipple of female breast in perpendicular section. × 6. (After Schaffer.)

converging upon the nipple has a local dilatation, the *sinus lactiferus*. Distal to this the duct narrows again and emerges at the end of the nipple as a separate opening 0.4 to 0.7 mm in diameter.

Each lobe is subdivided into lobules of various orders. The smallest consist of elongated tubules, the *alveolar ducts*, covered by small saccular evaginations, the *alveoli*. The interlobular connective tissue is more dense than the intralobular connective tissue. The latter is more cellular and contains fewer collagenous fibers and almost no fat. This loose intralobular stroma surrounding the system of ducts is believed to permit greater distensibility when the epithelial portions of the organ hypertrophy during pregnancy and lactation. The secretory portions of the gland, the alveolar ducts and alveoli, consist of cuboidal or low columnar secretory cells resting on a basal lamina and underlying processes of *myoepithelial cells*. The highly branched myoepithelial cells enclose the glandular alveoli in an open-meshed, basket-like network. They usually lie between the secretory cells and the basal lamina. The presence of myoepithelial cells is further evidence that mammary glands are morphogenetically related to sweat glands.

There are differences of opinion as to whether alveoli are present in the nonlactating human breast. According to most descriptions of the inactive gland, its epithelial com-

ponent consists only of ducts and their branches. Other authors, however, insist that a few small alveoli are present at the ends of the duct system and form miniature lobules. The question remains unresolved, owing in part to the rarity of opportunities to obtain normal human breast tissue at known phases of the menstrual cycle. Certainly the total mass of the epithelial elements is greatly reduced early in the cycle. A lumen is not evident and the cells seem to form more or less solid cords. In this condition, it is not easy to distinguish alveoli from primary ducts. Late in the menstrual cycle, the epithelial cells become cuboidal or low columnar, a lumen is apparent, and the surrounding connective tissue is highly vascular. Since both alveolar ducts and alveoli are potentially secretory, it is not important to make this distinction in the nonlactating breast. It is sufficient to note that there are microscopically detectable cyclic changes in the epithelial portions of the mammary gland, but these are relatively slight. The more obvious changes in breast size, and the sense of engorgement experienced by some women in certain phases of the cycle, are attributable to increased blood flow and a slight associated edema of the connective tissues of the breast.

Unlike many other glands, the mammary gland does not have a single excurrent duct. Each lobe is an independent compound alveolar gland whose primary ducts join and rejoin to form larger ducts that converge upon a single lactiferous duct, and lactiferous ducts of the several lobes open separately at the tip of the nipple. Thus, the mammary gland is a conglomerate made up of a variable number of independent units.

The myoepithelial cells are stellate in form, with long branching processes that occupy recesses in the bases of the glandular cells. The processes of neighboring myoepithelial cells join to form a cellular network that completely envelops the alveolus. These cells lie between the epithelial cells and the basal lamina. Their form and topographical relationships are seen to advantage in scanning electron micrographs of glands exposed during specimen preparation to collagenase to remove the basal lamina and associated reticular fibers (Figs. 33–2, 33–3).

The Active Mammary Glands

Pregnancy brings about changes in the levels of circulating hormones that result in profound changes in the mammary glands.

During the first half of gestation, there is a rapid growth and branching from the terminal portion of the duct system of the gland and a proliferation of alveoli. The growth of epithelial components of the gland takes place, at least in part, at the expense of the interstitial adipose tissue of the breast, which regresses concurrently with the growth of the glandular tissue. In this period of growth, there is also an increasing infiltration of the interstitial tissue with lymphocytes, plasma cells, and eosinophils. In the later months of pregnancy, the hyperplasia of the glandular tissue slows down, and the subsequent enlargement of the breasts is mostly a consequence of enlargement of the parenchymal cells and distention of the alveoli with a secretion rich in lactoproteins but relatively poor in lipid. This constitutes the *colostrum*, the first milk that comes from the breasts after birth. It has special laxative properties and contains antibodies that provide the newborn with some measure of passive immunity. During the first few days after delivery the degree of infiltration of the stroma of the

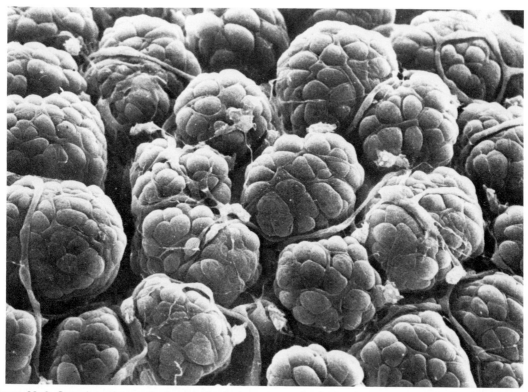

Figure 33–2. Scanning micrograph of acini of rodent mammary gland. The tissue was treated with enzymes during specimen preparation to digest away collagen fibrils, extracellular matrix, and basal lamina, thus exposing the bases of the epithelial and myoepithelial cells. (Micrograph from Nagato, T. Cell Tissue Res. *209*:1, 1980.)

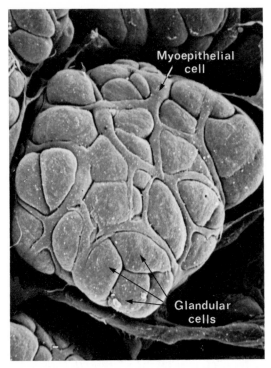

Figure 33–3. Scanning micrograph of an acinus of the mammary gland, clearly showing the branching myoepithelial cells occupying grooves between the bases of the secretory cells. Specimen prepared as described for Figure 33–2. (Micrograph from Nagato, T. Cell Tissue Res. *209*:1, 1980.)

gland by lymphoid elements becomes less intense, and the colostrum gives way to a copious secretion of milk rich in lipid.

The histological appearance of different parts of the active mammary gland varies considerably (Figs. 33–4, 33–5). Apparently, different areas are not all in the same functional state at the same time. In some places, the secretory portions are filled with milk; their lumen is wide and the walls are dilated and thin. In other areas, the lumen is narrow and the epithelium relatively thick.

The shape of the epithelial cells varies from flat to low columnar. The boundary between them is usually indistinct in histological sections. If the cells are tall, their distal ends are often separated and project into the lumen of the alveoli as rounded or dome-shaped protrusions. The nucleus may be round or oval and is at about the middle of the cell. If the cells are short, their free surface is usually more or less smooth.

In the cytoplasm are short, rod-shaped mitochondria, few in number in the flattened cells but more plentiful in the taller ones. The cells are generally acidophilic, but some basophilic substance may be found at the base of the cells. Droplets of lipid, often of large size, accumulate near the free surface and often project into the lumen (Fig. 33–6). After the extraction of fat in preparing histological sections, large clear vacuoles remain in place of the lipid droplets. In addition to the accumulations of lipid, small proteinaceous secretory granules can also be seen in the apical region of the cell. Cyclic changes in the Golgi apparatus during the different phases of secretion have been described. The lumen of the alveoli is filled with fine granules and lipid droplets similar to those that protrude from the cells (Figs. 33–6, 33–7).

The mammary gland was formerly believed to have a mode of release of its product that was intermediate between *merocrine* secretion, in which the secretory materials pass out through the cell apex without loss of cytoplasm, and *holocrine* secretion, in which the entire cell is given up in contributing its contents to the secretion. The cells of the mammary gland were believed to undergo a partial disintegration in which the lipid-filled apical portion of the cell, projecting into the lumen, was described as constricting from the base of the cell, which remained in place. It was believed that the remainder of the cell did not die but rapidly replaced the lost protoplasm and reaccumulated secretion. This mode of release was called *apocrine secretion*. Studies with the electron microscope have now radically changed our views as to the mechanisms of release of cell products, and the traditional concept of apocrine secretion is no longer applicable to the mammary gland.

In electron micrographs the main cytological features of the glandular cells are in accord with desriptions resulting from use of the light microscope. The chromophilic areas of the cytoplasm contain numerous cisternal profiles of the granular endoplasmic reticulum. There are a moderate number of mitochondria, a large supranuclear Golgi complex, and a few lysosomes. It is evident that the cell has two distinct secretory products, formed and released by different mechanisms. The protein constituents of the milk, like other protein secretions, are elaborated

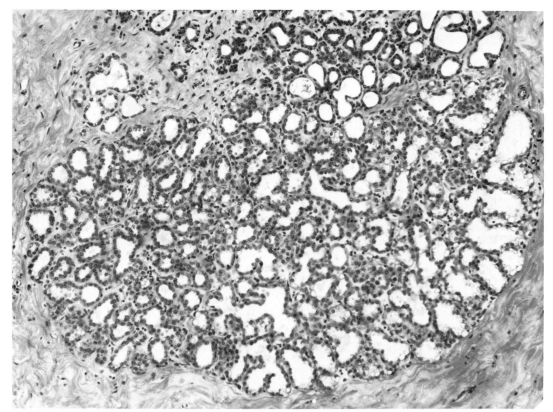

Figure 33–4. Photomicrograph of human mammary gland at eight months of pregnancy.

on the ribosome-studded membranes of the endoplasmic reticulum. They first become visible as multiple dense spherical granules about 400 nm in diameter in vesicles associated with the Golgi complex. They are transported to the cell surface in these membranous vesicles, which fuse with the plasmalemma and discharge their contents into the lumen of the acinus. The mode of formation and release of this particulate component of the milk is identical to that of other protein-secreting glands that are generally classified as *merocrine*.

The fatty components of the milk do not develop in association with the Golgi apparatus but arise as small lipid droplets free in the cytoplasmic matrix. These increase in size by fusion and move into the apical region, where they come to project into the lumen covered by the plasmalemma. These droplets are ultimately cast off, enveloped by a detached portion of the cell membrane (Fig. 33–8). This mode of release could be considered *apocrine* in the sense that it involves loss

of cell membrane and, in some instances, of a thin layer of cytoplasm, but the amount lost is certainly far less than envisioned by the classical cytologists who introduced the concept.

Lymphocytes are sometimes encountered among the alveolar epithelial cells. Between the epithelial cells and the basal lamina are occasional cells with pale cytoplasm rich in lipid droplets and vacuoles with highly heterogeneous granular and membranous contents. These have been interpreted by some as degenerating epithelial cells, but it seems more likely that they are macrophages.

The myoepithelial cells lie on the epithelial side of the basal lamina. Their processes are filled with parallel arrays of myofilaments 6 nm in diameter. There are spindle-shaped densities among the myofilaments like those found in smooth muscle cells. The cell organelles are concentrated in the perinuclear region of the cell body, but occasional mitochondria and profiles of the endoplasmic reticulum extend into the cell processes

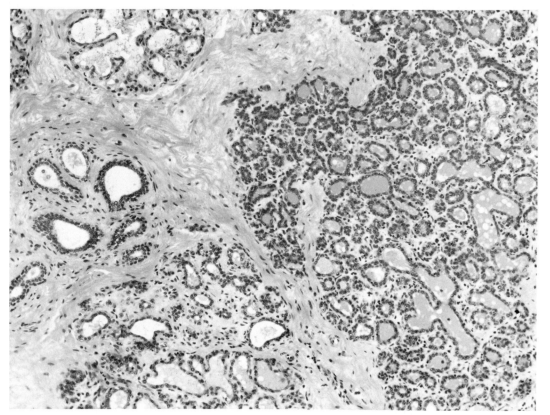

Figure 33–5. Photomicrograph of lactating human mammary gland. Notice the local variations within the gland. Alveoli in some areas have a large lumen and abundant secretion, whereas in other areas the lumen is very small.

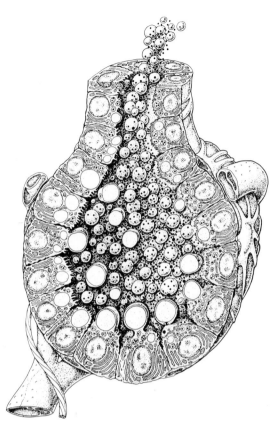

Figure 33–6. Drawing of rat mammary gland acinus, showing the relationships of the myoepithelial cells, the structure of the secretory cells, and the presence of small granules of casein and membrane-bounded lipid droplets in the lumen. (Drawing from Krstić, R. Die Gewebe des Menschen und der Säugetiere. Berlin, Springer-Verlag, 1978.)

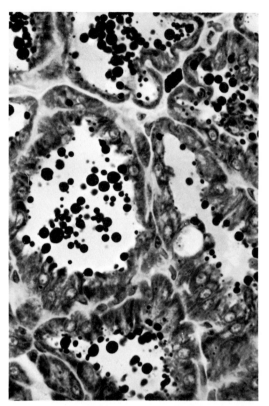

Figure 33–7. Photomicrograph of lactating mammary gland from a mouse, fixed in osmium tetroxide. The large droplets of lipid are preserved both in the apex of the cells and in the lumen of the acini. The smaller protein granules are not visible. × 560. (Preparation by N. Feder.)

Histophysiology of the Mammary Gland

The functioning of the mammary glands is dependent on multiple and complex neural and endocrine factors. Some are involved in the development of the glands to a functional state (*mammogenesis*), others in the establishment of milk secretion (*lactogenesis*), and still others are necessary for maintenance of lactation. Given a normal coordinated interplay of all the factors concerned, the average milk production of a mother breast-feeding a single infant is in excess of 1100 ml/24 hr for the first six months of lactation, and mothers breast-feeding twins may produce over 2100 ml/24 hr.

The duct system of the gland that develops in fetal life continues to grow after birth only in proportion to the growth of the body as a whole until puberty. Then, in the female, a more rapid extension of the duct system begins. This accelerated growth depends primarily on estrogen and progesterone from the ovaries, but also requires prolactin and somatotrophin from the pituitary.

In pregnancy the large quantities of estrogen secreted by the placenta stimulate further growth of the duct system. Increased levels of circulating progesterone from the corpus luteum of pregnancy acting together with hypophyseal and adrenal hormones induce development of alveoli and differentiation of their cells in preparation for lactogenesis. Secretion of prolactin by the pituitary steadily increases from the fifth week of pregnancy until full term, when it may reach levels ten times those of the nonpregnant state. Hypophyseal prolactin is the principal hormone stimulating milk production. Ad-

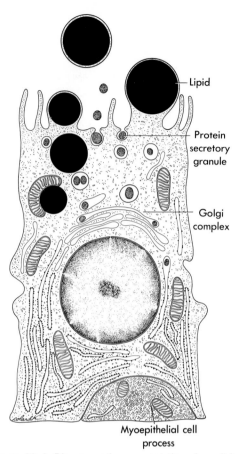

Figure 33–8. Diagrammatic representation of a cell from a lactating mammary gland, showing large lipid droplets being cast off enclosed in a layer of cytoplasm, and small granules of protein secretion being concentrated in the Golgi apparatus and released by coalescence of their small vesicles with the plasma membrane. A myoepithelial cell process is depicted in cross section between the epithelial cell and the basal lamina. (Drawing based on observations of Bargmann, W., and A. Knoop. Zeitschr. f. Zellforsch. *49*:344, 1959.)

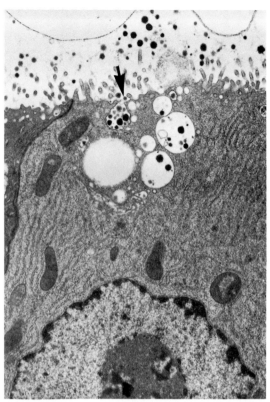

Figure 33–9. Electron micrograph of a mammary epithelial cell, showing several vacuoles containing granules of milk protein. One *(at arrow)* is in process of exocytosis. (Micrograph courtesy of A. Ichikawa.)

renal glucocorticoids and insulin also play a significant role in lactation. In the absence of insulin, the mRNA for synthesis of the milk protein casein fails to accumulate to normal levels in the mammary epithelium.

Although the mammary gland is fully developed late in pregnancy, very little milk is formed owing to inhibition of secretion by high levels of estrogen and progesterone. The small amount of fluid produced, called *colostrum*, is poor in lipid but rich in protein, and contains IgA. With the elimination of the placenta at birth, estrogen and progesterone levels in the mother fall dramatically. Without their inhibitory action on the mam-

mary glands, the high level of prolactin can exert its powerful lactogenic effect, and within a few days full lactation is established. Prolactin secretion by the pituitary falls to basal levels post partum, but each time the baby is breast-fed the stimulation of the nipples by suckling sends nervous impulses to the hypothalamus that are relayed to the hypophysis, resulting in a brief tenfold increase in release of prolactin. These frequently repeated surges of the hormone stimulating the cells of the mammary gland serve to maintain milk production. Frequent breast feeding is important to maintain lactogenesis. The tendency of mothers in developed countries to prolong the interval between feedings and to abandon nighttime feeding as soon as possible contributes to their poor lactational performance. In contrast, women of hunter-gatherer societies whose babies are always with them and feed on demand throughout the day and night are able to continue to

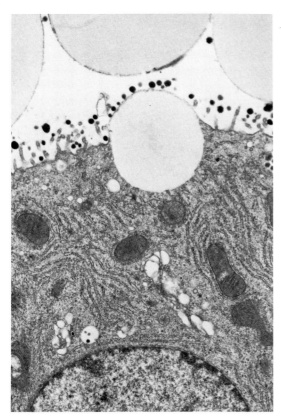

Figure 33–10. Micrograph of a mammary epithelial cell with a lipid droplet protruding into the lumen covered by a portion of the cell membrane. Secreted lipid droplets and granules of milk protein are visible in the lumen. (Micrograph courtesy of A. Ichikawa.)

breast-feed their babies for up to three and a half years.

In women breast-feeding their babies, there is usually a concurrent suppression of the menstrual cycle and ovulation—*lactational amenorrhea*. Its mechanism is not fully understood, but it is believed that neural inputs to the hypothalamus generated by suckling stimulate release of beta endorphin, which suppresses secretion of gonadotropin releasing hormone and results in diminished secretion of luteinizing hormone and failure of ovulation. Prolonged lactation is the only method of contraception practiced by the great majority of women in the developing countries.

The production of milk is a continuous process, but its delivery is episodic. The cells of the lactating mammary gland synthesize and release their product continuously into the lumen of the alveoli and alveolar ducts,

where it accumulates in the intervals between feedings. Flow of milk from the nipples requires participation of the baby. The stimulus of suckling generates afferent nerve impulses that ascend in the spinal cord to the hypothalamus. In addition to activating release of prolactin from the anterior pituitary, efferent impulses from the hypothalamus to the posterior lobe of the pituitary result in its secretion of the hormone *oxytocin*. Carried in the blood to the mammary gland, oxytocin stimulates contraction of the myoepithelial cells, resulting in ejection of milk from the alveoli into the ducts and the initiation of flow from the nipple.

The secretory cells of the mammary epithelium are unusual among glandular cells in that they produce multiple products using different biosynthetic pathways. The milk proteins are synthesized on ribosomes; segregated in the endoplasmic reticulum; and glycosylated, concentrated, and packaged in vesicles in the Golgi complex. Among the proteins produced is the enzyme *lactose synthetase*, which catalyzes the synthesis of the milk sugar *lactose* from glucose and UDP-galactose. The membrane of the Golgi vesicles is permeable to these precursor molecules but not to the product lactose, which accumulates and creates an osmotic gradient that draws water and monovalent ions into the vesicles. In other protein-secreting cells, large dense granules are formed and enclosed individually in a close-fitting membrane. In the mammary gland, multiple small granules of milk protein are sequestered in relatively large vesicles also containing lactose, water, and ions, which are extracted in specimen preparation. In micrographs, therefore, the secretion vesicles appear empty save for a few small protein granules (Fig. 33–9). Their contents are discharged into the lumen by exocytosis.

The lipid of the milk is not synthesized in a membrane-bounded organelle but appears as small droplets in the cytoplasmic matrix. These enlarge and coalesce into very large droplets that bulge into the lumen, covered only by the apical plasmalemma (Fig. 33–10). By a process of exocytosis that is unique and poorly understood, the cell membrane fuses behind the projecting droplets, which are thus cast off into the lumen invested in a detached portion of the plasmalemma.

The immunoglobulin of the milk follows a third transcellular path. It is synthesized by

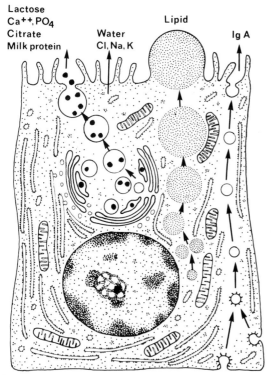

Lactose
Ca++, PO4
Citrate
Milk protein

Lipid

Water
Cl, Na, K

Ig A

Figure 33–11. Schematic representation of the transcellular pathways involved in milk secretion. Casein, lactate, calcium, and citrate are packaged in vacuoles arising in the Golgi complex and released by exocytosis. Water and ions diffuse freely through the cell membrane. Lipid droplets enclosed in detached portions of plasmalemma are released in a unique form of apocrine secretion. Immunoglobulin taken up at the basal and lateral surfaces by receptor-mediated endocytosis is transported in small vesicles across the cell and released into the lumen. (Redrawn and modified after Neville, M.C., et al. *In* Lactation: Physiology, Metabolism and Breast-feeding. New York, Plenum Press, 1983.)

plasma cells in the stroma of the mammary gland that were exposed to intestinal pathogens in the lamina propria of the mother's intestine and carried to the gland in the blood. There, IgA is taken up by receptor-mediated endocytosis at the basal and lateral surfaces of the glandular cells, transported in vesicles to the cell apex, and discharged into the lumen (Fig. 33–11). In the fourth and fifth months of lactation, a mother may be secreting in her milk as much as 0.5 g of antibody per day. The antibody in the lumen of the baby's gut combats enteric infections, a common cause of infant mortality. Early weaning and bottle feeding deprive the baby of this passive immunity.

Regression of the Mammary Gland

If regular suckling is permitted, lactation can be maintained for many months or even for several years. However, if milk is not removed, the glands become greatly distended and milk production quickly ceases. This is in part due to interruption of the neurohormonal reflex mechanism for maintenance of prolactin secretion, but the engorgement of the breasts may also compress the blood vessels, resulting in diminished access of oxytocin to the myoepithelial cells. After a few days the secretion remaining in the alveolar spaces and ducts is absorbed, and the glandular elements gradually return to the resting state. The gland, however, does not return completely to its original state, because many of the alveoli that had formed during the period of pregnancy do not disappear entirely, and the remains of the secretion may sometimes be retained in the mammary ducts for a considerable time. The gland remains in such a resting condition until the following pregnancy, when the same cycle of changes is repeated.

The process of mammary gland regression has been studied mainly in laboratory animals, but the changes are undoubtedly very similar in the human. A few days after weaning, the alveoli are greatly distended with secretory products, and the epithelium is correspondingly flattened. Later there is a gradual collapse of the alveoli and an associated increase in perialveolar connective tissue and adipose tissue. There is an increase in macrophages in the interstitial tissue but no true inflammatory reaction. By ten days after weaning, the glandular tissue is largely replaced by connective and adipose tissue, and the remaining alveoli appear as scattered solid cords of epithelial cells.

Examined in electron micrographs, the alveolar cells show an early accumulation of intracellular secretory protein in large vacuoles. There is also a marked progressive increase in the number of intraepithelial macrophages. Whereas autophagic vacuoles are rare in the alveolar epithelium of the lactating gland, they rapidly increase in number and size in the first few days after weaning. Their contents include mitochondria, granular reticulum, and secretory granules. There is a concomitant increase in the heterophagic activity of the intraepithelial macrophages. Since they may contain ingested secretory granules, it is concluded that they take up organelles and inclusions from regressing or degenerating epithelial cells. Some of the latter clearly slough in later stages of regression, and these are disposed of by macrophages.

Concomitant with the electron microscopic appearance of increases in autophagic and heterophagic vacuoles in the first few days after weaning, there is also a marked increase in activity of the lysosomal enzymes aryl sulfatase, cathepsin D, and acid phosphatase despite the fact that the activity of other nonlysosomal enzymes is declining. Thus, there is apparently a synthesis of new lysosomal enzymes during the early phases of regression.

In old age, the mammary gland gradually undergoes involution. The epithelium of the secretory portions, and partly also of the excretory ducts, atrophies, and the gland tends, in a general way, to return to the prepubertal condition, in which there are only a few scattered ducts. Equally striking changes occur in the interstitial connective tissue. This becomes decidedly less cellular; the number of collagenous fibrils decreases, and the whole mass becomes more homogeneous and stains much less intensely with eosin.

The mammary epithelium not infrequently is the site of pathological changes. The disorder known as chronic cystic disease is very common in women between 30 and 50 years of age. The terminal ducts and acini may lose their continuity with the remainder of the duct system and may form fluid-filled cysts of varying size. The breast is the most common site of cancer among women. About one in every 17 newborn girls (6 per cent) may be expected to develop breast cancer at some time during her life—an incidence three times that of cancer of the colon, the second most common type.

Blood and Lymphatic Vessels

The arteries of the mammary gland arise from the anterior thoracic (internal mammary) artery, the thoracic branches of the axillary artery, and the intercostal arteries. They pass mainly along the larger ducts and break up into dense capillary networks on the external surface of the basal lamina of the secretory portions. The veins drain into the axillary and anterior thoracic veins.

The lymphatic vessels begin with capillary networks located in the connective tissue layers surrounding separate alveoli. They collect along the course of the mammary ducts into a subpapillary lymphatic network. From here several large vessels drain the lymph mainly into the lymph nodes in the axilla and subclavicular area, but they also have connections with the lymphatics that penetrate the intercostal spaces to reach parasternal lymph nodes. Understanding the lymphatic drainage of the gland is of clinical importance owing to the necessity of removing the regional lymph nodes in radical mastectomy for breast cancer.

Innervation

Norepinephrine-containing nerve fibers are abundant among the smooth muscle cells of the nipple and at the interface between media and adventitia of the arteries of the breast. This is in accord with physiological observations indicating that the efferent nerves of these structures are sympathetic adrenergic. There seems to be no evidence that cholinergic fibers supply any part of the gland.

Most mammary nerves follow the arteries and arterioles and supply these structures. A few fibers leave the perivascular networks and lie near the walls of the ducts. They may correspond to sensory fibers for sensing milk pressure, which have been postulated on the basis of behavioral and electrophysiological studies. There is no morphological evidence of a nerve supply to the secretory cells or myoepithelial cells.

REFERENCES

Bauman, D. E., and C. L. Davis: Biosynthesis of milk fat. *In* Larson, B. L., and V. R. Smith, eds.: Lactation: A Comprehensive Treatise. Vol. II. New York, Academic Press, 1974, pp. 31–75.

Cowie, A. T., and S. J. Folley: The mammary gland and lactation. *In* Young, W. C., ed.: Sex and Internal Secretions, 3rd ed. Baltimore, Williams & Wilkins Co., 1961, p. 590.

Dempsey, E. W., H. Bunting, and G. B. Wislocki: Observations on the chemical cytology of the mammary gland. Am. J. Anat. *81*:309, 1947.

Foote, F. W., and F. W. Stewart: Comparative studies of cancerous versus non-cancerous breasts. I. Basic morphological characteristics. Ann. Surg. *121*:6, 1945.

Gardner, W. U., and G. van Wagenen: Experimental development of the mammary gland in the monkey. Endocrinology *22*:164, 1938.

Hebb, C., and J. L. Linzell: Innervation of the mammary gland. A histochemical study in the rabbit. Histochem. J. *2*:491, 1970.

Helminen, H. J., and J. L. E. Ericsson: Studies on mammary gland involution. I. On the ultrastructure of the lactating mammary gland. J. Ultrastruct. Res. *25*:193, 1968.

Helminen, H. J., and J. L. E. Ericsson: Studies on mammary gland involution. II. Ultrastructural evidence for auto- and heterophagocytosis. J. Ultrastruct. Res. *25*:214, 1968.

Helminen, H. J., J. L. E. Ericsson, and S. Orrenius: Studies on mammary gland involution. IV. Histochemical and biochemical observations on alteratons in lysosomes and lysosomal enzymes. J. Ultrastruct. Res. *25*:240, 1968.

Hollmann, K. H.: Cytology and fine structure of the mammary gland. *In* Larson, B. L., and V. R. Smith, eds.: Lactation: A Comprehensive Treatise. Vol. I. New York, Academic Press, 1974, pp. 1–91.

Kon, S. K., and A. T. Cowie: Milk; The Mammary Gland and Its Secretion. New York, Academic Press, 1961.

Kurosumi, K., Y. Kobayashi, and N. Baba: The fine structure of mammary glands of lactating rats with special reference to the apocrine secretion. Exp. Cell Res. *50*:177, 1968.

Linzell, J. L., and M. Peaker: Mechanism of milk secretion. Physiol. Rev. *51*:564, 1971.

Mayer, G., and M. Klein: Histology and cytology of the mammary gland. *In* Kon, S. K., and A. T. Cowie, eds.: Milk: The Mammary Gland and its Secretion. Vol. 1. New York, Academic Press, 1961.

Miller, M. R., and M. Kasahara: Cutaneous innervation of the human female breast. Anat. Rec. *135*:153, 1959.

Mills, E. S., and Y. J. Topper: Some ultrastructural effects of insulin, hydrocortisone and prolactin on mammary gland explants. J. Cell Biol. *44*:310, 1970.

Montagna, W.: Histology and cytochemistry of human skin. XXXV. The nipple and areola. Br. J. Dermatol. *83*(Suppl.):2, 1970.

Mostov, K. E., J. P. Krakenbuhl, and G. Blobel: Receptor-mediated transcellular transport of immunoglobulin: synthesis of secretory component as multiple and larger transcellular forms. Proc. Natl. Acad. Sci. U.S.A. *77*:7257, 1980.

Neville, M. C., J. C. Allen, and C. Watters: The mechanism of milk secretion. *In* Neville, M. C., and M. R. Neifert, eds.: Lactation: Physiology, Nutrition, and Breast Feeding. New York, Plenum Press, 1983, pp. 49–103.

Richardson, K. C.: Contractile tissues in the mammary gland, with special reference to myoepithelium in the goat. Proc. R. Soc. B *136*:30, 1949.

Short, R. V.: Breast feeding. Sci. Am. *250*:23, 1984.

Tindal, J. S.: Hypothalamic control of secretion and release of prolactin. J. Reprod. Fertil. *39*:437, 1974.

Vorherr, H., ed.: Human Lactation. New York, Grune & Stratton, 1979.

Wellings, S. R., K. B. DeOme, and D. R. Pitelka: Electron microscopy of milk secretion in the mammary gland of the C3H/Crgl mouse. I. Cytomorphology of the prelactating and the lactating gland. J. Natl. Cancer Inst. *25*:393, 1960.

Wellings. S. R., B. W. Grunbaum, and K. B. DeOme: Electron microscopy of milk secretion in the mammary gland of the C3H/Crgl mouse. II. Identification of fat and protein particles in milk and in tissue. J. Natl. Cancer Inst. *25*:423, 1960.

Wellings, S. R., and J. R. Phelp: The function of the Golgi apparatus in lactating cells of the BALB/cCrgl mouse: an electron microscopic and autoradiographic study. Zeitschr. f. Zellforsch. *61*:871, 1964.

34

THE EYE

The ability to react to light is a widespread property of living matter. Plants use solar energy for photosynthesis and exhibit phototropic responses. Primitive invertebrates have scattered photoreceptor cells that detect varying intensities of light and enable them to position themselves favorably with respect to light or darkness. Vertebrates have evolved eyes—more efficient organs with a *lens* to concentrate light and focus an image on closely packed photoreceptors in a *retina*, which detects light intensity, color, form, and motion and encodes the various parameters of the image for transmission to the brain. The eyes of most vertebrates are placed on the sides of the head where they provide a nearly complete panoramic view of the environment. *Panoramic vision*, together with the evolution of muscles and reflexes for rotation of the eyes, provided early warning against predators. On the other hand, in many predatory mammals and birds the orbits gradually moved forward so that the uniocular fields of vision came to overlap in varying degree and the sector of the environment in front of the animal was seen by both eyes. Complex neural mechanisms developed to coordinate and fuse the slightly different images, thus achieving *binocular vision* and, in some instances, stereoscopic vision with perception of depth in a three-dimensional view of the environment essential to successful pursuit of prey. Acquisition of stereoscopic vision, evolution of a large brain to process the information, and freeing of the hands from a locomotor function enabled our hominoid ancestors to develop the manipulative skills that contributed to the ascendancy of humans.

STRUCTURE OF THE EYE IN GENERAL

The anterior segment of the eye, the *cornea*, is transparent, permitting the rays of light to enter. The rest of the wall of the eye is opaque and possesses a darkly pigmented inner surface, which absorbs light rays. The posterior segment of the eye is to a great extent lined with photosensitive nervous tissue, the *retina*, which develops as an outgrowth from the brain. The cavity of the eyeball is filled with transparent media arranged in separate bodies, which, together with the cornea, act as a system of convex lenses. These produce on the photosensitive layer of the retina an inverted and reduced image of the objects in the environment.

The wall of the eyeball is composed of three layers: the tough, fibrous, *corneoscleral coat*; the middle, vascular coat, or *uvea*; and the innermost layer, the photosensitive *retina*. The thick fibrous layer protects the delicate inner structures of the eye and, together with the intraocular fluid pressure, serves to maintain the shape and turgor of the eyeball. It is divided into a large opaque posterior segment, the *sclera*, and a smaller transparent anterior segment, the *cornea*. The uvea is concerned with the nutrition of the ocular tissues and also provides mechanisms for visual accommodation and control of the amount of light entering the eye. Its three regional differentiations are the *choroid*, the *ciliary body*, and the *iris*. The choroid is the highly vascular portion of the uvea that underlies the photosensitive retina. Extending forward from the scalloped anterior margin of the retina, called the *ora serrata*, to the corneoscleral junction is the *ciliary body*. It forms a belt 5 to 6 mm wide around the interior of the eyeball and contains the smooth muscle that makes this structure the instrument of accommodation, acting upon the lens to bring light rays from different distances to focus upon the retina. The iris is a thin continuation of the ciliary body projecting over the anterior surface of the lens, with its free edge outlining the *pupil*. The diameter of the iris is approximately 12 mm. Its opening, the pupil, can be reduced

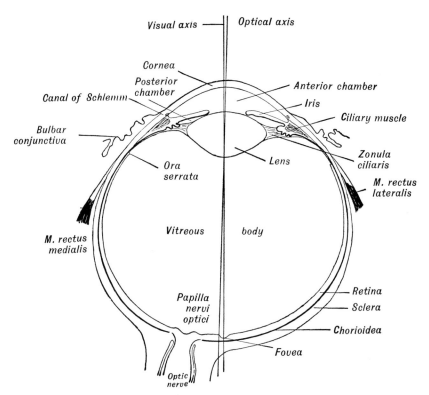

Figure 34–1. Diagram of horizontal meridional section through the right eye of man.

or expanded through the contraction or relaxation of the *constrictor* and *dilator muscles* of the pupil. In this way, the iris functions as an adjustable optic diaphragm regulating the amount of light entering the eye (Figs. 34–1, 34–2).

The innermost layer, the retina, contains in its sensory part the receptors for light and complex neural networks that encode the visual information and send impulses through the *optic nerve* to the brain. The spot where the nerve enters the eyeball, the *papilla* of the optic nerve, is a pink disc approximately 1.4 mm in diameter located about 3 mm medial to the posterior pole of the eye. The portion of the retina anterior to the ora serrata and lining the inner surface of the ciliary muscle (*ciliary portion* of the retina) and that lining the posterior surface of the iris (*iridial portion* of the retina) are not photosensitive. These will be discussed with the uvea and iris.

The transparent *dioptric media* include the cornea and the contents of the cavity enclosed by the tunics of the eye. Because of the considerable difference between the index of refraction of the cornea (1.376) and that of

the surrounding air (1.0), the cornea is the chief refractive element of the eye. Of the enclosed transparent media, the most anterior is the *aqueous humor*. It is contained in the *anterior chamber*, a small cavity bounded in front by the cornea and behind by the iris and the central portion of the anterior surface of the lens. The *posterior chamber*, also filled with aqueous humor, is a narrow, annular space enclosed anteriorly by the lens, the iris, and the ciliary body and posteriorly by the vitreous body (Figs. 34–1, 34–2).

The next of the transparent media is the *crystalline lens*. This is an elastic biconvex body suspended from the inner surface of the ciliary body by a circular ligament, the *ciliary zonule*. It is placed directly behind the pupil, between the aqueous humor of the anterior chamber and the vitreous body posteriorly. The lens is second in importance to the cornea as a refractive element of the eye, and is the dioptric organ of accommodation.

The greater portion of the cavity of the eye, situated between the posterior surface of the lens and ciliary body anteriorly and the retina posteriorly, is the *vitreal cavity*, filled with a viscous transparent substance,

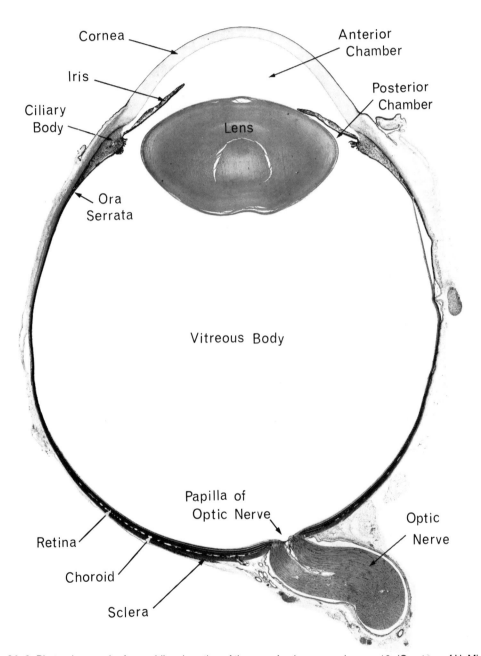

Figure 34–2. Photomicrograph of a meridional section of the eye of a rhesus monkey. × 10. (Courtesy of H. Mizoguchi.)

the *vitreous humor* or *vitreous body*. It permits light to pass freely from the lens to the photoreceptors.

The retina is transparent in the living state. Only its outermost layer, the *pigment epithelium*, is opaque and forms the first barrier to the rays of light.

DIMENSIONS, AXES, PLANES OF REFERENCE

The adult human eyeball is a roughly spherical body about 24 mm in diameter and weighing 6 to 8 g. The center of the cornea is the *anterior pole*; the *posterior pole* is located between the optic papilla and the *fovea*, a thin depression in the retina providing the most distinct vision. The line connecting the two poles is the *anatomical axis*. The *visual axis* is the line drawn from the center of the fovea to the apparent center of the pupil (Fig. 34–1). The *equatorial plane* is vertical and perpendicular to the visual axis, passing through the greatest width of the eyeball, the *equator*. Other planes passing through the axis determine the *meridians* of the eye. The two most important are the vertical and the horizontal meridians. The vertical passes through the fovea and divides the eyeball, including the retina, into nasal and temporal halves. The plane of the horizontal meridian divides the eyeball and retina into an upper and a lower half. These two planes divide the eyeball and the retina into four quadrants, an upper nasal, an upper temporal, a lower nasal, and a lower temporal.

The *anteroposterior diameter* along the axis of the eye is 24 mm, or a little more. The *inner axis*, the distance between the inner surface of the cornea and the inner surface of the retina at the posterior pole, measures a little less than 22 mm. The *optical axis* passes through the optical centers of the refractive media and is almost identical with the anatomical axis. The visual axis, where it touches the retina, is from 4 to 7 degrees lateral and 3.5 degrees below the optical axis.

The *radius of curvature* of the large posterior segment at the fundus measures somewhat less than 13 mm, and gradually decreases toward the corneoscleral junction. The cornea has the smallest radius of curvature, approximately 7.8 mm (outer corneal surface).

The eyeball is lodged in a soft tissue cushion filling the bony orbit of the skull and made up of loose connective and fatty tissue, muscles, fasciae, blood and lymphatic vessels, nerves, and a gland. This soft tissue cushion permits the eye to move freely around its *center of rotation*. The eye is connected to the general integument by the *conjunctiva*, which lines the lids and continues over the eyeball to the margins of the cornea. The lids are a mechanical protection against external noxious agents.

FIBROUS TUNIC

Sclera

The sclera is 1 mm thick at the posterior pole, 0.4 to 0.3 mm at the equator, and 0.6 mm toward the edge of the cornea. It consists of flat collagenous bundles that run in various directions parallel to the surface. Between these bundles are networks of elastic fibers. The cells of the sclera are flat, elongated fibroblasts. Melanocytes also can be found in the deeper layers, especially in the vicinity of the entrance of the optic nerve.

The tendons of the eye muscles are attached to the outer surface of the sclera, which in turn is connected with a dense layer of connective tissue—the *fascial sheath* of the eye, or *capsule of Tenon*—by an exceedingly loose system of thin collagenous membranes separated by clefts—the *episcleral space*, or *space of Tenon*. The eyeball and the capsule of Tenon rotate together in all directions on a bed of orbital fat.

Between the sclera and the choroid is a layer of loose connective tissue with elastic networks and numerous melanocytes and fibroblasts. When these two tunics are separated, part of this loose tissue adheres to the choroid and part to the sclera as its *suprachoroid lamina*.

Cornea

The cornea is slightly thicker than the sclera, measuring 0.8 to 0.9 mm in the center and 1.1 mm at the periphery. In the human the refractive power of the cornea, which is a function of the index of refraction of its tissue (1.376) and of the radius of curvature of its surface (7.8 mm), is twice as high as that of the lens.

In a cross section through the cornea, the following layers can be seen: (1) the corneal epithelium, (2) the membrane of Bowman,

(3) the stroma, or substantia propria, (4) the membrane of Descemet, and (5) the endothelium (Fig. 34–3).

Epithelium. The epithelium is stratified squamous, with an average thickness of 50 μm. It consists, as a rule, of five layers of cells. The outer surface is quite smooth and is composed of large squamous cells. As in other types of stratified squamous epithelium, the cells are connected with one another by many short interdigitating processes that adhere at desmosomes. The cytoplasm contains numerous mitochondria and scattered profiles of granular endoplasmic reticulum in a cytoplasmic matrix filled with randomly oriented fine filaments.

The epithelium of the cornea is extremely sensitive and contains numerous free nerve endings. It is endowed with a remarkable capacity for regeneration. Minor injuries heal rapidly by a gliding movement of the adjacent epithelial cells to fill the defect. Mitoses in the basal epithelial cells appear later and may be found at considerable distances from the wound. A few mitoses can be found in the basal cell layer under normal conditions.

Bowman's Membrane. The corneal epithelium rests on a faintly fibrillar lamina 6 to 9 μm thick. This structure is not actually a membrane but the outer layer of the substantia propria of the cornea, from which it cannot be separated. It is nevertheless distinguishable with the optical microscope because its fibers are not so well ordered. With the electron microscope it is seen to consist of a feltwork of randomly arranged collagen fibrils, about 18 nm in diameter, which may show a periodic banding. It does not contain elastin and ends abruptly at the margin of the cornea. Bowman's membrane is not present in all mammals; in rabbits the corneal epithelium rests on a simple basal lamina.

Stroma or Substantia Propria. This layer forms about 90 per cent of the thickness of the cornea (Fig. 34–3). It is a transparent, regular connective tissue whose bundles form thin lamellae arranged in many layers. In each layer the direction of the bundles

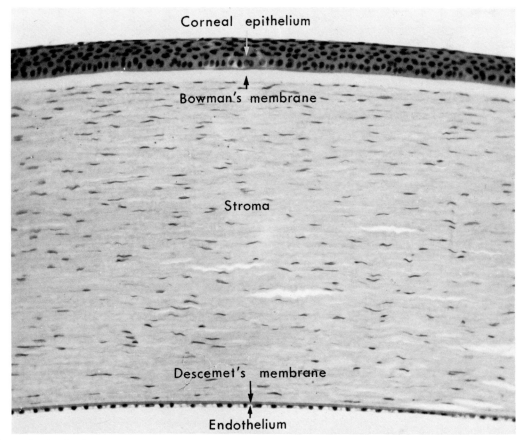

Figure 34–3. Photomicrograph of a section of human cornea. × 160. (After Kuwabara, T. In Greep, R. O., ed.: Histology. 2nd ed. New York, McGraw-Hill Book Co., 1966.)

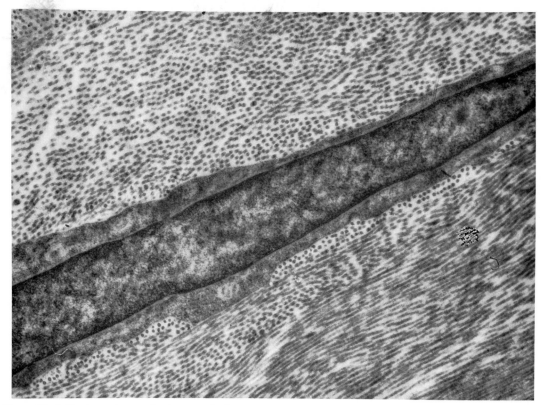

Figure 34–4. Electron micrograph of a part of a keratocyte in the cornea and the surrounding layers of collagen fibrils oriented at right angles to one another. (Micrograph courtesy of M. Jakus.)

changes and those in successive layers cross at various angles (Figs. 34–3, 34–4). The lamellae everywhere interchange fibers and thus are kept tightly together. The collagen fibrils are somewhat thicker than those in Bowman's membrane, measuring about 23 nm on the average. Between the fibrils, the bundles, and the lamellae, there is a metachromatic ground substance. The molecules responsible for its metachromasia are chondroitin sulfate and keratan sulfate. The cells of the stroma are long slender fibroblasts (keratocytes) lodged in narrow clefts among the parallel bundles of collagen fibrils. In addition, the stroma always contains a number of lymphocytes, which migrate from the blood vessels of the corneal limbus. In inflammation, enormous numbers of neutrophilic leukocytes and lymphocytes penetrate between the lamellae.

Membrane of Descemet and Corneal Endothelium. This homogeneous-appearing lamella, 5 to 10 μm thick, can be isolated from the posterior surface of the substantia propria. At the periphery of the cornea, Descemet's membrane continues as a thin layer on the surface of the trabeculae of the limbus. In its structure it is essentially a very thick basal lamina elaborated by the corneal endothelium, which rests upon it (Figs. 34–3, 34–5). It appears homogeneous under the light microscope, but when examined with the electron microscope, Descemet's membrane of older individuals may show an apparent cross striation, with bands about 107 nm apart, connected by filaments less than 10 nm in width and about 27 nm apart (Fig. 34–6A). Tangential sections reveal a two-dimensional array of nodes, about 107 nm apart and connected by filaments to form hexagonal figures (Fig. 34–6B). The diagram in Figure 34–7 shows the relationship between the images seen in the two planes. Histochemical data, chemical analyses, and x-ray diffraction studies support the conclusion that the filaments forming this hexagonal array are an atypical form of collagen. In young individuals, Descemet's membrane is more homogeneous in appearance. It is suggested that the hexagonal pattern of fibers forms with advancing age by aggregation of collagen that is normally dispersed in the

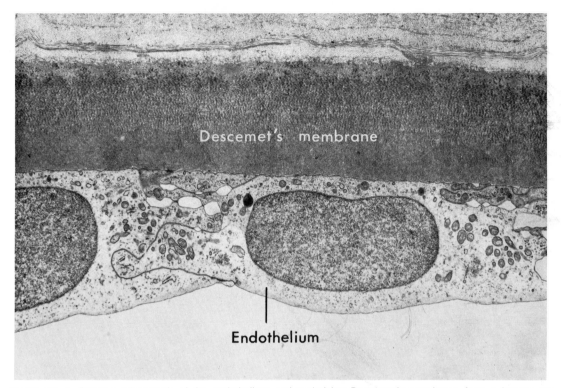

Endothelium

Figure 34–5. Electron micrograph of the endothelium and underlying Descemet's membrane from a human eye. (Courtesy of T. Kuwabara.)

A

Figure 34–6. Electron micrographs of Descemet's membrane, showing the unusual configuration of collagen, characteristic of this layer. *A*, Cross section with its striated appearance. *B*, Tangential section, illustrating hexagonal arrangement of nodes connected by filaments. (Courtesy of M. Jakus.)

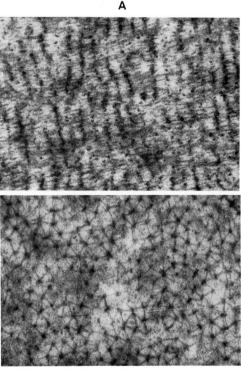

B

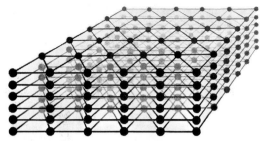

Figure 34–7. Diagram of structure of Descemet's membrane based on electron micrographs. See text for explanation. (Courtesy of M. Jakus.)

amorphous ground substance as tropocollagen. This and other atypical forms of collagen occur in the membrane at the periphery of the cornea, where randomly oriented fibrous bands with a 100-nm periodicity are frequently encountered. These are particularly common in *Hassall-Henle bodies* or *warts*, dome-shaped protrusions from the periphery of Descemet's membrane into the anterior chamber, which occur with increasing frequency in human eyes after the age of 20.

The inner surface of the membrane of Descemet is covered by a layer of large squamous cells (Fig. 34–5); the intercellular spaces between these endothelial cells permit free exchange of fluid between corneal stroma and anterior chamber.

Histophysiology of the Cornea

The transparency of the cornea is great, although less than that of the aqueous humor. It is due, at least in part, to the uniform diameter and regular spacing of its collagen fibrils, so that scattered rays cancel each other by destructive interference. Proteoglycans of the ground substance may be responsible for the orderly arrangement of the fibrils. An increase in the amount of the interfibrillar fluid, such as occurs in swelling, causes cloudiness of the cornea.

The cornea is avascular, and its central region depends on diffusion from the aqueous humor for its nourishment. The blood vessels of the limbus supply the peripheral cornea by diffusion and account for the presence, in the corneal stroma, of leukocytes and substances that are excluded from the aqueous humor. Oxygen for the corneal epithelium comes directly from the atmosphere. The contribution of tears to corneal nourishment seems to be negligible.

The cornea is one of the few organs that can be successfully transplanted into allogeneic recipients. One possible explanation for this phenomenon is that the lack of blood vessels protects the transplanted cornea from the host's immune system.

The Limbus

The *limbus*, or sclerocorneal junction, is an important region of the eye because it represents a valuable landmark for the ophthalmologist and contains the apparatus for the outflow of the aqueous humor (Figs. 34–8, 34–9). About 1.5 to 2 mm wide, its outer surface displays a shallow depression called the *external scleral sulcus*, where the gently curving sclera is continuous with the more convex cornea. On its inner aspect, the sclerocorneal stroma is marked by a circular depression, the *internal scleral sulcus*, which is filled in by the *trabecular meshwork* and the *canal of Schlemm*, specialized tissues constituting the outflow system for the aqueous humor. On the posterior lip of the internal scleral sulcus, the scleral stroma projects toward the interior of the eye, forming a small circular ridge, the *scleral spur*; this affords attachment to the trabecular meshwork anteriorly and to the ciliary muscle posteriorly.

At the limbus, there is a gradual transition of the corneal epithelium into that of the conjunctiva of the bulb (Fig. 34–8). The membrane of Bowman terminates and is replaced by the conjunctival stroma and the anterior margin of the capsule of Tenon. In the connective tissue underlying the epithelium, the conjunctival vessels form arcades that extend radially into the cornea for about 0.5 mm beyond the limbal edge. These vessels nourish the periphery of the cornea and are the source of the occasional lymphocytes found in the corneal stroma. The blood vessels that invade the corneal stroma in chronic inflammation arise from these loops. When the limbus is examined in a living subject with the slit-lamp microscope, *aqueous veins*, veins containing aqueous humor instead of blood, may be seen emerging from the limbal stroma and contributing to the plexus of the episcleral veins. At the limbus, the collagenous sclera gradually continues into the corneal stroma, and its collagenous bundles progressively acquire the uniform small diameter and orderly arrangement typical of the cornea. Deep to the stroma of the limbus, Descemet's membrane ends and gives way to the spongy tissue of the *trabecular meshwork*, situated between the anterior chamber, the root

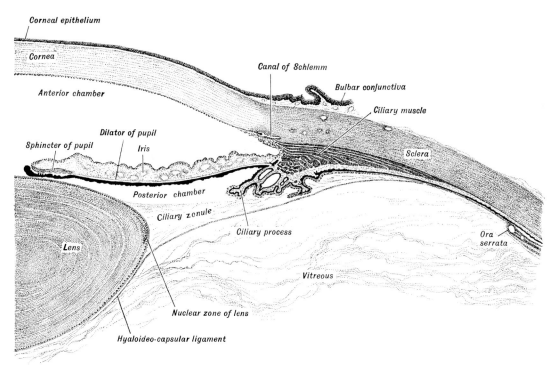

Figure 34–8. Part of meridional section of human eye. × 14. (Modified from Schaffer.)

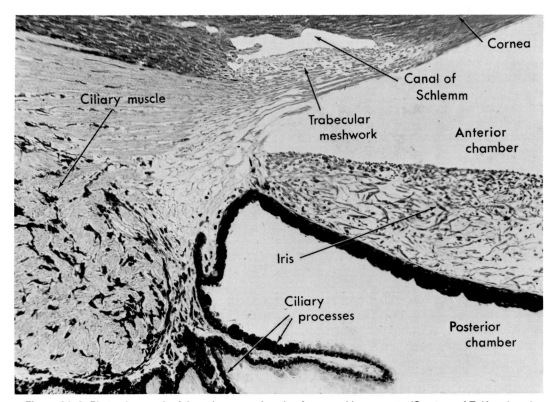

Figure 34–9. Photomicrograph of the sclerocorneal angle of a normal human eye. (Courtesy of T. Kuwabara.)

of the iris, the limbal stroma, and the scleral spur (Figs. 34–9, 34–10). The trabecular meshwork is composed of a large number of flattened, fenestrated connective tissue sheets and branching and anastomosing beams or trabeculae. These are completely invested by an attenuated endothelium, continuous with the corneal endothelium (Fig. 34–11). They bound a labyrinthine system of minute passages, the intertrabecular spaces, which communicate with the anterior chamber and are filled with aqueous humor.

Interposed between the trabecular meshwork and the limbal stroma is the *canal of Schlemm*, a flattened vessel that extends around the entire circumferene of the limbus. The canal of Schlemm has a varicose outline and in places breaks up into irregular branches that coalesce again. The wall of the canal consists of endothelium, a discontinuous basal lamina, and a thin layer of connective tissue. On the outer wall of the canal—that is, toward the limbal stroma—the endothelium is extremely attenuated (Fig. 34–12); on the inner wall of the canal—toward the trabecular meshwork—the endo-

thelium varies greatly in thickness with different techniques of specimen preparation and may display large intra- or intercellular vacuoles. Great importance has been attributed to these "giant vacuoles," for it is believed that they are involved in the process of aqueous humor reabsorption from the anterior chamber.

The lumen of the canal does not communicate directly with the spaces of the trabecular meshwork but is separated from them by the following layers: (1) the endothelium that invests the internal wall of the canal; (2) the connective tissue adventitia of the canal, which here becomes especially rich in stromal cells and is usually referred to as juxtacanalicular connective tissue; and (3) the endothelial lining of the trabecular spaces.

From the outer wall of the canal, 25 to 35 *collector channels* arise, which join the deep veins of the limbus; these in turn pass to the surface of the limbal stroma and empty into the episcleral veins.

The aqueous humor contained in the anterior chamber permeates the maze of minute intercommunicating passages of the tra-

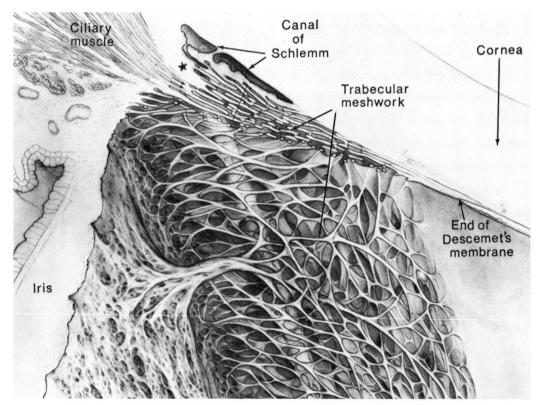

Figure 34–10. Diagram of the outflow system of the aqueous humor. Star indicates scleral spur. (After Hogan, M. Y., J. A. Alvarado, and J. E. Weddell: Histology of the Human Eye. Philadelphia, W. B. Saunders Co., 1971.)

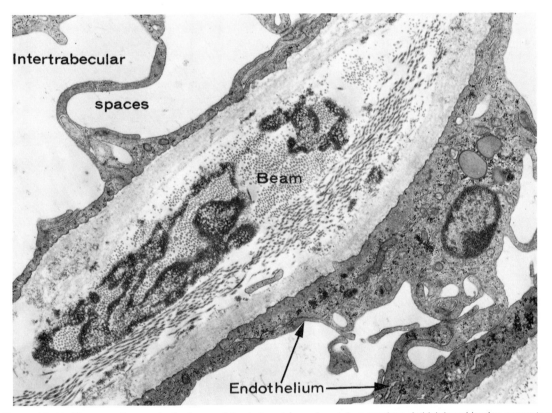

Figure 34–11. Electron micrograph of a beam of the trabecular meshwork in a monkey. A thick basal lamina separates the connective tissue core of the beam from the investing endothelium. The intertrabecular spaces are crisscrossed by processes of the endothelial cells. × 8600. (From Raviola, G. Invest. Ophthalmol. *13*:828, 1974.)

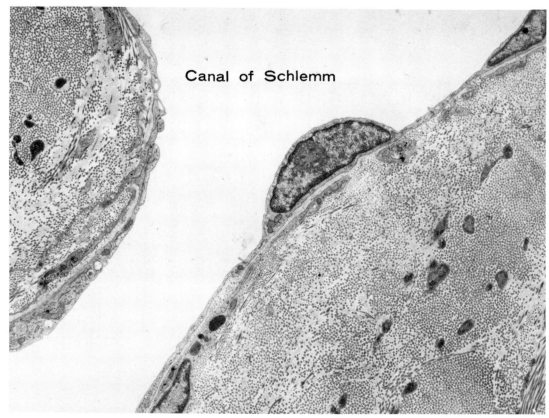

Figure 34–12. Canal of Schlemm in a monkey. The external wall of the canal consists of an attenuated endothelium, a discontinuous basal lamina, and an adventitial layer of flattened fibroblasts. The collagen fibrils of the limbal stroma are seen in cross section. × 6200. (From Raviola, G. Invest. Ophthalmol *13*:828, 1974.)

becular meshwork; thence, it reaches the lumen of the canal of Schlemm and is finally drained by the episcleral veins. The precise pathway followed by the aqueous humor from the intertrabecular spaces to the lumen of the Schlemm canal is poorly understood. The Schlemm canal usually contains aqueous humor, but it may rarely fill with blood when there is stasis and back pressure in the venous system. Obstruction to the filtration of aqueous humor through the intertrabecular spaces or to its drainage via the canal of Schlemm results in the rise in intraocular pressure characteristic of the serious eye disease *glaucoma*.

THE VASCULAR TUNIC: THE UVEA

Choroid

The choroid is a thin, soft, brown layer adjacent to the inner surface of the sclera.

Between the sclera and the choroid is a potential cleft, the *perichoroidal space*, which is traversed by thin lamellae that run obliquely from the choroid to the sclera and form a loose, pigmented tissue layer—the *suprachoroid lamina*. This is composed of fine, transparent sheets, with fibroblasts on their surface and with a rich network of elastic fibers. Large flat melanocytes are scattered everywhere between and within the connective tissue lamellae. In the suprachoroid, as in the rest of the uvea, there are also scattered macrophages. The lamellae of the suprachoroid pass without a distinct boundary into the substance of the choroid proper. This tunic can be subdivided into three main layers; from outside inward, they are (1) the vessel layer, (2) the choriocapillary layer, and (3) the glassy membrane, or *Bruch's membrane* (Fig. 34–13).

Vessel Layer. This layer consists of a multitude of large and medium-sized arteries and veins. The spaces between the vessels are filled with loose connective tissue rich in melanocytes. The lamellar arrangement here is much less distinct than in the suprachoroid.

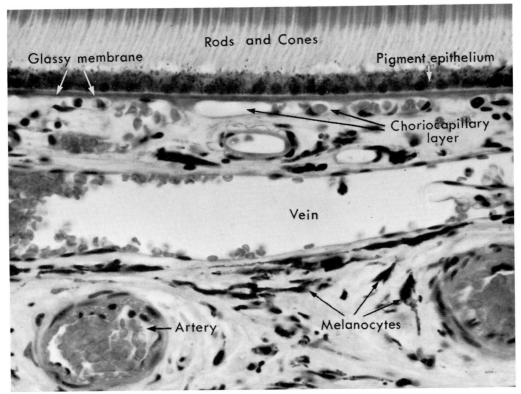

Figure 34–13. Photomicrograph of choroid and outermost layers of the retina. (After Kuwabara, T. *In* Greep, R. O., ed.: Histology. 2nd ed. New York, McGraw-Hill Book Co., 1966.)

According to some, the vessel layer contains strands of smooth muscle that are independent of the walls of blood vessels.

Choriocapillary Layer. This is a capillary network arranged in one plane. In places this layer is connected with the vessel layer. The individual capillaries have a large and somewhat irregular caliber; toward Bruch's membrane their endothelium is fenestrated. The layer is thicker and the capillary network denser in the region underlying the fovea. Anteriorly it ends near the ora serrata.

Bruch's Membrane (Glassy Membrane). This is a refractile layer 1 to 4 μm thick between the choroid and the pigment epithelium of the retina. The electron microscope has shown that this so-called membrane is not a homogeneous structure but consists of five different components: (1) the basal lamina of the endothelium of the capillaries of the choriocapillary layer; (2) a first layer of collagen fibers; (3) a network of elastic fibers; (4) a second layer of collagen fibers; and (5) the basal lamina of the pigment epithelium of the retina.

Ciliary Body

If the eyeball is cut across along its equator, and its anterior half is inspected from within after removal of the vitreous, a sharply outlined, dentate border is seen running around the inner surface of the wall in front of the equator (Fig. 34–14). This is the *ora serrata* or *ora terminalis* of the photosensitive retina. The zone between the ora and the edge of the lens is the *ciliary body*, a thickening of the vascular tunic. Its surface is covered by the darkly pigmented, nonphotosensitive ciliary portion of the retina. In a meridional section through the eye bulb, the ciliary body appears as a thin triangle with its small base facing the anterior chamber of the eye and attached by its anterior and outer angle to the scleral spur. The long, narrow posterior angle of its triangular section extends backward and merges with the choroid (Fig. 34–8). The inner aspect of the ciliary body is divided into a narrow anterior zone, the *ciliary crown*, and a broader posterior zone, the *ciliary ring*. Seen in surface view, the inner

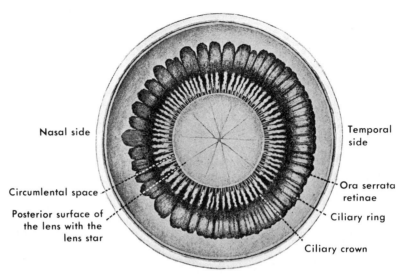

Nasal side

Temporal side

Circumlental space

Posterior surface of the lens with the lens star

Ora serrata retinae

Ciliary ring

Ciliary crown

Figure 34–14. Anterior half of right eye, seen from within. × 3. (After Salzmann.)

surface of the ring has shallow grooves, *ciliary striae*, which run forward from the teeth of the ora serrata. On its inner surface, the ciliary crown has 70 radially arranged ridges, the *ciliary processes* (Figs. 34–8, 34–9, 34–14).

The bulk of the ciliary body, exclusive of the ciliary processes, consists of the muscle of accommodation, the *ciliary muscle*. It is smooth muscle and is composed of three portions. Closest to the sclera is the *muscle of Brücke*, whose bundles are deployed chiefly in the meridional direction. This outer part of the ciliary muscle stretches the choroid and is also called the *tensor muscle of the choroid*. In the next inward portion of the ciliary muscle, the bundles of muscle cells radiate fanlike from the region of the scleral spur toward the cavity of the eyeball. This is the *radial* or *reticular portion* of the ciliary muscle. The third or *circular portion* of the ciliary muscle (*Müller's muscle*) is usually absent in the newborn, appearing in the course of the second or third year. The contraction of this portion relaxes the tension on the lens and thus is important in accommodation for near vision. The classical subdivision of the ciliary muscle into three portions has been challenged as too schematic, for, in fact, the muscle fibers seem to be interwoven in a tridimensional network but with regions where fibers of meridional, radial, and circular orientation predominate. The interstices between the muscular bundles are filled with a small amount of connective tissue containing abundant elastic fibers and melan-

ocytes (Fig. 34–9). The latter become especially numerous toward the sclera.

The inner, *vascular layer* of the ciliary body consists of connective tissue and numerous blood vessels. In the ciliary ring it is the direct continuation of the same layer of the choroid. In the region of the ciliary crown it covers the inner surface of the ciliary muscle and forms the core of the ciliary processes. The vessels are almost exclusively capillaries and veins of varying caliber. The corresponding arteries ramify in the peripheral layers of the ciliary body. The capillary endothelium is fenestrated and freely permeable to plasma proteins. The connective tissue is dense, especially near the root of the iris, and contains abundant elastic fibers. In old age it often shows hyaline degeneration.

The ciliary portion of the retina continues forward beyond the ora serrata as the *ciliary epithelium* investing the inner surface of the ciliary body. Its function is the production of the aqueous humor. The ciliary epithelium consists of two layers of cells, an inner layer of nonpigmented elements bounding the posterior chamber, and an outer pigmented layer, which rests on the stroma of the ciliary body (Fig. 34–15). Toward the root of the iris, the cells of the inner epithelial layer gradually accumulate pigment granules. Because of the embryonal origin of the ciliary epithelium from the edge of the double-walled optic cup, the pole of the nonpigmented cells directed toward the interior of the eye is usually referred to as the cell base,

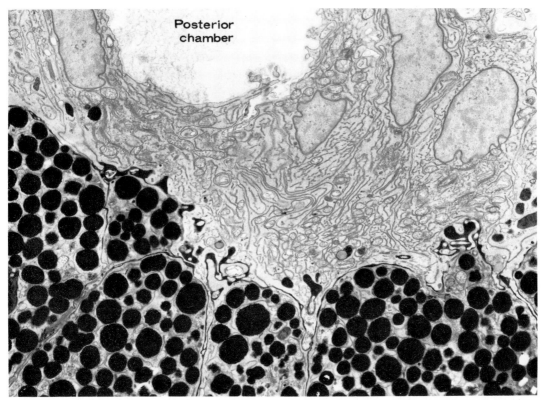

Figure 34–15. Ciliary epithelium in a monkey that was injected intravenously with horseradish peroxidase. The ciliary epithelium consists of two cell layers, one nonpigmented *(above)*, which bounds the posterior chamber; the other pigmented *(below)*, which rests on the stroma of the ciliary body. The tracer escaped through the permeable walls of the vessels of the ciliary body and has permeated the intercellular clefts between pigmented and nonpigmented cells, but its further progression toward the posterior chamber is blocked by an impermeable tight junction, which connects the apices of the nonpigmented cells. × 6400. (From Raviola, G. Invest. Ophthalmol. *13*:828, 1974.)

whereas the base of the pigmented cells is the end that adjoins the stroma of the ciliary body. Thus, the apices of the pigmented and nonpigmented epithelial cells face each other. At intervals, they are separated by discontinuous intercellular spaces called *ciliary channels*.

A basal lamina invests both surfaces of the ciliary epithelium; that toward the stroma of the ciliary body is continuous with the basal lamina of the pigment epithelium of the retina; the other is continuous with the inner limiting membrane of the retina.

The basal and lateral regions of the nonpigmented cells are occupied by a labyrinth of interdigitating processes formerly described as "membrane infoldings" (Fig. 34–16). In this respect, the nonpigmented cells resemble other epithelia actively engaged in transport of ions and water. Between the central nucleus and the cell apex is the cell center, consisting of a well-devel-

oped Golgi apparatus, a centriole, and occasionally a cilium, which protrudes from the cell surface in a channel bounded by the plasma membrane. The cytoplasm is permeated by flat cisternae of the granular endoplasmic reticulum, tubules of the agranular reticulum, and bundles of filaments radiating from the desmosomes that join adjacent cells. The mitchondria are not especially numerous, nor do they appear to be arranged in an orderly manner with respect to the plasmalemmal invaginations, as is the case for the convoluted tubules of the kidney or the striated ducts of the salivary glands. Especially prominent in the pigmented epithelial cells are the melanin granules, which completely fill the cytoplasm, leaving but little space for a moderate number of mitochondria and thin bundles of filaments. The nucleus is located toward the apex of the cell, being separated from it by a small Golgi apparatus. The plasma membrane at the base

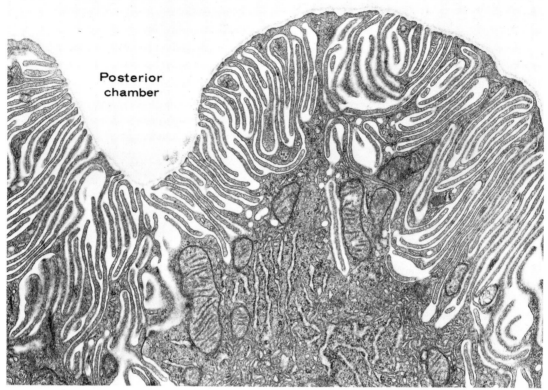

Figure 34–16. Electron micrograph of the ciliary epithelium of a rabbit. The base of the nonpigmented cells is occupied by a complex labyrinth of interdigitating processes. The basal lamina that separates the ciliary epithelium from the content of the posterior chamber is barely visible. × 18,000. (Courtesy of G. Raviola.)

of the cell is repeatedly invaginated, but the basal labyrinth is not as complex as in nonpigmented cells.

The ciliary epithelium is exceptional among actively transporting epithelia because it consists of two layers of cells, both provided with a basal labyrinth of interdigitating processes. These structural specializations suggest that the ciliary epithelium represents a unique biological device, consisting of two pumps working in series. This might result in a considerable amplification of the transport efficiency, but it requires accurate synchronization of the cells' activity. Gap junctions probably ensure such a precise coordination of the function of the myriad independent cell units; they connect adjacent pigmented cells, adjacent nonpigmented cells, and the confronted apices of the pigmented and nonpigmented cells. Furthermore, the lateral surfaces of the nonpigmented cells are connected to each other by an elaborate zonula occludens, a zonula adherens, and a few desmosomes.

Aqueous Humor and the Blood-Aqueous Barrier

Proper eye functioning requires a precise spatial arrangement of the retina with respect to the refractive media and a special chemical composition of the intraocular fluids, optimally adjusted to the metabolic needs of the retina, lens, and cornea. The aqueous humor subserves both of these functions. An accurate balance between its rates of production and reabsorption is responsible for maintenance of the intraocular pressure, which confers mechanical stability upon the ocular structures. Its specific composition, differing from plasma and somewhat resembling cerebrospinal fluid, cooperates with the blood-retinal barrier in generating an extracellular environment best suited to the functional requirements of the cells of the retina, lens, and cornea. Finally, it nourishes the lens, which lacks a blood supply.

The aqueous humor is a clear, watery fluid of slightly alkaline reaction with an index of refraction of 1.33, contained in the anterior and posterior chambers of the eye. In its chemical composition, the aqueous humor differs from blood plasma in its lower content of proteins; higher content of ascorbate, pyruvate, and lactate; and lower content of urea and glucose. Also, its electrolyte content is slightly different from that of the plasma. Continuously secreted by the ciliary epithelium, probably through a process of active transport, it fills the posterior chamber, nourishes the lens, and permeates the vitreous body. From the posterior chamber, it flows into the anterior chamber through the pupil and is finally drained through the trabecular meshwork and canal of Schlemm. The flow of the aqueous humor is determined by the difference in pressure between the fluids within the eye (about 20 mm Hg) and the pressure in the episcleral veins (about 13 mm Hg). In turn, the intraocular pressure is generated by an accurate adjustment of the rate of aqueous humor secretion by the ciliary epithelium and its rate of reabsorption at the limbus. When this balance is disrupted, as in glaucoma, the intraocular pressure increases, with devastating effects on the function of the eye.

Secretion of a fluid such as the aqueous humor, with a composition different from that of the plasma, is possible only if free diffusion of solutes between blood and the chambers of the eye is prevented. This is the role of the so-called *blood-aqueous barrier*, the peculiar physiological mechanism that limits the exchange of materials between the vascular compartment and the interior of the eye. When an ultrastructural tracer, such as horseradish peroxidase, is injected into the bloodstream, it rapidly diffuses across the permeable walls of the vessels of the ciliary body, permeates the stroma underlying the ciliary epithelium, and is finally blocked by the tight junctions that connect the apices of the nonpigmented cells (Fig. 34–15). These junctions, which limit free movement of molecules between ciliary body stroma and posterior chamber, are therefore believed to represent the major anatomical site of the blood-aqueous barrier.

Iris

The posterior surface of the iris near the pupil rests on the anterior surface of the lens; in this way the iris separates the anterior chamber from the posterior chamber. The margin of the iris connected with the ciliary body is called the *ciliary margin*, or the root of the iris. The pupil is surrounded by the *pupillary margin of the iris*. The iris diminishes in thickness toward both margins. Besides its individually varying color, the anterior surface of the iris presents certain distinct markings. About 1.5 mm from the pupil, a jagged line concentic with the pupillary margin separates the anterior surface into a *pupillary zone* and a wider *ciliary zone*. Near the pupillary and the ciliary margins the anterior surface has many irregular excavations, the *crypts*, which may extend deep into the tissue. In addition, there are oblique, irregularly arranged contraction furrows, which are especially marked when the pupil is dilated.

The main mass of the iris consists of a loose, pigmented, highly vascular connective tissue. The anterior surface of the stroma is lined with a discontinuous layer of fibroblasts and melanocytes. A thin layer of stroma immediately beneath this cell investment, the *anterior stromal sheet* or lamella, is devoid of blood vessels. Deep to this is a layer containing numerous vessels; their walls consist of endothelium, pericytes, and an unusually thick connective tissue adventitia. The posterior surface of the iris is covered with a double layer of heavily pigmented epithelium, the iridial portion of the retina (Figs. 34–9, 34–17).

The anterior stromal sheet or lamella contains a few collagenous fibers and many fibroblasts and melanocytes in a homogeneous ground substance. The color of the iris depends on the quantity and the arrangement of the pigment and on the thickness of the lamella. If this layer is thin and its cells contain little or no pigment, the black pigment epithelium on the posterior surface, as seen through the colorless tissue, gives the iris a blue color (Fig. 34–18). An increasing amount of pigment brings about the different shades of gray and greenish hues. Large amounts of dark pigment cause the brown color of the iris. In albinos, the pigment is absent or scanty, and the iris is pink because of its rich vascularity.

The epithelial pigment layer on the posterior surface of the iris is a direct continuation of the ciliary portion of the retina and, like it, originally consists of two layers of epithelium. The inner, nonpigmented layer of the ciliary portion of the retina becomes heavily pigmented in the iridial region with dark brown melanin granules that obscure the cell

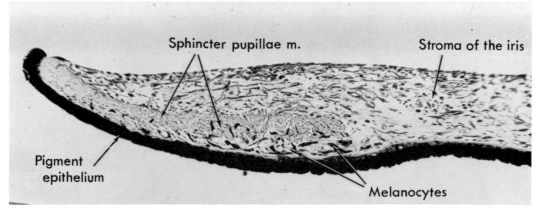

Figure 34–17. Photomicrograph of a transverse section of human iris. (Preparation by T. Kuwabara.)

outlines. The posterior or inner surface is covered by the *limiting membrane of the iris*, a typical basal lamina. The outer or anterior pigmented layer becomes less pigmented. These outer epithelial cells derived from the outer wall of the embryonic optic cup undergo a remarkable transformation into contractile elements—the *myoepithelium of the dilator pupillae*.

Being an adjustable diaphragm, the iris contains two muscles that keep the membrane stretched and hold it against the surface of the lens. The contraction of the circular *sphincter of the pupil* reduces the diameter of the pupil. It is a thin, flat ring surrounding the margin of the pupil. Its breadth changes, according to the contraction of the iris, from 0.6 to 1.2 mm. Its smooth muscle fibers are arranged in thin, circumferentially oriented bundles (Fig. 34–17). The *dilator of the pupil* opens the pupil and consists of radially arranged myoepithelial elements, which form a thin membrane between the vessel layer and the pigment epithelium (Fig. 34–19).

The innervation of the two muscles is quite different. The dilator is innervated by sympathetic postganglionic neurons located in the superior cervical ganglion Their axons pass to the trigeminal ganglion and thence into the ophthalmic branch of the latter, and finally reach the dilator muscle through the long ciliary nerves. The sphincter muscle is innervated by parasympathetic fibers from postganglionic neurons located in the ciliary ganglion, and their axons reach the sphincter

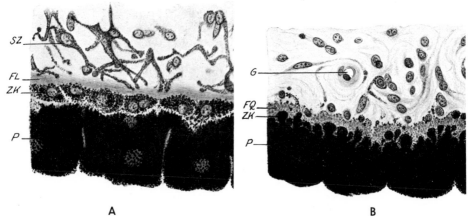

A   B

Figure 34–18. Sections of human iris. *A,* Posterior part of a radial (meridional) section of a dark human iris, from an enucleated eyeball. *FL,* Fibrillae of the dilator muscle in longitudinal section; *P,* pigment epithelium of the inner (posterior) layer of the iridial portion of the retina; *SZ,* pigment-containing connective tissue cells (melanocytes) of the vascular layer; *ZK,* pigment-containing cell bodies of the dilator muscle (outer or anterior layer of the iridial portion of the retina). *B,* Tangential section of a light human iris. *FQ,* Fibers of the dilator muscle in cross section; *G,* blood vessel in the stroma; other symbols as in *A.* × 380. (After Schaffer.)

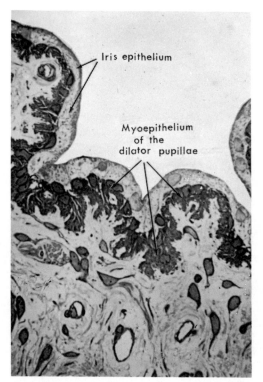

Iris epithelium

Myoepithelium
of the
dilator pupillae

Figure 34-19. Photomicrograph of transverse section through the posterior surface of albino rabbit iris, showing the pale cuboidal iris epithelium and the underlying dark-staining myoepithelium of the dilator pupillae muscle. × 480. (After Richardson, K. C. Am. J. Anat. *114*:173, 1964.)

with the short ciliary nerves. The sympathetic and parasympathetic divisions of the autonomic nervous system thus have opposite effects upon the pupil. On the other hand, the sphincter and the ciliary muscles, which are both innervated by the short ciliary nerves, work in concert. When the eye accommodates for near vision by contraction of the ciliary muscle, there is always a simultaneous contraction of the pupillary sphincter.

In electron micrographs, the axons among the contractile elements of the sphincter pupillae are seen to be packed with synaptic vesicles typical of cholinergic axons. Axons associated with the dilator muscle contain a mixture of dense-cored and agranular vesicles typical of the endings of adrenergic sympathetic nerve fibers.

An accurate adjustment of the size of the pupil modifies the amount of light entering the eye, thus permitting useful vision over a wide range of light intensities. Furthermore, as the pupil constricts in brilliant light, the depth of focus of the dioptric media is increased and aberrations are minimized.

The blood vessels of the iris in the rhesus monkey, and possibly in the human, are unusual in that their walls have the same structure irrespective of their diameter and cannot be classified according to the traditional morphological criteria for distinguishing arterioles, capillaries, and venules (Fig. 34-20). No smooth muscle is found in any of these vessels. Their wall consists of a continuous layer of endothelium on a thin basal lamina; pericytes enclosed between two layers of the basal lamina; and an adventitia of fibroblasts, melanocytes, and occasional macrophages. The intercellular clefts of the endothelium are closed by tight junctions that prevent paracellular escape of macromolecules from the blood, and plasmalemmal vesicles do not transport any significant amount of blood-borne peroxidase across the endothelium. However, if this tracer is perfused through the anterior chamber, it freely enters the iridial stroma and reaches the lumen of the blood vessels by transcellular vesicular transport. The luminal and abluminal plasma membranes of the endothelium seem to bear a different electrical charge, for anionic molecules are readily transported to the lumen but cationic substances are excluded. It is suggested that in the iridial vessels there is a unidirectional vesicular transport that selectively moves anionic organic substances from the anterior chamber to the bloodstream. The importance of this pathway in aqueous humor dynamics has yet to be evaluated.

REFRACTIVE MEDIA OF THE EYE

The cornea and the anterior and posterior chambers of the eye have been described. The other components of the refractive apparatus of the eye are the crystalline lens and vitreous body.

Lens

The lens is a transparent, biconvex body situated immediately behind the pupil. Its shape changes during the process of accommodation. Its outer form varies somewhat in different persons and also with age. Its diameter ranges from 7 mm in a newborn to 10 mm in an adult. Its thickness is approximately 3.7 to 4 mm, increasing during accommodation to 4.5 mm and more. The posterior surface is more convex than the anterior, the

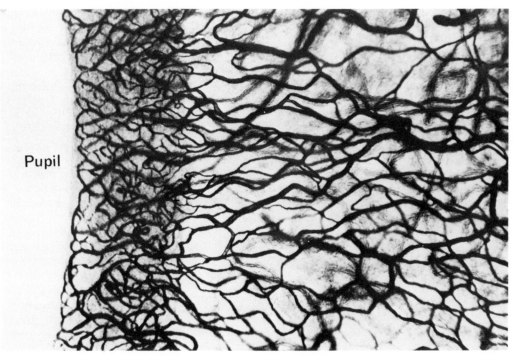

Pupil

Figure 34–20. A whole mount of an injected preparation of the iris of *Macaca mulatta* in moderate mydriasis. A series of large radial vessels gives rise to a complex network of intermediate and small vessels throughout the length of the iris. A continuous arcade of small vessels is seen at the pupillary margin. (Photomicrograph from Freddo, T., and G. Raviola. Invest. Ophthalmol. Vis. Sci. 22:279, 1982.)

respective radii of curvature being 6.9 and 10 mm. The index of refraction is 1.36 in the peripheral layers and 1.4 in the inner zone. The lens weighs 0.2 g and is slightly yellow.

The lens is covered with a homogeneous, highly refractive *capsule*, an 11- to 18-μm coating, rich in collagen and proteoglycans, which invests the outer surface of the layer of cuboidal cells that make up the epithelium of the lens (Figs. 34–21, 34–22). Toward the equator of the lens these cells approach a columnar form and become arranged in meridional rows. Becoming progressively elongated, the cells at the equator are transformed into *lens fibers* that constitute the bulk of the substance of the lens. In this transitional or *nuclear zone* the cells have a characteristic arrangement. The epithelial cells are of prime importance for the normal metabolism of the lens. The capsule covering the posterior surface of the lens has no underlying epithelium.

In the human lens, each cell, commonly called a lens fiber, is a six-sided prism, 7 to 10 mm long, 8 to 12 μm wide, and only 2 μm thick (Fig. 34–23). In the region of the nucleus, the thickness may reach 5 μm. The prismatic fibers of the cortical zone of the lens are hexagonal in cross section. The cell surfaces are about 15 nm apart and attached by numerous gap junctions. The cells of the lens epithelium and the fibers of the equatorial region both exhibit complex interdigitations of their surfaces. This is particularly marked at the "sutures," where cortical fibers from opposite sectors of the lens converge (Fig. 34–23). Since these interdigitations occur principally in the anterior curvature, periaxial zone, and equator—those regions that undergo the greatest dimensional changes—it has been suggested that their presence may be associated with changes of fiber shape in the mechanism of intracapsular accommodation.

The lens fibers have a finely granular cytoplasm, with a few small vesicles scattered through the ectoplasmic region of the cell and occasional mitochondria in the vicinity of the sutures, but in general the organelles and inclusions are exceedingly sparse. Their cytoskeleton consists of abundant intermediate filaments (Fig. 34–24).

The lens is held in position by a system of fibers constituting the *ciliary zonule*. The zonule fibers (Fig. 34–8) arise from the epithe-

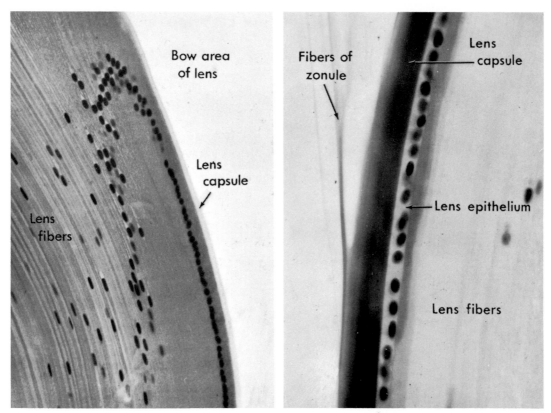

Figure 34–21

Figure 34–22

Figure 34–21. Photomicrograph of the bow area of the human lens, where the epithelial cells become greatly elongated to form lens fibers. (Courtesy of T. Kuwabara.)

Figure 34–22. Photomicrograph at higher magnification of human lens stained with the periodic acid–Schiff reaction. The lens capsule overlying the epithelium stains strongly. Zonule fibers merge with the capsule. (Preparation by T. Kuwabara.)

lium of the ciliary portion of the retina. Near the ciliary crown they fuse into thicker fibers and finally form about 140 bundles. At the anterior margin of the ciliary processes they leave the surface of the ciliary body and radiate toward the equator of the lens. The larger ones are straight and reach the capsule in front of the equator of the lens (*anterior zonular sheet*). The thinner fibers assume a slightly curved course and are attached to the posterior surface of the lens (*posterior zonular sheet*). All zonular fibers break up into a multitude of finer fibers, which fuse with the substance of the outermost layer of the lens capsule (Fig. 34–22). With the electron microscope, the zonular fibers appear as bundles or sheets of exceedingly fine filaments, 11 to 12 nm in diameter, which have a hollow appearance in cross section (Fig. 34–25). They are digested with elastase, but not by collagenase, and have an amino acid composition different from collagen. They are iden-

tical to the microfibrils embedded in the elastic fibers of other organs. Where the vitreous body touches the lens capsule, it forms the *hyaloideocapsular ligament*.

The radii of curvature of the surfaces of the several dioptric media of the normal eye, especially of the lens, and their indices of refraction are such that light rays coming from a remote point form an inverted and real image of the object in the layer of the photoreceptive cones and rods in the retina. If the object is approaching, the light rays diverge more and more, and the image moves backward in the retina. A change of position of an object from infinite distance to about 5 m causes the image to shift about 60 μm backward in the retina. Since this image is still within the outer segments of the rods and cones, accommodation is not needed. For nearer distances, accommodation is necessary.

In a camera, the focusing of objects that

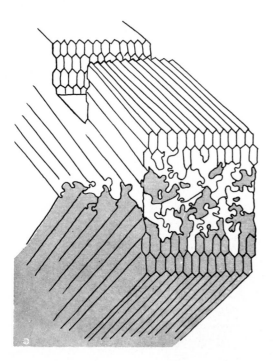

Figure 34–23. Schematic drawing of the arrangement of lens fibers in rows and their prevailing hexagonal cross-sectional form, except in the suture area, where there may be considerable irregularities and interdigitation of fibers converging from opposite sectors of the lens. (After Wanko, T., and M. Gavin: The Structure of the Eye. New York, Academic Press, 1961.)

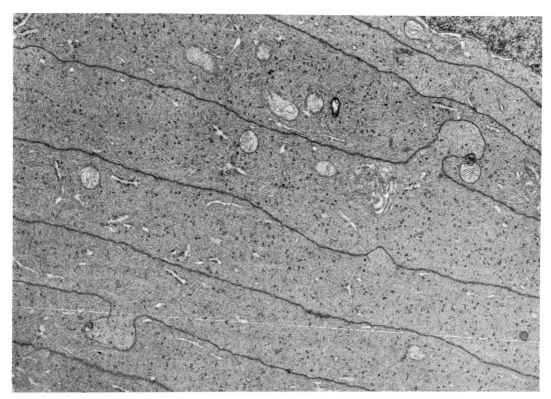

Figure 34–24. Electron micrograph of cortical fibers of the human lens. A few profiles of granular endoplasmic reticulum, occasional mitochondria, and numerous polyribosomes are distributed in an otherwise homogeneous and concentrated cytoplasmic matrix. (Courtesy of T. Kuwabara.)

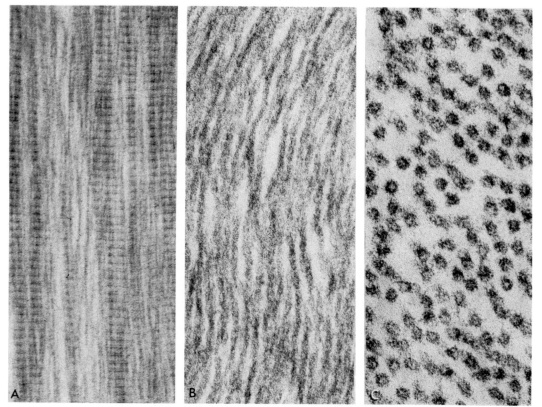

Figure 34–25. Electron micrograph of ciliary zonule in monkeys. *A, B,* Zonular fibers, which consist of exceedingly fine fibrils, 11 to 12 nm in diameter. When fibrils are tightly packed *(A)*, the zonular fibers display a cross striation. *A,* × 40,000; *B,* × 160,000. *C,* In cross section, the fibrils have a hollow appearance. *C,* × 200,000. (From Raviola, G. Invest. Ophthalmol. *10*:851, 1971.)

move nearer to the lens is effected by moving the ground glass plate away from the lens. In the higher vertebrates and in the human, the curvature of the lens is changed. When the eye is at rest, the lens is kept stretched by the ciliary zonule in the plane vertical to the optic axis. When the eye has to focus on a near object, the ciliary muscle contracts—its meridional fibers pull the choroid and the ciliary body forward, whereas its circular fibers, acting as a sphincter, move the ciliary body toward the axis of the eye. This relieves the tension on the zonule; the lens gets thicker, and its surface, especially at the anterior pole, becomes more convex. This increases the refractive power of the lens and keeps the focus within the photoreceptor layer.

Vitreous Body

The vitreous body fills the vitreal cavity between the lens and the retina. It adheres everywhere to the optical portion of the ret-

ina, and the connection is especially firm at the ora serrata. Farther forward, it gradually recedes from the surface of the ciliary portion of the retina.

The fresh vitreous body is a colorless, structureless, gelatinous mass with a glasslike transparency. Its index of refraction is 1.334. Nearly 99 per cent of the vitreous body consists of water. A liquid and a solid phase can be distinguished in it; the liquid phase contains hyaluronic acid in the form of long, coiled molecules enclosing large amounts of water; the solid phase is collagen in the form of thin fibrils that lack the usual 64-nm periodicity and are arranged in a random network. The hyaluronate of the liquid phase is joined to the collagen network by weak bonds. The peripheral region of the vitreous body or cortex has more collagen fibrils and hyaluronate than the central region and contains cells, called *hyalocytes,* which may be concerned with the synthesis of collagen and hyaluronic acid. Macrophages also are occasionally found.

Extending through the vitreous body from the papilla of the optic nerve to the posterior surface of the lens is the *hyaloid canal* (canal of Cloquet). It is a residue remaining after the resorption of the embryonic hyaloid artery. It has a diameter of 1 mm and is filled with liquid. In the living, especially in young persons, it is visible with the help of the slit lamp microscope.

THE RETINA

The retina is the innermost of the three coats of the eyeball and is the photoreceptor organ. It arises in early embryonic development from a bilateral evagination of the prosencephalon, the *primary optic vesicle*. Later it is transformed by local invagination into the *secondary optic vesicle*. Each optic cup remains connected with the brain by a stalk, the future optic nerve. In the adult, the derivatives of the bilaminar secondary optic vesicle consist of an outer pigmented epithelial layer, the *pigment epithelium*, and an inner sheet, the *neural retina* or *retina proper*. The latter contains elements similar to those of the brain, and it may be considered to be a specially differentiated part of the brain.

The *optical* or functioning portion of the retina lines the inner surface of the choroid and extends from the papilla of the optic nerve to the ora serrata anteriorly. At the papilla, where the retina is continuous with the tissue of the nerve, and at the ora serrata, the retina is firmly connected with the choroid. In the retina, exclusive of the fovea, the papilla, and the ora serrata, ten parallel layers can be distinguished from outside inward (Figs. 34–27, 34–28): (1) the pigment epithelium; (2) the layer of rods and cones; (3) the outer limiting membrane; (4) the outer nuclear layer; (5) the outer plexiform layer; (6) the inner nuclear layer; (7) the inner plexiform layer; (8) the layer of ganglion cells; (9) the layer of optic nerve fibers; and (10) the inner limiting membrane. About 2.5 mm lateral to the border of the optic papilla, the inner surface of the retina shows a shallow, round depression, the *fovea* (Figs. 34–26, 34–45). This is surrounded by the *central area*, distinguished by the great number of ganglion cells and by the general refinement and even distribution of the structural elements, especially of the rods and cones. The smallest and most precisely ordered sensory elements of the retina are in the fovea, where they are accumulated in greatest numbers. In the retinal periphery, the elements are fewer, larger, and less evenly distributed.

When detached from the pigment epithelium, the fresh retina is almost perfectly transparent. It has a distinctly red color because of the presence in its rod cells of *visual purple*, or *rhodopsin*. Light rapidly bleaches the visual purple; in darkness the color gradually reappears. The fovea and its immediate vicinity contain yellow pigment and are called the *macula lutea*. Large blood vessels circle above and below the central fovea, whereas only fine arteries, veins, and capillaries are present in it. In the very center of the fovea, in an area measuring 0.5 mm across, even the capillaries are absent, greatly increasing its transparency.

Only the portion of the image of an external object that falls upon the fovea is seen sharply. Accordingly, the eyes are moved so as to bring the object of special attention into this central part of the visual field. Photoreceptors are absent from the optic papilla. This is the "blind spot" of the visual field.

Pigment Epithelium

This sheet of heavily pigmented epithelial cells is derived from the outer layer of the cuplike outgrowth of the embryonic nervous system that gives rise to the retina, and it has traditionally been included as one of the layers of the retina (Figs. 34–27, 34–29). Bruch's membrane, on the other hand, has been considered part of the choroid. The demonstration that this latter structure includes the basal lamina of the pigment epithelium makes it illogical to assign the pigment epithelium to the retina and its basal lamina to the choroid. Some authors therefore prefer to consider the pigment epithelium as a component of the choroid. Although the cells of this layer extend processes that interdigitate with the retinal rods and cones, there is no actual anatomical connection between the photosensitive and the pigmented layers, except at the head of the optic nerve and at the ora serrata. An artifactitious separation is found between the two layers in most histological preparations, and in the "retinal detachment" that is a common cause of partial blindness, the separation occurs along this plane of cleavage between the photosensitive elements of the retina and the pigment epithelium.

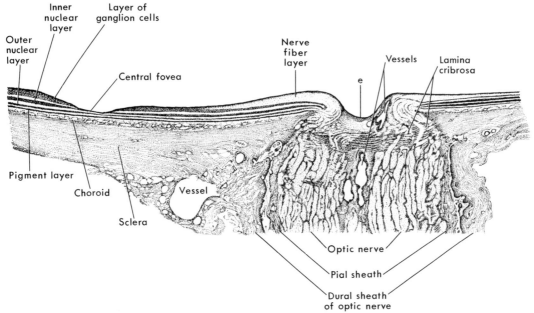

Figure 34–26. Central fovea and place of entrance of the optic nerve as seen in a horizontal meridional section of an enucleated human eye. *e,* Excavation. × 18. (Redrawn and slightly modified from Schaffer.)

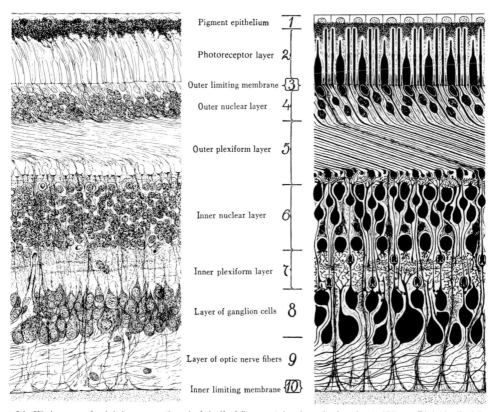

Pigment epithelium   *1*

Photoreceptor layer   *2*

Outer limiting membrane   *3*

Outer nuclear layer   *4*

Outer plexiform layer   *5*

Inner nuclear layer   *6*

Inner plexiform layer   *7*

Layer of ganglion cells   *8*

Layer of optic nerve fibers   *9*

Inner limiting membrane   *10*

Figure 34–27. Layers of adult human retina. Left half of figure stained routinely, about 400 ×. Right half of figure is a schematic reconstruction from sections stained with Golgi's method. (Slightly modified from Polyak.)

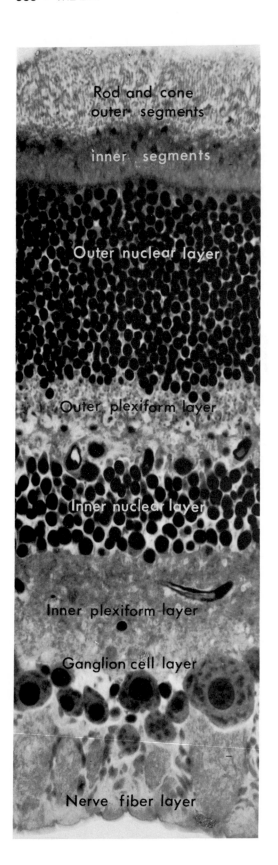

Figure 34–28. Photomicrograph of cat retina. (Courtesy of A. J. Ladman.)

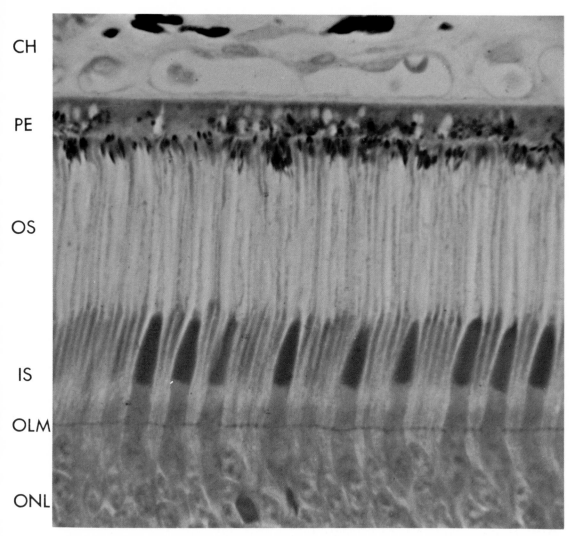

Figure 34–29. Light micrograph of the outermost retinal layers in a monkey. Cones are easily distinguished from rods, for their inner segment is larger and the ellipsoid intensely stained. *CH,* choroid; *PE,* pigment epithelium; *OS,* outer segments; *IS,* inner segments; *OLM,* outer limiting membrane; *ONL,* outer nuclear layer. (Courtesy of J. Rostgaard.)

Pigment epithelial cells have a remarkably regular shape, appearing as hexagonal prisms about 14 μm wide and 10 to 14 μm tall; toward the ora serrata, they increase in diameter. The cell base, which rests on Bruch's membrane, displays the labyrinth of interdigitating processes typical of actively transporting epithelia, whereas the lateral cell surface has only a slightly undulating course. Adjacent cells are connected to each other by a junctional complex consisting of apical gap junctions, followed by an elaborate tight junction and a zonula adherens. The cell apex, which faces the rods and cones, gives rise to two sorts of processes: cylindrical sheaths, which invest the tip of the photoreceptor outer segments, and slender microvilli, which occupy the interstices between the photoreceptors. The cell nucleus is displaced toward the cell base, and numerous mitochondria intervene between the nucleus and basal labyrinth of interdigitating processes. The most prominent feature of the apical cytoplasm is the presence of numerous melanin granules, elliptical or rounded in shape. A second important component of the apical cytoplasm consists of residual bodies filled with lamellar debris, which represents the partially digested residue of the phagocytized tips of the rod outer segments. Another prominent feature of the cytoplasm of these cells is a highly developed agranular endoplasmic reticulum in the form of a rich network of branching and anastomosing tubules that permeate the interstices among the melanin granules and residual bodies. Cisternae of the granular endoplasmic reticulum and a supranuclear Golgi apparatus complete the list of the cytoplasmic organelles.

The pigment epithelium has many important functions. The tight junctions that seal the intercellular spaces between adjoining epithelial cells protect the retina proper from undesirable metabolites that may be present in the stroma of the choroid. The pigment granules absorb light after it has traversed the photoreceptor layer, thus preventing its reflection from the external ocular tunics. In retinas of lower vertebrates, it has been shown that the pigment granules migrate along cell processes among the photoreceptors upon illumination, thus effectively screening scattered light, and they return to the cell body in the dark. The pigment epithelial cells participate in the turnover of the photoreceptors, continuously engulfing and digesting the growing tips of the rod outer segments. Finally regeneration of rhodopsin after exposure to light occurs only if photoreceptors maintain an intimate relationship with the pigment epithelium. Vitamin A, a precursor of rhodopsin and one of the products of rhodopsin degradation upon light absorption, moves to the pigment epithelium after maximal light adaptation and returns to the photoreceptors during dark adaptation. Vitamin A is a fat-soluble hydrocarbon and may be stored in the membranes of the agranular endoplasmic reticulum found throughout the cytoplasm of the cells of the pigment epithelium.

Neural Retina

The retina proper contains six types of neurons: (1) *photoreceptor cells*, (2) *horizontal cells*, (3) *bipolar cells*, (4) *amacrine cells*, (5) *interplexiform cells*, and (6) *ganglion cells*. Photoreceptor, horizontal, and bipolar cells synapse with each other in the *outer plexiform layer*; bipolar, amacrine, and ganglion cells synapse with each other in the *inner plexiform layer*. Interplexiform cells provide a centrifugal pathway for transfer of signals from inner to outer plexiform layer. The axons of the ganglion cells leave the retina to become fibers of the optic nerve. The retinal neurons are supported by neuroglial elements called *radial cells of Müller*.

Photoreceptor Cells

There are two kinds of visual cells, the *rod cells* and the *cone cells*. Their outer segments are the parts sensitive to light, and the light rays, before reaching them, must first penetrate most of the retina.

Rod Cells. The rod cell is a long, slender, highly specialized cell with its outer portion vertical to the retinal layers (Figs. 34–29, 34–30, 34–31). The parallel arrangement of these elements is responsible for the regular striation of the layer of rods and cones. The scleral part of the rod cell, the *rod proper*, is situated between the outer limiting membrane and the pigment epithelium, its outward third being embedded in the pigment-containing processes of the pigment epithelial cells. The vitreal end of the rod proper extends through the so-called outer limiting membrane into the outer nuclear layer. The rods are fairly uniform in appearance, although their dimensions vary somewhat from region to region. Their thickness in the central area is 1 to 1.5 μm, gradually increasing to 2.5 or 3 μm near the ora serrata. Their length decreases from approximately 60 μm near the fovea to 40 μm in the far periphery. Each rod proper consists of an outer and an inner segment. The *outer segment* is a slender cylinder of uniform thickness, which appears homogeneous in the fresh condition. It possesses a peculiarly brillant refractility and is positively birefringent in polarized light. The *inner segment* contains the usual co185lement of cytoplasmic organelles.

The finer structure of the rod cells has been greatly clarified by electron microscopy. The outer segment in longitudinal section is seen to be composed of a very large number of parallel lamellae oriented transverse to the axis of the rod (Figs. 34–32A, 34–33). Each lamella is in fact a closed, membrane-limited sac flattened into a disc approximately 2 μm in diameter and about 14 nm thick. In section, therefore, the profile of each lamella or disc appears as a pair of parallel membranes continuous with one another at the ends and enclosing an exceedingly narrow cavity about 8 nm across. The outer segment is joined to the inner segment by a slender stalk, which contains nine longitudinally oriented doublet microtubules terminating in a centriole or basal body in the distal end of the inner segment. In transverse sections, the stalk has the appearance of a defective cilium, having

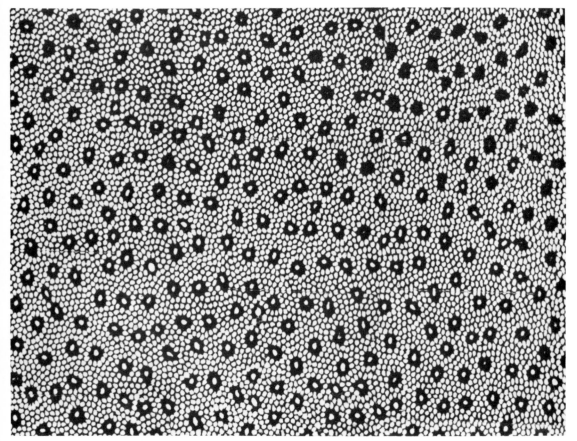

Figure 34–30. Light micrograph of a cross section through the outer segments of the photoreceptor cells in the retinal periphery of a monkey. The large diameter of cone inner segments keeps the rods at a distance from cone outer segments. Toluidine blue, printed as a negative. × 800. (Courtesy of E. Raviola.)

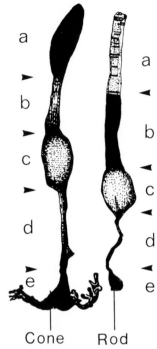

a

b

c

d

e

a

b

c

d

e

Cone   Rod

Figure 34–31. A cone cell and rod cell from a rabbit retina stained with the Golgi technique and drawn with a camera lucida. *a,* Outer segment; *b,* inner segment; *c,* cell body; *d,* inner fiber; *e,* synaptic ending (pedicle in cone; spherule in rod). (Courtesy of G. Sacchi and E. Raviola.)

the nine peripheral doublets but lacking the central pair of singlet microtubules. Studies on the development of the photoreceptors have shown that the outer segments of the rods do in fact develop by modification of cilia. The inner segment consists of two portions, the *ellipsoid* toward the sclera and the *myoid* toward the vitreous. The ellipsoid contains a great number of mitochondria. Cross-striated fibrous rootlets may extend downward from the basal body of the rod outer segment among the mitochondria. The myoid contains the Golgi apparatus, free ribosomes, and cisternae of both agranular and granular endoplasmic reticulum. Microtubules are abundant throughout the rod inner segment.

Autoradiographic studies with the light and electron microscopes demonstrate that the outer segments of rod cells are being renewed constantly. Protein is first synthesized on the ribosomes of the myoid; after moving through the Golgi apparatus, it migrates to the base of the outer segment, where it is used in the assembly of the membranous discs. As new discs are continuously

added at the vitreal end of the outer segments, the old ones move sclerally toward the tip of the rods till they are phagocytized and destroyed by the cells of the pigment epithelium (Fig. 34–35). In the rat, rod outer segments are totally renewed in about ten days.

The rest of the rod cell is made up of the *outer fiber,* the *cell body,* the *inner fiber,* and the rod synaptic ending or *spherule* (Fig. 34–31). The rod outer fiber is a slender protoplasmic process, 1 μm or less in thickness, that extends from the base of the inner segment of the rod proper deep into the outer nuclear layer. Here it joins a spherical cell body containing the rod nucleus, which is smaller and stains more intensely than the cone nucleus. The rod nuclei represent the majority of the nuclei of the outer nuclear layer in all retinal regions except in the fovea, where rods are few, and in its center, where they are absent. The rod inner fiber, rich in microtubules, connects the body to a pear-shaped spherule, rich in synaptic vesicles, located in the outer plexiform layer. In the central area, the rod inner fibers assume a slanting-to-horizontal course, while in the more peripheral retinal regions they are vertical. The rod proper, along with the outer fiber, is the homologue of a dendrite of a neuron; the inner rod fiber corresponds to the axon, and through its terminal spherule this fiber is connected to bipolar and horizontal cells.

All rod cells, except those in a zone 3 to 4 mm wide at the ora serrata, contain visual purple or rhodopsin, the substance responsible for absorption of light. The rhodopsin molecules are localized in the interior of the membrane of the outer segment discs, where they appear as intramembrane particles in freeze-fractured specimens (Fig. 34–34).

As there are only a few rods in the periphery of the fovea and none in its center, this area appears devoid of rhodopsin. When the retina is exposed to light, rhodopsin breaks down, but it is constantly produced anew. This regeneration occurs only as long as the close relation of the rods with the pigment epithelium is preserved.

Cone Cells. These neurons (Figs. 34–29, 34–30, 34–31) are made up of essentially the same parts as the rod cells, but they differ in certain details. There is no visual purple in the cones but instead there are different types of pigments sensitive to blue, green,

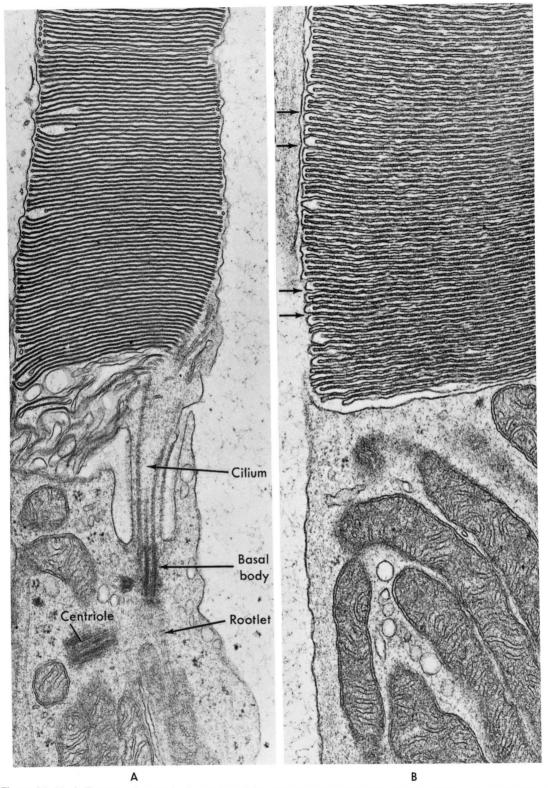

A   B

Figure 34–32. *A,* Electron micrograph of a portion of the outer and inner segment of a rod, showing the connection of the two by a modified cilium. *B,* Corresponding region of a cone. Notice that some of the discs are open to the extracellulr space *(arrows).* (Courtesy of T. Kuwabara.)

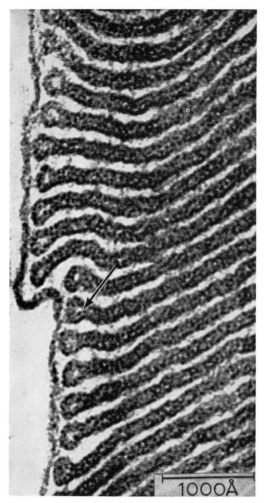

Figure 34–33. Electron micrograph showing profiles of the membranous discs of the outer segment of a rod cell from frog retina. They exhibit a compact granular fine structure *(arrow)* when prepared with very-low-temperature and osmium fixation (osmium-cryofixation), low-temperature dehydration, and embedding. (Courtesy of H. Fernández-Morán.)

possibly significant difference between rods and cones.

The cone outer segment is also connected to the inner segment by an eccentrically placed modified cilium, terminating in a basal body set in the distal end of the inner segment. The other member of the diplosome is usually oriented at a right angle to the basal body, and striated rootlets extend from it downward among the longitudinally oriented mitochondria that crowd the ellipsoid. Cone inner segments resemble in fine structure those of rod cells (Figs. 34–36, 34–37).

The cones vary considerably in different regions of the retina. In the central fovea, they measure 75 μm or more in length and from 1 to 1.5 μm in thickness. Their length gradually decreases to 45 μm in the periphery. The relative length of the outer and the inner segments is usually 3:4. In the fovea the two segments are approximately the same length. The proximal end of the inner cone segment occupies an opening in the "outer

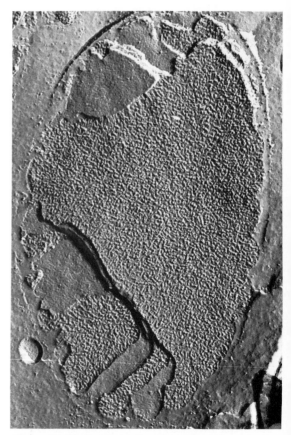

Figure 34–34. Freeze-fracture appearance of a rod outer segment in a monkey. The membranes of the discs contain a large number of particles, which probably are rhodopsin. × 82,500. (Courtesy of E. Raviola.)

and red light. Instead of a slender cylinder, the cone outer segment is a long conical structure, considerably wider than a rod at its base and tapering down to a blunt rounded tip. As in the rod, the outer segment is made up of a large number of discs stacked one above the other. Each of these consists of a pair of membranes. In most of the discs the two membranes are continuous at their margins and enclose a narrow space. In the discs close to the inner segment, the two membranes are continuous with the plasma membrane, and the narrow cleft between them is open to the extracellular space (Fig. 34–32B). This appears to be a consistent and

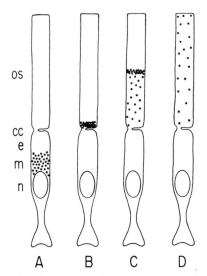

OS

CC

e

m

n

A   B   C   D

Figure 34–35. Diagram illustrating the turnover of rod outer segments. After injection of a radioactive amino acid, electron microscope autoradiography shows that the label is first concentrated in the myoid of rod cells *(A),* where ribosomes and the Golgi apparatus are contained. Later, labeled protein moves to the membranous discs at the base of the outer segments *(B)* and ascends progressively toward the tip of the rods *(C).* Finally, it disappears from rod cells *(D)* and becomes localized in the residual bodies contained in the cytoplasm of the pigment epithelium cells. *OS,* outer segments; *CC,* connecting cilium; *e,* ellipsoid; *m,* myoid; *n,* nucleus. (From Young, R. W., and D. Bok. J. Cell Biol. *42*:392, 1969.)

limiting membrane," and protrudes slightly into the fourth layer.

In teleostean fishes and amphibians the inner cone segment is contractile. It shortens in bright light and stretches in dim light or darkness. The displacement of these cones is, accordingly, opposite in direction to that of the rod.

In contrast to rods, the turnover of cone outer segments involves neither continuous movement of the discs toward the pigment epithelium nor phagocytosis of the growing tips by the pigment epithelium cells. Proteins found in the inner segment are inserted randomly into the disc membrane throughout the outer segment. The reason for this difference is not clear.

Proximal to the outer limiting membrane, the inner cone segment merges with its *body,* containing a nucleus, which is larger and paler-staining than the rod nucleus. The bodies and nuclei of the cones, in contrast to those of the rods, are arranged in a single row immediately beneath the outer limiting membrane. Exceptional in this regard are the cones in the outer fovea, whose nuclei are accumulated in several rows. Only in this

region do the cones have an *outer fiber.* But from the body of all cones, a stout, smooth *inner fiber* descends to the middle zone of the outer plexiform layer, where it terminates with a thick triangular or club-shaped synaptic ending, the *cone pedicle.* Up to a dozen short, barblike processes emanate from the base of each pedicle, except in the fovea, where there are usually none. These outgrowths are deployed horizontally in the outer plexiform layer. The length and course of the inner cone fibers may vary considerably, depending on the region, the longest (600 μm) and most nearly horizontally placed being those in the central area, where the inner rod and cone fibers form a thick fiber layer at the boundary between outer nuclear and outer plexiform layers, called the *outer fiber layer of Henle.* The inner cone fibers have all the characteristics of an axon, while the cone pedicle has those of the synaptic ending of a neuron and makes synapses with bipolar and horizontal cells.

The number of cones in the human retina is estimated at 6 to 7 millions. The ratio of the number of nerve fibers of the optic nerve (438,000) to the number of cones of one eye is 1:6 or 1:7.

The relative number and distribution of the rods and cones in different vertebrates present great variations, depending on the mode of life. In diurnal birds the cones are more numerous than the rods. In most diurnal reptiles, rods are exceedingly rare. In many nocturnal vertebrates, only rods are present, although in others a few rudimentary cones can be found among numerous rods. On similar comparative data M. Schultze (1866) based his assumption that there is a difference in function of the two kinds of photoreceptors.

Outer Limiting Membrane. The dense staining line traditionally called the *outer limiting membrane* is not a membrane at all. Instead, it is found in electron micrographs to be a row of zonulae adherentes where the photoreceptor cells are attached to the Müller cells, which surround and support all the neural elements (Fig. 34–38). Distal to this row of zonulae adherentes, tufts of microvilli project from the free surface of the Müller cells into interstices between the rod and cone inner segments.

Horizontal Cells

These cells are typical neurons whose bodies form the uppermost one or two rows of

Figure 34–36

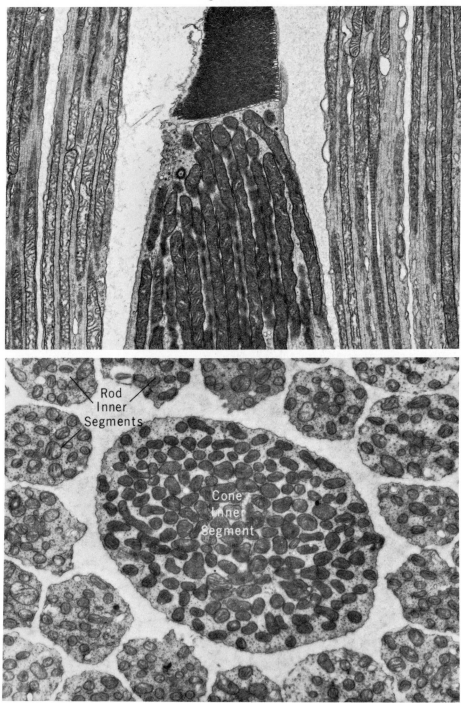

Figure 34–37

Figure 34–36. Vertical section of the inner segments of a cone and several neighboring rods in the human retina, illustrating the larger size of the cone and the high concentration of longitudinally oriented mitochondria in the ellipsoid. (Courtesy of T. Kuwabara.)

Figure 34–37. Horizontal section through the inner segments of the photoreceptor elements in rat retina. Notice the larger size of the cone ellipsoid and its great number of mitochondria. (After Marchesi, V. T., M. L. Sears, and R. J. Barrnett. Invest. Ophthalmol. 3:1, 1964.)

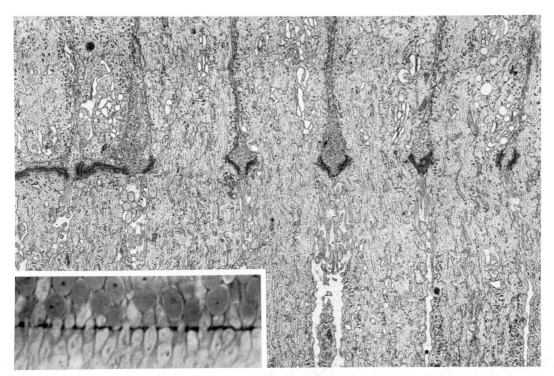

Figure 34–38. Electron micrograph of the region of the "outer limiting membrane" of the retina, showing that it is not a membrane, as it appears to be with the light microscope *(inset)*, but a row of zonulae adherentes between the rod and cone cells and the surrounding Müller cells. (Courtesy of T. Kuwabara.)

the inner nuclear layer. From the scleral end of the body arise short dendritic twigs, which produce several tufts deployed in the outer plexiform layer. Each dendritic tuft is connected to a single cone pedicle. The axon takes a horizontal course in the outer plexiform layer, and its terminal twigs come into contact with rod spherules (Fig. 34–39). In mammals such as the cat and rabbit, horizontal cells without an axon are also found.

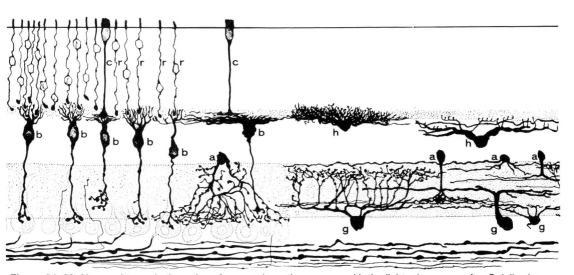

Figure 34–39. Neuronal types in the retina of mammals as they appear with the light microscope after Golgi's chromo-argentic impregnation. *r,* Rod cells (dog); *c,* cone cells (dog); *b,* bipolar cells (dog); *h,* horizontal cells (dog); *a,* amacrine cells (dog and ox); *g,* ganglion cells (ox). In rod and cone cells, the photoreceptor proper is not represented. (After Cajal, 1893, modified.)

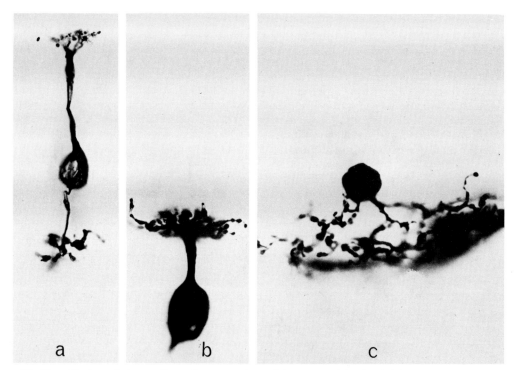

Figure 34–40. *a,* Bipolar cell; *b,* ganglion cell; *c,* amacrine cell impregnated by the Golgi technique. The bipolar and ganglion cells are from the retina of *Macaca mulatta;* the amacrine cell is from rabbit retina. (Photomicrograph courtesy of E. Raviola.)

Bipolar Cells

These neurons extend from the outer to the inner plexiform layer and therefore stand approximately upright with respect to the retinal layers (Figs. 34–39, 34–40). Their body is located in the inner nuclear layer and gives rise to one or more primary dendrites, which ascend to the outer plexiform layer, where they branch and connect with the photoreceptor cell terminals. The single, inwardly directed axon of the bipolar cells ramifies in the inner plexiform layer, where it is synaptically related to ganglion and amacrine cells. Four types of bipolar cells can be distinguished in the primate retina: (1) *rod bipolar cells,* which connect to rod cells; (2) and (3) *invaginating midget bipolar cells* and *flat midget bipolar cells,* each synapsing with a single cone pedicle; and (4) *flat* or *diffuse cone bipolar cells,* connected to many cone pedicles. The precise synaptic relationships of the axon terminals of the four types of bipolar cells with the various types of amacrine and ganglion cells are poorly understood.

Outer Plexiform Layer

This is the region of synaptic interplay between photoreceptor, bipolar, and horizontal cells. The synaptic terminals of cone cells or pedicles are large pyramidal endings containing synaptic vesicles and mitochondria, whose flattened base is invaginated at many points to enclose the tips of the dendrites of the horizontal and invaginating midget bipolar cells. The remaining free surface of the base of the pedicle makes hundreds of superficial or basal contacts with the dendrites of the flat midget and diffuse cone bipolars. With a high degree of consistency and geometrical order, each of the 12 to 25 synaptic invaginations of a cone pedicle contains the tip of two horizontal cell dendrites and one dendrite of an invaginating midget bipolar cell (a "*triad*"). The horizontal cell dendrites may contain synaptic vesicles, are deeply inserted, and lie on either side of a wedge-shaped projection of the pedicle, called the *synaptic ridge.* The dendrite of the invaginating midget bipolar cell lies centrally and more superficially, separated from the apex of the ridge by the cleft intervening between adjoining horizontal cell dendrites. The synaptic ridge is bisected by a dense lamella or synaptic ribbon, surrounded by a halo of synaptic vesicles; the ribbon sits at a right angle to the apex of the ridge, separated from the pedicle membrane by a trough-shaped body, the acriform density (Fig.

34–41*B*). The significance of the synaptic ribbon is poorly understood, but it is probably instrumental in capturing synaptic vesicles and positioning them near the plasma membrane. The superficial or basal contacts of cone pedicles do not display prominent junctional specializations; the synaptic cleft is slightly enlarged and the adjoining membranes of the pedicle and bipolar dendrites bear a layer of fluffy cytoplasmic material.

Rod spherules have a single synaptic invagination and no basal contacts. In their invaginating synapse, two deeply inserted axonal endings of the horizontal cells lie on either side of a ridge containing a ribbon and vesicles (Fig. 34–41*A*). The tips of one to four dendrites belonging to the rod bipolar cells lie centrally and less deeply inserted. The axonal endings of the horizontal cells often contain synaptic vesicles.

Using Golgi's chromo-argentic impregna-tion and electron microscopy, the neural interconnections in the outer plexiform layer of the primate retina have been worked out in great detail. Both invaginating and flat midget bipolars are "private" cone bipolars; that is, each of them is contacted by a single cone pedicle. The invaginating variety, however, sends its dendrites to the invaginating synapses, whereas the flat variety makes basal contacts with the cone pedicles. The diffuse cone bipolars, on the other hand, touch about six cone pedicles at superficial contacts. The rod bipolar cells connect exclusively with rod cells; their dendritic terminals end as slightly inserted processes in the invaginations of numerous spherules. Horizontal cells contact cone cells with their dendrites and rod cells with their axon; both dendritic and axonal terminals of these cells end as deeply inserted processes in the invaginating synapses (Fig. 34–42).

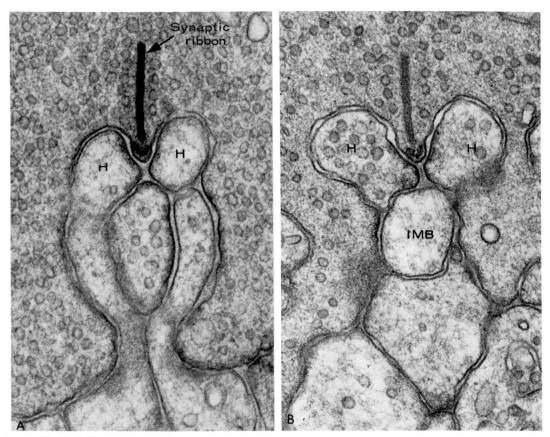

Figure 34–41. *A,* Electron micrograph of the invaginating synapse of a rod spherule in the retina of a rabbit. Two deeply inserted processes *(H),* probably arising from the axon of the horizontal cells, lie on either side of a wedge-shaped projection of the spherule (synaptic ridge), which contains the synaptic ribbon, surrounded by a halo of synaptic vesicles, and the arciform density. The dendrites of the rod bipolar cells cannot be identified in this micrograph. ×65,000. *B,* Invaginating synapse of a cone pedicle in the retina of a monkey. A typical "triad" consists of two deeply invaginated dendrites of the horizontal cells *(H)* and a slightly inserted, centrally positioned dendrite of an invaginating midget bipolar cell *(IMB).* Notice the synaptic vesicles in the horizontal cell dendrites. ×65,000. (Micrographs courtesy of E. Raviola.)

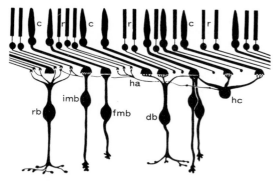

Figure 34–42. Diagram of the synaptic connections in the outer plexiform layer of the primate retina. For explanation, see text. *c,* Cone cells; *r,* rod cells; *rb,* rod bipolar cell; *imb,* invaginating midget bipolar cell; *fmb,* flat midget bipolar cell; *db,* diffuse cone bipolar cell; *ha,* horizontal cell axon; *hc,* horizontal cell. (From Kolb, H. Phil. Trans. R. Soc. Lond. B 258:261, 1970.)

Amacrine Cells

These neurons have numerous dendrites but lack an axon (Figs. 34–39, 34–40c). Their body lies in the vitreal part of the inner nuclear layer, and their dendrites spread in the inner plexiform layer. They connect with each other, with the axonal endings of the bipolar cells, and with the dendrites of the ganglion cells. The primate retina contains numerous varieties of amacrine cells; these are classified as *diffuse* and *stratified*. Diffuse amacrine cells send their dendritic branches throughout the thickness of the inner plexiform layer, whereas the ramifications of the stratified amacrine cells are confined to different sublaminae of the inner plexiform layer.

Interplexiform Cells

Interplexiform cells have their perikaryon in the inner nuclear layer and send their processes to both plexiform layers. In the inner plexiform layer, their processes are both pre- and postsynaptic to amacrine cell dendrites. In the outer plexiform layer, their processes are exclusively presynaptic to horizontal and bipolar cells. Thus, the input to these cells is confined to the inner plexiform layer, whereas their output is in both plexiform layers.

Ganglion Cells

Ganglion cells represent the terminal link of the neural networks of the retina. With their dendrites, they connect with bipolar endings and amacrine dendrites in the inner plexiform layer; their body is located in the ganglion cell layer; their axon, which becomes a fiber of the optic nerve, conducts to the brain the results of the complex neural activity that takes place in the retina. The primate retina contains numerous varieties of ganglion cells, classified according to the shape of their dendritic tree and the mode of distribution of their dendritic branches in the inner plexiform layer. In the central area the most common type of ganglion cell is represented by the *midget ganglion cell,* characterized by a single dendritic shaft that ascends into the inner plexiform layer, where it ends with a minute basket of short secondary and tertiary dendrites. *Diffuse ganglion cells* send their dendrites throughout the thickness of the inner plexiform layer, whereas *stratified ganglion cells* have their dendritic arborization confined to one or more levels of the inner plexiform layer. Intermediate forms between diffuse and stratified ganglion cells are also described.

Inner Plexiform Layer

This is the region of synaptic interplay between bipolar, amacrine, and ganglion cells. Two kinds of synaptic contacts are found in this layer: the ribbon synapse, characterized by a dense lamella, surrounded by a halo of vesicles in the presynaptic process; and a more conventional type of synaptic contact, which lacks ribbon and is characterized by clustering of vesicles against the presynaptic membrane (Fig. 34–43). At ribbon synapses, the axonal endings of the bipolar cells are presynaptic to amacrine and ganglion cell dendrites. Amacrine cell dendrites, in turn, make conventional synapses with bipolar endings, ganglion cell dendrites, and dendrites of other amacrine cells. Reciprocal synapses between bipolar terminals and amacrine dendrites frequently occur in this layer, with the bipolar contacting the amacrine cell as the presynaptic element of a ribbon synapse, and the amacrine cell returning a conventional feedback synapse onto the bipolar. Thus, amacrine cell dendrites have the unusual property of containing synaptic vesicles and behaving as presynaptic elements of *dendroaxonic* and *dendrodendritic* synapses. The existence of dendrodendritic synapses was originally described in the olfactory bulb, where the granule cells, which lack an axon, establish reciprocal dendrodendritic synapses with the dendrites of the mitral cells.

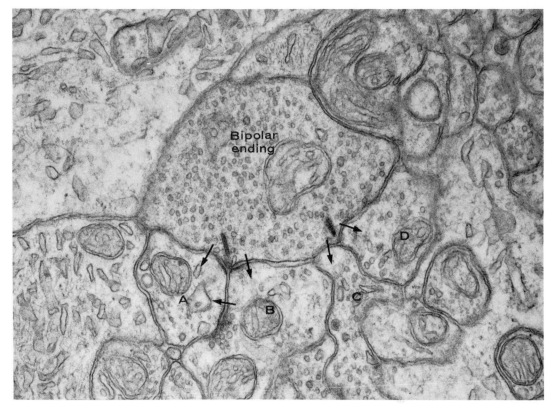

Figure 34–43. Electron micrograph of a portion of the inner plexiform layer in the retina of a monkey. An axonal ending of a bipolar cell makes two ribbon synapses with four processes, labeled *A, B, C,* and *D*. Processes *B, C,* and *D* contain synaptic vesicles and may represent dendrites of amacrine cells. Process *B* makes a conventional type of synaptic contact with process *A*, whose identity is unknown. Arrows indicate the direction of the synaptic influences. × 38,400. (Courtesy of E. Raviola.)

The precise pattern of neural interconnections in the inner plexiform layer is poorly understood. Sublayers can be distinguished in it, for the axonal arborizations of the bipolar cells and the dendritic expansions of the stratified amacrine and ganglion cells are distributed at different levels within the layer. This and recent findings in nonprimate retinas suggest that the various types of bipolar, amacrine, and ganglion cells establish specific synaptic connections with each other. However, the details of their "wiring" have not yet been worked out for the primate retina.

Optic Nerve Fibers in the Primate Retina

Because of the presence of the central fovea, the optic nerve fibers have a special course. In general they converge radially toward the optic papilla. However, those originating in the upper temporal quadrant of the retina circle above the central area, while those originating in the lower temporal quadrant circle below it on their way to the papilla. They follow the larger retinal vessels fairly closely. A line connecting the fovea with the temporal circumference of the retina separates the optic nerve fibers of the upper from those of the lower temporal quadrant. This separation is preserved along the central visual pathway as far as the cortex.

In primates, each retina is divided into two halves along the vertical meridian passing through the center of the fovea. The fibers from the nasal half cross in the optic chiasma and pass to the optic tract of the opposite side; those from the temporal half enter the tract on the same side. Each optic tract is, therefore, composed of fibers from the temporal half of the retina of the same side and the nasal half of the retina of the opposite eye. This arrangement remains in the visual radiation in the occipital lobes of the brain. It accounts for the blindness in the opposite halves of the two fields of view (homonymous hemianopsia) when the optic tract or the visual radiation of one side is interrupted.

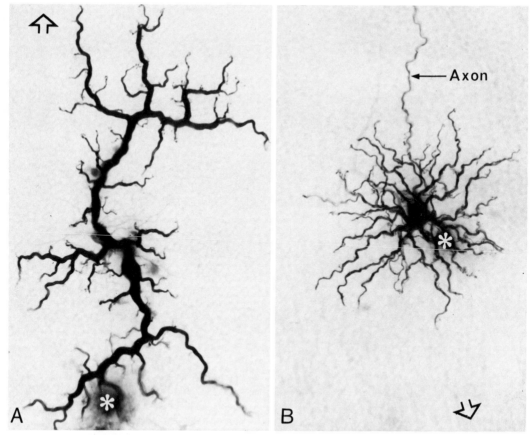

Figure 34–44. Horizontal cells of rabbit retina. *A,* An axonless horizontal cell injected with horseradish peroxidase. The cell has a small number of stout, tortuous dendrites, which branch sparsely and have minute terminal branchlets. At the asterisk, a Müller cell has been stained by peroxidase that leaked from the electrode during penetration. *B,* The somatic end of an axon-bearing horizontal cell. The cell has numerous wavy dendrites radiating in all directions. These carry clusters of fine terminal branchlets. The site of electrode penetration is marked by an asterisk. Open arrows indicate the direction to the optic nerve head. (Photomicrographs from Dacheux, R. F., and E. Raviola. J. Neurosci. 2:1486, 1982.)

Inner Limiting Membrane

This traditional term is no longer appropriate. It is not a membrane but merely the basal lamina of the Müller cells. It separates their inner conical ends from the vitreous body.

Supporting, or Neuroglial, Elements of the Retina

The retina, being a modified part of the brain, contains supporting elements of neuroglial character. The most important are the radial cells of Müller. These are present throughout the central area, including the fovea, as well as in the periphery.

Their oval nuclei lie in the middle zone of the inner nuclear layer. The cell body is a slender pillar that extends radially from the outer to the inner limiting membrane. In the two plexiform layers the radial pillars give off many branches, which form a dense neuroglial network in whose meshes are lodged the ramifications of the neurons described earlier. In the nuclear layers, the Müller cells are beset with excavations that envelop the bodies of the retinal neurons.

At the limit between the outer nuclear layer and the layer of the rods and cones, Müller cells, as described, have prominent zonulae adherentes that produce the linear density formerly interpreted as an outer limiting membrane.

Central Area and Fovea ("Macula")

Slightly lateral to the papilla is the place of most distinct vision. This region, the central area, is characterized by the presence of

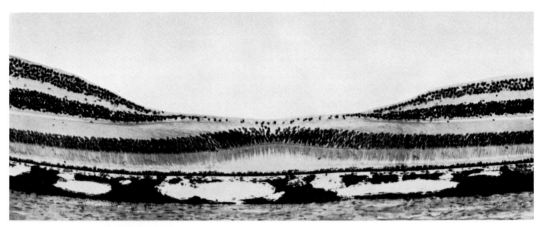

Figure 34–45. Photomicrograph of the fovea of a macaque retina, showing the marked reduction in thickness in this area of maximal visual acuity. (Courtesy of H. Mizoguchi.)

cones and other nervous elements in numbers greater than elsewhere and by their structural specialization and synaptic perfection. In the center of this area, the layers inward to the outer nuclear layer are displaced laterally, producing a shallow depression on the vitreal surface of the retina, called the central fovea. This permits an almost free passage of rays of light to the layer of photoreceptors, and it is here that the visual axis touches the retina.

The fovea is a shallow bowl with its concavity toward the vitreous (Fig. 34–45). It is in the middle of the central area, 2 to 2.5 mm on the temporal side of the papilla. In its center a *floor* or *fundus* can be distinguished, together with the *slopes* and a *margin of the fovea*. The width of the entire foveal depression measures 1.5 mm.

In the fundus of the fovea, the cones are thinner and longer than elsewhere in the retina. The central *rod-free* area, where only cones are present, measures 500 to 550 μm in diameter and contains up to 30,000 cones.

Capillaries are present in the foveal slopes to the very edge of the foveal floor, or 275 μm from the very center. The *avascular central territory* is almost as large as the rodless area (450 to 500 μm).

HISTOPHYSIOLOGY OF THE RETINA

The eye is essentially a camera obscura provided with dioptric media: the cornea, the aqueous humor, the adjustable crystalline lens, and the vitreous body. The inner surface of this dark chamber is lined with the photosensitive retina. The rays of light emanating from each point of an illuminated object impinging on the cornea are refracted by it and converge on the lens. In the lens, the rays are further refracted and focused in the photosensitive layer of the retina. In relation to the object, the retinal image is inverted (because of the crossing of the rays in the pupil's aperture); it is a real image, and is very much reduced in size.

In the retina, the quanta of incident light are converted or transduced by the photoreceptor cells into nerve signals; these are elaborated by the networks of retinal neurons and finally translated into a code of nerve impulses, which is conducted to the brain by the fibers of the optic nerve.

The transduction process can be conveniently subdivided into primary and secondary steps. The primary step is a photochemical reaction and consists in the absorption of a quantum of light by one of the visual pigments contained in the discs of the photoreceptor outer segments, and a subsequent configurational change in the absorbing molecule. The secondary step consists of changes in the concentration of internal transmitters within the cytoplasm of the outer segments, which influence the ionic permeability of the plasma membrane and cause the hyperpolarization of the photoreceptor cell.

Rod and cone cells differ in their sensitivity to intensity and wavelength of light. Rod cells are active in dim illumination (scotopic vision) and contain a single visual pigment, rhodopsin, which absorbs light of various wavelengths, although most efficiently in the blue-green. In the human retina there are three types of cones, containing different visual pigments that absorb maximally red, blue, or green light; furthermore, cone cells are active under the conditions of diurnal illumination (photopic vision).

Visual pigments consist of a combination of vitamin A aldehyde, known as *retinal*, with a protein of the class called *opsins*. Opsins are hydrophobic proteins with one retinal group per molecule, a carbohydrate side chain, no phospholipid, and a molecular weight of about 27,000 daltons. They are buried within the membrane of the discs of the photoreceptor outer segments. When retinal is combined with opsin in the dark-adapted retina, it has a bent and twisted form (*11-cis*). When the pigment moleule absorbs a quantum of light, the retinal shape becomes straight (*all-trans*) and separates from opsin, which in turn undergoes a conformational change. This leads to activation of various enzymes and the lowering of the concentration of cGMP in the outer segment. At the same time, calcium ions are released into the cytoplasm. Either cGMP, calcium, or both may represent the internal transmitters that regulate the patency of the ion channels in the plasma membrane. In the dark, sodium ions are continuously pumped out of the cell in the inner segment and reenter the cell through sodium channels located in the plasma membrane of the outer segment. Light diminishes or suppresses this "dark current" by blocking the sodium channels of the outer segment, and thus causes the hyperpolarization of the photoreceptor cell. Meanwhile the cell is recombining retinal and opsin into the light-absorbing form of the pigment molecule.

Most present knowledge on the electrophysiology of retinal neurons stems from intracellular recordings in nonprimate retinas. Stripped of many important details, the complex story of the interneuronal relationships in the retina is as follows. Most retinal neurons generate slow, graded potentials; spikes first appear in amacrine cells and are especially typical of the ganglion cell response. The photosensitive rod and cone cells are depolarized and release transmitter in the dark; the light-induced hyperpolarization decreases the output of transmitter by their synaptic endings. In cold-blooded vertebrates, there are two physiological classes of horizontal cells: *luminosity* horizontal cells, which respond to illumination of the photoreceptors by hyperpolarization; and *chromat-icity* horizontal cells, which may hyperpolarize or depolarize, depending on the wavelength of the stimulating light. In the retina of the turtle, the hyperpolarization of luminosity horizontal cells causes depolarization of cone cells; it has therefore been suggested that cones receive from horizontal cells a feedback synapse. In all vertebrates, there are two physiological classes of bipolar cells, one depolarizing, the other hyperpolarizing, upon light stimulation. Bipolar cells are the first elements in the chain of retinal neurons that show a "center-and-surround" organization of their receptive field; that is, the cell response to stimulation of neighboring photoreceptors is antagonized by the stimulation of distant photoreceptors. Furthermore, some bipolars are color-coded; that is, they respond to light of specific wavelength. The neuronal circuitry that underlies the bipolar activity is not well understood; the response of bipolars to stimulation of the photoreceptors in the center of their receptive field may be mediated by a photoreceptor-to-bipolar synapse. The "surround effect" is probably due to the activity of the horizontal cells, which are activated by the photoreceptors and in turn antagonize the center response of the bipolar cells. The precise mechanism of this interaction, however, is unknown; horizontal cells may feed back onto photoreceptors or may influence directly the bipolar cells. Thus, the function of the synapses in the outer plexiform layer is to signal the intensity and color of the retinal image and at the same time to accentuate its contrast through the activity of the horizontal cells.

The signals of bipolar cells are further processed in the inner plexiform layer by the amacrine and ganglion cells before their transmittal to the brain in the form of changes in frequency of the nerve impulses traveling along the fibers of the optic nerve.

The function of the amacrine cells is poorly understood; there are many varieties of them, both morphological and physiological, and they modulate the transfer of signals from bipolar to ganglion cells. In the monkey retina two main types of ganglion cells were identified by intracellular recordings, one responding to the onset, the other to the cessation, of a light stimulus applied to the center of their receptive field; the response was inverted upon stimulation of the periphery of their receptive field. Among the on-center cells, some are not color-coded and phasic—that is, they discharge transiently to sustained stimuli of any wavelength; others are color-coded and tonic—that is, they discharge continuously to sustained stimuli of either green or red light. The tonic cells are thought to correspond to the midget ganglion cells. It has been speculated that the neural interactions in the inner plexiform layer may be concerned with codification of the dynamic or temporal aspects of the visual image, but much work remains to be done before the significance of the synaptic interactions among bipolar, amacrine, and ganglion cells is fully elucidated.

BLOOD VESSELS OF THE EYE

These arise from the ophthalmic artery and can be subdivided into two groups, which are almost completely independent and anastomose with each other only in the region of the entrance of the optic nerve. The first group, the *retinal system*, represented by the central artery and vein, supplies a part of the optic nerve and the inner retina. The second, the *ciliary system*, is destined for the uveal tunic; through the uvea, it provides for the nourishment of the outer retina. Like the brain, the retina is protected from circulating macromolecules by a *blood-retina barrier*; its structural counterpart is chiefly represented by the zonulae occludentes that seal the intercellular spaces between the cells of the pigment epithelium and those between the endothelial cells of the retinal blood vessels.

LYMPH SPACES OF THE EYE

True lymph capillaries and lymph vessels are present only in the scleral conjunctiva. In the eyeball they are absent.

A mass injected into the space between the choroid and sclera penetrates along the walls of the vortex veins into the space of Tenon. The latter continues as the *supravaginal space* along the outer surface of the dural sheath of the optic nerve to the optic foramen. Again, it is possible to inject into Tenon's space from the subarachnoid space of the brain. From the anterior chamber the injected liquid passes into the posterior chamber and also into Schlemm's canal. All these spaces cannot, however, be regarded as belonging to the lymphatic system.

NERVES OF THE EYE

These are the optic nerve, originating from the retina, and the ciliary nerves, supplying the eyeball with motor, sensory, and sympathetic fibers.

The optic nerve, an evagination of the prosencephalon, is not a peripheral nerve like the other cranial nerves, but is a tract of the central nervous system. It consists of about 1200 bundles of nerve fibers whose myelin sheaths are produced by oligodendroglial cells.

The meninges and the intermeningeal spaces of the brain continue into the optic nerve. The outer sheath of the nerve is formed by the dura, which continues toward the eyeball and fuses with the sclera. The intermediate sheath is formed by the arachnoid and the inner sheath by the pia mater. The pia mater forms a connective tissue layer that is closely adherent to the surface of the nerve and fuses with the sclera at the entrance of the optic nerve. This pial layer sends connective tissue partitions and blood vessels into the nerve. Inflammatory processes can extend from the eyeball toward the meningeal spaces of the brain through the spaces between the sheaths.

The optic nerve leaves the posterior pole of the eyeball in a slightly oblique direction and continues into the entrance canal of the optic nerve. Just after leaving the eye through the openings in the lamina cribrosa, the fibers acquire their myelin sheaths. The central artery and central vein reach the eyeball through the optic nerve; they penetrate the nerve on its lower side at a distance from the eyeball varying from 5 to 20 mm, but usually 6 to 8 mm.

ACCESSORY ORGANS OF THE EYE

In an early stage of embryonic development the anterior segment of the eyeball projects freely on the surface. Later a circular fold of integument encircles the cornea. From its upper and lower parts the upper and lower lids grow toward each other over the surface of the cornea. In this way, the conjunctival sac is formed, which protects and moistens the free surface of the eye, especially the cornea. The part lining the inner surface of the lids is the *palpebral con-*

junctiva, and that covering the eyeball is the *bulbar conjunctiva*. The reflection of the palpebral onto the bulbar conjunctiva forms deep recesses between the lids and the eyeball, the *superior* and the *inferior fornices*.

Eyelids

The outermost layer of the eyelids is the skin. It is thin and provided with a few papillae and many small hairs with sebaceous and small sweat glands (Fig. 34–46). The dermis contains a varying number of pigment cells with yellow or brown granules. The loose subcutaneous layer is rich in fine elastic fibers, and in Caucasians is almost completely devoid of fat. Toward the edge of the lid the dermis becomes denser and has higher papillae.

The *eyelashes* are large hairs obliquely inserted in three or four rows along the edge of the lid. With their follicles they penetrate deeply into the tissue. The sebaceous glands connected with the eyelashes are small, and arrector muscles are missing. The eyelashes are replaced every 100 to 150 days.

Between and behind the follicles of the eyelashes are peculiar sweat glands, the *glands of Moll*. Unlike ordinary sweat glands, the terminal portion here is generally straight or only slightly coiled. The ducts open, as a rule, into the follicles of the eyelashes. The epithelium of the terminal portions consists of an indistinct, outer myoepithelial layer and an inner layer of pyramidal, apocrine glandular elements. The lumen is often considerably dilated, and the glandular cells are flattened. In the ducts the epithelium consists of two distinct cell layers. The nature of the secretion of these glands is not known.

The next layer of the eyelid inward consists of the thin, pale, striated fibers of the palpebral portion of the ring of facial muscle surrounding the eye (*orbicularis oculi*). The part behind the follicles of the eyelashes is the *ciliary muscle of Riolan*.

Deep to the orbicular muscle is a layer of connective tissue, the *palpebral fascia*, a continuation of the tendon of the palpebral levator (*levator palpebrae*) muscle. In the upper part of the upper lid, strands of smooth muscle, the *superior tarsal muscle of Müller*, are attached to the edge of the *tarsus*, a plate of dense connective tissue that forms the skeleton of the lid. In the upper lid its breadth is about 10 mm, in the lower only 5 mm. The *glands of Meibom* are embedded in its sub-

stance. They are elongated and arranged in one layer, parallel to one another and perpendicular to the length of the tarsal plate. Their openings form a single row immediately in front of the inner free edge of the lid, at the line of transition from the skin into the conjunctiva.

The meibomian glands are sebaceous but have lobated alveolar terminal portions. They are connected by short lateral ducts with a long central excretory duct lined with stratified squamous epithelium.

The innermost layer of the lid is the *conjunctiva*. At the inner edge of the margin of the lid, the epidermis continues into the inner surface of the lid. Here the superficial cells become thicker, the number of layers decreases, and the epithelium assumes a stratified columnar character, which is typical of the whole conjunctiva and varies only in the thickness in different places. The superficial cells have a short prismatic form. Goblet cells are scattered between them (Fig. 34–47).

At the upper edge of the tarsus the epithelium is sometimes reduced to two cell layers, and its surface presents many irregular invaginations. Some of them are lined with mucous cells and are described as glands. In the conjunctiva of the fornix, the epithelium is thicker.

The lamina propria of the conjunctiva is dense connective tissue. In the region of the fornix it is very loosely attached to the intraorbital fat tissue, permitting the free motion of the eyeball in the conjunctival sac.

In the region of the corneal limbus the epithelium of the conjunctiva assumes a stratified squamous character and continues as such onto the surface of the cornea. It may still contain a few scattered mucous cells.

The rudimentary *third eyelid*, or *semilunar fold* (the homologue of the nictitating membrane of the lower vertebrates), is formed by the scleral conjunctiva at the inner palpebral commissure, lateral to the lacrimal caruncle. It consists of connective tissue that contains smooth muscle fibers and is covered with conjunctival epithelium, which, on the outer surface, contains many mucous cells.

Lacrimal Gland

Opening into the conjunctival space there is a system of glands whose secretion moistens, lubricates, and flushes the surface of the eyeball and of the lids. Of these glands, only the *lacrimal gland* reaches a high degree

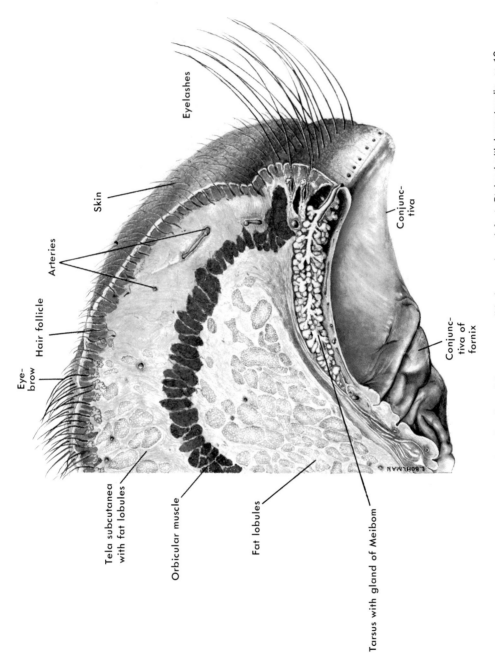

Figure 34–46. Camera lucida drawing of a slice of the upper eyelid of a newborn infant. Stained with hematoxylin. × 12.

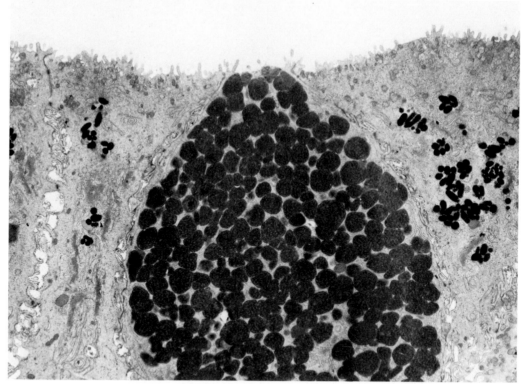

Figure 34–47. Photomicrograph of the superficial portion of the conjunctival epithelium of *Macaca mulatta,* showing a goblet cell and clusters of melanosomes in the neighboring epithelial cells. (Photomicrograph courtesy of G. Raviola.)

of development. It has the size and shape of an almond and is lodged beneath the conjunctiva at the lateral upper side of the eyeball. It consists of a group of separate glandular lobules and has six to 12 excretory ducts, which open along the upper and lateral quadrant of the superior conjunctival fornix.

The lacrimal gland is of the tubuloalveolar type. Its terminal portions are provided with a relatively large lumen and with irregular, saccular outpocketings. The basal lamina is lined with glandular cells resembling those of the serous salivary glands. They have, however, a narrower columnar shape and contain, in addition to small lipid droplets, large, pale secretion granules whose number changes according to the functional conditions. These cells are provided with secretory canaliculi. Between their bases and the basal lamina are well-developed myoepithelial cells. The smallest intralobular ducts are lined with a layer of low columnar or cuboidal cells and have a few myoepithelial cells. The larger intralobular ducts have a two-layered epithelium.

On the inner surface of the lids, especially the upper one, near the upper edge of the tarsus, there are a varying number of small accessory lacrimal glands—the *tarsal lacrimal glands.*

After having washed the conjunctival cavity, tears reach the region of the inner palpebral commissure (internal canthus). Here the two eyelids are separated by a triangular space, the *lacrimal lake*, in which the secretion accumulates temporarily. From here it passes through two tiny orifices called *lacrimal points*, one on the margin of each eyelid, into the *lacrimal ducts*. The latter converge medially into the *lacrimal sac*, whence the *nasolacrimal duct* leads into the inferior meatus of the nasal cavity.

The wall of the excretory lacrimal passages is formed by connective tissue lined with epithelium. The epithelium of the lacrimal ducts is stratified squamous. The lacrimal sac and the nasolacrimal duct are lined with a pseudostratified, tall columnar epithelium.

From the bottom of the lacrimal lake, between the two lacrimal ducts, there bulges a small, soft mass of tissue, the *lacrimal caruncle*.

The top is covered with a thick, squamous epithelium in which only the uppermost layers are flattened, although not cornified. It contains mucous cells, and gradually merges into the conjunctival epithelium. The lamina propria contains bundles of striated muscles, sweat glands, abortive lacrimal glands, and tiny hairs with sebaceous glands. These are the source of the whitish secretion that often collects in the region of the inner palpebral commissure.

Blood and Lymph Vessels of the Eyelids

The arteries in each lid form two archlike anastomoses, which run in front of the tarsus, one near the free margin of the lid, the other near the other margin of the tarsus. The palpebral conjunctiva is provided with dense, subepithelial capillary networks that can be easily studied in living condition with the aid of the slit lamp microscope. Branches of the blood vessels in the scleral conjunctiva anastomose with the marginal blood vessels of the cornea and with the branches of the anterior ciliary arteries.

The lymphatics form a dense plexus in the conjunctiva behind the tarsus. In front of the latter there is another, thinner, pretarsal net. A third net can be distinguished in the skin and the subcutis. All these networks communicate with one another. The lymphatic capillaries of the scleral conjunctiva end blindly near the corneal margin.

The abundant supply of the conjunctiva with blood and lymph capillaries accounts for the rapid absorption of solutions introduced into the conjunctival sac.

HISTOGENESIS OF THE EYE

The stalk of the optic vesicle growing out of the brain is transformed into the optic nerve (Fig. 34–48). The double-walled vesicle gives rise to the retina. Where the optic vesicle touches the ectoderm, the latter forms an invagination with a greatly thickened bottom, the *primordium of the lens*. It apparently develops as the result of inductive stimulation of the ectoderm by the optic vesicle. In amphibian larvae, after excision of the optic vesicle, the lens is not formed. The lens primordium comes to lie in the invagination of the optic vesicle. Simultaneously, mesenchyme and blood vessels grow into the choroidal fissure, in the lower part of the optic vesicle. Simultaneously, mesenchyme and blood vessels grow into the choroidal fissure, in the lower part of the optic vesicle. These vessels give rise to the hyaloid and retinal vascular systems. The opposite margins of the fissure, which received the vessels, soon grow together, and the secondary optic vesi-

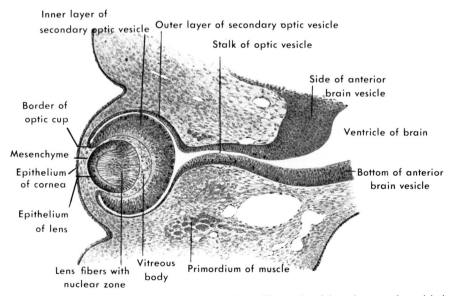

Figure 34–48. Primordium of the eye of an 8-mm mouse embryo. The cavity of the primary optic vesicle is reduced to a thin cleft. × 70. (After Schaffer.)

cle assumes the form of a double-walled cup, while the stalk is transformed into a solid strand, the optic nerve.

The lens primordium soon becomes detached from the ectoderm, and the space between the two is filled by a layer of mesenchyme—the primordium of the substantia propria of the cornea and of the connective tissue of the iris. The lens, surrounded by vascular mesenchyme, acquires a solid, spherical form, while the original cavity disappears. The inner, thicker sheet of the double wall of the optic cup differentiates into the retina proper. It remains permanently in direct continuation with the optic nerve. The outer sheet of the cup is transformed into the pigment epithelium. The surrounding mesenchyme comes into close relation with the optic cup and gives rise to the two outer tunics of the eyeball, the uveal and fibrous tunics. The structural differentiation of the retina proceeds in a way similar to that of the wall of the neural tube. The eyeball attains full size toward the end of the first decade. The structure of the retina, including the central fovea, matures toward the end of the first year.

REFERENCES

GENERAL

Davson, H.: The Physiology of the Eye. New York, Academic Press, 1972.

Duke-Elder, S., and K. C. Wybar: *In* Duke-Elder, S., ed.: The Anatomy of the Visual System. System of Ophthalmology. Vol. 2. St. Louis, C. V. Mosby Co., 1961.

Fine, B. S., and M. Yanoff: Ocular Histology. New York, Harper & Row, 1972.

Hogan, M. J., J. A. Alvarado, and J. E. Weddell: Histology of the Human Eye. Philadelphia, W. B. Saunders Co., 1971.

Walls, G. L.: The Vertebrate Eye and its Adaptive Radiation. Bloomfield Hills, MI, Cranbrook Press, 1943.

CORNEA

Hay, E. D.: Development of the vertebrate cornea. Int. Rev. Cytol. *63*:263, 1980.

Jakus, M. A.: Studies on the cornea. II. The fine structure of Descemet's membrane. J. Biophys. Biochem. Cytol. (Suppl.) *2*:243, 1956.

IRIS

Freddo, T. F., and G. Raviola: Homogeneous structure of blood-vessels in the vascular tree of *Macaca mulatta* iris. Invest. Ophthalmol. Vis. Sci. *22*:279, 1982.

Gregersen, E.: The spongy structure of the human iris. Acta Ophthalmol. *36*:522, 1958.

Raviola, G., and J. M. Butler: Unidirectional transport mechanism of horseradish peroxidase in the vessels of the iris. Invest. Ophthalmol. Vis. Sci. *25*:827, 1984.

Richardson, K. C.: The fine structure of the albino rabbit iris with special reference to the identification of adrenergic and cholinergic nerves and nerve endings in its intrinsic muscles. Am. J. Anat. *114*:173, 1964.

CILIARY BODY

Fine, B. S.: Structure of the trabecular meshwork and the canal of Schlemm. Trans. Am. Acad. Ophthalmol. Otolaryngol. *70*:777, 1966.

Inomata, H., A. Bill., and G. K. Smelser: Aqueous humor pathways through the trabecular meshwork and into Schlemm's canal in the cynomolgus monkey (*Macaca irus*). Am. J. Ophthalmol. *78*:760, 1972.

Ishikawa, T.: Fine structure of the human ciliary muscle. Invest. Ophthalmol. *1*:587, 1962.

Raviola, G.: The fine structure of the ciliary zonule and ciliary epithelium. Invest. Ophthalmol. *10*:851, 1971.

Raviola, G.: The structural basis of the blood-ocular barriers. Exp. Eye Res. (Suppl.) *25*:27, 1977.

Raviola, G., and E. Raviola: Intercellular junctions in the ciliary epithelium. Invest. Ophthalmol. Vis. Sci. *10*:958, 1978.

Raviola, G., and E. Raviola: Paracellular route of aqueous outflow in the trabecular meshwork and Schlemm canal. Invest. Ophthalmol. *21*:52, 1981.

Toates, F. M.: Accommodation function of the human eye. Physiol. Rev. *52*:828, 1972.

Tormey, J. McD.: Fine structure of the ciliary epithelium of the rabbit with particular reference to "infolded membranes," "vesicles," and the effects of Diamox. J. Cell Biol. *17*:641, 1963.

LENS AND VITREOUS BODY

Farnsworth, P. N., S. C. Fu, P. A. Burke, and I. Bahia: Ultrastructure of rat eye lens fibers. Invest. Ophthalmol. *13*:274, 1974.

Swann, D. A.: Chemistry and biology of the vitreous body. Int. Rev. Exp. Pathol. *22*:2, 1980.

Wanko, T., and M. A. Gavin: Electron microscopic study of lens fibers. J. Biophys. Biochem. Cytol. *6*:97, 1959.

RETINA

Dacheux, R. F., and E. Raviola: Horizontal cells in the retina of the rabbit. J. Neurosci. *2*:1486, 1982.

Dowling, J. E.: Organization of vertebrate retinas. Invest. Ophthalmol. *9*:665, 1970.

Polyak, S.: The Retina. Chicago, University of Chicago Press, 1941.

Raviola, E.: Intercellular junctions in the outer plexiform layer of the retina. Invest. Ophthalmol. *15*:881, 1976.

Raviola, E., and N. B. Gilula: Intramembrane organization of specialized contacts in the outer plexiform layer of the retina. J. Cell Biol. *65*:192, 1975.

Raviola, G., and E. Raviola: Light and electron microscopic observations on the inner plexiform layer of the rabbit retina. Am. J. Anat. *120*:403, 1967.

Rodieck, R. W.: The Vertebrate Retina. San Francisco, W. H. Freeman, 1973.

Schwartz, E. A.: First events in vision: the generation of responses in vertebrate rods. J. Cell Biol. *90*:271, 1982.

Young, R. W.: Visual cells and the concept of renewal. Invest. Ophthalmol. *15*:700, 1976.

Young, R. W., and D. Bok: Participation of the retinal pigment epithelium in the rod outer segment renewal process. J. Cell Biol. *42*:392, 1969.

35

THE EAR

The organ of hearing is divisible into three parts, each of which differs from the others not only in its gross anatomy but also in its histology and in the functions that it subserves in the translation of sound waves into meaningful information that can be processed in the central nervous system. The first part, the *external ear*, receives the sound waves. In the second part, the *middle ear*, the waves are transformed into the mechanical vibrations of bony *auditory ossicles*. These, in turn, by impinging upon the fluid-filled spaces of the third part, the *internal ear* (or labyrinth), generate specific nerve impulses that are conveyed by the acoustic nerve to the central nervous system. In addition to organs for analysis of sound, the internal ear contains vestibular organs, which are concerned chiefly with the function of maintaining eqiulibrium.

EXTERNAL EAR

Auricle

The *auricle*, or *pinna*, consists of a single, highly irregular plate of elastic cartilage, 0.5 to 1 mm thick, overlain by a flexible perichondrium containing abundant elastic fibers. The covering skin has a distinct subcutaneous layer only on the posterior surface of the auricle and is provided with a few small hairs and associated sebaceous glands, the latter sometimes being of considerable size. In old age, especially in men, large stiff hairs develop on the dorsal edge of the auricle and on the ear lobe. Sweat glands are scarce, and when present are small.

External Auditory Meatus

The outer portion of the external auditory meatus is a medial continuation of the auricular cartilage, and the inner portion is a canal

in the temporal bone (Fig. 35–1). It forms an S-shaped curve coursing for about 2.5 cm medially and inferiorly, and is bounded at its medial end by the eardrum or *tympanic membrane*. The skin lining the meatus is thin and is firmly attached to the underlying perichondrium and periosteum. Numerous hairs in the lining of the outer cartilaginous portion of the meatus tend to prevent entrance of foreign bodies. In old age these hairs enlarge considerably, as do those on the auricle. Sebaceous glands connected with the hair follicles are exceptionally large. In the bony portion of the meatus, small hairs and sebaceous glands are found only along the upper wall. No eccrine sweat glands are present in the meatus.

The external meatus contains *cerumen,* a brown, waxy secretion that protects the skin from desiccation and presumably from invasion by insects. It is a mixture of the secretion of the sebaceous glands and *ceruminous glands* of the skin of the meatus. Ceruminous glands are a special variety of coiled tubular apocrine sweat gland. In cross section, they appear to be aggregated into discrete lobules invested by connective tissue. Each glandular tubule is surrounded by a thin network of myoepithelial cells. In the resting state, the gland lumen is large and the epithelial cells lining it are cuboidal. In the active state, however, the cells are columnar and the lumen is constricted. Ducts of ceruminous glands open either onto the free surface of the skin or, with the sebaceous glands, into the necks of hair follicles.

MIDDLE EAR

The middle ear comprises the *tympanic cavity* and its contents, the auditory ossicles; the *eustachian tube*; and the *tympanic membrane,* which closes the tympanic cavity externally.

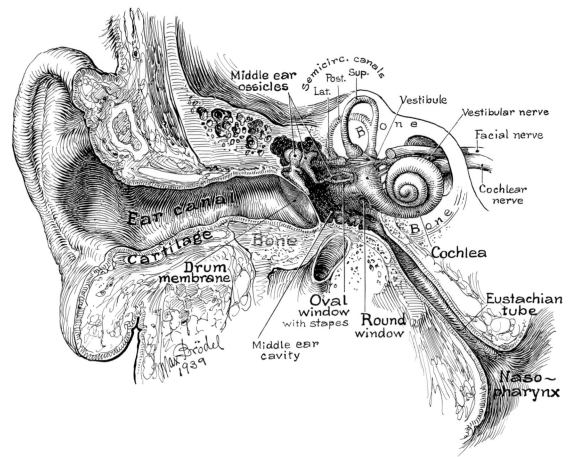

Figure 35–1. Schematic representation of the anatomical relations of the various parts of the human ear. (After Brödel, M. *In* Malone, Guild, and Crowe. Three Unpublished Drawings of the Human Ear. Philadelphia, W. B. Saunders Co., 1946.)

TYMPANIC CAVITY

The tympanic cavity is an irregular, air-filled space in the temporal bone. Its lateral wall is formed largely by the tympanic membrane and its medial wall by the lateral aspect of the bony wall of the internal ear (Fig. 35–2). Anteriorly it continues into the *auditory tube* and posteriorly it is connected, through the tympanic antrum, with air-filled cavities in the mastoid process of the temporal bone. The cavity contains the *auditory ossicles;* the tendons of two small muscles (the *tensor tympani* and the *stapedius*) connected with the ossicles; and the *chorda tympani nerve* (Fig. 35–2).

The epithelium lining the tympanic cavity is simple squamous, for the most part, but near the opening of the auditory tube and near the edge of the tympanic membrane it is cuboidal or columnar and provided with cilia. The presence of glands associated with the lining of the cavity is generally denied.

Auditory Ossicles

Three small bones—the *malleus*, the *incus*, and the *stapes*—extend from the attachment of the malleus on the tympanic membrane to the medial wall of the tympanic cavity, where the footplate of the stapes fits into the *fenestra vestibuli*, or *oval window*, a hiatus in the wall of the osseous labyrinth (Figs. 35–1, 35–2). The footplate is maintained in the fenestra by means of an annular fibrous ligament. The three bones are connected to one another by means of typical diarthrodial joints and are supported in the cavity by minute connective tissue ligaments. Small patches of hyaline cartilage are usually found on the manubrium of the malleus and on the footplate of the stapes. The mucosa lining the

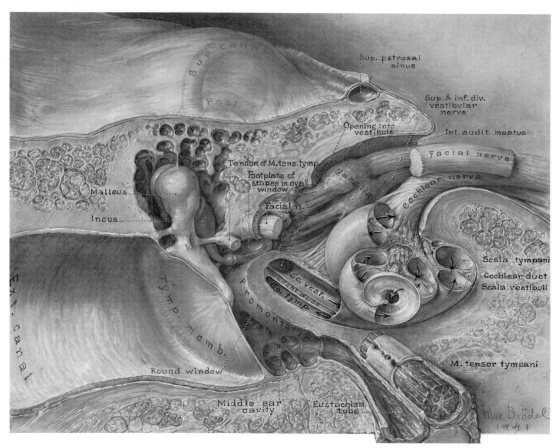

Figure 35–2. Drawing of some of the anatomical features of the external, middle, and inner ear. (After Brödel, M. *In* Malone, Guild, and Crowe. Three Unpublished Drawings of the Human Ear. Philadelphia. W. B. Saunders Co., 1946.)

tympanic cavity is reflected over the ossicles and is firmly attached to their periosteum.

TYMPANIC MEMBRANE

This oval, semitransparent membrane is shaped like a very flat cone with its apex directed medially (Figs. 35–1 to 35–3). Its conical form is maintained by the insertion, onto its inner surface, of the manubrium of the malleus, which tends to pull the center of the membrane medially. The tympanic membrane is formed of two layers of collagenous fibers and fibroblasts that are similar to those of a flat tendon (Fig. 35–3). However, there is a flaccid portion in its anterosuperior quadrant, *Shrapnell's membrane*, that is devoid of collagenous fibers. In the outer layer of the membrane the collagen fibers have a radial arrangement, whereas those in the inner layer are disposed circularly. There are also thin networks of elastic fibers, located mainly in the central and peripheral parts of the membrane. Externally the membrane is covered by a very thin (50 to 60 μm) layer of skin devoid of hairs and other appendages. Its inner surface is lined by the mucosa of the tympanic cavity, here only 20 to 40 μm thick and consisting of simple squamous epithelium overlying a lamina propria of sparse collagenous fibers and capillaries. Over the manubrium of the malleus is a layer of connective tissue through which vessels and nerves reach the center of the tympanic membrane.

AUDITORY TUBE

From its origin in the anterior wall of the tympanic cavity, the auditory, or eustachian, tube extends anteromedially and inferiorly for about 4 cm to an opening on the posterolateral wall of the nasopharynx. The rostral two thirds of the tube is supported medially by cartilage, and the portion near the tympanic cavity is supported by bone.

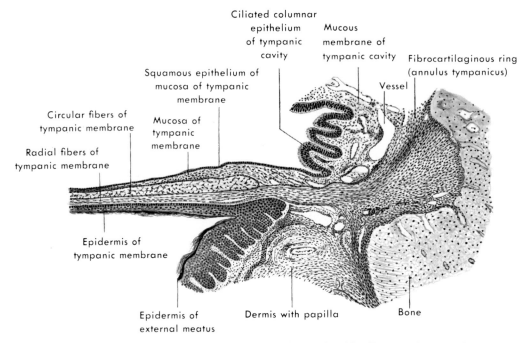

Figure 35–3. Cross section of edge of tympanic membrane of a child. (Redrawn from von Ebner.)

The cartilage supporting the auditory tube lies mainly medial to the lumen, but a ridge of cartilage running longitudinally for most of the length of the tube curves superolaterally, so that in cross section the cartilage has the appearance of a shepherd's crook (Fig. 35–4). The cartilage is elastic throughout most of its length, but at the isthmus it loses its elastic fibers and becomes hyaline. The lumen of the tube, flattened in the vertical plane, is largest at its pharyngeal end, decreases to a mere slit (the isthmus) at the junction of the cartilaginous and bony portions, and then expands again in its course through the temporal bone. The tube is lined by a mucosa, of variable thickness, plicated into rugae at both the pharyngeal and tympanic ends. In the bony portion of the auditory tube, it is relatively thin and is composed of low columnar ciliated epithelium resting on a thin lamina propria firmly bound to the periosteum. The epithelium in the cartilaginous portion of the tube is pseudostratified and composed of tall columnar cells, many of which are ciliated. The underlying lamina propria is much more complex here than in the bony portion. Toward the pharyngeal orifice, it contains many compound tubuloalveolar glands that secrete mucus via ducts opening into the tubal lumen. In this vicinity, also, goblet cells are interspersed among the columnar epithelial cells.

There is considerable individual variation in number and distribution of ciliated cells and goblet cells, and in the degree of development of the glandular elements. Throughout the lamina propria, in both portions of the tube, a great many lymphocytes can be found, the number varying with age and from one individual to another. Near the pharyngeal opening there are often discrete collections of lymphoid tissue forming the *tubal tonsils.* Usually the auditory tube is closed. During the acts of swallowing and yawning, the lumen is opened for a short interval, allowing the pressure in the tympanic cavity to equalize with that outside.

INTERNAL EAR

The internal ear, called the labyrinth because of its complex structure, is composed of a series of fluid-filled sacs and tubules in cavities of corresponding form in the petrous portion of the temporal bone (Fig. 35–5).

The canals and cavities in the bone constitute the *osseous labyrinth.* Occupying this system of cavities are the thin-walled, fluid-filled tubules and saccules of the *membranous labyrinth,* which constitute the *endolymphatic system.* This is surrounded by the cells and fluid of the *perilymphatic system.*

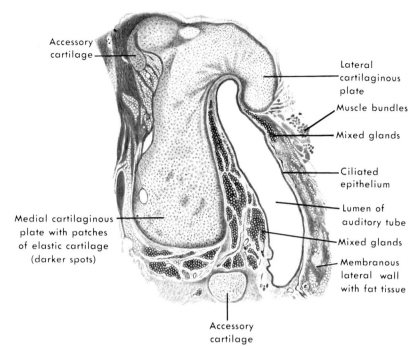

Figure 35–4. Transection of cartilaginous portion of the auditory tube near its opening into the pharynx. × 11. (Redrawn from von Ebner.)

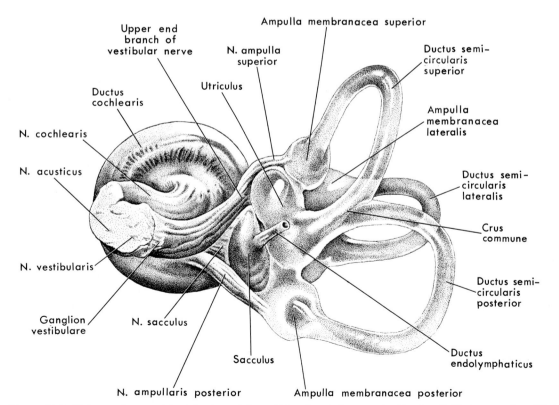

Figure 35–5. Right membranous labyrinth of an adult; medial and posterior aspects. About × 5. (Redrawn and modified from Spalteholz.)

THE BONY LABYRINTH

There are two major cavities in the bony labyrinth: the *vestibule,* which houses the *saccule* and *utricle*; and anteromedial to it, the spirally coiled *cochlea,* which contains the *organ of Corti* (Figs. 35–1, 35–2).

The Vestibule

The vestibule is an irregularly ovoid cavity located medial to the tympanic cavity. Its wall facing the tympanic cavity is penetrated by the fenestra vestibuli, and certain recesses in its wall produce characteristic bony protrusions on the medial wall of the tympanic cavity in relationship to the fenestra. For a more detailed description, the student is referred to a textbook of gross anatomy. Three *semicircular canals* arise from recesses in the wall of the vestibule and return to it. According to their position, they are named the superior, posterior, and lateral semicircular canals. Two of the recesses located anterosuperiorly accommodate the dilated *ampullae* of the superior and lateral *semicircular ducts* of the membranous labyrinth, and posteriorly a third recess houses the *posterior ampulla.* Given off from these recesses are the superior (or anterior), the lateral, and the posterior *semicircular canals.* The lateral canal curves laterally around the vestibule and rejoins it behind the posterior ampullary recess. The superior and posterior canals join each other superior to the vestibule in the recess for the *crus commune,* which opens into the medial part of the vestibule. From the medial wall of the vestibule a thin canal, the *vestibular aqueduct,* extends to the posterior surface of the petrous portion of the temporal bone.

The Cochlea

The bony cochlea is anteromedial to the vestibule (Figs. 35–1, 35–2, 35–5). It consists of a complex bony canal that makes two and three quarter spiral turns around an axis formed by the conical pillar of spongy bone called the *modiolus.* The base of the modiolus forms the deep end of the *internal acoustic meatus.* Blood vessels and the central processes of nerve fibers belonging to the cochlear division of the eighth cranial nerve pass through numerous openings into the bony substance of the modiolus. The cell bodies of these bipolar afferent neurons are found in the *spiral ganglion,* which courses spirally within the modiolus along the inner wall of the cochlear canal (Fig. 35–11). Their peripheral processes traverse the remaining distance to the cochlear hair cells that they innervate.

The lumen of the canal of the osseous cochlea (about 3 mm in diameter) is divided along its whole course (about 35 mm in the human) into an upper and a lower section by the *spiral lamina.* The lamina is divided into two zones: an inner zone containing bone (the *osseous spiral lamina*) and a fibrous outer zone (the *membranous spiral lamina*). The latter is also called the *basilar membrane* (Figs. 35–11, 35–13, 35–14). At the attachment of the basilar membrane to the outer wall of the cochlea, the periosteum is thickened and forms a structure that has been called the *spiral ligament,* although histologically it does not have the characteristics of a ligament. The cochlear canal is further subdivided by a thin membrane, the *vestibular membrane (Reissner's membrane),* which extends obliquely from the spiral lamina to the outer wall of the bony cochlea (Fig. 35–11). Thus, a cross section of the bony cochlea will show three compartments: an upper cavity, the *scala vestibuli;* a lower cavity, the *scala tympani;* and an intermediate cavity, the *scala media* (Fig. 35–11). The latter is the *cochlear duct,* a portion of the endolymphatic system that connects with the vestibular part of the membranous labyrinth by way of the small *ductus reuniens.*

The scala tympani and scala vestibuli are perilymphatic spaces. The scala vestibuli extends into and through the perilymphatic cistern of the vestibule and reaches the inner surface of the *fenestra ovalis.* The scala tympani ends at the *fenestra rotundum.* At the apex of the cochlea the two scalae communicate through a small opening, the *helicotrema.*

THE MEMBRANOUS (OR ENDOLYMPHATIC) LABYRINTH

The fluid-filled sacs of the membranous labyrinth arise embryologically from a single otic vesicle of ectodermal origin. Although the semicircular ducts are derived from the utricle, and the cochlear duct and the endolymphatic sac are derived from the saccule, all these parts of the labyrinth are in communication and all are filled with *endolymph.*

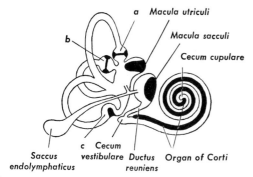

a *Macula utriculi*

Macula sacculi

Cecum cupulare

b

c *Cecum*
vestibulare *Ductus* *Organ of Corti*
reuniens

Saccus
endolymphaticus

Figure 35–6. Diagram of membranous labyrinth with neuroepithelial area in black. *a, b,* and *c* respectively designate the ampullae of the superior, lateral, and posterior semicircular canals. (Modified from von Ebner.)

Utricle, Saccule, and Ampullae

In the vestibule, the oblong utricle lies superior and then posterior to the roughly spherical saccule and communicates via five orifices with the three semicircular ducts and their ampullae (Fig. 35–5). The semicircular ducts are eccentrically placed in the bony canals and are lined by a simple squamous epithelium. Each ampulla has a flattened floor and a hemispherical roof bulging on the concave side of the duct. Both the saccule and utricle give off ducts medially, which join and form the slender *endolymphatic duct* (Fig. 35–5), which in turn courses under the utricle and then medially through the vestibular aqueduct to end on the posterior surface of the petrous portion of the temporal bone as a small dilation, the *endolymphatic sac.* The sac is located between layers of the meninges and is richly surrounded by blood vessels and connective tissue.

The epithelium lining the membranous structures in the vestibule is of simple squamous type, similar to that found in the semicircular ducts except in the immediate vicinity of sensory areas. The sensory areas and cells just peripheral to them, however, are specialized and in many respects highly complex.

Crista Ampullaris and Maculae. The epithelium in the floor of the three ampullae is raised into a transverse ridge, the *crista,* which is covered with the sensory epithelium and is bounded at either end by cells of the *planum semilunatum* (Figs. 35–8, 35–9). The latter are perpendicular to the long axis of the crista.

Sensory epithelium on the cristae is histologically the same as that composing the *mac-*

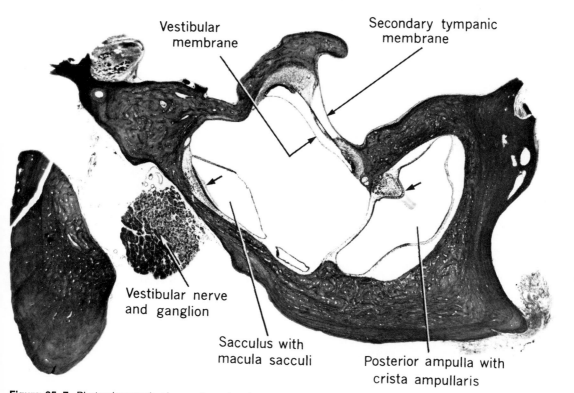

Vestibular
membrane

Secondary tympanic
membrane

Vestibular nerve
and ganglion

Sacculus with
macula sacculi

Posterior ampulla with
crista ampullaris

Figure 35–7. Photomicrograph of a section of a rhesus monkey inner ear, including the sacculus with the macula sacculi *(at arrow)* and the posterior ampulla with the crista ampullaris *(at arrow).* (Courtesy of H. Mizoguchi.)

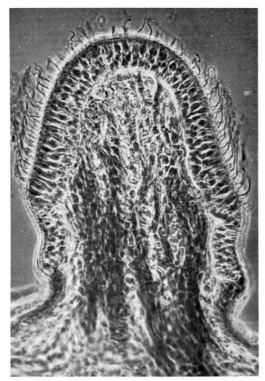

Figure 35–8. Phase-contrast photomicrograph of an unstained section in plastic of guinea pig crista ampullaris, showing the hairs projecting from the hair cells of the neuroepithelium. (Courtesy of H. Enström.)

ulae of the utricle and saccule, with variation apparently only in the relative number of different cell types. Classically, sensory epithelia in the vestibular portion of the internal ear are described as possessing two cell types, *hair cells* and *supporting cells*. Recent investigations have shown, however, that among the hair cells two morphological types can be distinguished.

HAIR CELLS. Hair cells of type I are flask-shaped cells with a rounded base and constricted neck region (Fig. 35–9). The round nucleus is located basally and surrounded by a more or less dense population of mitochondria. Mitochondria also are found congregated at the apex of the cell immediately beneath the free surface, which bears specialized microvilli, or hairs, of considerable length, and a single cilium. From its constricted neck inferiorly the hair cell is enclosed in a chalice-like nerve terminal.

Hair cells of type II are simple columnar cells innervated by numerous small synaptic endings that are difficult to see with the light microscope (Fig. 35–9). Nuclei of type II hair cells are round and regular in outline, like those of type I hair cells. They can be found at various levels in the cell, but usually form a row at a higher level in the epithelium than those of the type I hair cells and the supporting cells.

Seen with the electron microscope, the luminal border of both type I and type II hair cells is characterized by the presence of a single cilium and 50 to 110 straight *hairs*. These are actually highly specialized microvilli more appropriately described as *stereocilia*. The hairs are covered by plasma membrane and are noticeably constricted at their bases. They have an axial core, which is composed of longitudinally arranged fine filaments. This core continues downward from the narrow base of the hair and is embedded in the thickened terminal web, which extends across the cell immediately below its specialized free border. The hairs are arranged upon the cell surface in regular hexagonal array, and in successive rows show a progressive increase of length from less than 1 μm on one side to 100 μm on the other, the longest hairs being located at the side of the cell bearing the cilium (Fig. 35–20). The cilium originates from a basal body located in a terminal web-free area of the apical cytoplasm. The cilium has the typical nine outer doublet tubules and two central tubules found in cilia elsewhere, but the central tubules end shortly after leaving the basal body. A rootlet extends from the basal body into the cytoplasm on the side opposite the stereocilia aggregate. Although the cilium is considered to be nonmotile, it is commonly called a *kinocilium*. The existence of a gradient of stereocilia length, the eccentric location of the kinocilium, and the arrangement of the rootlet result in a morphological polarization of the hair cell, which is reflected in its physiological responses to stimuli. Both sensory cell types have a very dense terminal web or *cuticular plate* just below the apical plasmalemma. This structure may extend 0.5 μm or more into the cell cytoplasm, but is discontinuous in the area of the basal body of the cilium.

In both types of hair cells there are scattered profiles of granular endoplasmic reticulum, but smooth-surfaced tubules and vesicles are more abundant. Vesicles about 20 nm in diameter are present in greatest profusion in the type II hair cells. The supranuclear Golgi complex is also more extensively developed in this type. Characteristic of the type I cell is the occurrence of a great

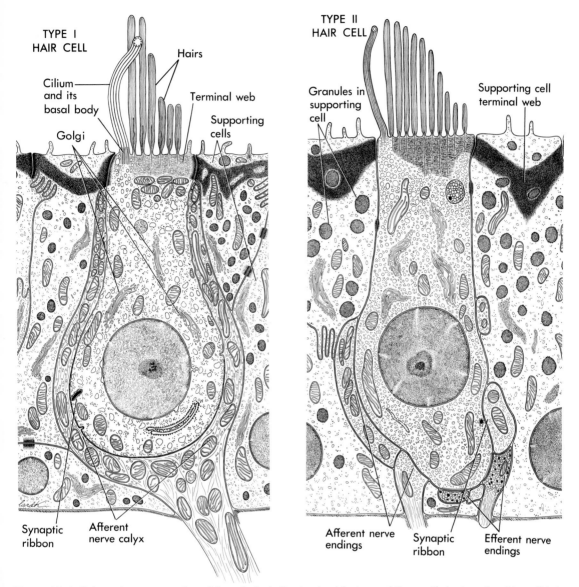

TYPE I
HAIR CELL

Cilium
and its
basal body

Golgi

Hairs

Terminal web

Supporting
cells

Synaptic
ribbon

Afferent
nerve calyx

TYPE II
HAIR CELL

Granules in
supporting
cell

Supporting cell
terminal web

Afferent nerve
endings

Synaptic
ribbon

Efferent nerve
endings

Figure 35–9. Schematic representation of the principal ultrastructural features of the vestibular type I and type II hair cells and their supporting cells. (Drawn by Sylvia Colard Keene.)

many microtubules, mostly concentrated in the apical cytoplasm just beneath the terminal web.

The nature of the synaptic contact between the two types of hair cells and the terminations of the vestibular nerve fibers is quite different (Fig. 35–9). In the case of type I, the afferent nerve envelops the hair cell in a cuplike ending called the calyx. At the base of the cell, the intercellular space between the plasmalemma and the axolemma is about 30 nm wide. Dense linear structures with an associated halo of small vesicles (resembling the so-called *synaptic ribbons* in the retina) are

found in varying numbers in the hair cell cytoplasm immediately opposite the nerve calyx. These specializations are characteristic of chemical synapses. Additionally there are certain discrete areas where the pre- and postsynaptic membranes are only about 5 nm apart. These resemble low-resistance contacts found at electrical synapses. At present, however, there are no physiological data relevant to this question. Nearer the rim of the cuplike ending around the upper part of the hair cell, there are in the axoplasm large numbers of vesicles 50 to 200 nm in diameter, some with dense cores.

The type II hair cell is not enveloped by a chalice-like ending, but a large number of separate *terminal boutons* impinge upon its surface. Synaptic ribbons are often found in the hair cell opposite sparsely granulated boutons, and the bouton membrane may be thickened at such synaptic sites. A second type of bouton is distinguished by its dense packing of small synaptic vesicles. It is believed that these boutons are efferent in nature. In addition to contacting type II hair cell bases directly, such boutons also contact nerve chalices of type I hair cells, other afferent boutons, and passing nerve fibers. However, the pre- and postsynaptic membrane thickenings traditionally considered indicative of synapses are only rarely noted at points of apposition between these vesiculated boutons and hair cells. They are more common where the vesiculated efferents contact other neural structures. It is clear that the synaptic relationships are far more complicated than was imagined from light microscope studies, and their exact nature remains unsettled.

The effective stimulus for vestibular hair cells is movement of the head in one or another plane. This presumably sets up movement of the endolymph, which acts in some manner to trigger an impulse in the afferent vestibular nerve. The transducers of the original mechanical stimulus into electrical signals are presumably the hair-bearing surfaces of the hair cells. Exactly how a receptor potential is set up in the hair cell and how it, in turn, influences the afferent nerve are unsolved problems. Some evidence seems to indicate that bending of the hairs initiates the process, but so little is known of their physiological properties that this is still speculative.

SUPPORTING CELLS. The supporting cells have their nuclei near the base of the sensory epithelium and extend to its free surface, but their cell bodies are so contorted that the full extent of any given cell can never be seen in a single section (Fig. 35–9). One usually sees a mosaic of sections of many cells cut at different levels. With the light microscope little can be resolved in their cytoplasm, but in electron micrographs they are found to possess a cytoskeleton of bundles of microtubules running from the basal cytoplasm to a dense terminal web, which is far more elaborately developed in these cells than in the hair cells. They have a prominent Golgi complex and the cytoplasm is crowded with membrane-limited granules resembling secretory granules. Little is known about the function of the supporting cells. They may contribute to the nutrition of the hair cells or may be involved in some way in the metabolism of the endolymph. Toward the periphery of the sensory region, there is a gradual transition to the cells making up the *planum semilunatum.*

The planum semilunatum is generally composed of columnar cells with slightly infolded lateral membranes. Investigations using ^{35}S and colloidal iron implicate these cells in the elaboration and secretion of sulfated mucopolysaccharide components of the cupula.

On the sloping sides of the crista ampullaris are very complex cells with highly infolded basal membranes and a dense cytoplasmic matrix with large vacuoles containing a flocculent material. These "dark cells" are reminiscent of other cells known to be involved in ion movement, and it has been speculated that they maintain the high K^+ level in endolymph.

CUPULAE AND OTOLITHS. Overlying the hairs in maculae are a multitude of minute (3 to 5 μm) crystalline bodies, *otoliths.* These are a complex of calcium carbonate and a protein. In life, they are suspended within the jelly-like glycoprotein substance that surrounds the sensory areas of the maculae.

The *cupulae* are gelatinous bodies located above the cristae. In life, these are composed of glycoprotein that is evidently much more viscous than the rest of the endolymph. This component is often lost or deformed during specimen preparation, and in the past this led some otologists to question its reality. That a cupula does exist is no longer doubted, but there is very little substantial information about its origin or functions.

Endolymphatic Sac

The cell types encountered in different parts of the vestibular system are basically similar from one region to the other. In the endolymphatic sac, however, one finds cells that appear to be specialized for an absorptive function, and these are structurally different from other cells in the vestibular membranous labyrinth. Unlike the other membranous sacs, the endolymphatic sac usually contains cellular debris of one sort or another. The electrolyte concentration in its endolymph also differs from that elsewhere in the inner ear.

Histologically, there is a transition from

the squamocuboidal cells of the endolymphatic duct to tall columnar cells in the sac. The latter have been variously described as covering protruding papillae or occupying crypts. Whichever is the case, there are two distinct columnar cell types present. One is a dense cell with a large irregularly shaped nucleus, a relatively unspecialized free surface, and a cell base with slightly infolded membranes. The other is a less dense cell characterized by long microvilli on its surface and many pinocytotic vesicles and vacuoles. Basally the cell membrane is smooth, but laterally it interdigitates extensively with other cells. There is good evidence that the endolymphatic sac acts as a site for absorption of endolymph and that free phagocytic cells, which appear to be macrophages and neutrophils, may cross the epithelium here to engulf and digest cellular debris and foreign material that may gain access to the endolymph.

The Cochlear Duct

The cochlear duct is a highly specialized diverticulum of the saccule. It contains the *organ of Corti*—the effective organ of hearing—and a number of other specialized areas subserving different functions and having their own special histological characteristics. This is a very complex area, and in order to facilitate understanding the different regions will be described individually in the following order: *vestibular membrane, stria vascularis, spiral prominence, organ of Corti*, and *tectorial membrane*. It can be seen in Figure 35–11 that this order of description proceeds in a counterclockwise direction around the circumference of the cochlear duct.

Vestibular Membrane. The vestibular membrane is a delicate bilaminar structure extending across the cochlea from medial to lateral. Its inner surface is lined by cells that are differentiated in a manner suggesting that they may be involved in water and electrolyte transport. The bulging perinuclear region of the cells is readily apparent in the light microscope, but peripherally the cell body is highly attenuated. Toward the scala media the surface of these cells bears many short, clavate microvilli similar to those found on cells in the choroid plexus. At the basal surface, the membranes are highly infolded and interdigitate extensively with those of the neighboring cells. A distinct basal lamina is found along this basal surface. Directly apposed to these cells, with little or no intervening collagen, is a layer of squamous peri-

lymphatic cells of the scala vestibuli, so attenuated that they can scarcely be seen with the light microscope.

Stria Vascularis. The epithelial covering of the vestibular membrane becomes continuous, at the outer wall of the cochlea, with the basal layer of cells in the specialized band of striatified epithelium called the *stria vascularis* (Figs. 35–10 to 35–12). With the light microscope it is possible to distinguish two cell types in this epithelium—a layer of light-staining *basal cells* and a darker-staining superficial layer of *marginal cells* possessing numerous mitochondria. In electron micrographs some workers have identified a third cell type, the *intermediate cells*. Although these latter are intermediate between marginal and basal cells in their location, they are difficult to distinguish cytologically from basal cells. The convex free surface of the marginal cells apparently varies with the species and may be smooth or have microvilli, as it does in the human. The basal portion of these cells is partitioned by deep infoldings of the plasmalemma into a labyrinthine system of narrow compartments occupied by numerous mitochondria. The intermediate and basal cells have relatively few mitochondria and numerous processes that interdigitate with each other and with the marginal cells. Ascending processes of the basal cells form cuplike structures surrounding and partially isolating each marginal cell from neighboring areas of the epithelium (Fig. 35–12). Capillaries penetrate into the stria vascularis and course longitudinally within the epithelium, surrounded by processes of the intermediate and marginal cells. The stria vascularis is presumed to be involved in the secretion of the endolymph, and the resemblance of the elaborate basal compartmentation of the marginal cells to similar basal specializations of other cells involved in ion transport has led to the suggestion that these cells may help maintain the unusual ionic composition of the endolymph.

Spiral Prominence. The stria vascularis ends inferiorly, and its basal cell layer is continuous with the cells overlying the *spiral prominence* (Fig. 35–13). This prominence extends the whole length of the cochlear duct and rests on a very richly vascularized thickening of the underlying periosteum. The epithelium of the spiral prominence continues downward and is reflected from the outer wall of the cochlea onto the basilar membrane, forming at its line of reflection the *external spiral sulcus*. The cells here take on a

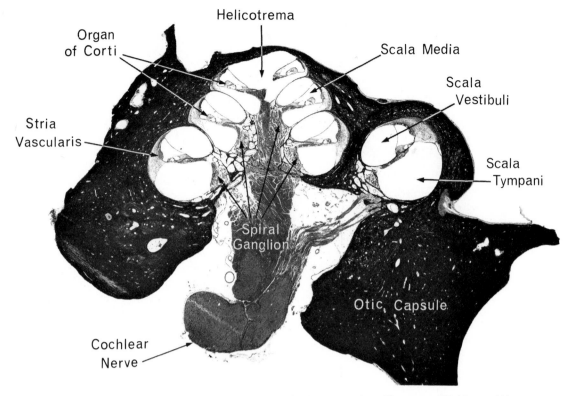

Figure 35–10. Photomicrograph of the cochlea of a rhesus monkey. (Courtesy of H. Mizoguchi.)

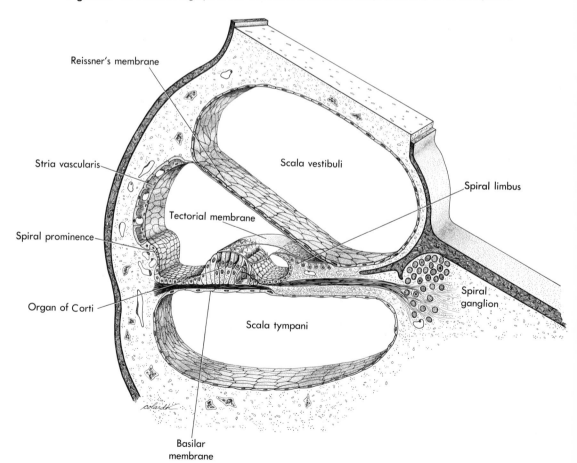

Figure 35–11. Schematic representation of a section through one of the turns of the cochlea. (Drawn by Sylvia Colard Keene.)

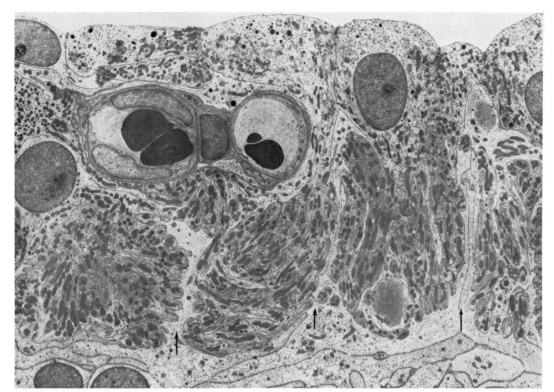

Figure 35–12. Electron micrograph of the stria vascularis of the cat inner ear, illustrating the intraepithelial capillaries, the ascending process of the basal cells *(at arrows)*, and the elaborately infolded bases of the marginal cells. (After Hinojosa, R., and E. Rodriguez-Echandia. Am. J. Anat. *118*:631, 1966.)

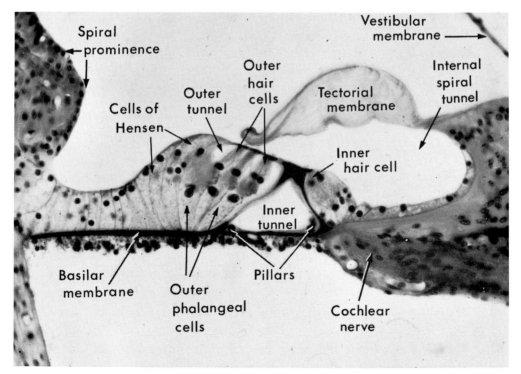

Figure 35–13. Photomicrograph of the organ of Corti of a cat. The tectorial membrane has been lifted away from the inner hair cells in specimen preparation. (Courtesy of H. Engström.)

cuboidal shape, and those continuing onto the pars pectinata of the basilar membrane are known as the *cells of Claudius*. In the basal coil of the cochlea, small groups of polyhedral cells (*cells of Boettcher*) are interposed between the basilar membrane and the cells of Claudius (Fig. 35–14). These cells have large spherical nuclei, and their cytoplasm is denser than that of the adjoining cells of Claudius. The plasma membrane of the lower half of these cells gives rise to numerous microvilli, which may either interdigitate extensively with those of adjacent cells or protrude into the intercellular space. Such specializations suggest that the Boettcher cells have a secretory or absorptive function.

Organ of Corti

Over the pars pectinata and pars arcuata the cells become columnar and bulge into the cochlear duct, forming the epithelial ridge called the *organ of Corti* (Figs. 35–10, 35–11, 35–13). This highly specialized complex of epithelial cells extends throughout the length of the cochlea and is composed of *hair cells*, the receptors of stimuli produced by sound, and various *supporting cells*.

Supporting Cells. The several types of supporting cells have certain characteristics in common. They are tall, slender cells extending from the basilar membrane to the free surface of the organ of Corti, and they contain conspicuous tonofibrils. Although the cells are separated by large intercellular spaces, their upper surfaces are in contact with each other and with the hair cells to form a continuous free surface for the organ. This surface is called the *reticular membrane*. The supporting cells include *inner* and *outer pillars, inner* and *outer phalangeal cells, border cells*, and *cells of Hensen*.

Within the organ of Corti is the *inner tunnel*, a canal extending the length of the cochlea and bounded below by extensions of the pillar cells, which lie on top of the basilar membrane, and above by the bodies of the inner and outer pillar cells. The bodies of the pillars are separated by clefts through which the tunnel communicates with the other intercellular cavities in the organ of Corti, including the *outer tunnel* or *space of Nuel*.

INNER PILLARS. The inner pillars have a broad base that rests on the basilar membrane and a conical cell body with its apex extending upward (Figs. 35–14, 35–16). The cytoplasm of the pillar cell contains the nucleus at the inner angle of the roughly triangular tunnel. The most distinctive feature of these cells is the darkly staining tonofibrils that course from the cell base through the cylindrical body of the pillar to end in the junctional complexes at the apex, where the cell expands into a flat flange to contact neighboring pillar cells and the inner hair

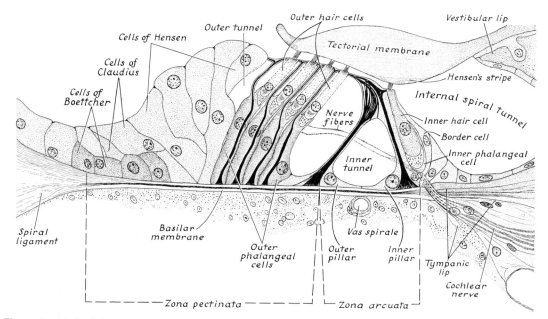

Figure 35–14. Radial transection of the organ of Corti, from the upper part of the first coil of human cochlea. (Slightly modified from Held.)

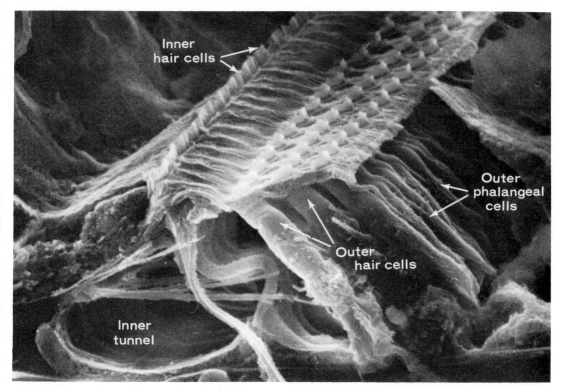

Figure 35–15. Scanning electron micrograph of guinea pig organ of Corti. For further orientation, see Figure 35–14. (Courtesy of H. Engström.)

cells. The contact between inner and outer pillar cells is of particularly large area and forms a structurally sound supporting mechanism. What appear to be tonofibrils with the

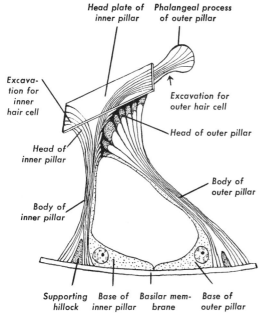

Figure 35–16. Diagram of inner and outer pillars of organ of Corti. (Modified from Kolmer.)

light microscope are found in electron micrographs to be a highly organized array of unusually large microtubules, with an outside diameter of 27 nm and a wall thickness of about 6 nm. Interspersed among these are 6-nm microfilaments (Fig. 35–25). This array of tubules and filaments runs from the base of the pillar cell to the apex of the cell at the top of the organ of Corti.

OUTER PILLARS. The outer pillars are longer than the inner ones (Figs. 35–14, 35–16). Their base is situated on the basilar membrane at the junction of the pars pectinata and pars arcuata, adjoining the base of the inner pillar. The cell body is similar to that of the inner pillar, but the free surface of the cell has a somewhat different shape. The head of the outer pillar abuts the head of the inner pillar and sends out a phalangeal process that forms a junction with the outer hair cells. The outer pillars, in fact, form the first row of phalanges.

The inner pillars number approximately 5600, the outer ones 3800. On an average, three inner pillars are connected with two outer pillars.

INNER PHALANGEAL CELLS. These cells are arranged in a row on the inner surface of the inner pillars and completely surround the inner hair cells. In contradistinction to the outer phalangeal cells there is no enlarged extracellular space between the supporting cells and the hair cells. Afferent and efferent nerve fibers travel through and are supported by the inner phalangeal cells. The relationship between supporting cells and inner hair cells is completely analogous to that between the supporting and hair cells of the vestibular system.

OUTER PHALANGEAL CELLS (of Deiters). The outer phalangeal cells act as supporting elements for the three to four rows of outer hair cells (Figs. 35–17 to 35–19). These phalangeal cells are columnar, with their bases resting on the basilar membrane. Apically they surround the inferior third of the outer hair cell and also enclose the afferent and efferent nerve bundles traveling to the hair cell base. This portion of the cell does not reach the free surface of the organ of Corti, but on the side of the cell away from the outer pillar cells, it gives off a slender finger-like process internally reinforced by a bundle of microtubules. This phalanx expands at the surface of the organ of Corti to form a flat apical plate joined at its edges to the hair cell that it is supporting and to the hair cell in the row next to it. The platelike expansion at the surface also contains abundant supporting microtubules.

The upper two thirds of the outer hair cells are not surrounded by other cells but are exposed within a fluid-filled space (the space of Nuel) that is in communication with the inner tunnel through the clefts between the pillars. The fluid that bathes the hair cells and occupies the space of Nuel and inner tunnel is apparently separated from the endolymphatic or perilymphatic spaces, and thus may be of a composition different from that of either perilymph or endolymph.

BORDER CELLS. The inner phalangeal cells continue into a row of slender cells, termed border cells, that delimit the inner boundary of the organ of Corti (Fig. 35–14). There is a gradual transition in height from these to the squamous cells lining the inner spiral sulcus.

CELLS OF HENSEN. Adjacent to the last row of outer phalangeal cells are the tall cells of Hensen that constitute the outer border of the organ of Corti. They are arranged in several rows decreasing rapidly in height and laterally abutting the cells of Claudius.

Cochlear Hair Cells. In the cochlea, as in the vestibule, two types of hair cells are present (Figs. 35–11, 35–13, 35–19). The *inner hair cells* are arranged in a single row along the whole length of the cochlea. The *outer hair cells* form three rows and are lodged between the outer pillars and the outer pha-

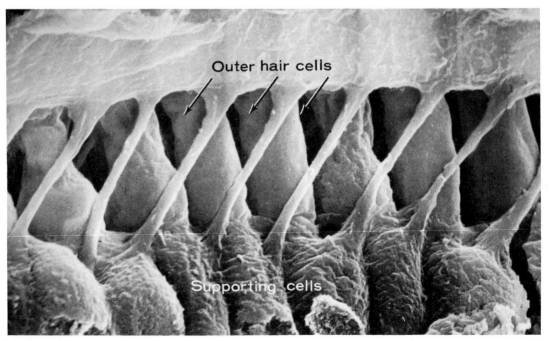

Figure 35–17. Scanning electron micrograph of outer hair cells and slender processes of supporting cells of Deiters. For orientation, see Figure 35–18. (Courtesy of H. Engström.)

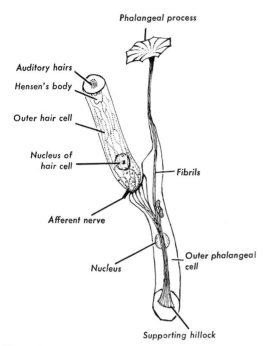

Figure 35–18. Diagram of supporting cells of Deiters and the associated outer hair cell. (Modified from Kolmer.)

of the cochlear nerve. Many of these run beside the hair cell up to the level of its nucleus, though not all the area of apposition is synaptic. Pre- and postsynaptic membrane thickenings and synaptic ribbons are considered to demarcate sites of synaptic transmission. In addition, small neuronal profiles containing many synaptic vesicles, some of which are dense-cored, make contact with inner hair cells, though this is rather rare. More often, contacts with pre- and postsynaptic membrane thickenings are seen between these heavily vesiculated fibers and the afferent fibers just before the latter make contact with the inner hair cell. Many such vesiculated fibers are found beneath the inner hair cell, and they are considered efferent in nature.

Outer hair cells have a different structure from that of inner hair cells and this has led to speculation that the two cell types have different functions. Outer hair cells, as pre-

langeal cells. In the human, a fourth and sometimes a fifth row of outer hair cells may appear toward the apex, though these supernumerary rows may not be as regular as the first three.

Inner hair cells resemble type I cells in the vestibular labyrinth in many respects. They are relatively short, goblet-shaped cells with a slightly constricted neck region. The surface of the cell bears hairs similar in structure to those on vestibular hair cells, but in the adult there is no associated cilium. However, a basal body and an associated typical centriole persist as the only remnants of the ciliary apparatus. The hairs are arranged on the cell surface in the form of a letter W or U (Fig. 35–23). The rootlets of the hairs extend down into, and at times through, the dense terminal web or cuticular plate. The cell body contains scattered ribosomes and 20-nm vesicles interspersed among larger vesicular profiles, presumably representing the smooth endoplasmic reticulum. Mitochondria are aggregated under the terminal web and at the cell base, but are scattered in smaller numbers throughout the cytoplasm. The synaptic area of the inner hair cell extends from the base of the cell to the level of the nucleus. The vast majority of the endings contacting the inner hair cell are sparsely vesiculated and are considered to be endings

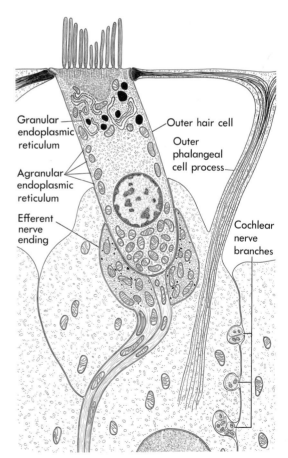

Figure 35–19. Schematic representation of the relationship of the outer hair cells to the outer phalangeal cells, as revealed in electron micrographs. (Drawn by Sylvia Colard Keene.)

viously stated, are supported on the apices of outer phalangeal cells and receive innervation from the cochlear nerve at their bases (Figs. 35–14, 35–27). The hairs on the apex of these cells form a distinctive W similar to that of the inner hair cells, but here there are more rows of hairs, and the length of the hair varies from long at the perphery to short centrally (Figs. 35–20, 35–24). Again, no cilium is present, although a basal body can be found at the base of the W. Immediately deep to the terminal web are dense, lipid-like inclusions interspersed with elongated, highly convoluted elements of the granular endoplasmic reticulum. Mitochondria are generally aggregated in the basal cytoplasm and line up along the sides of the cell in relation to one or more rows of smooth-surfaced vesicles that are aligned parallel to the plasmalemma. A single row of such smooth-surfaced vesicles is also found along the nonsynaptic plasmalemma of the inner hair cell. At present the function of these vesicular aggregates is unknown.

The basal part of the outer hair cell receives synapses from both efferent and afferent nerve fibers. Here, however, the afferent fibers from the cochlear nerve frequently

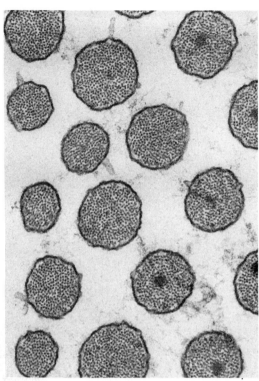

Figure 35–21. Transverse sections through the hairs on a guinea pig outer hair cell, showing the large number of filaments in their interior. (Courtesy of H. Engström.)

give rise to the smaller endings. Such synapses exhibit pre- and postsynaptic membrane thickenings and, in some species, synaptic ribbons, but they are not heavily

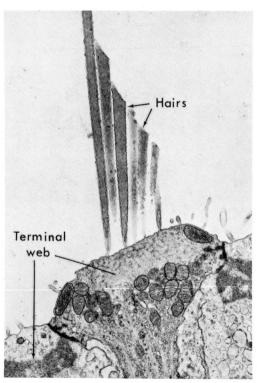

Figure 35–20. Electron micrograph showing the hairs on a hair cell. Notice their narrow base and the continuation of their fibrous core into the terminal web. (Courtesy of D. Hamilton.)

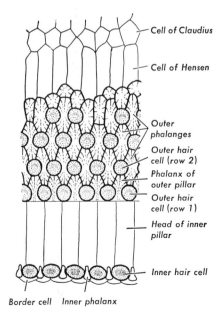

Figure 35–22. Diagram of the organ of Corti viewed from above, showing the relationship of the phalanges of the supporting cells to the hair cells. (Modified from Retzius, Kolmer, Schaffer.)

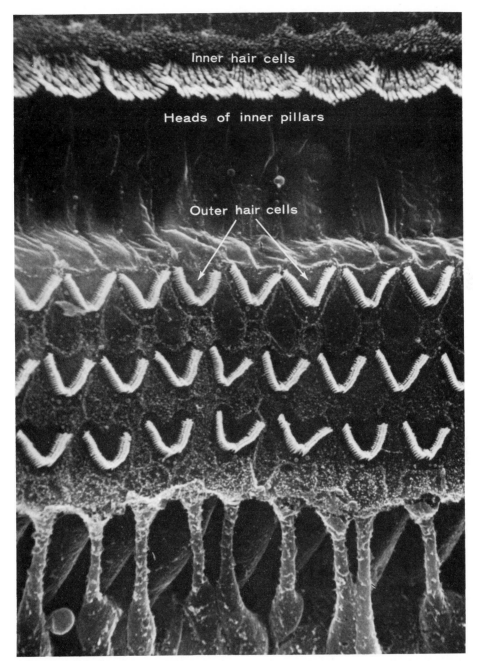

Figure 35–23. Scanning micrograph of guinea pig organ of Corti, middle turn, seen from above. For orientation, see Figure 35–22. (Courtesy of H. Engström.)

vesiculated. The efferent endings on the outer hair cells are larger than those of the afferent fibers and contain many densely packed vesicles. In the hair cell cytoplasm, parallel to the plasmalemma and extending the entire length of the efferent synapse, is found a single continuous flattened cisterna, the "subsynaptic cisterna."

Spiral Limbus. In the inner angle of the scala media, the periosteal connective tissue of the upper surface of the osseous spiral lamina bulges into the scala media as the *spiral limbus* (Figs. 35–11, 35–13, 35–14). Its edge overhangs the internal spiral sulcus. The two margins of the sulcus are the *vestibular lip* and *tympanic lip*. The collagenous fibers of the limbus continue laterally, via the tympanic lip, into the pars arcuata of the basilar membrane. Within the body of the limbus the fibers are arranged vertically to produce the distinctive *auditory teeth* (of Huschke). Between these collagenous fibers

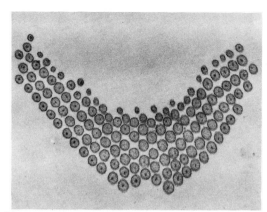

Figure 35–24. Electron micrograph of the W configuration of the hairs or stereocilia on the outer sensory cells of the human organ of Corti. × 10,500. (Courtesy of R. Kimura.)

are stellate fibroblasts. Uniformly spaced along the upper margin of the limbus, between the auditory teeth, are the so-called *interdental cells*, which secrete the tectorial membrane. The bases of interdental cells are firmly embedded in the connective tissue of the limbus, but their apices spread out over the upper surface of the limbus, interdigitating and joined by junctional complexes. These form a continuous sheet over the upper surface of the limbus and complete the cellular investment of the cochlear duct.

Tectorial Membrane. The tectorial membrane is secreted from the luminal surfaces of the interdental cells and overlies these cells as a cuticle. It extends laterally beyond the vestibular lip of the limbus to overlie the hairs on the hair cells of the organ of Corti (Figs. 35–11, 35–13). Recent evidence indicates that the tips of the hairs are embedded within or are firmly bound to the membrane. If this is so, micrographs showing a space between the hairs and the tectorial membrane must be artifactitious. The tectorial membrane is composed primarily of a protein having a number of similarities to epidermal keratin. In fixed preparations numerous fibrils are observed within it, forming patterns suggesting a highly ordered structure.

THE PERILYMPHATIC LABYRINTH

The perilymphatic system surrounds the whole of the membranous labyrinth and provides support for its epithelium lining. The distinct scalae vestibuli and tympani in the cochlea have been mentioned, but it must be

remembered that similar, though less specialized, perilymphatic spaces surround the structures in the vestibule.

Histologically the perilymphatic tissue is described as a reticulum, and close examination with the electron microscope shows that this reticulum is composed primarily of highly attenuated processes of many stellate cells. Except close to the periosteum of the bony labyrinth and to the membranous labyrinth, there are few extracellular fibers associated with these reticular cells. Immediately surrounding the membranous labyrinth, however, extracellular fibers are formed and, in some species, make up a relatively dense, stable sheath 1 or 2 μm thick, composed of multitudes of short fibers. In the vicinity of the cells of the perilymphatic system, both in the cochlea and in the vestibule, are fiber bundles that have a characteristic form different from that of any other known extracellular fiber. The bundles are composed of a variable number of dense 10-nm filaments, which can be shown to be composed of four 5-nm subunits that appear to be helically wound around one another. The dense fibers that form the bundles are embedded in an amorphous matrix.

Numerous blood capillaries course throughout the perilymphatic tissue destined to supply the metabolic needs of the labyrinthine epithelium.

Scala Vestibuli and Scala Tympani

The cells that line these two scalae usually are extremely attenuated squamous cells with very little obvious cellular differentiation. At times, however, especially in the vicinity of the basilar membrane, the cells do become somewhat cuboidal, although they possess few structural features of note.

Basilar Membrane. The most elaborate specialization of perilymphatic tissue is the basilar membrane, which provides a supporting base for the cells of the organ of Corti and which by its movement presumably transmits vibrations to the hair cells. The basilar membrane is a highly organized layer of fibers. There is some indication that the perilymphatic cells may actively secrete the basilar membrane, but this has not been clearly established. It is divided into two distinct zones: one, running from the osseous spiral lamina approximately one third of the way to the outer cochlear wall, is termed the *pars arcuata (tecta)*; the other, approximately two thirds of the width of the basilar membrane, is termed the *pars pectinata* and contains, as can be seen even at the light microscopic level, distinct parallel striations termed the *auditory strings*. In fact, both portions of the membrane are composed of transversely oriented filaments (8 to 10 nm thick) embedded in an amorphous matrix. In the pars pectinata the filaments are aggregated into bundles that run in two strata: one immediately beneath the organ of Corti, composed of small bundles, and another situated more deeply in the lamina, composed of larger bundles. At the outer wall of the cochlea, these two layers again merge, to pass into the connective tissue of the spiral ligament. Blood vessels penetrate into the pars arcuata but not into the pars pectinata.

The term *spiral ligament* is an unfortunate designation for the lateral insertion of the basilar membrane, because this component does not have the histological structure of ligaments found elsewhere in the body (Fig. 35–11). It is merely a local differentiation of periosteal connective tissue containing numerous fibroblasts and blood vessels. A better term would be *spiral crest*.

ENDOLYMPH AND PERILYMPH

The spaces delimited by the membranous labyrinth are filled with the viscous fluid called endolymph, and the labyrinth is surrounded by the perilymph, which occupies the perilymphatic spaces. The two fluids are amazingly different in their chemical composition. The most striking difference is in their electrolyte composition. Whereas perilymph to some degree resembles extracellular fluid in general, endolymph has the characteristics of intracellular fluid in having high K^+ and low Na^+ concentrations (Table 35–1).

Table 35–1. ELECTROLYTE COMPOSITION OF BODY FLUIDS (mEq/l)*

	Plasma	CSF	Perilymph	Endolymph
Protein	6000–8000	10–38	75–100	10
K	20	12–17	15	140
Na	140	150	148	26
Cl	600	750	120	140
Sugar	70–120	40–80		
Mg	1.0–3.0	2.0	2.0	0.9
Ca	7.0	3.0	3.0	3.0

*From F. C. Ormerod.

It was recognized early in this century that endolymph was a product of secretion, although the actual site or sites of its elaboration were not known. It was supposed that the stria vascularis, the spiral prominence, and the extrasensory cells around the maculae and cristae were primarily responsible. Recent evidence would indicate that these areas do indeed take part in elaboration of endolymph, but the electron microscope has made it clear that many of the cells lining the membranous labyrinth have cytological characteristics compatible with synthetic and secretory activity and might therefore participate in endolymph metabolism. Specifically, autoradiographic studies have implicated the planum semilunatum in elaboration of sulfated mucopolysaccharides, and measurement with microelectrodes has shown that the high DC potential of the scala media is produced in the vicinity of the stria vascularis, which would indicate that some sort of ion secretion is taking place there.

The site of absorption of endolymph has been thought to be the endolymphatic sac. However, electron micrographs of cells of the membranous labyrinth show many instances of micropinocytotic activity, which would suggest that absorption may be going on in other areas of the labyrinth.

Although it is well established that endolymph is a secretion, the genesis of perilymph is still being debated. Some feel that it is an ultrafiltrate of plasma, others that it is derived from cerebrospinal fluid. There is no doubt that the perilymphatic spaces are functionally connected to the subarachnoid space, but the exact functional significance of this relationship is not yet clear.

NERVES OF THE LABYRINTH

The eighth cranial nerve supplies the sensory areas of the labyrinth. It consists of two parts of quite different functional nature and central connections—the *vestibular* and the *cochlear* nerves (Figs. 35–5, 35–28). Each is composed of primary afferent fibers from the sense organs and efferent feedback fibers from the central nervous system. The cell bodies of the afferent fibers are bipolar cells and form two peripheral ganglia, the *spiral* or *cochlear ganglion* in the modiolus and the *vestibular* or *Scarpa's ganglion* in the internal auditory meatus of the temporal bone.

The vestibular nerve divides into a superior and an inferior branch. The superior

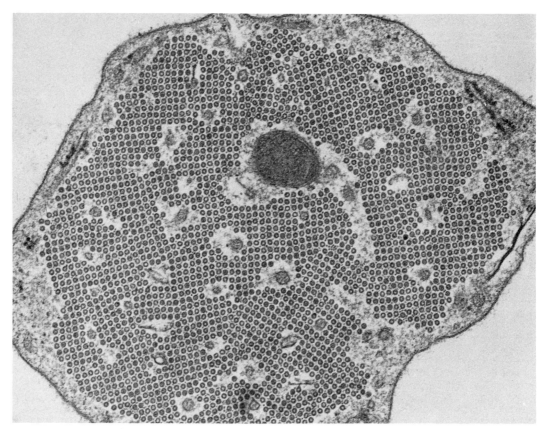

Figure 35–25. Electron micrograph of an inner pillar cell in transverse section, showing the highly ordered bundle of thick walled microtubules and microfilaments. (Courtesy of H. Engström.)

branch supplies the horizontal crista ampullaris, the superior crista ampullaris, the macula utriculi, and a small part of the macula sacculi. The inferior branch supplies the posterior crista ampullaris and the major portion of the macula sacculi, and it sends a small anastomosing branch to the cochlear nerve.

The bipolar cell bodies, both in the vestibular ganglion and in the cochlear ganglion, are invested by a thin layer of myelin, and this continues onto the axons. The axons of the cochlear nerve lose their myelin as they run through the openings of the osseous spiral lamina beneath the inner hair cells. In the vestibular nerve, myelin persists until the nerve enters the sensory area.

The cochlear nerve contains two morphological kinds of afferent nerve fibers. The more numerous ones radiate from the spiral ganglion in parallel bundles to the nearest segments of the organ of Corti. Because of their course, they are called the *radial acoustic fibers*. The second category of fibers, usually thicker and fewer than the first, are also arranged radially at the outset, but after

reaching the outer hair cells of the organ of Corti, they turn sharply and follow a spiral course. These are the *spiral fibers* (Fig. 35–26).

The functional implications of these two patterns of distributions are not clear. Although the relationship between the peripheral receptors and acoustic neurons is not as individualized as the monosynaptic relationship of the foveal cones, it is sufficiently restricted to permit the reception of localized stimuli impinging upon small segments of the cochlea.

The vestibular nerve terminates centrally in the reflex centers of the medulla oblongata and cerebellum. Its cortical connections are unknown, although it mediates reflex movements of the eyes through its thalamic connections. The cochlear nerve synapses in the cochlear nucleus, whence fibers ascend in the lateral lemniscus to the medial geniculate body of the thalamus and thence to the temporal lobe gyri of the cortex.

Both the vestibular and cochlear divisions of the eighth cranial nerve contain appreciable numbers of efferent fibers that originate

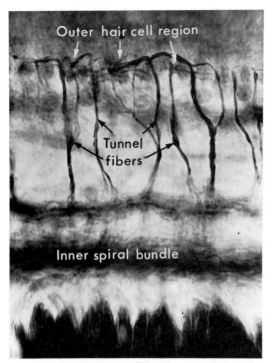

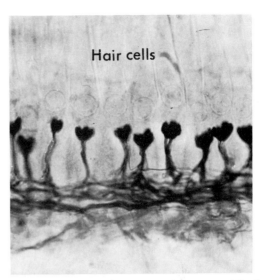

Figure 35–27. Longitudinal section of the organ of Corti, showing the efferent nerve fibers ending about bases of the outer hair cells. (Courtesy of H. Engström.)

Figure 35–26. Optical section of guinea pig organ of Corti viewed from above, showing nerve fibers traversing the tunnel to reach the region of outer hair cells. Modified Maillet nerve stain using zinc iodide and osmium tetroxide. (From Engström, H., H. W. Ades, and A. Andersson: Structural Pattern of the Organ of Corti. Stockholm, Almqvist and Wiksell, 1966.)

bilaterally from the vicinity of the superior olive. Initially these fibers travel in the vestibular nerve, but within the internal auditory meatus some efferent fibers reach the cochlear nerve by way of the anastomosis between the vestibular and cochlear nerves. The peripheral terminations of the efferent component are presumably at the hair cells, but incontrovertible evidence for the position and mode of ending of these fibers is still lacking. Stimulation of the efferent bundle results in suppression of auditory nerve activity, and anatomical evidence derived from sectioning the bundle indicates that the "granulated" endings are efferent, for they apparently degenerate after sectioning (Figs. 35–9, 35–19).

BLOOD VESSELS OF THE LABYRINTH

The labyrinthine artery is a branch of the inferior cerebellar artery. It enters the internal auditory meatus and divides into two branches, the *vestibular* artery and the *common cochlear* artery. The latter divides into the *vestibulocochlear* artery and the *cochlear* artery proper.

The vestibular artery supplies the upper and lateral parts of the utricle and saccule and parts of the superior and lateral semicircular ducts. It forms dense networks of capillaries in the region of the maculae; in the thin perilymphatic tissue of these structures, the capillary networks are relatively loose.

The vestibulocochlear artery supplies, with its vestibular branch, the lower and medial parts of the utricle and saccule, the crus commune, and the posterior semicircular duct. Its cochlear branch supplies the lowest part of the first cochlear coil.

The cochlear artery proper penetrates the cavities of the modiolus, where its tortuous branches run spirally to the apex. This is the so-called "spiral modiolar artery." From it, branches go to the spiral ganglion and, through the periosteum of the scala vestibuli and the osseous spiral lamina, to the inner parts of the basilar membrane. Here the capillaries are arranged in arcades in the tympanic covering layer under the tunnel and the limbus. The vascular stria and the spiral crest receive their blood through branches of the spiral modiolar artery, which run in the roof of the scala vestibuli. They do not form connections with the vessels of the basilar membrane. The lower wall of the scala tympani receives its own small arteries from the same source.

The course of the veins of the labyrinth is quite different from that of the arteries.

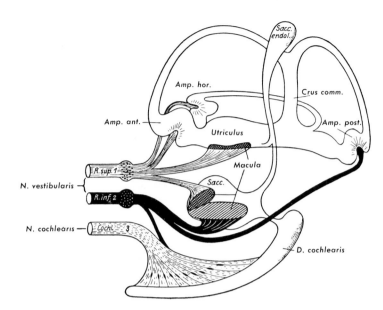

Figure 35–28. Diagram of distribution of nerves in the membranous labyrinth of the rabbit. (After deBurlet, from Kolmer.)

There are three main venous drainage channels. In the cochlea, veins originate in the region of the spiral prominence and run downward and inward through the periosteum of the scala tympani to the spiral vein, which is found under the spiral ganglion. Upper and lower spiral veins, belonging to the corresponding coils of the cochlea, receive branches from the osseous spiral lamina and the spiral ganglion. Above the spiral vein is the small vein of the spiral lamina, which receives a part of the blood from the spiral lamina and spiral ganglion and is connected by anastomoses with the spiral vein. These cochlear veins form a plexus in the modiolus, which empties the blood partly into the internal auditory vein and partly into the vein of the cochlear aqueduct, which drains into the jugular vein. The veins of the vestibule empty into the veins of the vestibular and cochlear aqueducts.

This arrangement of the vessels in the internal ear seems to ensure the best possible protection of the sound receptors from the arterial pulse wave. The arteries are arranged for the most part in the wall of the scala vestibuli, while the wall of the scala tympani contains the veins. The course of the spiral arteries in the modiolus probably also contributes to the damping of pulsations. In certain mammals the coiling of these arteries is so prominent that the convoluted regions suggest glomeruli.

True lymphatics are absent from the labyrinth. Instead the fluid is drained into the perilymphatic spaces, which are connected with the subarachnoid space. A certain amount of drainage may be effected through perivascular and perineural connective tissue sheaths.

FUNCTIONAL CONSIDERATIONS

Functions of the various structural components of the ear have already been mentioned briefly in the descriptions under specific headings. It is impossible, of course, to consider in detail the functioning of the ear in a textbook of histology, but there are certain physiological considerations that suggest new problems and approaches to research on this organ.

The external and middle ears lend themselves quite well to physiological research and have been intensively studied for some time. The vibrations of the tympanic membrane are transmitted through the chain of auditory ossicles to the fenestra ovalis and thence to the perilymph filling the scala tympani. The organ of Corti is the receptor for sound stimuli, but this function depends to a large degree on the properties of the basilar membrane. This membrane may be compared to an unstressed gelatinous plate with varying resistance to displacement related to its uniformly varying width. The deformation of this membrane produced by movement of the stapes resembles a traveling wave. Regions of observed maximal displacement change with frequency but are rather broad. As the stimulus frequency rises, the length of the basilar membrane responding becomes shorter, and progressively more of the distal area becomes inactive. The pitch-discriminating ability of the ear is only partly due to this physical separation of the responding areas along the basilar membrane.

Nerve impulses elicited by stimulation of the maculae and the cristae play an important role in the regulation and coordination of the movements of equilibrium and locomotion. The stimuli to the vestibular end organs are *angular acceleration* for the semicircular ducts and *linear acceleration* for the maculae. These impulses exert their influences upon coordinated muscular contraction, upon muscular tonus, and upon eye movement through the brain stem and cerebellum.

The ear is essentially a biological transducer. The transduction in the external and middle ears is relatively easily monitored. The extreme anatomical complexity of the internal ear, however, has hindered attempts at understanding the transducer phenomenon by which mechanical energy (the stimulus) is transferred into electrical energy (the nerve impulse). It is generally believed that the transduction process takes place in the apex of the hair cells. Indications are that the mechanism in vestibular and cochlear hair cells probably does not differ significantly, even though there are considerable anatomical differences in the cells.

It has been possible to show very clearly in the ampulla of Lorenzini in fish, where the sensory cells are in many respects anatomically similar to vestibular hair cells, that bending of the hairs toward the kinocilium results in depolarization of the cell. Bending in the opposite direction hyperpolarizes the cell, while bending normal to these directions has no appreciable ionic effect. Since mammalian vestibular hair cells are morphologically polarized, the same functional responses to stimuli that bend the hair cells toward or away from the kinocilium would probably occur. The polarization of the hair cells of the maculae varies regularly from one part of these organs to the other, covering within each organ a full 360 degrees. Thus a movement of the head in any direction will be a sufficient stimulus to excite some of the hair cells and inhibit others. Furthermore, the stepwise lengthening of the hairs may provide a built-in biological amplifier. How the transduction process takes place remains

unexplained, however, for the hairs extend into the endolymph with its highly unusual ionic composition. Thus, with equal K^+ and Na^+ inside and outside the cell, the $Na^+ = K^+$ movements that are known to be involved in excitation in other excitable cells would not take place. Nevertheless, it has been shown that a nerve cell membrane put into the same ionic conditions as the hairs responds to pressure changes by transient potential changes across the membrane, and although the mechanism for this is equally unclear, it is possible that this experimental system is analogous to the hairs. In the near future it may help to explain how hair cells function.

REFERENCES

GENERAL

Bast, T. H., and B. J. Anson: The Temporal Bone and the Ear. Springfield, IL, Charles C Thomas, 1949.

Békésy, G. von: Experiments in Hearing. New York, McGraw-Hill Book Co., 1960.

Dallas, P.: The Auditory Periphery. New York, Academic Press, 1973.

Davis, H.: Mechanisms of the inner ear. Ann. Otol. 77:644, 1968.

Engström, H., H. Ades, and A. Anderson: Structural Pattern of the Organ of Corti. Stockholm. Almqvist & Wiksell, 1966.

Iurato, S., ed.: Submicroscopic Structure of the Inner Ear. New York, Pergamon Press, 1967.

EXTERNAL EAR

Perry, E. T.: The Human Ear Canal. Springfield, IL, Charles C Thomas, 1957.

Sophian, L. H., and B. H. Senturia: Anatomy and histology of the external ear in relation to the histogenesis of external otitis. Laryngoscope 64:772, 1954.

EUSTACHIAN TUBE

Graves, G. O., and L. F. Edwards: The eustachian tube. A review of its descriptive, microscopic, topographic and clinical anatomy. Arch. Otolaryngol. 39:359, 1944.

Ladman, A. J., and A. J. Mitchell: The topographical relations and histological characteristics of the tubulo-acinar glands of the eustachian tube in mice. Anat. Rec. 121:167, 1955.

COCHLEA

Bredberg, G.: Cellular pattern and nerve supply of the human organ of Corti. Acta Otolaryngol. (Suppl.) 236:1, 1968.

Engström, H., H. Ades, and J. Hawkins: Structure and function of the sensory hairs of the inner ear. J. Acoust. Soc. Am. 34:1356, 1962.

Fernandez, E.: The innervation of the cochlea (guinea pig). Laryngoscope 51:1152, 1951.

Flock, A.: Transduction in hair cells. In Loewenstein, W. R., ed.: Handbook of Sensory Physiology. Vol.

1. Principles of Receptor Physiology. Berlin, Springer-Verlag, OHG, 1971.

Kimura, R. S.: Hairs of the cochlear sensory cells and their attachment to the tectorial membrane. Acta Otolaryngol. *61*:55, 1966.

Kimura, R. S., H. F. Schuknecht, and I. Sundo: Fine morphology of the sensory cells of the organ of Corti in man. Acta Otolaryngol. (Stockh.) *58*:390, 1965.

Rodriguez-Echandia, E. L., and M. H. Burgos: The fine structure of the stria vascularis of the guinea pig inner ear. Zeitschr. f. Zellforsch. *67*:600, 1965.

Spoendlin, H.: The organization of the cochlear receptor. *In* Advances in Oto-Rhino-Laryngology. Vol. 13. Basel, S. Karger, 1968.

VESTIBULAR ORGAN

Citron, L., D. Exley, and C. S. Hallpike: Formation, circulation, and chemical properties of the labyrinthine fluids. Br. Med. Bull. *12*:101, 1956.

Flock, A.: The ultrastructure of the macula utriculi with special reference to directional interplay of sensory response as revealed by morphological polarization. J. Cell Biol. *22*:413, 1964.

Guild, S. R.: Observations upon the structure and normal contents of the ductus and saccus endolymphaticus in the guinea pig. Am. J. Anat. *39*:1, 1927.

Guild, S. R.: Circulation of the endolymph. Am. J. Anat. *39*:57, 1927.

Kimura, R. S., P. G. Lundquist, and J. Wersäll: Secretory epithelial linings in the ampullae of the guinea pig labyrinth. Acta Otolaryngol. *57*:517, 1964.

Lundquist, P. G.: The endolymphatic duct and sac in the guinea pig. Acta Otolaryngol. Suppl. 201:1, 1965.

Ormerod, F. C.: The physiology of the endolymph. J. Laryngol. Otol. *74*:659, 1960.

Wersäll, J., and A. Flock: Physiological aspects on the structure of reticular end organs. Acta Otolaryngol. Suppl. 192:85, 1963.

Index

Note: Page numbers in *italics* refer to illustrations, and page numbers followed by (t) refer to tables.